OXFORD HANDBOOK OF CLINICAL SPECIALTIES

ELEVENTH EDITION

Edited by
ANDREW BALDWIN

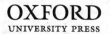

OXFORD
UNIVERSITY PRESS

OXFORD
UNIVERSITY PRESS

Great Clarendon Street, Oxford, OX2 6DP,
United Kingdom

Oxford University Press is a department of the University of Oxford.
It furthers the University's objective of excellence in research, scholarship,
and education by publishing worldwide. Oxford is a registered trade mark of
Oxford University Press in the UK and in certain other countries

© Oxford University Press 2020

The moral rights of the authors have been asserted

First published 1987	Seventh edition 2006	Translations:	
Second edition 1989	Eighth edition 2008	Spanish	Romanian
Third edition 1991	Ninth edition 2013	German	Russian
Fourth edition 1995	Tenth edition 2016	Hungarian	Portuguese
Fifth edition 1999	Eleventh edition 2020	Greek	Polish
Sixth edition 2003			

Impression: 1

Published in the United States of America by Oxford University Press
198 Madison Avenue, New York, NY 10016, United States of America

British Library Cataloguing in Publication Data
Data available

Library of Congress Control Number: 2019955812

ISBN 978-0-19-882719-1

Printed in Italy by
L.E.G.O. S.p.A.

Drugs

Except where otherwise stated, recommendations are for the **non-pregnant
adult** who is **not breastfeeding** and has reasonable **hepatic and renal** function.

We have made every effort to check this text, but it is still possible that drug or
other errors have been missed. oup makes no representation, express or implied,
that doses are correct. Readers are urged to check with the most up-to-date
product information, codes of conduct, and safety regulations. The authors and
the publishers do not accept responsibility or legal liability for any errors in the
text, or for the misuse or misapplication of material in this work.

For updates/corrections, see oxfordmedicine.com/ohcs11updates.

Contents

Each chapter's contents are detailed on its first page.

Preface to 11th edition

Rotations through medical school or Foundation Programme training may fill you with conflicting emotions. If your heart is set on a career in cardiology, you may wonder what the value is in studying ophthalmology. However, qualifying as a doctor requires knowledge of all the specialties. Just as an artist needs to link or combine every colour of the palette to complete their picture, so a doctor needs that entire palette of medical knowledge to view the whole picture. Budding cardiologists who study ophthalmology may find their eyes opened, as the eye is host to many diseases, and in some cases a window to diseases of the heart.

We trust this book will equip you with the relevant facts and knowledge, but we also aim to motivate and inspire you. At the start of each chapter we include stories of individuals or inventions that have helped shape healthcare. It is from these anecdotes, and the daily quirks we encounter from practising medicine, that we recall easily forgotten facts. We also include a brand-new chapter on your health, focusing on managing stress, avoiding burnout, and improving resilience. It is an unsettling paradox that when we study or practise medicine, we may neglect our own health.

We welcome a dose of 8 new authors to this edition. Each has worked tirelessly to update every page. They bring fresh knowledge and experience from their area of expertise to ensure that every chapter gives a concise overview of exactly what you need to know. The global spread of our authors and international reach of this book remind us that the discipline of medicine round the world feeds off the same root system.

ANDREW BALDWIN—*Preface to the 11th edition*—East Sussex, 2020

Preface to 1st edition

When someone says that he is 'doing obstetrics'—or whatever, this should not hide the fact that much more is being done besides, not just a little of each of medicine, psychiatry, gynaecology, and paediatrics, but also a good deal of work to elicit and act upon the patient's unspoken hopes and fears. At the operating table he must concentrate minutely on the problem in hand; but later he must operate on other planes too, in social and psychological dimensions so as to understand how the patient came to need to be on the operating table, and how this might have been prevented. All the best specialists practise a holistic art, and our aim is to show how specialism and holism may be successfully interwoven, if not into a fully watertight garment, then at least into one which keeps out much of the criticism rained upon us by the proponents of alternative medicine.

We hope that by compiling this little volume we may make the arduous task of learning medicine a little less exhausting, so allowing more energy to be spent at the bedside, and on the wards. For a medical student coming fresh to a specialty the great tomes which mark the road to knowledge can numb the mind after a while, and what started out fresh is in danger of becoming exhausted by its own too much. It is not that we are against the great tomes themselves—we are simply against reading them too much and too soon. One starts off strong on 'care' and weak on knowledge, and the danger is that this state of affairs becomes reversed. It is easier to learn from books than from patients, yet what our patients teach us may be of more abiding significance: the value of sympathy, the uses of compassion, and the limits of our human world. It is at the bedside that we learn how to be of practical help to people who are numbed by the mysterious disasters of womb or tomb, for which they are totally unprepared. If this small book enables those starting to explore the major specialties to learn all they can from their patients, it will have served its purpose—and can then be discarded.

JABC & JML—*Preface to the 1st edition*—Ferring, 1987

Contributors

Sanju Arianayagam
ST5 Dermatology
Churchill Hospital
Oxford University Hospitals NHS
Foundation Trust
Oxford, UK
Dermatology

Andrew Baldwin
GP Partner
The Lighthouse Medical Practice
Eastbourne, UK
*General practice; Eponymous
syndromes; Doctors' health and
performance*

Simon Buckley
Specialty Registrar ST8
Paediatrics
Guy's and St Thomas'
NHS Foundation Trust
London, UK
Paediatrics

Juliet Clutton
Specialty Registrar ST6
Trauma & Orthopaedics
University Hospital of Wales
Cardiff, UK
Trauma; Orthopaedics

Terry Collingwood
Specialty Registrar ST7
Intensive Care & Pre-Hospital
Emergency Medicine
East Anglian Air Ambulance
Norwich, UK
Pre-hospital emergency medicine

Alastair Denniston
Consultant Ophthalmologist
(Uveitis and Medical Retina)
University Hospitals Birmingham
NHS Foundation Trust
Birmingham, UK
Ophthalmology

Charlotte Goumalatsou
Specialty Registrar ST7
Obstetrics & Gynaecology
Royal Surrey County Hospital
NHS Foundation Trust
Guildford, UK
Obstetrics; Gynaecology

Blair Graham
Specialty Registrar Emergency
Medicine
RCEM Doctoral Research Fellow
Plymouth Hospitals NHS Trust
Plymouth, UK
Emergency medicine

Nina Hjelde
ST4 Anaesthesia
Salford Royal NHS Foundation Trust
Manchester, UK
Anaesthetics

Priscilla Mathewson
Adnexal Fellow
Moorfields Eye Hospital
NHS Foundation Trust
London, UK
Ophthalmology

Gil Myers
Consultant Child and Adolescent
Psychiatrist
Paediatric Mental Health Liaison
Whittington Health NHS Trust
London, UK
*Psychiatry; Doctors' health and
performance*

Nicholas Steventon
Consultant Otolaryngologist
Southern Cross Hospital
New Plymouth, New Zealand
Ear, nose, and throat

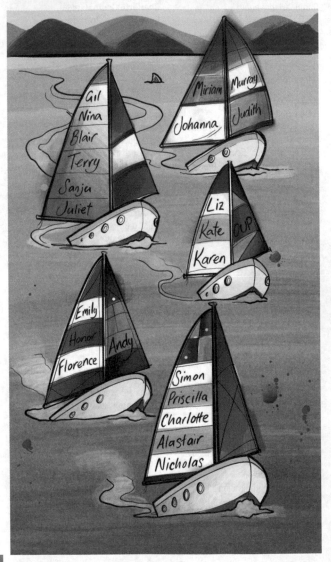

Artwork by Gillian Turner.

'He who studies medicine without books sails an uncharted sea,
but he who studies medicine without patients does not go to sea at all.'
William Osler
Canadian physician, 1849–1919

Acknowledgements

This book was conceived and inspired by Judith Collier and Murray Longmore, who as lead authors presided over it for more than 25 years—from publication of the first edition in 1987, until publication of the 9th edition in 2013. Their knowledge, wisdom, creativity, and holistic approach to medicine live on in the pages of this edition and their work has been loved and trusted by generations of doctors.

We thank all the authors who have contributed to previous editions: Judith Harvey, Tim Hodgetts, Duncan Brown, Peter Scally, Mark Brinsden, Ahmad R. Mafi, Tom Turmezei, and Keith Amarakone.

Specialist and junior readers We are hugely indebted to our specialist and junior readers for their advice, encouragement, and constructive criticism. Each chapter in this book has benefitted from their trustworthy oversight. They are thanked individually at the beginning of each chapter.

Reader participation We have been very fortunate to receive so many well-considered suggestions and corrections to the book from readers all over the globe. Their contributions have enhanced the book and we are grateful. If you would like to give us feedback, correct a mistake, or make a suggestion, you can do so at www.oup.com/uk/academic/ohfeedback.

References Every reference has an individual identification indicated by a pink superscript number. The details of every reference are held online at oxfordmedicine.com/ohcs11references

Symbols and abbreviations

▶▶.............don't dawdle!—prompt action saves lives
▶...............this phrase is important
1,2,3..........references at oxfordmedicine.com/ohcsl1references
☞...............controversial subject
☺...............an opportunity for holistic/non-reductionist thinking
#................fracture
ΔΔ.............differential diagnosis; Δ diagnosis
♂:♀...........male to female ratio
↓................decreased; ↑ increased; ↔ normal; → leading to
~................about; ≈ approximately equal
−ve............negative; +ve positive
∵...............on account of; ∴ therefore
A&E...........emergency department
ABC...........airway, breathing, circulation
ABR...........audiological brainstem responses
ABX...........antibiotics
ADHD.........attention deficit hyperactivity disorder
AED...........antiepileptic drug
AFP...........α-fetoprotein (α=alpha)
AIDS..........acquired immunodeficiency syndrome
AION.........anterior ischaemic optic neuropathy
AKI............acute kidney injury
ALS...........advanced life support
ANS...........autonomic nervous system
AP.............anteroposterior
APH...........antepartum haemorrhage
APLS.........advanced paediatric life support
ARM..........artificial rupture of membranes
ASD...........atrioseptal defect/autistic spectrum disorder
AVM...........arteriovenous malformation
BD.............twice daily
βhcg..........β-human chorionic gonadotrophin
BNF...........British National Formulary
BNFC.........British National Formulary for Children
BP.............blood pressure
BVM...........bag valve mask
CBRN.........chemical, biological, radiological, nuclear
CBT...........cognitive behavioural therapy
CCF...........congestive cardiac failure
CGA...........corrected gestational age
CHC...........combined hormonal contraceptive
CI..............contraindications
CIN............cervical intraepithelial neoplasia
CM.............congenital malformation
CMPA.........cows' milk protein allergy
CMV...........cytomegalovirus
CNS...........central nervous system
COC(P).......combined oral contraceptive (pill)
CPAP.........continuous +ve airways pressure
CPR...........cardiopulmonary resuscitation
CRP...........c-reactive protein
CRPS.........complex regional pain syndrome
CS.............caesarean section
CSF...........cerebrospinal fluid
CT.............computed tomography
CTG...........continuous cardiotocography
CVB/S........chorionic villus biopsy/sampling
CVP...........central venous pressure
CVS...........cardiovascular system
CXR...........chest x-ray
D&C...........dilatation (cervix) & curettage
D&V...........diarrhoea and vomiting
DB.............decibel
DHS...........dynamic hip screw
DIC............disseminated intravascular coagulation
DIP............distal interphalangeal
DKA...........diabetic ketoacidosis
DL.............decilitre
DM.............diabetes mellitus
DMSA.........dimercaptosuccinic acid
DNA...........deoxyribonucleic acid
DSM-5........Diagnostic & Statistical Manual, 5e

DUB...........dysfunctional uterine bleeding
DVT...........deep venous thrombosis
EBM...........evidence-based medicine
EBV...........Epstein–Barr virus
ECG...........electrocardiogram
ECT...........electroconvulsive therapy
ECV...........external cephalic version
ED.............emergency department
EEG...........electroencephalogram
EFM...........electrical fetal monitoring
ENT...........ear, nose, and throat
ERPC.........evacuation (of) retained products (of) conception
ESR...........erythrocyte sedimentation rate
ET.............endotracheal
FB.............foreign body
FBC...........full blood count
FBS...........fetal blood sampling
FCR...........flexor carpi radialis
FDP...........flexor digitorum profundus
FDS...........flexor digitorum sublimis
FH.............family history
FM.............fetal movement
FNA...........fine needle aspiration
FNT...........fetal nuchal translucency
FSE...........fetal scalp electrode
FSH...........follicle-stimulating hormone
G...............gauge
g...............gram(s)
G6PD.........glucose-6-phosphate dehydrogenase
GA.............general anaesthesia
GCS...........Glasgow Coma Scale/Score
GFR...........glomerular filtration rate
GH.............growth hormone
GI..............gastrointestinal
GORD.........gastro-oesophageal reflux disease
GP.............general practitioner
h...............hour
HB.............haemoglobin
HBsAg........hepatitis B surface antigen
HBV...........hepatitis B virus
HCG...........human chorionic gonadotrophin
HFOV.........high-frequency oscillatory ventilation
HIV............human immunodeficiency virus
HLA...........human leucocyte alleles
HPO...........hypothalamic–pituitary–ovarian
HPV...........human papilloma virus
HRT...........hormone replacement therapy
HSCT.........haematopoietic stem cell transplantation
HSP...........Henoch–Schönlein purpura
HUS...........haemolytic uraemic syndrome
HVS...........high vaginal swab
ICP...........intracranial pressure
Ig..............immunoglobulin
IHD............ischaemic heart disease
IM.............intramuscular
INR............international normalized ratio
IOP...........intraocular pressure
IP.............interphalangeal
IPPV..........intermittent positive pressure ventilation
IPT............interpersonal therapy
IQ.............intelligence quotient
ITP............idiopathic thrombocytopenic purpura
ITU...........intensive therapy unit
IU.............international unit
IU(C)D.......intrauterine (contraceptive) device
IUGR.........intrauterine growth restriction
IUI............intrauterine insemination
IUS...........intrauterine system
IV.............intravenous
IVF............in vitro fertilization
IVI............intravenous infusion
IVIg..........intravenous immunoglobulin
IVM...........in vitro maturation

IVU	intravenous urography	PIP	proximal interphalangeal
JIA	juvenile idiopathic arthritis	PKU	phenylketonuria
JVP	jugular venous pressure	PMB	postmenopausal bleeding
K⁺	potassium	PMH	past medical history
kg	kilogram	PO	*per os* (Latin for by mouth)
kPa	kilopascal	PONV	postoperative nausea and vomiting
L	litre	POP	progesterone-only pill/plaster of Paris
LBC	liquid-based cytology	PPH	postpartum haemorrhage
LBW	low birth weight (<2500g)	PROM	premature rupture of membranes
LDH	lactate dehydrogenase	PR	*per rectum*
LFT	liver function test	PTA	pure tone audiogram
LH	luteinizing hormone	PUO	pyrexia of unknown origin
LHRH	luteinizing hormone-releasing hormone	PUVA	psoralen-ultraviolet A
LLETZ	large loop excision of the transformation zone (of the cervix)	PV	*per vaginam* (via the vagina)
		PVD	posterior vitreous detachment
LMP	last menstrual period	R̠	treatment (prescribing drugs)
LMWH	low-molecular-weight heparin	RBC	red blood cell
LP	lumbar puncture	RCGP	Royal College of General Practitioners
LSCS	lower segment caesarean section	RCOG	Royal College of Obstetricians and Gynaecologists
LVH	left ventricular hypertrophy		
MAOI	monoamine oxidase inhibitor	RCT	randomized controlled trial
MC&S	microscopy, culture, & sensitivity	REM	rapid eye movement
mcg	microgram(s)	RMO	registered medical officer
MCI	mass casualty incident	RR	relative risk
MCP	metacarpophalangeal	RSI	repetitive strain injury; rapid sequence induction
MCV	mean cell volume		
MDT	multidisciplinary team	RTC	road traffic collision
mg	milligram(s)	RUQ	right upper quadrant
MHA	Mental Health Act	SAD	seasonal affective disorder/supraglottic airway device
MI	myocardial infarction		
mL	millilitre(s)	SALT	speech and language therapist
mmHg	millimetres of mercury	sao₂	arterial blood O₂ saturation
MRI	magnetic resonance imaging	sc	subcutaneous
MSU	midstream sample (of) urine (for culture)	SCBU	special care baby unit
MTP	metatarsophalangeal	SE	side effect(s)
mu	milliunit(s)	sec	second(s)
NaCl	sodium chloride	SERM	selective (o)estrogen receptor modulator
NAI	non-accidental injury	SFH	symphysis fundal height
NBM	nil by mouth	SGA	small-for-gestational age
NGT	nasogastric tube	SIADH	syn. of inappropriate antidiuretic hormone secretion
NICE	National Institute for Health and Care Excellence		
		SNHL	sensorineural hearing loss
NICU	neonatal intensive care unit	spo₂	pulse oximetry estimated sao₂
NIHL	noise-induced hearing loss	SSRI	selective serotonin reuptake inhibitor
NMJ	neuromuscular junction	stat	*statim* (Latin for once); single dose
NOF	neck of femur	STI	sexually transmitted infection
NSAID	non-steroidal anti-inflammatory drug	SUFE	slipped upper femoral epiphysis
NT	nuchal translucency	syn	syndrome
OAE	otoacoustic emissions	T°	temperature (degrees Centigrade)
OD	once daily	T3	triiodothyronine; T4 thyroxine
OHSS	ovarian hyperstimulation syndrome	TB	tuberculosis
OM	otitis media	TCA	traumatic cardiac arrest
OME	otitis media with effusion	TENS	transcutaneous electrical nerve stimulation
OMV	open mouth view		
ON	*omni nocte* (take at night)	TFT	thyroid function tests
OOH	out of hours/out of hospital	TGNB	transgender/non-binary
ORh−ve	blood group O, Rh negative	TIA	transient ischaemic attack
ORIF	open reduction and internal fixation	TOP	termination of pregnancy
OT	occupational therapist	TPH	transplacental haemorrhage
OTC	over the counter	TSH	thyroid-stimulating hormone
PA	posteroanterior	TSOH	transient synovitis of the hip
paco₂	partial pressure of co₂ in arterial blood	TTTS	twin–twin transfusion syndrome
pao₂	partial pressure of oxygen in arterial blood	U	unit(s)
		U&E	urea and electrolytes
PCOS	polycystic ovarian syndrome	UPSI	unprotected sexual intercourse
PCR	polymerase chain reaction/protein–creatinine ratio (urinary)	URTI	upper respiratory tract infection
		us(s)	ultrasound (scan)
PCV	packed cell volume	UTI	urinary tract infection
PDA	patent ductus arteriosus	UV	ultraviolet
PE	pulmonary embolus	VA	visual acuity
PEA	pulseless electrical activity	VSD	ventriculoseptal defect
PEP	post-exposure (to HIV) prophylaxis	VTE	venous thromboembolism
PET	positron emission tomography	VUR	vesico-ureteric reflux
PGD	preimplantation genetic diagnosis	WCC	white blood cell count
PICU	paediatric intensive care unit	wks	weeks
PID	pelvic inflammatory disease	wt	weight
		yrs	years

1 Obstetrics
Charlotte Goumalatsou

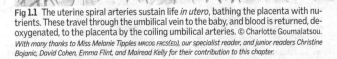

Fig 1.1 The uterine spiral arteries sustain life *in utero*, bathing the placenta with nutrients. These travel through the umbilical vein to the baby, and blood is returned, deoxygenated, to the placenta by the coiling umbilical arteries. © Charlotte Goumalatsou.

With many thanks to Miss Melanie Tipples MRCOG FRCS(ED), our specialist reader, and junior readers Christine Bojanic, David Cohen, Emma Flint, and Mairead Kelly for their contribution to this chapter.

☼ Women and childbirth in the 21ˢᵗ century

Obstetrics is perhaps as much of an art as a science, and concerns pregnancy, labour, and the postpartum period. As doctors, our role is to help navigate the most dangerous, yet shortest journey a person can take. This voyage is made riskier by underlying maternal medical conditions, pregnancy-specific diseases, conditions affecting the fetus, and insults during labour. Pre-pregnancy and pregnancy itself present opportunities to modify these risks, educate women, and promote health in pregnancy and the puerperium.

Maternal mortality in the UK is thankfully rare but often highlights missed opportunities for intervention. We know from serial MBRACE reports that many of these women had substandard antenatal care, that pre-existing medical conditions are common, prevalence of obesity is ever-increasing, and perinatal mental health problems are strongly associated with suicide.[1] These women need early review by obstetricians and access to obstetric physicians (a growing subspecialty of medicine). Psychiatry, specialist midwives, and anaesthetists are all important—use them.

If an obstetrician could be granted one wish, it would be to make every pregnancy *planned* and *desired by the mother*. Worldwide, a woman dies every minute from the effects of pregnancy, and most of these women never wanted to be pregnant in the first place—but either had no means of contraception, or were without the skills, authority, and self-confidence to negotiate with their partners. So the real killers are poverty, ignorance, and the sexual desires of men, and the real solutions entail literacy, economic growth, and an equality of dialogue between the sexes. Any obstetric or governmental initiatives in reproductive health which do not recognize these facts are doomed.[2]

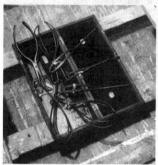

Fig 1.2 The birth of forceps begins in the 16th century with the Chamberlen brothers—French Huguenots—whose family fled to England following a ban on Protestant physicians. Both brothers—Peter 'the elder' and Peter 'the younger' had significant roles in the practice of 'man-midwifery'. Their quest to protect their invention and use of forceps led to extensive means of concealment—forceps were only revealed once the woman had been blindfolded, the birth taking place under blankets and with only the Chamberlens in attendance. Through these elaborate measures, and with their sons continuing in the practice, the Chamberlens were able to keep the secret of forceps for nearly a century. Hugh, son of Peter the younger and physician to King Charles II, fled to Holland after the King's forced abdication and is said to have sold some instruments to a Dutch obstetrician named Van Roonhuysen, whose family again kept the secret for many years. The original Chamberlen instruments were only discovered in 1813 under the floorboards of their Essex home and bear a remarkable resemblance to modern-day instruments.[3] Consider the Chamberlen's ingenuity as you approach problems, being mindful and thankful for advances in patient autonomy, and in the collaborative working of professionals.

Reproduced from Dunn PM, *Arch Dis Child Fetal Neonatal Ed* 1999;81(3):F232–F235, copyright Royal College of Paediatrics and Child Health 1999, with permission from BMJ Publishing Group Ltd.

Useful resources

NICE and RCOG guidelines (www.nice.org.uk, www.rcog.org.uk).

MBRACE maternal mortality reports (www.npeu.ox.ac.uk).

For safety of medicines when pregnant or breastfeeding: www.medicinesinpregnancy.org (part of UK teratology information service).

This can seem complicated at first and takes practice. There are more components than for a normal medical history but each step is important. Remember to use a translator if needed (not a family member) and bring out your sensitive side. Privacy and confidentiality are of utmost importance and the woman may not be willing to divulge intimate details with family members present. If you can, read her pregnancy notes before you see her (hospitals are phasing out handheld notes in favour of interactive apps which both the woman and clinician can access from a two way interface).

Current pregnancy Include name, age, occupation, relationship status, gravidity and parity, LMP, and EDD (preferably dated by 1st-trimester scan). See BOX 'Definitions and obstetric shorthand'. Irregular cycles, long cycles, and hormonal contraception make dating by LMP inaccurate. Ask about how the pregnancy is going, general health and symptoms, and fetal movements if >20 weeks. Ask about admissions or problems in this pregnancy as well as tests and scans. The woman may not know if everything is normal—this information is found in the pregnancy health record. Every woman will usually have had routine blood tests, a 1st-trimester scan, and an anomaly scan at 20 weeks.

Past obstetric history This should include details of all previous pregnancies including miscarriages and terminations (plus reason for termination eg fetal abnormality). Antenatal problems eg pre-eclampsia, date and place of delivery, mode and gestation at delivery, sex, birth weight, delivery complications Including shoulder dystocia, haemorrhage, and stillbirth. Don't forget to ask about the postnatal period and neonatal life.

Gynaecological, medical, and surgical history Ask about contraception, preconception, difficulties with conception, smear history, and previous gynaecological problems or procedures. Establish any pre-existing medical disorders eg asthma, diabetes, epilepsy, or heart disease and if under the care of other medical specialists or GP. Psychiatric history is also important. Surgical history may impact antenatal care or mode of delivery eg midline laparotomy for bowel resection for Crohn's or hip surgery limiting hip abduction.

Drug history Always check allergies and reaction. Include regular and as-required medication, as well as over-the-counter drugs. Some drugs may not be safe in pregnancy or breastfeeding (see resources on p. 1).

Family history Taking a family history of diseases or congenital abnormalities enables adequate screening and antenatal care. Remember to ask about problems with any children the woman already has. Ask about consanguinity 'Are you and your partner related in any way?'

Social history Drug and alcohol use, smoking, support at home. 'Ask the question' about domestic violence (p. 834) at each visit (domestic violence affects women of each social class equally). Domestic violence often escalates in pregnancy.

Definitions and obstetric shorthand

Gravidity Refers to the number of pregnancies that a woman has had, to any stage, including the current one.

Parity Refers to pregnancies that resulted in delivery beyond 24 weeks' gestation. An example of the shorthand way of expressing pregnancies before and after 24 weeks is para 2+1. This means that she has had 2 pregnancies beyond 24 completed weeks' gestation, and 1 which ended prior to 24 weeks. If she is not pregnant at the time of taking the history she is gravida 3, but if she is pregnant now she is gravida 4. Twins present a problem as there is controversy as to whether they count as 1 for both parity and gravidity or should count as 2 for parity.

In general, aim to use proper English rather than the shorthand described, which is open to ambiguity. For example, when presenting a patient try something like: 'Mrs Cottard is a 32-year-old lady who is 15 weeks into her 4th pregnancy; the 3rd ended in a miscarriage at 17 weeks, and the others came to term with normal deliveries of children who are now 2 & 8.' The bold statement 'Para 2+1' is ambiguous, incomprehensible to the patient, and misses the point that the patient is now approaching the time when she lost her last baby.

Dating a pregnancy Normal pregnancy is 40 weeks from the LMP. Naegele's rule: expected delivery date (EDD) ≈1yr and 7 days after LMP minus 3 months (not if last period was a withdrawal bleed). For cycles shorter than 28 days, subtract the difference from 28; if longer, add the difference. A revised rule suggests the addition of 10 days rather than 7 is more accurate. In the UK, pregnancies are dated in the 1st trimester by ultrasound (US); this is accurate and based on the premise that the fetus grows at a known rate.

The labour ward This runs on a combination of shorthand, acronyms, and many, many cups of tea. This list should help for your first few shifts:

APH: Antepartum haemorrhage: bleeding >24/40.

ARM: Artificial rupture of membranes.

CTG: Cardiotocography.

FM: Fetal movements.

GBS: Group B *Streptococcus*.

GDM: Gestational diabetes mellitus.

IOL: Induction of labour.

IUD: Intrauterine death or stillbirth.

MEC: Meconium-stained liquor, either significant or insignificant.

MROP: Manual removal of placenta.

NND: Neonatal death.

NVD: Normal vaginal delivery.

OC: Obstetric cholestasis.

PET: Pre-eclampsia (used to be known as pre-eclamptic toxaemia).

PIH: Pregnancy-induced hypertension.

PPH: Postpartum haemorrhage: bleeding >500mL postpartum.

PPROM: Preterm prelabour rupture of membranes <37/40.

PROM: Usually refers to prelabour rupture of membranes.

SFH: Symphysis–fundal height.

SPD: Symphysis pubis dysfunction.

SROM: Spontaneous rupture of membranes.

SVD: Spontaneous vaginal delivery.

VBAC: Vaginal birth after caesarean section.

The uterus occupies the pelvis and cannot be felt *per abdomen* until ~12 weeks' gestation. By 16 weeks, its fundus lies half way between the symphysis pubis and the umbilicus. By 20–24 weeks it reaches the umbilicus. In a primip, the fundus is under the ribs by 36 weeks. At term, the uterus lies a bit lower than at 36 weeks, as the head descends into the pelvis. From 16 weeks the SFH increases ~1cm/week (see table 1.1).

Table 1.1 The symphysis fundal height during pregnancy

As a rule of thumb, at:	16–26 weeks	the SFH (cm) ≈ dates (in weeks)
	26–36 weeks	the SFH (cm) ± 2cm ≈ dates
	36 weeks to term	the SFH (cm) ± 3cm ≈ dates

SFH is used as a screening tool to find babies small for gestational age (SGA) (p. 54). Suspect this if the measurement lies >1–2cm outside these ranges given previously. NB: more false positives will occur with the simpler rule of *weeks of gestation = cm from pubic symphysis to fundus*. The SFH should be plotted on a customized growth chart (p. 55).

Other reasons for discrepancy between fundal height and dates
• Inaccurate menstrual history • Multiple gestation • Fibroids • Polyhydramnios • Adnexal mass • Maternal size • Hydatidiform mole.

On inspecting the abdomen Note size, asymmetry, and fetal movements. Signs consistent with pregnancy include a line of pigmentation, the linea nigra, extending in the midline from pubic hair to umbilicus. This darkens during the 1st trimester (the first 13 weeks). Striae gravidarum (stretch marks) can either be purple (new) or silvery-white (old). Note surgical scars, particularly from previous caesarean, laparotomy, and laparoscopy.

Palpating the abdomen *Measure the SFH* after 20 weeks (palpate <20 weeks). *Estimate number of fetuses.* Then *assess fetal lie* (longitudinal, oblique, transverse) in relation to the uterus. *Presentation* is the part of the fetus overlying the pelvic brim and is most commonly cephalic or breech. *Engagement* of the head is measured in fifths palpable eg by Pawlik's grip (examining the lower pole of the uterus between the thumb and index fingers of the right hand). Watch the patient's face during palpation and stop if it causes pain. Obesity, polyhydramnios, and tense muscles make it difficult to feel the fetus. Midwives are skilled at palpation, and under 32 weeks of pregnancy it is often difficult, so ask them if you need help. See table 1.2 and figs 1.3 & 1.4 for abdominal palpation of fetal position, although this is not helpful unless the woman is in labour.

Auscultation The fetal heart may be heard by Doppler us (eg Sonicaid™) from ~12 weeks and with a Pinard stethoscope from ~24 weeks. Listen over the anterior shoulder of the fetus for rate and rhythm for 1 minute.

Fetal movements First noted by mothers at 18–20wks, movements ↑ until 32wks then plateau at average 31/h. Fetuses sleep for 20–40min cycles day and night (rarely >90min). Maternal posture affects detection (lying > sitting > standing). If fetal movements are reduced, the woman should contact her midwife or obstetric unit for assessment[4] (see p.70).

Engagement The level of the head is assessed in 2 ways: engagement, or fifths palpable abdominally. Engagement entails passage of the biggest diameter of the presenting part through the pelvic inlet. Fifths palpable abdominally states what you can feel, and makes no degree of judgement on degree of engagement of the head. In primigravida, the head usually enters the pelvis by 37 weeks, otherwise causes must be excluded (eg placenta praevia or fetal abnormality). In multips, the head may not enter the pelvis until onset of labour.

Table 1.2 Position—ie which way is the fetus facing?

Occipitoanterior	Occipitolateral	Occipitoposterior
Back easily felt	Back can be felt	Back not felt
Limbs not easily felt	Limbs lateral	Limbs anterior
Shoulder lies 2cm from midline on opposite side from back	Midline shoulder	Shoulder 6–8cm lateral, same side as back
Back from midline = 2–3cm	6–8cm	>10cm

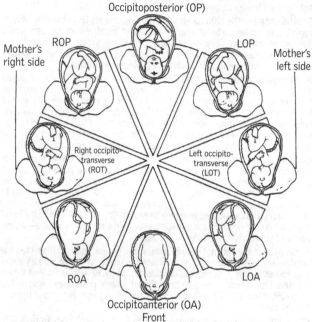

Occipitoposterior (OP)

ROP   LOP

Mother's right side   Mother's left side

Right occipito-transverse (ROT)   Left occipito-transverse (LOT)

ROA   LOA

Occipitoanterior (OA)
Front

Fig 1.3 Fetal positions.

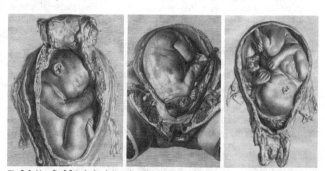

Fig 1.4 Use fig 1.3 to help determine the lie, the presentation, and the position from these dissections by William Hunter (1718–1783): *Anatomia uteri humani gravidi tabulis illustrata* (The anatomy of the human gravid uterus exhibited in figures).

Courtesy of the U.S. National Library of Medicine.

1 Obstetrics

Hormonal changes Progesterone, synthesized by the corpus luteum until 35 post-conception days and by the placenta mainly thereafter, decreases smooth muscle excitability (uterus, gut, ureters) and raises body temperature. *Oestrogens* (90% oestriol) increase breast and nipple growth, water retention, and protein synthesis. The maternal thyroid often enlarges due to increased colloid production. See 'Thyroid disease in pregnancy', p. 28. Pituitary secretion of *prolactin* rises throughout pregnancy. Maternal *cortisol* output is increased but unbound levels remain constant.

Genital changes The 100g non-pregnant uterus weighs 1100g by term. Muscle hypertrophy occurs up to 20 weeks, with stretching after that. The cervix may develop an ectropion ('erosion') (p. 164). Late in pregnancy, cervical collagen reduces. Vaginal discharge increases due to cervical ectopy, cell desquamation, and ↑ mucus production from a vasocongested vagina.

Haemodynamic changes *Blood:* From 10 weeks, the plasma volume rises until 32 weeks when it is 3.8 litres (50% > non-pregnant). Red cell volume rises from 1.4 litres when non-pregnant to 1.64 litres at term if iron supplements are not taken (↑ 18%), or 1.8 litres at term (↑ 30%) if supplements are taken—hence Hb falls due to dilution (physiological 'anaemia'). wcc (mean 10.5×10^9/L), platelets, ESR (up 4-fold), cholesterol, β-globulin, and fibrinogen are raised. Albumin and gamma-globulin decrease. Urea and creatinine decrease (see table 1.3, p. 9).

Cardiovascular: Cardiac output rises from 5 litres/min to 6.5–7 litres/min in the first 10 weeks by increasing stroke volume (10%) and pulse rate (by ~15 beats/min). Peripheral resistance falls (due to hormonal changes). BP, particularly diastolic, falls during the 2nd trimester by 10–20mmHg, then rises to non-pregnant levels by term. With increased venous dispensability, and raised venous pressure (as occurs with any pelvic mass), varicose veins may form. Vasodilation and hypotension stimulate renin and angiotensin release—an important feature of BP regulation in pregnancy.

Aortocaval compression: From 20 weeks, the gravid uterus compresses the inferior vena cava (and to a lesser extent the aorta) in supine women, reducing venous return. This reduces cardiac output by 30–40% (so-called supine hypotension). ►Placing the woman in the left lateral position or wedging her tilting 15° to the left relieves the pressure and restores cardiac output to more normal levels.

Other changes Ventilation increases 40% (tidal volume rises from 500 to 700mL), the increased depth of breath being a progesterone effect. O_2 consumption increases only 20%. Breathlessness is common as maternal $PaCO_2$ is set lower to allow the fetus to off-load CO_2. Gut motility is reduced, resulting in constipation, delayed gastric emptying, and, with a lax lower oesophageal sphincter, heartburn. Renal size increases by ~1cm in length during pregnancy.

Frequency of micturition emerges early (glomerular filtration rate ↑ by 60%), later from bladder pressure by the fetal head. The bladder muscle is lax but residual urine after micturition is not normally present. Skin pigmentation (eg in linea nigra, nipples, or as chloasma—brown patches of pigmentation seen especially on the face), palmar erythema, spider naevi, and striae are common. Hair shedding from the head is reduced in pregnancy but the extra hairs are shed in the puerperium.

Pregnancy tests Increasingly sensitive and may be positive from 9 days post conception (or from day 23 of a 28-day cycle). The false +ve rate is low. They detect the β-subunit of human chorionic gonadotrophin in early-morning urine, so are positive in trophoblastic disease (pp. 128–9).

The aim is to minimize the risks to the mother, neonate, or fetus by modifying pre-pregnancy conditions and risk factors. This may involve advising against pregnancy or delaying conception until a safer time. Babies conceived 18–23 months after a live birth have the lowest rate of perinatal problems.

Ensure rubella immune.

Stop smoking Smoking reduces ovulation and Fallopian tube function, causes abnormal sperm production (less penetrating capacity), ↑ rates of miscarriage (×2), and is associated with preterm labour and fetal growth restriction, placenta praevia, and abruption. Women should be encouraged and supported to stop smoking (p. 825), and if this is not possible, to reduce the amount they smoke.

Weight loss For both partners increases conception rate and reduces risks (p. 43). Aim for BMI >18.5 and <30kg/m².

Exercise Should be encouraged. It improves fitness and self-esteem. Avoid contact sports and sports where abdominal trauma is possible.

Folic acid supplementation To prevent neural tube defects (NTDs) and cleft lip, all should have folate-rich foods + folic acid 0.4mg daily >1 month preconception till 13wks (5mg/day if past NTD, on antiepileptics, diabetic, pp. 26–7, obese (BMI >30), HIV+ve on co-trimoxazole prophylaxis, or sickle cell disease, p. 6). Avoid liver & vit. A (vit. A embryopathy) & limit caffeine to 200mg/day (roughly 2 cups of tea or coffee); cook meat thoroughly, avoid pâté, soft cheese, shellfish, and raw fish.

Vitamin D supplementation For all women, but check particularly that at-risk ethnic groups, the obese, and those with chronic medical disease and reduced mobility are taking it.

Alcohol High levels of consumption are known to cause fetal alcohol syndrome. Minimal drinking eg 1–2u/wk has not been shown to adversely affect the fetus but alcohol does cross the placenta and may affect the fetal brain. Miscarriage rates are higher among drinkers of alcohol. NICE recommends <1u/24h. Binge drinking (>5u/session) is especially harmful. To cut consumption: see 'Managing alcohol consumption', pp. 826–7.

Recreational drug use Associated with miscarriage, preterm birth, poor fetal development, and intrauterine death; refer the woman for help early.

Pre-existing medical disorders May worsen during pregnancy, or be worsened by pregnancy. This may be transient or permanent. As a general rule, poorly controlled disease will remain the same or worsen with poorer outcomes, and well-controlled disease remains the same or improves, with a better outcome. Refer for specialist help early: this enables optimal control of the disease and reduces risk (eg fetal malformation in diabetes mellitus, or deterioration with SLE). If the disease is severe or pregnancy involves risk to life, conception may be discouraged (eg pulmonary hypertension, end-stage renal failure). If the woman is already pregnant, termination may be offered.

Medication Should be changed prior to conception to reduce the risk of teratogenesis eg antiepileptic drugs (AEDs), ACEI, immune-modulators. Seek expert help and use lowest effective dose with minimal polypharmacy. Don't forget over-the-counter preparations, including homeopathic or herbal (eg St John's wort).

Genetic counselling Should be offered at a regional centre if relevant personal or family history.

Spontaneous miscarriage (SM) Risk of miscarriage: 15–20% of all pregnancies, rising at extremes of age (>3 consecutive miscarriages = recurrent miscarriage, p. 125).

The placenta is the organ of respiration, nutrition, and excretion for the fetus. It produces hormones for maternal well-being. It immunologically protects the fetus from rejection and allows the passage of maternal IgG antibodies.

Development The placenta develops when the blastocyst implants into the decidua and forms from trophoblastic cells. Some of these cells are invasive, penetrating endometrial blood vessels, forming sinuses (lacunae). These trophoblastic cells become primitive villi, then secondary and tertiary villi, the core being fetal blood vessels. Villi formation starts at 6 weeks, and stem villi are established by 12 weeks. The placenta continues to grow both in circumference and thickness until 16 weeks (hence the need to start aspirin in those at risk by 16 weeks to prevent pre-eclampsia), and after this, circumferentially.

Placental villi: These are the functional units of the placenta (fig 1.5). Each placenta has around 60, grouped into cotyledons containing 3–4 villi. On the maternal (outer or uterine) surface is the syncytiotrophoblast which is in direct contact with maternal blood, then cytotrophoblast, basement membrane, mesenchymal stroma, and then the basement membrane of fetal blood vessels. The maternal surface looks raw, rough, and spongy. The fetal surface is smooth and shiny, covered by the amnion, and the umbilical cord is attached at the centre. Look for the branching of the umbilical vessels to and from the placenta. A monochorionic twin placenta is more interesting—examine closely to see if any vessels interconnect (as with twin-to-twin transfusion syndrome).

Circulation In the placenta, this consists of two different systems: uteroplacental and fetoplacental. *Uteroplacental* circulation is maternal blood travelling through the intervillous spaces. The uterus at term receives 500–600mL/min of blood, with the potential for torrential blood loss either as antepartum or postpartum haemorrhage. The circulation is set up so as to favour transfer of oxygen and other nutrients to the fetus. The spiral arteries become dilated and low-pressure, high-flow vessels to maximize blood flow. The first change occurs in the 1st trimester with structural modification, and the second wave in the 2nd trimester with myometrial segments of these spiral arteries being invaded. If this mechanism fails for some reason, and the uteroplacental circulation becomes high resistance with low flow, the result is varying degrees of IUGR and pre-eclampsia. The *fetoplacental* circulation consists of two *umbilical arteries* which carry deoxygenated blood from the fetus to the placenta. These arteries subdivide into many branches, entering the stem of the chorionic villus, then into arterioles and capillaries. The blood is then oxygenated and picks up nutrients, flowing into its relevant venous drainage system, eventually becoming the singular *umbilical vein*. The maternal and fetal circulations coexist as a form of countercurrent, and never mix.

Functions The placenta attaches the fetus, is the organ of gaseous and nutrient exchange, and produces many substances (hCG, growth factors, oestrogens, progestogens, PAPP-A), as well as a barrier (infection, drugs). At term the placenta weighs 1/6th the weight of the baby. The placenta changes throughout pregnancy as calcium is deposited in the villi and fibrin on them. Excess fibrin may be deposited in diabetes and rhesus disease, so ↓ fetal nutrition.

After delivery Examine the placenta for abnormalities (clots, infarcts, vasa praevia, single umbilical artery). Blood may be taken from the cord for pH (especially if abnormal CTG pre-delivery), Hb, Coombs' test, LFTs, and blood group (eg for rhesus disease), or for infection screens, if needed.

For placenta praevia, see p. 80.

1 Obstetrics

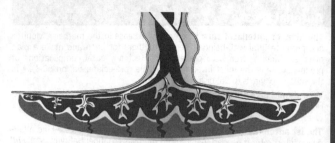

Fig 1.5 The placenta and umbilical cord. Seven spiral arteries are here seen to have been successfully invaded by trophoblast and they are now flooding the vast intervillous spaces with hot maternal blood—producing the slow whooshing crescendos heard by the us probe as the backdrop to the faster fetal heartbeat. To get to the fetus proper, nutrients have a 6-part journey: maternal blood space → syncytiotrophoblast → trophoblast basement membrane → capillary basement membrane → capillary endothelium → fetal blood.

In pre-eclampsia, trophoblast invasion is too shallow: there is no progress beyond the superficial portions of the uterine spiral arterioles. So these spiral arterioles retain their endothelial linings and remain narrow-bore, high-resistance vessels, resulting in poor maternal blood flow. The mother may raise her blood pressure to compensate for this—but the price may be eclampsia (pp. 50-1).

Plasma chemistry in pregnancy

Table 1.3 Plasma chemistry values in pregnancy

	Non-pregnant		Trimester 1		Trimester 2		Trimester 3	
Centile	2.5	97.5	2.5	97.5	2.5	97.5	2.5	97.5
Na^+ mmol/L	138	146	135	141	132	140	133	141
Ca^{2+} mmol/L	2	2.6	2.3	2.5	2.2	2.2	2.2	2.5
*corrected	2.3	2.6	2.25	2.57	2.3	2.5	2.3	2.59
Albumin g/L	44	50	39	49	36	44	33	41
AST IU/L	7	40	10	28	11	29	11	30
AST IU/L	0	40	6	32	6	32	6	32
TSH	0	4	0	1.6	1	1.8	7	7.3

*Calcium corrected for plasma albumin (онсм p676)

Other plasma reference intervals (not analysed by trimester)

	Non-pregnant	Pregnant
Alk phos IU/L	3–300	≤450 (can be ↑↑ in normal pregnancies)
Bicarbonate mmol/L	24–30	20–25
Creatine μmol/L	70–150	24–68
Urea mmol/L	2.5–6.7	2–4.2
Urate μmol/L	150–390	116–276 (24wks), 110–322 (32wks), 120–344 (36wks)

c-reactive protein does not change much in pregnancy.
Platelets ≥150×10⁹/L (beware if <120×10⁹/L see pp. 50-1).
For anaemia in pregnancy, see p21.
TSH may be low <20wks in normal pregnancy (suppressed by hCG); see earlier & p. 28.
Protein s falls in pregnancy, so protein s deficiency is difficult to diagnose.
Activated protein c (APC) resistance is found in 40% of pregnancies so special tests are needed when looking for this. Genotyping for factor v Leiden and prothrombin G20210A are unaffected by pregnancy.

The aims of antenatal care • Detect any disease in the mother • Monitor and promote fetal well-being • Prepare mothers for birth and make a plan of care • Monitor trends to prevent or detect any early complications of pregnancy: BP is the most important variable (pre-eclampsia, pp. 50–1). • Is thromboprophylaxis (p. 36) or aspirin needed?

Who should give antenatal care? Midwives manage care, calling in obstetricians if risks *or specific needs are identified*. Book by 12 weeks: see within 2 weeks if already ≥12 weeks pregnant.

The 1st antenatal (booking) visit This is very comprehensive. ►Find a language interpreter if needed. Avoid using relatives (confidentiality issues). *Full obstetric history:* (See p. 2.) Particularly, is there a family history of diabetes, BP ↑, fetal abnormality, inheritable disease, or twins?

- Does she have concurrent illness? Has she been 'cut' (FGM p. 111)? Risk assess for venous thromboembolism and if high risk refer to obstetrics; may need antenatal and postnatal low-molecular-weight heparin (LMWH) (p. 36).
- Is gestational diabetes (GDM) a risk? Screen (75g glucose tolerance test) at 28wks if BMI >30, previous baby >4.5kg, 1st-degree relative diabetic, family origin (FO) from area of high risk for diabetes. If previous GDM, screen at 16 & 28wks.
- Past mental illness? If serious (schizophrenia, bipolar disorder, self-harm) or past postnatal depression, get antenatal assessment by perinatal mental health team and put management plan in notes.
- Women born outside the UK are at higher risk of haemoglobinopathies, blood-borne viruses, and pre-existing cardiac disease.
- *Unsupported women:* those with unplanned pregnancies or unemployed are likely to need more support. Always *ask the question* about domestic violence (p. 834). Check for *substance abuse* (pp. 828–9). 'Healthy Start Vitamins for Women'—folic acid + vitamins C & D (10mcg/d) are free to some during pregnancy and for 1 year after birth (Healthy Start Scheme[UK]).

Examination: Check heart, lungs, BP, weight (record BMI), and abdomen. Cervical smears: 3 months postnatal (if due).

Tests: Blood: Hb, blood group, and rhesus antibody screen, syphilis & rubella (± chicken-pox) serology, HBsAg HIV test; sickle test depending on family origin, Hb electrophoresis and 25-hydroxyvitamin D if relevant.[5] Take an MSU (protein; bacteria). If she is from an area endemic for TB or a TB contact, consider referral for Mantoux test and CXR.

Screening for chromosomal and structural abnormalities should be offered at booking. The 12-week scan also confirms EDD (p.12).

Advise on: Smoking, alcohol, diet, correct use of seat belts (above or below the bump, not over it). Offer antenatal classes, information on maternity benefits, including free dental care. Usual exercise and travel are OK (avoid malarious areas) up to 36 weeks (singleton)[6] but check with airline; many require a 'fit to fly' letter beyond 32 weeks. Intercourse OK if no vaginal bleeding.

Later visits Discuss screening results and treat anaemia or UTI. At each visit, check urine for protein; BP; fundal height. Visits are at <12 weeks then at 16, 25, 28, 31, 34, 36, 38, 40, and 41 weeks (primip).

- 28wks: do Hb and Rh antibodies at 28 weeks and give anti-D if needed (p. 11). Weigh only if clinically indicated.
- 34wks: discuss labour and birth, pain relief.
- 36wks: discuss breastfeeding, neonatal vitamin K, postnatal care, postnatal depression, and the baby blues.
- 40wks: discuss post-dates pregnancy and its management (p.56).
- 41wks: offer membrane sweep and book IOL by 42 weeks.

If a pregnant woman with rhesus-negative blood is exposed to rhesus-positive blood from the fetus, she may produce antibodies against the RhD antigen (sensitization—from miscarriage, placental bleeding, or injury). The immune response does not usually harm this pregnancy but future RhD positive pregnancies are at risk (anti-RhD antigens cross the placenta and cause fetal anaemia and haemolytic disease of the newborn). Give anti-D IM in the deltoid as soon as possible after the sensitizing event and within 72h (some protection if by 10 days). From 20^{+0} weeks test for fetal maternal haemorrhage (FBC bottle of maternal blood; counts fetal RBCs = Kleihauer test). Don't give anti-D if already sensitized ie antibodies to anti-D are present.[7]

Use of anti-D in miscarriage in Rh−ve women

1. Anti-D should be given to all having surgical or medical terminations of pregnancy, evacuation of molar pregnancy (p. 128), and ectopic pregnancies, unless they are already sensitized. Give 250u if <20 weeks; 500u (and Kleihauer) if $>20^{+0}$ weeks' gestation.
2. Anti-D should always be given for medical or surgical management of miscarriage or retained products of conception.
3. Anti-D should be given where spontaneous miscarriage occurs after 12^{+0} weeks' gestation.
4. Threatened miscarriage $\geq12^{+0}$ weeks give anti-D; if bleeding continues intermittently give anti-D 6-weekly until delivery.
5. Routine anti-D is not recommended with threatened miscarriage before 12 weeks' gestation (but consider if viable fetus, heavy or repeated bleeding, and abdominal pain).

Routine antenatal anti-D prophylaxis for all Rh−ve women

1. Give anti-D 500u at 28 weeks as the single-dose regimen or 28 and 34 weeks in the 2-dose regimen. Take 28-week blood sample for blood group and antibody screen before 28-week anti-D is given.
2. When significant transplacental haemorrhage (TPH) may occur: with chorionic villus sampling; external cephalic version, APH; uterine procedures (eg amniocentesis, fetal blood sampling); abdominal trauma; intrauterine death (within 72h of fetal death, not delivery).

Postnatal use 500u is the normal dose after 20^{+0} weeks' gestation. 37% of Rh−ve women give birth to Rh−ve babies and these women do not need anti-D.

• Anti-D should be given to all Rh−ve women where the baby's group cannot be determined.

• Do a Kleihauer test on all eligible for anti-D. 500u anti-D can suppress immunization by up to 4mL of fetal red cells (8mL of fetal blood), but 1% of women have TPH of >4mL, especially after manual removal of placenta, and with caesarean section. A Kleihauer test is especially important in stillbirth, as massive spontaneous transplacental haemorrhage can be the cause of fetal death. Where >4mL TPH is suggested by the Kleihauer screen, a formal estimation of the TPH volume is required and 500u anti-D given for every 4mL fetal cells transfused (maximum 5000u anti-D at 2 IM sites/24h). Note: Kleihauer tests can be negative where there is ABO incompatibility as fetal cells are rapidly cleared from the maternal circulation. Liaise with the transfusion service. Check maternal blood every 48h to determine clearance of cells and need for continuing anti-D.

Role of cell-free fetal DNA (cffDNA) testing

• Approximately 40% of Rh D negative women will be carrying a Rh D negative fetus, equating to around 40,000 women who are receiving unnecessary prophylaxis. Some UK units are now offering cffDNA testing at 16 weeks to Rhesus negative women. Those carrying a negative fetus do not need anti-D. Overall this is thought to be cost-neutral to the NHS.

'The first half of pregnancy can become a time of constant "exams" to see if the baby can be allowed to graduate to the second half of pregnancy'. Congenital abnormalities, including aneuploidy, affect 2% of newborns. They are responsible for 21% of perinatal mortality and the outcome may involve physical and/or mental disability. Most congenital abnormalities are in low-risk patients with uncomplicated pregnancies. Women at higher risk are those with a previously affected fetus or child, pre-existing diabetes, epilepsy (even if not on AEDs). Everyone in the UK should be offered screening tests for structural and chromosomal abnormalities. Prenatal identification of problems allows decision-making for timing, mode, and place of delivery; meeting the neonatal team; ongoing fetal surveillance; time for the parents to come to terms with having an affected child; and in cases in which the problem would have a major impact on the child, termination of pregnancy may be offered. Remember that screening is not diagnostic, and can be declined by the woman.

Ultrasound This can detect a pregnancy from ~5 weeks' gestation. *Early pregnancy scans* at <11 weeks are used to determine location, viability, and dating of the pregnancy. These are not routinely carried out unless there is bleeding, pain, or hyperemesis gravidarum (to exclude a molar pregnancy or twins). To *date a pregnancy,* crown–rump length between 6 and 12 weeks is most accurate—the growth is constant across the population. After 14 weeks, biparietal diameter (BPD) is the most accurate up to 20 weeks. After 34 weeks, BPD is unreliable. A woman who books for the first time in the 3rd trimester will require 2 growth scans, 2 weeks apart, to give the best estimate of gestation.

The dating scan: This is carried out at 11^{+0}–13^{+6} weeks and determines viability (excludes miscarriage), dates pregnancy, and diagnoses multiple pregnancy and chorionicity (p. 66). 59% of those with major structural abnormalities can be detected at this stage eg anencephaly, and up to 81% with the later anomaly scan.[8] Screening for chromosomal abnormalities is carried out using the nuchal fold measurement (nuchal translucency (NT) + blood test (pp. 16–7). Increased NT may reflect fetal heart failure,[9] and be seen in serious anomaly of the heart and great arteries.[10] The fetus should be in the neutral position as degree of neck flexion influences measurements. Taking the 99th percentile as a cut off for cardiac screening enables 33% of heart abnormalities to be detected antenatally.[11] Referring 99th percentile fetuses for echocardiography may show 106 cardiac abnormalities per 1000 fetuses examined.[12] There is a strong association between chromosomal abnormality and NT. In one study, 84% of karyotypically proven trisomy 21 fetuses had a NT >3mm at 10–13 weeks' gestation (as did 4.5% of chromosomally normal fetuses). The greater the extent of NT, the greater the risk of abnormality. Together with the blood screening tests, NT screening is used to calculate risk of chromosomal abnormality and if high risk (<1:150), invasive testing is offered (p. 17). Of all chromosomally normal fetuses (euploid) with significant nuchal thickening, 70–90% have normal outcome, 2.2–10.6% miscarry, 0.5–12.7% have neurodevelopmental problems, and 2.1–7.6% of malformations were undiagnosed before birth.[13]

The anomaly scan: This is a detailed US undertaken at 18–22 weeks' gestation to detect structural malformations. It takes ~30 minutes to complete and sensitivity varies depending on gestation, maternal BMI, operator skill, quality of the US machine, and the fetal structure involved (eg fetal heart defects are harder to detect than CNS defects).

Anomaly scan requirements

- *Skull shape and internal structures* including the cerebellum, ventricular size, and nuchal fold.
- *Spine* in longitudinal and transverse views.
- *Abdomen* for shape and content at the level of the stomach, kidneys, umbilicus/abdominal wall, and bladder.
- *Arms and legs* for 3 long bones per limb, and a hand or foot.
- *Heart* in 4-chamber view, with outflow tracts, and lungs.
- *Face and lips.*

Lethal anomalies: Anencephaly (absence of skull and cerebral cortex), bilateral renal agenesis, some major cardiac abnormalities, and trisomies 13 and 18. Offer a second opinion in a fetal medicine unit. Some anomalies have better survival rates than others and counselling must be supportive and informative no matter what the decision.

Fetal echocardiography: Offered to those at high risk of fetal cardiac abnormality: family or personal history, NT of >3.5mm, suspected abnormality, drugs in pregnancy eg lithium, pre-existing diabetes, monochorionic twins. It is carried out in tertiary centres or by fetal medicine specialists.

Soft markers: Findings on the anomaly scan that are in themselves of little significance, but are slightly more common in chromosomally abnormal fetuses. Choroid plexus cysts are seen in 1% of 20-week scans and are not significant; weak association with trisomy 18. Echogenic bowel has echogenicity similar to adjacent bone with the same US settings and is associated with an increased risk of chromosomal abnormalities, congenital infection, CF, and bowel obstruction. Others include 2-vessel umbilical cord, echogenic intracardiac foci, and mild renal pelvic dilatation.

Fetal growth scans: Require accurate gestational age. Head circumference and abdominal circumference (sometimes with femur length) are used to calculate estimated fetal weight. Along with liquor volume (single deepest vertical pocket or amniotic fluid index) this is used to determine pattern of growth. Scans should be at least 2 weeks apart and used when there is an increased risk of growth abnormality eg previous growth restriction, pre-eclampsia, measuring small for dates. A scan finding of a SGA fetus (p. 54) should prompt umbilical artery Doppler to distinguish between a fetus who is small and coping from those who are beginning to decompensate and require early delivery.

Doppler US: Measures blood flow in the uterus, placenta, and fetus. In an unselected population, it has not been shown to be of value but it is useful in high-risk pregnancies. *Uterine artery Doppler* measures resistance within the placenta. It is usually carried out at 23 weeks. High resistance increases risk of maternal pre-eclampsia and fetal growth restriction and requires extra maternal and fetal surveillance during pregnancy. *Umbilical artery Doppler* measures resistance in the placenta. High resistance indicates placental failure, and these fetuses are at higher risk of intrauterine death. If very preterm (<28 weeks), this can be used to time delivery. In absent or reversed end-diastolic flow, urgent delivery by caesarean section should be considered, depending on gestation. Dopplers of fetal vessels (middle cerebral artery (MCA) and ductus venosus) may be used to time delivery. MCA Dopplers are also used to detect fetal anaemia eg with rhesus disease and parvovirus infection. Computerized CTG is helpful in monitoring of the compromised fetus (p. 46).

1 Obstetrics

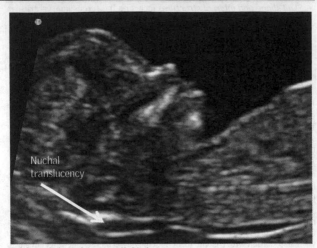

Fig 1.6 Nuchal translucency at 11–14wks uss.
Reproduced from Collins *et al. Oxford Handbook of Obstetrics and Gynaecology* (2013) with permission from OUP.

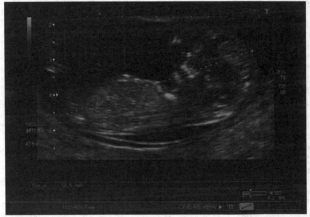

Fig 1.7 us image of a 12wk fetus measuring the crown–rump length.
Reproduced from Collins *et al. Oxford Handbook of Obstetrics and Gynaecology* (2013) with permission from OUP.

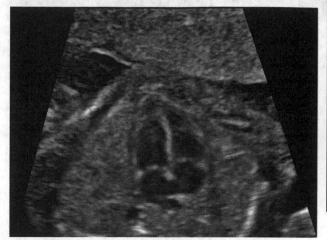

Fig 1.8 USS of a normal cardiac 4-chamber view.
Reproduced from Collins *et al. Oxford Handbook of Obstetrics and Gynaecology* (2013) with permission from OUP.

Screening in the UK NHS is offered to all women at booking. Most units use the combined test for trisomy 21 (Down syndrome) screening, which has a detection rate of 75% with a false +ve rate of <3%. A risk of 1:150 or less is high risk and the woman is offered invasive testing eg amniocentesis. Screening tests estimate risk of trisomies 21, 13, and 18 taking into account results from NT, blood tests, and the woman's age. Results are modified further by smoking status, multiple pregnancy, IVF, maternal weight, ethnicity, and diabetes.

Trisomy 21 This is the commonest cause of learning disability and the most common chromosomal abnormality. 10% die before age 5, and life expectancy is ~55 years. More fetuses at 16 weeks will have T21 than at term due to the increased rate of spontaneous miscarriage. Prevalence increases with increasing maternal age, and most occur secondary to non-disjunction of chromosome 21 at meiosis. Congenital cardiac malformations are common and 46% have VSD or ASD. Duodenal atresia is also common. **Trisomy 18** (Edwards syndrome, p. 846.) This the second most common trisomy after T21. Most die soon after birth and survival after 1 year is rare. Features include small chin, low-set ears, rocker-bottom feet, and VSD. **Trisomy 13** (Patau syndrome, p. 854.) This is rare, and babies die soon after birth. Features include microcephaly, holoprosencephaly, exomphalos, and cleft lip and palate.

Risk of trisomy 21 with rising maternal age	
<25 years: 1:1500	
30 years: 1:910	
35 years: 1:380	
40 years: 1:110	
45 years: 1:30	

The combined test This is the recommended screening test in the UK. It uses NT + free human chorionic gonadotrophin (hCG) + pregnancy-associated plasma protein (PAPP-A) + the woman's age. Used between 11 and 13 weeks + 6 days. It achieves detection rates of 90% of all aneuploidies, 86% trisomy 21, and higher for trisomy 18 and trisomy 13. PAPP-A levels are ~19.6% lower in smokers.[14] In multiple pregnancy, risk is calculated per pregnancy if monochorionic; or per fetus when dichorionic or trichorionic.[15]NICE Absent or hypoplastic nasal bone, and significant tricuspid regurgitation modifies the risk. A high risk screening result is followed up with counselling for either NIPT (p. 17) or an invasive test for diagnosis (p. 17).

The integrated test This is a better screening test than the combined test but expensive and rarely used. It involves NT + PAPP-A in the 1st trimester + the quadruple test in the 2nd trimester. Do not use 2nd-trimester tests for triplets.[15]NICE

The quadruple test This is a blood test at 16 weeks and uses a dating scan (not a NT scan) plus maternal α-fetoprotein (AFP) + unconjugated estriol + free βhCG or total βhCG + inhibin-A + the woman's age in the 2nd trimester. Use between 15 weeks + 0 days and 20 weeks + 0 days, so useful for women presenting in the 2nd trimester.

Alpha-fetoprotein AFP is a glycoprotein synthesized by the fetal liver and GI tract. In 10% with a high AFP there is a fetal malformation eg an open neural tube defect (but closed defects are missed), exomphalos, posterior urethral valves, nephrosis, GI obstruction, teratomas, Turner syndrome (or normal twins). In ~30% of those with no malformation, there is an adverse outcome eg IUGR, preterm delivery, placental abruption, and 3rd-trimester deaths.

Pregnancy-associated plasma protein A (PAPP-A) This is a large glycoprotein produced by the placenta that may have functions including matrix mineralization and angiogenesis. Therefore, low levels (<0.4 multiples of the median (MoM)) reflect poor early placentation. Low levels in 1st-trimester screening are associated with trisomies 18 and 21, pre-eclampsia, growth restriction, preterm delivery, and fetal demise.

Preimplantation genetic diagnosis

Preimplantation genetic diagnosis (PGD) is an early form of prenatal diagnosis in which embryos created *in vitro* are analysed for well-defined genetic diseases eg monogenic disorders such as CF or beta-thalassaemia, or chromosome structural abnormalities. One to two cells are extracted at the 6–10-cell stage of the embryo. Fluorescence *in situ* hybridization (FISH) is used for analysis of chromosomes and polymerase chain reaction (PCR) for analysis of genes in monogenic diseases. One or two disease-free embryos are then used for implantation.

PGD selection of embryos by HLA type so that a child born after using this technology can be used as a stem cell donor to save a sibling from certain conditions (eg with Fanconi anaemia, thalassaemia, or leukaemia) is possible. Sex selection, unless to avoid sex-linked diseases, is illegal in the UK.

Pregnancy rates following PGD are 17% after testing for structural chromosome abnormality (including translocations), 16% after sexing, 21% after testing for monogenic diseases. This is lower than the expected rate of 20–25% expected for regular IVF.

Invasive testing This is offered if screening suggests an increased risk of aneuploidy (and may therefore be declined). DNA can be analysed for single-gene disorders such as CF or sickle cell disease.

Chorionic villus biopsy: Carried out at 10–13 weeks. The placenta is sampled by a transabdominal or occasionally a transcervical approach under continuous US control. Karyotyping takes 2 days, enzyme and gene probe analysis 3 weeks, so termination for abnormality is earlier, safer, and is done before the pregnancy is apparent, compared with amniocentesis. Risks are an excess miscarriage rate of 1–2%, increased transmission of blood-borne viruses (HIV, hepatitis B & C), rarely contamination by maternal cells, and false positives or negatives from placental mosaicism (1%). It is not recommended in dichorionic multiple pregnancy. Is anti-D needed (p. 11)?

Amniocentesis: Undertaken from 16 weeks onwards and involves the aspiration of fluid containing fetal cells shed from skin and gut. A small needle is passed transabdominally under continuous US, preferably not transplacentally. Fetal loss rate is ~1% at ~16 weeks' gestation. Anti-D is needed in all Rh–ve women (p. 11). Amniocentesis has the advantage of being able to diagnose fetal infections such as CMV and the excess miscarriage rate is lower than for CVS. Full cell culture for karyotyping may take as long as 3 weeks, but rapid results are possible within 2 days by FISH and PCR.

Cell-free fetal DNA (cffDNA) This is a method of non-invasive prenatal testing (NIPT) for chromosomal abnormalities. Fetal DNA is produced by the placenta from the 1st trimester, released into the maternal circulation, and is cleared rapidly following delivery. Current methods cannot completely extract fetal DNA from maternal blood, and so the primary focus is on differing certain sequences eg Y chromosome of the male fetus, or Rh-D sequences in a Rh–ve woman (see p. 11). It can also be used to guide the need for invasive testing in x-linked diseases—no need for invasive testing in female fetuses. There are good data to show that detection of trisomies 18 and 21 have sensitivity and specificity rates approaching 100%.

Dichorionic twins, maternal obesity, gestation <10 weeks, and placental mosaicism are known to affect results due to lower levels of cffDNA in maternal blood. The use of cffDNA is likely to be offered in the future within the NHS to high-risk women (high-risk combined screening, previous affected fetus) and has clear advantages in reducing the risks associated with invasive testing.[18,RCOL]

▶Before prescribing any drug, think—is it safe? Check (eg *BNF*, and see p. 1).

Symptoms and signs in the first 12 weeks Early symptoms are amenorrhoea, nausea, vomiting, and bladder irritability. Breasts engorge, nipples enlarge (darken at 12 weeks), Montgomery's tubercles (sebaceous glands on nipples) become prominent. Vulval vascularity increases and the cervix softens and looks bluish (4 weeks). At 6–10 weeks the uterine body is more globular. Basal body temperature rises (<37.5°c).

Headaches, palpitations, and fainting These are all commoner in pregnancy. Dilated peripheral circulation ↑ sweating and feeling hot. *Management:* Increase fluid intake. If she feels faint from postural hypotension, stand slowly.

Urinary frequency Due to pressure of the fetal head on the bladder in later pregnancy. GFR also increases, increasing urine output. Exclude UTI (p. 31).

Abdominal pain See p. 42.

Breathlessness Common. Are there risk factors for VTE? See p. 37.

Constipation Tends to occur as gut motility decreases. Adequate oral fluids and a high-fibre diet help combat it. Avoid stimulant laxatives—they increase uterine activity in some women. Increased venous distensibility and pelvic congestion predispose to *haemorrhoids* and *varicose veins*. Resting with feet up and properly worn elastic stockings help.

Gastro-oesophageal reflux (heartburn) Occurs as progesterone-mediated pyloric sphincter relaxation allows irritant bile to reflux into the stomach. This is then worsened week-by-week from an ever-enlarging fetus pressing on the upper GI tract. Cigarettes and spices should be avoided; cold, small meals, and antacids and H2-receptor antagonists or proton pump inhibitors may be used. Use more pillows, and a semi-recumbent position.

Musculoskeletal Symphysis pubis dysfunction (SPD), due to pelvic ligament and muscle relaxation may affect 10% (usually mild). *Management:* Simple analgesia, physiotherapy. Not an indication for IOL or CS. Backache is common—manage as for SPD.

Carpal tunnel syndrome (p. 555) In pregnancy, this is due to fluid retention. Advise wrist splints until delivery.

Itch/itchy rashes These are common (up to 25%) and may be due to the usual causes or to pruritic eruption of pregnancy (PEP—an intensely itchy papular/plaque rash on the abdomen and limbs). PEP is most common in first pregnancies beyond 35 weeks' gestation. Emollients and weak topical steroids ease it. Delivery cures it. If vesicles are present, think of *pemphigoid gestationis* (PG): a rare (1:50,000) condition which may cause fatal heat loss and cardiac failure; the baby may be briefly affected; refer early (prednisolone may be needed). PG may recur in later pregnancies.

Ankle oedema This is a very common, almost normal, manifestation of pregnancy. Measure BP and check urine for protein (pre-eclampsia, pp. 50-1). Check legs for DVT. It often responds to rest and leg elevation. Reassure that it is harmless (unless pre-eclampsia).

Leg cramps 33% get cramp, often in the latter half of pregnancy, which is severe in 5% and worse at night. Anecdotally, good hydration, consumption of bananas, and tonic water can help. Restless leg syndrome is rarer but very difficult to treat, and poorly understood. Try measures for cramp.

Chloasma This is a patch of darker pigmentation, usually on the face: p. 436.

Nausea Affects ~80%. **Vomiting** Occurs in ~50%. It may start by 4 weeks and decline over the following weeks. At 20 weeks 20% may still vomit. Most respond to frequent small meals, reassurance, and a stress-free environment. It is associated with good outcome (fewer fetal losses). Hyperemesis: p. 19.

1 Obstetrics

This is persistent nausea and vomiting in pregnancy causing weight loss (>5%), dehydration, and electrolyte imbalance. It is rare and affects 0.3–3.6% of pregnant women. Risk is increased in multiple pregnancies, molar pregnancies, and those with previous HG. May be fatal if no access to help (Charlotte Bronte died from it). It is thought to be related to high levels of hCG.

Presentation Nausea, vomiting, hypersalivation, spitting, loss of weight, inability to tolerate food and fluids, effect on quality of life. Quantify severity using PUQE score (based on frequency of nausea, vomiting, and retching). Exclude other causes of nausea and vomiting: ask about abdominal pain, urinary symptoms, infection, drug history, and chronic *Helicobacter pylori* infection. Examine her and take a full set of observations. Weigh her, and look particularly for signs of dehydration and muscle wasting.

Tests Urine dip for ketones and UTI (send MSU). FBC may reveal raised haematocrit; U&E to exclude hypokalaemia or hyponatraemia. Transaminases may be abnormal and albumin low. If refractory HG, check TFTs, LFTs (to exclude hepatitis/gallstones), calcium and phosphate, amylase to exclude pancreatitis, and ABGs to exclude metabolic disturbance/monitor severity. US should be carried out to diagnose multiple pregnancy and exclude trophoblastic disease.

Treatment Take the woman seriously. Ginger and acupressure may help mild to moderate nausea and vomiting. Rest, assess mental health status, and prescribe oral antiemetics when required, using combinations if single-line therapy is ineffective. Admit to hospital if unable to keep anything down despite oral antiemetics, for rehydration and correction of metabolic disturbance, or if coexisting morbidity such as UTI. Aggressively fluid replace with either 0.9% NaCl + K or Hartmann's. Glucose can precipitate Wernicke's encephalopathy. Daily U&E to guide potassium and sodium replacement. Antiemetics regularly eg promethazine or cyclizine. Metoclopramide PO/IV/IM (risk of extrapyramidal SE) and ondansetron PO/IV (limited safety data but so far reassuring) are second-line therapy. If vomiting still intractable, consider a course of corticosteroids eg **prednisolone** 40–50mg daily or **hydrocortisone** 100mg/12h IV. Some women are so badly affected by HG that they opt for ToP. Prescribe high-dose **folic acid** 5mg/day and **thiamine** to prevent Wernicke's encephalopathy (50mg PO TDS or IV B vitamins eg Pabrinex®). These women are high risk for VTE and while in hospital should have daily thromboprophylaxis (eg **enoxaparin** 40mg/24h SC) and anti-thromboembolic stockings. If HG continues into the 2nd and 3rd trimester, arrange serial growth scans.

Hyperemesis gravidarum: Amy's story

Suffering from hyperemesis was worse than anything I had experienced. I vomited every single day from 6 weeks' gestation until 4 hours after my baby was born.

I was admitted 5 times for fluid rehydration and that was while taking 4 different antiemetics. Some days rolling over in bed caused continuous vomiting. I couldn't work for 2 months and even after that I only managed mornings. Despite working in the medical profession, some people didn't understand the illness and thought I was using pregnancy as an excuse to lighten the workload.

I felt like nothing was ever going to help. I was scared every day and became isolated. My son is 100% worth it but my pregnancy felt like a lifetime! Even now I worry about the effects of so many medications on my baby but as Charlotte Bronte died of hyperemesis I took all medical advice, admissions, and medications to get myself and my son to term!

1 Obstetrics

Further reading

RCOG (2016). *The Management of Nausea and Vomiting of Pregnancy and Hyperemesis Gravidarum* (Green-top Guideline No. 69). London: RCOG.

Sickle cell disease (SCD) is caused by a group of haemoglobin disorders (single-gene recessive) which predispose to 'sickling' of red cells in low oxygen conditions causing vaso-occlusion in small vessels, and cells prone to increased haemolytic breakdown. There are increased risks of painful crises, perinatal mortality, premature labour, and fetal growth restriction.[17] Some studies suggest ↑ spontaneous miscarriage, maternal infection, thromboembolic events, pre-eclampsia, and APH. Most prevalent in those of African descent, it is also prevalent in the Caribbean, Middle East, Mediterranean, parts of India, and South and Central America. There are 100–200 pregnancies in women with SCD in the UK annually.

Preconception Women with SCD should be under annual clinic review to monitor disease. Arrange sickle specialist preconception review. Advice should cover factors affecting sickling crises (cold, hypoxia, dehydration—hence nausea and vomiting of pregnancy, over-exertion, stress). Pregnancy worsens anaemia, so ↑ risk of crises and acute chest syndrome—chest pain, cough, tachypnoea, and new infiltrates on CXR: treat as for pneumonia + blood transfusion. Screen for red cell antibodies (if present ↑ risk of haemolytic disease of newborn). Pregnancy ↑ risks of infection (especially UTI). Address chance of fetus being affected (partner's blood to check carrier/haemoglobinopathy status: genetic counselling if needed). Assess current disease: echocardiography if not done in last year to exclude pulmonary hypertension (tricuspid regurgitant jet velocity >2.5m/sec high risk); BP & urinalysis, U&E, LFTS; retinal screening (proliferative retinopathy common); screen for iron overload if multiply transfused (if significantly overloaded, preconception chelation therapy is advised). SCD is a hyposplenic state; advise daily penicillin or erythromycin and update vaccines: hepatitis B, single-dose haemophilus influenza B & meningococcal C, 5-yearly pneumococcal, and annual H1N1 with seasonal influenza. Stop ACE/A2A drugs & hydroxycarbamide ≥3 months, preconceptually. Give 5mg folic acid daily (p.7) preconceptually and throughout pregnancy.

Antenatal care Ensure preconception measures addressed. Manage by specialist multidisciplinary team if possible; if not, by 'high-risk' team using protocols. If fetus has haemoglobinopathy risk, offer prenatal testing by 8–10 weeks. From 12 weeks give 75–150 mg aspirin daily to reduce risk of developing pre-eclampsia. Suggest TEDS in pregnancy. If hospitalized, give heparin thromboprophylaxis. Check BP at all antenatal visits and an MSU monthly. Offer viability scan at 7–9 weeks, dating scan at 11–14, anomaly scan at 20, and growth scan 4-weekly from 24 weeks. Only supplement iron if proven deficiency. Blood transfusion is not routine; if needed for sickling complication use fully compatible rhesus C,D,E and Kell typed CMV-negative blood (if so, transfusion regimen may be needed for rest of pregnancy). Top up transfusions may be needed if Hb falls to 60g/L. *Crises:* Affect 27–50%. Admit if fever, severe or atypical pain, chest pain, or breathless. If pain needs IV opiates use morphine/diamorphine (not pethidine, it risks fits); give nasal O₂ if oxygen sats <95% (take to ITU if O₂ sats not maintained), and adequate fluid intake 60mL/kg/h PO/IV unless pre-eclampsia (then specialist advice). Exchange transfusion is needed for acute chest syndrome or if stroke.

Intrapartum and postpartum care Aim for delivery at 38–40 weeks at hospitals able to manage SCD.[17] Keep warm and hydrated in labour/postpartum. Continuous monitoring of fetus, and maternal O₂ sats. Avoid pethidine (as for antenatal care). Give 7 days of heparin thromboprophylaxis post vaginal delivery, 6 weeks if CS. Progestogenic contraception is first choice; oestrogen-containing contraceptives are used as second-line agents.

Further reading

RCOG (2011). *Management of Sickle Cell Disease in Pregnancy* (Green-top Guideline No. 61). London: RCOG.

1 Obstetrics

Cardiac disease is the leading indirect cause of maternal death in the UK, but affects <1% of pregnant women. Examine the heart in all pregnancies, but especially in those from an immigrant population.

The key is preconception counselling to identify and address risks, but much heart disease is undiagnosed, along with pregnancies being unplanned. Risk depends on presence of pulmonary hypertension, effect on haemodynamics, NYHA functional class, and presence of cyanosis. Also, history of arrhythmia, TIA, heart failure, left heart outflow tract obstruction (mitral or aortic stenosis with valve area <2cm^2 and 1.5cm^2 respectively), and ejection fraction <40% predict poorer outcome. *Never ignore* even asymptomatic cases of Marfan syndrome, pulmonary hypertension, and mitral stenosis.

Cardiac diseases *Pulmonary hypertension:* Has a mortality rate of 25–40% in pregnancy. Due to lung disease, connective tissue disease, veno-occlusive disease, and Eisenmenger syndrome. Advise of very significant risks of pregnancy. Manage pregnancy in a tertiary centre. *Congenital heart disease:* More women survive to adulthood. Most commonly PDA, ASD, and VSD. If cyanotic and uncorrected, ↑ risk of IUGR. Refer for fetal echocardiography. *Marfan syndrome:* Autosomal dominant with 80% cardiac involvement with mitral valve prolapse, regurgitation, and/or aortic root dilatation. Risk of aortic dissection and rupture (esp. if root >4cm). Offer root replacement pre-pregnancy and LSCS if root >4.5cm. *Mitral stenosis:* Can be dangerous. Watch for dyspnoea, orthopnoea, and PND. Monitor with echo, aggressively treat AF (digoxin and β-blockers safe), treat pulmonary oedema. Valve area <1cm^2 has poor prognosis. *Arrhythmias:* If sinus tachycardia, exclude anaemia and hyperthyroidism. SVT is the commonest arrhythmia and can be treated with vagal manoeuvres and/or adenosine. *Artificial heart valves:* Warfarin risks fetal harm; heparin risks valve thrombosis. Difficult decisions may have to be made. Options include warfarin throughout pregnancy (INR 2.5–3.5), treatment-dose LMWH 6–12 weeks then warfarin, or LMWH throughout. *Ischaemic heart disease:* Increasingly common with rising maternal age and obesity. Symptoms may be atypical and go unrecognized or be mistaken for PE. ECG, troponin, and manage as for non-pregnant women. *Peripartum cardiomyopathy:* Rare and defined as heart failure without known cause and no previous history of heart disease. Onset 1 month pre- and 5 months postpartum. Diagnosis by echocardiography. Manage with elective delivery if antenatal, anticoagulants, conventional treatment for heart failure, and may require intra-aortic balloon pumps/left ventricular assist devices and/or cardiac transplantation. *Cardiac failure:* This is managed with diuretics, vasodilators, cardioselective β-blockers, inotropes, and once delivered, ACEI. Beware new-onset asthma in a pregnant woman—pulmonary oedema causes wheezing too.

Antenatal management Regular visits to cardiologist/obstetric combined clinic. Prevent anaemia, obesity, and smoking. Treat hypertension. Examine to exclude pulmonary oedema and arrhythmias at all visits.

Labour Outcome is worst for mothers unable to ↑ their cardiac output (rare). Have O$_2$ and drugs to treat cardiac failure to hand. Aim for vaginal delivery at term. Shorten 2nd stage if fixed cardiac output state and offer LSCS as per cardiology advice. Epidurals are safe if hypotension is avoided. Beware IV fluids. Avoid ergometrine (use oxytocin). Most cardiac deaths are in immediate postpartum period.

Normal findings in pregnancy Ejection systolic murmur in >90% of pregnant women. CXR: slight cardiomegaly, ↑ pulmonary vascular markings. ECG: ectopics, Q-wave and inverted T in lead III, and T-wave inversion in lateral leads. The QRS shows left shift.

Further reading

Nelson-Piercy C (2015). *Handbook of Obstetric Medicine* (5th ed). Boca Raton, FL: CRC Press.

1 Obstetrics

Decisions about medication in pregnancy and breastfeeding should take into account the risks and benefits of treatment versus no treatment. Whilst fetal toxicity and anomalies are a concern, the primary duty is to protect and treat the mother. Have a higher threshold for drug treatment and use psychotherapy and counselling. Use the lowest effective dose and consider drugs which have previously been effective. Few drugs are regarded as contraindicated, but none can be regarded as entirely safe due to a lack of good-quality data. Older drugs have traditionally been favoured as the evidence base is greater. With severe depression, bipolar affective disorder, schizophrenia, or other mental health diagnoses requiring specialist input, do not stop or change medication without their help. Remember the high risk of rapid postpartum relapse with significant associated risks to mother and infant, particularly in women with bipolar disorder (up to 50%).

Antidepressants See p. 712. Ante- and postnatal depression are common. Try to wait until the 2nd trimester before prescribing but do not delay if severe symptoms. 1st-line therapy is with SSRIs (usually sertraline); available data suggest risk of fetal anomaly similar to that of obese mothers. There is a very small risk of persistent fetal pulmonary hypertension and neonatal withdrawal (breastfeeding can ease this). Avoid paroxetine (1st trimester use may be associated with cardiac malformations, and increased risk of neonatal withdrawal). Breastfeeding should be supported where it is not detrimental to maternal well-being (eg worsening sleep deprivation and stress). Fluoxetine and citalopram are present in relatively high concentrations in breast milk. Sertraline, paroxetine, imipramine, and nortriptyline have low concentrations. For all drugs, exposure through breastfeeding is lower than that *in utero*.

Mood stabilizers (AEDs) These have varying malformation rates (also used as antiepileptics). Valproate and carbamazepine should **not** be prescribed to women of childbearing age and urgent advice sought with a view to stopping them if a woman taking them is pregnant. Valproate has the highest malformation rate (10%) with NTDs, craniofacial abnormalities, and neurodevelopmental problems (30–40%). Carbamazepine (2.2%) is also known to have increased rates of NTDs. Lamotrigine has a malformation rate of 2.1%, check blood levels regularly. All should be avoided in breastfeeding.

Lithium (p. 716) This is linked with teratogenicity (heart defects, including Ebstein anomaly), neonatal thyroid abnormalities, and floppy baby syndrome. Lithium should only be prescribed to women of childbearing age when alternatives have been ineffective and with appropriate counselling regarding risks. Offer specialist fetal echocardiography in those women electing to stay on lithium. Monitor drug levels 4-weekly to 36wks, then weekly, aiming for the individual's therapeutic window. Do not change brands (bioavailability varies). Signs of toxicity are tremor, drowsiness, visual disturbance. Stop lithium during labour. Check a 12h post-dose level and restart lithium based on this result. Women with bipolar disorder are at high risk of postpartum relapse which can evolve rapidly and is associated with morbidity and mortality for mother and infant. Breastfeeding is contraindicated due to the risk of neonatal toxicity.

Antipsychotics NB: rates of fetal abnormality are increased in schizophrenia, even in those taking no drugs. NICE warns of possible raised prolactin levels with amisulpride, sulpiride, and risperidone. Women taking antipsychotics associated with weight gain should have an OGTT. Women taking clozapine should not breastfeed due to the risk of fetal agranulocytosis. Depot medication should be avoided where possible in women of childbearing age.

Benzodiazepines May be linked to cleft lip and palate and should be avoided. Avoid diazepam during delivery, as neonatal withdrawal may occur.

ACKNOWLEDGEMENTS *With thanks to Dr Sarah Ashurst-Williams MRCPsych.*

►Even a small PPH (p. 96) may become life-threatening if the mother is anaemic. Anaemia predisposes to PPH, infection, makes heart failure worse, and is the main cause of perinatal problems associated with malaria. Above all, anaemia is a leading mechanism by which poverty exacts its morbid toll in pregnancy.

Definition of anaemia of pregnancy Hb <105g/L. The fall in Hb is steepest around 20 weeks' gestation, and is physiological (p. 6).

Who is prone to anaemia? Those who start pregnancy anaemic eg from menorrhagia, hookworm, malaria, with haemoglobinopathies; those with frequent pregnancies, twin pregnancy, or a poor diet.

Antenatal screening Includes Hb estimation at booking and at 28 weeks. In black patients do sickle-cell tests; in others at risk consider Hb electrophoresis for other haemoglobinopathies. From malarious areas consider malaria, and thick films. See p. 30.

Investigation Should include FBC (MCV reduced, and later MCHC). Serum iron, TIBC, and serum ferritin are low in iron deficiency. In folate deficiency, MCV is raised, serum and red cell folate reduced.

Causes By far the most common is iron deficiency—many women enter pregnancy with low iron stores. The next most common is folate deficiency. Also consider coeliac disease, chronic kidney disease, and autoimmune disease.

Treatment Pregnancy increases iron needs by 700–1400mg (throughout pregnancy), due to a pregnancy-induced 9-fold increase in iron absorption. Iron and folate supplements (and prevention against hookworm and malaria) are recommended in many developing countries.

Offer *oral iron* (eg **ferrous sulfate** 200mg BD PO); there is good evidence that once-daily dosing taken together with orange juice is as good as more frequent ingestion[18]; women should also avoid taking it with tea, calcium, or any other metal-containing supplements. Alternate-day dosing or even twice weekly may prevent gastrointestinal side effects and improve Hb. In women who would refuse blood transfusion (see BOX 'Managing those refusing blood transfusion in pregnancy', p. 97), prevention is key so prescribe iron. *Parenteral iron* may be given (to those with iron deficiency anaemia not tolerating oral iron) as iron dextran or iron sucrose. Beware anaphylaxis. Use only if cardiopulmonary resuscitation facilities to hand. Hb rises by 8g/L/week over 6 weeks, so late severe anaemia (Hb <90g/L) may need blood transfusion. One unit of blood increases the Hb by ~7g/L.

Thalassaemias (*OHCM* p342) These globin chain production disorders are found in Mediterranean, Indian, and South-east Asian populations. Although anaemic, never give parenteral iron as iron levels are usually high. Seek expert advice as to use of oral iron and folate. β-thalassaemia does not affect the fetus but in homozygotes regular transfusions sustain life only until young adulthood. There are α chains in fetal HbF, so in α-thalassaemias the fetus may be anaemic or, if severe, stillborn. Mothers carrying lethally affected hydropic fetuses risk severe pre-eclampsia, and delivery complications due to a large fetus and bulky placenta. Prenatal diagnosis is possible by chorionic villus sampling (p. 17) for thalassaemias anticipated by parental blood studies.

Sickle cell disease See p. 20. *Sickle cell/haemoglobin c disease* is a milder variant of SCD. Hb levels are usually near normal so women may be unaware they are affected. They are still susceptible to sickling crises in pregnancy and the puerperium, so antenatal diagnosis is essential. Prenatal sickle-cell diagnosis is possible by chorionic villus sampling.

►Aim for diagnosis at birth (cord blood) at the latest so that penicillin pneumococcal prophylaxis may be started (*OHCM* p340).

Without intervention, ~15% of babies acquire HIV if the mother is +ve (↑ risk in Africa). ►2/3 vertical transmission occurs during vaginal delivery but breast-feeding doubles transmission rate. Membrane rupture for >4h doubles risk. Transmission also ↑ with viral load >400 copies/mL, seroconversion during pregnancy, advanced disease, preterm labour, hepatitis C. Maternal antiretro-viral use, elective caesarean delivery, and bottle feeding attains ≤1% risk.

Antenatal care Offer HIV tests at booking; if declined, again at 28wks. If HIV status unknown in labour, rapid (20min) tests are recommended. If positive in labour, use drugs to reduce maternal–fetal transmission (see later in topic; seek expert advice). If HIV+ve arrange multidisciplinary care with HIV physician to monitor viral loads, drug regimens, and toxicity monitoring. Check for hepatitis B & C, varicella zoster, measles, & toxoplasmosis antibodies. Offer hepatitis B, pneumococcal, and influenza vaccines (safe in pregnancy). Screen for genital infections at booking and at 28wks. Treat infections, even if asymptomatic (to reduce risk of preterm birth). Women needing highly active antiretroviral treat-ment (HAART) for their own health (symptomatic HIV/falling or low CD4 lympho-cyte count <350 × 10⁶/L) should continue treatment throughout pregnancy and postpartum. If on HAART at booking, screen for gestational diabetes and warn of ↑ risk of premature labour. If on co-trimoxazole for *Pneumocystis jirovecii* prophylaxis (CD4 <200 × 10⁶/L), add pre-pregnancy/1st-trimester 5mg **folic acid**/day. Women not needing antiretrovirals for their own health should start HAART by 24wks, taking until delivered. (If good CD4 levels, viral load <10,000 copies/mL, and elective caesarean delivery planned, zidovudine monotherapy orally from 20–28wks, IV in labour is an alternative.) Plan mode of delivery by 36wks.

Premature labour If membranes rupture >34wks, expedite delivery, what-ever the maternal viral load. If membranes rupture <34wks, give steroids (pp.52-3), give erythromycin, ensure mother takes usual HAART regimen, seek HIV specialist advice on how to optimize her regimen to reduce fetal transmission eg maternal nevirapine crosses placenta with long fetal plasma concentration, plus zidovudine infusion. Determine delivery balancing risks of prematurity, and infection. Manage preterm labour without membrane rupture as if HIV-ve.

Intrapartum care *Vaginal delivery:* Offer to women with viral loads <50 copies/mL (<400 copies/mL if on HAART).[19] Continue HAART in labour. Avoid fetal blood sampling/scalp electrodes. Avoid amniotomy unless delivery imminent. Oxytocin can be used for augmentation. Low cavity forceps are preferred over ventouse (less fetal trauma). Avoid mid-cavity or rotational forceps. *Caesarean section:* Offer elective caesarean section at 38 weeks' gestation to women if on zidovudine monotherapy (see earlier), if on HAART with viral loads > those previ-ously mentioned, or if co-infected with hepatitis C and not on HAART. If viral load is <50 copies/mL, and elective section needed, plan for 39+ weeks.

Postpartum Avoid breastfeeding in resource-rich countries (breastfeeding doubles HIV transmission risk, and the undetectable=untransmissable statement applies only to sexual transmission due to a lack of data). Cabergoline 1mg PO within 24h of birth is recommended to suppress lactation. Newborns are treated within 4h of birth eg zidovudine twice daily for 4 weeks; HAART if high risk eg untreated mothers; mother with viral loads >50 copies/mL despite being on HAART. Co-trimoxazole (PCP prophylaxis) is given to babies at high risk of transmission. Babies are tested at day 1, 6wks, and 12wks for HIV with confirmatory test at 18 months. Affected women should have annual smears. Condoms, intrauterine systems (eg Mirena®), and depot progesterone injections are all suitable for women on HAART. Some antiretrovirals are enzyme inducers and may affect efficiency of progesterone only, and combined pills. Check if maternal MMR vaccine (if CD4 count >200/mL, contraindicated if lower), and varicella zoster vaccine (only if CD4 count >400/mL) required.

Further reading

BHIVA (2019). *Guidelines for the Management of HIV in Pregnancy and Postpartum 2018 (2019 second interim update)*. London: BHIVA.

Approximately 5% of women in the UK who give birth every year have either pre-existing (type 1 or type 2) or gestational diabetes (GDM). Of these, 87% have GDM, 7% have type 1 diabetes, and the remaining 5% type 2 diabetes. With rising obesity and age of pregnant women, the prevalence of both gestational and type 2 diabetes has increased in recent years.

Risks of diabetes in pregnancy

- *Maternal:* Hypoglycaemia unawareness (T1DM esp. 1st trimester) so warn about it. Increased risk of pre-eclampsia and infection, as well as higher rates of LSCS.
- *Fetal:* Miscarriage, malformation rates ↑ × 3 but this is reduced with good glycaemic control (fetal sacral agenesis, pathognomonic of pre-existing maternal diabetes, is rare; CNS & CVS malformations much commoner). With any type of diabetes, babies may be macrosomic (risk of shoulder dystocia and birth injury) or growth restricted. Polyhydramnios (?fetal polyuria), preterm labour, stillbirth.

Preconception counselling for women with pre-existing diabetes

One of the cornerstones of diabetes education in women of childbearing age is to avoid unplanned pregnancy. Establishing good blood glucose control before pregnancy and continuing this throughout pregnancy reduces (but does not eliminate) risks of miscarriage, congenital malformation, stillbirth, and neonatal death. *Recommendations:*

- Use contraception until good blood glucose control has been achieved—HbA1c of ≤48mmol/mol (avoid pregnancy if HbA1c >86mmol/mol). In women with pre-existing diabetes, aim for capillary blood glucose targets which are the same as for all patients with type 1 diabetes (fasting glucose of 5–7mmol/L on waking and plasma glucose before meals of 4–7mmol/L at all other times of the day).
- Women should be offered a structured education programme if they have not already attended one.
- Take **folic acid 5**mg daily until 12 weeks' gestation.
- Aim for a BMI <27kg/m^2.
- Stop oral hypoglycaemics (except metformin), statins, ACE and A2A inhibitors (use other antihypertensive p. 35, if needed).
- Treat retinopathy pre-pregnancy. Retinopathy screen; ≤20% develop proliferative retinopathy in pregnancy. Nephropathy may worsen antenatally; if severe, avoid pregnancy.

Gestational diabetes (Fasting glucose >5.6mmol/L or OGTT glucose ≥7.8mmol/L.) *Incidence:* 3–6% depending on population studied. 50% develop T2DM—this is an opportunity for the woman to make long-term positive lifestyle and dietary changes.[20] Check fasting glucose 6 weeks postpartum or HbA1c at 13 weeks postpartum and screen annually.

Screen with the 2h 75g oral glucose tolerance test (OGTT) if:
- 1st-degree relative with diabetes.
- Previous baby >4.5kg.
- BMI >30kg/m^2.
- Ethnicity with high prevalence of diabetes (South Asian, Caribbean, Middle Eastern).

If previous GDM, offer either early blood glucose monitoring or OGTT as soon after booking as possible. If this is negative, repeat at 24–28 weeks. *Do not* screen using fasting plasma glucose (GDM is predominantly a disease of insulin resistance), HbA1c (due to the relatively short duration of a pregnancy), or urinalysis (glycosuria unrelated to DM is common (GFR ↑ and tubular glucose reabsorption ↓)). However, glycosuria of 2+ on 1 occasion or 1+ on 2 occasions should be investigated to rule out GDM. All women diagnosed with GDM should have an HbA1c at booking to identify those with type 2 diabetes.

Treatment of GDM Involves early referral to the joint diabetes–antenatal clinic, dietician (low glycaemic index diet), and 30 minutes of exercise per day. If targets not met within 1–2 weeks of diagnosis, offer metformin. If blood glucose targets still not met, offer addition of insulin. In those in whom fasting glucose values are above 7mmol/L, start insulin immediately. Fetal macrosomia and/or polyhydramnios are also indications for commencement of insulin (4-weekly scans from 28 weeks). Glibenclamide can be used in women who cannot tolerate metformin or if blood glucose targets are not achieved using metformin and the woman declines insulin.

Antenatal care of women with pre-existing diabetes Use care plan & review in joint clinic with diabetologist, obstetrician, diabetes specialist nurse, and midwife.
- Give **folic acid** 5mg from preconception and **aspirin** 75mg from 1st trimester to reduce the risk of developing hypertension (especially pre-eclampsia).
- Measure HBA1C at booking to assess level of risk of complications and consider repeating in 2nd and 3rd trimesters.
- Insulin: rapid-acting analogues have benefits over human insulin (quicker onset of action with less hypoglycaemia).
- Educate about benefits of normoglycaemia. Aim for home-monitored glucose 1h after every meal (postprandial) and before bed. Insulin needs increase by 50–100% as pregnancy progresses so review regularly. Aim for fasting level <5.3mmol/L without problematic hypoglycaemia; 1h post-prandial level <7.8mmol/L and 2h post-prandial level <6.4mmol/L.
- Admit if adequate control unachievable at home and consider conversion to insulin pump (CSII) if adequate control is not achievable.
- Hypoglycaemia unawareness increases particularly in the 1st trimester partly due to tighter blood glucose targets and women should be warned of this.
- Give GlucoGel* and glucagon kit (ensure partner knows how to use).
- Exclude ketoacidosis if unwell (poorly tolerated by fetus)—give capillary blood ketone strips to all women with type 1 diabetes at the start of pregnancy. Assess renal function; refer to nephrologist if creatinine >120μmol/L, protein excretion >2g/24h (use thromboprophylaxis if >5g/24h).
- Ultrasound: confirm gestation with early US at 7–9 weeks; offer combined screening at 12 weeks; detailed anomaly scan at 18–20 weeks including fetal heart; monitor fetal growth by growth scans every 4 weeks from 28 to 36 weeks.

Delivery Should take place in hospital with round-the-clock obstetric and neonatal facilities. NICE recommends elective delivery from 37–38[+6] weeks with pre-existing diabetes, and by 40[+6] weeks with uncomplicated GDM. Women should have a discussion regarding the risks and benefits of induction of labour, vaginal birth, and caesarean section if the fetus is macrosomic (2–4 times higher risk of shoulder dystocia).[21][NICE] If preterm labour, corticosteroids should be given to promote fetal lung maturity (use sliding scale for 24h after last dose of steroid).

In labour: Continuous fetal monitoring. Avoid hyperglycaemia (causes neonatal hypoglycaemia) and use sliding scale if DM on insulin, or CBG >7mmol/L in GDM. Aim for glucose level of 4–7mmol/L. Halve rate of insulin infusion on delivery of placenta in T1DM. Insulin needs fall as labour progresses and immediately postpartum. Stop infusions at delivery in GDM and T2DM if not on insulin pre-pregnancy. Return to pre-pregnancy regimen.

Postnatal • Encourage breastfeeding (insulin, metformin, and glibenclamide are compatible with breastfeeding) • Breastfeeding increases risk of maternal hypoglycaemia • Encourage pre-pregnancy counselling *before* next pregnancy • If preproliferative retinopathy, review ophthalmologically for 6 months • Discuss contraception.

Further reading

NICE (2015). Diabetes in Pregnancy: Management from Preconception to the Postnatal Period (NG3). London: NICE.

1 Obstetrics

▶Whenever a mother isn't quite right postpartum, check her TSH & free T₄—but note that any apparent hypothyroidism may be transitory.

Biochemical changes in normal pregnancy NB: normal pregnancy mimics hyperthyroidism (pulse ↑, warm moist skin, slight goitre, anxiety).

- Thyroid binding globulin & T₄ output rise to maintain free T₄ levels.
- High levels of hcg mimic TSH.
- There is reduced availability of iodine (in iodine-limited localities).
- TSH may fall below normal in the 1st trimester (suppressed by hcg).
- The best thyroid tests in pregnancy are free T₄, free T₃, and TSH.

Pre-pregnancy hyperthyroidism Treatment options include antithyroid drugs (but 60% relapse on stopping treatment), radioactive iodine (contraindicated in pregnancy or breastfeeding: avoid pregnancy for 4 months after use), or surgery. Fertility is reduced by hyperthyroidism.

Hyperthyroidism in pregnancy (Usually Graves disease.) If severe, it is associated with infertility. There is ↑ risk of prematurity, fetal loss, and, maybe, malformations. Severity of hyperthyroidism often falls in pregnancy. Transient exacerbations may occur (1st trimester & postpartum). Carbimazole and propylthiouracil (PTU) are commonly used. PTU crosses the placenta less and is used in newly diagnosed thyrotoxicosis in pregnancy. Monitor ≥ monthly. PTU is preferred postpartum (less concentrated in breast milk). Partial thyroidectomy can be done in the 2nd trimester—most commonly for dysphagia, stridor, large goitre, suspected carcinoma, or antithyroid drug allergy.

TRAb (TSH-receptor stimulating antibodies): ↑ levels can cause *fetal thyrotoxicosis* (1%) after 24wks causing premature delivery; fetal goitre and polyhydramnios from oesophageal obstruction; extended neck in labour and fetal tachycardia. If mother has been on antithyroid drugs signs may not be manifest until the baby has metabolized the drug (7–10 days postpartum). Test thyroid function in affected babies frequently. Antithyroid drugs may be needed. It resolves spontaneously at 2–3 months, but perceptual motor difficulties, and hyperactivity can occur later in childhood.

Note labour, delivery, surgery, and anaesthesia can precipitate *thyroid storm* (fever, tachycardia, altered mental state—agitation, psychosis, coma) requiring urgent treatment.

Hypothyroidism Untreated hypothyroidism is associated with infertility, oligomenorrhoea or menorrhagia, ↑ rates of miscarriage, stillbirth, anaemia, pre-eclampsia, and IUGR. Also, reduced IQ and neurodevelopmental delay in offspring. Optimize T₄ preconception. Monitor replacement by T₄ and TSH measurement in each trimester or 6 weeks post dose adjustment. Use pre-pregnancy levothyroxine doses postpartum.

Postpartum thyroiditis Prevalence: 5%. Hyperthyroidism is followed by hypothyroidism (~4 months postpartum). The hyperthyroid phase does not usually need treatment as it is self-limiting. If treatment is required, β-blockers are usually sufficient. Antithyroid drugs are ineffective as thyrotoxicosis is from thyroid destruction releasing thyroxine, rather than increased synthesis. Monitor the hypothyroid phase for >6 months, and treat if symptomatic. Withdraw treatment after 6–12 months for 4 weeks to see if long-term therapy is required. 90% have thyroid antiperoxidase antibodies; 5% of antibody-positive women become permanently hypothyroid each year so monitor annually. Hypothyroidism may be associated with postpartum depression, so check thyroid status of women with postpartum depression.

Further reading

Nelson-Piercy C (2015). *Handbook of Obstetric Medicine* (5th ed). Boca Raton, FL: CRC Press.

►Get expert help *promptly*. Jaundice in pregnancy may be lethal. Know exactly what drugs were taken and when (*prescribed* or *over the counter*). Where has she travelled to? Jaundice occurs in 1:1500 pregnancies. Viral hepatitis and gallstones may cause jaundice in pregnancy and investigation is similar to the non-pregnant. Those with Gilbert and Dubin–Johnson syndromes do well in pregnancy (jaundice may be exacerbated with the latter).

Tests Urine tests for bile and protein (to diagnose pre-eclampsia), FBC, serology, LFTs, clotting if LFTs deranged, and US. Bile acids are a test usually only requested in pregnancy and if raised, diagnose obstetric cholestasis. See *OHCM* p272.

Obstetric cholestasis Incidence: 0.7% pregnancies in UK.[22] There is pruritus, especially of palms and soles in the second half of pregnancy, without a rash and worse at night. Diagnosis of exclusion—test for viral hepatitis, autoimmune screen, and US of liver. Liver transaminases are mildly ↑ (<300U/L) in 60%, ↑ bilirubin in 25%, and ↑ bile acids. There is risk of preterm labour, fetal distress, meconium, and stillbirth (but recent research suggests risk of stillbirth lower than previously thought)—offer IOL from 37–38 weeks. Give **vitamin k** 10mg PO/24h to the mother if abnormal clotting screen, and 1mg IM to the baby at birth. Ursodeoxycholic acid reduces pruritus and abnormal LFTs. Symptoms resolve within days of delivery. It can recur with oestrogen-containing contraceptive pills and in 40–70% of subsequent pregnancies.

Acute fatty liver of pregnancy Incidence: 1:6600–13,000 deliveries—so it is rare but extremely serious. The mother develops abdominal pain, jaundice, headache, vomiting, ± thrombocytopenia and pancreatitis. There is associated pre-eclampsia in 30–60% (±postpartum). It usually occurs after 30 weeks. There is hepatic steatosis with micro-droplets of fat in liver cells. Deep jaundice, uraemia, severe hypoglycaemia, and clotting disorder may develop causing coma and death. Manage in HDU or ITU (may need tertiary centre support). Monitor BP. Give supportive treatment for liver and renal failure and treat hypoglycaemia vigorously (CVP line). Correct clotting disorders. Enlist haematologist's help. Expedite delivery. Epidural and regional anaesthesia are CI. Monitor postpartum. Beware PPH and neonatal hypoglycaemia. ►Maternal mortality is 18% (higher with delayed diagnosis) and 23% for the fetus.

Some other causes of jaundice in pregnancy

• Viral hepatitis; ALT ↑, eg >200U/L; maternal mortality ↑ (~20%) in E virus,[19] treatment is supportive. Hepatitis C is thought to affect <1% of women in the UK at present. Vertical transmission affects about 5% of babies. Elective caesarean delivery is only recommended for those with coexistent HIV not on HAART.[19] Passive antibodies transferred from the mother wane by 18 months. Check baby for HCV RNA at 2–3 months (& 12 months, and anti HCV antibody at 12–18 months), refer baby to paediatric hepatologist if HCV RNA positive.[23] Refer infected women for specialist treatment to clear the viral infection after birth (*OHCM* p402).

• Jaundice of severe pre-eclampsia (hepatic rupture and infarction can occur); ALT <500U/L; bilirubin <86µmol/L.

• Hepatitis may occur if halothane is used for anaesthesia (so avoid it).

• HELLP syndrome (pp. 90–1) (haemolysis, elevated liver enzymes, and low platelet count). Incidence in pregnancy: 0.1–0.6%; in pre-eclampsia: 4–12%. It causes upper abdo pain, malaise, vomiting, headache, jaundice, microangiopathic haemolytic anaemia, DIC, LDH ↑, ALT ↑ <500U/L, bilirubin <86µmol/L. It recurs in 20%. *Treatment*: get expert help. Admit; deliver if severe.

Hepatitis B Check HBsAG in all women with jaundice and look for IgM anti-HBc to detect acute infection. Babies need immunoglobulin and vaccination at birth. Offer vaccination to all the family. Avoid FSE/FBS.

In any woman who presents with odd behaviour, fever, jaundice, sweating, DIC, fetal distress, premature labour, seizures, or loss of consciousness, always ask yourself: ►*Could this be malaria?* If so, do thick and thin films. Confirm (or exclude) pregnancy. Seek expert help.

Plasmodium falciparum malaria is dangerous (and complicated) in pregnancy, particularly in those with no malaria immunity. Cerebral malaria has a 50% mortality rate in pregnancy. 3rd-stage placental autotransfusion may lead to fatal pulmonary oedema. Hypoglycaemia may be a feature (both of malaria itself and secondary to quinine). There is ↑ susceptibility to sepsis. Women with coexistent HIV have less good pregnancy outcomes (fetal and maternal).

Other associations between *falciparum* malaria and pregnancy are anaemia, miscarriage, stillbirth, low birth weight, and prematurity. PPH is also more common. Hyperreactive malaria splenomegaly (occurs typically where malaria is holoendemic) may contribute to anaemia via ↑ haemolysis.

Vivax malaria is less dangerous, but can cause anaemia and ↓ birth weight.

Treating malaria ►*OHCM* p418. ►►Cerebral malaria, *OHCM* p480. In severe *falciparum* **artesunate** 2.4mg/kg IV at 0, 12, & 24h then daily until can take oral **artesunate + clindamycin** as 1st line, if available (tel. 08451 555000 tropical medical registrar for advice/supply), or load with **quinine** 20mg/kg IVI over 4h in 5% glucose (max. 1.4g) (do not load if on quinine/mefloquine). Then 10mg/kg IVI over 4h in 5% glucose every 8h with 450mg **clindamycin**/8h IV. Beware hypoglycaemia with quinine. Switch to artesunate regimen as soon as it is available.▨▨When severe, treat on ITU. If haematocrit <20% give slow transfusion of packed cells, with 20mg furosemide. Include the volume of packed cells in fluid balance calculations. Consider exchange transfusion. Beware hyperpyrexia (fan, give paracetamol); renal failure; pulmonary oedema; and sepsis (if shock do blood cultures, give IV ceftriaxone). Get expert help. Uncomplicated *falciparum* and resistant *vivax* are treated for 7 days with **quinine** 600mg with **clindamycin** 450mg/8h PO. Non-resistant *vivax, ovale,* and *malariae* are treated with chloroquine orally over 3 days with weekly dose to prevent relapse during pregnancy. 3 months after delivery (and G6PD testing) primaquine is then given for *ovale* and *vivax* prevention of relapse.

If infection peripartum, anticipate fetal distress, fluid-balance problems, and hypoglycaemia in labour. Monitor appropriately. After any infection send placenta for histology and placental, cord, and baby blood (weekly ×4) for blood films to check if baby infected (0.3–4% are), and treat baby if infected.

Prevention in UK women Advise against malarious areas. If it is unavoidable, give prophylaxis (*OHCM* p419). Emphasize importance of preventive measures such as mosquito nets and insect repellents. Normal-dose chloroquine and proguanil if *P. falciparum* strains are sensitive. With proguanil, give concurrent **folic acid** 5mg/day. If chloroquine resistance, mefloquine is best.

Mefloquine is recommended for 2nd- and 3rd-trimester use.[25] Heed strict contraindications (eg epilepsy, neuropsychiatric disorder). If unsuitable atovaquone–proguanil (eg Malarone®), with folic acid is an alternative in 2nd and 3rd trimesters for chloroquine- or mefloquine-resistant areas. 1st-trimester prophylaxis is a problem. Seek expert advice (eg tel. National Travel Health Network and Centre 0845 602 6712).

Mothers living in endemic areas Chemoprophylaxis improves birthweight (by ~250g, with fewer very low birthweight babies). Red cell mass also rises. WHO advises intermittent preventive treatment (IPT) eg with 2 or 3 doses of sulfadoxine–pyrimethamine (SP) during pregnancy, but monthly doses are better if HIV +ve.[26] But SP causes Stevens–Johnson syndrome in 1:7000, and resistance to SP has spread fast, so new IPT regimens need urgent evaluation in pregnancy.[27] Dihydroartemisinin–piperaquine (eg Artekin®) is a good candidate.[28]

►If in doubt, phone an expert—eg in the UK, at Liverpool (tel. 0151 705 3100).

Note Values considered normal when not pregnant may reflect decreased renal function in pregnancy. ▸▸Creatinine >75µmol/L and urea >4.5mmol/L merit further investigation. See table 1.3 on p. 9. Glycosuria in pregnancy usually reflects altered renal physiology rather than hyperglycaemia.

Asymptomatic bacteriuria Found in 2% of sexually active women, it is commoner (up to 7%) during pregnancy—especially in diabetics and in those with renal transplants. With the dilatation of the calyces and ureters that occurs in pregnancy, 30% will go on to develop pyelonephritis, which can cause fetal growth restriction, fetal death, and premature labour. This is the argument for screening all women for bacteriuria at booking. If present on MSU, treatment is given (eg **cefalexin** 500mg TDS PO for 5d). Trimethoprim and nitrofurantoin are safe alternatives but avoid trimethoprim in the 1st trimester (antifolate action) and nitrofurantoin in the 3rd (neonatal haemolytic anaemia). Check MSU on a regular basis eg at each visit to ensure eradication. 15% develop recurrent asymptomatic bacteriuria. Acute cystitis affects 1%, characterized by urinary frequency, urgency, dysuria, haematuria, and lower abdominal pain. Most infections are due to *E. coli* and urine dip positive for nitrites and leucocytes suggests UTI. Send MSU and treat as per asymptomatic bacteriuria.

Pyelonephritis Affects 1–2% of pregnant women and is more common due to dilatation of upper renal tract in pregnancy. Also more common in congenital renal abnormalities, neuropathic bladder, and stones. This may present as malaise with urinary frequency or as a more florid picture with raised temperature, tachycardia, vomiting, and loin pain. Urinary infections should always be excluded in those with hyperemesis gravidarum and those admitted with premature labour. After blood and urine culture give IV antibiotics (eg **cefuroxime** 1.5g/8h IV, awaiting sensitivities, and if septic consider stat dose of gentamicin). Continue IV antibiotics for at least 24h and orals for 2–3 weeks. MSUs should be checked for eradication of infection. Check renal function regularly and carry out US of renal tract to exclude stones and abnormalities. In those who suffer repeated infection, low-dose oral amoxicillin or cefalexin may prevent recurrences. If 2 or more confirmed UTIs in pregnancy, perform renal US and consider antibiotic prophylaxis for the rest of pregnancy.

Chronic renal disease With mild renal impairment (pre-pregnancy creatinine <125mmol/L) without hypertension there is little evidence that pregnancy accelerates renal disorders. Patients with marked anaemia, hypertension, retinopathy, or heavy proteinuria should avoid pregnancy as further deterioration in renal function may be expected. Risks include miscarriage, pre-eclampsia, fetal growth restriction, preterm delivery, and fetal death.

Pregnancy for those on dialysis is fraught with problems (fluid overload, hypertension, pre-eclampsia, polyhydramnios). A 50% increase in dialysis is needed. Live birth outcome is 50%. Outcome is better for those with renal transplants, but up to 10% of mothers die within 7 years of giving birth.

Obstetric causes of acute kidney injury Most commonly occurs postnatally and is rare. Anuria is uncommon—check for retention, blocked catheters, and ureteric damage.

- Sepsis (septic miscarriage, puerperal sepsis, urinary).
- Haemolysis (eg HELLP syndrome, acute fatty liver, sickle cell crisis, malaria).
- Hypovolaemia (blood loss from PPH or abruption).
- Volume contraction (pre-eclampsia, hyperemesis gravidarum).
- Don't forget drugs—especially NSAIDs.

Whenever these situations occur, monitor urine output and fluid balance carefully (catheterize the bladder). Aim for >30mL/h output. Monitor renal function (U&E, creatinine). Management depends on the cause. Avoid using diuretics unless under specialist advice. Dialysis may be needed (*OHCM* p306).

Epilepsy affects ~0.5% of women of childbearing age and is the commonest neurological condition in this age group. It is categorized according to seizure type: primary generalized epilepsy (tonic–clonic seizures, absences, myoclonic jerks), and partial or focal seizures which may progress to secondary generalization (complex partial seizures) of which temporal lobe epilepsy is a part.

Other causes of seizures in pregnancy Eclampsia is the most important (pp. 90-1); cerebral vein thrombosis, intracranial mass, stroke, hypoglycaemia, hyponatraemia, drugs and withdrawal, infection, postdural puncture, non-epileptic attack disorder (may overlap with epilepsy). Two-thirds of women have no change in seizure frequency in pregnancy and those without a high risk of unprovoked seizures can be managed as 'low risk'. Poorly controlled epilepsy is most likely to deteriorate (check drug compliance). Status epilepticus is a medical emergency and dangerous for both mother and fetus, and complicates 1.8% of pregnancies. Overall, the risk of seizure is highest peripartum (1–2% fit intrapartum).[29]

Preconception
- Neurologist involvement to confirm diagnosis.
- Optimize treatment, aim for seizure control on lowest dose to minimize risk of congenital malformation (CM). Note—CM rate depends on AED used but is increased even if on no treatment. Can consider withdrawing (under expert supervision) if no seizures for 2 years. See p. 22 for risks of AEDs.
- **Folic acid** 5mg daily for >3 months prior to conception.
- Increased risk of epilepsy in offspring (4–5% but higher risk with maternal, and 15–20% if both parents affected).

Antenatal care
- Attendance at consultant-led obstetric clinic with aim for vaginal delivery; do not change drugs without expert advice from an epilepsy specialist.
- If she has an unplanned pregnancy and is taking AEDs, urgent discussion is required with an epilepsy specialist.
- Attendance at NT and anomaly scans (may need fetal echocardiography) and then serial growth scans in the 3rd trimester (higher risk of SGA fetus).
- 5mg **folic acid** daily until end of 1st trimester.
- Routine drug level testing is not indicated.
- Epilepsy is not an indication for induction of labour or planned LSCS. Stress and sleep deprivation increase seizure risk and this should be avoided wherever possible (including in labour).

Intrapartum care
- Aim for vaginal delivery unless obstetric indications occur for LSCS. A fit in labour is not an indication for LSCS unless in status.
- Delivery should take place in a hospital and AEDs continued in labour.
- Pain relief is a priority; epidural anaesthesia is safe.
- Benzodiazepines if seizure not self-terminating (**lorazepam** 4mg IV, **diazepam** 10–20mg rectally or IV). Seizures are more common intrapartum and postpartum due to sleep deprivation and reduced drug absorption.

Postnatal care
- Give baby **vitamin K** 1mg IM to reduce haemorrhagic disease of the newborn.
- Avoid early discharge: stay in hospital for 24 hours when seizure risk highest.
- Strategies for avoiding dropping the baby during a seizure ie changing the baby on the floor.
- Encourage breastfeeding especially if she is taking AEDs, and review AED dose within 10 days of delivery to avoid toxicity. Discuss contraception (copper/Mirena® coil and injected progestogens should be promoted if taking enzyme-inducing AED, but all forms can be given if on non-enzyme-inducing AEDs). Oestrogen-containing contraception increases seizure risk in women taking lamotrigine due to reduced drug levels.

Oxygen demand increases significantly in pregnancy, due to raised metabolic rate and consumption. Tidal volume increases more than respiratory rate. Arterial po_2 increases, and pco_2 falls, along with bicarbonate, giving a compensated respiratory alkalosis. This is normal. PEFR is unchanged in pregnancy, along with FEV1. Breathlessness is a common symptom affecting 75% of women and is usually worse in the 3rd trimester.

Asthma Common, affecting up to 7% of women in pregnancy and is due to reversible bronchoconstriction of airways from smooth muscle spasm, along with inflammation and increased mucus production. *Symptoms:* Include cough, breathlessness, wheeze, and chest tightness, often with a diurnal variation (worse at night and early morning). Coexistent atopy (hay fever, eczema) is common. *Diagnosis:* Based on history, >20% diurnal variation in PEFR for 3+ days/week during 2-week period, or >15% improvement in FEV1 after inhaled bronchodilators. For most women asthma remains unchanged or improved, but it may worsen (especially if poorly controlled to start with). Severe and/or poorly controlled asthma may result in fetal growth restriction and preterm labour. *Management:* Should focus on preventing acute attacks. Follow British Thoracic Society guidelines and use a stepwise approach. Most medication is safe in pregnancy (but do not start leukotriene receptor antagonists). Remember to check inhaler technique and give smoking cessation advice. Asthma attacks in pregnancy are rare due to endogenous steroid production; continue usual medication and treat as for non-pregnant patient. In PPH use carboprost with caution unless life-threatening haemorrhage.

Pneumonia This is no more common than in non-pregnant women, but has a higher mortality rate, especially with varicella zoster pneumonia. Smokers, those with chronic lung disease, and the immunosuppressed are more at risk. *Symptoms:* Often start with a dry cough, progressing to productive, fever, rigors, breathlessness, and pleuritic chest pain. Listen for coarse crackles on auscultation and look for signs of consolidation. Take FBC, U&E, CRP, sputum culture, ABG, and CXR (very small dose of radiation—a fraction of the maximum dose allowed in pregnancy). *Management:* Maintain o_2 sats >96%, ensure hydrated, arrange chest physiotherapy, and give antibiotics (**amoxicillin 500mg** TDS or **clarithromycin 500mg** BD (unlicensed)). Severe pneumonia requires IV treatment with **cefuroxime 1.5g** TDS ± **clarithromycin 500mg** BD. Treat for 7 days. Call for help if adverse features: RR >30/min, sats <92% or po_2 <8kPa, systolic BP <90mmHg, acidosis; bilateral or multiple lobe involvement on CXR.

Tuberculosis (TB) On the increase in the UK, Europe, and America partly due to HIV+ve patients having higher susceptibility. In the UK, ethnic minority women in pregnancy are most commonly affected. *Onset:* Insidious, with cough, haemoptysis, weight loss, and night sweats, and may cause coarse crackles in the upper lobes and lymphadenopathy. *Diagnosis:* Confirmed on sputum for acid-fast bacilli, but culture takes 6 weeks. The Mantoux test is not affected by pregnancy. Congenital infection via placenta is rare. Refer to a respiratory physician. *Treatment:* Rifampicin, isoniazid (plus pyridoxine), and pyrazinamide and/or ethambutol. Infectious until 2 weeks of treatment. The baby should be given the BCG ± isoniazid in high-risk cases. Encourage breastfeeding.

Cystic fibrosis (CF) Has improving life expectancy (47 years at present—www.cysticfibrosis.org), so pregnancy is more common. Prenatal genetic counselling is important and paternal screening should be carried out. Obstetric care jointly with CF physicians, dietician, and physiotherapist. Optimize status pre-pregnancy. Cardiac echo, admit for o_2 if sats <90%, and treat infections aggressively. Increased risk of IUGR due to hypoxia therefore growth scans every 4 weeks from 28 weeks. Maintain high-calorie diet and screen for GDM. Aim for vaginal delivery but limit second stage (increased risk of pneumothorax).

Rheumatoid arthritis A systemic inflammatory disorder affecting predominantly synovial joints. 75% of women have an improvement in pregnancy (but exacerbations occur in 90% in the puerperium). 70% are rheumatoid factor or anti-CCP positive. ESR (to monitor disease activity) in pregnancy is unreliable because it is usually elevated. Anti-Ro antibodies confer a risk of neonatal lupus.

Paracetamol is first line for analgesia. Non-steroidal anti-inflammatories can be used but are not recommended in the 3rd trimester as they can cause premature closure of the ductus arteriosus and late in pregnancy have been associated with renal impairment in the newborn (but this is reversible after discontinuation of NSAIDs). Corticosteroids can be continued in pregnancy (prednisolone does not cross the placenta) and are a better option than NSAIDs (but note increased risk of GDM). Long-acting intramuscular steroids are also safe in pregnancy. Azathioprine is safe in pregnancy (fetal liver lacks the enzyme used to convert it into its active form). Hydroxychloroquine and sulfasalazine are safe to use in both pregnancy and breastfeeding. Mycophenolate mofetil, penicillamine, gold salts, and leflunomide should be avoided due to teratogenicity. TNF-α antagonists can be used if all else fails to control symptoms but ideally stopped by 32 weeks to minimize levels in the neonate.

Systemic lupus erythematosus 96% of patients are antinuclear antibody (ANA) positive and titres are unchanged regardless of disease activity. SLE exacerbations are commoner in pregnancy and the puerperium. Most are mild to moderate involving skin, but those with renal involvement and hypertension have increased rates of fetal loss, pre-eclampsia, and IUGR. Women in remission with no antiphospholipid syndrome, renal involvement, or hypertension have similar rates of pregnancy loss and pre-eclampsia to the general population, therefore planned pregnancies during remission have better outcomes.

Disease flares should be actively managed with corticosteroids (symptoms, rising anti-DNA antibody titres, red blood cells or casts in urine, fall in complement levels). Hydroxychloroquine is safe (see earlier) and discontinuing could lead to a flare. The woman should be monitored throughout in a high-risk antenatal clinic for disease activity, hypertension, and fetal growth (including uterine artery Dopplers at 20–24 weeks to predict pre-eclampsia and IUGR risk). **Aspirin** 75-150 mg daily from positive pregnancy test should be continued until delivery. If the mother is Ro-positive, risk of congenital heart block is 2% and transient neonatal cutaneous lupus 5%.

Antiphospholipid syndrome Antiphospholipid antibodies (lupus anticoagulant and/or anticardiolipin antibodies on 2 tests taken >8 weeks apart) ± past arterial thrombosis, venous thrombosis, or recurrent miscarriage, 1 or more fetal death >10 weeks' gestation, or premature birth due to severe pre-eclampsia or placental insufficiency. It may be primary, or follow other connective tissue disorder (usually SLE in which it occurs in 10%).

Outcome: Untreated, <20% of pregnancies proceed to a live birth due to 1st-trimester loss or placental thrombosis (causes placental insufficiency, leading to IUGR and fetal death).

Management: Women should have uterine artery Dopplers at 20–24 weeks to predict those with a higher chance of developing pre-eclampsia and IUGR. Higher-risk women should have 4-weekly fetal growth scans including umbilical artery Dopplers from 28 weeks. **Aspirin** 75-150 mg daily if no previous adverse outcomes (live birth rate 70–80%). Add prophylactic LMWH eg **enoxaparin** 40mg sc/24h from when fetal heart identified (~6 weeks) if previous fetal loss. Those who have suffered prior thromboses receive treatment-dose LMWH throughout pregnancy. See p. 36. Postpartum, use either heparin or warfarin (breastfeeding safe) as risk of thrombosis is high.

BP falls in early pregnancy until 24 weeks due to a fall in vascular resistance. Stroke volume then increases after this time, leading to a rise in BP. It tends to fall again after delivery (often tricking doctors into stopping antihypertensives too early), peaking again at day 3–4 postpartum. Use the correct cuff size—using a small cuff on a large arm leads to a falsely elevated reading. Automated BP monitors tend to under-record BP; best practice is to use a sphygmomanometer. Hypertensive disorders in pregnancy account for a significant proportion of maternal morbidity and mortality due to stroke, as well as neonatal problems from iatrogenic prematurity. ►A BP of >160/110mmHg in pregnancy is a medical emergency (p. 90). If proteinuria develops, this is superimposed pre-eclampsia (pp. 50–1).

Chronic hypertension Affects 3–5% pregnancies and predates the pregnancy. Women who develop hypertension before 20 weeks' gestation or have a high booking BP (130–140/80–90mmHg) are more likely to have chronic hypertension. These women have a higher risk of developing pre-eclampsia (double if on treatment), fetal growth restriction, and placental abruption. If it is a new finding, exclude other causes of hypertension (coarctation, renal artery stenosis, other renal disease, rarely Cushing syndrome, Conn syndrome, and phaeochromocytoma). *Preconception:* ACE inhibitors, A2A blockers, and thiazide risk congenital abnormality so change these prior to conception to labetalol or methyldopa. *Antenatal:* Ensure suitable antihypertensive is being used (see earlier). Aim for BP <150/90 (140/90 if end-organ damage), but with diastolic ≥80mmHg. If hypertension is secondary to another disorder involve a specialist in hypertensive disorders. Give aspirin 75–150 mg/24h/PO from conception until the baby is born. Admit if BP >160/110. Fetal US every 4 weeks from 28 weeks to assess fetal growth, amniotic fluid volume, and umbilical artery Dopplers. Aim for induction of labour around the EDD if BP if well controlled. *Intrapartum:* During labour, monitor BP hourly if BP <159/109, continuously if ≥160/100. If severe hypertension does not respond to treatment, advise operative delivery. Give oxytocin alone at 3rd stage of labour (ergometrine causes severe hypertension, risking stroke). *Postnatally:* Check BP on days 1, 2, and once on days 3–5 and at 2 weeks. Change methyldopa to another antihypertensive post delivery as risk of postnatal depression. Avoid diuretics if breastfeeding (labetalol, atenolol, metoprolol, captopril, and enalapril are safe).

Pregnancy-induced hypertension (PIH) Affects 6–7% of pregnancies. It is defined as hypertension in the second half of pregnancy (BP >140/90) in the absence of proteinuria or other features of pre-eclampsia. There is an increased risk of developing pre-eclampsia (15–26%) especially with earlier onset of hypertension. *Management:* Assessment in secondary care, with urine testing for proteinuria with automated reagent strip readings or urine protein/creatinine ratio testing to rule out pre-eclampsia. Check urine and BP weekly if mild (BP 140/90–149/99) but start treatment eg with labetalol PO if >150/100 and check BP and urine twice weekly. If BP ≥160/110 admit to hospital, measure BP 4 times daily, and check urine daily and check FBC, U&E, AST/ALT, and bilirubin at presentation and weekly. If hypertension is mild do 4-weekly fetal growth scans; if severe and cannot stabilize on oral treatment make plans for delivery. Aim for delivery after 37 weeks unless pre-eclampsia (pp. 50–1) supervenes. During labour continue antihypertensives, monitor BP hourly (continuously if >160/110). If BP is outside target range despite antihypertensives (>160/110) advise operative delivery. Continue antenatal antihypertensives postnatally (as above), reducing treatment if BP <130/80. Review at 2 and 6 weeks. If treatment is still needed at 6 weeks, arrange review with specialist in hypertensive disorders.

Further reading

NICE (2010). *Hypertension in Pregnancy: Diagnosis and Management* (CG107). London: NICE.

Venous thromboembolism (VTE) is a leading cause of morbidity and mortality in pregnancy in developed countries and is preventable. It includes deep vein thrombosis (DVT) of the legs, pelvis, and pulmonary embolism (PE). Every woman should have VTE risk assessed at booking, each antenatal admission, in labour, and postnatally. Basic steps should also be taken to reduce VTE: avoid immobility and dehydration (don't forget hyperemesis). Pregnancy alone is a risk factor due to a combination of venous stasis, trauma to pelvic veins at delivery, procoagulant changes to the clotting cascade (higher levels of factors X, VIII, and fibrinogen, reduced endogenous anticoagulation activity, and reduction in protein s activity). These changes occur from early in the 1st trimester until 6 weeks postpartum. LMWHs are drugs of choice in pregnancy and safer than unfractionated. If in doubt as to whether a woman needs it, seek senior advice or refer to haematology.

Risk factors for VTE *High risk (give antenatal LMWH prophylaxis):* History of >1 VTE, unprovoked or oestrogen-related VTE, single provoked VTE + thrombophilia or family history, antithrombin III deficiency (30% risk of VTE in pregnancy). *Intermediate risk (consider antenatal LMWH prophylaxis):* Thrombophilia but no VTE, single provoked VTE, medical comorbidities eg cancer, inflammatory conditions, significant cardiac or respiratory conditions, SLE, sickle cell disease, nephrotic syndrome, IV drug user, any antenatal surgery. *Other risk factors:* If 3 or more, consider antenatal prophylaxis: age >35, obesity, parity 3 or more, smoker, large varicose veins, current infection, pre-eclampsia, immobility, dehydration, multiple pregnancy, assisted reproduction techniques.

Indications for LMWH thromboprophylaxis See list for VTE risk factors. For any woman requiring antenatal LMWH it must be given for 6 weeks postpartum. Any woman undergoing emergency LSCS needs 7 days' postpartum LMWH. If other risk factors are also present it may need to be given for longer. Other postpartum risk factors include mid-cavity or rotational instrumental delivery, postpartum haemorrhage, and blood transfusion. Check local trust guidelines. Often the postnatal drug chart or notes will have a colour-coded VTE risk assessment which will help you assess need for thromboprophylaxis.

Dosing of LMWH Depends on body weight. **Enoxaparin** 40mg sc/24h if 50–90kg, 60mg sc/24h if 91–130kg, 80mg/24h if 131–170kg. Postnatally, enoxaparin can be given as soon as possible as long as no ongoing postpartum haemorrhage, and >4h since epidural sited or removed.

Thrombophilia in pregnancy

Thrombophilia is the tendency to increased clotting and there are many underlying causes. Whether or not women need antenatal LMWH depends on the presence of other risk factors and expert advice. *Factor v Leiden* (4% population) increases risk 5–8 times if heterozygote and 10–34 times if homozygote. *Protein c deficiency* (0.3% population) risk increased by 2–4.8 times. *Protein s deficiency* (2% population) increases risk 3.2 times. *Antithrombin III deficiency* (0.02%) increases risk 4.7–10 times. *G20210A prothrombin gene mutation* (1% population) increases risk 3–10 times in heterozygotes and 26 times in homozygotes. *Acquired thrombophilia* is lupus anticoagulant ± cardiolipin antibody and increases risk of both arterial and venous thrombosis.

Screening Should occur if there is a past history of VTE and should be carried out when the woman is not pregnant. Screen those with a personal/family history of 2nd-trimester pregnancy loss and early-onset pre-eclampsia.

Further reading

RCOG (2015). *Reducing the Risk of Venous Thromboembolism during Pregnancy and the Puerperium* (Green-top Guideline No. 37a). London: RCOG.

RCOG (2015). *Thromboembolic Disease in Pregnancy and the Puerperium: Acute Management* (Green-top Guideline No. 37b). London: RCOG.

1 Obstetrics

▶ *This is a medical emergency and is one of the leading causes of maternal morbidity and mortality in the UK.* VTE can happen in any trimester and occurs in 1–2:1000 pregnancies. Symptoms may be atypical; DVT is 3 times more common than PE and a DVT will lead to PE in 16% of untreated patients. Overall, VTE is most common in the postnatal period.

Symptoms and signs of VTE

Deep vein thrombosis: Leg swelling (left more often than right), pain, redness. Look for swelling (2cm greater diameter than other leg), tenderness, pyrexia, erythema, oedema, and in pelvic DVT lower abdominal pain. WBC count may be raised.

Pulmonary embolism: Shortness of breath, chest pain, haemoptysis. Think of PE in any collapsed pregnant or postpartum woman. She may feel faint, have a raised JVP, and also have symptoms or signs of DVT. On auscultation there may be a pleural rub or fine crepitations, but more likely no chest signs at all. She may be hypoxic with a raised respiratory rate. In massive PE there is hypoxia, low blood pressure, tachycardia, and collapse leading to cardiac arrest.

Investigations Should include FBC, U&E, LFTs, and a clotting screen. Thrombophilia screens may be falsely positive in pregnancy. If PE is suspected carry out ECG (look for signs of right heart strain) and CXR.

Imaging Imaging for DVT is by compression or duplex US of the deep veins. If there is high clinical suspicion of DVT or PE and investigations are negative, continue treatment dose LWMH and repeat imaging in 1 week. Seek expert advice from haematology in these cases. In PE, if there are symptoms and/or signs of DVT, arrange compression or duplex US of the legs (if positive, PE can be presumed if chest symptoms, and further radiation of chest avoided). If negative, or no DVT symptoms/signs, and CXR is normal, perform ventilation/perfusion lung scanning (V/Q) (small increase in risk of childhood cancer for the fetus). If the CXR is abnormal, CTPA is the recommended next option (CTPA increases lifetime breast cancer risk by up to 13%, but the radiation dose to the fetus is low).[30] Women should have the opportunity to discuss the risks and benefits of imaging for PE.

D-dimers Tricky in pregnancy. Generally speaking, they are not helpful as they are commonly raised due to changes in the coagulation system. False negatives are possible in pregnancy and D-dimer should not be used to rule out VTE.

Treatment Should start as soon as there is clinical suspicion of VTE and only stopped once it is ruled out. *Massive PE:* Necessitates immediate expert help. The woman may need thrombolysis or percutaneous catheter thrombus fragmentation. Embolectomy can only be carried out in centres with cardiothoracics. Consider unfractionated heparin (loading dose 5000IU then 1000–2000IU/h). Take blood for APTT 6h post loading dose, aiming for 1.5–2.5× laboratory control value. *LMWH:* is more effective and safer than unfractionated heparin. Treat twice daily eg enoxaparin or dalteparin—see *BNF* and local guidelines. Refer to haematologist for follow up—they will want anti-X_a activity measuring 3h post injection to ensure correct dosage. Continue anticoagulation for 6 months and 6 weeks postpartum. Consider switching to warfarin post delivery (safe in breastfeeding). Remember that in the next pregnancy, the woman needs thromboprophylaxis throughout, and for 6 weeks postpartum. *During labour:* LMWH should be stopped. Keep well hydrated. Avoid regional anaesthesia (spinal/epidural) until at least 12h after last dose of prophylactic, and 24h after therapeutic LMWH. Wait >4h until epidural catheter removed until next dose, and do not remove catheter until >12h after last dose. Those at high risk on stopping anticoagulation: consider unfractionated heparin; can also consider IVC filter.

Investigating rash in pregnancy Rashes can be either infectious or non-infectious.[31] Investigate maculopapular rashes for rubella and parvovirus B19 (p. 204) (both can infect the fetus) and measles. Also consider causes of rash such as *Streptococcus*, meningococcus, Epstein–Barr virus, and syphilis.

Measles This is unfortunately on the increase due to reduced uptake of the MMR vaccine. Measles in pregnancy can be dangerous, leading to mortality and severe morbidity from encephalitis and pneumonia. It is an RNA paramyxovirus, spread by respiratory droplets and is highly infectious. Incubation is 9–12 days, with the infectious period 2–5 days before and after the rash develops. Symptoms include fever, generalized maculopapular erythematous rash, Koplik's spots (pathognomonic, see p. 204). Look for cough, coryza, and conjunctivitis as well as corneal scarring. Diagnosis is on serology with paired samples in the acute and convalescent phase (10–14 days later). IgM in serum is positive >4 days but <1 month after the rash, and viral RNA in saliva. Measles in pregnancy is associated with fetal loss and preterm delivery, but not congenital infection or abnormality. If maternal rash appears 6 days pre or post delivery, give human normal immune globulin immediately after birth or exposure, to prevent neonatal subacute sclerosing panencephalitis.

Rubella Childhood vaccination prevents rubella susceptibility and routine antenatal screening has been withdrawn. Ensure 2 MMR doses prior to conception (avoid pregnancy for 1 month: vaccine is live). Spread is by respiratory droplets, with an incubation period of 14–21 days. Symptoms (p. 28) are absent in 50%. The fetus is most at risk in the 1st 16 weeks' gestation. 80% of fetuses are affected if maternal primary infection is in the 1st 12 weeks of gestation: <5% are affected if infection is after 16 weeks. Risk of fetal damage is much lower (<5%) with reinfection. Cataract is associated with infection at 8–9 weeks, deafness at 5–7 weeks (can occur with 2nd-trimester infection), cardiac lesions at 5–10 weeks. *Other features*: purpura, jaundice, hepatosplenomegaly, thrombocytopenia, cerebral palsy, microcephaly, IQ ↓, cerebral calcification, microphthalmia, retinitis, growth disorder. Miscarriage or stillbirth may occur. If suspected in the mother, seek expert help. Take antibody levels 10 days apart and look for IgM antibody 4–5 weeks from incubation period or date of contact. If infection is confirmed in the 1st trimester, TOP is offered without invasive prenatal diagnosis.

Cytomegalovirus (CMV) In the UK, CMV causes more motor and cognitive impairment than rubella. Maternal infection is mild (or ↑ T°, lymphadenopathy, rash, & sore throat). Up to 5:1000 live births are infected; with primary maternal infection, 40% fetuses are infected irrespective of gestation. Of these, 90% are normal at birth of which 20% develop late and usually minor problems. Of the 10% symptomatic babies, 33% will die and 67% have long-term problems. CMV-associated congenital defects include IUGR, microcephaly, hepatosplenomegaly and thrombocytopenia, jaundice, chorioretinitis. Later-onset problems include motor and cognitive impairment and sensorineural deafness. Δ: (Tricky; ask lab.) Paired sera. Are IgM and IgG antibodies found? Amniocentesis at >20wks + shell viral culture can detect fetal transmission. Also do throat swab, urine culture, and baby's serum after birth. Reducing exposure to toddlers' urine (the source of much infection) in pregnancy limits spread. NB: reactivation of old CMV may occur in pregnancy; it rarely affects the baby. One way to know that +ve serology does not reflect old infection is to do serology (or freeze a sample) pre-pregnancy.

Toxoplasmosis 40% of fetuses are affected if the mother has the illness (2–7:1000 pregnancies); the earlier in pregnancy, the more the damage but the lower the transmission rate. Symptoms are similar to glandular fever. Fever, rash, and eosinophilia also occur. If symptomatic, the CNS prognosis is poor. Diagnose by reference laboratory IgG and IgM tests. *Maternal, R (Royal College regimen):* Start **spiramycin** promptly in infected mothers eg 1.5g/12h PO. In symptomatic non-immune women test every 10 weeks through pregnancy. If infected, consider amniocentesis to see if the fetus is infected. If the fetus is infected, give the mother **pyrimethamine** 50mg/12h as loading doses on day 1, then 1mg/kg/day + **sulfadiazine** 50mg/12h + **calcium folinate** 15mg twice weekly all until delivery. *Affected babies:* (Diagnose by serology—>90% asymptomatic.) Intracranial calcification, hydrocephalus, chorioretinitis if severely affected. Encephalitis, epilepsy, mental and physical developmental delay, jaundice, hepatosplenomegaly, thrombocytopenia, and skin rashes occur. Treat with 4-weekly courses of pyrimethamine, sulfadiazine, and calcium folinate ×6, separated by 4 weeks of spiramycin. Prednisolone is given until signs of CNS inflammation or chorioretinitis abate. *Prevention:* Avoid eating raw meat, wash hands if raw meat touched, wear gloves if gardening or dealing with cat litter, and avoid sheep during lambing time.

Parvovirus B19 is a DNA virus, spread by respiratory droplets with a 4–20-day incubation period. 50% of women in the UK are immune. In pregnancy often no symptoms occur, but may include 'slapped cheek' rash, a maculopapular rash, fever, and arthralgia. Diagnosis is again on paired samples in the acute and convalescent phases (>10 days apart). IgM antibodies appear and IgG titres increase. Consequences in the woman herself are minimal unless she is immuno-compromised, in which case watch for sudden haemolysis requiring blood transfusion. 30% fetuses are infected, causing fetal suppression of erythropoiesis and cardiac toxicity. This leads to cardiac failure and fetal hydrops. 10% of fetuses infected at <20 weeks' gestation will die. Parvovirus is not teratogenic. Manage with serial US looking for signs of fetal anaemia (fetal hydrops and abnormal middle cerebral artery Dopplers). If the fetus does develop anaemia, manage in a tertiary fetal medicine unit and consider *in utero* red cell transfusion.

Intrauterine syphilis Maternal screening occurs (UK screen 55,700 to prevent 1 case. In some parts of London 2:1000 women are infected); if infection found, treat the mother with **benzylpenicillin** 600mg/24h IM daily for 10 days. ~⅓ are stillborn. Neonatal signs: rhinitis, snuffles, rash, hepatosplenomegaly, lymphadenopathy, anaemia, jaundice, ascites, hydrops, nephrosis, meningitis, ± keratitis, and nerve deafness. Nasal discharge exam: spirochetes; x-rays: perichondritis; CSF: ↑ Monocytes and protein with +ve serology. *Neonatal treatment:* Give **benzylpenicillin** 30mg/kg/12h IV for 7 days then 8h for 10 days.

Listeria Affects 6–15:100,000 pregnancies. Maternal symptoms: fever, shivering, myalgia, headache, sore throat, cough, vomiting, diarrhoea, vaginitis. Miscarriage (can be recurrent), premature labour, and stillbirth may occur. Infection is usually via infected food (eg milk, soft cheeses, pâté). ►Do blood cultures in any pregnant patient with unexplained fever for ≥48h. Serology, vaginal and rectal swabs do not help (can be commensal). See *OHCM* p389.

Perinatal infection usually occurs in 2nd or 3rd trimester. 20% of affected fetuses are stillborn. Fetal distress in labour is common. An early postnatal feature is respiratory distress from pneumonia. There may be convulsions, hepatosplenomegaly, pustular or petechial rashes, conjunctivitis, fever, leucopenia. Meningitis is commoner after perinatal infection. Diagnose by culture of blood, CSF, meconium, and placenta. Infant mortality: 30%. Isolate baby (nosocomial spread can occur). Treat with **ampicillin** 50mg/kg/6h IV and **gentamicin** 3mg/kg/12h IV until 1 week after fever subsides. Monitor levels.

Further reading

Health Protection Agency (2011). *Guidance on Viral Rash in Pregnancy*. London: HPA.

Hepatitis B virus (HBV) All mothers should be screened for HBsAg. Carriers have persistent HBsAg for >6 months. High infectivity is associated with HBeAg so anti-HBe antibodies are negative. Without immunization 95% of babies born to these mothers might develop hepatitis B, and 93% of the babies would be chronic carriers at 6 months. If the mother develops acute infection in the mid- or 3rd trimester there is high risk of perinatal infection. Her risk of death is 0.5–3%. Most neonatal infections occur at birth but some (especially in the East) are transplacental; hence the seeming failure of vaccination in up to 15% of neonates adequately vaccinated. Most infected neonates will develop chronic infection and in infected ♂ lifetime risk of developing hepatocellular cancer is 50%; 20% for ♀. Most will develop cirrhosis, so immunization is really important. ▶Give immunoglobulin (200u IM) and vaccinate babies of carriers and infected mothers at birth. In uncomplicated hepatitis, HBV DNA is cleared, anti-core antibodies develop, followed by anti-HBe antibodies with the decline and disappearance of HBeAg and HBsAg at 3 months. Do serology of vaccinated baby at 12–15 months old. If HBsAg–ve and anti-HBs is present, the child is protected.

Hepatitis C See p. 29.

Hepatitis E Risk of maternal mortality is ↑ (25% if in 3rd trimester); death is usually postpartum, preceded by fulminant hepatic failure, coma, and massive PPH. 33–50% of babies become infected. A vaccine is being developed.

Herpes simplex (HSV) Neonatal infection can cause blindness, IQ ↓, epilepsy, jaundice, respiratory distress, DIC, and death (in 30%, even if treated).

Prevalence of past (2°) HSV infection is ~25% and recurrence in pregnancy is not usually a problem thanks to maternal antibodies. If a mother develops primary (first-ever) genital herpes in pregnancy, refer to a genitourinary clinic to screen her for other infections and confirm it is 1°. If in last trimester, give her oral aciclovir or valaciclovir ± elective caesarean if 1° infection within 6 weeks of her due date. Type-specific HSV diagnosis: PCR.

If active 1° infection lesions at time of delivery, LSCS is recommended, even if membranes have ruptured up to 4h previously. If a mother with 1° lesions does deliver vaginally, risk of infection to the baby is 41%, so give mother (by IVI in labour) and newborn high-dose aciclovir (do PCR at birth). Try to avoid fetal blood sampling, scalp electrodes, and instrumental delivery. Neonatal infection usually appears at 5–21 days with grouped vesicles/pustules on a red base eg at the presenting part or sites of trauma (eg scalp electrode) ± periocular and conjunctival lesions. Non-vesicular rashes also occur.

Varicella zoster If mothers develop chickenpox near delivery, aim for delivery after 7 days, give babies varicella immune immunoglobulin (VZIG) at birth, and monitor for 28 days; and treat with aciclovir if neonate develops chickenpox. Babies of non-immune mothers also need VZIG if contacts in 1st 7 days of life. Earlier in pregnancy, if women with no personal history of chickenpox have had significant (eg 15min) chickenpox contact; check blood for varicella antibodies; if none, give VZIG, and manage as still potentially infectious 8–28 days later and notify doctor if develops rash. Women developing chickenpox in pregnancy should avoid contact with pregnant women, and have oral aciclovir 800mg 5× daily PO for 7 days if >20wks pregnant if presenting within 24h of rash. Hospitalize if chest, CNS symptoms, dense/haemorrhagic rash, or immunocompromised. Fetal varicella syndrome (FVS) complicates ~1% fetuses of mothers infected at 3–28 weeks of pregnancy by reactivation *in utero*. FVS features: skin scarring, eye defects (microphthalmia, chorioretinitis, cataracts), neurological abnormalities (microcephaly, cortical atrophy, IQ ↓, bowel and bladder sphincter disturbances). Refer to fetal medicine specialist for detailed US at 16–20wks, or 5wks post infection.⁊

(margin, vertical text) 1 Obstetrics

Chlamydia trachomatis Associations: low birthweight, premature membrane rupture, fetal death. ~30% of infected mothers have affected babies. Conjunctivitis develops 5–14 days after birth and may show minimal inflammation or purulent discharge. The cornea is not usually involved. *Complications:* Chlamydia pneumonitis, pharyngitis, or otitis media. *Tests: Special swabs are available but may be unreliable.* See p. 133. *Treatment:* Local cleansing of eye + **erythromycin** 12.5mg/kg/6h PO for ~3 weeks eliminates lung organisms. Give parents/partners **erythromycin**[33] or **azithromycin** 1g PO single dose.

Gonococcal conjunctivitis Occurs within ~4 days of birth, with purulent discharge and lid swelling, ± corneal hazing, corneal rupture, and panophthalmitis. Note, 50% will also have concurrent chlamydial infection. *Treatment:* Infants born to those with known gonorrhoea should have **cefotaxime** 100mg/kg IM stat, and **chloramphenicol** 0.5% eye-drops within 1h of birth. For active gonococcal infection give **benzylpenicillin** 50mg/kg/12h IM and 3-hourly 0.5% **chloramphenicol** drops for 7 days. Isolate the baby.

Ophthalmia neonatorum This is purulent discharge from the eye of a neonate <21 days old. The most common cause is self-limiting—blocked lacrimal ducts. Infective causes: *Chlamydia*, herpes virus, staphylococci, streptococci, pneumococci, *E. coli*. *Tests:* Swab for bacterial and viral culture, microscopy (look for intracellular gonococci), and *Chlamydia* (eg immunofluorescence). Treat gonococcus and *Chlamydia* as previously described. Bathe eyes with cool boiled water or expressed breast milk. Other infections should be treated with broad-spectrum antibiotics eg chloramphenicol.

Clostridium perfringens Suspect this in any complication of illegal termination of pregnancy and when intracellular encapsulated Gram+ve rods are seen on genital swabs. It may infect *in utero* deaths or any other anaerobic site (eg haematomas). *Signs:* Endometritis→septicaemia/gangrene→myoglobinuria→renal failure→death. *Treatment:* • Surgically debride all devitalized tissue • Hyperbaric O_2 • High-dose IV benzylpenicillin (erythromycin if serious penicillin allergy). The use of gas gangrene antitoxin is controversial. Seek expert help.

TB All babies born into households with TB, to mothers from areas with a high TB prevalence, or who will travel to such areas should have BCG (Bacillus Calmette–Guérin) vaccination after birth, 0.05mL intradermally at deltoid's insertion: 0.03mL if using a multiple puncture gun. Babies not vaccinated in hospital are unlikely to be vaccinated in the community.[34] Give other vaccinations as usual, avoiding the BCG vaccinated arm for 3 months. Separate babies from mothers with active or open TB until she has had 2 weeks of R_x and is sputum –ve. Vaccinate the baby with BCG and treat with isoniazid until he or she has a +ve skin reaction (Mantoux). Consider CXR in pregnant women with cough, fever, or weight loss. Encourage breastfeeding.

Group B *Streptococcus* (GBS)

GBS is a common bowel commensal carried by up to 20% of women vaginally. There is no screening for it in the UK but it may be found on routine high vaginal swabs or on urine culture. Neonatal risks include severe, early-onset infection which has 20% mortality, presenting as pneumonia, meningitis, and/or septicaemia. **In labour** Give all women IV antibiotics if: • +ve GBS high vaginal swab at any time in this/previous pregnancy • Any baby previously infected with GBS • Any documented GBS bacteriuria in this pregnancy • Gestation <37wks • Any intrapartum fever • If a woman is GBS+ve (swab or bacteriuria), with prelabour rupture of membranes at term, treat with GBS antibiotic prophylaxis and induce labour • If culture result unknown and membranes are ruptured at term for >18h: GBS prophylaxis (eg penicillin).[35] Give **benzylpenicillin** 3g IV as loading dose then 1.5g 4-hourly throughout labour. If penicillin allergic, give **clindamycin** 900mg IV 8-hourly.

►With any pain in pregnancy think, is this labour? If pain is in the second half of pregnancy, is this pre-eclampsia (pp. 50–1)? ►Women with chest, back, or epigastric pain severe enough for opiates need full investigation: cardiac causes (ECG, CXR, troponin, echocardiography, CT angiography + CT/MRI chest scan).

Abdominal pain may be from ligament stretching or from symphysis pubis strain. In early pregnancy, remember miscarriage (pp. 124-5) and ectopics (pp. 126-7).

Abruption The triad of abdominal pain, uterine rigidity, and vaginal bleeding suggests this. It occurs in between 1 in 80 and 1 in 200 pregnancies. Fetal loss is high if >50% of placenta affected. A tender uterus is highly suggestive. US is poor at diagnosis—rely on clinical signs. A live viable fetus merits rapid delivery as demise can be sudden. Prepare for DIC, which complicates 33–50% of severe cases, and beware PPH, which is also common. See pp. 92 & 96.

Uterine rupture See p. 95.

Uterine fibroids For torsion and red degeneration, see p. 138.

Uterine torsion The uterus rotates axially 30–40° to the right in 80% of normal pregnancies. Rarely, it rotates >90° causing acute uterine torsion in mid or late pregnancy with abdominal pain, shock, a tense uterus, and urinary retention (catheterization may reveal a displaced urethra in twisted vagina). Fibroids, adnexal masses, or congenital asymmetrical uterine anomalies are present in 90%. Diagnosis is usually at laparotomy. Deliver by LSCS.

Ovarian tumours Torsion, rupture, see pp. 172-3. **Pyelonephritis** See p. 31.

Appendicitis Incidence: ~1:1000 pregnancies. It is not commoner in pregnancy but mortality is higher (esp. from 20wks). Perforation is commoner (15–20%). Fetal mortality is ~1.5% for simple appendicitis; ~30% if perforation. The appendix migrates upwards, outwards, and posteriorly as pregnancy progresses, so pain is less well localized (often para-umbilical or subcostal—but right lower quadrant still commonest) and tenderness, rebound, and guarding less obvious. Peritonitis can make the uterus tense and woody-hard. ►Don't delay surgery!— Laparotomy over site of maximal tenderness with patient tilted 30° to the left by an experienced general surgeon (laparoscopy also appears to be safe).

Cholecystitis Incidence 1–6 per 10,000 pregnancies. Pregnancy encourages gallstone formation due to biliary stasis and increased cholesterol in bile. Symptoms are similar to the non-pregnant with subcostal pain, nausea, and vomiting. Jaundice is uncommon (5%). US confirms the presence of stones. The main differential diagnosis is appendicitis, and laparotomy or laparoscopy is mandatory if this cannot be excluded. Surgery should be reserved for complicated non-resolving biliary tract disease during pregnancy as in >90% the acute process resolves with conservative management. For patients requiring surgery, laparoscopic cholecystectomy can be a safe and effective method of treatment, but miscarriage/preterm labour is a risk.

Rectus sheath haematoma Very rarely, bleeding into the rectus sheath and haematoma formation can occur with coughing (or spontaneous) in late pregnancy causing swelling and tenderness. US is helpful. ΔΔ: Abruption. *Management:* Laparotomy (or perhaps laparoscopy—but not in late pregnancy) is indicated if the diagnosis is in doubt or if there is shock.

Pancreatitis In pregnancy is rare, but mortality is high (37% maternal; 5.6% fetal). Diagnose by serum amylase.

Urinary tract infection See p. 31.

Gastroenteritis Common and symptoms may be severe. If otherwise well, try and manage at home. Most settle with rehydration salts and rest. Always think—could diarrhoea and vomiting be a symptom of severe sepsis (pp. 88–9)?

☺Pregnancy and obesity (BMI >30 at booking)

Maternal obesity is continually increasing in the developed world, such that 1 in 5 pregnant women are now obese in the UK. A normal body mass index (BMI) is 18.5–24.9, overweight 25–29.9, and obesity is defined as a BMI over 30kg/m^2. Obesity is known to carry a higher risk of maternal death but also of every obstetric complication.

►Ideally, women should lose weight to a healthy BMI pre-pregnancy. The woman should not diet as such once pregnant, but should be discouraged to gain further weight and encouraged to eat a balanced diet, as well as take regular exercise. 'Eating for two' is a myth and calorie intake only needs to increase a small amount from the 2nd trimester.

Maternal and fetal risks

Pregnancy-induced hypertension and pre-eclampsia: Twice as likely, especially if there is excessive weight gain. *Gestational diabetes:* Three times more common. *Venous thromboembolism:* Risk is doubled. *Other risks include:* Subfertility, miscarriage, stillbirth, maternal cardiac disease, induction of labour, failed induction, caesarean section, instrumental delivery, macrosomia, shoulder dystocia, 3rd- and 4th-degree perineal tears, difficulty siting regional anaesthesia, higher risks during general anaesthetic, higher failure rate of VBAC, wound infection, endometritis, chest infection, postpartum haemorrhage, and higher rates of postnatal depression.

Management of all pregnant woman with obesity

2010 CMACE/RCOG guidelines recommend:

- Referral for consultant-led care.
- 5mg **folic acid** from 1 month before conception and for the 1st trimester to prevent increased risk of NTDs.
- Obese women are more prone to vitamin D deficiency so ensure they are taking 10mcg **vitamin D** supplementation while pregnant and breastfeeding.
- Screen for diabetes eg OGTT at 24–28 weeks and consider LMWH thromboprophylaxis for 7 days postnatally if one additional thrombotic risk factor (p. 36).
- Mobilize as soon as possible after vaginal or delivery by caesarean section.
- If women with BMI ≥30 require caesarean section and if subcutaneous fat is >2cm thick, suture that separately, to reduce risk of infection.
- Consider serial growth scans if BMI >35kg/m^2 (SFH measurement may not be accurate).
- *Women with BMI >40* should always receive 7-day postnatal heparin prophylaxis and TED stockings whatever the mode of delivery. They should have an antenatal consultation with an obstetric anaesthetist with an anaesthetic plan made for labour and delivery, and need 3rd-trimester assessment to plan manual handling requirements and provision of appropriate TED stockings. When in labour, inform anaesthetist. They should have continuous midwifery care and should have an IV sited early in labour. If operative delivery is required, the attending anaesthetist should be a consultant (or signed off obese-competent) obstetric anaesthetist.

The ideal pelvis This has a rounded brim, a shallow cavity, non-prominent ischial spines, a curved sacrum with large sciatic notches, and sacrospinous ligaments >3.5cm long. The angle of the brim is 55° to the horizontal, the AP diameter at least 12cm, and transverse diameter at least 13.5cm. The subpubic arch should be rounded and the intertuberous distance at least 10cm. A *clinically favourable* pelvis is one where the sacral promontory cannot be felt, the ischial spines are not prominent, the subpubic arch and base of supraspinous ligaments both accept 2 fingers, and the intertuberous diameter accepts 4 knuckles when the woman is examined.

The true pelvis Anteriorly there is the symphysis pubis (3.5cm long) and posteriorly the sacrum (12cm long). See fig 1.9.

Zone of inlet: Boundaries: anteriorly lies the upper border of the pubis, posteriorly the sacral promontory, laterally the ileopectineal line. Transverse diameter 13.5cm; AP diameter 11.5cm.

Zone of cavity: This is the most roomy zone. It is almost round. Transverse diameter 13.5cm; AP diameter 12.5cm.

Zone of mid-pelvis: Boundaries: anteriorly, the apex of the pubic arch; posteriorly, the tip of the sacrum; laterally the ischial spines (the desirable distance between the spines is >10.5cm). Ovoid in shape, it is the narrowest part.

Zone of outlet: The pubic arch is the anterior border (desirable angle >85°). Laterally lie the sacrotuberous ligaments and ischial tuberosities, posteriorly the coccyx.

Head terms The *bregma* is the anterior fontanelle. The *brow* lies between the bregma and the root of the nose. The *face* lies below the root of the nose and supraorbital ridges. The *occiput* lies behind the posterior fontanelle. The *vertex* is the area between the fontanelles and the parietal eminences. For presenting diameter see table 1.4.

Moulding The frontal bones can slip under the parietal bones which can slip under the occipital bone so reducing biparietal diameter. The degree of overlap may be assessed vaginally.

Movement of the head in labour (normal vertex presentation)

1 Descent with increased flexion as the head enters the cavity. The sagittal suture lies in the transverse diameter of the brim.
2 Internal rotation occurs at the ischial spine level due to the grooved gutter of the levator muscles. Head flexion increases. (The head rotates 90° if occipitolateral position, 45° if occipitoanterior, 135° if occipitoposterior.)
3 Disengagement by extension as the head comes out of the vulva.
4 Restitution: as the shoulders are rotated by the levators until the bisacromial diameter is anteroposterior, the head externally rotates the same amount as before but in opposite direction.
5 Delivery of anterior shoulder by lateral flexion of trunk posteriorly.
6 Delivery of posterior shoulder by lateral flexion of trunk anteriorly.
7 Delivery of buttocks and legs.

Table 1.4 Presenting diameters

Presentation	Relevant diameter presenting	
Flexed vertex	Suboccipitobregmatic	9.5cm
Partially deflexed vertex	Suboccipitofrontal	10.5cm
Deflexed vertex	Occipitofrontal	11.5cm
Brow	Mentovertical	13cm
Face	Submentobregmatic	9.5cm

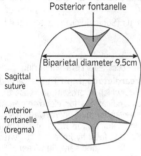

Posterior fontanelle

Biparietal diameter 9.5cm

Sagittal suture

Anterior fontanelle (bregma)

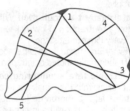

1 Sub occipitobregmatic 9.5cm
  flexed vertex presentation
2 Suboccipitofrontal 10.5cm
  partially deflexed vertex
3 Occipitofrontal 11.5cm deflexed vertex
4 Mentovertical 13cm brow
5 Submentobregmatic 9.5cm face

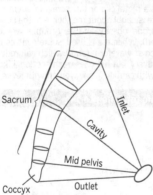

Sacrum

Inlet

Cavity

Mid pelvis

Coccyx

Outlet

Fig 1.9 Pelvic diameters vs fetal head.
'Life forced her through this gate of suffering.' DH Lawrence, Sons and Lovers.

Fetal monitoring in labour aims to detect signs of fetal compromise and is carried out either by intermittent auscultation (IA) or by continuous cardiotocograph (CTG), also known as electronic fetal monitoring (EFM). Approximately 10% of cerebral palsy is due to intrapartum hypoxia. Uterine contractions restrict the blood supply to the fetus, especially those in the second stage. A healthy, well-grown fetus with a good reserve should withstand labour, but one that has started to decompensate pre-labour (eg in absent or reversed end-diastolic flow in umbilical artery Dopplers, p. 13) is unlikely to manage the stress of regular contractions and reduction in blood supply.

Intermittent auscultation With Doppler US (Sonicaid™) for a full minute after a contraction in low-risk women:
• Every 15min in 1st stage.
• Every 5min throughout 2nd stage.
• If abnormality noted or intrapartum problems occur, start CTG monitoring.

Electronic fetal monitoring/continuous cardiotocograph This is carried out for certain maternal and fetal risk factors which, if present, increase the risk of fetal compromise in labour (see BOX 'Indications for electronic fetal monitoring'). It results in higher rates of intervention and operative delivery (instrumental and LSCS) without a convincing reduction in rates of cerebral palsy. CTG is sensitive but not specific in detecting fetal hypoxia: a fetus with an abnormal CTG will be hypoxic (acidotic) on fetal blood sampling (FBS) 50% of the time. The interpretation of CTG is probably another factor, and doctors and midwives working on the labour ward should undergo yearly CTG training with regular group teaching to maintain skills. The monitoring itself is carried out either through an abdominal probe (US) or via a fetal scalp electrode (FSE, producing a fetal ECG). FSE is a metal clip or tiny screw in direct contact with the fetus and is useful if there is doubt about the source of the heartbeat, poor contact of the abdominal probe, obesity, and very mobile women (requires membranes to have ruptured). When FSE is used, some centres have the facility to measure the fetal ECG ST waveform (STAN) which can reduce the need for FBS and instrumental delivery, but not caesarean section. Like FBS (p. 48), STAN should be approached with caution in any woman with fever.

Indications for electronic fetal monitoring

• Induction of labour
• Post-maturity (>42 weeks)
• Previous LSCS
• Maternal cardiac problems
• Pre-eclampsia or hypertension
• Prolonged rupture of membranes >24h
• Prematurity <37 weeks
• Diabetes of any type
• Antepartum or intrapartum haemorrhage
• Small for gestational age
• Oligohydramnios
• Abnormal umbilical artery Dopplers
• Multiple pregnancy
• Meconium-stained liquor
• Abnormal lie (eg breech)
• Oxytocin augmentation
• Epidural anaesthesia
• Pyrexia
• Abnormality heard on intermittent auscultation

Terms used to describe the CTG

The language used should be standardized and you may be asked to describe a trace using 'DR C BRAVADO'. This useful mnemonic is broken down as follows: *DR*, determine risk; why is the woman having EFM? *C* for contractions; how many in 10 minutes? *BRA* meaning baseline rate; *V* for variability, *A* for accelerations, *DE*celerations, and *O*verall (normal, suspicious, pathological). See table 1.5.

Baseline rate (BR) The average level of the fetal heart rate when any accelerations or decelerations have been excluded. It appears as a straight-ish line between other features on the trace. Normal is 110–160bpm. Bradycardia is a baseline of <100bpm; tachycardia >160bpm can be associated with maternal fever. BR >180bpm is abnormal.

Variability Best thought of as the 'bandwidth' of the baseline. Take a small square on the CTG; each one should contain a variation in FHR of >5bpm. Reduced variability is <5bpm (but this can be normal if <30min and can happen when the baby is sleeping). Other causes of reduced variability include fetal hypoxia, malformation, magnesium, and prematurity <28 weeks.

Accelerations An upward spike of >15bpm for >15 seconds. They are a reassuring feature and commonly occur when the fetus is moving.

Decelerations Appear as downward spikes of >15bpm for >15 seconds. These may be a normal feature of labour, and how concerning they are depends on the shape of them, and when they appear relative to a contraction. *Early* decelerations mimic the shape and timing of the contraction and are caused by head compression. They are therefore seen in breech presentation in labour and the second stage. *Late* decelerations reach their nadir after the peak of the contraction has passed and are a sign of acidosis especially with other abnormal features. *Shallow* decelerations together with reduced variability represent an abnormal trace that warrants intervention *Typical variable* decelerations are v-shaped with shoulders on either side, and are associated with cord compression and are not usually associated with hypoxia. *Atypical* variables have loss of shouldering, last >60 seconds, >60 beats from the baseline, may be slow to recover, be a 'w' shape, and lose variability within the deceleration. They may be a sign of fetal hypoxia. See figs 1.10–1.14 on pp. 48–9.

Table 1.5 Classification of the CTG

	Baseline (bpm)	Variability (bpm)	Decelerations	Accelerations
Reassuring	110–160	>5	None or early	Present
Non-reassuring	100–109 161–180	<5 for 30–50min	Variable decelerations for >50% contractions for >90min, taking <60s to recover, or drop from BR of >60 beats, or taking >60 seconds to recover, for <30min	
Abnormal	<100 >180	<5 for >50min	Late decelerations for >50% contractions for >30min Single prolonged deceleration for >3min	

Source: data from NICE 2014. Intrapartum care: cg190. https://www.nice.org.uk/guidance/cg190

Normal All 4 features are in the reassuring category.

Suspicious 1 non-reassuring feature, and 2 reassuring features.

Pathological 2 or more non-reassuring or 1 abnormal feature.

1 Obstetrics

Improving a CTG Correct any possible insults: left lateral position to shift weight off maternal vessels and correct cord compression; IV fluids; reduce or stop oxytocin infusion if contracting >5 contractions in 10min or bradycardia. **Terbutaline** 250mcg SC can be used as an emergency tocolytic to stop or reduce contractions. If the CTG is abnormal offer *fetal scalp stimulation* (VE—a positive response is reflected by an acceleration on the CTG). If this fails offer FBS, or consider expediting delivery.

Fetal blood sampling Used to improve the specificity of CTG in detecting fetal hypoxia with an abnormal CTG, unless immediate delivery is required (eg bradycardia >3min, suspected LSCS scar rupture). The woman is placed in the left lateral position. A specialized speculum with a light is placed against the fetal scalp. A small scratch is made on the fetal scalp and fetal blood collected in a capillary tube and analysed in a blood gas machine. The woman should be at least 4cm dilated with ruptured membranes. If FBS fails, the baby should be delivered as soon as possible—by LSCS if not fully dilated. Do not attempt FBS/FSE if the woman has suspected ITP, any blood-borne viruses, and use with caution in pyrexia. In units where STAN is used (p. 46) a normal FBS result is required prior to this method of EFM commencing when the CTG is abnormal.

- Normal pH: >7.25 (repeat in 1h if CTG remains abnormal).
- Borderline pH: 7.21–7.24 (repeat in 30min if CTG remains abnormal).
- Abnormal pH: <7.20 (immediate delivery).

1 Obstetrics

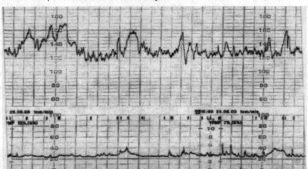

Fig 1.10 Normal CTG. All characteristics (see p. 47) are within normal limits.
Reproduced from Sarris *et al. Training in Obstetrics and Gynaecology* (2009) with permission from OUP.

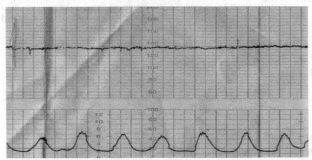

Fig 1.11 Significantly reduced variability (almost a pencil line). This can be normal in sleep-cycling but if >90min is ominous; can also occur with narcotic agents.
Reproduced from Sarris *et al. Training in Obstetrics and Gynaecology* (2009) with permission from OUP.

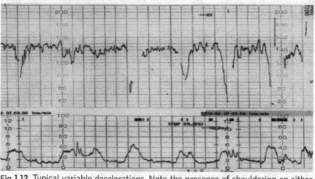

Fig 1.12 Typical variable decelerations. Note the presence of shouldering on either side of the deceleration, and the clear 'v' shape. These are usually a sign of cord compression, head, or eyeball compression during labour and are due to a fetal reflex and are not ominous.

Reproduced from Sarris *et al. Training in Obstetrics and Gynaecology* (2009) with permission from OUP.

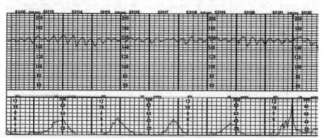

Fig 1.13 Sinusoidal pattern which if >10min can indicate fetal anaemia but if <10min could be due to thumb-sucking.

Reproduced with permission from periFACTS OB/GYN Academy.

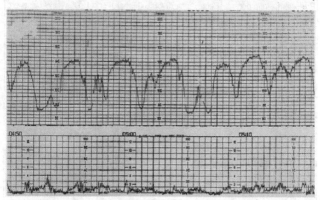

Fig 1.14 Abnormal CTG with reduced variability and atypical variable decelerations. There is loss of shouldering, reduced variability within the decelerations, and some have a 'w' shape.

Reproduced from Sarris *et al. Training in Obstetrics and Gynaecology* (2009) with permission from OUP.

Pre-eclampsia This is characterized by hypertension in a pregnant woman which occurs after 20 weeks, with either proteinuria or evidence of systemic involvement which resolves by 6 weeks postpartum. It occurs in 5–8% of pregnancies. It is associated with failure of trophoblastic invasion of spiral arterioles leaving them vasoactive and therefore is also associated with fetal growth restriction and placental failure. Increasing BP partially compensates for this. Pre-eclampsia also affects hepatic, renal, and coagulation systems. Pre-eclampsia is a major cause of maternal morbidity (from cerebral haemorrhage, multiorgan failure, and adult respiratory distress syndrome) and mortality, as well as iatrogenic prematurity (the only cure is delivery of the baby).

Risk factors (See table 1.6.) *High risk:* • Previous severe or early-onset pre-eclampsia (<20 weeks) • Chronic hypertension (p. 35) or hypertension in previous pregnancy • Chronic kidney disease • Diabetes mellitus • Autoimmune disease (SLE, antiphospholipid, thrombophilia). *Moderate risk:* • 1st pregnancy • ≥40yrs • Pregnancy interval >10yrs • BMI ≥30kg/m² • FH pre-eclampsia • Multiple pregnancy • Low PAPP-A (p. 16) • Uterine artery notching on Doppler US at 22–24 weeks. If 1 high-risk or 2 moderate-risk factors take **aspirin** 75-150 mg/24h PO from 12th week of pregnancy until delivery to prevent pre-eclampsia. *Fetal:* Hydatidiform mole; multiple pregnancy; fetal hydrops (eg rhesus disease).

Symptoms May be absent, especially with mild pre-eclampsia. Ask about headache, flashing lights, epigastric or right upper quadrant pain, nausea and vomiting, and swelling of face, fingers, and lower limbs. *Signs:* May include pregnancy-induced hypertension, proteinuria, epigastric or right upper quadrant tenderness, brisk reflexes, >2 beats of clonus, confusion, fits, placental abruption, IUGR, and stillbirth.

Table 1.6 Effect of risk factors on pre-eclampsia

Risk factor	Effect on pre-eclampsia
Primiparity	Risk doubled compared with multips
New paternity	Protective effect of multiparity lost
Pre-eclampsia in previous pregnancy	Recurrence 10–50% (higher if onset <30 weeks or severe disease, lower if late onset or mild)
Family history	Risk 25% if mother had it; 33% if a sister had it. Genetics are thought to play a part in its development
BMI >30kg/m²	Increased risk with increasing BMI
Age >35 years	Increased risk with extremes of age but especially >35 and 40 years (4× a 25-year-old woman) possibly related to more comorbidities and reduced adaptability
Multiple pregnancy	Morbidity and mortality higher from pre-eclampsia than singleton pregnancies
Subfertility	Risks higher despite accounting for increased maternal age and other risk factors. With a donor embryo risk is almost 50%
Gestational/chronic hypertension	At least 25% of these women will develop pre-eclampsia
Autoimmune disease	Risk increased especially with antiphospholipid syndrome. Can be difficult to distinguish flare of autoimmune disease from pre-eclampsia. Both conditions may become severe, causing a critically unwell patient
Renal disease	25% incidence of pre-eclampsia

1 Obstetrics

Diagnosis Traditionally based upon:
- Systolic BP >140mmHg or diastolic >90mmHg *and* urine PCR >0.3mg/dL.
- However, there is now a shift towards also including the following, in the absence of proteinuria:
  - Thrombocytopenia (platelets <100 × 10⁹/L).
  - Serum creatinine >88μmol/L or doubling of serum creatinine in the absence of other renal disease.
  - Impaired liver function with elevated liver transaminases to twice normal concentration.
  - Pulmonary oedema.
  - Cerebral or visual disturbance.

This shift is to reflect the multisystem disease that is pre-eclampsia. In a minority of patients, proteinuria develops very late or not at all but evidence of other system involvement can present much earlier.

Investigations Urinalysis (reagent strip testing) and PCR; fetal ultrasound including umbilical artery Dopplers to provide information on growth and well-being of the baby; fetal CTG at diagnosis then twice weekly; FBC particularly for detection of anaemia and thrombocytopenia; LFTS; renal function; coagulation screen (may be abnormal if pre-eclampsia is severe).

The triage PIGF (placental growth factor) test can be used from 20–34⁺⁶/40 in conjunction with clinical judgement and other tests to help diagnose suspected pre-eclampsia and the level of risk for associated delivery within 14 days of testing.[36]

Management Depends on disease severity. All women with pre-eclampsia should deliver on a labour ward. NICE recommends admission of all women with pre-eclampsia, but units are increasingly managing mild disease as out-patients.
- *Mild pre-eclampsia:* BP 140–149/90–99mmHg. Urine PCR >0.3mg/dL is diagnostic in the presence of hypertension and does not need to be repeated—it is not reflective of severity of pre-eclampsia. 4-hourly BP; twice-weekly bloods to monitor renal function, LFTS, FBC. Fetal growth scans every 2 weeks. Do not start antihypertensives unless BP >150/100mmHg. IOL after 37/40.
- *Moderate pre-eclampsia:* BP 150–159/100–109mmHg. Admit to hospital until delivery. Measure BP 4-hourly; check bloods 3 times per week; fortnightly fetal growth scans, and twice-daily CTG. Start antihypertensives. Aim for IOL at 37/40.
- *Severe pre-eclampsia:* BP >160/110mmHg, or symptoms/signs (eg clonus), or end-organ damage. Call for senior help from obstetrics, anaesthetic, and midwifery staff. Stabilize BP with antihypertensives eg **nifedipine** 10mg PO twice 30 min apart. If BP still remains high, start IV antihypertensives (labetalol or hydralazine). Prophylactic **magnesium sulfate** 4g IV loading dose then 1g IV/hour. Bloods every 12–24h. Maintain strict fluid balance, catheterize, give steroids for fetal lung maturity and if >34 weeks deliver. For women <34 weeks, time delivery according to senior advice but will generally need to be once woman is stable, but ideally within 24–48h.

Effects of pre-eclampsia Plasma volume ↓; peripheral resistance ↑; placental ischaemia. If the BP is >180/140mmHg microaneurysms develop in arteries. DIC may develop. Oedema may develop suddenly. The liver may be involved (contributing to DIC)—and HELLP syndrome may be present with placental infarcts.

Severe complications: Eclampsia, HELLP syndrome (pp. 90–1), cerebral haemorrhage, IUGR, renal failure, and placental abruption.

Further reading

ACOG (2013). Task Force on Hypertension in Pregnancy. *Obstet Gynecol* 122:1122–31.

NICE (2010). *The Management of Hypertensive Disorders during Pregnancy* (CG107). London: NICE.

►This is a leading cause of perinatal mortality and morbidity: 5–10% births but 50% of perinatal deaths. Premature infants are those born before 37 weeks' gestation. Prevalence: ~6% of singletons, 46% of twin, 79% of triplet or higher-order deliveries. About 1.4% are before 32^{+0} weeks—when neonatal problems are greatest. In 25%, delivery is elective (p. 60). 10% are due to multiple pregnancy; 25% are due to APH, cervical incompetence, chorioamnionitis, uterine abnormalities, diabetes, polyhydramnios, pyelonephritis, or other infections. In 40% the cause is unknown, but abnormal genital tract colonization (bacterial vaginosis) with *Ureaplasma* and *Mycoplasma hominis* is implicated, as either a risk factor or risk marker.

Risk factors Previous preterm birth, multiple pregnancy, cervical surgery (eg LLETZ or cone biopsy), uterine anomalies, pre-existing medical conditions, pre-eclampsia, IUGR, and abnormal genital tract colonization (see earlier).

Managing preterm rupture of membranes (PROM)
Admit for 48h (highest risk of preterm labour); rule out any evidence of chorioamnionitis and sepsis. If there is evidence of chorioamnionitis, expedite delivery irrespective of gestation. Take T°, MSU, and HVS—using a sterile bivalve speculum. Signs such as raised CRP develop late and should not be relied upon. Give corticosteroids for fetal lung maturity (see p. 53) and **erythromycin** 500mg PO QDS for 10 days (reduces neonatal morbidity). In 80%, membrane rupture initiates labour. The problem with the 20% who do not go into labour is balancing advantages of remaining *in utero* (maturity and surfactant ↑) against the threat of infection (causes 20% of neonatal deaths). Intrauterine infection supervenes after membranes have ruptured in 10% by 48h, 26% by 72h, 40% by >72h. If infection develops, take blood cultures and give IV antibiotics (include cover for group B *Streptococcus*) and expedite labour (p. 60). The risks to the fetus from PROM are those of prematurity, infection, pulmonary hypoplasia, and limb contractures. If labour does not occur spontaneously, discharge after 48h and manage as an out-patient avoiding intercourse, tampons, and swimming, with weekly follow-up in the day unit for FBC and CRP. Aim for IOL at 34–36 weeks if cephalic.

Management of preterm labour In 50% contractions cease spontaneously. Treating the cause (eg pyelonephritis) may help it cease. Give corticosteroids (p. 53). Trials of tocolytic drugs have shown them to be of almost no clinical benefit, and only nifedipine is associated with improvement of fetal outcome. It is quite reasonable not to use tocolytic drugs; though they may be considered desirable in certain circumstances eg to give time for corticosteroids to work, or for *in utero* transfer. Consider transfer to hospital with NICU facilities. Check presentation (breech more common with increasing prematurity). Check FBC, CRP, HVS, MSU. Speculum to rule out PROM, take fetal fibronectin (see p. 53) and if no PROM gentle vaginal exam to assess dilatation. If in labour, give IV antibiotics to prevent GBS (eg **benzylpenicillin** 3g loading dose followed by 1.5g 4-hourly). Call paediatrician to attend to the baby at birth. See cord-cutting recommendations on p. 53.

Tocolytics Absolute CI: chorioamnionitis, fetal death or lethal abnormality, condition (fetal or maternal) needing immediate delivery. Relative CI: fetal growth restriction or distress, pre-eclampsia, placenta praevia, abruption, cervix >4cm. Atosiban (licensed in Europe) has fewer maternal effects, but has not been shown to benefit the fetus. Nifedipine is as effective, and associated with less newborn respiratory distress and admission to intensive care. Regimen: **nifedipine** 20mg PO then 10–20mg/6–8h according to uterine activity (unlicensed use). Use up to 48h. SE: ↓ BP; headache; flushing; pulse ↑ (transient); myocardial infarction (very rare); CI: heart disease (use with caution in diabetes, and multiple pregnancy as pulmonary oedema risk).

Fetal fibronectin A protein not usually detected in vaginal secretions between 22 and 35 weeks. It is used to rule out preterm labour and is a bedside test. Those with positive fFN have a 10% chance of preterm delivery and should be admitted and given corticosteroids. Falsely positive if intercourse, significant bleeding, speculum, or vaginal exam within 48 hours.

Glucocorticoids *Dose:* **Betamethasone** 12mg IM with a 2nd dose 12–24h later (or **dexamethasone** 6–12mg in 2–4 doses totalling 24mg over 24h).

These help fetal surfactant production, lowering mortality (by 31%) and complications of RDS (p. 304) by 44%. They also help close patent ductuses and protect against periventricular malacia, a cause of cerebral palsy.

- Use in all women at risk of iatrogenic or spontaneous preterm birth between ~24[+0] and ~34[+6] weeks.[37][RCOG]
- If growth restriction too, use up to 35[+6] weeks.
- If risk at 23[+0]–23[+6] weeks use only on senior advice.
- Consider using before elective CS under 39 weeks.
- Consider use at 35–36 weeks if delivery expedited for pre-eclampsia (NICE).[37][RCOG]
- If diabetic, monitor glucose (may need admission and insulin infusion).

Benefit occurs within 24h. Repeat doses are not beneficial. A further 'rescue' dose is only recommended if the first course was given before 26 weeks and a new obstetric indication arises.[37][RCOG]

Magnesium sulfate Studies show a neuroprotective effect if given antenatally for babies <34 weeks' gestation. It is estimated that 63 women will need treatment to prevent 1 case of cerebral palsy. Australian draft national clinical guidelines recommend a maternal loading dose of 4g IV over 20–30 minutes followed by 1g/h maintenance infusion for up to 24h (or birth, if earlier), and use if fetus <30 weeks' gestation.[38]

Delivery Babies delivered at <28 weeks' gestation should be delivered in a room with temperature of 26°C, wrapped in food-grade plastic wrap or bag without drying after birth, and be placed under heat while stabilizing (keep wrapped until temperature checked in NICU).[39] Older babies are wrapped in dry towels. A 3min delay in cutting the cord (if premature babies are vigorous and not needing active resuscitation), and holding the baby 20cm below the introitus, results in higher haematocrit levels, and reduces transfusion and oxygen supplement requirements in premature babies, and reduces rates of intraventricular haemorrhage, but increases the need for phototherapy.[39]

Prematurity, survival, and disability—the figures

- Cerebral palsy is present in 20% of surviving babies born at 24–26 weeks' gestation (compared with 4% at 32 weeks) in a large French study.[40]

Viability thresholds for very premature babies have reduced by 1 week per decade for the last 40 years. Survival before 22 weeks is very rare. In 1995, 1% of babies born at 22–23 weeks survived to leave hospital, 11% at 23–24; 26% at 24–25; 44% at 25–26. Of surviving babies born between 23–24 weeks, two-thirds had moderate or severe disability; by 25 to 26 weeks, two-thirds had no or only mild disability. These figures have led to guidelines for consideration of treatment at different gestations eg not resuscitating babies of <22 weeks' completed gestation unless specifically requested by parents after discussion with senior paediatrician; but normally admitting babies of >23 weeks' completed gestation to neonatal intensive care.[41] More recent figures for England, Wales, and Northern Ireland were that 17% of babies born at 22–22[+6] weeks' gestation survived the neonatal period, increasing to 35% at 23–23[+6] weeks; 59% at 24–24[+6], 74% for 25–25[+6], 83% for 26–26[+6], to 98% at 31–31[+6] weeks.[42]

Further reading

RCOG (2010). *Antenatal Corticosteroids to Reduce Neonatal Morbidity and Mortality* (Green-top Guideline No. 7). London: RCOG.

►All women should be assessed at booking for risk factors for the sᴄᴀ fetus in order to identify those at increased risk who require increased monitoring. At booking, every woman should have a customized growth chart for sꜰʜ which takes into account maternal age, parity, ʙᴍɪ, ethnicity, and birthweights of previous children. A single sꜰʜ measurement <10th centile or static growth should prompt referral for fetal us (fig 1.15). Those women at high risk (see later) should be referred for consultant-led care and have serial us measurement of fetal size including umbilical artery Doppler from 26–28 weeks. Women with 3 or more minor risk factors should have uterine artery Doppler at 20–24 weeks, and if abnormal, serial growth scans. Identifying the sᴄᴀ fetus is important because they have a higher mortality (both intra-uterine and neonatal), higher incidence of cerebral palsy, and are more likely to have intrapartum fetal distress, meconium aspiration, and emergency ʟsᴄs.

Definition Estimated fetal weight <10th centile for their gestational age or abdominal circumference <10th centile. *Placental factors:* Abnormal trophoblast invasion eg pre-eclampsia, infarction, abruption. Tends to cause asymmetrical growth restriction with head sparing and reduced abdominal circumference. *Fetal factors:* Genetic abnormalities especially trisomies 13, 18, and 21, and Turner syndrome; congenital anomalies and infection such as ᴄᴍᴠ, rubella; multiple pregnancy. Usually causes a symmetrically small fetus.

Major risk factors • Maternal age >40yrs • Smoker • Cocaine use • Previous sᴄᴀ baby • Previous stillbirth • Maternal/paternal sᴄᴀ • Chronic hypertension • Diabetes • Renal impairment • Antiphospholipid syndrome • Heavy antepartum bleeding • Echogenic bowel • Pre-eclampsia • Low ᴘᴀᴘᴘ-ᴀ (p. 16). **Minor risk factors** • Maternal age >35yrs • Nulliparity • ʙᴍɪ <20 • ɪᴠꜰ • Pregnancy-induced hypertension.

Management Once a fetus is identified as sᴄᴀ, if the umbilical artery Dopplers are normal, growth scans should be carried out every 2–3 weeks. If Dopplers remain normal, aim for ɪᴏʟ at 37 weeks. If abnormal Dopplers and preterm, delivery depends on other indices such as ductus venosus Doppler (<32 weeks). If absent or reversed end-diastolic flow in umbilical artery Doppler, consider delivery by ʟsᴄs. Offer corticosteroids for fetal lung maturity up to 35^{+6} weeks. Growth-restricted fetuses are more susceptible to hypoxia and even if Dopplers are normal, intervention rate in labour is higher. After birth, temperature regulation may be a problem, so ensure a warm welcome and encourage skin-to-skin contact with the mother. Neonates have little stored glycogen so are prone to hypoglycaemia. Feed within 2h of birth. *Effects of ɪᴜɢʀ in adult life:* As adults, higher risk of hypertension, coronary artery disease, type 2 diabetes, and autoimmune thyroid disease.

Large for gestational age

These are babies above the 95th centile in weight for gestation.

Causes Constitutionally large (usually familial—the largest 10% of the population); maternal diabetes (pp. 26–7); obesity is a major cause (as much as ᴅᴍ).

Labour and aftercare Large babies risk birth injury (see 'Shoulder dystocia', p. 94) but ɪᴏʟ does not reduce it. They are prone to hypoglycaemia and hypocalcaemia. Polycythaemia may result in jaundice. They are also prone to left colon syndrome: a self-limiting condition clinically mimicking Hirschsprung disease (p. 222) whereby temporary bowel obstruction (possibly also with meconium plug) occurs.

Further reading

ʀᴄᴏɢ (2013). *The Investigation and Management of the Small-for-Gestational-Age Fetus* (Green-top Guideline No. 31). London: ʀᴄᴏɢ.

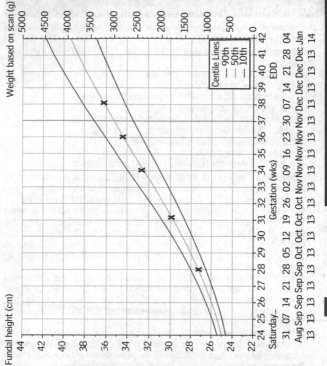

Fig 1.15 Customized antenatal growth chart. The sfh should follow the same centile throughout pregnancy. Deviation from this should prompt referral for a fetal growth scan.

With permission from the Perinatal Institute, www.perinatal.org.uk.

Definition Prolonged pregnancy is defined as that exceeding 42 completed weeks of pregnancy.

Incidence 5–10% of pregnancies (30% if previous prolonged pregnancy).

Problems
- Intrapartum deaths 4 times more common.
- Early neonatal deaths 3 times more common.
- Increased rates of induction of labour and operative delivery.
- Possible placental insufficiency.
- Macrosomia (25% >4000g), shoulder dystocia, and fetal injury.
- Fetal skull more ossified so less mouldable.
- Increased meconium passage in labour (25–40%) (p.70).
- Increased fetal distress in labour.
- Increased caesarean rates for labours after 41 completed weeks.

Management Confirm EDD. At 38-week visit discuss what is recommended if spontaneous labour does not occur by 41 completed weeks, including membrane sweep and induction. Arrange for visit at 41 weeks if not delivered.

1 Membrane sweep. On vaginal examination as much membrane is swept from the lower segment as possible by a finger inserted through the cervix. It is thought to induce natural prostaglandins. This may cause discomfort and a little bleeding but may induce labour 'naturally'. 8 women are membrane swept for 1 formal induction avoided. Offer at 40- and 41-week visit in nullips, at 41 weeks in multips.

2 A policy of induction after 41 completed weeks' pregnancy does reduce fetal death rate. NICE says to offer induction between 41^{+0} and 42^{+0} weeks.[43] Induction is with vaginal prostaglandin followed by oxytocin (p. 60). After induction, monitor the fetus in labour (p46). It is estimated that 500 inductions are needed to prevent 1 perinatal death.

3 If the woman declines induction then arrange twice-weekly CTG (p. 46), and us estimation of amniotic fluid depth to try to detect fetuses who may be becoming hypoxic. Doppler studies of cord blood flow may be used to look for absent end-diastolic flow as a predictor of fetal compromise.

Signs of postmaturity in the baby: Dry, cracked, peeling, loose skin; decreased subcutaneous tissue; scaphoid (hollow) abdomen; meconium staining of nails and cord.

1 Obstetrics

This is rupture of the membranes prior to the onset of labour in women at or over 37 completed weeks' gestation. It occurs in 8–10% of term pregnancies.

Causes Mostly unknown; infection of the lower genital tract or amnion is a known aetiological factor; polyhydramnios; multiple pregnancy; malpresentation.

When there is PROM, risk of serious infection is increased (1% vs 0.5% for women with intact membranes). 60% of women will go into spontaneous labour within 24h. After 24h chorioamnionitis and endometritis are more common, and the baby is more likely to be admitted to SCBU.

Conservative management Appropriate up to 24h post membrane rupture if the liquor is clear, the mother is well, and there are no fetal concerns (see following 'Indications for immediate induction of labour'). She should regularly take her temperature, report to labour ward if any change in fetal movements, colour, or smell of liquor, and avoid sexual intercourse.

Induction of labour If spontaneous labour has not commenced by 24h then NICE recommends induction of labour.[43] Vaginal prostaglandin is the preferred method of trying to induce labour eg **dinoprostone gel** 1–2mg for 6h followed by an oxytocin infusion if contractions have not started. Those giving birth after 24h of ruptured membranes should deliver where there are neonatal care facilities, and advised to stay in hospital for 12h after birth.

Routine prophylactic use of IV antibiotics in labour is not recommended. However, if there is clinical evidence of infection, IV antibiotics should be commenced and should include cover for group B *Streptococcus* with broad-spectrum antibiotics. Take HVS, send MSU and blood cultures before starting antibiotics. *If induction of labour is declined:* Offer advice from a senior midwife or doctor. Monitor fetal heart rate at 1st contact and every 24h after membrane rupture while the woman is not in labour. Ask her to report if there are reduced fetal movements.

Indications for immediate induction of labour Group B *Streptococcus* carriers; HIV carriers aiming for a vaginal delivery; signs of chorioamnionitis; concerns regarding fetal movements; meconium-stained liquor; herpes simplex genital infection.

Management of the neonate Babies are most susceptible to infection within 12h of birth. Observe at 1h, 2h, and then 2-hourly for a further 10h. Observations should include general well-being, chest movement and nasal flare, capillary refill, feeding, muscle tone, temperature, respirations, and heart rate. If there is any suggestion of sepsis in the baby, call a neonatal care specialist. Mothers should also be advised to report any health concerns about the baby in the 1st 5 days of life.

'Labour is one of the shortest yet most hazardous journeys humans make in their lifetime.' From the 1st trimester, the uterus has Braxton Hicks contractions (ie non-painful 'practice' contractions eg to ≤15mmHg pressure; in labour, pressure is ~60mmHg). They are commonest after 36 weeks.

Normal labour (fig 1.16) ~60% of births are normal and need no intervention. Normal labour occurs after 37wks' gestation and results in spontaneous vaginal delivery of the baby within 24h of the onset of regular spontaneous contractions. It is often heralded by a 'show', ie a plug of cervical mucus and a little blood as the membranes strip from the os (membranes may then rupture).

The first stage of labour *Latent phase:* There are painful, often irregular contractions, the cervix initially *effaces* (becomes shorter and softer) then dilates to 4cm. *Established phase:* Regular contractions with dilatation from 4cm. A satisfactory rate of dilatation from 4cm is 0.5cm/h. The 1st stage generally takes 8–18h in a primip, and 5–12h in a multip. During the 1st stage check maternal BP, and T° 4-hourly, pulse hourly; assess the contractions every 30min, their strength (you should not be able to indent the uterus on abdominal examination during a contraction) and their frequency (ideally 3–4 per 10min, lasting up to 1min). Note frequency of bladder emptying. Offer vaginal examination eg every 4h to assess the degree of cervical dilatation, the position, and the station of the head (measured in cm above or below the ischial spines) and note the degree of moulding and caput (p. 44). Note the state of the liquor (p. 70). Auscultate fetal heart rate (if not continuously monitored), by Pinard or Doppler every 15 min, listening for 1 min after a contraction. For fetal monitoring, see p. 46.

The second stage *Passive stage:* This is complete cervical dilatation but no pushing. This is seen particularly in women with epidural anaesthesia where 1–2h of passive stage is recommended to reduce the instrumental delivery rate. *Active stage:* Maternal pushing uses abdominal muscles and the Valsalva manoeuvre until the baby is born (see 'Movement of the head in labour', p. 44). Discourage supine maternal position in 2nd stage. Encourage mother to adopt a comfortable position. Check BP and pulse hourly, T° 4-hourly, assess contractions half-hourly, auscultate for 1min after a contraction every 5 min, offer vaginal examination hourly, and record urination during 2nd stage. If contractions wane, oxytocin augmentation may be needed.

As the head descends, the perineum stretches and the anus gapes. Expect birth within 3h from active 2nd stage in primips (refer to obstetrician if not imminent at 2h); expect birth within 2h in a multip (refer if birth not imminent at 1h). Prevent a precipitate delivery (and so intracranial bleeding) by pressure over the perineum. 1min delay in clamping the cord is recommended in healthy term babies. 3min delay benefits premature babies (↓ anaemia)."

The third stage Delivery of the placenta. As the uterus contracts to a <24-week size after the baby is born, the placenta separates from the uterus through the spongy layer of the decidua basalis. It then buckles and a small amount of retroplacental haemorrhage aids its removal.

Signs of separation: Cord lengthening → rush of blood (retroplacental haemorrhage) *per vaginam* → uterus rises → uterus contracts in the abdomen (felt with hand as a globular mass). Physiological (natural) 3rd stage takes ≤1h.

Use of Syntometrine® (**ergometrine maleate** 500mcg IM + **oxytocin** 5u IM) as the anterior shoulder is born decreases third stage time (to ~5min), and decreases the incidence of PPH. It can precipitate myocardial infarction and is contraindicated in those with pre-eclampsia, severe hypertension, severe liver or renal impairment, and severe heart disease. If BP not measured in labour give just oxytocin. Examine the placenta to check it is complete.

►Is thromboprophylaxis needed (p. 36)?

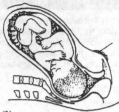

(1)
First stage of labour. The cervix
dilates. After full dilatation
the head flexes further and
descends further into the pelvis.

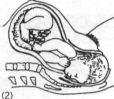

(2)
During the early second
stage the head rotates at
the level of the ischial spine
so the occiput lies in the
anterior part of pelvis.
In late second stage the
head broaches the vulval ring
(crowning) and the perineum
stretches over the head.

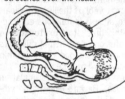

Fig 1.16 Normal labour.

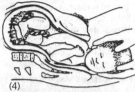

(4)
Birth of the anterior shoulder.
The shoulders rotate to lie in the
anteroposterior diameter of the
pelvic outlet. The head rotates
externally, 'restitutes', to its
direction at onset of labour.
Downward and backward traction
of the head by the birth attendant
aids delivery of the anterior shoulder.

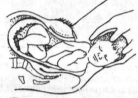

(5)
Birth of the posterior
shoulder is aided by lifting
the head upwards whilst
maintaining traction.

(3)
The head is born. The shoulders still lie
transversely in the midpelvis.

~20% of UK labours are induced artificially, usually because it has been decided that to remain *in utero* is relatively more risky for the fetus than to be born, but in some it is because of risk to the mother. 75% of inductions are for hypertension, pre-eclampsia, prolonged pregnancy, or rhesus disease. Other indications are diabetes, previous stillbirth, abruption, fetal death *in utero*, and placental insufficiency.

▶Inducing mothers at 41+ weeks aims to reduce stillbirth rates.

Contraindications Malpresentations (including breech), fetal distress, placenta praevia, cord presentation, vasa praevia, pelvic tumour eg cervical fibroid.

Cervical assessment When an induction is being planned the state of the cervix will be assessed. If primips are induced with an unripe cervix (Bishop score ≤3, see table 1.7) the rates of prolonged labour, fetal distress, and caesarean section are increased. This is less marked in multips.

Table 1.7 Modified Bishop score

Score	0	1	2
Cervical dilation (cm)	0	1–2	3–4
Length of cervix (cm)	>2	1–2	<1
Station of head (cm above ischial spines)	–3	–2	–1
Cervical consistency	Firm	Medium	Soft
Position of cervix	Posterior	Middle	Anterior

A score of >5 is favourable and if >7, induction with artificial rupture of membranes should be possible, thereby avoiding prostaglandins. Induction of labour is carried out using **dinoprostone** in the form of a 10mg/24h pessary or vaginal gel 1–3mg 6-hourly. The fetus should be monitored on CTG prior to prostaglandin use, and for 30min post insertion. PGE2 may stimulate uterine contractions or precipitate labour. Failed induction prompts reassessment of the cervix by someone senior. If rupture of membranes is not possible, induction can be reconsidered 48 hours later or LSCS offered.

After artificial or spontaneous rupture of membranes (amniotomy), start intrapartum fetal heart rate monitoring using CTG (p. 46). If the liquor is clear, allow the woman to mobilize for 2–4 hours to allow spontaneous contractions to start. If she is not contracting after this time, start **oxytocin** IV in 0.9% saline using a pump system (eg Ivac®). Infusions start at 1–4 milliunits (MU) per min, increasing every 30min until 4 contractions occur every 10min (usually at a rate of 4–10MU/min: occasionally 20MU/min may be needed).

Monitor the fetal heart and stop if fetal distress or uterine hyperstimulation (>5 contractions in 10min with fetal compromise). Beware using large volumes of IV fluid (if >4 litres, there is risk of water intoxication—ie confusion, seizures, and coma). Use standard strength solutions as per *BNF*. Induction of labour in a woman with a previous caesarean section is controversial and senior advice should be sought due to the increased risk of scar rupture with prostaglandins and oxytocin infusions. **Misoprostol** (a prostaglandin E1 analogue) PO or PV is as effective at cervical ripening and inducing labour as PGE2 and oxytocin. Oral route (eg 50mcg 4-hourly) has fewer problems with uterine hyperstimulation.[45] NICE says to only use this for labour induction after intrauterine death.[43]

Problems with induction • Failed induction (15%) • Uterine hyperstimulation (1–5%) • Iatrogenic prematurity • Infection • Bleeding (vasa praevia) • Cord prolapse (eg with a high head at amniotomy) • Caesarean section (22%) and instrumental delivery rates (15%) are higher • Uterine rupture (rare).

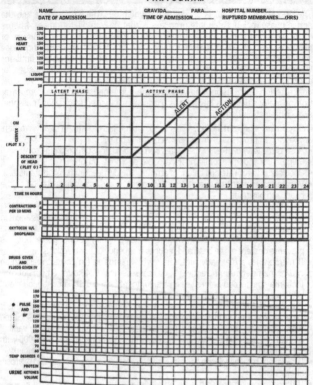

Fig 1.17 Example of a partogram. It has a steep x/y gradient of ratio 1:1. Less steep ratios (eg 2:1) may predispose to premature intervention, as does inclusion of the 'latent' phase on the partogram.

Reproduced from Collins *et al. Oxford Handbook of Obstetrics and Gynaecology* (2013) with permission from OUP.

The first stage of labour is divided into two stages: the latent phase and the active phase (p. 58). Adequate progress is that of 2cm dilatation per 4 hours of active labour (also see partogram, fig 1.17). However, other markers of progress are descent of the head and effacement of the cervix and these should also be taken into consideration. There is no absolute time limit for labour and progress is assessed dynamically throughout. The causes of poor progress are described according to *power, passenger, and passage*; poor uterine contractions (power) are the commonest cause; malpresentation or malposition or a large fetus (passenger); inadequate pelvis (passage) or a combination thereof.

Delay in 1st stage of labour This is <2cm/h dilatation in 4h in any woman; or slowing in progress in 2nd or subsequent labours.
- *Assess the woman:* Review her notes and obstetric/past obstetric history.
- Palpate her abdomen for lie, head palpable, and contractions.
- Check fetal heart rate and colour of amniotic fluid (meconium, blood stained).
- Vaginal assessment of dilatation, effacement, caput, moulding, station of the head, and position.
- Does she need analgesia and rehydration?
- *Management:* Offer artificial rupture of membranes (ARM) and reassessment in 2 hours. Empty the bladder if she is unable to do so due to compression of the head: a full bladder is not only at greater risk of injury during labour, but also prevents descent of the head and reduces frequency of contractions.
- If membranes are already ruptured, oxytocin infusion (to correct malposition and/or inefficient uterine activity) and reassessment in 4 hours. 8 hours of oxytocin may be needed before seeing a significant change. Start continuous fetal heart rate monitoring with oxytocin infusion.
- If the woman is multiparous or has had a previous LSCS, get senior advice; this is because oxytocin use in a multiparous uterus with no previous LSCS is associated with increased rates of rupture. Oxytocin use in a woman attempting vaginal birth after caesarean section also increases uterine rupture (from 50:10,000 with spontaneous labour to 8:1000 with oxytocin and 24:1000 with prostaglandin).
- If there are fetal heart rate concerns, perform FBS prior to commencing oxytocin augmentation.
- If there is slow progress after the above-listed steps, consider LSCS.
- Offer epidural before starting oxytocin; also change maternal position to upright or left lateral if she is lying flat on her back!

Delay in 2nd stage of labour The active 2nd stage starts when the woman starts pushing. There is delay in a primip if delivery is not imminent after 2 hours of active pushing. If delivery not imminent at this point, she requires obstetric review for consideration of instrumental delivery or LSCS. A multiparous woman requires review after 1 hour of active pushing for consideration of instrumental delivery or LSCS.

Causes of delay are as for delay in the first stage, but also maternal exhaustion. For instrumental delivery, see pp. 72–3.

Delay in 3rd stage of labour Retained placenta, see p. 71.

Further reading

NICE (2014). *Intrapartum Care for Healthy Women and Babies* (CG190). London: NICE.

Pregnant women in the UK have a choice of giving birth at home, in midwifery-led units (MLU), or in a hospital. For those women wanting a home or MLU birth, they must have a low-risk pregnancy. Those women with risk factors are safer having a hospital delivery. Overall, home birth now accounts for ~2% of births in the UK, compared with 80% in the 1930s, but this varies significantly by area.

Reasons to choose a home birth
- Own home where the woman is more likely to feel relaxed.
- Fear of hospitals.
- Continuity of care with a named midwife (labour wards are not staffed with community midwives as a rule, whereas her community midwife would be on call for her as part of a team).
- Support from family members (hospitals limit the number of people allowed to be in the labour room and/or present for delivery).
- Previous home birth.
- Previous bad experience in a hospital setting or with a hospital delivery.
- To avoid intervention.

If a woman is booked for a home birth
- 29% change to consultant-led care (eg she develops a risk factor such as hypertension, or the baby is SGA).
- 30% of nulliparous woman and 15% of multiparous women transfer to hospital in labour, mostly for slow progress or pain relief.
- Should there be an acute complication such as fetal hypoxia or maternal haemorrhage, the delay caused by transfer to hospital could lead to a worse outcome.
- Neonatal resuscitation facilities are more limited at home.
- Overall, perinatal mortality is slightly increased.
- Maternal mortality is the same.
- Obstetric intervention is lower, even in women transferred to hospital (but remember they are low risk and so at lower risk of intervention to start with).
- Apgar scores are higher with fewer neonatal respiratory problems.

Other things to consider include that the home environment is clean and that there is easy access for an ambulance. Midwives at a home delivery usually work as a pair, especially during the second stage.

►Pain relief in labour is our greatest gift to womankind; labour is painful, especially if it has been induced or is being augmented with oxytocin. In the antenatal period, educating women on what to expect in labour, and the options for pain relief, help to reduce fear. The ideal analgesia must be harmless to mother and baby, must allow good maternal cooperation, and must not affect uterine contractility or maternal mobility.

Non-pharmacological methods

Education about labour reduces fear; breathing exercises and relaxation techniques teach the mother ways to cope with pain herself. The presence of a supportive *birth partner* reduces the need for pain relief as well as intervention. *Acupuncture, homeopathy, and hypnosis* may be helpful, but are not offered by the NHS. *Transcutaneous electrical nerve stimulation (TENS)* is safe and useful especially in shorter labours, and postpones use of stronger analgesia. NICE does not recommend its use in established labour. A TENS machine is a small, battery-operated device that connects to electrodes, which attach to the skin via self-adhesive pads. *Water birth* as labouring in water has been shown to reduce the need for regional anaesthesia. It is recommended by NICE with the advice that water temperature be checked hourly and kept <37.5°c to prevent maternal pyrexia. However, it is usually not possible for a high-risk woman on continuous monitoring to labour in water due to technical difficulties with CTG equipment underwater. Newer machines have waterproof attachments or remote monitoring facilities; not every room on a labour ward has a birthing pool.

Pharmacological methods

Nitrous oxide: (50% in O_2 = Entonox®.) Can be inhaled throughout labour and is self-administered using a demand valve. CI: pneumothorax. It has a short onset of action and half-life, but SE include nausea, vomiting, and feeling faint.

Opiate analgesia: Should be available in all birth settings eg pethidine and diamorphine. They can provide limited pain relief during labour but may have significant SE for both mother (drowsiness, nausea, vomiting) and baby (short-term respiratory depression, and drowsiness which may last several days). They may also interfere with breastfeeding, and if given intramuscularly or intravenously should be given with an antiemetic. Narcotic analgesia is a contraindication to entering the birthing pool within 2 hours of administration. **Pethidine** 50–150mg IM given with **cyclizine** 50mg IM is most commonly used. If regional anaesthesia is contraindicated (sepsis, low platelets, recent LMWH), consider setting up a PCA eg remifentanil, which is rapidly metabolized and unable to cross the placenta—get anaesthetic advice.

Pudendal nerve block: (Sacral nerve roots 2, 3, and 4.) Uses 8–10mL of 1% lidocaine injected 1cm beyond a point just below and medial to the ischial spine on each side. It is used with perineal infiltration for instrumental delivery, but analgesia is insufficient for rotational forceps.

Local anaesthetic (lidocaine): This is infiltrated into the perineum and used before episiotomy at the time of delivery, and before suturing vaginal tears.

Regional anaesthesia

Epidural analgesia: (fig 1.18) See also pp. 680–1. Pain relief is by anaesthetizing pain fibres carried by T10–S5. The woman should be fully consented before regional anaesthesia is given due to the small complication rate. Epidurals are safe and offer effective analgesia. There is reduced maternal catecholamine secretion. Epidurals can be regularly topped up (a catheter is left in the epidural space) and can help lower BP in pre-eclampsia. *Complications* include failure to site, patchy block, hypotension, dural puncture (<1:100) and post-dural puncture headache, transient or permanent nerve damage (extremely rare), and increased risk of operative vaginal delivery. Before siting an epidural, check platelet count is >75×10⁹, insert wide-bore IV access, and gain consent. It can be inserted with the woman sitting or lying on her side. Full aseptic technique must be followed and L3/4 space is usually used. Once the epidural has been inserted, monitor BP every 5min for 20min, and record block height and density. Continuous electronic fetal monitoring is required. It is not uncommon to see a fetal bradycardia following epidural insertion due to maternal hypotension. Give IV fluids—it almost always recovers. Top-ups are required ~2-hourly (unless it is patient-controlled epidural anaesthesia (PCEA)). Recall anaesthetist if inadequate pain relief within 30min. If the epidural is used for LSCS, remember that the block will take longer to establish compared with spinal.

Epidurals, spinals, and LMWH: Wait 12h after heparin dose before inserting block or removing catheter (24h if on therapeutic rather than prophylactic dose of heparin). Wait at least 4h after block siting before next dose of LMWH.

Combined spinal epidural (CSE) anaesthesia: Gives quicker pain relief, with the option of prolonging the anaesthesia with the epidural. CSE is sometimes used to cover a caesarean section with the potential to take more time than usual eg placenta praevia, or previous difficult surgery.

Spinal anaesthesia: (fig 1.18) Used for most LSCS performed in the UK. They are relatively easier to insert than epidurals, produce a reliably dense block, but because they are a single injection, may wear off if the procedure is prolonged (>2h) and can cause more profound hypotension compared with epidural.

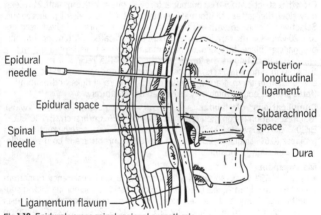

Epidural needle

Posterior longitudinal ligament

Epidural space

Subarachnoid space

Spinal needle

Dura

Ligamentum flavum

Fig 1.18 Epidural versus spinal regional anaesthesia.
Reproduced from Allman *et al. Oxford Handbook of Anaesthesia* (2011) with permission from OUP.

Further reading
NICE (2014) *Intrapartum Care for healthy women and babies* (CG190). London: NICE.

Incidence[UK] Twins: 3:200 pregnancies; triplets: 1:5000.

Predisposing factors Previous twins; FH of twins (dizygotic only—these women are 'superovulators'); ↑ maternal age (<20yrs 6.4:1000, >25yrs 16.8:1000); induced ovulation and IVF (1% of all UK pregnancies of which 25% are ≥twins); race origin (1:150 pregnancies for Japanese, 1:23 in Nigerian Yoruba women). The worldwide rate for monozygotic (of which 75% monochorionic ie shared placenta) twins is constant at ~4:1000. *Features* Early pregnancy: uterus large for dates; hyperemesis. Later there may be polyhydramnios. The signs are: >2 poles felt; a multiplicity of fetal parts felt; 2 fetal heart rates heard (reliable if rates differ by >10 beats/min). US confirms diagnosis (at 11[+0]–13[+6] weeks distinguishes monochorionic from dichorionic twins by placental masses, lambda sign in dichorionic).

Complications during pregnancy • Polyhydramnios • Pre-eclampsia (10% in singleton pregnancies; 30% in twins) • Anaemia commoner (iron and folate requirements ↑) • APH incidence rises (6% for twins vs 4.7% for singletons) from both abruption and placenta praevia (large placenta) • Gestational diabetes • Operative delivery.

Fetal complications Perinatal mortality ↑ (8:1000 singletons; 36.7:1000 for twins; 73:1000 for triplets; 204:1000 for higher multiples). The main problem is prematurity. Mean gestation for twins is 37 weeks, for triplets 33 weeks. Growth restriction (p. 54) is commoner (growth rate=singletons until 24 weeks, may slow thereafter). Malformation rates ↑ ×2–4, especially if monozygotic. Selective feticide (eg with intracardiac potassium chloride)[1] is best used before 20 weeks in the rare instances where it is indicated. With monochorionic pregnancies, placental vascular anastomoses may result in disparate twin size and one twin acting as the 'donor' and the other the 'recipient' ie twin–twin transfusion syndrome (TTTS).[1] Placental anastomoses can be ablated by laser coagulation *in utero*. Rarely, a fetus dying *in utero* shrinks and mummifies (fetus papyraceus) which may be delivered prematurely.

Complications of labour PPH (4–6% in singletons, 10% in twins). Malpresentation is common (cephalic (Ce)/Ce 40%, Ce/breech (Br) 40%, Br/Br 10%, Ce/transverse (Tr) 5%, Br/Tr 4%, Tr/Tr 1%). Vasa praevia rupture; cord prolapse (0.6% singleton, 2.3% twins); placental abruption and cord entanglement (especially monoamniotic).

Management
- US at 11[+0]–13[+6] weeks for viability, chorionicity, nuchal translucency, malformation: monthly from 20wks (2-weekly if monochorionic: membrane folding suggests TTTS). Name twins eg left, right. Discordant growth of ≥25% (suggests TTTS) indicates tertiary centre referral. Check FBC at 20–24 weeks. Give aspirin >12wks if other risks for pre-eclampsia.
- High-risk pregnancy—for consultant-led care.
- More antenatal visits eg weekly from 30 weeks (risk of pre-eclampsia ↑).
- Tell the mother how to identify preterm labour, and what to do.
- Offer elective birth at 37[+0] wks for uncomplicated dichorionic twins; at 36[+0] wks (+steroids p. 53), for uncomplicated monochorionic twins; at 35[+0] weeks (+steroids) for uncomplicated triplets. Use IV access in labour and anaesthetist availability at delivery. Have paediatricians (1 per baby) present at delivery in case resuscitation needed (2nd twins have a higher risk of asphyxia). Most women spontaneously deliver before these dates.
- Postnatal support groups for multiple pregnancy eg for breastfeeding.

Terminology *Monochorionic* twins or triplets share the placenta. If *monoamniotic* they share one amniotic sac; if diamniotic there are 2 sacs, triamniotic, there are 3. One placenta risks fetofetal transfusion, 1 sac risks entanglements.

IVF babies, and psychological consequence of triplets

With >4 million IVF babies born worldwide since 1978, it is apparent that there are increased problems for pregnancy and offspring, not merely those of multiple pregnancy.[47] These are:

- Multiple birth: affects 1 in 4 IVF pregnancies. Monozygotic twins are also commoner. The rate of triplets was 5× pre-IVF rates by 1998 but are now only twice, as only 2 embryos are implanted into women <40 years old. Meta-analysis shows that 1 fresh embryo transfer with a frozen embryo months later if unsuccessful gives as good results as 2-embryo transfer.[48]
- Older mother effects: so more pre-eclampsia, pregnancy-induced hypertension, caesarean section delivery, and diabetes in the mothers (all of which have implications for offspring).
- Donor egg problems: pregnancy-induced hypertension is 7.1 times more common if nulliparous women receive donated eggs than for standard IVF.
- Genetic defects: Beckwith–Wiedemann syndrome is 6 times commoner in IVF babies and there is concern that intracytoplasmic sperm injection (ICSI) techniques could encourage chromosomal abnormalities or CF in offspring of men with azoospermia or oligospermia. Men with low sperm counts are now screened for CF carrier status and chromosomal abnormalities before referral for ICSI.
- Low birthweight is 1.75 times commoner for singleton IVF babies compared to naturally conceived babies (and very low birthweight 2.7–3 times commoner). Part of this is due to prematurity, part to growth restriction. Interestingly low birthweight is particularly correlated to the number of gestation sacs at earliest scan, even if a baby ends up as a singleton. IVF twins are less commonly low birthweight compared to naturally conceived twins. There is also some evidence to suggest a slightly higher rate of stillbirth.
- Vasa praevia (p. 8) rates increased, possibly up to 1:300.[49]
- Prematurity is twice as common in IVF singleton babies compared to those naturally conceived, 3 times more common for prematurity <32 weeks. Again it is commoner if there was originally >1 gestation sac. There is less difference between IVF and naturally conceived twins.
- Perinatal mortality is ↑60% in IVF conceived singletons (but natural conception after delay ↑ mortality ×3 compared to quick conception).
- Abnormality rates are slightly increased (in singletons too).

Bringing up one child is difficult: twins are often very very difficult—but triplets are more than very very very difficult—and are frequently a source of significant psychopathology. Even 4 years after their birth, all mothers in one triplets study[50] suffered from exhaustion and emotional distress. One-third of mothers had sufficient depression to require psychotropic medication, and one-third spontaneously expressed regrets about having triplets. If triplets are reduced to twins *in utero*, subsequently one-third of mothers will suffer emotional problems (persistent sadness and guilt) up to 1 year. However, adjustment had occurred in ~90% by 2 years after birth.[51]

Legislation in most developed countries is trying to limit the numbers of embryos that may be implanted at IVF in order to reduce higher-order pregnancies (already there has been a reduction by 25% since 1998). The UK current practice is moving to single embryo transfer in mothers <35yrs.

1 In monochorionic twins, total cord coagulation is required to avoid haemorrhage from the co-twin into the dying fetus. Potassium is CI (could pass to other twin).[71] Ethical and legal considerations are complex.

Breech presentation The commonest malpresentation: 40% of babies are breech at 20 weeks, 20% at 28 weeks, but only 3% at term. In pregnancy, it is normal for the buttocks to come to lie in the fundus.

Causes and associations: • Idiopathic • Uterine abnormalities eg bicornuate uterus, fibroids • Prematurity • Placenta praevia • Oligohydramnios • Fetal abnormalities eg hydrocephalus. US may show the cause and influence the management.

Extended breech presentation is commonest (70%)—hips flexed but knees extended. *Flexed breeches* (15%) sit with hips and knees both flexed so that the presenting part is a mixture of buttocks, external genitalia, and feet. *Footling breeches* (15%) have the greatest risk of cord prolapse (5–20%).

Diagnosis of breech presentation Try to diagnose antenatally, but 30% present undiagnosed in labour. The mother may complain of pain under the ribs. On palpation the lie is longitudinal, no head is felt in the pelvis, and in the fundus there is a smooth round mass (the head) which can be balloted, a sensation akin to quickly sinking an apple in water. Ultimately the diagnosis is made by US, or if the woman is labouring, feeling the breech vaginally.

External cephalic version (ECV) Turning the breech by manoeuvring it through a (usually forward) somersault. Turn the baby only if vaginal delivery planned, after 36–37 weeks. Success rate 40% primips, 60% multips.[RCOG] *ECV contraindications:* • Placenta praevia • Multiple pregnancy (except delivery of 2nd twin) • APH in last 7 days • Ruptured membranes • Growth-restricted babies • Abnormal CTG • Mothers with uterine scars, uterine abnormality • Fetal abnormality • Pre-eclampsia, or hypertension (risk of abruption is increased). Monitor CTG (p. 46). Give anti-D (500U) to Rh–ve patients (see p. 11). Emergency caesarean rate after ECV is 1:200.

Mode of delivery The risk of fetal hypoxia and birth trauma is increased with vaginal delivery but is very dependent on the experience of birth attendants. Neonatal morbidity and mortality are increased irrespective of mode of delivery, possibly due to higher risk of congenital abnormalities and preterm babies being breech. Planned caesarean section may provide better outcome for the fetus and evidence suggests that the neonate is less likely to go to SCBU (but no difference at 2 years of age). Most breeches are delivered by LSCS and as a result, there is less experience with vaginal breech delivery. Evidence is less clear for preterm singletons and twins. (RCOG recommends caesarean if 1st twin breech; vaginal delivery if 2nd twin breech.) If vaginal delivery occurs, attendants experienced at breech delivery should be present. Contraindications to vaginal breech include inexperienced clinician, footling or kneeling breech, estimated fetal weight >3800 or <2000g, previous LSCS, and hyperextended fetal neck.

Vaginal breech delivery The most important thing is to call for help from an experienced midwife or obstetrician. You will see them approach with a 'hands-off' technique: the baby is not touched until the scapulae are visible. The baby is encouraged to remain so that the spine is anterior. The body may need to be rotated in each direction to allow delivery of the arms. Once the nape of the neck is visible, place two fingers of the right hand over the maxilla, and two fingers from the left hand over the occiput to flex the head (Mauriceau–Smellie–Veit manoeuvre). Suprapubic pressure from an assistant can also help. If this fails, forceps are used to deliver the head. A neonatal doctor should be present for a vaginal breech delivery because the most difficult and risky part is delivery of the head, and once the baby has delivered to the umbilicus, the cord is compressed and blood flow to the fetus interrupted. ►Check baby for hip dislocation at birth and by US at 6 weeks (↑ incidence): also, if vaginal delivery, for Klumpke's paralysis (p. 556) and signs of CNS injury.

Occipitoposterior position (OP) In 50% of patients the mothers have a long 'anthropoid' pelvis. Diagnosis may be made antenatally by palpation (p. 4). On vaginal examination the posterior fontanelle will be found to lie in the posterior quadrant of the pelvis. Labour tends to be prolonged because of the degree of rotation needed, so adequate hydration and analgesia (consider epidural) are important. During labour, 65% rotate 130° so that the head is occipitoanterior at the time of birth, 20% rotate to the transverse and then arrest ('deep transverse arrest'), 15% rotate so that the occiput lies truly posterior and birth is by flexion of the head from the perineum. Although in 73% delivery will be a normal vaginal delivery, 22% will require forceps and 5% a caesarean section.

Face presentation (fig 1.19b) Incidence 1:600–1:1500. 15% are due to congenital abnormality such as anencephaly, tumour of or shortened fetal neck muscles. Most occur by chance as the head extends rather than flexes as it engages. On early vaginal examination, the nose and eyes may be felt but later this will not be possible because of oedema. Most engage in the transverse (mentobregmatic diameter ≈9.5cm). 90% rotate so that the chin lies behind the symphysis (mentoanterior) and the head can be born by flexion. If the chin rotates to the sacrum (mentoposterior), caesarean section is indicated. Ventouse is contraindicated but forceps delivery is possible if the head is well below the spines.

Brow presentation (fig 1.19a) This occurs in 1:1000–1:3500 deliveries. The head is between full flexion and full extension, and may revert to either. If it persists, vaginal delivery is not possible. Most of the time, it is diagnosed in advanced labour. On vaginal examination the anterior fontanelle and supra-orbital ridges may be felt. Management is expectant; if progress is slow or brow presentation persists, delivery by LSCS is indicated.

Transverse lie (compound shoulder presentation) Antenatal diagnosis: ovoid uterus wider at the sides, the lower pole is empty, the head lies in one flank, the fetal heart is heard in variable positions. On vaginal examination with membranes intact, no distinguishing features may be felt, but if ruptured and the cervix dilated, ribs, shoulder, or a prolapsed hand or cord may be felt. The risk of cord prolapse is high. If malpresentation persists or ECV at 37 weeks fails, caesarean section will be necessary. Those with persistent instability of lie need hospital admission from 37 weeks (to prevent cord prolapse at home when the membranes rupture) and decision as to elective caesarean section.

Typical causes
• Multiparity
• Multiple pregnancy
• Polyhydramnios
• Placenta praevia
• Arcuate/septate uterus
• Contracted pelvis

(a)   (b)

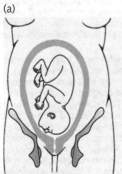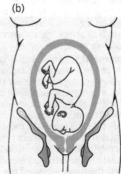

Fig 1.19 (a) Brow presentation; (b) face presentation.
Reproduced from Collins *et al. Oxford Handbook of Obstetrics and Gynaecology* (2013) with permission from OUP.

In late pregnancy, it is normal for some babies to pass meconium (bowel contents), which stains the amniotic fluid a dull green. This is not significant. During labour, fresh meconium, which is dark green, sticky, and lumpy, may be passed. This may be a response to the stress of a normal labour, or a sign of distress, so transfer to a consultant-led unit and commence continuous fetal heart rate monitoring (p. 46). Prelabour rupture of membranes with meconium-stained liquor requires immediate induction of labour in an obstetric-led unit with advanced neonatal life support available.

Aspiration of fresh meconium can cause severe pneumonitis (meconium aspiration syndrome) and occurs in 1:1000 deliveries. Routine suction of nasopharynx and oropharynx prior to birth is not recommended. Only suction airway if there is thick meconium in oropharynx and the baby requires resuscitation. Have a healthcare professional trained in advanced neonatal support in attendance to suck out pharynx and trachea under direct vision using a laryngoscope if the baby has depressed vital signs. Observe babies for 12 hours.

Reduced fetal movements

Movements should first be apparent to the mother at between 18 and 20 weeks' gestation, increasing in strength and frequency until about 32 weeks, and then staying in a pattern particular to that fetus until delivery. Any reduction in fetal movements is potentially an important clinical sign of impending fetal demise—55% of women who have had a stillbirth experienced reduced fetal movements (RFM) prior to diagnosis. When a woman reports RFM it should be taken seriously—an inappropriate response by UK and Norwegian clinicians was found to be a contributory factor in stillbirth.[13]

What is normal? There is no universally agreed definition of RFM, but most women are aware of fetal movements (FM) by 20 weeks' gestation. Movements tend to plateau by 32 weeks; after this there is no reduction in frequency (a common misconception is a 'quiet baby' awaiting the onset of labour—this should alert the woman, her friends and family to urge her to seek urgent midwifery and/or obstetric review). Perception of FM may be influenced by being busy (the woman should try sitting in a quiet room), an anterior placenta prior to 28 weeks, and a fetus whose back is laying anteriorly. Cigarette smoking, administration of corticosteroids to promote fetal lung maturity, and sedating drugs may reduce fetal activity but evidence is unconvincing.

Assessment of fetal movements This is primarily by the mother's own perception of them and if she feels they are reduced after 28 weeks, she should contact her local maternity unit and be assessed that same day. If unsure regarding FM, the woman should lie in the left lateral position and focus on FM for 2 hours. If 10 or more movements are not felt in that time, she should contact her local maternity unit immediately.

Management The initial goal is to exclude fetal death. After this, the woman should be risk assessed for factors associated with adverse pregnancy outcome. Firstly, take a history: key risk factors are fetal growth restriction, the SGA fetus (p. 54), placental insufficiency, and congenital malformations. If no risk factors are present, FM are normal and the fetal heart has been heard, no further intervention is required. However, if FM still reduced and/or risk factors identified, a CTG is required if the woman is >28+0 weeks' gestation. If the CTG is normal, and FM still reduced, or risk factors present, refer for fetal growth scan and amniotic fluid volume within 24 hours. This approach has been shown to reduce the incidence of stillbirth in Norway. In recurrent RFM, senior review is advised; there is an increased risk of poor perinatal outcome in these women and ultimately a decision needs to be taken regarding timing of delivery. In RFM after 40 weeks IOL is recommended.

The third stage of labour (p. 58) is considered delayed if not complete by 30min with active management, by 60min with physiological 3rd stage. A placenta not delivered by then will probably not be expelled spontaneously. The danger with retained placenta is haemorrhage. Associations: • Previous retained placenta or uterine surgery • Preterm delivery • Maternal age >35yrs • Placental weight <600g • Parity >5 • Induced labour • Pethidine used in labour.

Management If the placenta does not separate readily, avoid excessive cord traction—the cord may snap or the uterus invert. Check that the placenta is not in the vagina. Palpate the abdomen. Rub up a contraction, and encourage breastfeeding (stimulates oxytocin production). Give 20iu **oxytocin** in 20mL saline into umbilical vein and clamp the cord proximally to the injection site. Empty the bladder (a full bladder causes atony). If the placenta still does not deliver within further 30min, offer examination to see if manual removal is needed (delay may precipitate a PPH). Stop if examination is painful.⁵⁴ Insert iv access and take FBC and G&S. Take written consent. Transfer to theatre for regional anaesthesia (or epidural top-up) and manual removal of the placenta.

Manual removal (fig 1.20) With the mother in the lithotomy position, using aseptic technique, place 1 hand on the abdomen to stabilize the uterus. Insert the other hand through the cervix into the uterus. Following the cord assists finding the placenta. Gently work round the placenta, separating it from the uterus using the ulnar border of the hand. When separated it should be possible to remove it by cord traction. Check that it is complete. Give oxytocic drugs and 1 dose of antibiotic eg **cefuroxime** 1.5g and **metronidazole** 500mg iv.

Rarely, the placenta will not separate (placenta accreta)—call for senior help. A more experienced pair of hands can sometimes separate the placenta (also their fresh arm—because MROP can be physically demanding especially if the cervix tries to contract shut against the operator's forearm).

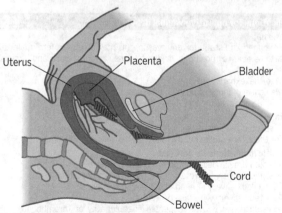

Fig 1.20 Manual removal of placenta.
Reproduced from Sarris *et al. Training in Obstetrics and Gynaecology* (2009) with permission from OUP.

1 Obstetrics

Operative vaginal delivery (the use of an instrument to aid delivery) occurs in 10–15% of births in the UK. A companion in labour, an upright or lateral position for delivery, and delay in pushing with epidural, reduce the need for operative deliveries. If an instrumental delivery is not possible or fails, LSCS in the 2nd stage of labour becomes the only method to deliver the baby, and this is associated with increased morbidity to the mother and fetus. Forceps and ventouse have different characteristics and uses, and the woman should be fully informed and verbally consented before undertaking this type of delivery. Only an experienced operator may undertake an instrumental delivery. The term 'trial' may be used and refers to a situation where the operator is uncertain if instrumental vaginal delivery will be successful. A trial therefore takes place in theatre where immediate LSCS can be carried out. This requires written consent, and failure is more likely if BMI >30, suspected large baby, OP position, and with a mid-cavity delivery (head at or 1cm below spines). 2nd-stage LSCS requires senior support.

Criteria for use

- Consent for and explain the procedure.
- 1/5th or less head palpable per abdomen (fig 1.21).
- Ruptured membranes.
- Adequate analgesia: epidural or pudendal block.
- Adequate contractions.
- Bladder empty and catheter balloon deflated.
- Fully dilated cervix with head at ischial spines or below.
- Check presentation (must be cephalic) and position of head.
- Check instrument ie forceps lock.
- Once instrument applied, recheck position and that no maternal tissues are caught.
- Neonatal doctor in attendance.

> ### Indications for operative vaginal delivery
>
> **Maternal**
> - Prolonged 2nd stage for any reason; this may be due to fetal malposition such as OP or OT positions, or due to dense epidural block and diminished urge to push.
> - Maternal exhaustion.
> - Medical avoidance of pushing eg severe cardiac disease.
> - Pushing not possible eg tetraplegia or paraplegia.
>
> **Fetal**
> - Suspected fetal distress.
> - For the after-coming head in a breech delivery.
>
> **Specific indications for forceps**
> - Assisted breech delivery, forceps to deliver head.
> - Assisted delivery of preterm infant <34 weeks' gestation.
> - Controlled delivery of head at caesarean section.
> - Assisted delivery with face presentation.
> - Assisted delivery with suspected coagulopathy or thrombocytopenia in fetus (but note coagulopathy is a relative CI to forceps).
> - Instrumental delivery where maternal condition precludes pushing (eg cardiac disease, respiratory disease).
> - Cord prolapse in second stage of labour.
> - Instrumental delivery under GA.
> - Presence of significant caput (fetal head swelling secondary to labour).
>
> ▶Abandon operative vaginal delivery if no progression with each pull and delivery not imminent with 3 pulls by experienced operator.

1 Obstetrics

Forceps

These consist of curved blades designed to fit around the fetal head, allowing traction to be applied via handles. They require much less maternal effort for successful delivery than ventouse and are therefore less likely to fail. There are several different type of forceps (see fig 1.23). Forceps may be safer for the baby, but can cause significant maternal genital tract trauma (and they add 1cm to the diameter of the head).

Low cavity forceps (eg Wrigley's) are used for 'lift out' deliveries, when the head is on the perineum. They have a short shank and are lighter in weight. They are sometimes used at LSCS to help control delivery of the head.

Mid-cavity non-rotational forceps (Neville-Barnes; Simpson) have a long shank, cephalic and pelvic curves, and must only be used when the sagittal suture lies in the AP diameter. The blades are placed one by one in-between contractions.

Mid-cavity rotational forceps (Kjelland) have a reduced pelvic curve, making them suitable for rotation (only in experienced hands).

Ventouse (vacuum extraction)

This technique uses a suction device to suck fetal scalp tissues into a ventouse cup. The artificial caput (swelling) created is called a chignon, and takes 24–48 hours to resolve (and is something the mother should be warned of). The baby must be >34 weeks' gestation with no maternal coagulopathy. Ventouse is associated with less genital tract trauma than forceps but is more likely to cause fetal trauma (cephalohaematoma and retinal haemorrhage) and more likely to fail. Like with forceps, there are different types of ventouse available (fig 1.24) including the metal cup, soft cup, and most commonly, the Kiwi® OmniCup (a single-use cup with hand pump).

See figs 1.23 & 1.24 on p. 75 for images.

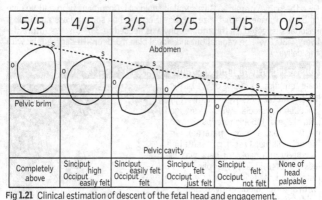

Fig 1.21 Clinical estimation of descent of the fetal head and engagement.

Reproduced from Collins *et al. Oxford Handbook of Obstetrics and Gynaecology* (2013) with permission from OUP.

1 Obstetrics

Complications of operative vaginal delivery
- Maternal genital tract trauma, especially with forceps; includes obstetric anal sphincter injury.
- Spiral vaginal tears with rotational forceps deliveries.
- Fetal injuries with forceps (rare):
  - Facial nerve palsy.
  - Skull fractures.
  - Orbital injury.
  - Intracranial haemorrhage.
- Fetal injuries with ventouse:
  - Cephalhaematoma (most common).
  - Retinal haemorrhage.
  - Scalp lacerations and scalp avulsions (more common if >3 pulls used).

▶The use of sequential instruments should be avoided where possible because the rate of complications is increased, hence the need for choosing the initial instrument wisely. Women in labour and in their birth plans frequently ask for forceps to be avoided—but a well-planned and straightforward forceps delivery is much better for both mother and baby than a failed ventouse followed by a forceps.

When to abandon an operative vaginal delivery
- No descent with each subsequent pull.
- Delivery not imminent after 3 pulls when the instrument is correctly applied and the operator is experienced.
- Proceeding to emergency LSCS: the head may be impacted in the pelvis and difficult to deliver.

After delivery
Give the baby vitamin κ. Give regular analgesia. Document time and volume of 1st void urine (catheterize for 12h if epidural or spinal). Pass catheter if residual suspected. Is thromboprophylaxis needed (p. 36)? Discuss future delivery; >80% will be vaginal but individual plan if 3rd- or 4th-degree tear with this delivery.

Obstetric brachial plexus injury (OBPI)

OBPI complicates <0.5% of live births.

Risk factors Large birthweight; shoulder dystocia with prolonged 2nd stage of labour; forceps delivery; vacuum extraction; maternal diabetes mellitus; breech presentation. Formerly, the cause of OBPI was excessive lateral traction applied to the fetal head at delivery, in association with anterior shoulder dystocia.

Instrumental-associated OBPI may arise because of nerve stretch injuries after rotations of >90° or from direct compression of the forceps blade in the fetal neck.[55] Not all cases of brachial plexus palsy are attributable to traction. Intrauterine factors may play some role.[56]

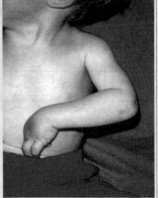

Management 10–20% need surgical intervention for optimal results.[57] Some injuries will be permanent.[58] See p. 556 for orthopaedic insights.

Fig 1.22 Brachial plexus injury.

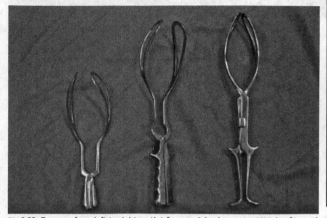

Fig 1.23 Forceps, from left to right: outlet forceps (also known as Wrigley forceps) for use during an outlet vaginal delivery or at cs; non-rotational forceps (Neville-Barnes or Simpson) for direct oa or op vaginal delivery and have a pelvic curve; and rotational forceps (Kjelland) which have no pelvic curve, to enable rotation without damaging maternal tissues. Rotational forceps also have a sliding lock mechanism.
Reproduced from Collins *et al. Oxford Handbook of Obstetrics and Gynaecology* (2013) with permission from OUP.

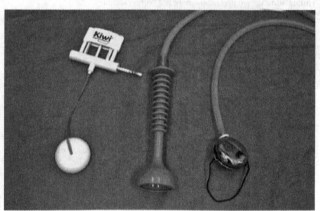

Fig 1.24 Ventouse, from left to right: the Kiwi®, a plastic hand-held device with a hand pump, commonly used in units around the uk. The silicone cup, which is attached to a separate suction pump and foot pedal, and the metal cup, which is again attached to a separate pump and foot pedal.
With permission of Clinical Innovations Europe Ltd, 2008, and Menox AB, Goteborg, Sweden, 2008.

This is the delivery of a fetus through an incision in the abdominal wall and uterus. In the UK, 24% of nulliparous women deliver by CS (<5% in a multip with no previous CS). Having a previous caesarean is the biggest predictor of having another (67% in the next pregnancy, mostly elective).

Maternal mortality ~1 per 100,000. Morbidity is higher with emergency operations—eg infection, ileus, and thromboembolism. For 1st operations 25% are due to failure to progress, 28% for fetal distress, 14% for breech. Use of support in labour, induction at 41 weeks, and consultant involvement in decision to section all help reduce the incidence of CS. 9:1000 will require ITU care.

Types of caesarean section

Lower uterine segment incision: Joel Cohen skin incision (straight incision 3cm above symphysis pubis) with blunt dissection thereafter is recommended (reduces blood loss). Transverse incision in the lower segment is associated with reduced adhesion formation, less blood loss, and lower risk of scar dehiscence in subsequent pregnancies. Fetal laceration rate is 1–2%.

Classical cs: (Vertical incision on uterus, with either transverse or vertical skin incision.) Rarely used. Indications: • Very premature fetus, lower segment poorly formed • Fetus lies transverse, with ruptured membranes • Structural abnormality makes lower segment use impossible • Fibroids positioned such that lower segment incision is not possible • Some anterior placenta praevias when lower segment abnormally vascular • Maternal cardiac arrest and rapid birth desired (but LSCS may be quicker if operator more experienced with this method). A classical CS is associated with more adhesion formation and infection, and is a contraindication to attempting vaginal delivery subsequently.

Indications Varied and many; here are some examples:
• Repeat CS.
• Fetal compromise such as fetal bradycardia, scalp pH <7.20, cord prolapse.
• Failure to progress in labour, or failed induction of labour.
• Malpresentation eg breech, transverse lie.
• Severe pre-eclampsia and induction of labour unlikely to be successful.
• IUGR with absent or reversed end-diastolic flow.
• Twin pregnancy with non-cephalic presenting twin.
• Placenta praevia.

Category of CS Determines the timing and is dependent on the indication. *Category 1* (crash) is for immediate threat to life of woman or fetus and the baby should be delivered within 30min of the decision being made; eg placental abruption, fetal bradycardia. *Category 2* is for maternal or fetal compromise, not immediately life-threatening (30–60min) eg failure to progress. *Category 3* is also thought of as semi-elective eg pre-eclampsia, or failed induction of labour, and *Category 4* is elective eg term singleton breech. Elective CS should be carried out after 39 weeks, unless maternal or fetal indications arise, to reduce the incidence of transient tachypnoea of the newborn. If elective delivery is planned for <39 weeks, corticosteroids should be considered for fetal lung maturity.

Complications These are most common with emergency CS (which itself may be considered by some to be a complication of failed vaginal delivery). *Intraoperative* complications include blood loss >1L (7–9%), uterine lacerations/extensions beyond the uterine incision, blood transfusion (2–3%), bladder laceration (0.5%), bowel injury (0.05%), ureteral injury (0.03–0.09%), and hysterectomy (0.2%). Haemorrhage is more likely with placenta praevia or abruption, extremes of birth weight, and maternal obesity.

Postoperative complications most commonly involve wound infections, endometritis, and UTI. Venous thromboembolism is more common and every woman with emergency CS should have 7 days of prophylactic LMWH. High BMI is independently associated with infection, along with chorioamnionitis, pre-eclampsia, and increased surgical blood loss. *Before undertaking any CS:* Check placental site to exclude praevia, and if previous LSCS, accreta, or percreta.

Before an emergency section ▶Explain to the mother what is to happen and take written consent. Most emergency CS happen under regional anaesthesia.

- Activate the anaesthetist, theatre staff, and paediatrician.
- Get senior help—in the daytime, senior obstetric staff should be present.
- If GA is planned, neutralize gastric contents with 20mL of 0.3 molar **sodium citrate**, and promote gastric emptying with **metoclopramide** 10mg IV. (NB: there is no time for H₂ agonists to work; **omeprazole** is kept for elective sections eg 40mg PO 2h before surgery.) The stomach should be routinely emptied prior to extubation to minimize risk of postoperative aspiration. See *Mendelson syndrome*, p. 95.
- Take blood for group and save and/or crossmatch eg 2u; if for abruption; if placenta praevia insert 2nd IV line and cross-match 6u.
- Take to theatre (awake); set up IVI.
- Catheterize the bladder before giving GA, or after regional anaesthesia. Tilt 15° to her left side on operating table.
- Ensure neonatologist is present before starting.
- Offer prophylactic antibiotics and give before skin incision.[19][NICE]

▶In reducing maternal mortality, the importance of having an experienced anaesthetist is vital. When appropriate, offer regional anaesthesia. Document indication for and urgency of operation. Note: in 2002–3 only 8% of caesarean sections were under GA.

Management of women already on thromboprophylaxis: If on high dose or 75% of weight-adjusted therapeutic dose prophylaxis (see p. 36), halve to same dose/24h as was previously being given/12h, on the day before planned CS.[46][RCOG] For all on prophylaxis, omit dose on morning of CS and give 3h postoperatively unless epidural used: see pp. 64–5. 2% of women will get a wound haematoma.

After CS Give one-to-one support in recovery unit.[59][NICE] Aim for baby/mother skin to skin contact (beware chilling baby). Check pulse, respiratory rate (RR), BP, and sedation levels at least half hourly for 1st 2h, then 4-hourly for 24h. Use MEOWS (modified early obstetric warning score chart). After epidural, remove urinary catheters when mobile or 12h after delivery (whichever is later). After GA, give extra midwife support to help establish breastfeeding. Mobilize early. Remove wound dressing at 5d. Give analgesia (ibuprofen + paracetamol with morphine for breakthrough pain). Average hospital stay is 2–3 days but mothers can be discharged after 24h if they wish and are well. Discuss reason for CS, birth options in future, and contraception.

Long-term effects of CS In subsequent pregnancies, there is a higher incidence of placenta praevia and accreta. The risk of uterine rupture is also increased to 1:200 with spontaneous labour (almost unheard of in nulliparous UK women). Risk of antepartum stillbirth in the next pregnancy doubles, and the cause is unclear. In those undergoing multiple CS, surgical risks increase with each subsequent CS.

1 Obstetrics

Stillbirths are those babies born dead after (but were alive at) 24 weeks completed gestation (see BOX 'Helping parents after stillbirth'). Rate: 1:200 total births. Death *in utero* can occur at any stage of pregnancy or labour. Delivery can be understandably emotionally very difficult for the mother, family, and attendant staff.

Some hours after a fetus has died *in utero* the skin begins to peel. At delivery such fetuses are described as *macerated*, as opposed to *fresh* stillbirths. If left, spontaneous labour usually occurs (80% within 2 weeks, 90% within 3 weeks). Coagulopathy (p. 99) occurs in 10% within 4 weeks of late IUD: 30% thereafter.

Causes of stillbirth (CMACE 2009.) No cause found (28%), placental cause (12%), ante- or intrapartum haemorrhage (11%), major congenital anomaly (9%), infection (5%), hypertension in pregnancy (6%), maternal disease (renal, diabetes 5%), IUGR (7%), mechanical eg cord prolapse, knot in cord (8%). Multiple pregnancy ↑ risk (16.6:1000). Social deprivation, increasing maternal age, smoking, previous CS, IVF, and obesity increase incidence.

Diagnosis The mother may report absent or reduced fetal movements. No fetal heart sounds on handheld Doppler (unreliable). Diagnose by absent fetal heart beat on US by 2 different practitioners. It may help the mother to see lack of heart beat. Mothers sometimes feel passive movements after death. Repeat US, if mother requests. If mother alone at diagnosis; offer to call a companion.

Management ▶If mother Rh−ve give anti-D (see BOX 'Using anti-D Immunoglobulin', p. 11). Do Kleihauer on *all* women to diagnose fetomaternal haemorrhage (FMH)—a cause of stillbirth; and to determine anti-D dose. If large FMH diagnosed; repeat Kleihauer at 48h to check fetal cells cleared. Check maternal T°, BP, urine for protein, and blood clotting screen if fetus not thought recently demised. Advise delivery if pre-eclampsia, abruption, sepsis, coagulopathy, or membrane rupture. If safe, the mother may want to go home after diagnosis to reflect, collect things, and make arrangements. If not induced in 48h check for coagulopathy twice weekly. Labour is induced using mifepristone orally, adding prostaglandin vaginally. Oxytocin augmentation may be needed later. If uterine scar, seek consultant advice re induction/augmentation. Deliver away from sounds of babies, if possible.

Ensure good pain relief in labour (if epidural, check clotting tests all normal and no sepsis). Do not leave the mother unattended. When the baby is born, wrap it (as with any other baby) and offer to the mother to see and to hold—if she wishes. Photographs should be taken for her to take home, a lock of the baby's hair and palm-print given (keep in notes for later if not wanted). Unseen babies can be difficult to grieve for. Naming the baby and holding a funeral service may help with grief. Remember thromboprophylaxis if needed (p. 36). Discuss lactation suppression and contraception.

Tests to establish cause *Maternal tests:* Kleihauer (see earlier); FBC, CRP, LFT, TFT, HbA1c, glucose, blood culture, viral screen (TORCH (Toxoplasmosis, Other, Rubella, CMV, Herpes) etc. screen), thrombophilia screen, antibodies (anti-red cell, anti-Ro, anti-La, alloimmune antiplatelet, if indicated♀☉), MSU, urine for cocaine (if indicated and permission given), cervical swabs.♀☉

Fetal tests: Fetal and placental swabs. Cord blood in lithium heparin tube for infection. Thorough examination of the baby. Take time to talk to parents about how helpful a postmortem may be to them, in understanding what happened, and planning further pregnancies. If postmortem is refused, MRI (may miss significant pathology and is not routinely available), cytogenetics (use fetal skin, cartilage, and placenta, this can also be used for sexing babies which may be difficult in macerated and very premature stillbirths) ± small volumes of tissue for metabolic studies, and placental histology may be acceptable but are less informative and still need written parental consent.

Helping parents after stillbirth

- Give parents a follow-up appointment to discuss causes found by the tests described on p. 78. Consider a home visit if parents prefer. Refer for genetic counselling if appropriate.
- In England, a *Certificate of Stillbirth* is required (issued by obstetrician or midwife attending birth), that the mother or father is required to take to the Registrar of Births and Deaths within 42 days (21 days in Scotland, 5 days in Northern Ireland) of birth for fetuses born after 24 weeks' completed gestation. If there is developmental or us evidence that the fetus was not alive at 24 completed weeks' gestation (eg in cases of fetus papyraceous, or after selective fetal reduction before 24 weeks), then such a certificate is not issued,[61][RCOG] but evidence for the fact why the fetus is not believed to have been alive at 24 completed weeks should be written in the woman's notes. The father's name only appears in the register if the parents are married, or if both parents make the registration, or the father signs a Form of Declaration (available from Registrar). Registration can be delegated to a healthcare professional or hospital bereavement officer.
- The Registrar then issues a Certificate of Burial or Cremation which the parents then give to the undertaker (if they have chosen a private funeral—in which case they bear the cost of the funeral), or to the hospital administrators if they have chosen a hospital funeral—for which the hospital bears the cost. Parents are issued with a Certificate of Registration to keep which has the name of the stillborn baby (if named), the name of the informant who made the registration, and the date of stillbirth.
- uk hospitals are directed by the Department for Work and Pensions to offer 'hospital' funerals for stillborn babies (arranged through an undertaker). If the parents offer to pay for this, the hospital may accept. The hospital should notify the parents of the time of the funeral so that they may attend, if they wish. With hospital funerals a coffin is provided and burial is often in a multiple-occupancy grave in a part of the graveyard set aside for babies. The hospital should inform parents of the site of the grave. Graves are unmarked, so should the parents not attend the funeral and wish to visit later it is recommended that they contact the graveyard attendants for the grave to be temporarily marked. Parents may buy a single occupancy grave, if they wish, on which they can later erect a headstone. Hospitals can arrange cremations, but the parents pay for this. Tell parents that there may not be any ashes after cremation.
- Arrange a follow-up appointment with the obstetrician to discuss implications for future pregnancy, and the cause (if known) of the stillbirth. Give parents the address of a local branch of an organization for bereavement counselling eg SANDS.[62] Grief may take a long time to resolve and parents may find it difficult to contact ordinary medical staff.

Each maternity unit should have a specialist bereavement midwife to support the parents, and help guide them through the formalities, as well as ensuring they are aware of the resources and support available.

In the uk, statutory maternity pay and the maternity allowance and social fund maternity payments are payable after stillbirth.

After stillbirth Be vigilant to possible depression. In next pregnancy after stillbirth recommend obstetrician antenatal care and delivery, and screen for diabetes. If there was evidence of growth restriction, assess growth by serial us biometry in subsequent pregnancies.[60][RCOG]

1 Obstetrics

Further reading

RCOG (2010). *Late Intrauterine Fetal Death and Stillbirth* (Green-top Guideline No. 55). London: RCOG.
SANDS offers free support to anyone in the uk affected by the death of a baby (www.sands.org.uk).

Placental types

- *Velamentous insertion:* (1%.) Umbilical vessels travel within the membranes before placental insertion.
- *Placenta succenturia:* (5%.) There is a separate (succenturiate) lobe away from the main placenta which may fail to separate normally and cause a PPH or puerperal sepsis.
- *Vasa praevia:* Fetal vessels from velamentous insertion or between lobes (succenturia, or bilobe placenta) risk damage at membrane rupture causing fetal haemorrhage. Caesarean delivery is needed (urgent if fetal compromise at membrane rupture, elective if detected antenatally by US).
- *Placenta membranacea:* (1:3000.) A thin placenta surrounds the baby. Some is in the lower segment so predisposes to APH. It may fail to separate in the 3rd stage.
- *Placenta accreta:* There is abnormal (morbid) adherence of all or part of the placenta to the uterus, termed *placenta increta* if myometrium infiltrated, *placenta percreta* if penetration reaches the serosa. These 3 types predispose to PPH and there is an increased need for caesarean hysterectomy. Incidence ↑ with the number of previous caesarean sections. Diagnose prenatally (colour Doppler US/MRI).

Placenta praevia The placenta lies in the lower uterine segment. It is found in ~0.5% of pregnancies. Risks are of significant haemorrhage by mother and fetus. Avoid digital PV examinations (speculum examination is safe), and advise against penetrative intercourse.

Associations: Caesarean section; sharp curette TOP; multiparity; multiple pregnancy; mother >40 years; assisted conception; deficient endometrium–manual removal of placenta, D&C, fibroids, endometritis. US at <24 weeks' gestation shows a low-lying placenta in 28% but with lower segment development only 3% lie low at term. Transvaginal US is superior to transabdominal for localizing placentas accurately, especially when the placenta is posterior, and, if combined with 3D power Doppler/MRI, diagnoses vasa praevia and placenta accreta. It has not been shown to increase bleeding. Repeat US at 32wks if major praevia, 36wks if minor.

Major placenta praevia (placenta covering the internal os) requires caesarean section for delivery. Minor placenta praevia (placenta in lower segment but does not cross the internal os): aim for normal delivery unless the placenta encroaches within 2cm of the internal os (especially if posterior or thick). Presentation may be as APH (separation of the placenta as the lower segment stretches causes bleeding) or as abnormal fetal lie. Problems are with bleeding and with mode of delivery as the placenta obstructs the os and may shear off during labour, or may be accreta (5%), especially after a previous CS (>24%). Poor lower segment contractility predisposes to postpartum haemorrhage. Caesarean section should be consultant-performed or supervised with consultant anaesthetic attendance at 36–7wks after a single course of corticosteroids[18]NICE, at a hospital with blood bank and level 2 critical care beds.[RCOG]If there has been a history of vaginal bleeding, consider late preterm delivery at 34+0–36+6 weeks. Women undergoing CS should be made aware of the risk of hysterectomy to control haemorrhage if pharmacological and surgical haemostatic techniques fail.

Further reading

RCOG (2018). *Placenta praevia and placenta accreta: diagnosis and management.* (Green-top Guideline No. 27a). London: RCOG.

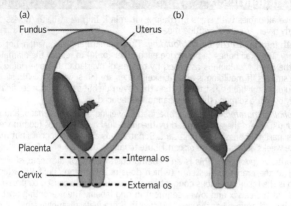

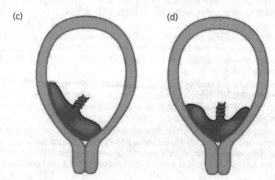

Fig 1.25 (a) Grade I placenta praevia, encroaches the lower segment but does not reach the os. (b) Grade II placenta praevia reaches the os but does not cover it. (c) Grade III placenta praevia partially covers the os and (d) Grade IV completely covers the os. Placenta praevia may also be classified minor (a and b) or major (c and d).

With permission from Angel RK Shere.

▶Give all babies with signs of trauma **vitamin k** 1mg IM at birth (unless already given as part of routine measures).

Birth injuries to the baby *Moulding:* This is a natural phenomenon, not an injury. The skull bones can override each other (p. 44) to reduce the diameter of the head. Moulding is assessed by degree of overlap of the overriding at the sutures. If moulding is absent, skull bones are felt separately. With slight moulding, the bones just touch, then they override but can be reduced; finally they override so much that they cannot be reduced.

Cephalhaematoma: This is a subperiostial swelling on the fetal head, and its boundaries are therefore limited by the individual bone margins (commonest over parietal bones). It is fluctuant. Spontaneous absorption occurs but may take weeks and may cause or contribute to jaundice.

Caput succedaneum: This is an oedematous swelling of the scalp, superficial to the cranial periosteum (which does not, therefore, limit its extent) and is the result of venous congestion and exuded serum caused by pressure against the cervix and lower segment during labour. The presenting part of the head therefore has the swelling over it. It gradually disappears in the first days after birth. When ventouse extraction is used in labour, a particularly large caput (called a chignon) is formed under the ventouse cup.

Erb's palsy: See fig 1.22, p. 74. This can result from shoulder dystocia (p. 94) (so ↑ ×10 in UK diabetic pregnancies)🔊.The baby's arm is flaccid and the hand is in the 'porter's tip' posture (p. 74). Exclude a fractured clavicle and arrange physiotherapy. Most resolve, but if it has not resolved by 6 months, it is unlikely to improve further.

Subaponeurotic haematoma: Blood lies between the aponeurosis and the periosteum. As haematoma is not confined to the boundaries of one bone, collections of blood may be large enough to result in anaemia or jaundice. They are associated with vacuum extractions.

Skull fractures: These are associated with difficult forceps delivery and may also occur after a difficult second-stage cs delivery where the head is impacted. They are commonest over parietal or frontal bones. If depressed fractures are associated with CNS signs, ask a neurosurgeon if the bone should be elevated.

Intracranial injuries: Intracranial haemorrhage is especially associated with difficult or fast labour, instrumental delivery, and breech delivery. Premature babies are especially vulnerable. Normally a degree of motility of intracranial contents is buffered by cerebrospinal fluid. Excessive moulding and sudden changes in pressure reduce this effect and are associated with trauma. In all cases of intracranial haemorrhage check babies' platelets. If low, check mother's blood for platelet alloantibodies (PLA1 system). Subsequent babies are at equal risk. IV maternal immunoglobulin treatment is being evaluated.

Anoxia may cause intraventricular haemorrhage (p. 306). Asphyxia causes intracerebral haemorrhage (often petechial) and may result in cerebral palsy. Extradural, subdural, and subarachnoid haemorrhages can all occur. Babies affected may have convulsions, apnoea, cyanosis, abnormal pallor, low heart rate, alterations in muscle tone, restlessness, somnolence, or abnormal movements. Treatment is supportive and expectant. See pp. 306-7.

Fetal laceration: Occurs in 1–2% of cs deliveries. It is more common with breech cs delivery and with cs after membrane rupture (the baby's skin may lie flush against the uterus). Most are superficial and heal without scarring but the parents should be warned of this risk when consent is taken for cs.

1 Obstetrics

Anal sphincter injury

Approximately 85% of vaginal deliveries are complicated by perineal trauma, and of these 60–70% will require suturing. The vast majority are 1st- and 2nd-degree tears (affecting perineal skin and/or muscles) but 3–4% will be 3rd- or 4th-degree injuries. A 3rd-degree tear is one affecting part or all of the anal sphincter muscle, and a 4th the anal mucosa (see p. 84). Primary repair of obstetric anal sphincter injuries (OASI) significantly reduces the risk of ongoing flatus and stool incontinence but doesn't alleviate it completely. Faecal incontinence is a source of misery, and requires expert attention.

Risk of mechanical injury is greatest after the first vaginal delivery. Traumatic stretching of the pudendal nerves occurs in >30% of primips, but is mostly asymptomatic, or mildly/transiently so. These patients are at ↑ risk in subsequent deliveries (cumulative pudendal nerve injury is well recognized). Other risk factors: • Baby >4kg • Persistent occipitoposterior position • Induced labour • Epidural • 2nd stage >1h • Midline episiotomy • Instrumental delivery (6–7% OASI in primip, 2.5% multip).

After repair, prescribe laxatives (eg **lactulose** 15mL OD or BD depending on stool softness) and antibiotics (**cefuroxime** 500mg PO/8h and **metronidazole** 400mg PO/8h for 7–10 days). Arrange follow-up at 6–12 weeks post delivery to check healing and continence. If flatus or faecal incontinence occurs, get expert help. Referral for specialist physiotherapy is essential, along with endoanal US. Whether symptomatic or not, there is an argument for elective CS delivery next time but the mother will need counselling. If asymptomatic, there is still an increased risk of repeat OASI. If symptomatic despite specialist help, the woman requires a secondary sphincter repair post delivery of any subsequent children—this fact will not be altered by offering elective CS. Elective caesarean may not protect against symptoms caused by pudendal nerve neuropathy.

Vesicovaginal fistula

This abnormal opening between bladder and vagina leading to urinary incontinence, a common sequel to obstructed labour, is thought to affect 3 million women worldwide,[65] now almost exclusively in developing countries.

Obstructed labour is particularly a problem for malnourished girls who become pregnant before full pelvic maturation. In obstructed labour, the pelvic head progressively compresses the soft tissues of vagina, bladder, and rectum against the pelvis causing ischaemic damage to these tissues and fetal asphyxiation. 2 days after the fetus dies it becomes macerated, softens, and can be vaginally expelled. A few days later, the mother passes sloughed ischaemic tissue leaving a fistula between bladder, urethra, and vagina or rectum and vagina (or both). Damaged tissues adjacent to the sloughed tissue heal poorly, often with fibrosis. Vagina and rectum may later stenose; chronic pyelonephritis and renal failure can ensue. Incontinent women are often shunned by family, divorced by their husbands, and stigmatized (especially in cultures where the affliction is believed to be punishment by a god).

Treatment is with continuous urinary drainage for 3 months if presenting with vesicovaginal fistula early (<3 months postpartum) or surgery if later. Operation is most successful for 1st operation and small defects (<2cm) with successful closure rates of up to 85% (but 16–32% of these women remain incontinent).

Good obstetric management of obstructed labour prevents fistulas. Early treatment can allow healing without recourse to surgery. Sadly it is those parts of the world where there is poor access to obstetric facilities where women develop fistulas and where the chance of having subsequent repair is also limited.

Further reading

Aliyu F *et al.* (2011). A patient's journey: living with obstetric fistula. *BMJ* 342:1360.

►Examine gently. Unless marked bleeding, allow the mother some bonding time with baby before examination and repair (but it should be completed within an hour of delivery; endorphins from delivery also help reduce pain).⁵⁴ₙᵢᴄᴇ

Perineal tears These are classified by the degree of damage caused. Risk factors for development are discussed in the box 'Birth injuries to the mother' on p. 83.

Labial tears Common; these heal quickly; suturing is required if both labia are torn to prevent them fusing together. These tears are particularly painful.

First-degree tears These tears are superficial and do not damage muscle. Suture unless skin edges are well apposed to aid healing.⁵⁴ₙᵢᴄᴇ

Second-degree tears These lacerations involve perineal muscle. Repair is similar to that of episiotomy (see later).

Third-degree tears Damage involves the anal sphincter muscle. Classification:

3a: External anal sphincter (circular fibres) thickness <50% torn.

3b: External anal sphincter thickness >50% torn.

3c: Both external and internal anal sphincters (longitudinal fibres) torn.

If anal/rectal mucosa also involved it is a *fourth-degree tear*. 3rd/4th-degree tears need repair by an experienced surgeon, under epidural or GA in theatre with intraoperative antibiotic cover. Rectal mucosa is repaired first using absorbable suture from above the tear's apex to the mucocutaneous junction. Muscle is interposed. Vaginal mucosa is then sutured. Internal anal sphincter is repaired with interrupted sutures. Overlap and repair severed ends of the external anal sphincter. Finally repair skin. Give antibiotic prophylaxis with 3rd- and 4th-degree tears. Advise high-fibre diet and laxatives, eg Laxido® 1 sachet 1–3 times daily, for 10 days to avoid constipation. Arrange pelvic floor physiotherapy and obstetric clinic follow-up at 6–12 weeks postnatally. If pain or incontinence refer to specialist gynaecologist or colorectal surgeon for endoanal US or manometry.

Episiotomy This is performed to enlarge the outlet eg to hasten birth of a distressed baby, for instrumental or breech delivery, and to try to prevent 3° tears (but anal tears are not reduced by more episiotomies in normal deliveries). Rates: 8% Holland, 12% England, 50% USA.

The tissues which are incised are vaginal epithelium, perineal skin, bulbocavernous muscle, superficial, and deep transverse perineal muscles. With large episiotomies, the external anal sphincter or levator ani may be partially cut, and ischiorectal fat exposed.

Technique: Hold the perineal skin away from the presenting part of the fetus (2 fingers in vagina). Infiltrate area to be cut with local anaesthetic eg 1% lidocaine. Still keeping the fingers in the introitus, cut medio-laterally towards the ischial tuberosity, starting midline (6 o'clock), so avoiding the Bartholin's glands.

Repair: (See fig 1.26.) NB: use resorbable suture—eg polyglactin 910. In lithotomy, and using good illumination, repair the vaginal mucosa first. Start above the apex using continuous non-locked stitches 1cm apart, 1cm from wound edges. Then repair muscles with continuous non-locked technique⁵⁴ₙᵢᴄᴇ to obliterate any dead spaces. Finally close the skin with subcuticular stitch. Perform rectal examination afterwards to check sutures have not penetrated the rectal mucosa.

Problems with episiotomy: Bleeding; infection, and breakdown; haematoma formation. For comfort some suggest ice packs, salt baths, cool hair dryer to dry perineum. 60% of women suffer perineal damage (episiotomy or tear) with spontaneous vaginal delivery; rectal diclofenac can provide effective analgesia. Superficial dyspareunia: see p. 137. If labia minora are involved in the skin bridge, the introitus is left too small.

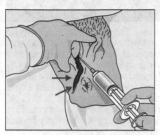

1. Swab the vulva towards the perineum. Infiltrate with 1% lidocaine (→ arrows).

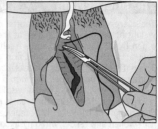

2. Place tampon with attached tape in upper vagina. Insert 1st suture above apex of vaginal cut (not too deep as underlying rectal mucosa nearby).

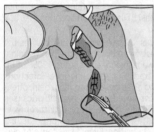

3. Bring together vaginal edges with continuous stitches placed 1 cm apart. Knot at introitus under the skin. Appose divided levator ani muscles.

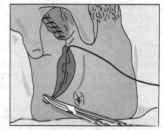

4. Close perineal skin (subcuticular continuous stitch is shown here).

5. When stitching is finished, remove tampon and examine vagina (to check for retained swabs). Do a **PR** to check that apical sutures have not penetrated rectum.

Fig 1.26 Repairing an episiotomy.

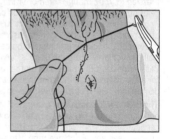

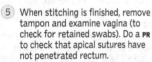

The puerperium is the 6 weeks after delivery. The uterus involutes, from 1kg weight at delivery to 100g. Felt at the umbilicus after delivery, it is a pelvic organ by 10 days. Afterpains are felt (especially while breastfeeding) as it contracts. The cervix becomes firm over 3 days. The internal os closes by 3 days, the external os by 3 weeks. Lochia (endometrial slough, red cells, and white cells) is passed *per vaginam*. It is red (*lochia rubra*) for the 1st 3 days, then becomes yellow (*lochia serosa*), then white over the next 10 days (*lochia alba*), until 6 weeks. The breasts produce milky discharge and colostrum during the last trimester. Milk replaces colostrum 3 days after birth. Breasts are swollen and tender with physiological engorgement at 3–4 days.

The first days Is thromboprophylaxis needed (p. 36)? If Rh–ve, give anti-D, within 72h (see BOX 'Using anti-D immunoglobulin', p. 11). Check T°, BP, breasts, legs, lochia, fundal height if heavy PV loss. Teach pelvic floor exercises. Persistent *red lochia*, failure of *uterine involution*, or *PPH* (p. 96) suggest endometritis or retained products. *Sustained hypertension* may need drugs (OHCM p140). ►Check rubella immunity. Vaccinate if non-immune (simultaneously but different limb from anti-D, or wait 3 months).[66]_NICE Discuss contraception (see BOX 'Contraception after a baby', p. 87).

Pyrexia in the first 14 days after delivery or miscarriage always requires full clinical assessment (sepsis p. 88-9)—chest, breasts, legs, lochia, and vaginal examination. Culture MSU, high vaginal swabs, blood, and sputum. 90% of infections will be urinary or of the genital tract. Superficial perineal infections occur around the second day. *Endometritis* gives lower abdominal pain, offensive lochia, and a tender uterus. Endometritis needs urgent IV antibiotics (see later). For breast infection give **flucloxacillin** 1g/6h PO early or **clarithromycin** 500mg/12h PO for ≥10 days, to prevent abscesses. Breastfeeding or breast expression should continue to prevent milk stagnation. Even if the cause of pyrexia is unknown, it is wise to treat with **cefalexin** 500mg/8h + **metronidazole** 400mg/8h.

Puerperal psychosis (1:500 births.) ►See p. 750-1. This is distinguished from the mild depression that often follows birth by a high suicidal drive, severe depression (p. 750), mania, and more rarely schizophrenic symptoms (p. 704) with delusions. Exclude puerperal infection causing delirium. Presentation is by day 7 postpartum in 50%, by 3 months in 90%. Onset is usually sudden and deterioration rapid. Refer to the perinatal psychiatry team. Out of hours you may need to contact the liaison psychiatrist on call (not all hospitals have access to specialist psychiatry, although there is currently a UK government drive to improve this). Admission to a specialist mother and baby unit may be needed. See p. 750 for a full discussion of postnatal depression. 10% of mothers develop postnatal depression; in ⅓–½ of these depression is severe.

The 6–8-week postnatal examination Gives a chance to: • See how mother and baby relate • Do BP & weight • Do FBC if anaemic postnatally • Arrange a cervical smear >3 months postnatally if due • Check contraceptive plans are enacted (see BOX 'Contraception after a baby', p. 87) • Ask about: depression, backache, incontinence. Ask: 'It's probably the last thing on your mind, but have you tried sex since having a baby?' Sexual problems are common: ~50% report that intercourse is less satisfactory than pre-pregnancy, with major loss of libido, and dyspareunia the chief complaints. Breastfeeding can cause temporary atrophic changes in the vagina so recommend lubricants (particularly silicone based). Sleep deprivation with a new baby is often a huge shock to a couple and will not help libido. It could be an evolutionary nudge to prolong inter-pregnancy interval (safest after 18–23 months—WHO 2007). At 1 year post delivery, there is no difference in dyspareunia between those who have had a vaginal versus CS delivery. Vaginal examination to check healing is *not* usually needed unless the woman has concerns or she reports incontinence.

Contraception after a baby

Up to 50% of women will have resumed sexual intercourse by 6 weeks post delivery, and ovulation can return as early as 3–4 weeks postnatally in those who aren't breastfeeding. 1 in 13 women presenting for termination of pregnancy had conceived within a year of childbirth.[67]

Lactational amenorrhoea (LAM)[68] This is nature's contraception. Breastfeeding delays return of ovulation (breastfeeding disrupts frequency and amplitude of gonadotrophin surges so that although there is gonadotrophin rise in response to falling placental sex steroids after delivery, ovulation does not occur). Women who are fully breastfeeding day and night, and are <6 months postpartum, and amenorrhoeic can expect this method to be 98% effective. Average 1st menstruation in a breastfeeding mother is at 28.4 weeks (range 15–48). Contraceptive efficacy of LAM is decreased after 6 months, if periods return, if breastfeeding frequency reduces, night feeding stops, there is separation from the baby (eg return to work), if the baby receives supplements, or if mother or baby become ill or stressed.

Progesterone-only pill (PoP, p. 156) These may be started any time postpartum but if started after day 21 additional precautions are needed for 2 days. They do not affect breast milk production. Low doses (<1%) of hormone are secreted in the milk but have not been shown to affect babies.

Combined pill If the woman is not breastfeeding: start at day 21 if no additional risk factors for venous thromboembolism; use additional contraception for 7 days. If later than day 21 and periods have returned, start as per any other woman wanting coc. If menstrual cycles have not returned, start as per any amenorrhoeic woman. If she is breastfeeding, start at between 6 weeks and 6 months as per a woman who is not breastfeeding (see earlier).[69] May affect early milk production and is therefore not recommended if breastfeeding until 6 weeks. Levels of hormone in breast milk are similar to that of ovulatory cycles.

Emergency contraception Use of emergency contraception (p. 151) is suitable for all. It is not needed before 21 days postpartum.

Depot injections and contraceptive implants Can be started at any time postpartum, independent of breastfeeding status. Additional contraceptive cover is not required if started <21 days postpartum. **Medroxyprogesterone acetate** 150mg given deep IM 12-weekly or **norethisterone enantate** 200mg into gluteus maximus 8-weekly (licensed for short-term use only, but can be given immediately postpartum when medroxyprogesterone use can cause heavy bleeding).

Intrauterine contraceptive devices (copper coil or levonorgestrel-releasing IUD) These should be inserted within the first 48h of a caesarean or vaginal birth, as early as 10 minutes after delivery of the placenta (postpartum intrauterine contraception, PPIUC), or after 4–6 weeks. For intra-caesarean insertion, the device is removed from its inserter and placed fundally, with the threads left untrimmed and left directed towards the os. Following vaginal delivery, a device can be inserted using long forceps. Expulsion rates with PPIUC are 0–17% with intra-caesarean and 10–34% with vaginal insertion. Infection and perforation rates are not increased. Intrapartum or postpartum sepsis or prolonged SROM are contraindications to PPIUC.[67]

Diaphragms and cervical caps The woman needs to be fitted at 6 weeks.

Sterilization Unless sterilization highly advisable at caesarean section (eg family complete), it is best to wait an appropriate interval as immediate postpartum tubal ligation has an increased failure rate (1:100 vs 1:200 outside of pregnancy) and is more likely to be regretted. See p. 157.

1 Obstetrics

Sepsis in pregnancy is one of the leading direct causes of maternal death in the UK, with many caused by group A *Streptococcus* caught in the community. The mortality rate of severe sepsis with organ dysfunction is 20–40%, reaching 60% with septic shock. In the non-pregnant population, surviving sepsis is clearly linked to its early recognition and treatment.

Definitions *Sepsis:* Infection plus systemic manifestations of infection. *Severe sepsis:* Sepsis with sepsis-induced organ dysfunction or evidence of tissue hypoperfusion. *Septic shock:* Persistent tissue hypoperfusion despite adequate fluid replacement. *Risk factors:* Obesity, impaired glucose tolerance/diabetes, impaired immunity, immunosuppressants, anaemia, vaginal discharge, pelvic infection, history of group B *Streptococcus*, invasive procedures such as amniocentesis, cervical cerclage, prolonged rupture of membranes (>24 hours), group A *Streptococcus* infection in close contacts, black or other ethnic minority group origin. *Organisms:* Lancefield group A beta-haemolytic *Streptococcus* and *E. coli* are most common. Mixed Gram-negative and Gram-positive organisms occur in chorioamnionitis. Coliforms are associated with UTI, preterm prolonged rupture of membranes, and cervical cerclage. Anaerobes such as *Clostridium perfringens* are less common, with *Peptostreptococcus* and *Bacteroides* predominating.

Clinical features Fever, rigors, diarrhoea or vomiting (may indicate endotoxin production), rash (generalized maculopapular streptococcal rash or purpura fulminans indicates toxic shock syndrome), abdominal or pelvic pain, offensive vaginal discharge (smelly suggests anaerobes; serosanguinous *Streptococcus*), productive cough, and urinary symptoms.

Diagnostic criteria for sepsis • Fever (>38°C) or hypothermia (<36°C) • Tachycardia • Tachypnoea • Systolic hypotension (<90mmHg) or mean arterial pressure <70mmHg • Impaired mental state • Significant oedema or positive fluid balance • Hyperglycaemia (plasma glucose >7.7mmol/L). *Inflammatory markers:* • Raised WCC (>12×10⁹/L) but be aware that leucocytosis is common in labour • Leucopenia (<4×10⁹/L) • CRP >7mg/L. *Tissue perfusion:* • Raised lactate (>4mmol/L) • Decreased capillary refill or mottling. *Organ dysfunction:* • Arterial hypoxaemia • Oliguria (<0.5mL/kg/h for 2h despite adequate fluid resuscitation) • Creatinine rise of >44μmol/L (severe sepsis if creatinine >176μmol/L) • INR >1.5; APTT >60 seconds • Thrombocytopenia (platelets <100×10⁹/L) • Hyperbilirubinaemia (>70umol/L) • Ileus. ▶These signs are often unreliable in the pregnant woman and develop late and far more rapidly than in the non-pregnant state.

Investigations Blood cultures are key—take before giving antibiotics. Other cultures (eg throat, high vaginal swab, mid-stream urine) should also be taken but should not delay therapy. Take FBC, U&E, CRP, LFTs and clotting as well as serum lactate to guide management. An ABG will determine if there is hypoxia. Do not delay imaging on the grounds of pregnancy.

Treatment Give IV broad-spectrum antibiotics (eg **piperacillin-tazobactam** 4.5g/8h) within 1h of recognition (fig 1.27: the 'Golden Hour of Sepsis')—see BOX 'Choice and limitations of antibiotic therapy' for alternatives. If lactate >4mmol/L and/or hypotensive, give an initial fluid bolus of 20mL/kg of crystalloid. Vasopressors may be given if BP does not respond to initial fluid bolus; aim for mean arterial pressure (MAP) of >65mmHg. Oxygen should be given. The woman may require central venous access. Immunoglobulin may be helpful in severe streptococcal or staphylococcal infection if other therapies have failed. It neutralizes exotoxin and inhibits production of tumour necrosis factor and interleukins. It has no effect on endotoxins. Use the multidisciplinary team and involve critical care outreach. Early consultant obstetrician, anaesthetic, and microbiologist review is recommended. Sepsis is associated with preterm labour so warn the neonatal unit. If chorioamnionitis is suspected, expedite delivery.

Transfer to intensive care If: • Persistent hypotension or raised lactate suggesting need for inotropes • Pulmonary oedema • The woman requires mechanical ventilation or airway adjuncts • Decreased conscious level • Renal dialysis • Hypothermia • Uncorrected acidosis • Multiorgan failure. Some units can manage high-dependency patients within the labour ward setting.

Fetal monitoring Continuous fetal monitoring in labour is recommended (neonatal encephalopathy and cerebral palsy is increased with intrauterine infection). If the mother is pyrexial, the fetus will be about a degree hotter leading to uncomplicated fetal tachycardia. Fetal blood sampling may be less reliable and results valid for a significantly shorter time period than usual due to increased fetal metabolic rate. Spinal and epidural anaesthesia should be avoided and general anaesthesia used for caesarean section. If preterm delivery is anticipated, consider giving maternal corticosteroids. Unless the source of sepsis is intrauterine, stabilize the woman first. At delivery of the baby, take arterial and venous cord blood gases.

Choice and limitations of antibiotic therapy

- *Cefuroxime:* Associated with *Clostridium difficile*; no cover for MRSA, *Pseudomonas*, or ESBL.
- *Metronidazole:* Anaerobic cover only.
- *Co-amoxiclav:* No MRSA or *Pseudomonas* cover, concern about increased risk of necrotizing enterocolitis in neonates exposed *in utero*.
- *Clindamycin:* Covers most streptococci and staphylococci. Switches off exotoxin production. Not renally excreted or nephrotoxic. Useful in penicillin-allergic patients.
- *Piperacillin–tazobactam and carbapenems:* Covers all except MRSA; renal sparing
- *Gentamicin:* Nephrotoxic with abnormal renal function; requires regular monitoring of levels after 3 doses.

---

1 Obstetrics

Sepsis in the puerperium The source is most commonly the genital tract and uterus, resulting in endometritis. Don't forget mastitis and breast abscess. Check caesarean and episiotomy wounds. If the degree of pain appears beyond clinical signs, consider necrotizing fasciitis. Organisms include group A *Streptococcus*, *E. coli*, *Staphylococcus aureus*, *Streptococcus pneumoniae*, and MRSA. Signs to look for are fever, rigors, diarrhoea, breast engorgement, abdominal pain, offensive vaginal discharge, cough, urinary symptoms, delay in uterine involution, heavy or offensive lochia (postpartum vaginal blood loss), lethargy, and reduced appetite. Investigate and treat as previously. The neonate may require treatment with IV antibiotics, especially if the mother is infected with group A *Streptococcus*.

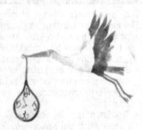

Fig 1.27 The Golden Hour of Sepsis.
© Charlotte Goumalatsou.

Further reading

RCOG (2012). *Bacterial Sepsis in Pregnancy* (Green-top Guideline No. 64a). London: RCOG.

RCOG (2012). *Bacterial Sepsis following Pregnancy* (Green-top Guideline No. 64b). London: RCOG.

1 Obstetrics

▸▸ **This is an obstetric emergency** It is a tonic–clonic seizure + pre-eclampsia. It occurs in 1% of pregnancies diagnosed with pre-eclampsia (pp. 50–1).

▸▸ 38% fit antenatally, 18% intrapartum, and 44% postnatally. It may be the first presentation of pre-eclampsia. If death occurs it is usually due to cerebral haemorrhage, HELLP, or organ failure.

▸▸ Call for help: senior obstetrics staff, senior midwives, anaesthetic registrar and consultant, a scribe, and neonatal team should delivery be required.

▸▸ Don't forget to manage airway, breathing, circulation, and IV access. Continuously monitor maternal oxygen saturation, and BP.

▸▸ **Magnesium sulfate** is used to prevent and treat seizures. Give 4g IV over 5–10min then 1g/h for 24h. Treat further fits with 2g bolus.

▸▸ Repeated seizures should be treated with diazepam and intracranial haemorrhage needs to be ruled out.

▸▸ Catheterize for hourly urine output (with urometer). HR, BP, respiratory rate, and oxygen saturations every 15min. FBC, U&E, LFTs, creatinine, and clotting studies every 12–24h.

▸▸ Stop magnesium sulfate IVI if respiratory rate <12/min or tendon reflex loss, or urine output <20mL/h. Have IV **calcium gluconate** ready in case of MgSO₄ toxicity: 1g (10mL) over 10min if respiratory depression.

▸▸ Restrict fluids to 80mL/h. Hourly urine output. Maintain fluid restriction until clinically and biochemically improving. Fluid restriction is inappropriate if there is haemorrhage—may need CVP line for accurate assessment.

▸▸ Monitor fetal heart rate with CTG.

▸▸ Deliver once the mother is stable; vaginal delivery is not contraindicated but LSCS is the quickest route as IOL is likely to take a long time eg if preterm.

▸▸ *Manage the third stage with oxytocin. Syntometrine® and ergometrine are contraindicated due to risk of severe hypertension leading to stroke.*

Treatment of hypertension Beware: automated BP devices underestimate BP.

▸▸ If BP >160/110mmHg or mean arterial pressure >125mmHg, use **labetalol** 20mg IV increasing after 10min intervals to 40mg then 80mg until 200mg total is given. Aim for BP <150/100mmHg. Alternative is **hydralazine** 5mg slowly/20min until 20mg given (unless pulse >120bpm).

▸▸HELLP syndrome

This is a severe variant of pre-eclampsia and consists of *H*aemolysis, *E*levated *L*iver enzymes, and *L*ow *P*latelets. Pregnancies affected by pre-eclampsia can develop HELLP in varying degrees, and liver enzymes usually rise first, followed by a drop in platelets (may be severe) and then haem-olysis. As with pre-eclampsia, cure is with delivery of the fetus.

• *Symptoms* are epigastric or right upper quadrant pain, nausea and vomiting, and dark urine due to haemolysis. The woman may have right upper quadrant tenderness and raised BP. It may be discovered after eclampsia.

• *Treatment* is as for eclampsia and is an indication for delivery. Involve the anaesthetist and senior help. Regional anaesthesia is contraindicated if platelets <80, and if platelets are <50 and surgery is required, cover with platelet transfusion.

Immediate resuscitation is key. Broadly speaking, follow the Advanced Life Support algorithm. Call for help, and put out a maternal collapse call via switchboard (2222 in the UK). Senior staff including obstetric and anaesthetic consultants and registrars, senior midwives, medical registrar, and neonatal teams as well as a porter should come quickly. Cardiac arrest in pregnancy is rare, occurring in 1 in 30,000 deliveries and the most common direct cause is thromboembolism. If appropriate, the aim is to defibrillate within 3 minutes of recognition of the arrest.

Airway Open the airway with head tilt and chin lift.

Breathing Look for chest movement and listen for breath sounds.

Circulation Check carotids for pulse; if pulse present check BP. If no pulse and/or no breathing, put out maternal cardiac arrest call and start CPR. CPR after 20 weeks should be carried out in left lateral position (place a wedge under the woman or tilt the table) or with manual uterine displacement to minimize aortocaval compression. After 20 weeks, if no return of spontaneous circulation after 4 minutes, perform LSCS aiming to have delivered the fetus by 5 minutes. This is not to save the fetus—it is essential for maternal resuscitation.

Drugs Think of overdose, drugs to maintain circulation or to dissolve massive thromboembolism. Remember to check blood glucose to exclude hypoglycaemia.

Environment Avoid injury of the patient and staff, especially if defibrillating.

The history may help ascertain the cause. Check observations every 15 minutes and catheterize for urine output. Take blood for FBC, U&E, LFTs, coagulation screen, group and save, and cross-match if suspicion or confirmed bleeding. Other investigations depend on the suspected cause but may include ABG, CXR, V/Q scan or CTPA, ECG, CT/MRI brain. Anaesthetic and general medical colleagues are invaluable in these situations especially if she has a cardiac arrest or is sick enough to require ITU.

Causes of maternal collapse

Obstetric causes

- Massive obstetric haemorrhage: may be ante- or postpartum (p. 92 & p. 96).
- Eclampsia (pp. 50–1).
- Intracranial haemorrhage (especially if preceding severe pre-eclampsia).
- Amniotic fluid embolism (p. 100).
- Uterine inversion causing neurogenic shock (p. 98).
- Post-surgical haemorrhage eg intra-abdominal following LSCS.
- Severe sepsis (pp. 88–9).
- Peripartum cardiomyopathy.

Non-obstetric causes

- Massive pulmonary embolism (p. 37).
- Pre-existing cardiac disease; never dismiss myocardial infarction as a possibility, or aortic dissection.
- Anaphylaxis (check the drug chart; could it be latex allergy?).
- Stroke.
- Meningitis.
- Overdose.
- Diabetic ketoacidosis; hypoglycaemia.
- Has the woman been abroad? Think about malaria (p. 30).

Further reading

Advanced Life Support Group (2011). Cardiopulmonary resuscitation in the non-pregnant and pregnant patient (MOET Manual, chapter 4) (www.alsg.org).

1 Obstetrics

Genital tract bleeding from 24^{+0} weeks' gestation complicates 3–5% of pregnancies. Any bleeding in pregnancy is associated with increased perinatal mortality. Severe bleeds can cause maternal death. Ask about domestic violence.

▶Speculum examination is safe in placenta praevia.

Dangerous causes Abruption, placenta praevia, vasa praevia (here the baby may bleed to death). *Lower genital tract sources:* Cervical polyps, erosions and carcinoma, cervicitis, vaginitis, vulval varicosities.

Placental abruption Part of the placenta becomes detached from the uterus. The outcome depends on the amount of blood loss and degree of separation. It may recur in subsequent pregnancies (4%: 19–24% if twice). *Associations:* Pre-eclampsia, smoking, IUGR (p. 54), PROM (p. 57), multiple pregnancy, polyhydramnios, ↑ maternal age, thrombophilia, abdo trauma, assisted reproduction, cocaine/amphetamine use, infection, non-vertex presentation. Bleeding may be well localized to one placental area and there may be delay before bleeding is revealed. See table 1.8 for the differences between bleeding from placental abruption and placenta praevia. *Consequences:* Placental insufficiency may cause fetal anoxia or death. Compression of uterine muscles by blood causes tenderness, and may prevent good contraction at all stages of labour, so beware a postpartum haemorrhage once the fetus has been delivered (occurs in ~25%). Posterior abruptions may present with backache. There may be uterine hypercontractility (>5 contractions per 10min). Thromboplastin release may cause DIC (10%). Concealed bleeding may cause maternal shock after which beware renal failure and Sheehan syndrome.

Placenta praevia (For terminology and complications, see p. 80.) The placenta lies in the lower uterine segment. Bleeding is always revealed (see fig 1.25, p. 81).

Management of APH *Admit* (unless spotting which has stopped, and the placenta is not low-lying). ▶▶If bleeding is severe, 2 large-bore cannulae, put up IVI, take bloods (FBC, U&E, G&S, x-match 2–6 units, clotting screen), and tilt bed head down. Give O$_2$ at 15L/min via mask with reservoir. Catheterize bladder; keep urine output >30mL/h. *Summon expert help urgently*—senior obstetrics team, anaesthetist, theatre team, haematologist, laboratory staff, porters, and if the fetus is alive, neonatal team. Definitive management in severe APH is by *delivery*—caesarean section if not fully dilated or she has placenta praevia. Beware PPH (active management of 3rd stage with Syntometrine®).

For milder bleeding, take bloods as described and insert large-bore cannula. Check pulse, BP, and blood loss regularly. If she is >28 weeks' gestation CTG 3–4 times per day and during active bleeding. Establish diagnosis (US for placental location, and speculum examination). If placenta praevia is the diagnosis, consider admission until delivery (caesarean section at 34–36^{+6} weeks). If pain and bleeding from a small abruption settles and the fetus is not compromised the woman may go home (after anti-D, if RhD –ve; 6-weekly if recurrent bleeds), but then treat as 'high-risk' pregnancy (serial scans). IOL if APH at term.

Table 1.8 Distinguishing *abruption* from *placenta praevia*

Abruption	Placenta praevia
Shock out of keeping with visible loss	Shock in proportion to visible loss
Pain constant	No pain
Tender, tense uterus	Uterus not tender
Normal lie and presentation	Both may be abnormal
Fetal heart: absent/distressed	Fetal heart usually normal
Coagulation problems	Coagulation problems rare
Beware pre-eclampsia, DIC, anuria	Small bleeds before large

Note: the risk of PPH is increased in both conditions. The lower segment may not contract well after a placenta praevia.

▶▶Cord prolapse

This is descent of the cord through the cervix, below the presenting part, after rupture of membranes (fig 1.28). It is an emergency because cord compression and vasospasm from exposure of the cord causes fetal asphyxia.

Incidence 0.1–0.6%; ↑ if: 2nd twin, footling breech, prematurity, polyhydramnios, unengaged head, transverse or unstable lie, male. If cord presentation is noted prior to membrane rupture, carry out caesarean section. Whenever you rupture membranes, remember that cord prolapse is possible eg if the presenting part is poorly applied.

Presentation The problem is obvious if the cord is at the introitus. But the only sign may be fetal bradycardia or variable fetal heart decelerations: always do a vaginal exam in this context to exclude prolapsed cord.

Action Get senior help. Activate alarms. Tell labour ward. Keep cord in vagina (minimal handling prevents spasm). Stop the presenting part from occluding the cord: The aim is to deliver the fetus as quickly as possible, either by LSCS or instrumental if the woman is fully dilated. The following steps are to minimize cord compression and vasospasm:

▶▶ Displace the presenting part by putting a hand in the vagina; push it back up (towards mother's head) during contractions. NB: there is little evidence that replacing the cord above the presenting part helps (*not* recommended).ᴿᶜᴼᴳ

▶▶ Knee-to-chest position so that her bottom is higher than her head.

▶▶ Infuse 500mL saline into bladder via an IVI giving set taped to a catheter (16G). Remember to empty the bladder before any attempt at delivery/extraction.

▶▶ Tocolysis (**terbutaline** 0.25mg sc) reduces contractions and helps bradycardia.

If cervix fully dilated and the presenting part is low in pelvis, delivery by ventouse/forceps (if cephalic) or by breech extraction (by an experienced obstetrician) is best if it leads to birth in <15min. The neonatal team should be present at delivery and paired cord blood samples taken for pH and base excess (if normal, intrapartum hypoxic brain injury is 'excluded').

1 Obstetrics

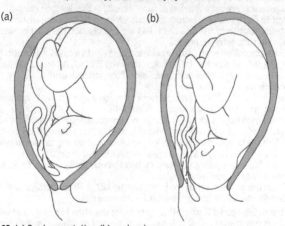

(a)   (b)

Fig 1.28 (a) Cord presentation; (b) cord prolapse.
Reproduced from Medforth *et al. Oxford Handbook of Midwifery* (2017) with permission from OUP.

Further reading
RCOG (2014). *Umbilical Cord Prolapse* (Green-top Guideline No. 50). London: RCOG.

RCOG definition A delivery requiring additional obstetric manoeuvres to release the shoulders after gentle downward traction has failed. The incidence is 1:200 deliveries (UK and USA). There can be high rate of fetal mortality and morbidity. Postpartum haemorrhage occurs in 11% of mothers and 3.8% get 4th-degree perineal tears whether or not manoeuvres are used. Brachial plexus injuries occur in 4–16% (1:2300 live births UK) of which 10% are left with permanent disability. A common cause of litigation: note which shoulder is anterior as posterior shoulder injuries are not considered due to the birth attendant (maternal propulsive forces may contribute to injuries).

Associations • Large/postmature fetus (but most babies >4800g do not develop it and 48% that do weigh <4000g), maternal BMI >30kg/m² • Induced or oxytocin augmented labours • Prolonged 1st or 2nd stage or secondary arrest • Assisted vaginal delivery • Previous shoulder dystocia (1–16%). Most occur in women with no risk factors. • Diabetes mellitus. ▶Suggest caesarean delivery to diabetic mothers with fetuses >4500g; discuss antenatally if previous shoulder dystocia.

Management The danger is death from asphyxia. ▶▶Speed is vital as the cord is usually squashed at the pelvic inlet; prompt and rehearsed shoulder dystocia drills (part of every labour ward mandatory training) improves outcome.

- *Help* from extra midwives, labour ward coordinator, senior obstetrician, neonatologist, anaesthetist, and a scribe for timing of manoeuvres.
- *Episiotomy* to give space for internal manoeuvres. The episiotomy itself won't relieve the shoulder dystocia.
- *Legs*—place in McRoberts (hyperflexed lithotomy) position. It is successful in 90%. Abduct, rotate outwards, and flex maternal femora so each thigh touches the abdomen (1 assistant to hold each leg). This straightens the sacrum relative to the lumbar spine and rotates the symphysis superiorly helping the impacted shoulder to enter the pelvis without manipulating the fetus.
- *Suprapubic pressure* with flat of hand laterally in the direction baby is facing, and towards mother's sacrum, continuously or with a rocking motion. Apply steady traction to the fetal head. This aims to displace the anterior shoulder allowing it to enter the pelvis.
- *Enter the pelvis* for internal manoeuvres; these aim to rotate the fetal shoulders to the oblique diameter. If this fails, rotation by 180° so posterior shoulder now lies anteriorly may work, as may *delivery of the posterior arm*.
- *Roll* the mother on to all fours if these fail.
- In practice, if McRoberts and suprapubic pressure fails, attempt whichever internal manoeuvre you are most confident with.
- *Other manoeuvres* include maternal symphysiotomy; or replacement of the fetal head by firm pressure of the hand to reverse the movements of labour and return the head to the flexed occipito-anterior position and caesarean delivery (Zavanelli). The baby is likely to be severely acidotic at this stage.
- If the baby dies prior to delivery, cutting through both clavicles (cleidotomy) with strong scissors assists delivery.
- Check the baby for damage eg Erb's palsy (fig 1.22, p.74) or fractured clavicle.
- Beware PPH or 3rd/4th-degree vaginal tears in the mother.

In the notes, record time of delivery of head; direction head faced after restitution; manoeuvres (timing & sequence); time of delivery of body; who and when present; Apgar of baby at birth; umbilical cord blood acid–base measurement. Debrief both the team and the mother.

Further reading

NICE (2017). *Intrapartum Care for Healthy Women and Babies* (CG190). London: NICE.
RCOG (2012). *Shoulder Dystocia* (Green-top Guideline No.42). London: RCOG.

1 Obstetrics

▸▸Uterine rupture

Ruptured uterus is rare in the UK (0.5–2:10,000 deliveries in an unscarred uterus but 1:100 deliveries in parts of Africa). Associated maternal mortality is 5%, and the fetal mortality 30%. ~70% of UK ruptures are due to dehiscence of CS scars. Lower-segment scars are far less likely to rupture (<0.74%) than the classical scars (2–9%)—see p. 76. Other risk factors: • Obstructed labour in the multiparous, especially if oxytocin is used • Previous cervical or uterine surgery • High forceps delivery (high station of head eg above the spines is a contraindication to instrumental delivery) • Internal version • Breech extraction. Rupture is usually during the 3rd trimester or in labour.

Vaginal birth after caesarean (VBAC) Vaginal birth will be successful in 72–76%. Endometritis, need for blood transfusion, uterine rupture, and perinatal death (↑ by 2–3:10,000 births—mainly due to increased stillbirth at around 39 weeks: this increases mortality to that of a firstborn) are commoner than with elective repeat caesarean. ₍ᵣcoₗ₎ Neonatal respiratory problems are, however, reduced. 24–28% undergo repeat emergency section. Of 9 ruptures in 4021 women undergoing VBAC there were no maternal or fetal deaths.[72] Use continuous electronic fetal monitoring in labour.[19,NICE]

Signs and symptoms Rupture is usually in labour. In a few (usually a caesarean scar dehiscence), rupture precedes labour. Pain is variable, some only having slight pain and tenderness over the uterus. In others, pain is severe. Vaginal bleeding is variable and may be slight (bleeding is intraperitoneal). Unexplained maternal tachycardia, sudden maternal shock, cessation of contractions, disappearance of the presenting part from the pelvis, and fetal distress are other presentations. *Postpartum indicators of rupture:* Continuous PPH with a well-contracted uterus; if bleeding continues postpartum after vaginal repair; and whenever shock is present.

Management If suspected in labour, perform category 1 CS (p. 76), and explore the uterus. ▸▸ • Give O₂ at 15L/min via a tight-fitting mask with reservoir • Set up IVI • Crossmatch 6U of blood and correct shock by fast transfusion. The type of operation performed should be decided by a senior obstetrician; if the rupture is small, repair may be carried out; if the cervix or vagina are involved in the tear, hysterectomy may be necessary. Care is needed to identify the ureters and exclude them from sutures. Give postoperative antibiotic cover eg **cefuroxime** 1.5g/8h IV and **metronidazole** 500mg/8h.

▸▸Mendelson syndrome

This is the name given to the cyanosis, bronchospasm, pulmonary oedema, and tachycardia that develop due to inhalation of gastric acid during general anaesthesia, especially during pregnancy. Clinically it may be difficult to distinguish from cardiac failure or amniotic fluid embolism. Preoperative H₂ antagonists, sodium citrate, gastric emptying, cricoid pressure (see fig 11.8, p. 670), the use of cuffed endotracheal tubes during anaesthesia, and pre-extubation emptying of stomach aim to prevent it.

Management ▸▸Tilt the patient head down. Turn her to one side and aspirate the pharynx. Give 100% O₂. Give **aminophylline** 5mg/kg by slow IVI and **hydrocortisone** 200mg IV stat.[73] The bronchial tree should be sucked out using a bronchoscope under general anaesthesia. Antibiotics should be given to prevent secondary pneumonia. Ventilation conducted on intensive care may be needed. Physiotherapy should be given during recovery.

Primary PPH This is the loss of >500mL in the first 24h after delivery. This occurs after ~6% of deliveries; major PPH (>1L) in 1.3%. *Causes (4 Ts): Tone:* uterine atony (90%); *Tissue:* retained products of conception; *Trauma:* genital tract trauma (7%); *Thrombin:* clotting disorders—p.99 (3%). Death rate: 2/yr in the UK; 125,000/yr worldwide. Massive obstetric haemorrhage is the loss of >1500mL and should prompt a hospital alert (2222 call, see BOX 'Management of postpartum haemorrhage').

Secondary PPH This is excessive blood loss from the genital tract after 24h from delivery. It usually occurs between 5 and 12 days and is usually due to retained placental tissue or clot, often with infection. Uterine involution may be incomplete. Treat with antibiotics, US to look for retained products (difficult to interpret postpartum).

Risk factors for PPH *Antenatal:* • Previous PPH or retained placenta • BMI >35kg/m² • Maternal Hb <85g/L at onset of labour • Antepartum haemorrhage • Multiparity >4 • Maternal age >35 • Uterine malformation or fibroids • A large placental site (twins, severe rhesus disease, large baby) • Low placenta • Overdistended uterus (polyhydramnios, twins) • Extravasated blood in the myometrium (abruption). *In labour:* • Prolonged labour (1st, 2nd, or 3rd stage) • Induction or oxytocin use • Precipitate labour • Operative birth or caesarean section. ▶Book mothers with risk factors for obstetric unit delivery.

Management of postpartum haemorrhage

- Call for help—this is a life-threatening emergency. Ask for senior midwife, obstetrics registrar and SHO, anaesthetic registrar, a scribe, and if massive haemorrhage put out 2222 call to alert haematologist, blood bank, porters, and theatres.
- High-flow oxygen.
- Assess airway and intubate if decreased conscious level.
- Insert two large-bore cannulae (14G/grey or above) and take blood for FBC, U&E, LFTs, clotting screen, and cross-match 4–6 units. If blood loss torrential and mother unstable use group O Rh−ve blood until cross-matched available. Transfuse 1 unit packed red cells to 1 unit fresh frozen plasma.
- Start IV fluids eg 1 litre Hartmann's stat.
- Catheterize and use urometer for hourly urine output.
- Deliver placenta, empty the uterus of clots or retained tissue.
- Massage uterus to generate contraction/perform bimanual compression.
- Give drugs to contract uterus (sequentially)
  - **Syntometrine®** IM 1 ampoule
  - **Oxytocin** infusion 40 units at 10 units/hour
  - **Ergometrine** 500mcg IV/IM
  - **Misoprostol** 1000mcg PR
  - **Carboprost** 250mcg every 15min up to 8 doses.
- Repair vaginal or cervical tears.
- If ongoing bleeding after 2nd dose of carboprost, or suspicion of uterine rupture or retained tissue, take to theatre for examination under anaesthesia, including laparotomy if necessary.
- In theatre, ensure no retained placenta. Insert Rusch balloon (fig 1.29—large balloon which sits inside the uterus, exerting direct pressure on placental bed).
- If uterus still atonic despite empty bladder and drugs, and bleeding responds to compression, insert a B-lynch suture (fig 1.30). This is a compression suture inserted through lower segment, over the top of the uterus including the posterior surface and looks like a belt and braces.
- If bleeding is still ongoing, consider internal iliac or uterine artery ligation.
- Uterine artery embolization helpful but not available in all units at all times.
- Subtotal or total hysterectomy: the decision should not be delayed because maternal death may result.

Managing those refusing blood transfusion in pregnancy

* Document maternal attitude to transfusion at booking.
* Give oral iron and folate to mother to maximize haemoglobin stores (parenteral iron if does not respond—p. 23 (not if thalassaemia)).
* Book for delivery where there are good facilities to deal with haemorrhage promptly (including facilities for hysterectomy, and interventional radiology techniques such as uterine artery embolization), and with critical care facilities and cell salvage if the mother is high risk eg if placenta praevia.
* Ensure consultant obstetrician and anaesthetist assess antenatally to make plans for labour.
* The woman should make an Advanced Directive, making clear her views on which blood products she will and won't accept.
* Arrange us to know placental site.
* Inform consultant when admitted in labour. Ensure experienced staff conduct labour. Give oxytocin as soon as the baby is delivered. Do not leave the mother alone for first hour post delivery.
* Consultant obstetrician and anaesthetist should perform caesarean section if required.
* Cell savers which wash the woman's own blood so that it may be returned may be acceptable to some women (suitable for intra-abdominal blood not contaminated by amniotic fluid).[62]
* Haemorrhage should be dealt with promptly, and clotting disorders excluded early. Involve a consultant obstetrician early (to decide if intervention may be needed eg embolization of uterine arteries, B-Lynch suture, internal iliac ligation, or hysterectomy), and a consultant anaesthetist (for help with fluid replacement and for use of intensive care facilities). Liaise with a consultant haematologist. Avoid dextran (adversely affects haemostasis), but Gelofusine® is useful. Erythropoietin is not an effective alternative to transfusion as it takes 10–14 days to work.
* Ensure the woman does not want to change her mind and receive a transfusion.
* Should the woman die of exsanguination, both bereaved relatives and distressed staff should be offered support.

1 Obstetrics

Fig 1.29 Bakri and Rusch balloons.
Reproduced from Georgiou, C. (2009), Balloon tamponade in the management of postpartum haemorrhage: a review. *BJOG: An International Journal of Obstetrics & Gynaecology*, 116: 748–757. doi: https://doi.org/10.1111/j.1471-0528.2009.02113.x. The Authors Journal compilation © RCOG 2009 BJOG: An International Journal of Obstetrics and Gynaecology.

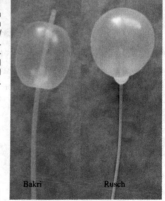

Bakri   Rusch

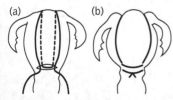

(a)   (b)

Fig 1.30 B-lynch suture.
Reproduced from Clyburn *et al. Obstetric Anaesthesia for Developing Countries* (2010) with permission from OUP.

Inversion of the uterus is rare. It may be due to mismanagement of the 3rd stage eg with cord traction in an atonic uterus (between contractions) and a fundal insertion of the placenta. It may be completely revealed, or partial when the uterus remains within the vagina. Even without haemorrhage the mother may become profoundly shocked, due to increased vagal tone.

Management The ease with which the uterus is replaced depends on the amount of time elapsed since inversion, as a tight ring forms at the neck of the inversion.
- Call for help: senior midwife, obstetrician and anaesthetist, and theatre staff.
- Immediate replacement: push the fundus through the cervix with the palm of the hand (fig 1.31).
- If this fails, insert 2 large-bore IV cannulae and take blood for FBC, U&E, clotting, and crossmatch 4–6 units (94% have postpartum haemorrhage).
- IV fluid.
- Transfer to theatre for anaesthesia.
- If the placenta is still attached, leave it there as removing it will increase the bleeding.
- Tocolytic drugs (eg terbutaline) to relax the uterus and make replacement easier. Agents used for general anaesthesia are also helpful.
- Try manual replacement but if this fails, replace using hydrostatic pressure: infuse warm saline into the vagina, sealing the labia with the other hand.
- If this fails, laparotomy to try and pull the uterus up.

1 Obstetrics

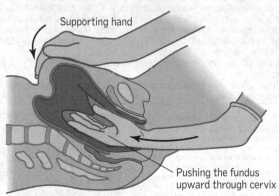

Supporting hand

Pushing the fundus
upward through cervix

Fig 1.31 Correction of uterine inversion.
Reproduced from Sarris *et al. Training in Obstetrics and Gynaecology* (2009) with permission from OUP.

DIC Occurs as the result of cytokine release related to many obstetric scenarios. Known triggers are delayed delivery of a stillbirth; pre-eclampsia, obstetric haemorrhage (eg from placental abruption or atonic PPH), toxic shock syndrome, amniotic fluid embolism, and acute fatty liver of pregnancy. *Pathogenesis:* Thromboplastins are released into the circulation, fibrin and platelets are consumed as intravascular clotting occurs. Consumption of clotting factors then predisposes to bleeding. Presentation may be as heavy bleeding and shock. *Tests:* Caution must be taken in interpreting test results—tests are unreliable and the clinical picture is paramount. FBC for platelet count ↓; prothrombin time (PT) ↑, fibrinogen ↓, D-dimer often raised in pregnancy anyway. In situations where you are highly suspicious of DIC, also send blood for cross-match. *Management:* Treat the underlying cause as quickly as possible which will correct the DIC eg treating massive haemorrhage will treat the DIC. 1. Treat shock—▶▶Give O₂ at 15L/min via a tight-fitting mask with reservoir. Set up 2 wide-gauge IVIs, take bloods as described earlier. 2. Blood product support (seek expert help from haematologist)—tranexamic acid, vitamin K (particularly if prolonged PT), single pool of platelets if <30–50; fibrinogen concentrates may be required to keep it above 1.5. 3. Frequent re-assessment of the clinical picture and laboratory tests due to the dynamic nature of the condition. *Mortality:* <1% if caused by placental abruption; 50–80% if infection.

Idiopathic thrombocytopenic purpura (ITP) Incidence 1–2:1000 pregnancies. A consumptive problem whereby normal platelets are made but prematurely destroyed by autoantibodies. Bone marrow platelet production increases with increased megakaryocytes in the bone marrow and larger immature platelets seen in peripheral blood. Maternal IgG antibodies can cross the placenta, and cause thrombocytopenia in ~10% of fetuses. Exclude systemic lupus erythematosus in the mother (thrombocytopenia may be an early presentation; do DNA binding, *OHCM* p554). Consider maternal HIV.

Early recognition is important to allow optimal timely management by haematology. Asymptomatic patients with platelet counts >30 can be monitored until the 3rd trimester. **Prednisolone** 1mg/kg (does not cross placenta) should be considered if platelets fall below 75 and response assessed frequently over a fortnight. IVIG is given if no adequate response. IVIG is a blood product and requires appropriate counselling, ideally avoided where possible. Splenectomy is no longer favoured.

Aim for non-traumatic delivery for both mother and baby: avoid FBS, FSE, ventouse, and rotational forceps delivery. Neonatal platelet count may fall further in the first days of life, then gradually rise to normal over 4–16 weeks. Treatment is not needed unless surgery is contemplated. Maternal mortality due to ITP is now negligible, but fetal mortality remains (due to intracranial bleeding). Take cord blood at delivery. If platelets <20×10⁹/L give baby IgG 1g/kg IVI at birth.

Causes of thrombocytopenia in pregnancy Spurious—platelets react with EDTA, so send repeat in citrated bottle; gestational thrombocytopenia—usually progressive from mid 2nd trimester. It is asymptomatic and self-limiting, and platelets rarely fall <70; ITP; pre-eclampsia (platelets may fall early, preceding clotting abnormality); consumption in DIC, haemolytic uraemic syndrome (HUS) or thrombotic thrombocytopenic purpura (TTP) (*OHCM* p315); folate deficiency; congenital (May–Heggin anomaly, hereditary macrothrombocytopenia); bone marrow disease incl. haematological malignancy; hypersplenism; HELLP syndrome (pp. 90–1).

ACKNOWLEDGEMENT With thanks to Dr Lucinda Blake MRCP, FRCPath, RAMC.

This condition is thankfully rare but carries a high mortality of up to 61% (20% in 2006–8 UK). 8% of direct maternal deaths were caused by AFE in the UK and of those who survive, 85% have permanent neurological damage. The incidence is 1:8000–1:30,000 births and it tends to occur with rupture of membranes (70%), at CS (19%), during delivery, and rarely during termination of pregnancy, manual removal of placenta, and amniocentesis.

Risk factors Include multiple pregnancy, maternal age >35yrs, CS, instrumental delivery, eclampsia, polyhydramnios, placental abruption, uterine rupture, and induction of labour.

Clinical features Symptoms and signs evolve rapidly and the first sign may be maternal collapse.

- Dyspnoea, chest pain, hypoxia and/or respiratory arrest leading to acute respiratory distress syndrome (ARDS) (*OHCM* p186).
- Hypotension.
- Fetal distress.
- Seizures (20%).
- Reduced conscious level.
- Cardiac arrest.
- Almost all women go on to develop DIC within 48h.

An anaphylactic type of response occurs to amniotic fluid in the maternal circulation.

Management

▶▶ The first priority is to prevent death from respiratory failure. Give high-flow oxygen (15L/min with non-rebreathe reservoir) and call an anaesthetist urgently. Endotracheal intubation and ventilation may be necessary. Set up IVI in case DIC should supervene. Cardiovascular collapse is due to left ventricular failure. DIC and haemorrhage then usually follow. Treatment is essentially supportive—important steps are detailed here. Diagnosis may be difficult: exclude other causes of maternal collapse (see BOX 'Causes of maternal collapse', p.91).

▶▶ Cardiopulmonary resuscitation if indicated.

▶▶ Give highest available O₂ concentration. If unconscious, ventilate and use 100% inspired O₂. This is to prevent neurological sequelae from hypoxia.

▶▶ Monitor for fetal distress.

▶▶ If hypotensive, give fluids rapidly IVI to increase preload. If still hypotensive consider inotropes: **dobutamine** (a better inotrope than dopamine) eg in a dose range of 2.5–10mcg/kg/min IVI may help.

▶▶ Pulmonary artery catheterization (Swan-Ganz catheter if available) helps guide haemodynamic management.

▶▶ After initial hypotension is corrected, give only maintenance requirements of fluid to avoid pulmonary oedema from ARDS. Transfer to intensive care unit as soon as possible.

▶▶ Treat DIC with fresh whole blood or packed cells and fresh frozen plasma. Use of heparin is controversial; there are insufficient data to warrant routine heparinization.

▶▶ If the mother has a cardiac arrest, it is recommended to deliver the baby via CS. Perimortem CS within 5 minutes aids resuscitation of the mother.

Most mortality occurs in the first hour. Mortality rates reported: 26.4–61%. (In 2006–8, there were 13 deaths in England and Wales.) Report suspected cases to National Amniotic Fluid Embolism Register (at UKOSS).[2] Should the woman die, perform autopsy as soon as possible. Specifically request that the lungs be examined for amniotic squames or lanugo hair to confirm the diagnosis.

2 UKOSS The National Perinatal Unit, Old Road Campus, Old Road, Headington, Oxford, OX3 7LF, www.npeu.ox.ac.uk

1 Obstetrics

1 Obstetrics

Worldwide perspective In North Europe, a woman's lifetime risk of dying in pregnancy or childbirth is 1:30,000; in the world's poorest parts it is 1:6.[74]

Definition The death of a mother while pregnant or within 42 days of the pregnancy ending, from any cause related to or aggravated by the pregnancy or its management, but not from accidental or incidental causes. *Direct deaths:* Result from obstetric complications of the pregnant state (including pregnancy, labour, and the puerperium) from interventions, omissions, incorrect treatment, or a chain of events resulting from any of these eg eclampsia, haemorrhage, or amniotic fluid embolism. *Indirect death:* A death which has arisen from pre-existing disease or disease that developed during pregnancy which was not due to direct obstetric causes, but which was aggravated by pregnancy eg diabetes, heart disease, epilepsy, or hormone-dependent malignancies. *Coincidental death:* Accidental or incidental death which would have happened even if the woman was not pregnant eg domestic violence or road traffic accidents. *Late deaths:* Those occurring between 42 days and 1 year after termination, miscarriage, or delivery that are due to direct or indirect maternal causes.

History Since 1952 there have been confidential enquiries into maternal deaths, which are reported by the obstetric unit involved and investigated by a team of experts. Reports allow analysis, reflection, and recommended actions so each death should improve future care. Maternal mortality has reduced since reports started: (deaths per 100,000 *maternities* were 67.1 in 1955–7, 33.3 in 1964–6, & 8.76 in 2013–15 of which direct deaths were 3.82/100,000).

Currently In 2013–15 (MBRACE-UK report from 2017[1]), 240 women died during, or within 6 weeks of the end of their pregnancy, 202 of which were from direct (44%) or indirect causes (56%). 38 women died from coincidental causes. There has been no significant decrease in the maternal death rate since the last report which is concerning, but there has been a reduction in indirect causes which is primarily due to fewer deaths from influenza—each pregnant woman in the UK is offered the flu vaccine.

In 2013–15, thrombosis was the chief cause of direct death in the UK, followed by obstetric haemorrhage (due to more women having abnormal placentation), and then suicide. Suicide is the leading direct cause of maternal death up to 1 year.

Cardiac disease was the leading cause of indirect deaths. Neurological disease is the third-highest and also remains static. 25% of mothers were still pregnant at the time of their deaths, and 59% were <20 weeks' gestation. 78% of infants survived. Of the 36 babies delivered by perimortem cs, 14 survived. Maternal mortality rates remain highest in older women, those from the most deprived areas, and from some ethnic minorities. Just under a quarter of women were born outside the UK. 68% had pre-existing medical conditions, 16% mental health problems, and 8% a cardiac history. There is a known correlation between pre-existing medical comorbidities and maternal death. 34% were obese, 19% overweight and almost a quarter smoked during pregnancy. Only 36% received the level of antenatal care recommended by NICE (only 26% of those with mental illness and 4% with epilepsy).

Key messages from the report: • In the women who died there were multiple opportunities to intervene and improve outcomes • Pre-pregnancy advice for women with pre-existing medical or mental health problems • Early involvement of senior clinicians • Clear leadership where multiple specialties are involved • Early access to (joint) specialist antenatal care.

Further reading

MBRACE-UK (2017). *Saving Lives, Improving Mothers' Care* (www.npeu.ox.ac.uk).

This is the number of stillbirths and deaths in the 1st week of life (early neo-natal deaths)/1000 births. Stillbirths only include those fetuses of >24 weeks' gestation; if a fetus of <24 weeks' gestation is born showing signs of life, and then dies, this is counted as a perinatal death in the UK (if dying within the 1st 7 days). Neonatal deaths are those infants dying up to and including the 28th day after birth. Other countries use different criteria—including still-births from 20 weeks and neonatal deaths up to 28 days after birth, so it is not always easy to compare statistics.

Perinatal mortality is affected by many factors. Rates are high for *small* (61% of deaths are in babies <2500g) and *preterm* babies (70% of deaths occur in the 10% who are preterm). See p. 52-3 & p. 298. Congenital abnor-malities contribute to 1 in 6 perinatal deaths. *Regional variation* in the UK is quite marked. There is a *social class variation* with rates being higher in those with lower socioeconomic status. *Teenage mothers and those >35yrs* have higher rates than mothers aged 20–29. *Second babies* have the lowest mortality rates. Mortality rates are doubled for 4th and 5th children, trebled by 6th and 7th. Rates are lower for *singleton births* than for multiple (↑ ≈10 for triplets vs singletons).[75] Time to conception also has an influence with mortality rates being 3 times more if it has taken a long time to conceive compared with a short time.[76] Perinatal mortality in UK* (*figures exclude Scotland) is twice as high in offspring of mothers of black ethnicity; 1.5 times commoner if of Asian ethnicity.[77]

Perinatal mortality rates in the UK have fallen over the years from 62.5:1000 in 1930–5 to 5.6:1000 in 2015 for UK*. Declining mortality reflects improvement in standards of living, improved maternal health, and declining parity, as well as improvements in medical care.

The RCOG introduced the 'Each Baby Counts' initiative in 2015 with the aim of halving the number of deaths or severe brain injuries caused by prevent-able events in term labour by 2020. The first report was published in 2018 into all deaths and brain injuries occurring during term labour in 2015. Each case was investigated and found that in most, different care would have re-sulted in a different outcome. This sobering statement identified that no one single factor was responsible but a complex mixture of factors concerning team working and communication issues, CTG interpretation, neonatal care, management of labour, delay in delivery, patient factors, risk recognition, and human factors (eg stress, fatigue, lack of leadership) to name but a few.[78]

Examples of how changed medical care may reduce mortality

- Worldwide, treatment of syphilis, antitetanus vaccination (of mother during pregnancy), and clean delivery (especially cord techniques) have the greatest influence in reducing perinatal mortality.
- Antenatal detection and termination of malformed fetuses.
- Reduction of mid-cavity procedures and vaginal breech delivery.
- Detection of placenta praevia antenatally.
- Prevention of rhesus incompatibility.
- Preventing progression of preterm labour.
- Better control of diabetes mellitus in affected mothers.
- Antenatal monitoring of 'at-risk' pregnancies.

∴ While we must try to reduce morbidity and mortality still further, this must not blind us to other problems that remain, such as the 'over-medicalization' of birth; the problem of reconciling maternal wishes to be in charge of her own delivery with the immediate needs of the baby; and the problem of explaining risks and benefits in terms that both parents under-stand, so that they can join in the decision-making process.

*With many thanks to Miss Melanie Tipples MRCOG FRCS and Mr George Goumalatsos MRCOG MSC, our specialist
readers, and junior readers Grace Castronovo and Sophie Howarth for their contribution to this chapter.*

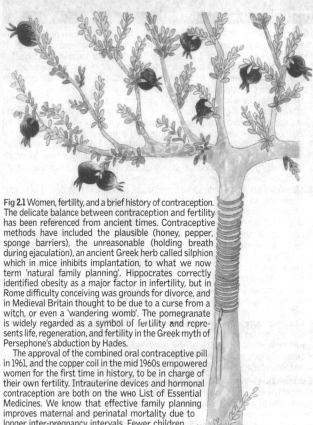

Fig 2.1 Women, fertility, and a brief history of contraception. The delicate balance between contraception and fertility has been referenced from ancient times. Contraceptive methods have included the plausible (honey, pepper, sponge barriers), the unreasonable (holding breath during ejaculation), an ancient Greek herb called silphion which in mice inhibits implantation, to what we now term 'natural family planning'. Hippocrates correctly identified obesity as a major factor in infertility, but in Rome difficulty conceiving was grounds for divorce, and in Medieval Britain thought to be due to a curse from a witch, or even a 'wandering womb'. The pomegranate is widely regarded as a symbol of fertility and represents life, regeneration, and fertility in the Greek myth of Persephone's abduction by Hades.

The approval of the combined oral contraceptive pill in 1961, and the copper coil in the mid 1960s empowered women for the first time in history, to be in charge of their own fertility. Intrauterine devices and hormonal contraception are both on the WHO List of Essential Medicines. We know that effective family planning improves maternal and perinatal mortality due to longer inter-pregnancy intervals. Fewer children results in better family economic resources, as does delaying starting a family until being in a better financial position. Unplanned births are associated with unhappier intimate relationships, more depression and anxiety in mothers, and reduced access to education (eg a pregnant teenager is less likely to finish school or go to university).

While some countries appear to be taking backwards steps regarding contraceptive access (particularly the USA), we can hope that globally, access to effective contraception and safe abortion improves. As Margaret Sanger, a nurse who opened the first birth control clinic in America once said, 'No woman can call herself free who does not control her own body'.

© Charlotte Goumalatsou.

History Introduce yourself. Let her tell the story and use open questions. She may be reluctant to discuss some problems, particularly in front of relatives. If required, use a professional translator. A frustration for the medical student is that the story you are told is different to the one elicited by the consultant or the GP. But sometimes the first telling is the most valid. ► It is also true that none of us (doctors and patients) can tell the same story twice.[1]

1 *Symptoms:* If she has *pain* what is it like? Uterine pain may be colicky and felt in the sacrum and groins. Ovarian pain tends to be felt in the *iliac fossa* and radiates down front of the thigh to the knee. Ask about *dyspareunia* (painful intercourse). Is it superficial (at the entrance) or deep inside? If she has *vaginal discharge* what is it like (amount, colour, smell, itch)? When does she get it? Ask about *prolapse* and *incontinence*. Is incontinence stress or urge? How does it affect quality of life? Ask about bowel symptoms (irritable bowel can cause pelvic pain), and faecal incontinence.

2 *Menstrual history:* ►Date of last menstrual period (LMP; 1st day of bleeding) or menopause. Was the last period normal? Cycles: number of days bleeding/number of days from day 1 of one period to day 1 of next (eg 5/26). Are they regular? If heavy, are there clots or floods? Are periods painful? If so, does the pain precede the start of the period? Are there any associated bowel symptoms? Is bleeding intermenstrual (IMB), postcoital (PCB), or postmenopausal (PMB)? Age at menarche?

3 *Sex and contraception:* Is she sexually active? Are there problems with sex (see p.107)? What contraception is she using and is she happy with it? What has she tried previously? Has she had problems conceiving? If so, has she had treatment for subfertility? What about sexually transmitted infections? Date and result of last cervical smear, and history of abnormal smears.

4 *Obstetric history:* How many children? For each pregnancy: antenatal problems, delivery, gestation, outcome; weights of babies; puerperium? Terminations/miscarriages—at *what* stage, *why*, and *how*?

5 *Other:* General health, past medical history, profession, drug history, smoking, and alcohol use. Previous gynaecological treatment or surgery.

Examination ►Women may find pelvic examination painful, undignified, and embarrassing. Explain what you are going to do and stop if it is too painful. Be gentle. Use of a trained chaperone is mandatory; this is to support the patient but also to protect yourself medicolegally. A family member or friend cannot chaperone. Let the woman undress in privacy and provide a sheet to cover.

General: Is she well or ill? If the woman looks unwell, start with ABC.

Abdomen: Inspect the abdomen. Palpate for tenderness and peritonism. If there is a mass, could it be a pregnancy? If distended, percuss for ascites.

Vaginal examination: Inspect the vulva, and use a *speculum* to examine the vagina and cervix and your *fingers* to assess the uterus and adnexae bimanually. Examination is usually done with the patient on her back or in the left lateral position (best for detecting prolapse). *Sims' speculum* has 2 right-angle bends, and is used for inspecting the vaginal walls in left lateral position, eg for prolapse and incontinence.

Cusco's (bivalve) speculum: Used for inspecting the cervix with the aid of a light. Lubricate with jelly (unless taking a smear, in which case use warm water). Insert closed, with blades parallel to the labia, usually up to the hilt and aim for the sacrum. Rotate it, open it, and usually the cervix pops into view. If it does not, do a bimanual to check the position of the cervix (pp.132-3), and try again. Take swabs (pp.132-3) and a cervical smear (p.165) if needed. Close the speculum gradually, under direct vision, as you withdraw it, to avoid trapping the cervix.

---

1 The first telling awakes memories which colour or transform the next telling, which itself influences the next telling in an infinite regression in which one telling becomes the audience for the next.

Sex requires the participation of the mind and body and when there is a problem, or sexual dysfunction, it often involves both. It affects 20% of women attending gynaecology clinics and may present overtly with the woman wanting help, or covertly with a different complaint (such as pelvic pain or dissatisfaction with genitalia).

What is 'normal'? The pioneers of research into sexual function were Masters and Johnson, who studied the sexual response of men and women between 1957 and the 1990s. They characterized female sexual arousal, proved that lubrication is vaginal, not cervical, and that some women are capable of multiple orgasms and unlike men, have no refractory period. Importantly, they also did much to promote sex as a normal and healthy activity. They described the four-stage model of sexual response: arousal/excitement, plateau, orgasm, and resolution. However, this type of linear model is thought by some to better reflect the male sexual response. Basson proposed an intimacy-based cyclical model which reflects the importance of other factors including emotional and physical satisfaction, biological, psychological, and sexual stimuli, and sexual drive.

Hypoactive sexual desire disorder (HSDD) Presents with loss of libido and decline in overall sexual desire, affecting personal relationships and causing distress. Most have a psychosexual cause but organic causes include menopause, depression, chemotherapy, and radiotherapy. When did it start? For example, does she have concerns about what is 'at the end of her vagina' after hysterectomy? What is normal sexual function to her? Is this realistic and is this at odds with her partner's beliefs? Are there any relationship problems? Testosterone supplementation may help (especially if symptoms started following oophorectomy) but psychosexual counselling is recommended.

Sexual pain *Dyspareunia* (p. 137) may be superficial or deep. Superficial dyspareunia can be due to infections, or skin conditions such as lichen sclerosis. Treat the underlying cause—but pain can start a cycle of fear, anticipation, and avoidance. Lubricants and local anaesthetic gel may also help break the cycle. *Vaginismus* is the difficulty of the woman to allow vaginal penetration despite wanting to; it involves involuntary contraction of the pelvic floor muscles and thigh adductors and is a symptom or sign, not a diagnosis. It is usually precipitated by another cause, be it physical or psychological, or a combination. Exclude anatomical problems such as vaginal septa. It may be so severe that vaginal penetration is not possible. Using vaginal dilators may help eliminate the pubococcygeal reflex, but encouraging the woman to use her own fingers in combination with relaxation exercises may be more useful. *Vulvodynia* is described as a burning pain, occurring in the absence of relevant visible findings or a specific, clinically identifiable neurological disorder. It can be difficult to treat; use a team-based approach with physiotherapy, psychosexual medicine, and pain management. Explain the diagnosis. 1st-line treatment is with pelvic floor exercises, internal and external perineal massage, and topical anaesthetic. Tricyclic antidepressants or gabapentin may help.

Treatment What does the woman want? *Motivation is important*, as is the quality of the non-sexual component of the relationship. *Lifestyle:* Diet, exercise, stress reduction, exploration of relationship problems/body image issues. *Education:* About body function, encourage exploration; sexual education material, lubricants. *Hormonal:* Oestrogen replacement in menopausal women; testosterone if oophorectomy and hypoactive sexual desire disorder. *Behavioural therapy:* Using a range of psychotherapeutic techniques. *Devices:* Such as for anorgasmia or vaginismus eg dilators or clitoral stimulators.

Further reading

Cowan F *et al.* (2015). The management of common disorders in psychosexual medicine. *TOG* 17:47–53.
Institute of Psychosexual Medicine: www.ipm.org.uk

2 Gynaecology

Vulva (fig 2.2) The vulva comprises the entrances to the vagina and urethra, the structures which surround them (clitoris, labia minora, and fourchette), and the encircling labia majora and perineum. The hymen, when broken (by tampons or intercourse) leaves tags at the mouth of the vagina (*carunculae myrtiformes*). *Look for:* Rashes; atrophy; ulcers; lumps (p. 130); deficient perineum (back wall of the vagina is visible); incontinence, discharge.

Vagina The vagina is a potential space with distensible folded muscular walls. The contents of the rectum, which runs behind the posterior wall, are palpable through the vagina. The cervix projects into the vault at the top which forms a moat around it, deepest posteriorly, conventionally divided into anterior, posterior, and 2 lateral fornices. From puberty until the menopause, lactobacilli in the vagina keep it acidic (pH 3.8–4.4), discouraging infection.

Look for: Inflammation; discharge (pp. 132–3); prolapse (p. 160).

Cervix The cervix is mostly connective tissue. It feels firm, and has a dent in the centre (the os of the cervical canal). Mucin-secreting glands of the endocervix lubricate the vagina. The os is circular in nulliparous women, but is a slit in the parous.

Look for: Pain on moving the cervix (excitation—p. 126 & p. 134); cervical ectropion; cervicitis and discharge; polyps, carcinoma (p. 167).

Uterus The uterus has a thick muscular-walled *body* made from myometrium, lined internally with columnar epithelium (the endometrium) connected to the cervix or neck. It is supported by the uterosacral, cardinal, and round ligaments. The peritoneum is draped over the uterus. The valley so formed between it and the rectum is the rectovaginal pouch (of Douglas), and the fold of peritoneum in which the fallopian tubes lie is known as the broad ligament. The *size* of the uterus is described by comparison with its size at different stages of pregnancy. Estimates are approximate: non-pregnant—plum-sized; 6 weeks—egg; 8 weeks—small orange; 10 weeks—large orange.

The uterus is *anteverted in most women*, ie its long axis is directed forward in relation to the vagina. The body then flops forwards on the cervix—*anteflexed* (the relation of the long axis of the uterus in relation to the cervix). An anteverted uterus can be palpated between the hands on bimanual examination (unless she is obese, or tense, or the bladder is full). In 20% it is retroverted, retroflexed, and mobile. It rarely causes problems but is more difficult to palpate on bimanual examination and may fail to lift out of the pelvis after 12 weeks of pregnancy, causing urinary retention. A fixed retroverted uterus is not normal and may be due to endometriosis or previous pelvic inflammatory disease.

Look for: Position (important to know for practical procedures); mobility (especially if retroverted); size (including fibroids); tenderness (p. 126 & p. 134).

Adnexae These are the *fallopian tubes, ovaries*, and associated connective tissue (*parametria*). They are palpated bimanually in the lateral fornices, and if normal may not be felt. The ovaries are the size of a large grape and may lie in the rectovaginal pouch.

Look for: Masses (pp. 172–3) and tenderness (p. 134, pp. 140–1).

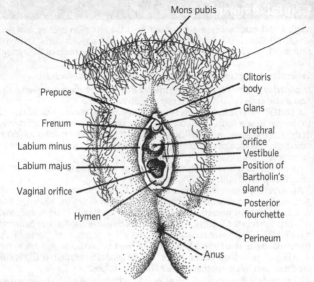

Fig 2.2 Gynaecological anatomy.

Labels (top to bottom, clockwise):
- Mons pubis
- Clitoris body
- Glans
- Urethral orifice
- Vestibule
- Position of Bartholin's gland
- Posterior fourchette
- Perineum
- Anus
- Hymen
- Vaginal orifice
- Labium majus
- Labium minus
- Frenum
- Prepuce

Clinically useful anatomy

The abdominal wall below the arcuate line (ie where an incision for cae-sarean section is made) consists of skin, subcutaneous fat containing Camper's and Scarpa's fascias, anterior layer of rectus sheath (made from aponeuroses of external and internal oblique and tranversus), pyramidalis in some, the rectus muscle (posterior wall of rectus sheath is absent below ar-cuate line), and then the peritoneum. The pudendal nerve (s2-4) supplies sen-sation to the perineum, and motor supply to the external anal sphincter and urethral sphincter. The inferior epigastric artery is a branch of the external iliac artery, and is seen between the insertion of the round ligament and the obliterated umbilical artery—lateral ports for laparoscopy are carefully placed to avoid these. The umbilicus is at the level of the junction between L3 and L4 (dermatome T10); the aorta bifurcates at L4; the ureter lies under the uterine artery (water under the bridge).

Vagina and uterus These are derived from the Müllerian duct system and urogenital sinus and formed by fusion of the right and left parts. Different degrees of failure to fuse lead to duplication of any or all parts of the system (fig 2.3).

Vaginal septa are quite common (and often missed on examination).

Duplication of the cervix and/or uterus may also be missed, eg until the woman becomes pregnant in the uterus without the IUCD!

A partially divided (*bicornuate*) uterus or a uterus where one side has failed to develop (*unicornuate*) may present as recurrent miscarriage, particularly in the 2nd trimester, or as difficulties in labour. Such abnormalities are diagnosed by *hysterosalpingogram, ultrasound/MRI, or on hysteroscopy and/or laparoscopy.*

An absent uterus or a rudimentary uterus with absent endometrium is rare. They present with primary amenorrhoea.

An absent or short vagina is uncommon but can be corrected by plastic surgery. The membrane at the mouth of the vagina where the Müllerian and urogenital systems fuse (the hymen) may be imperforate. There is apparent primary amenorrhoea, with a history of monthly lower abdominal pain and swelling, and the membrane bulging under the pressure of dammed up menstrual blood (haematocolpos). It is relieved by a cruciate incision in the membrane. NB: in some communities, female genital mutilation (p. 111) is still practised, and this is another cause of haematocolpos.

▶Renal system abnormalities often coexist with genital ones, so IVU and US should be considered.

Ovary Thin, rudimentary 'streak' ovaries are found in Turner syndrome (p. 859). Ovaries are absent in testicular feminization syndrome, but primitive testes are present. Remnants of developmental tissue (eg the Wolffian system) may result in cysts around the ovary, broad ligament, and vagina.

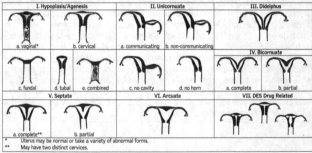

Fig 2.3 ASRM classification of uterine anomalies.

Reprinted by permission from the American Society for Reproductive Medicine (*Fertility and Sterility*, 1988, 49(6), pp.944–55).

Female genital mutilation (FGM), circumcision, or cutting, is the removal or partial removal of external female genitalia or injury to other internal female genital organs, for cultural or non-therapeutic reasons. It is illegal in the UK under the 2003 Female Genital Mutilation Act and more recently has been openly recognized as a form of child abuse. 140 million women are believed to be affected (2 million/year). It is traditionally practised mainly in Africa, but also in some parts of India and Indonesia. In the UK, most affected women come from Somalia, Sudan, Kenya, Eritrea, Ethiopia, and the Yemen. It is common in Mali, Guinea, and Egypt. It is not limited to any particular cultural or religious group. The type of mutilation varies between countries, with 90% types I, II, and IV and the remaining 10% type III (see BOX 'Summary of WHO classification of types of FGM').

Summary of WHO classification of types of FGM

Type I Partial or total removal of the clitoris and/or prepuce (clitoroidectomy).

Type II Partial or total removal of the clitoris and labia minora, with or without excision of the labia majora.

Type III Narrowing of the vaginal orifice with the creation of a covering seal by cutting and appositioning of the labia minora and/or the labia majora, with or without excision of the clitoris (infibulation).

Type IV Any other harmful procedures to the female genitalia for non-medical purposes eg pricking, piercing, cauterization, incising, and scraping.

Reprinted with permission from *Classification of female genital mutilation* 2008, WHO, Copyright 2008. https://www.who.int/reproductivehealth/topics/fgm/overview/en/

When talking to women about FGM, it is important to remember that they did not choose it. It occurred in childhood when they were too young to consent, often in a society where the practice is traditional and may be viewed as normal, even by themselves. Where FGM is illegal, families may seek a traditional circumciser, take the girl 'on holiday', or try and approach a healthcare worker. It is illegal in the UK to undertake or assist with FGM, as well as re-infibulation. There is also a duty of child safeguarding. ▶New cases in those <18yrs (eg divulged or observed) must be reported to the police. Suspected cases and those considered at high risk should be discussed via local safeguarding procedures. Social expectations are changing in countries that practise 'cutting' but parents believe the social harm of not cutting is greater than the physical, psychological, and legal risk of doing so.

Acute complications Include death, blood loss, sepsis, pain, urinary retention, tetanus, hepatitis, and HIV. It is carried out in unhygienic conditions, by a traditional circumciser, birth attendant, or midwife, usually using no anaesthesia and shared blades. **Long-term sequelae** Include apareunia, superficial dyspareunia, anorgasmia, sexual dysfunction, chronic pain, keloid scar, very slow urination, urinary tract infections, haematocolpos, subfertility, increased susceptibility to HIV and other blood-borne diseases, as well as emotional trauma. Maternal consequences include fear of childbirth, increased risk of cs, postpartum haemorrhage, episiotomy, severe vaginal lacerations and fistula, and difficulty in examining and catheterization.

Management Defibulation may be performed before marriage, antenatally, or in the 1st stage of labour. If not corrected antenatally, deliver in a unit with emergency obstetric care, having planned labour after expert advice. If vaginal examination is poorly tolerated, or anterior episiotomy anticipated, offer epidural. Women with FGM should be screened for hepatitis C. Repair post delivery should control bleeding but re-infibulation is illegal, and must not result in a vaginal opening making intercourse difficult or impossible. In 2003–2005, female genital cutting affected 1.4% of UK maternities and was implicated in 4 maternal deaths.[1]

Further reading

RCOG (2015). *Female Genital Mutilation and its Management* (Green-top Guideline No. 53). London: RCOG.

Puberty The development of adult sexual characteristics. The sequence: breast buds→growth of pubic hair→axillary hair→menses begin (*menarche*) from ~10yrs onwards (mean ~12.7yrs and falling—earlier if low birth weight; African; short & overweight in childhood; urban environment; various fascinating pheromone-related family events mediating anti-inbreeding strategies).[2]

Investigate if no periods by ~16yrs (p. 114) or no signs of puberty by 14. A growth spurt is the 1st change in puberty and is usually completed 2yrs after menarche when the epiphyses fuse.

The menstrual cycle (fig 2.4) The cycle is controlled by the 'hypothalamic-pituitary–ovarian' (HPO) axis. Pulsatile production of gonadotrophin-releasing hormones (GnRHs) by the hypothalamus stimulates the pituitary to produce the gonadotrophins: follicle-stimulating hormone (FSH) and luteinizing hormone (LH). These stimulate the ovary to produce oestrogen and progesterone. The ovarian hormones modulate the production of gonadotrophins by feeding back on the hypothalamus and pituitary.

Day 1 of the cycle is the 1st day of menstruation. Cycle lengths vary greatly (eg 20–45 days in adolescence); only 12% are 28 days. Cycles soon after menarche and before the menopause are most likely to be irregular and anovulatory. In the 1st 4 days of the cycle, FSH levels are high, stimulating the development of a primary follicle in the ovary. The follicle produces oestrogen, which stimulates the development of a glandular 'proliferative' endometrium and of cervical mucus which is receptive to sperm. The mucus becomes clear and stringy (like raw egg white) and if allowed to dry on a slide produces 'ferning patterns' due to its high salt content. Oestrogen also controls FSH and LH output by positive and negative feedback.

14 days before the onset of menstruation (on the 16th day of the cycle of a 30-day cycle) the oestrogen level becomes high enough to stimulate a surge of LH. This stimulates ovulation. Having released the ovum, the primary follicle then forms a corpus luteum and starts to produce progesterone. Under this influence, the endometrial lining is prepared for implantation: glands become convoluted ('secretory phase'). The cervical mucus becomes viscid and hostile to sperm and no longer ferns. If the ovum is not fertilized the corpus luteum breaks down, so hormone levels fall. This causes the spiral arteries in the uterine endothelial lining to constrict and the lining sloughs—hence menstruation.

Menstruation The loss of blood and uterine epithelial slough; it lasts 2–7 days and is usually heaviest at the beginning. Normal loss is 20–80mL (median 28mL). In practical terms, menstrual loss is not measured unless for research purposes. For reference, a normal-sized tampon or sanitary towel holds 5mL blood. For menorrhagia, see p. 117.

Menopause The ovaries fail to develop follicles. Without hormonal feedback from the ovary, gonadotrophin levels rise. Periods cease (menopause), usually at ~52 years of age in the UK (p. 120-1).

Postponing menstruation (eg on holiday) Try **medroxyprogesterone** 10mg BD from 3 days before the period is due until bleeding is acceptable, or **norethisterone** 5mg TDS from 3 days before, or if taking the combined pill, take 2 packets consecutively without a break.

2 *The socioendocrinology of family life:* presence in the household of the biological father *delays* sexual maturation—as does having a sister at home (esp. an elder sister). Brothers have no influence, but half- or step-brothers at home are associated with an *earlier* menarche. In addition, stressful life events such as immigration for adoption are associated with early menarche (risk of precocious puberty ↑×20, p. 254).

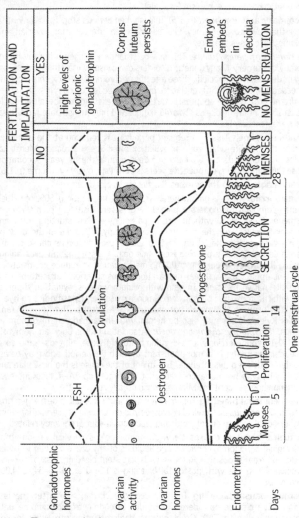

Fig 2.4 The menstrual cycle.

Primary amenorrhoea (p. 145) This is failure to start menstruating. It needs investigation in a 16-year-old, or in a 14-year-old who has no signs of puberty. For normal menstruation to occur she must be structurally normal with a functioning control mechanism (HPO axis).

Secondary amenorrhoea (p. 115) This is when periods stop for >6 months, other than due to pregnancy. HPO axis disorders are common, ovarian and endometrial causes are rare.

Ovarian insufficiency/failure: This may be secondary to chemotherapy, radiotherapy, or surgery. Many genetic disorders can cause ovarian follicle dysfunction or depletion—especially those affecting x chromosomes. 1 x chromosome is needed for ovarian differentiation, but 2 are needed by oocytes. In Turner syndrome (xo), oocyte apoptosis starts at 12 weeks and numbers deplete in the 1st 10yrs of life. Mosaics 45,xo/46,xx pp. 120–1 may menstruate for several years after menarche.

Oligomenorrhoea This is infrequent periods. It is common at the extremes of reproductive life when regular ovulation often does not occur. Menstrual cycles in adolescents are typically <45 days, even in the 1st year. A common cause throughout the reproductive years is polycystic ovary syndrome (p. 116).

Menorrhagia (p. 117) This is excessive menstrual blood loss.

Dysmenorrhoea This is painful periods (± nausea or vomiting). 50% of British women complain of moderate pain, 12% of severe disabling pain. *Primary dysmenorrhoea:* Pain without organ pathology—often starting with anovulatory cycles after the menarche. It is crampy with ache in the back or groin, worse during the 1st day or two. Excess prostaglandins cause painful uterine contractions, producing ischaemic pain. R: NSAIDs inhibit prostaglandins, eg **ibuprofen** 400mg/8h PO during menstruation to reduce contractions and hence pain. No particular preparation seems superior. Paracetamol is a good alternative to NSAIDs. In pain with ovulatory cycles, ovulation suppression with the combined pill can help. Smooth muscle antispasmodics eg **hyoscine butylbromide** (20mg/6h PO) give unreliable results. The Mirena® (and smaller Kyleena®) IUS may also be helpful with the added benefit of contraception. *Secondary dysmenorrhoea:* Associated pathology: adenomyosis (pp. 140–1), endometriosis, pelvic inflammatory disease, fibroids—and so it appears later in life. It is more constant through the period, and may be associated with deep dyspareunia. Treatment of the cause is the best plan and this may be with hormonal contraception or surgery pp. 176–7. IUCDs increase dysmenorrhoea, except the Mirena® which usually reduces it.

Intermenstrual bleeding This may follow a mid-cycle fall in oestrogen production. *Other causes:* Cervical polyps; ectropion; carcinoma; cervicitis/vaginitis; hormonal contraception (spotting); IUCD; chlamydia; pregnancy related.

Postcoital bleeding *Causes:* Cervical trauma; polyps; cervical, endometrial, and vaginal carcinoma; cervicitis and vaginitis of any cause. Screen for chlamydia and treat if positive. Refer all with persistent bleeding. Risk of cervical carcinoma in those with postcoital bleeding is 1:2400 aged 45–54; 1:44,000 aged 20–24.[3]

Postmenopausal bleeding This is bleeding occurring >1yr after the last period. ▶It must be considered to be due to endometrial carcinoma until proven otherwise (p. 170). *Other causes:* Vaginitis (often atrophic); foreign bodies, eg pessaries; carcinoma of cervix or vulva; endometrial or cervical polyps; oestrogen withdrawal (hormone replacement therapy or ovarian tumour). She may confuse urethral, vaginal, and rectal bleeding.

►*Always ask yourself 'Could she be pregnant?'* See *Pregnancy tests* (p. 6).

Primary amenorrhoea This may cause great anxiety. In most patients puberty is just late (often familial), and reassurance is all that is needed. In some, the cause is structural or genetic, so check:

• Has she got normal external secondary sexual characteristics? If so, are the internal genitalia normal (p. 110)—arrange transabdominal US to look for presence of uterus and ovaries (if virgo intacta do not examine internally).

• Causes can be the same as for secondary amenorrhoea: consider tests (see later in topic).

• If she is not developing normally, examination and karyotyping may reveal Turner syndrome (p. 859) or androgen insensitivity syndrome. The aim of treatment is to help the patient to look normal, to function sexually, and, if possible, to enable her to reproduce if she wishes.

Causes of secondary amenorrhoea

• *Hypothalamic–pituitary–ovarian causes:* Common (34% of cases) as control of the menstrual cycle is easily upset, eg by stress (emotions, exams), ↑ exercise, weight loss. Up to 44% of competitive athletes have amenorrhoea.

• *Hyperprolactinaemia:* (14%; 30% have galactorrhoea.) Other hormonal imbalances (hypo- or hyperthyroidism). Severe systemic disease, eg renal failure. Pituitary tumours and necrosis (Sheehan syndrome) are rare.

• *Ovarian causes:* Polycystic ovarian syndrome (p. 116) is common (28%); tumours; ovarian insufficiency/failure (premature menopause: the cause in 12%, it affects ~1% of women under 40).

• *Uterine causes:* Pregnancy related, Asherman syndrome (uterine adhesions after a D&C: consider also TB). 'Post-pill amenorrhoea' is generally oligomenorrhoea/secondary amenorrhoea masked by regular withdrawal bleeds so, if need be, investigate (see later).

Tests • βhCG (eg urinary) to exclude pregnancy • FSH/LH (low if hypothalamic–pituitary cause but may be normal if weight loss or excessive exercise the cause: raised eg FSH >20IU/L if premature menopause, in which case, if age <30 and concerns for future fertility, refer for karyotyping) • Prolactin (↑ by stress, hypothyroidism, prolactinomas, and drugs, eg phenothiazines, domperidone, metoclopramide). If level >1000IU/L do MRI scan. 40% of those with hyperprolactinaemia have a pituitary tumour • TFT (4% of women with amenorrhoea have abnormal thyroid function) • Testosterone level: levels >5nmol/L may indicate androgen secreting tumour or late-onset congenital adrenal hyperplasia so need more investigation, eg dehydroepiandrosterone sulfate level.

Treatment Related to cause. Premature ovarian failure cannot be reversed but hormone replacement (p. 144) is necessary to control symptoms of oestrogen deficiency and protect against osteoporosis. Pregnancy can be achieved with oocyte donation (not available on NHS) and IVF techniques.

Hypothalamic–pituitary axis malfunction: If mild (eg stress, moderate weight loss), there is sufficient activity to stimulate enough ovarian oestrogen to produce an endometrium (which will be shed after a progesterone challenge, eg **medroxyprogesterone acetate** 10mg/24h for 10 days), but the timing is disordered so cycles are not initiated. If the disorder is more severe the axis shuts down (eg in anorexia). FSH and LH and hence oestrogen levels are low. Reassurance and advice on diet or stress management, or psychiatric help if appropriate, and time may solve the problem. She should be advised to use contraception as ovulation may occur at any time. If she wants fertility restored now, or the reassurance of seeing a period, mild dysfunction will respond to clomifene but a shut-down axis will need stimulation by GnRH (see p. 144 for both).

PCOS comprises hyperandrogenism, oligomenorrhoea, and polycystic ovaries on US in the absence of other causes of polycystic ovaries eg as seen with later-onset adrenal hyperplasia and Cushing's. The cause is unknown. It is one of the most common endocrine disorders in women of childbearing age, affecting 5–20%. Many women are obese and it is associated with metabolic syndrome (hypertension, dyslipidaemia, insulin resistance, and visceral obesity) and there is an adverse cardiovascular risk profile with higher prevalence of type 2 diabetes and sleep apnoea. Darkened skin (acanthosis nigricans) on neck and skin flexures reflects hyperinsulinaemia.

Presentation Usually with oligomenorrhoea, with or without hirsutism, acne, and subfertility.

Diagnosis This is made using the Rotterdam criteria (2 out of 3 must be present):
- Polycystic ovaries (12 or more follicles or ovarian volume >10cm^3 on US).
- Oligo-ovulation or anovulation.
- Clinical and/or biochemical signs of hyperandrogenism.

Other causes of irregular cycles should be excluded before the diagnosis is made if there is clinical suspicion eg thyroid dysfunction, hyperprolactinaemia, congenital adrenal hyperplasia, androgen secreting tumours, and Cushing syndrome (*OHCM* p224). If clinically hyperandrogenic and total testosterone >5nmol/L check 17-hydroxyprogesterone and exclude androgen secreting tumours. LH is raised in 40%, testosterone in 30%.

Management *Weight loss* and exercise are the mainstay of treatment and increase insulin sensitivity. Advise smoking cessation. Treat diabetes, hypertension, dyslipidaemia, and sleep apnoea. *Metformin* improves insulin sensitivity in the short term and may improve menstrual disturbance and ovulatory function but does not have a significant impact on hirsutism or acne (it does not cause weight loss). It is not licensed for use in treating PCOS so the risks and benefits should be fully discussed. *Clomifene citrate* induces ovulation (50–60% conceive in 1st 6 months of treatment; but it should only be used by a specialist and in conjunction with fertility investigations, in women with a BMI <35 and for no more than 6 cycles). Risk of multiple pregnancy and ovarian cancer (pp. 174–5). Monitor response by US in at least 1st cycle. Women with PCOS are at ↑ risk of ovarian hyperstimulation (p.146) with assisted conception. *Ovarian drilling* (needlepoint diathermy to ovary with the intent of reducing steroid production) is recommended by NICE[4]~NICE~ for those not responding to clomifene (though it may be useful as primary treatment). 65% conceive. It does not increase risk of multiple pregnancy. Preterm birth, pre-eclampsia, gestational diabetes, and large babies are more common. The COCP (p. 152) will control bleeding and reduce risk of unopposed oestrogen on the endometrium (risk of endometrial carcinoma). Recommend *regular withdrawal bleeds* if not taking the pill eg 3-monthly, eg induced with **medroxyprogesterone** 10mg BD PO for 7–10 days in those in whom oestrogen use is not wanted or is contraindicated. *Hirsutism* may be treated cosmetically, or with an antiandrogen, eg **cyproterone** 2mg/day, as in co-cyprindiol, eg Dianette®. Depilatory creams, electrolysis, waxing, shaving, and laser help (laser is not funded by the NHS). Eflornithine facial cream is antiandrogenic and can also help with acne. **Spironolactone** 25–200mg/24h/PO (unlicensed use) is also antiandrogenic (avoid pregnancy as teratogenic).

Long-term consequences Gestational diabetes (screen in pregnancy at 24–28wks), type 2 diabetes (screen if overweight or other RF), cardiovascular disease, endometrial cancer (3–4-monthly withdrawal bleeds reduce risk). There is no ↑ risk of ovarian or breast cancer.

Further reading

RCOG (2014). *Long-term Consequences of Polycystic Ovarian Syndrome* (Green-top Guideline No. 33). London: RCOG.

2 Gynaecology

This is heavy menstrual bleeding (HMB) that interferes with quality of life. Historically it had been defined as menstrual blood loss >80mL/cycle but this is meaningless as it is impossible to measure unless in a research setting (or possibly a menstrual cup). What makes a woman consult may be a change in volume (clots, floods, etc.), or a worsening impact on her life. Ask about both. It is the most common gynaecological symptom.

Causes Most is due to dysfunctional uterine bleeding (DUB), which is heavy and/or irregular bleeding in the absence of recognizable pelvic pathology—this is a diagnosis of exclusion. Also: IUCD, fibroids, endometriosis and adenomyosis, pelvic infection, polyps, hypothyroidism, and coagulation disorders. With increasing age and RF, endometrial cancer.

Symptoms and signs Heavy, prolonged vaginal bleeding, often worse at the extremes of reproductive life, dysmenorrhoea, symptoms of anaemia, pallor. IMB and PCB are abnormal too and also need investigation—check smear history and rule out infection. An enlarged uterus suggests fibroids or adenomyosis, and speculum examination may reveal a cervical polyp.

Investigations Exclude pregnancy. FBC, haematinics if anaemic, TSH if clinically aneuthyroid, cervical smear if due, STI screen. Consider starting pharmacological treatment while awaiting investigations. If risk factors for endometrial cancer (obesity, PCOS, failed treatment) or history suggests endometrial pathology refer straight to 'see and treat' outpatient hysteroscopy. This involves use of tiny 3.5mm hysteroscopes (patient takes simple analgesia beforehand) to identify endometrial pathology and if possible, remove it and/or take biopsies. Ultrasound is 1st line in those with a pelvic mass, abdominally palpable uterus, obesity, dysmenorrhoea, suspected adenomyosis, or declining hysteroscopy. Do not obtain 'blind' endometrial biopsies for HMB—hysteroscope.

Medical management *Mirena®* IUS should be considered 1st-line treatment. It reduces bleeding (by up to 86% at 3 months, 97% at 1yr) and 30% are amenorrhoeic at 12 months. It releases levonorgestrel into the endometrial cavity, leading to atrophy. Side effects include irregular bleeding for the 1st 4–6 months and progestogenic effects. *Antifibrinolytics*—taken during bleeding, they reduce loss (by 49%)—eg **tranexamic acid** 1g/6–8h PO (for up to 4 days). CI: thromboembolic disease—but this is no more common in those on tranexamic acid. Useful in those trying to conceive as non-hormonal. *NSAIDs,* eg **ibuprofen** 400mg/8h PO pc (CI: peptic ulceration) taken during days of bleeding particularly help if there is also dysmenorrhoea. They reduce bleeding by 29%. The *COCP* is effective (20–30% reduction in blood loss and improvement in dysmenorrhoea) but see CI (p. 152). 3rd-line recommendation is *progestogens* IM (p. 156). **Medroxyprogesterone** 10mg/12h PO FOR 7–10 days to stop heavy bleeding in the short term. Rarely, *gonadotrophin-releasing hormone agonists* (GnRHa) are used in treating very anaemic women quickly but induce a temporary menopausal state (p. 138).

Surgery If fibroids >3cm diameter (see p. 138), or inadequate response to previous treatments, or declined medical management. *Endometrial ablation* (p. 177) involves destruction of the endometrium by microwave, thermal balloon, or electrical impedance. About 30% become amenorrhoeic and 80–90% of the remainder have reduced flow. Contraception is still required (risk of severe placentation problems therefore must have completed family). Treat as with uterus for HRT (pp. 120–1). For women wishing to retain fertility who have fibroids >3cm consider *myomectomy* (p. 138).

Women not wishing to retain fertility and fibroids >3cm may benefit from *hysterectomy* (p. 176).

Further reading

NICE (2018). *Heavy Menstrual Bleeding: Assessment and Management* (NG88). London: NICE.

2 Gynaecology

PMS is common and about 40% of women experience symptoms, with 5–8% of these being affected severely. Symptoms tend to be worse in those who are obese, perform less exercise, and have lower academic achievement. Incidence is lower in those on hormonal contraception.

Causes See BOX 'Classification of PMS and aetiology'.

Definition A condition which manifests with distressing physical, behavioural, and psychological symptoms in the absence of organic or psychiatric disease, regularly occurring during the luteal phase of the menstrual cycle and with significant improvement by the end of menstruation. The timing of symptoms and degree of impact on daily activity supports a diagnosis of PMS.

Symptoms Mood swings, irritability, depression; bloating and breast tenderness; headache; reduced visuospatial ability, increase in accidents. Almost any symptom may feature.

Diagnosis Use symptom diary filled in over 2 prospective cycles (eg Daily Record of Severity of Problems)—recall of symptoms retrospectively is unreliable. This should be completed before starting any treatment.

Treatment
- General health measures regarding increasing exercise, improving diet, stress reduction, smoking cessation, and weight loss should be addressed.
- Symptom diaries should be used to assess the effect of treatment.
- When simple measures have failed, consider referral to a gynaecologist, who may also involve a psychiatrist and dietician.

1st line: Exercise, cognitive behavioural therapy (CBT), **pyridoxine (vitamin B6)** 10mg/24h (unlicensed use) PO; combined pill containing drospirenone continuously or cyclically; luteal-phase or continuous low-dose SSRI with newer agents eg **citalopram** 10mg. CBT has been shown to be as effective as an SSRI, with effects possibly lasting longer when assessed at 12 months and should be considered routinely. *2nd line:* **Estradiol patches** (100mcg) + lowest possible dose of micronized progesterone (cg **Utrogestan®** 100mg PO/PV day 17–28 or Mirena®). Micronized progesterone should be considered 1st line for opposition as less likely to cause PMS-like SE. The Mirena® can cause PMS-type SE and women should be counselled accordingly. Higher-dose SSRIs continuously or luteal-phase eg **citalopram** 20–40mg. *3rd line:* (Specialist only)GnRH analogues (+ addback HRT if >6 months eg **goserelin** 3.6mg sc every 28 days with **tibolone** 2.5mg PO daily or **estradiol patch** 50–100mg + **micronized progesterone** 100mg/day). These are highly effective at treating severe PMS symptoms, and adding tibolone or continuous combined HRT ameliorates bone thinning from GnRH agonists. If long-term treatment, organize yearly DXA scan and stop if bone density falls significantly. *4th line:* Total hysterectomy plus bilateral salpingo-oophorectomy (laparoscopic because recovery is quicker than with abdominal hysterectomy) with HRT. This should not be carried out without preoperative GnRH agonist to ensure PMS is cured and HRT tolerated. *Physical symptoms:* Treat with spironolactone (teratogenic; steroid receptor antagonist and improves mood as well; unlicensed so specialist prescription only). *Pregnancy* will relieve symptoms and therefore drug treatment should stop. *Complementary therapies* may be of benefit, but studies are often small and under-powered and remedies are not licensed for use in treating PMS. Having said that, most women benefit from an integrated approach, but access to alternative therapies is not funded on the NHS. The best evidence exists for calcium with vitamin D, magnesium, and *Agnus castus*. Interestingly, there is no evidence for the benefit of vitamin B6. Evening primrose oil may benefit those with mastalgia but not for other PMS symptoms.

Further reading
RCOG (2016). *Management of Premenstrual Syndrome* (Green-top Guideline No. 48). London: RCOG.

Classification (from the ISPMD consensus)[5]

Core premenstrual disorders (PMDS) are the most common. Symptoms must be severe enough to affect ability to function eg at work, school, or in a relationship. Symptoms are varied and non-specific, recurring in ovulatory cycles. They must be present in the luteal phase and cease with menstruation. Symptoms can be predominantly somatic, psychological, or a mixture.

Variant PMDS do not fit the criteria for core PMDS and fit into four subtypes:
• Premenstrual exacerbation of an underlying disorder eg diabetes, migraine, epilepsy.
• Non-ovulatory PMDS occur when there is ovarian activity without ovulation but is poorly understood with lacking evidence.
• Progestogen-induced PMDS are from exogenous progestogens present in HRT and the COCP. These women may be particularly sensitive to progestogens.
• PMDS with absent menstruation occur in those with a functional ovarian cycle but do not menstruate due to hysterectomy, an IUS, or endometrial ablation.

Aetiology
PMS is intrinsically linked to the ovarian cycle, evidenced from a lack of symptoms before puberty, during pregnancy, and after the menopause.
   Some physiological and pharmacological observations:[6,7]
• Serum concentrations of circulating oestrogen and progesterone are the same in those with and without PMS—suggesting that some women are especially 'sensitive' to progesterone.
• Artificially altering circulating progesterone and oestradiol (estradiol) does not induce premenstrual symptoms in previously well women—only in those already prone to PMS.
• Studies with psychoactive compounds suggest that the key events are occurring in the brain, not the ovary—eg an abnormal CNS response to normal progesterone excursions occurring in the luteal phase.
• Serotonin and GABA seem to be implicated and serotonin receptors are responsive to both oestrogen and progesterone.
• GABA levels can be altered by allopregnanolone (a metabolite of progesterone) and in women with PMS, allopregnanolone levels are reduced.
• This may explain why SSRIS are an effective treatment for PMS.

2 Gynaecology

The menopause is the time of waning fertility leading up to the last period. It is a retrospective diagnosis, having said to have occurred 12 months after the last period. Average age in the UK is 52yrs. Although it causes symptoms, it is not a disease, and part of a natural process. As far as we know, only killer whales, short-finned pilot whales, and humans go through the menopause. Problems are related to falling oestrogen levels:

- Menstrual irregularity as cycles become anovulatory, before stopping.
- Vasomotor disturbance—sweats, palpitations, and flushes (brief, nasty, and may occur every few minutes for >10yrs, disrupting life and sleep).
- Atrophy of oestrogen-dependent tissues (genitalia, breasts) and skin. Vaginal dryness can lead to vaginal and urinary infection, dyspareunia, traumatic bleeding, stress incontinence, and prolapse.
- Osteoporosis: the menopause accelerates bone loss which predisposes to fracture of femur neck, radius, and vertebrae in later life.

Management ≥20% of women seek medical help.

- Is it the menopause? Thyroid and psychiatric problems may present similarly. 2 consecutive FSH levels >30IU/L is suggestive of menopause but NICE does not recommend testing—levels vary and it is unreliable if taking hormones.
- Diet and exercise can help relieve symptoms.
- Menorrhagia responds to Mirena® coil. Consider referral for hysteroscopy if symptoms suggest endometrial pathology (p253).
- Use contraception until >1yr amenorrhoea if >50yrs; 2yrs if <50yrs (see later).
- Vaginal dryness responds to oestrogen eg **oestrogen cream** 0.1% PV every night for 2 weeks, and twice per week thereafter as required (may be used indefinitely).

Hormone replacement therapy (HRT) There are many preparations of HRT, consisting of different strengths, hormones, routes of administration, and combinations. It can be given systemically (eg tablets or patches) or locally (oestrogen creams). The first thing to establish is the presence or absence of a uterus: those with a uterus should be given combined HRT; those without can have oestrogen only. Use of unopposed oestrogens is a major risk factor for developing endometrial cancer and should therefore be avoided.

- Use oestrogen-only HRT in women without a uterus.
- Use oestrogen plus progestogen HRT in women with a uterus:
  - Use oestrogen and cyclical progestogen in women who are still having periods, or who are within 12 months of a period. This usually results in regular withdrawal bleeding.
  - Use continuous-combined HRT in postmenopausal women eg Kliofem®, **estradiol** 2mg and **norethisterone** 1mg. Oestrogen can be administered orally, transdermally, subcutaneously, and vaginally.
- Progestogens can be administered orally, transdermally, and via the intrauterine system (Mirena®).

Contraception ▶HRT does not provide contraception and a woman is considered potentially fertile until 2yrs after her LMP if <50yrs, and for 1yr if >50yrs. If any potentially fertile woman needs HRT, contraception is required (condoms, or POP plus combined sequential HRT, or Mirena® plus oestrogen-only HRT).[8]

HRT contraindications: • Oestrogen-dependent cancer • Past pulmonary embolus • Undiagnosed PV bleeding • LFT↑ • Pregnancy • Breastfeeding • Phlebitis. Avoid or monitor closely in Dubin–Johnson/Rotor syndromes (*OHCM* p698). If past spontaneous DVT/PE: is there thrombophilia (*OHCM* p374)?

Side effects: Fluid retention, bloating, breast tenderness, nausea, headaches, leg cramps, and dyspepsia. Mood swings, depression, acne, and backache are thought to be due to progestogens. Irregular breakthrough bleeding on combined HRT may need further investigation.

Annual check-up: Breasts; BP (stop if BP >160/100mmHg pending investigation and treatment). Weight; any abnormal bleeding?

Alternatives to HRT SSRIs can help treat vasomotor symptoms (clonidine used to be the mainstay for this but its effect is limited). Osteoporosis should be treated with calcium and vitamin D, bisphosphonates, or selective oestrogen receptor modulators (SERMS); HRT should not be used 1st line for osteoporosis unless menopausal symptoms need to be treated. If vaginal dryness is the most prominent symptom, local treatment with vaginal oestrogen eg Vagifem® helps and does not require systemic progestogens; if local treatment with vaginal oestrogens is contraindicated or the woman wishes to avoid hormones, try lubricants (eg Replens®); for improvement in dryness; for sexual intercourse, use a lubricant containing silicone eg Yes® or Astraglide® (water-based lubricants are absorbed too quickly).

Benefits of HRT
- Reduction of vasomotor symptoms is brought about by oestrogen, and improvement is usually evident by 4 weeks and maximum effect by 3 months. HRT should be continued for at least 1 year to minimize symptom recurrence.
- Improvement in urogenital symptoms and sexual function via systemic or vaginal oestrogens may take several months and needs to be long term.
- Osteoporotic fractures are reduced but studies suggest that treatment needs to be lifelong and sustained for HRT to be an effective treatment.
- Reduced risk of colorectal cancer by about a third (but prevention of colorectal cancer is not an indication for HRT).

Risks of HRT
- Breast cancer risk is increased by 2.3% per year and risk is dependent on duration of HRT. 5 years after stopping, risk returns to that of a woman who has never had HRT. The risk is also dependent on the regimen used and is greatest with oral combined oestrogen–progestogen therapy. Combined HRT probably leads to 3 extra cases of breast cancer per 1000 women who start at age 50 and continue for 5 years. This effect is not seen in those who start HRT for premature menopause. Transdermal oestrogen with Mirena® or Utrogestan® is thought to confer lowest risk of both breast cancer and VTE; oestrogen alone in those without a uterus lowest risk of all.
- Unopposed oestrogens increase risk of endometrial cancer (RR 2.3); this remains for 5 or more years after stopping.
- HRT more than doubles risk of VTE, but the absolute risk remains small. It is most likely to occur in the 1st year of taking HRT and risk is lower with transdermal preparations compared with oral. Risk also increases with age; the number of additional VTE events in healthy women on HRT >5 years is 4:1000 women aged 50–59 years, and 9:1000 women aged 60–69 years.

Uncertainties concerning HRT: Include its role in cardiovascular disease, dementia, and ovarian cancer. Women in the Women's Health Initiative study who started HRT within 10 years of the menopause had a lower risk of coronary heart disease than those starting later. Oestrogen may delay or reduce onset of Alzheimer disease, but has no effect once the disease has become apparent. Unopposed oestrogens seem to increase the risk of ovarian cancer in the long term, but this is unresolved and not seen with continuous combined therapy.

Recommendations for use
- Consider diet, exercise, and local treatments before systemic therapy.
- Starting HRT close to the menopause is safer than waiting 5 or 10 years.
- Discuss the benefits and risks of HRT with each patient.
- Encourage breast awareness and to report breast change. Attend breast screening.
- Use the lowest effective dose, for the shortest time possible.
- Be wary about HRT in those with a family history of breast cancer.

Further reading
NICE (2015). *Clinical Knowledge Summaries: Menopause.* http://cks.nice.org.uk/menopause

Incidence Worldwide, >20% of pregnancies are terminated and in the UK ⅓ of women have had a TOP by age 45. 190,000 TOP/yr in England.

Legal (GB) constraints The Abortion Act 1967 (amended 2002) and Human Fertilisation and Embryology Act 1990 allow termination if:

(a) that the pregnancy has not exceeded its 24th week and that the continuance of the pregnancy would involve risk, greater than if the pregnancy were terminated, of injury to the physical or mental health of the pregnant woman or any existing children of her family; or

(b)* that the termination is necessary to prevent grave permanent injury to the physical or mental health of the pregnant woman; or

(c)* that the continuance of the pregnancy would involve risk to the life of the pregnant woman, greater than if the pregnancy were terminated; or

(d)* that there is a substantial risk that if the child were born it would suffer from such physical or mental abnormalities as to be seriously handicapped.

*There is no time limit on the term of the pregnancies to which grounds (b)–(d) may apply.

At present, 2 doctors must sign certificate HSA1. If <16yrs try to get patient's consent to involve her parents or other adult. <1% of TOPs are done after 20 weeks, usually after amniocentesis, or when very young or menopausal mothers have concealed, or not recognized, pregnancy. TOPs after 24 weeks may only be carried out in NHS hospitals. Evidence suggests that women undergoing TOP are no more or less likely to suffer psychological sequelae than if they continued the pregnancy.

Before TOP
- Offer counselling and support with both verbal and written information.
- US to confirm gestation and identify non-viable or ectopic pregnancies.
- Screen for chlamydia ± other STIs.
- Give antibiotic prophylaxis to reduce postoperative infection rate (10% without) eg **metronidazole** 1g PR/800mg PO at TOP and **azithromycin** 1g PO same day.
- Discuss contraception (IUCD or sterilization at operation needs planning).
- If RhD–ve she needs anti-D (all gestations, whatever method see BOX 'Using anti-D immunoglobulin', p. 11). Bloods for HB, ABO + RhD group and antibodies; ± HIV, hepatitis B & C, and haemoglobinopathies, if relevant.

Methods Depends on gestation of pregnancy and the woman's choice, as well as which resources are available locally.

Medical termination: Uses the antiprogestogen mifepristone, followed by a prostaglandin eg misoprostol. For doses see BOX 'Regimens for terminating intrauterine pregnancies'. It is highly effective from ≥6 weeks (98% effective at ≤7 weeks, 95% for weeks 7–9) and is also used for 2nd-trimester terminations. Misoprostol can be used orally or vaginally and can now be taken at home. 5% will need surgical evacuation. Give NSAID pain relief; opiate analgesia may also be needed, especially if gestation >13 weeks (not suitable for home TOP in 2nd trimester due to risk of heavy bleeding and pain). *Surgical termination:* (Suction or dilatation and evacuation.) Consider need for preoperative cervical preparation to reduce difficulty with cervical dilatation (particularly gestation >10 weeks, women <18 years of age) in all women, eg with **misoprostol** 400mcg PV 3h or PO 2–3h preoperatively. Osmotic dilators provide superior dilatation from 14 weeks, but misoprostol can be used up to 18 weeks. Surgical TOP >13 weeks requires skilled practitioners; there is a greater risk of bleeding, incomplete evacuation, and perforation. Offer NSAID pain relief during TOP (paracetamol is ineffective). Bleeding and pain is less than with medical termination. *Vacuum aspiration:* Used from 7 to 14 weeks. Local anaesthesia or GA. If <7 weeks check for gestational sac in aspirate, follow-up with βhCG if not seen. Access to US is desirable. *Dilatation & evacuation:* Surgical forceps may be used at 13+0–24+0wks after cervical priming. Real-time US reduces uterine perforation rates and is recommended.

Early medical terminations ≤9 weeks' gestation

At ≤49 days' gestation use mifepristone 200mg PO + misoprostol 400mcg orally 24–48h later. At ≤63 days' gestation mifepristone 200mg PO + misoprostol 800mcg (4×200mcg tablets) PV/buccal or sublingual 24–48h later. For women at 50–63 days' gestation, if not successful 4h after misoprostol give a further 400mcg PO/PV (route depending on preference and amount of bleeding).

Medical terminations 9–13 weeks' gestation

Check local guidelines. Mifepristone 200mg PO + misoprostol 800mcg vaginally 36–48h later. A maximum of 4 further doses of misoprostol 400mcg may then be given 3-hourly PV/PO.

Medical terminations 13–24 weeks' gestation

Check local guidelines. Mifepristone 200mg PO followed 36–48h later by misoprostol 800mcg PV: then misoprostol 400mcg PV/PO every 3h to a maximum of 4 further doses. If abortion does not occur, mifepristone can be repeated 3h after the last dose of misoprostol and 12h later misoprostol recommenced. If there is clinical evidence that TOP is incomplete, surgical evacuation of the uterus will be needed.

Feticide

In terminations later than 21 weeks[+6] days (eg for abnormality, see p14) it is essential that the fetus is born dead (unless it is a lethal fetal abnormality). This may be achieved by use of 3mL intracardiac 15% **potassium chloride** (± anaesthetic and/or muscle relaxant instillation beforehand to abolish fetal movement. Confirm asystole with us. (Intra-amniotic digoxin is a less effective alternative requiring less expertise.) If born after 24 weeks the dead fetus is a stillbirth and needs registering (p. 79). If there are signs of life then a death certificate is required.[RCOG]

Complications of termination (terminology of risk)[3, 11][RCOG]

- Failed TOP (<1:100, medical TOP failure rate is higher than surgical.)
- Infection (~2:100); see 'Before TOP', p. 122.
- Haemorrhage (<1:1000) (4:1000 if at ≥20 weeks).
- Uterine perforation (1–4:1000), surgical terminations only.
- Uterine rupture (mid-trimester medical TOP): <4:1000.
- Cervical trauma (1:100). Risk less if early abortion: if experienced operator.
- Retained products of conception (1:100).

After termination

Has she had anti-D (p. 11)? (500IU if <20 weeks; 500IU +Kleihauer if later.) Is contraception arranged? (Can start pill same day. Advise that long-acting methods are more effective.) Give letter with sufficient information for practitioners elsewhere to manage complications. Give written and verbal information on symptoms to be expected, those requiring emergency care, and of symptoms of ongoing pregnancy. Give 24h telephone helpline number. Offer follow-up. Refer women requiring emotional support/at mental health risk. Women having medical terminations not confirmed as successful at time of procedure need follow-up to ensure no ongoing pregnancy (rate 0.5–1%). Misoprostol risks teratogenicity. Decision to arrange uterine surgical evacuation is made on clinical signs and symptoms.

Worldwide

It is estimated there are 210 million pregnancies at any one time, and 1 in 5 are terminated. Over three-quarters of women live in developing countries, where 97% of the estimated 20 million unsafe terminations are carried out. 68,000 women die annually after unsafe termination. Accessible contraception reduces need for termination. Legalization of termination reduces the number of unsafe terminations and subsequent maternal death.

3 *The language of risk*: 1:1–1:10 is very common; 1:10–1:100 is common; 1:100–1:1000 uncommon; 1:1000–1:10,000 is rare; < 1:10,000 is very rare.

Miscarriage is the loss of a pregnancy before 24 weeks' gestation. 15–20% of pregnancies miscarry, mostly in the 1st trimester. Most present with bleeding PV. Diagnosis may not be straightforward (consider ectopics p. 22): have a low threshold for doing an US. Pregnancy tests remain +ve for several days.

Management of early pregnancy bleeding Consider the following:

▶Is she haemodynamically shocked? There may be blood loss, or products of conception in the cervical canal (remove them with sponge forceps).

- Has pain and bleeding been worse than a period? Have products of conception been seen? (Clots may be mistaken for products.)
- Is uterine size appropriate for dates?
- Is she bleeding from a cervical lesion and not from within the uterus?
- For use of anti-D immunoglobulin in miscarriage see p. 11.

If symptoms are mild and the cervical os is closed it is a *threatened miscarriage*. 75% will settle. If symptoms are severe and the os is open it is likely to be an *inevitable miscarriage* or, if most of the products have already been passed, an *incomplete miscarriage*. If bleeding is profuse, consider **ergometrine** 0.5mg IM. If there is unacceptable pain or bleeding, or significant retained products on US, arrange surgical management of miscarriage (SMM, previously called evacuation of retained products of conception, ERPC).

Missed miscarriage: The fetus dies or never properly develops, but remains *in utero*. There may have been bleeding and/or pain or no symptoms, and the cervix is closed. Confirm with US: fetal pole ≥7mm with no fetal heart activity, or mean gestation sac diameter ≥25mm with no fetal pole or yolk sac. Mifepristone and misoprostol may be used as medical management of miscarriage. *Pregnancy of uncertain viability:* Intrauterine gestation sac <25mm with no fetal pole or yolk sac, or crown-rump length <7mm with no fetal heart activity. Arrange rescan in 10–14 days.

Expectant management: Appropriate if the woman is not bleeding heavily; effective for incomplete miscarriage but less so for missed miscarriage. Offer rescan in 2 weeks to ensure complete if there has been no significant bleeding. *Medical management:* Misoprostol either orally or vaginally (may need 2nd dose)—can be managed as out-patient. If 2nd trimester, use mifepristone (an antiprogestogen) to prime, and then 24–48h start misoprostol and admit. Bleeding may continue for 2 weeks following medical management. 80–90% successful in those <9 weeks gestation. Risk of heavy bleeding requiring urgent SMM. *Surgical management:* If heavy or persistent bleeding >2 weeks or patient choice. Suction evacuation is used, usually under GA and <13 weeks.

2nd (mid)-trimester miscarriage This may be due to mechanical causes, eg cervical weakness (rapid, painless delivery of a fetus), uterine abnormalities, chronic maternal disease (eg DM, SLE), infection (eg CMV p. 38), fetal cause or no cause identified. Cervical cerclage[12]_RCOG at ~14 weeks of pregnancy (eg if 3+ premature deliveries/mid-trimester losses, or previous loss/preterm delivery and US proven cervical shortening) may help. It is removed prior to labour. Mid-trimester loss should be investigated to ensure that any treatable factors are identified to reduce risk in the next pregnancy.

After a miscarriage ▶Miscarriage is a bereavement. Give the parents space to grieve, to ask why it happened, and if it will recur.[4] Offer follow-up.[13]_RCOG Fetal products should be incinerated but if the mother requests alternative disposal (to bury herself) respect her wishes. Give in opaque container.[14]_RCOG Most early pregnancy losses are due to aneuploidy and abnormal fetal development; 10% to maternal illness eg pyrexia. Most subsequent pregnancies are normal although at increased risk.

---

4 The Miscarriage Association can provide extra support: http://www.miscarriageassociation.org.uk

This is the loss of 3 or more consecutive pregnancies before 24 weeks' gestation with the same biological father. It affects 1% of women. Prognosis for future successful pregnancy is affected by the previous number of miscarriages, and maternal age. (Rates of miscarriage are greatest when maternal age is ≥35 years, and paternal age ≥40 years.) They may follow a successful birth and approximately half are unexplained.

Possible causes

Endocrine: Well-controlled endocrine disease (eg thyroid or DM) does not increase miscarriage risk, and neither does PCOS.

Infection: Bacterial vaginosis (p. 132) is associated with 2nd-trimester loss. Screening (and treatment) was previously recommended for those with previous mid-trimester miscarriage or preterm birth (benefit unproven).

Parental chromosome abnormality: 2–5%. It is usually a balanced reciprocal or Robertsonian translocation (p. 272). The parent is phenotypically normal but 50–75% of gametes will be unbalanced. Refer to a clinical geneticist. Genetic counselling offers prognosis for future pregnancy, familial chromosome studies, and appropriate advice for subsequent pregnancy. Pre-implantation genetic diagnosis (see BOX, 'Preimplantation genetic diagnosis', p. 17—involving *in vitro* fertilization) has lower rates of achieving healthy pregnancy outcome compared to natural conception (30% vs 50%).

Uterine abnormality: It is uncertain how much abnormality is associated with recurrent miscarriage or if hysteroscopic correction of abnormality contributes to successful pregnancy outcome, though septum division may help. Open uterine surgery increases chance of uterine rupture.

Antiphospholipid syndrome: Lupus anticoagulant, phospholipid, and anticardiolipin antibodies—these are present in 15% of women with recurrent miscarriage. Defined as presence of antibodies on 2 occasions plus 3 or more consecutive miscarriages <10 weeks, 1 fetal loss 10 weeks or older, or 1 or more births of a normal fetus >34/40 with severe pre-eclampsia or growth restriction. Give **aspirin** eg 75–150 mg/24h PO from the day of positive pregnancy test + LMWH, eg **enoxaparin** 40mg/24h SC[15] as soon as the fetal heart is seen (eg at 5 weeks on vaginal US) until delivery.[16] Get expert advice. Resulting pregnancies are at high risk of repeated miscarriage, pre-eclampsia, fetal growth restriction, and preterm birth so need special surveillance. Live birth rate is approximately 80%.

Thrombophilia: In those with inherited thrombophilia (eg factor V Leiden and prothrombin gene mutations, and protein C and S deficiency), heparin helps reduce risk of miscarriage.

Alloimmune causes: The theory is that these women share human leucocyte antigen (HLA) alleles with their partners and do not mount the satisfactory protective response to the fetus. Immunotherapy has not been found to increase live birth rate, is potentially dangerous, and should not be offered.

Recommendation[17]

- Offer referral to specialist recurrent miscarriage clinic.
- Test all women for antiphospholipid antibodies: positive if 2 tests +ve, taken 12 weeks apart.
- Thrombophilia screening.
- Pelvic US to assess uterus; further tests eg 3-D US/laparoscopy/hysteroscopy if anatomy abnormal.
- Karyotype fetal products (3rd and subsequent fetal losses). If an unbalanced chromosome abnormality is identified in the products of conception then karyotype the peripheral blood of both parents.

Further reading

RCOG (2011). *The Investigation and Treatment of Couples with Recurrent First-Trimester and Second-Trimester Miscarriage* (Green-top Guideline No. 17). London: RCOG.

The fertilized ovum implants outside the uterine cavity. The UK incidence is 11.1:1000 pregnancies and rising; worldwide rates are higher. ~7% of maternal deaths are due to ectopics (1.8 deaths/1000 ectopic pregnancies).

Predisposing factors Anything slowing the ovum's passage to the uterus increases risk: damage to the tubes (pelvic inflammatory disease; previous surgery); previous ectopic; endometriosis; IUCD; the POP (p. 156), subfertility and IVF (p.144), smoking. Pregnancy after tubal ligation is 9 times more likely to be ectopic.

Site 97% are tubal, mostly in ampulla; 25% in the narrow inextensible isthmus (presents early; risk of rupture ↑). 3% implant on ovary, cervix, caesarean section scar, or peritoneum.

Symptoms and signs ► Always think of an ectopic in a sexually active woman with abdominal pain; bleeding; fainting; or diarrhoea and vomiting.
• Often no symptoms or signs; uncertain LMP.
• Amenorrhoea 6–8 weeks.
• Pain; may be non-specific lower abdominal pain, but classically unilateral.
• Vaginal bleeding.
• Diarrhoea, loose stools, and/or vomiting.
• Dizziness.
• Shoulder tip pain from diaphragmatic irritation from haemoperitoneum.
• Collapse.
• Normal-sized uterus.
• Cervical excitation with or without adnexal tenderness.
• Rarely an adnexal mass.
• Peritonism.

Vaginal and speculum examinations do not rupture ectopic pregnancies! Failure to examine a woman with a suspected ectopic is indefensible.

Investigations Should include FBC, group and save (if unstable—cross match 6 units of blood, insert 2 large-bore IV cannulas, give IV fluids, and call senior help), serum progesterone to help identify a failing pregnancy, and hCG to guide management options. These hormones do not distinguish where the pregnancy is—only transvaginal ultrasound (TVS) can do that and is the primary diagnostic modality. US scan is looking for an adnexal mass which moves separately to the ovary if tubal. A further hCG in 48h may help decide management (see also 'Pregnancy of unknown location (PUL)', p. 127).

Management As long as the woman is stable, the woman should be offered the options of expectant and medical management according to strict selection criteria:
• Asymptomatic or mild symptoms.
• hCG <3000IU.
• Ectopic pregnancy <3cm on scan with no fetal heart activity.
• No haemoperitoneum on TVS.
• The woman must understand the diagnosis and risks of an ectopic pregnancy and must be willing to undertake regular follow-up and live close to the hospital with support at home.

Expectant: Falling hCG ideally <1500IU and the above-listed criteria; take serum hCG every 48h until confirmed fall, then weekly until <15IU. Plateauing or slowly rising hCG needs senior clinician involvement in the management plan.

Medical: Methotrexate (unlicensed use) is used (50mg/m² IM) as a single dose with the earlier-listed criteria, followed by hCG levels on days 4 and 7. If hCG has fallen by <15% a repeat dose is given (up to 25% cases). Methotrexate is teratogenic and the woman should use reliable contraception for 3 months afterwards. Side effects include conjunctivitis, stomatitis, diarrhoea, and abdominal pain. If the pain does not improve with simple analgesia she should come to hospital immediately. hCG level is not predictive of rupture, which may occur at any time.

Surgical: Laparoscopy is the preferred surgical treatment option due to reduced operating time, reduced length of hospital stay, reduced analgesia requirements, and less blood loss with a quicker recovery. Do not delay seeking senior help (registrar, consultant, and anaesthetist plus the senior ward nurse) in an unstable patient with a suspected ruptured ectopic pregnancy.
Salpingotomy vs salpingectomy: If the contralateral tube is healthy, RCOG guidelines recommend salpingectomy (removal of the tube) over salpingotomy (removal of the ectopic through a tubal incision). Subsequent intrauterine pregnancy rates are no different after salpingectomy, and salpingotomy has higher rates of persistent trophoblast (8% vs 4%) and subsequent ectopic pregnancy (18% vs 8%). Salpingotomy should be primary treatment if the other tube is not healthy to preserve chance of future intrauterine pregnancy (49%), but warn of risk of future ectopic pregnancy.[18][RCOG] Women with salpingotomy should be followed up with serum hCG to detect and treat persistent trophoblast early (methotrexate may be considered if the woman is stable). *Non-tubal ectopics:* Require multidisciplinary input.

Pregnancy of unknown location (PUL)

Definition There is no sign of intrauterine or ectopic pregnancy or retained products of conception in the presence of a positive pregnancy test, or serum hCG >5IU. Approximately 10% of attendances to the early pregnancy clinic are given this as their 1st diagnosis. The outcomes are as follows:
• Early intrauterine pregnancy (too early to see on scan).
• Complete miscarriage (no previous scan to prove that it was intrauterine).
• Failing PUL which will never be seen on scan but will resolve on its own.
• Ectopic pregnancy (10% of PULs).
• Persistent PUL.
• Extremely rarely, from an hCG-secreting tumour.
• History is unreliable in diagnosing location of pregnancy, and even if the history suggests complete miscarriage, classify it as a PUL until there is proof that it isn't.

Management Primarily according to symptoms because the most dangerous option for diagnosis is ectopic pregnancy. If the woman has significant pain and haemoperitoneum then laparoscopy is appropriate. If she is well with no haemoperitoneum, hCG and progesterone on the day of the 1st scan, followed by repeat 48h later and follow-up is appropriate. Check local guidelines but the following plan is reasonable:
• Progesterone <20nmol/L suggests failing pregnancy. If asymptomatic, repeat hCG in 7 days' time.
• hCG rise >66% in 48h: arrange a rescan when it is likely to be >1500IU or in 10–14 days' time.
• hCG rise <66% in 48h or plateau: monitor until <15IU, or consider rescan with more senior clinician to make diagnosis.
• hCG plateauing or fluctuating: senior advice after 2–3 serial hCGs. If asymptomatic can continue expectant management or offer methotrexate.

hCG levels and use in early pregnancy In a normal intrauterine pregnancy, hCG rises >66% every 48h. There is no hCG level that will correspond to weeks of gestation. The 'discriminatory zone' (the level at which a normal pregnancy should be visible on TVS) is not absolute and also relies upon experienced sonographers and quality of equipment. hCG should not be used in following up intrauterine pregnancies or women who are symptomatic—they should be managed clinically. It is unreliable in those who have multiple pregnancies and after assisted conception with hCG support.

Further reading
RCOG (2016). *Diagnosis and Management of Ectopic Pregnancy* (Green-top Guideline No. 21). London: RCOG.

2 Gynaecology

This comprises premalignant hydatidiform mole, and the malignant conditions of choriocarcinoma and the rare (0.23%) placental site trophoblastic tumour. Complete moles are diploid and androgenic, 75–80% following duplication of a single sperm after fertilization of an 'empty ovum', 20–25% after dispermic fertilization of an 'empty' ovum so no maternal nuclear DNA although mitochondrial DNA is maternal. Partial moles usually follow dispermic fertilization of an ovum and are triploid (2 sets paternal haploid genes, 1 haploid maternal set so 69 chromosomes rather than the usual 46) but 10% are tetraploid or mosaic conceptions. Partial moles usually have evidence of fetal parts or red cells. They are 3× commoner, grow slower (so present later), and are less often malignant (1% vs 15%).

Hydatidiform moles (fig 2.5) Tumours consist of proliferating chorionic villi which have swollen and degenerated. Derived from chorion, it makes lots of hCG, giving rise to exaggerated pregnancy symptoms and strongly +ve pregnancy tests. *Incidence:* 1.54:1000 pregnancies (UK). It is commoner at extremes of child-bearing age, after a previous mole, and in Asian women. A woman who has had a past mole is at ↑ risk for future pregnancies; 0.8–2.9% after one mole, and 15–28% after 2 moles. <1% have familial recurrent moles (recessive) with <1:50 chance of normal pregnancy.[iv] *Signs:* Most present with early pregnancy failure, eg failed miscarriage or signs on US. Bleeding may be heavy; molar tissue may look like frogspawn. US may show 'snowstorm

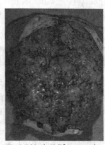

Fig 2.5 Hydatidiform mole.
Courtesy of Prof. J. Carter.

effect'. Severe morning sickness or 1st-trimester pre-eclampsia are rarer presentations. If twin pregnancy, proceed, if wished (40% viable baby outcome without ↑ persisting neoplasia or adverse treatment results).

Abdominal pain may be due to huge theca-lutein cysts in both ovaries. These may rupture or tort. They take ~4 months to resolve after molar evacuation. hCG resembles TSH, and may cause hyperthyroidism. ►Tell the anaesthetist as thyrotoxic storm can occur at evacuation. *Treatment:* Molar tissue is removed from the soft, easily perforated uterus by gentle suction. Send to histology for confirmation of diagnosis. Give anti-D if Rh−ve (see BOX 'Using anti-D immunoglobulin', p. 11). Pregnancy should be avoided until hCG normal for 6 months. Register the woman at specialist centre for hCG monitoring. Levels should return to normal within 6 months. If levels drop rapidly to normal, oral contraceptives may be used after 6 months. If they do not, either the mole was invasive (myometrium penetrated) or has given rise to choriocarcinoma (10%). Invasive moles may metastasize, eg to lung, vagina, brain, liver, and skin. Both conditions respond to chemotherapy. See BOX 'Indications for chemotherapy'.

Choriocarcinoma ►*Investigate all persistent post-pregnancy PV bleeding to exclude choriocarcinoma.* This highly malignant tumour occurs in 1:40,000 deliveries. The chief contexts are following a benign mole (50%), miscarriage (20%), or a normal pregnancy (10%). *Presentation: May be years after pregnancy,* with general malaise (due to 'malignancy' and ↑hCG) or uterine bleeding; signs and symptoms from metastases (may be very haemorrhagic, eg haematoperitoneum); nodules on CXR. Pulmonary artery obstruction via tumour emboli may cause pulmonary artery hypertension (haemoptysis; dyspnoea). *Treatment:* Choriocarcinoma in the UK is treated at 3 specialist centres; it is extremely responsive to combination chemotherapy based on methotrexate. Outlook is good if non-metastatic and fertility is usually retained.

Placental site trophoblastic tumour These grow slower, present later, produce less hCG. Post chemotherapy residual disease is excised (eg womb and nodes).

Indications for chemotherapy

- hCG ≥20,000 IU/L 4 weeks post evacuation.
- Static or rising hCG after evacuation in absence of new pregnancy.
- ↑hCG 6 months post evacuation, even if levels dropping.
- Heavy vaginal bleeding, or gastrointestinal or intraperitoneal bleeding.
- Evidence of brain, liver, or gastrointestinal metastases, or lung opacities >2cm (smaller lesions may regress spontaneously).
- Histology of choriocarcinoma.

Further reading

RCOG (2010). *The Management of Gestational Trophoblastic Neoplasia* (Green-top Guideline No. 38). London: RCOG.

Pruritus vulvae Genital itch is distressing and embarrassing. *Causes:* There may be a disorder causing general pruritus (pp. 436-7) or skin disease (eg psoriasis, lichen sclerosis). The cause may be local: infection and vaginal discharge (eg candida); allergy eg to washing powder, fabric dyes; infestation (eg scabies, pubic lice, threadworms); or vulval dystrophy (lichen sclerosis, leucoplakia, carcinoma). Psychosexual sequelae may ensue. Obesity and incontinence exacerbate symptoms. Postmenopausal atrophy does not cause itch.

The history may suggest the cause. Ask about autoimmune disorders and atopy. Examine general health and look for wider spread skin conditions. Examine the vulva and genital tract, under magnification if possible, and take a cervical smear, if due. Consider taking vaginal and vulval swabs and tests for diabetes and thyroid disease. If vulval dermatitis check serum ferritin and dermatology patch tests. Biopsy if diagnosis in doubt, if there is no response to treatment, or vulval intraepithelial neoplasia or carcinoma is suspected.

▶Scratching, self-medication, and the disease may have changed the appearance.

Treatment: This is often unsatisfactory. Treat the cause if possible. Avoid sensitizers (patch testing may reveal sensitizing agents eg 26–80% in vulval dermatitis studies). Reassurance can be very important. Vulval care advice (see BOX 'Vulval care'), may help. A short course of topical steroids, eg betamethasone valerate cream 0.1% may help. Avoid any topical preparation which may sensitize the skin.

Lichen sclerosis Thought to be an autoimmune disorder (40% develop other autoimmune disorders), elastic tissue turns to collagen (usually after middle age—or, occasionally, before puberty). The 'bruised' red, purpuric signs may appear, to the unknowing, to suggest abuse—particularly if there are bullae, erosions, and ulcerations. The vulva gradually becomes white, flat, and shiny. There may be an hourglass shape around the vulva and anus. It is intensely itchy. It may be premalignant and long-term surveillance is desirable if unresponsive to treatment. *Treatment:* Clobetasol propionate cream, eg Dermovate® daily for 28 days, then alternate days for 4 weeks, then twice weekly for 8 weeks, then as needed. The 4–10% who are steroid unresponsive may respond to topical tacrolimus (off licence, use in specialist clinic only, for <2 years). In children, 50% resolve by menarche.

Leucoplakia (White vulval patches due to skin thickening and hypertrophy.) It is itchy. It should be biopsied as it may be a premalignant lesion. *Treatment:* Topical corticosteroids (problems: mucosal thinning, absorption); psoralens with ultraviolet phototherapy; methotrexate; ciclosporin.

Lichen planus Of unknown cause, this is more likely to present with pain than itching (remember difference with lichen sclerosis by 'p for pain'). In mouth & genital area it can be erosive, appearing with a well-demarcated glazed appearance around the introitus. It can affect all ages.

Lichen simplex This presents with chronic intractable itching, especially at night, in those with sensitive skin or eczema. There is non-specific inflammation of vulva (± mons pubis and inner thighs). Stress, sensitizing chemicals, and low body iron stores can exacerbate symptoms. Treatment is with vulval care (see BOX 'Vulval care'), using steroids to break the itch/scratch cycle, if needed. Antihistamines or antipruritics (see earlier) can help.

Vulvovaginitis Think of fixed drug reactions (NSAIDs, statins); stop for 2 weeks. Desquamative inflammatory vaginitis, of unknown cause, characterized by shiny erythematous patches ± petechiae. It responds to 2–4 weeks of intravaginal clindamycin cream with hydrocortisone to the vulva.

2 Gynaecology

Vulval intraepithelial neoplasia

Vulval malignancy has a preinvasive phase, vulval intraepithelial neoplasia (VIN, fig 2.6, note white areas with surrounding inflammation). It may be itchy. **Cause** Often HPV, p. 162 (esp. HPV16); there may not be visible warts but 5% acetic acid stains affected areas white. If VIN is found on biopsy, examine cervix, anal canal if within 1.5cm,[20RCOG] natal cleft skin, and breasts (>10% have coexistent neoplasia elsewhere, most commonly cervical). **Treating VIN** Surveillance is the key with biopsy of suspicious lesions. Painful or irritating lesions can be removed but vulvectomy or laser ablation is not recommended as a general rule due to high recurrence rate and poor functional outcome. Histology reveals 12–17% unrecognized invasion in wide excision samples. Medical treatments have used 5% imiquimod cream with regression of grade 2–3 disease in 77% (it

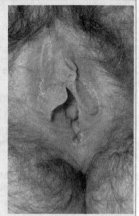

Fig 2.6 Vulval intraepithelial neoplasia (VIN).

is also used in the treatment of genital warts). It stimulates monocytes and macrophages, which secrete cytokines resulting in T-helper cell coordination of a cell-mediated immune response. Apply the cream 2–3 times per week for 12 weeks. Therapeutic use of human papilloma virus vaccine, photodynamic therapy, interferon use, and cavitron ultrasonic surgical aspiration techniques have been tried but none are currently recommended treatments.[21RCOG] Recurrence is common so follow-up regularly.

Vulval care for those with vulval disorders

- Use soap substitute with water for washing (eg aqueous cream, less drying than water alone).
- Shower, bath (with emollient), or clean vulva once daily only.
- Wash vulva with hand (not sponge/flannel); dab dry or blow dry with hairdryer on cool setting held well away from the skin.
- Wear loose-fitting silk or cotton white or light-coloured underwear (blue/black dyes can be irritant). Sleep without underwear.
- Avoid tight jeans/cycling trousers but wear loose trousers, dresses, or skirts. At home, wearing skirts without underwear may be more comfortable.
- Avoid soap, bubble bath, shower gels, biological washing powders, fabric conditioners, vulval creams or douches, antiseptics, regular sanitary towel or panty liner wear, baby wipe use, coloured toilet paper, & nail varnish.
- Also beware scented sanitary items.
- Regular emollient use (throughout day) can soothe and reduce flare ups.
- For irritated skin, dabbings of aqueous cream kept in the fridge can soothe.

Discharge may be physiological (eg pregnancy; sexual arousal; puberty; cocp).
Most discharges are smelly, itchy, and due to infection. Foul discharge may be
due to a foreign body (eg forgotten tampons, or beads in children). Note the
details of the discharge. Could it be a sexually transmitted disease (STD)? See
OHCM p412. If so, refer to a sexual health clinic. Do a speculum examination
and take swabs: vulvovaginal/endocervical samples for chlamydia and gonorrhoea. ►Discharges rarely resemble their classical descriptions.

Thrush (candidiasis)

The 2nd commonest cause of discharge (1st is bacterial vaginosis), 95% is due
to *C. albicans*, 5% *C. glabrata* (harder to treat). Vulva and vagina may be red,
fissured, and sore, especially if allergic component; discharge is non-offensive,
classically white curds. Her partner may be a carrier who is asymptomatic.
Pregnancy, contraceptive and other steroids, immunodeficiencies, antibiotics,
and diabetes are risk factors—check glucose. *Candida* elsewhere (eg mouth,
natal cleft) in both partners may cause reinfection. Thrush is not necessarily
sexually transmitted. *Diagnosis:* Microscopy (shows mycelia or spores) and culture. *Treatment:* Topical treatment (eg **clotrimazole** 500mg pessary + cream for
the vulva) gives similar cure rates to oral **fluconazole** 150mg PO as a single dose.
C. glabrata may require topical nystatin or 7–14-day course of an imidazole. Use
topical regimen alone if pregnant (7 day course[22]) or breastfeeding. Recurrent
infection may be treated by **fluconazole** 150mg PO every 72h for 3 doses.[23]

Trichomoniasis

Trichomonas vaginalis (TV; fig 2.7; sexually
transmitted) produces vaginitis and a bubbly,
thin, fish-smelling discharge. Cervix may have
'strawberry' appearance. Exclude gonorrhoea
(often coexists). Motile flagellates are seen on
wet films (×400), or cultured. *R:* (treat partner
too) **metronidazole** 2g PO stat or 400mg/12h PO
for 5 days (eg if pregnant).

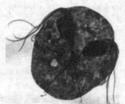

Fig 2.7 TV. © Prof S Upton;
Kansas Univ.

Bacterial vaginosis

Prevalence ~10% mostly asymptomatic. Any
discharge has a fishy odour, from cadaverine &
putrescine. Vaginal PH is >4.5. The vagina is not
inflamed and pruritus is uncommon. Mixed with
10% potassium hydroxide on a slide, a whiff of
ammonia may be detected. Stippled vaginal
epithelial 'clue cells' may be seen on wet microscopy (fig 2.8, top). There is altered bacterial
flora—overgrowth, eg of *Gardnerella vaginalis,*
Mycoplasma hominis, peptostreptococci,
Mobiluncus, and anaerobes, eg *Bacteroides*
species—with too few lactobacilli. There is ↑
risk of preterm labour, chorioamnionitis, susceptibility to HIV,[24] and post-termination sepsis.
Δ: By culture. *R:* **Metronidazole** 2g PO once, gel
PV, or **clindamycin** 2% vaginal cream, 1 appli-
cator full/night PV 7 times. If recurrent, treating
the partner may help. If pregnant, use **metronidazole** 400mg/12h PO for 5 days. Balance
Activ® vaginal acidic gel can be a useful (more
natural) alternative. Avoid douching—this
causes BV.

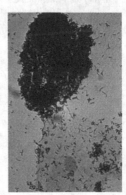

Fig 2.8 Clue cells.
Reproduced from Warrell, Cox,
et al., *The Oxford Textbook of
Medicine* (2010) with permission
from OUP.

2 Gynaecology

Discharge in children

May reflect infection from *faecal flora*, associated with alkalinity from lack of vaginal oestrogen (prepubertal atrophic vaginitis). *Staphs* and *streps*, as well as *scratching* may cause pus. *Threadworms* cause pruritus. Always consider *sexual abuse*.

Tests: Vulval ± vaginal swab (hard to know if result is normal flora). MSU: *is there glycosuria?* For prolonged or bloody discharge, examine under anaesthesia (paediatric laryngoscopes can serve as specula) ± US or x-rays.

Management: Discuss hygiene. If an antibiotic is needed, erythromycin is a good choice. An oestrogen cream may be tried (≤1cm strip).

Chlamydia

Chlamydia is the most common bacterial STI in the UK and is an important cause of tubal infertility. 70% cases are asymptomatic, but symptoms may include dysuria, vaginal discharge, and/or intermenstrual or postcoital bleeding. In the UK, the National Chlamydia Screening Programme tests over a million people per year, and has caused an estimated 20% drop in prevalence in those <25 years old. *Complications:* Include pelvic inflammatory disease (p. 134) in 10–40% of those infected, perihepatitis (Fitz-Hugh–Curtis syndrome) p. 134, reactive arthritis (a triad of arthritis, conjunctivitis, and urethritis is more common in men), tubal infertility, and increased risk of ectopic pregnancy. *Diagnosis:* Vulvovaginal or endocervical swab for nucleic acid amplification test (NAAT) using a special medium. Swabs may be self-taken. *Treatment:* GUM clinic referral advised. **Doxycycline** 100mg BD for 7 days (CI in pregnancy); if doxycycline contraindicated or not tolerated, **azithromycin** 1g stat followed by 500mg once daily on days 2 and 3 (resistance increasing). It is essential to treat partners and abstain from intercourse until this happens. Chlamydia in pregnancy is treated with azithromycin (see earlier) or **erythromycin** 500mg BD for 10–14 days, untreated, there is an increased risk of preterm rupture of membranes and premature delivery, and neonatal conjunctivitis and pneumonia.

Gonorrhoea

Full name *Neisseria gonorrhoeae*, a Gram –ve diplococcus. It is the 4th most common STI in the UK, and there is increasing antibiotic resistance. There are often no symptoms, but it may present with lower abdominal pain, vaginal discharge, & intermenstrual or postcoital bleeding. *Complications:* Include PID (10% of those infected), Bartholin's or Skene's abscess, tubal infertility, and increased risk of ectopic pregnancy. Disseminated gonorrhoea leads to fever, pustular rash, migratory polyarthralgia, and septic arthritis. *Diagnosis:* This is by vulvovaginal or endocervical swab for NAAT using a special medium. Swabs may be self-taken. Urethral, pharyngeal, and rectal swabs should be taken if appropriate. If NAAT +ve, take further swabs for culture for sensitivities prior to treatment due to high rates of antibiotic resistance (35% strains resistant to ciprofloxacin and 70% to tetracyclines). *Treatment:* (Refer to specialist sexual health clinic.) Treatment is with **ceftriaxone** 500mg IM stat. If this is unsuitable or unavailable, contact microbiology or sexual health clinic for advice. Treat partners and contact trace. Treatment is the same in pregnancy (untreated, gonorrhoea in pregnancy is associated with preterm rupture of membranes, preterm delivery, and chorioamnionitis, and to the baby, ophthalmia neonatorum).

Further reading

National Chlamydia Screening Programme: https://www.gov.uk/government/collections/national-chlamydia-screening-programme-ncsp

2 Gynaecology

Pelvic inflammatory disease (PID) is defined as infection of the upper genital tract. Many cases probably go undetected due to lack of symptoms, so prevalence is difficult to ascertain.

Causes
- Usually from ascending infection from the endocervix:
  - STIs.
  - Uterine instrumentation eg hysteroscopy, insertion of IUCD, TOP.
  - Postpartum.
- Can descend from other infected organs eg with appendicitis.
- 25% due to chlamydia and gonorrhoea.
- Remainder may be due to anaerobes and endogenous bacteria.

Age <25 years, previous history of STIs, and new or multiple sexual partners increase risk. Protective factors are use of barrier contraception, Mirena® IUS and the COCP.

History and examination The woman may give a history of lower abdominal pain which may be uni- or bilateral, which is constant or intermittent. There may be deep dyspareunia, vaginal discharge, intermenstrual or postcoital bleeding, dysmenorrhoea, and/or fever. On examination, vaginal discharge may be evident. There is cervical motion tenderness (cervical excitation) on vaginal examination, with or without adnexal tenderness. In mild or chronic PID she will be afebrile.

Investigations Take vulvovaginal/endocervical swabs for chlamydia and gonorrhoea, and MC&S. If the woman is acutely unwell, check FBC (elevated WCC) and CRP and take blood cultures if sepsis. If tubo-ovarian abscess is suspected, arrange TVS. Laparoscopy is not indicated unless diagnosis is uncertain eg right iliac fossa pain and possible appendicitis, drainage of tubo-ovarian abscess is required, or there is no response to treatment with IV antibiotics.

Complications
- Tubo-ovarian abscess.
- Fitz-Hugh–Curtis syndrome (liver capsule inflammation with perihepatic adhesions) (fig 2.9).
- Recurrent PID (can be instigated by gynaecological procedures).
- Ectopic pregnancy.
- Subfertility from tubal blockage (8% after 1 episode; 40% after 3 episodes).

Management ▶Prompt treatment and contact-tracing minimizes complications. Start treating with antibiotics before culture results are available. Well patients can be treated as outpatients and should be reviewed 72h later to check response. Admit for IV antibiotics if symptoms severe, there is sepsis, or symptoms fail to respond to oral treatment.

Outpatient management:
- **Ceftriaxone** 500mg IM stat or **azithromycin** 1g PO STAT, plus **doxycycline** 100mg PO BD for 14 days and **metronidazole** 400mg PO BD for 14 days.
- If gonorrhoea suspected, discuss with microbiologist due to high rates of antibiotic resistance.

Inpatient management:
- **Ceftriaxone** 2g IV OD plus **doxycycline** 100mg IV BD, followed by oral **doxycycline** 100mg BD for 14 days + **metronidazole** 400mg PO BD for 14 days.

Chronic PID Unresolved, unrecognized, or inadequately treated infection. Inflammation leads to fibrosis, so adhesions develop between pelvic organs. The tubes may be distended with pus (pyosalpinx) or fluid (hydrosalpinx).

Pelvic pain, menorrhagia, secondary dysmenorrhoea, discharge, and deep dyspareunia are some of the symptoms. Look for tubal masses, tenderness, and fixed retroverted uterus. Laparoscopy differentiates infection from endometriosis. Difficult to manage pain; antibiotics are generally not helpful.

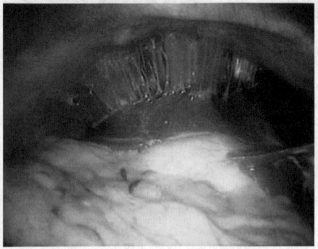

Fig 2.9 Laparoscopic view of perihepatic adhesions seen in Fitz-Hugh–Curtis syndrome.

Reproduced from Sarris *et al., Training in Obstetrics and Gynaecology* (2009) with permission from OUP.

Endometritis Uterine infection is uncommon unless the barrier to ascending infection (acid vaginal pH and cervical mucus) is broken eg after miscarriage, TOP and childbirth, IUCD insertion, or surgery. Infection may ascend further to involve fallopian tubes and ovaries. *Presentation:* Lower abdominal pain and fever; uterine tenderness on bimanual palpation, offensive vaginal discharge. *Tests:* Take high vaginal swabs and blood cultures if septic. Remove IUCD if not responding to antibiotics. *Treatment:* Give antibiotics (eg **cefalexin 500mg/8h** PO with **metronidazole** 400mg/8h PO for 7 days).

Endometrial proliferation Oestrogen stimulates endometrial proliferation in the 1st half of the menstrual cycle; it is then influenced by progesterone and is shed at menstruation. A particularly exuberant proliferation is associated with heavy menstrual bleeding and polyps.

Continuous high oestrogen levels (eg with obesity) make the endometrium hyperplastic (endometrial hyperplasia with or without atypia—a histological diagnosis after endometrial biopsy). It eventually breaks down, causing irregular heavy bleeding. *Treatment:* Address the cause; if no atypia on histology, treat with progestogens eg Mirena® coil and re-biopsy in 6–12 months. In older women proliferation may contain foci of atypical cells which may eventually lead to endometrial carcinoma (p. 170).

Pyometra This is a uterus distended by pus eg associated with salpingitis or secondary to outflow blockage. *Treatment:* Drain the uterus, treat the cause.

Haematometra This is a uterus filled with blood due to outflow obstruction. It is rare. The blockage may be an imperforate hymen in the young (p. 110); carcinoma; or iatrogenic cervical stenosis, eg after LLETZ.

Endometrial tuberculosis Genital tract tuberculosis is rare in Britain, except among high-risk groups (eg immigrants). It is blood-borne and usually affects first the fallopian tubes, then the endometrium.

It may present with acute salpingitis if disease is very active, or with subfertility, pelvic pain, and menstrual disorders (40%) eg amenorrhoea, oligomenorrhoea. There may be pyosalpinx. Send peritoneal fluid at laparoscopy, and/or endometrial curettings for culture and histology. Exclude lung disease by CXR. *Treatment:* Medical with antituberculous therapy (*OHCM* p394). Repeat endometrial histology after 1yr. Total abdominal hysterectomy with bilateral salpingo-oophorectomy is treatment of choice if there are adnexal masses and the woman is >40yrs.

Pelvic US Transvaginal US gives better resolution than transabdominal. Homogeneity, echoes of low intensity and presence of a linear central shadow are associated with absence of endometrial abnormality. *Normal cycle thickness:* <5mm early cycle, 11mm in proliferative phase; 7–16mm late cycle. Endometrial cancer should be ruled out by endometrial biopsy ± hysteroscopy if endometrial thickness >20mm (4mm if postmenopausal), heterogeneous appearance, and hypoechoic areas. Polyps have cystic appearance (also with hyperechoic endometrium) and are most clearly seen in the early days of the cycle.

If postmenopausal and not on HRT, endometrial thickness should be 4mm or less p. 170. HRT, tibolone, and tamoxifen all increase endometrial thickness. In practice, bleeding on HRT or tamoxifen is investigated as a 2 week rule referral (p. 170).

US is useful for detecting fibroids, assessing ovaries and adnexal masses. It is operator dependent, and obesity can hinder the view. It is unable to detect endometriotic deposits (unless ovarian endometrioma).

Chronic pelvic pain

This is a symptom, not a diagnosis, and describes intermittent or constant lower abdominal pain of >6 months' duration not associated exclusively with menstruation, intercourse, or pregnancy. Pain may cause, or be exacerbated by, emotional problems. She may be depressed. Adequate time needs to be given to allow the woman to tell her story and express her views as to the cause of pain, and explore psychological aspects. A past history of abuse is more common. A multidisciplinary approach effects most all round improvement.

Laparoscopy may reveal a cause but is normal in 30%: chronic pelvic infection, endometriosis, adenomyosis, adhesions (eg residual ovary syndrome and trapped ovarian syndrome).[25]_{RCOG} Consider also irritable bowel syndrome (*OHCM* p266), and interstitial cystitis.

If pain is cyclical, ovarian suppression may help. cocp can be used cyclically or by running packs together (see pp. 154–5). GNRH analogues are used to induce a temporary menopause and assess if pain is hormone dependent prior to more definitive surgery eg oophorectomy or hysterectomy.

Pelvic congestion Controversial diagnosis. Congested lax pelvic veins (seen at laparoscopy) cause pain worse on standing, walking, and premenstrually. Typically variable in site and intensity, there may be unpleasant postcoital ache. Deep palpation reveals maximal tenderness over ovaries. Vagina and cervix may look blue from congestion. Look for associated posterior leg varicosities.

Remedies include explanation ('pelvic migraine'), ovarian suppression, migraine remedies (*OHCM* p458), and relaxation techniques. For severe symptoms bilateral ovarian vein ligation, radiological embolization, or hysterectomy with salpingo-oophorectomy (±HRT) may cure.

Mittelschmerz This is mid-cycle menstrual pain which may occur in teenagers and older women around the time of ovulation—from the German *mittel* (=middle) and *Schmerz* (=pain).

Dyspareunia

This means pain during intercourse. There may be a vicious circle in which anticipation of pain leads to tense muscles and lack of lubrication, and so to further pain. ▶*The patient may not volunteer the problem so ask about intercourse.* Her attitude to pelvic examination may tell you as much as the examination itself. Ask her to show you where the problem is. If the problem is actually vaginismus do not insist on examination and consider counselling and psychosexual therapy (p. 107). Was there female genital mutilation (p. 111)?

Dyspareunia may be superficial (introital) eg from infection, so look for ulceration and discharge. Vaginal dryness may be caused by oestrogen deficiency (especially postmenopausal or with breastfeeding) or lack of sexual stimulation (p. 107). Has she had a recent postpartum perineal repair? A suture or scar can cause well-localized pain which is cured by massage or by removing the suture and injection of local anaesthetic. If the introitus has been rendered too narrow, she may need surgery. Deep dyspareunia is felt internally (deep inside). It is associated with endometriosis and pelvic infection; treat the cause if possible.

Dermatographism is a rare cause of dyspareunia: look for itchy vulval wheals some minutes after calibrated dermatographometer application. It is the commonest physical cause of urticaria, and the clue to its presence is linear wheals with a surrounding bright red flare (but no angio-oedema). Cause is unknown. Relief of dyspareunia in these cases has been achieved by 2% **adrenaline** (epinephrine) cream, and **cetirizine** 10mg/24h PO.

Further reading

RCOG (2012). *Chronic Pelvic Pain, Initial Management* (Green-top Guideline No. 41). London: RCOG.

2 Gynaecology

Fibroids are benign smooth muscle tumours of the uterus (leiomyomas) (fig 2.10). They are often multiple, and vary in size from seedlings to tumours occupying a large part of the abdomen. They start as lumps in the wall of the uterus but may grow to bulge out of the wall so that they lie under the visceral peritoneum (subserosal, 20%), intramurally, under the endometrium (submucosal, 5%), or become pedunculated. Fibroids are common (20–40% of women of reproductive age have fibroids), increasing in frequency with age, in Afro-Caribbean women, and those with a family history of fibroids.

Associations Mutation in the gene for fumarate hydratase can cause fibroids and a rare association with skin & uterine leiomyomata, and renal cell cancer.[26]

Natural history Fibroids are oestrogen dependent. Consequently they enlarge in pregnancy and on the combined pill and atrophy after the menopause. They may degenerate gradually or suddenly (red degeneration, see BOX 'Fibroids in pregnancy'). Occasionally they calcify ('womb stones'). Rarely, they undergo sarcomatous change—usually causing pain, malaise, bleeding, and increase in size in a postmenopausal woman.

Presentation Many are asymptomatic:

Menorrhagia: Fibroids often produce heavy and prolonged periods (± anaemia). They do not generally cause intermenstrual or postmenopausal bleeding. *Fertility problems:* Submucosal fibroids may interfere with implantation. Large or multiple tumours which distort the uterine cavity may cause miscarriage should pregnancy occur but this is unproven. *Pain:* This may be due to torsion of a pedunculated fibroid, producing symptoms similar to that of a torted ovarian cyst. 'Red degeneration' following thrombosis of the fibroid blood supply: see BOX 'Fibroids in pregnancy'. *Mass:* Large fibroids may be felt abdominally. They may press on the bladder, causing frequency, or on the veins, causing oedematous legs and varicose veins. Pelvic fibroids may obstruct labour or cause retention of urine.

Treatment If symptoms are minimal, no treatment is needed.

- *GnRH analogues* eg **goserelin** 3.6mg sc monthly, for 3–6 months prior to surgery can be used to shrink the fibroids. However, these are not a long-term option due to demineralization of bone.
- *Ulipristal acetate* is a selective progesterone receptor modulator (Esmya®) given for 3 months to shrink fibroids and induce amenorrhoea. It should not currently be used pending further safety investigations due to risk of serious liver injury. (NB: Use of ulipristal as emergency contraception (as EllaOne®, p. 151) is not affected by this safety regulation.)
- *Myomectomy* can be hysteroscopic, laparoscopic, or open, depending on size and location. Submucosal fibroids are better removed hysteroscopically, and laparoscopic myomectomy demands advanced minimal access skills as well as an isolated, subserous fibroid. Open myomectomy has a 10% risk of hysterectomy due to bleeding, and is less straightforward. If the endometrial cavity is breached at laparoscopic or open myomectomy, resulting pregnancies require elective CS for delivery to prevent uterine rupture in labour.
- *Uterine artery embolization (UAE)* is undertaken by an interventional radiologist after assessment by MRI. The uterine artery is catheterized and then embolized. It avoids a general anaesthetic but can be extremely painful in the recovery period, and may lead to a necrotic, infected uterus. Pregnancy outcomes are better after myomectomy than UAE, and UAE is not recommended by fertility specialists for women wishing to retain fertility.
- *Hysterectomy* is reserved for women who have completed their family or have no wish for preserving fertility.

2 Gynaecology

Fibroids in pregnancy

5:1000 Caucasian women have fibroids in pregnancy. They are commoner in Afro-Caribbean women. They increase in size in pregnancy—especially in the 2nd trimester. US aids diagnosis. Colour flow Doppler distinguishes fibroids from myometrium. If pedunculated they may tort. Red degeneration is when thrombosis of capsular vessels is followed by venous engorgement and inflammation, causing abdominal pain (± vomiting & low-grade fever), and localized peritoneal tenderness—usually in the last half of pregnancy or the puerperium. 'Here, a certain feverishness leads them to their final degeneration', and imitating the course of all grand passions, 'they grow big and tender, and then die'. DH Lawrence Sons & Lovers

Treatment is expectant (rest, analgesia) with resolution over 4–7 days.

Most fibroids arise from the body of the uterus and do not therefore obstruct labour, as they tend to rise away from the pelvis throughout pregnancy. If large pelvic masses of fibroids are noted prior to labour, caesarean section may be required.

2 Gynaecology

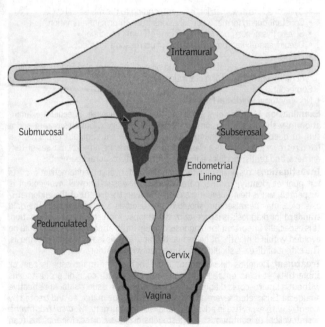

Fig 2.10 Diagram demonstrating the potential locations of uterine fibroids: pedunculated, subserosal, intramural, and submucosal.

Reproduced from Sarris *et al.*, *Training in Obstetrics and Gynaecology* (2009) with permission from OUP.

Endometriosis is defined as the presence of endometriotic tissue outside the uterus (figs 2.11 & 2.12). It is hormonally driven, principally by oestrogen, and therefore affects women of reproductive age. Adenomyosis refers to the presence of endometrial tissue within the myometrium. There is wide variation in severity of disease and its impact on pain. Some women are relatively asymptomatic with extensive disease, while others have only superficial endometriotic deposits with debilitating symptoms.

Cause Unknown. Three main theories exist: the first is retrograde menstruation, leading to adherence, invasion, and growth of tissue; the second is metaplasia of mesothelial cells (which may explain how it can develop in unusual places such as the lung and nasal cavity); the third, impaired immunity, suggests that endometrial cells from retrograde menstruation fail to be destroyed by the immune response. 10–12% of the general female population are estimated to have the disease, 20–50% of those undergoing fertility or chronic pain investigation and 40–60% of those with dysmenorrhoea.

Presentation
- Pain:
  - Cyclical due to endometrial tissue responding to the menstrual cycle.
  - Constant due to formation of adhesions from chronic inflammation.
  - Severe dysmenorrhoea leading to time off work or school.
  - Deep dyspareunia from involvement of uterosacral ligaments.
  - Dysuria.
  - Dyschezia (pain on defaecation) and/or cyclical rectal bleeding (rectovaginal nodules with invasion of rectal mucosa).
- Subfertility.
- No symptoms; incidental finding.

Examination May be normal if there is minimal disease. Speculum examination may show visible lesions in the vagina or cervix, but this is rare and a sign of deep infiltrating endometriosis. On bimanual vaginal examination, a fixed retroverted uterus is a classic sign. There may be adnexal masses or tenderness, and tender nodules palpable over the uterosacral ligaments.

Investigations TVS is useful for diagnosis of ovarian endometriotic cysts but poor at identifying other parameters of disease. If bowel involvement is suspected, MRI is being used increasingly to map the extent of the endometriosis. CA125 may be raised but should not be used as a screening test. The gold standard for diagnosis is laparoscopy with biopsy for histological confirmation. It is especially important for diagnosis of deep infiltrating lesions and should be avoided within 3 months of hormonal therapy, as this leads to underdiagnosis. The extent of disease should be documented with photographs.

Treatment Depends on symptoms and whether the main issue is pain or subfertility. It is acceptable to treat empirically with COCP or progestogens without a laparoscopic diagnosis if fertility is not the issue. NSAIDs are effective analgesia. Suspected severe endometriosis should be managed and treated by a centre with expertise in advanced laparoscopic surgery. *Medical treatment:* COCP (cyclical or continuous); progestogens orally, IM or SC; Mirena® IUS (can be inserted at laparoscopy); GnRH analogues eg goserelin short-term <6m and should be used with add-back HRT eg tibolone. *Surgical treatment:* Indicated once medical treatment has failed or fertility is a priority. Laparoscopy is the mainstay of management using ablation or excision. Nodules should be excised and endometriomas removed rather than drained (otherwise high recurrence). In mild–moderate disease, spontaneous pregnancy rates are increased after surgical removal of endometriotic lesions. Severe disease + subfertility: excision may not alter pregnancy outcome and could reduce ovarian reserve. Hysterectomy is a last resort.

Endometriosis and chronic pelvic pain There are high rates of relapse after stopping treatment such as COCP, and some patients with deep or superficial endometriosis, and those with adenomyosis (endometriotic tissue is largely inaccessible by surgery) will be left with chronic pain. This can be difficult to treat and ideally should be undertaken by an endometriosis specialist, in a centre where there is access to other support such as a clinical specialist nurse and a chronic pain team. Multiple repeat laparoscopies are not usually the answer unless there is evidence of recurrence. Consider other non-gynaecological causes which may coexist, eg irritable bowel syndrome, constipation, neuropathic pain from previous surgery or endometriosis, and fibromyalgia. Manage with analgesia (opiates may be required but if needed regularly should be managed with the help of a pain clinic), neuropathic treatments such as gabapentin, and hormonal treatments. If she is requesting a hysterectomy, a successful trial of GnRH analogues predicts successful pain relief. Also consider support groups (www.endo.org.uk) and if depression is also present, it should be treated.

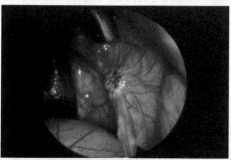

Fig 2.11 Endometriotic nodule. Note raised appearance with scarred peritoneum. Deep infiltrating endometriosis is more commonly found in the pouch of Douglas and the uterosacral ligaments, but may also involve the bladder, bowel, and ureters.
Reproduced with permission from Dan Martin, www.danmartinmd.com.

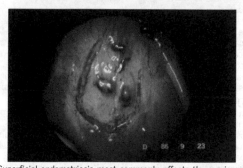

Fig 2.12 Superficial endometriosis most commonly affects the ovaries and pelvic peritoneum (particularly the pouch of Douglas and uterosacral ligaments).
Reproduced with permission from Dan Martin, www.danmartinmd.com.

Further reading

ESHRE (2013). *Management of Women with Endometriosis*. www.eshre.eu/Guidelines-and-Legal/Guidelines/Endometriosis-guideline/Guideline-on-the-management-of-women-with-endometriosis.aspx

NICE (2017). Endometriosis: Diagnosis and Management (NG73). London: NICE.

2 Gynaecology

▶*This can be devastating to both partners* and its investigation a great strain. Sympathetic management is crucial. 84% of couples having regular intercourse conceive within a year (92% by 2 years). Offer secondary care referral after 1yr of trying (earlier if ♀ aged ≥36 years, amenorrhoea, oligomenorrhoea, or past PID, undescended testes, or cancer treatments which may affect fertility). Fertility decreases with age: girls are born with ~300,000 potential eggs; by 30yrs, only 12% are left (by 40yrs, just 3%).

Causes
- Anovulation: 21%.
- Male factor: 25%.
- Tubal factor: 15–20%.
- Unexplained: 28%.
- Endometriosis: 6–8%.

Anovulation may be caused by premature ovarian failure, Turner syndrome, surgery or chemotherapy, as well as PCOS, excessive weight loss or exercise, hypopituitarism, Kallman syndrome, and hyperprolactinaemia.

History It takes 2 to be infertile (♀ causes ≈67%); see both partners. Note age and duration of subfertility. Have they had any previous pregnancies and does either partner have children? Menstrual history, regularity, pelvic pain, history of STIs, previous surgery (tubal or for ectopic pregnancy) are all important. Smoking reduces fertility, as does drinking more than the recommended amount of alcohol per week—in both partners. Check the medical history and drugs to optimize both. Ask about frequency of sexual intercourse and any problems during sex including erectile dysfunction. Ask the man about history of undescended testes, mumps as an adult, and check his medical, drug history, and smoking and alcohol use.

Examination BMI (obesity has an adverse effect on fertility, and there are BMI ranges above which treatment cannot be started). Are there signs of endocrine disorders eg PCOS? Exclude pelvic pathology eg endometriosis or fibroids, take a cervical smear if due, and high vaginal and chlamydia swabs. Surgical treatment of a scrotal varicocele has no effect on pregnancy rate.

Investigations
Primary care:
- Chlamydia screening.
- Baseline hormonal profile (day 2–5 FSH (should be 2–8.9IU/L) and LH (1–12IU/L).
- TSH, prolactin, and testosterone and rubella status (vaccinate if non-immune).
- Mid-luteal progesterone level to confirm ovulation (7 days before expected period eg day 21 if 28-day cycle, >30nmol/L is indicative of ovulation).
- Semen analysis (p. 145). Repeat in 3 months if abnormal, after making lifestyle changes and starting a multivitamin containing selenium, zinc, and vitamin C.

Secondary care:
- TVS to rule out adnexal masses, submucosal fibroids or endometrial polyps, or help confirm PCOS.
- Hysterosalpingogram (HSG) uses x-ray and contrast injected through a small cannula in the cervix to demonstrate uterine anatomy and tubal patency. May cause period-like cramps and tubal spasm, giving false positive. Only perform once *Chlamydia* swabs negative and give **azithromycin** 1g PO stat.
- Hysterosalpingo-contrast sonograph (HYCOSY) is similar to the above mentioned, but using US contrast and TVS.
- Laparoscopy and dye test is a day-case procedure and the gold standard for assessing tubal patency. Methylthioninium chloride (methylene blue) dye is injected thought the cervix while the tubes are visualized with a laparoscope. Used 1st line if strong clinical suspicion of tubal abnormality or needs a laparoscopy for other reasons. Used 2nd line if HSG or HYCOSY abnormal. Pelvic pathology can be treated at the same time.

2 Gynaecology

Subfertility options: abbreviations, problems, and ethics

DI	Donor insemination is used when the male partner has azoospermia with failed surgical sperm retrieval, in those at high risk of transmitting a genetic disorder, and those at high risk of transmitting HIV. It is also used for women with no (male) partner.
ICSI	Intracytoplasmic sperm injection (directly into an egg). Sperm may be taken from the ejaculate, or surgically from the testis or epididymis. This technique is used when the semen parameters are severely abnormal or failed fertilization has occurred with IVF cycles. There is some concern that genetic mutations (especially Y chromosome deletions) will be propagated by transmission to the offspring.
IUI	Intrauterine insemination: useful in mild male factor subfertility, co-ital difficulties, unexplained subfertility, and same-sex couples. It can be combined with ovarian stimulation, but if >3 follicles develop, the treatment cycle should be cancelled due to a high chance of multiple pregnancy (>25%).
IVF	*In vitro* fertilization: see p. 67 & p. 144.
IVM	*In vitro* maturation: immature eggs are collected from the ovaries, matured in the lab before sperm injection (ISCI). Avoids expensive ovulation-inducing drugs and risk of ovarian hyperstimulation, it may be especially suitable for women with polycystic ovaries.
OT/ NT(P)	Ooplasmic transfer/nuclear transfer procedure: the baby has 2 mothers: one (too old to conceive normally) gives a nucleus; the other gives fresher cytoplasm (+mitochondrial DNA) for the ovum. This is an example of human germline modification. 30 babies have been born worldwide using this technique.
PESA	Percutaneous epididymal sperm aspiration (uses a needle inserted into the epididymis, so scrotal exploration is not needed).
POT	Pregnancy by ovary transplant has been reported (autologous transplant, 1 between identical twin sisters, another between sisters).

Various national embryology authorities exist and pronounce on the ethics of fertility options, and their edicts can appear to be set in stone (although being mutually contradictory with those from other countries). One problem with this approach is that fertility options are constantly changing, as are society's views on what is acceptable. It is not clear whether these views should lead, or simply be taken into account (an opaque phrase) or be trumped by appeal to some higher authority (God, or the conscience of a quango).

Methods such as PGD allow embryos to be sexed and screened for genetic diseases with implantation only for those with the desired characteristics, eg offering a perfect match for stem cell transplantation to an older sibling, with Fanconi's anaemia. Controversies surrounding creating an individual expressly for the purposes of another might seem to be new, but mythology has, since before the dawn of time,[5][27] acclimatized us to this activity—which is why it is gaining acceptance.

Further reading

NICE (2013). Fertility: Assessment and Treatment of People with Fertility Problems (CG156). London: NICE. www.nice.org.uk/guidance/cg156

5 According to *Paradise Lost*, the First Operator, in a controversial act of vivisection, 'opened my left side, and took from thence a rib, with cordial spirits warm, and life-blood streaming fresh: wide was the wound, but suddenly with flesh filled up and healed: the rib he formed and fashioned with his hands; under his forming hands a creature grew, manlike, but different sex, so lovely fair, that what seemed fair in all the world, seemed now mean, or in her summed up: Thus was Eve made, not for herself, but simply to delight Adam and keep him company.

Lifestyle modification Treatment of subfertility is directed at the cause. The couple should lose or gain weight to a normal BMI, eat a healthy diet, stop smoking ± recreational drugs, reduce alcohol consumption to less than the recommended limits, take regular exercise, folic acid (the woman), aim to have regular intercourse every 2–3 days (avoid timed intercourse), and avoid ovulation monitors (they increase stress and there is no evidence of benefit). Couples who time intercourse for the day of ovulation may be too late—ideally there should be some sperm available for fertilization whenever ovulation occurs.

Ovulation induction There are several methods by which to induce ovulation. PCOS is the most common cause of anovulatory subfertility, accounting for 80%.
- *Weight loss or gain.*
- *Clomifene citrate:* 50mg days 2–6 of cycle.
  - Anti-oestrogen, which increases endogenous FSH via negative feedback to the pituitary.
  - 10% multiple pregnancy rate (higher if used inappropriately).
  - Can cause hot flushes, labile mood. If severe headache or visual disturbance, stop immediately.
  - Should only be used for 6–12 cycles (possible link with ovarian cancer).
  - Needs follicular monitoring by US (risk of hyperstimulation).
  - Should be prescribed by a specialist, ideally after tubal patency confirmed and semen count normal or near-normal and BMI <30–35.
- *Laparoscopic ovarian drilling:*
  - Used in patients with PCOS only (see p. 116).
  - Small holes are drilled into each ovary using needlepoint diathermy with the aim of reducing LH and restoring feedback mechanisms.
  - Successful in 50% and effects last for 12–18 months.
- *Gonadotrophins:* Used in specialist fertility units for clomifene-resistant PCOS or low oestrogen with normal FSH. Injected, expensive, and needs US monitoring.
- *Metformin:* Controversial and is used in women with PCOS. There is a possible small increase in ovulation rates but it is not licensed and weight loss is more effective.

Surgical techniques *Tubal disease:* Proximal blocks may respond to tubal catheterization or hysteroscopic cannulation. High rates of ectopic pregnancy. *Endometriosis:* pp. 140–1. *Intrauterine adhesions:* Use hysteroscopic adhesiolysis.

In vitro fertilization *Indications:* Include tubal disease, male factor subfertility, endometriosis, anovulation not responding to clomifene, subfertility due to maternal age, unexplained subfertility >2yrs. *Success:* This depends on many factors including age, duration of subfertility, previous pregnancy (higher success rate), smoking, and high BMI (lower success). Low anti-Müllerian hormone (AMH) levels predict poorer response. Women with hydrosalpinges should have salpingectomy prior to IVF to ↑chance of live birth. Screen couple for HIV, hepatitis B & C. Ovaries are stimulated (see 'Ovarian hyperstimulation syndrome', p. 146), ova collected (by transvaginal aspiration under transvaginal US guidance), fertilized, and 3–5 days later, 1–2 embryos returned under US guidance to the uterus as an outpatient procedure. Luteal support is given in the form of progestogens, and 2 weeks later the woman should do a pregnancy test. *NHS-funded assisted conception:* Inclusion criteria vary between regions but generally is limited to couples with no children, non-smokers, BMI <30, under 42yrs of age (35 in some counties), and who do not require gamete donation. *Egg donation:* Can offer women a chance of pregnancy when previous IVF attempts have failed, in ovarian failure, and in women >45yrs. Adoption and fostering are also options and this can be arranged locally.

We acknowledge Dr Gillian Coyle MRCOG for her contribution to this section.

(margin: 2 Gynaecology)

Spermatogenesis takes place in the seminiferous tubules. Undifferentiated diploid germ cells (spermatogonia) multiply and are then transformed into haploid spermatozoa, a process taking 74 days. FSH and LH are both important for initiation of spermatogenesis at puberty. LH stimulates Leydig cells to produce testosterone. Testosterone and FSH stimulate Sertoli cells to produce essential substances for metabolic support of germ cells and spermatogenesis.

Spermatozoa A spermatozoon has a dense oval head (containing the haploid chromosome complement) capped by an acrosome granule (contains enzymes essential for fertilization), and is propelled by the motile tail. Seminal fluid forms 90% of ejaculate volume and is alkaline to buffer vaginal acidity.

Normal semen analysis (WHO criteria 2009)

- Volume >1.5mL.
- Concentration >15×10⁶/mL.
- Progressive motility >32%.
- Total motility >40%.
- Normal forms >4%.

Male factors Male factors are the cause of subfertility in ~25% of subfertile couples. Only a small number of men have an identifiable treatable cause.
- Semen abnormality (85%):
  - Idiopathic oligoasthenoteratozoospermia, testicular cancer, drugs such as alcohol and nicotine, varicocele.
- Azoospermia (5%):
  - Pre-testicular, eg anabolic steroid use, hypogonadotropic hypogonadism, Kallmann syndrome.
  - Non-obstructive: cryptorchidism, orchitis, 47,XXY (Klinefelter syndrome), chemotherapy.
  - Obstructive: congenital bilateral absence of the vas deferens (CBAVD), vasectomy, chlamydia, gonorrhoea.
- Immunological (5%):
  - Anti-sperm antibodies, idiopathic, infective.
- Coital dysfunction (5%):
  - Erectile dysfunction with normal sperm function (remember drug causes such as beta-blockers, antidepressants).
  - Hypospadias, phimosis, disability.
  - Retrograde ejaculation.
  - Failure in ejaculation (multiple sclerosis, spinal cord injury).

Examination Look at body form and secondary sexual characteristics. Any gynaecomastia? Normal testicular volume is 15–35mL (compare with Prader orchidometer). Testicular US if the examination is abnormal. Rectal examination may reveal prostatitis.

Tests *Plasma FSH* is raised in testicular failure. *Testosterone and LH* levels are indicated if you suspect androgen deficiency. *Karyotype* to exclude 47,XXY and *cystic fibrosis screen* (associated with CBAVD).

Treatment Address lifestyle issues, such as alcohol and smoking. Optimize underlying medical conditions and consider stopping or changing medication. Consider starting a multivitamin containing zinc, selenium, and vitamin C. Repeat the semen analysis 3 months after making changes. *ICSI=intracytoplasmic sperm injection* (direct into egg) is the main tool for most male subfertility. The source of sperm is the epididymis or testis in men with obstructive azoospermia; even if the problem is non-obstructive, sperm can be retrieved in ~50%.

2 Gynaecology

Ovarian hyperstimulation syndrome (OHSS) is a complication of ovulation induction or superovulation. This is a systemic disease and vasoactive products (particularly vascular endothelial growth factor, VEGF) are central to its pathophysiology. It has an incidence of up to 33% in mild forms, and in 1:200 it is severe, requiring hospitalization. Higher risk of pre-eclampsia and preterm delivery if fertility treatment results in a pregnancy.

Characteristics
* Ovarian enlargement (figs 2.13 & 2.14).
* Fluid shift from intravascular to extravascular space:
  * This leads to the accumulation of fluid in peritoneal and pleural spaces.
  * Intravascular volume depletion causes haemoconcentration and hypercoagulability.

Risk factors Include young age, low BMI, polycystic ovaries, previous OHSS.

Presentation Abdominal discomfort, nausea, vomiting, and abdominal distension ± dyspnoea. Presentation is usually 3–7 days after hCG administration, or 12–17 days, if pregnancy has ensued.

Prevention Prediction and prevention are the key. Women should be given the lowest effective regimen of gonadotrophins. Cycle cancellation may be necessary, or elective embryo cryopreservation, for use in a further frozen-thawed cycle. In women with PCOS, *in vitro* maturation (IVM, p. 143), where immature eggs are collected, avoids ovarian stimulation and the risk of OHSS.

Management

Mild and moderate OHSS—abdominal bloating, mild to moderate pain, US evidence of ascites, and ovarian size usually 8–12cm:
* Outpatient management.
* Analgesia (paracetamol and/or codeine).
* Avoid NSAIDs (will worsen fluid shift and renal impairment).
* Drink to thirst, not to excess.
* Avoid strenuous activities and intercourse due to risk of ovarian torsion.
* Continue with progesterone luteal support, and avoid hCG.
* Review by the assisted conception unit every 2–3 days.

Severe OHSS—clinical ascites, oliguria, haematocrit is >45%, hypoproteinaemia, ovarian size >12cm:
* May be managed as an outpatient but may need admission to hospital.
* Analgesia and antiemetics (avoid NSAIDs).
* Daily FBC, U&E, LFTS, albumin.
* Strict fluid balance.
* Daily assessment of girth (ascites), weight, and legs (thrombosis).
* Thromboprophylaxis with compression stockings and LMWH—women should have a risk assessment and LMWH may need to extend beyond the period of OHSS.
* Paracentesis for symptomatic relief (± IV replacement albumin).
* Urinary catheter.

Critical OHSS—tense ascites, haematocrit >55%, WCC >25×10⁹/L, oligo- or anuria, thromboembolism, acute respiratory distress syndrome (OHCM p186):
* Get senior help early and consider ITU. Symptomatic pleural effusions may need drainage. Use antiembolic measures as above-listed. Pay meticulous attention to fluid balance. Aim to maintain intake at 3L/24h using normal saline if unable to tolerate oral fluids. Beware hyponatraemia. Note that severe or critical cases must be reported by the fertility centre to the HFEA.

Further reading

RCOG (2016). *The Management of Ovarian Hyperstimulation Syndrome* (Green-top Guideline No. 5). London: RCOG.

2 Gynaecology

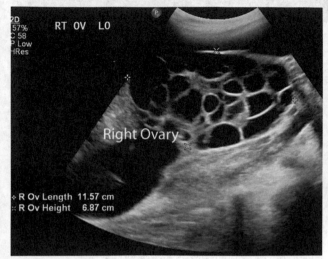

Fig 2.13 Doppler image of extremely enlarged right ovary. Numerous large cysts/follicles are present throughout. Normal ovarian vascularity is present. Large pelvic ascites is noted

Reproduced from Lockhart *et al. Genitourinary Radiology Cases* (2014) with permission from OUP.

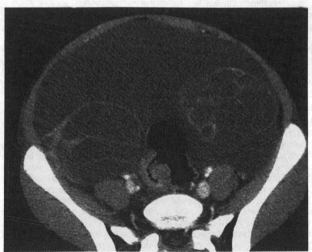

Fig 2.14 Contrast CT of massively enlarged ovaries containing numerous large cysts and large ascites.

Reproduced from Lockhart *et al. Genitourinary Radiology Cases* (2014) with permission from OUP.

2 Gynaecology

▶*Any method, even coitus interruptus, is better than none.* Without contraception about 85 of every 100 premenopausal sexually active women will become pregnant each year, and 1 in 3 pregnancies are unplanned. Properly used, contraception reduces this rate (see BOX 'The ideal contraceptive'). When dealing with under-16s use Fraser guidelines (see BOX 'Fraser guidelines'). After the menopause, stop contraception 2yrs after amenorrhoea if <50yrs, after 1yr if >50yrs.

Barrier methods ▶The main reason for failure is not using them. Condoms reduce transmission of most STDs but not those affecting the perineum. When failure has occurred (eg 'split condom'), remember postcoital emergency contraception (p. 151).

• *Condoms:* Effective when properly used, unroll onto the erect penis with the teat or end (if teatless) pinched to expel air. This prevents bursting at ejaculation. Use a new condom with each episode of sexual intercourse. Do not use with oil-based lubricants—this destroys the latex. Method failure rate 5%, typical user failure rate 15%/yr.

• *Caps:* Come in several forms.[6] [RCOL] Diaphragms stretch from pubic bone to posterior fornix. Check after insertion that the cervix is covered. Cervical caps fit over the cervix (so need a prominent cervix). Insert <2h before intercourse (keep in place >6h after sex). Use with a spermicide.* Problems: UTIs, latex sensitivity. They need professional fitting. 92–99% effective if perfect use.[7]

• *Cervical sponges:* Simple to use: spermicide* impregnated: unavailable in UK.

• *The female condom:* (eg Femidom®) Prescription and fitting are not needed. It has not proved popular. They can be noisy. 95% effective (TUFR 21%.).

• *Spermicide:* * Unreliable unless used with a barrier. Nonoxinol-9, the only spermicide available in UK is not recommended for those with or at high risk of HIV as it irritates vaginal epithelium and ↑ chance of HIV transmission.

Fertility awareness ('natural') methods Involve physiological monitoring to find fertile times (6 days prior to ovulation; the life of a sperm) to 2 days afterwards (the life of the ovum). Cervical mucus becomes clear and slippery prior to ovulation, and then abruptly thicker and tacky. No intercourse from the day mucus becomes slippery to 3 days after if becomes tacky. Basal body temperature ↑~0.3°c after ovulation (affected by fevers, drugs). Additional observations (mittelschmerz, p. 137 ± cervix changes) improve accuracy. Success is common if: • Regular cycles • Dedication • Self-control.

Lactational amenorrhoea See p. 87.

High-technology natural methods Devices eg Persona® use urine test sticks to measure *oestrone-3-glucuronide* (E3G—peaks 24h pre-ovulation) and luteinizing hormone (LH—ovulation occurs within 36h of LH surge and sperm penetration of cervical mucus drops after surge). Microtechnology builds a database of the woman's natural variability over time, to give her a green light (almost infertile), a red light (fertile—typically days 6–10), or an orange light (test early-morning urine for E3G and LH). Usually, only 8 urine tests are needed per cycle. She purchases sticks and monitor. A button is pressed the morning her period starts: she checks the monitor lights before passing urine each morning, in case a test is needed. *Reliability:* 93–95% (manufacturer's data, in motivated patients; it may be less in practice; results should be regarded as only preliminary; explain uncertainty). Phone apps tracking cycles are unreliable and should not be used for contraceptive purposes. Basal temperature can be affected by hormonal contraceptives, alcohol, illness, and oversleeping.

---

6 RCOG 2007 *FFPRHC* Guidance Female Barrier Methods. This paper gives great detail of all caps, diaphragms, etc. available.

7 But typical use failure rate (TUFR; user+method failure) = 16% in 1st year use of diaphragm (TUFR) for cervical caps: 9% nullips, 20% parous ♀.

2 Gynaecology

The ideal contraceptive—and the realities

An ideal contraceptive is: *100% effective*, with only desirable side effects (eg protection from sexually transmitted disease), and it must be *readily reversible*, and be usable *unsupervised by professionals* (table 2.1).[29] Find the best compromise for each person depending on age, health, and beliefs. Methods available:

- 'Natural methods' (no intercourse near time of ovulation): acceptable to Catholic Church; also, the simplest are free, requiring no 'pollution of the body' with drugs: see p. 148.
- Barrier methods (low health risk but need high user motivation & some protection from HIV). See p. 148.
- Hormonal (complex health interactions, but highly effective, p. 152).
- IUCD/IUS (convenient and effective—if not contraindicated—p. 150).
- Sterilization (very effective but effectively 'irreversible', p. 157).

Table 2.1 Failure rates % in 1st year with typical (T) and perfect (P) use

	85(T)	85(P)
No method	85(T)	85(P)
Cervical cap	16–32	9–20
Natural methods	25	1–9
Female condom	21	5
Withdrawal	27	4
Diaphragm + spermicide	16	6
Male condom	15	2
Pills (COC + POP)	8	0.3
Copper coil (for T-safe® CU380A)	0.8	0.6
Depo-Provera®	3	0.3
Tubal ligation	0.5	0.5
Vasectomy	0.15	0.1
Levonorgestrel IUS (Mirena®)	0.1	0.1

2 Gynaecology

'Is she pregnant already?'

This is a frequent question in family planning and other clinics. If a pregnancy test is not available, women who could be pregnant already will often be denied the contraception they need. Here, consider using this checklist to see if the patient may be pregnant. If she answers yes to *any* of these questions, and she is free from signs or symptoms of pregnancy, then pregnancy is very unlikely (negative predictive value >99%):

- Have you given birth in the past 4 weeks?
- Are you <6 months postpartum and fully breastfeeding, and your periods have not returned?
- Did your last menstrual period start within the last 7 days?
- Have you been using a reliable contraceptive consistently and correctly?
- Have you not had sex since your last period?[30]

Fraser guidelines

Those <16yrs may be prescribed contraception without parental consent if:
- They understand the doctor's advice.
- The young person cannot be persuaded to inform their parents that they are seeking contraceptive advice.
- They are likely to begin or continue intercourse with or without contraceptive treatment.
- Unless the young person receives contraceptive treatment their physical or mental health is likely to suffer.
- The young person's best interests require that the doctor gives advice and/or treatment without parental consent.
- Fraser guidelines and 'Gillick competence' are not interchangeable terms. Fraser guidelines are narrower than Gillick competence as they relate only to contraception, whereas Gillick competence relates to children aged <16 who have the legal capacity to consent to medical examination and treatment.

IUCDs (coils) are plastic shapes ~3cm long with copper winding, and a plastic thread for a tail. They inhibit fertilization, implantation, and sperm penetration of cervical mucus. Most need changing every 5–10 years. Use those with ≥300mm² copper eg T-safe® copper T380A (the most effective), for which pregnancy rate is 2.2 per 100 woman-years. Most of those who choose the IUCD (5%) are older, parous women in stable relationships, in whom the problem rate is low. They can be used for emergency contraception (p. 151).

Problems with IUCDs 1 They may be expelled (5%) by a uterus which is nulliparous or distorted (eg by fibroids). 2 They are associated with pelvic inflammatory disease up to 21 days following insertion. 3 They may cause dysmenorrhoea and menorrhagia (most common reason for discontinuation). 4 Risk of ectopic pregnancy is 1:20 should she become pregnant. *Contraindications:* Pregnancy; current pelvic infection/STD (including TB); allergy to copper; Wilson disease; heavy/painful periods; trophoblastic disease or gynaecological malignancy; undiagnosed abnormal uterine bleeding; distorted cavity. Use with caution if anticoagulated.

Insertion Screen for STD prior to insertion or use prophylactic antibiotics eg **azithromycin** 1g PO stat following insertion. Specialist training is required.

An IUCD can be inserted any time (and as emergency contraception), as long as she's not pregnant. Insert immediately after TOP/miscarriage or birth (see p. 87). Advise taking simple analgesia prior to insertion and warn her that this may cause cramps. Uterine perforation rate is <1:1000. Teach her to feel the threads: ask her to check after each period. ►Insertion of IUCDs may provoke 'cervical shock' (from increased vagal tone). Tip the woman head down with legs raised. Have IV atropine (and antiepileptics if patient epileptic) and resuscitation equipment to hand.

Follow-up Most expulsions are in the 1st 3 months. Follow-up after 1st period. Threads may be easier to feel than to see. Expulsion rate <1:20 in 5 years.

Lost threads The IUCD may have been expelled, so advise extra contraception and exclude pregnancy. Seek coil on US; if missing arrange x-ray to exclude extrauterine coils (surgical retrieval advised). If present and not due to be changed, leave *in situ*.

Infection Treat with the device in place, but if removed do not replace for 3 months. With symptomatic *Actinomyces*, remove coil, cut off threads, and send for culture. If positive, seek expert advice on treatment.

Pregnancy >90% are intrauterine. Remove coil, if you can as soon as pregnancy is diagnosed to reduce risk of miscarriage (20% if removed early, 50% if left), and to prevent miscarriage with infection. Exclude ectopic.

Removal Alternative contraception should be started (if desired) prior to removal, or abstinence for 7 days. At the menopause, remove after 2 years' amenorrhoea if age <50yrs (1yr's amenorrhoea if age >50yrs).

IUS, intrauterine systems eg Mirena® or Kyleena® (carries levonorgestrel). Local effect (reversible endometrial atrophy) makes implantation less likely, and periods lighter and less painful. 30% may experience reversible amenorrhoea (reliability equals sterilization, see p. 157). It lasts ~5yrs (Jaydess® lasts 3yrs). Risk of ectopic pregnancy and PID is reduced compared with copper IUCD. Can be used immediately postpartum, in breastfeeding, obesity, cardiovascular disease, and in women taking hepatic enzyme-inducing drugs. Warn about spotting ± heavy bleeding for the 1st few weeks following insertion; this usually settles within 3–6 months. Pregnancy rate <1:1000 over 5yrs. It may benefit women with endometriosis, adenomyosis, or simple endometrial hyperplasia without atypia. It is the first-line treatment for menorrhagia. It cannot be used as emergency contraception.

This is for use after isolated episodes of unprotected intercourse (UPSI), and should not be used regularly.[31] Tablets cover that UPSI only. Although usually given after UPSI, advance issue does not increase use and it may be sensible to 'be prepared'. ('Carrying an umbrella in the British climate is considered sensible, not a wish for rain.')[32] However, advance issue has not been shown to reduce pregnancy rates.

Management History of LMP; normal cycle; number of hours since unprotected intercourse. Any CI to later COCP use (p. 152)? Check BP. Explain that teratogenicity has not been demonstrated. Discuss future contraception. Give supply of oral contraceptives if day 1 start at next period is planned; if started immediately advise extra precautions as below. Offer infection screen and to cover HIV. Offer follow-up at 3–6 weeks if coil inserted; or if pregnancy or STI tests desired, or if she has contraceptive concerns.

Emergency IUCD More effective than tablet contraception (prevents 99% of expected pregnancies); a copper IUCD can be inserted within 120h of unprotected sex. If exposure was >5 days previously it can be inserted up to 5 days after likely ovulation, so is useful in women who present later. Screen for infection. Insert under antibiotic cover, eg **azithromycin** 1g PO if screening results unavailable. It is thought to inhibit fertilization by toxic effects and to inhibit implantation. If for long-term use, coils with 380mm^2 Cu have the lowest failure rates so should be used. Unaffected by enzyme inducers (p. 152), it is the method of choice for those taking them (but see later).

Ulipristal acetate (eg EllaOne®) Initiate within 120h of unprotected sex. Failure rate is ≤1.6% in non-inferiority (with levonorgestrel) trials. Efficacy is not reduced by obesity (levonorgestrel may be). It is thought to inhibit or delay ovulation. If vomiting ≤3h of taking the tablet, advise another (30mg). A progesterone receptor moderator, it is unsuitable for use if on, or within 28 days of taking, an enzyme inducer (p. 152), if on antacids or drugs raising gastric pH, for those with severe asthma uncontrolled by oral corticosteroids. Use with caution if liver dysfunction, hereditary galactose intolerance, Lapp lactase deficiency, glucose-galactose malabsorption. Avoid breastfeeding for 36h after use. Use only once per menstrual cycle. Periods average 2 days' delay (7 days in ≤20%). Advise extra contraceptive precautions for 14 days for combined pills, 16 days for Qlaira®, 9 days for progesterone only pills, if started or continued. Starting oral contraceptive immediately after ulipristal acetate is off licence. Should pregnancy occur, though no harm known, register via manufacturer.

Levonorgestrel Initiate within 72h of unprotected sex. Failure rates are ≤2.6%. Suitable for those with focal migraine and past thromboembolism, there are no medical contraindications to its use. **Levonorgestrel** 1.5mg preferably within 12h and no later than 72h after unprotected sex. If on, or within 28 days of, taking an enzyme inducer (p. 152), or with post-sexual exposure HIV prophylaxis, the dose is 3mg (consider 3mg higher dose if >70kg or BMI >26kg/m^2). If vomiting occurs within 2h of taking the dose, take another immediately. The earlier taken after UPSI, the fewer pregnancies occur. It is believed to inhibit ovulation. It can be used more than once in 1 cycle; and can be used (but may be less effective) in the same cycle after ulipristal acetate.

Warn that effective contraception should be used until the next period; and that she should return if she suffers any lower abdominal pain or the next period is abnormal. Advise pregnancy test if period >7 days late or unusually light, or after 21 days if 'quick start' contraception started. If immediate ('quick start') oral contraception started, or continuing, extra contraceptive precautions are needed for 7 days for combined pills (avoid immediate cocyprindiol start), 9 days for Qlaira®, 2 days for progesterone-only pills.

2 Gynaecology

Combined hormonal contraception (CHC) as vaginal ring, transdermal patch, or pills (COCP) contain oestrogen with a progestogen, either in fixed ratio or varying through the month (phased). Standard-dose pills (30mcg oestrogen) are the norm. Combined contraceptives inhibit ovulation, giving a withdrawal bleed in the pill-free interval. They can be taken in a variety of ways: traditionally, 21 days continuously followed by a 7-day break. This can be personalized to 'extended use' eg 3 packets with a 4–7-day break; continuously until a 3–4-day breakthrough bleed at which point a 4–7-day break is taken or for 21-days with shortened 4-day break.

COCP *Oestrogen content:* Most contain ethinylestradiol, but alternatives are estradiol valerate (Qlaira®) or mestranol (Norinyl-1®). Low-strength preparations contain 20mcg ethinylestradiol and are used if there are risk factors for circulatory disease, or oestrogenic side effects from a higher dose. The standard strength is 30–35mcg ethinylestradiol and is used for most women. *Progestogen type:* Most commonly, levonorgestrel and norethisterone are used. Consider using pills containing desogestrel, norgestimate, drospirenone, or gestodene if symptoms such as acne, headache, breakthrough bleeding. Co-cyprindiol is licensed for the treatment of acne—not licensed for contraception. Use for 3–4 months after resolution of symptoms. Higher risk of VTE compared with levonorgestrel.

Contraceptive patch (eg Evra®) Transdermal patch containing 20mcg ethinylestradiol and norelgestromin. Useful if compliance with taking daily tablets a problem. Apply patch on day 1 of cycle, change on days 8 and 15, and remove on day 22. Apply a new patch after 7-day patch-free interval to start the cycle again.

Contraceptive vaginal ring (eg NuvaRing®) Flexible ring which releases 15mcg/24h ethinylestradiol and etonogestrel. The woman inserts the ring into the vagina on day 1 of cycle, and leaves it in for 3 weeks. It is removed on day 22 for a 7-day ring-free interval.

Reasons to avoid combined hormonal contraception[8][33]
- *Venous disease:* Avoid if current/past VTE or sclerosing treatment to varicose veins. Use with caution if 1 risk factor, avoid if >1 of: age >35yrs, smoker (avoid if >35yrs and smokes >15/day), BMI >30kg/m² (avoid if BMI >35kg/m²), family history of VTE in 1st-degree relative <45yrs (avoid if known thrombophilia), immobility (avoid if bed-bound or in plaster), superficial thrombophlebitis.
- *Arterial disease:* Avoid if valvular or congenital heart disease with complications, or history of cardiovascular disease including stroke, TIA, IHD, peripheral vascular disease, hypertensive retinopathy. Risk factors for CVD (use with caution if 1, avoid if >1): age >35yrs, smoker (avoid if smokes >40/day), family history of arterial disease in 1st-degree relative <45yrs (avoid if atherogenic lipid profile), diabetes mellitus (avoid if vascular, renal, neurological, or eye complications), hypertension with BP >140/90mmHg (avoid if >160/95mmHg), migraine without aura (avoid if migraine with aura, migraine treated with ergot derivatives and those lasting >72h).
- *Liver disease:* Avoid if active or flare of viral hepatitis, liver tumours, severe cirrhosis, active gallbladder disease, and seek advice if history of contraceptive-associated cholestasis and avoid if previous obstetric cholestasis.
- *Cancer:* Avoid if current history of breast cancer. If no alternative and breast cancer >5yrs ago with no known gene mutation, seek specialist advice.
- *Previous pregnancy complications:* Avoid if pruritus in pregnancy, obstetric cholestasis, chorea, pemphigoid gestationis. Can be used from 6 weeks postpartum (including if breastfeeding) if other methods unacceptable.
- *Hepatic enzyme-inducing drugs:* Avoid if taking rifampicin or rifabutin. For others, increase the dose to 50mcg ethinylestradiol and shorten pill/patch/ring-free interval to 4 days. There is no evidence that broad-spectrum antibiotics decrease efficacy of combined contraceptives.

Migraine, ischaemic stroke, and combined hormonal contraceptives

The problem is ischaemic stroke. The background annual incidence is 2 per 100,000 women aged 20, and 20 per 100,000 for those aged 40. Migraine itself is a risk factor. For those with migraine and CHC use, incidence of ischaemic stroke becomes 8:100,000 if aged 20; and 80:100,000 in those aged 40. Low-dose COCPs only should be used. Those with migraine with aura are known to be at special risk precluding use of combined contraception in these women (however, there is no problem with them using progesterone only or non-hormonal contraception). Other risk factors for ischaemic stroke include smoking, age >35yrs, ↑BP, obesity (BMI >30), diabetes mellitus, dyslipidaemia, and family history of arterial disease <45yrs. Women known to have migraine should be warned to stop CHC immediately if they develop aura or worsening of migraine. If a woman has 1st migraine attack on CHC, stop it, observe closely: restart cautiously only if there are no sequelae and if migraine attack was without aura and there are no other risk factors (see earlier).[34]

Diagnosing migraine with aura

1 Slow evolution of symptoms (see later) over several minutes.
2 Duration of aura usually 10–30min, resolving within 1h, and typically before onset of headache.
3 Visual symptoms (99% of auras), eg:
   • Bilateral homonymous hemianopia.
   • Teichopsia and fortification spectra, eg a gradually enlarging C 𝒞 with scintillating edges.
   • Positive (bright) scotomata.
4 Sensory disturbance (31% of auras):
   • Usually associated with visual symptoms.
   • Usually in one arm spreading from fingers to face (leg rarely affected).
5 Speech disturbance (18% of auras): dysphasia; dysarthria; paraphasia.
6 Motor disturbances (6% of auras).

Both motor and speech disturbances are usually accompanied by visual and/or sensory disturbances.

Migraine without aura Includes symptoms of blurred vision, photophobia, phonophobia, generalized flashing lights affecting the whole visual field in both eyes, associated with headache.

Absolute contraindications to CHC use

• Migraine with aura.
• Migraine without aura in women with >1 risk factor for stroke (see earlier).
• Severe migraine or migraine lasting >72h (status migrainosus).
• Migraine treated with ergot derivatives.

8 UKMEC4 category denotes that use poses unacceptable health risk: UKMEC3=risk from use outweighs advantage; UKMEC2=advantage of use outweighs risk; UKMEC1=no restriction to use. UKMEC 2009.

Short-term side effects

Usually resolve within 2–3 cycles.

- *Oestrogenic:* Commonly include breast tenderness, nausea, cyclical weight gain, bloating, and vaginal discharge. Due to relative oestrogen excess.
- *Progestogenic:* Side effects include mood swings, PMT, vaginal dryness, sustained weight gain, decreased libido, and acne.
- *Headache:* Affects 2.9% of those taking CHC, and women should report increase in headache frequency or the development of focal symptoms. Discontinue immediately if focal symptoms occur and if not typical of migraine and last >1h, admit to hospital.
- *Breakthrough bleeding:* Most common in the 1st 6 months of use. If it persists >3 months, check compliance, exclude persistent diarrhoea/vomiting, and check for gynaecological causes. Screen for chlamydia, check cervix, check smear is up to date, exclude pregnancy and if >45yrs consider referral for hysteroscopy. Increase oestrogen content of COCP if on low-dose pill, if not change progestogen.
- *Risks and benefits of combined hormonal contraception:* See table 2.2.

Table 2.2 Risks and benefits of combined hormonal contraception

Risks	Benefits
VTE risk doubled (absolute risk low)	Improvement in acne
Ischaemic stroke (small ↑ risk)	↓ menorrhagia/dysmenorrhoea
Breast and cervical cancer (↑ risk small and disappears <10yrs after stopping)	↓ risk ovarian, endometrial, and bowel cancer (persists after stopping CHC)
Mood changes (no ↑ risk depression)	↓ menopausal symptoms

Start CHCS

Start on day 1 of cycle, on day of TOP, ≥21 days postpartum (>6 weeks if CHC and breastfeeding), or ≥2wks after fully mobile post major surgery. If starting CHC on day 1–5, cover is immediate, no other precautions (condoms) are needed. If later start (and not pregnant, p. 149), use condoms for 1wk. Qlaira*: start on day 1 (condoms for 9 days).

Stopping CHCS

Tell to stop at once if she develops: • Sudden severe chest pain • Sudden breathlessness (±cough/bloody sputum) • Severe calf pain • Unexplained leg swelling • Severe stomach pain • Unusual severe prolonged headache; sudden visual loss; collapse; dysphasia; hemi-motor/sensory loss; 1st seizure • Hepatitis, jaundice, liver enlargement • BP ≥160/95 • 4 weeks before leg or major surgery (p. 155) • Any CI (p. 152). On stopping, 66% menstruate by 6 weeks, 98% by 6 months; women amenorrhoeic post-CHC usually were before.

Missed pills

(Or severe diarrhoea.) Consult package inserts; advice varies. In general, if the start delay is ≥48h, or >48h since last pill continue pills but use condoms too for 7 days (+ days of diarrhoea); if this includes pill-free days, start next pack *without break* (omit inactive pills in 'ED' formulations). If ≥2 pills of 1st 7 days in pack forgotten, use emergency contraception if unprotected intercourse since end of last pack + condoms for 7d after restarting. Vomiting <2h post-pill: take another. Non-enzyme-inducing (p. 152) broad-spectrum antibiotics need extra precautions only if causing diarrhoea or vomiting. Postcoital options: p. 155. Diarrhoea and vomiting does not affect the contraceptive patch or ring.

Flying and high altitude

Avoid immobility if flight ≥3h. If trekking higher than 4500 metres for ≥1 week consider alternative.

Terminology

1st-generation pills are the original pills containing 50mcg oestrogen. *2nd-generation pills* are those containing ≤35mcg oestrogen and levonorgestrel, norethisterone, norgestimate, or cyproterone acetate. *3rd-generation pills* contain desogestrel or gestodene as the progesterone. Although designed to be more lipid friendly 3rd-generation pills have not been proven to be better in those with cardiac risk factors and are more thrombogenic.[35]

Risk of thromboembolism

Risk of thromboembolism is increased by combined hormonal preparations, whether pill, ring, or patch.[36][37col] Figures are not well known for progesterone-only preparations but they do not appear to be thrombogenic. Carriage of factor v Leiden mutation particularly increases risk of thrombosis (↑ risk ≈35). 3rd-generation

Table 2.3 Euras study 2007

Not on pill	44:100,000
Levonorgestrel	80:100,000
Drospirenone	91:100,000
Others	91:100,000
Pregnant	291:100,000

pills particularly increase resistance to our natural anticoagulant (activated protein c, APC), so increasing thrombosis. With antithrombin 3, protein c or s deficiency have thrombosis rates ↑ ≈5. Counsel those starting the pill that it does increase the risk of thrombosis, particularly in 1st year of use, but it is still a rare event (table 2.3).[37]

CHC and travel If immobile for >3h, the *BNF* recommends mid-journey exercises ± support stockings.

CHC and surgery Stop oestrogen-containing contraception 4wks preoperatively and arrange alternative contraception.

When to use emergency contraception (eg missed pill)

- CHC: if 2 or more 30–35mcg pills or 2 or more 20mcg pills forgotten in 1st 7 days of pack and unprotected sexual intercourse (UPSI) occurred in those 1st 7 days or pill-free week.
- POP: if 1 or more POPs have been missed or taken >3h late (>12h if desogestrel 75mcg, eg Cerazette®) and UPSI has occurred in the 2 days following this.
- IUCD IUS: if complete or partial expulsion identified or mid-cycle removal has been necessary and UPSI in the 7 days preceding this.
- Progesterone injection: if >12 weeks 5 days from last Depo-Provera® or >8 weeks from Noristerat® injection and UPSI occurred.
- Barrier method: failure of method (eg splitting, slippage).

Starting contraception after giving birth

- CHC: if not breastfeeding and no additional risk factors for VTE, CHC can be started on day 21 postpartum. Additional contraception is required for 7 days. If breastfeeding, CHC can be started after 6 weeks.
- POP (whether breastfeeding or not): start at any time. If >day 21 additional contraception is required for 48h.
- Progesterone injection/implant (whether breastfeeding or not): insert anytime. If >day 21 additional contraception required for 7 days (unless given days 1–5 of menstruation).
- IUD/IUS: fit <48h after delivery (effective immediately) or wait until >4 weeks postpartum, in which case IUD is effective immediately; IUS—additional contraception required for 7 days (or within days 1–7 of menstrual cycle).

Further reading

Family Planning Association: www.fpa.org.uk
Faculty of Sexual & Reproductive Healthcare: www.fsrh.org

Progestogen-only contraceptives thicken cervical mucus, reduce receptivity of the endometrium to implantation, and in some women, also inhibit ovulation. They have the advantage of reducing pelvic infection and are used where oestrogen-containing contraceptives are contraindicated. They can be initiated immediately postpartum and are safe with breastfeeding.

Reasons to avoid progestogen-only contraception Current breast cancer but may be used if >5yrs disease free, no other alternative, and after specialist advice; trophoblastic disease; liver disease; active viral hepatitis, severe decompensated cirrhosis, benign or malignant liver tumour; new symptoms or diagnosis of migraine with aura, IHD, stroke/TIA when taking progestogen-only contraception; avoid if SLE with antiphospholipid antibodies; any undiagnosed vaginal bleeding should be investigated before starting progestogen-only contraception.

Progestogen-only pill (POP) There are several brands available in the UK containing differing progestogens. Pills containing etynodiol, norethisterone, or levonorgestrel must be taken at the same time each day within a 3h window. Desogestrel-containing POPs (desogestrel 75mcg, eg Cerazette®) have a 12h window, and have a stronger ovarian suppressive effect than the others. *Side effects:* Higher failure rate than COCP, menstrual irregularities, increased risk of ectopic pregnancy and functional ovarian cysts, breast tenderness, depression, acne, reduced libido, and weight change. *Start:* On day 1–5 of the cycle (effective immediately) or any other time (use condoms for 2 days), or >3 weeks postpartum. Efficacy is affected by hepatic enzyme-inducing drugs— use alternative.

Depot progestogen (IM injection) 3 preparations are available: **medroxy-progesterone acetate** 150mg given deep IM 12-weekly; start during the 1st 5 days of a cycle (postpartum see p. 87); **norethisterone enantate** (Noristerat®) 200mg into gluteus maximus 8-weekly—licensed for 2 doses only; **Sayana Press®**—given SC every 13wks and can be self-administered (after 1st injection given and training received) thus reducing need for trip to GP surgery. Licensed for long-term use. Exclude pregnancy and use condoms for 7 days after injections >2wks late (consider emergency contraception if UPSI in last 5d). *Advantages:* Can be used up to age 50yrs if no other risk factors for osteoporosis, reduced risk of ectopic pregnancy, functional cysts, and sickle cell crises, reduced risk of endometrial cancer; may help PMS and menorrhagia. *Problems:* Menstrual disturbance usually settles with time, and amenorrhoea then supervenes. 33% amenorrhoeic after 6 months' use; 60% after 18 months. If very heavy bleeding occurs, exclude pregnancy; give injection early (but >8 weeks from previous dose) and give oestrogen if not CI. Fears of osteoporosis in users; recommend review after 2yrs' use and avoidance in adolescents unless the only acceptable method. Bone mass density increases when stopped. Other problems include weight gain (up to 2kg in 70% of women). There may be some delay in return of ovulation on stopping injections (median delay 10 months).

Implants Progesterone implants give up to 3yrs' contraception with one implantation. Nexplanon® is a radiopaque flexible rod containing **etonogestrel** 68mg which is implanted subdermally into the medial surface of the upper arm. Insert on day 1–5 of cycle (immediately effective), or any other time but use condoms for 7 days. Contraceptive effect stops when the implant is removed. It has no impact on bone density. <23% of users become amenorrhoeic after 12 months' use. Infrequent bleeding occurs in 50% in the 1st 3 months' use; 30% at 6 months. Prolonged bleeding affects up to 33% in 1st 3 months; frequent bleeding affects <10%. Effective contraception may not occur in overweight women (BMI >35kg/m²) in the 3rd yr, so consider earlier changing of implant. There is reduced efficacy with hepatic enzyme-inducing drugs.

Sterilization is permanent, irreversible contraception. There are no absolute contraindications provided that patients make the request themselves, are of sound mind, and are not acting under external duress. In the UK, funding on the NHS may depend on location; it is a 'low-priority procedure' and in some regions special funding needs to be agreed first and after alternative methods have failed or are contraindicated.

Ideally see both partners and consider the following

- *Alternative methods:* Do they know about depot progesterone injections, coils, and implants? Give written information (in relevant language) about alternative contraception and ♂ and ♀ sterilization.
- *Consent:* Is it the wish of both partners? Legally only the consent of the patient is required but the agreement of both is desirable. Those lacking mental capacity to consent require a High Court judgment.
- *Who should be sterilized?* Does she fear loss of femininity? Does he see it as being neutered? Is hysterectomy more appropriate (eg intractable menorrhagia)? Examine the one to be sterilized.
- *Irreversibility:* Reversal is only 50% successful in either sex and *never* funded by the NHS. Sterilization should be seen as an irreversible step. Sterilizations most regretted (3–10%) are those in the young (<30yrs), childless, at times of stress (especially relationship problems), or immediately after pregnancy (termination or delivery). For sterilization at CS, it should be discussed at least twice in the pregnancy (excluding the day of CS).
- *Warn of failure rates:* 1:200 for women (1:100 at CS), 1:2000 for men. In women, it is no better than the Mirena® coil. Advise seeking medical confirmation if future pregnancy suspected or abnormal vaginal bleeding or abdominal pain. If pregnancy occurs there is ↑ risk of ectopic (4.3–76%).
- *Side effect:* A women who has been on the COCP for many years may find her periods unacceptably heavy after sterilization. ▶Record in the notes: *Knows it's permanent, irreversible; lifetime failure rate discussed*, along with alternatives, eg 1:2000 for vasectomy, and 1:200 for ♀ sterilization.

Female sterilization The more the tubes are damaged, the lower the failure rate and the more difficult reversal becomes. In the UK, most sterilizations are carried out laparoscopically with general anaesthesia. Filshie clip occlusion is recommended with local anaesthetic applied to tubes (or modified Pomeroy operation at mini-laparotomy if postpartum or at CS). Do pregnancy test pre-operatively. Advise use of effective contraception until the operation and next period. Remove IUCD after the next period in case an already fertilized ovum is present. Alternatively, hysteroscopic sterilization using fallopian implants under local anaesthetic or IV sedation is endorsed by NICE.[38]

Vasectomy This is a simpler and safer procedure than female sterilization and can be performed as an outpatient under local anaesthetic. The vas deferens is identified at the top of the scrotum and is ligated and excised or the lumen cauterized. Fascial interposition improves effectiveness.[39] Bruising and haematoma are complications. No-scalpel techniques reduce these complications.[40] Late pain affects 3% from sperm granulomata, which are less common if thermal cautery (rather than electrical cautery) is used. Warn of risk of chronic testicular pain (up to 15%).

The major disadvantage of vasectomy is that it takes up to 3 months before sperm stores are used up. Obtain 1 semen sample 12 weeks and at least 20 ejaculates postoperatively and wait for negative result before stopping other methods of contraception (further samples may be required if there is doubt). Reversal is most successful if within 10 years of initial operation but this is never available on the NHS.

2 Gynaecology

Control of bladder function Continence in women is maintained in the urethra by the external sphincter and pelvic floor muscles maintaining a urethral pressure higher than bladder pressure. Micturition occurs when these muscles relax and the bladder detrusor muscle contracts.

Urinary history Incontinence is involuntary leakage of urine, which is divided into urge, stress, and mixed urinary incontinence. The woman may have waited for over 10yrs to seek help. Continuous urinary leakage is most commonly associated with a vesicovaginal fistula or congenital abnormality such as ectopic ureter. Ask about daytime voids (normal 4–7), nocturia (up to 70yrs, >1 night-time void is abnormal), nocturnal enuresis, urgency (most frequently due to detrusor overactivity), and voiding difficulties (hesitancy, straining, and slow or intermittent stream, most commonly seen with neurological conditions). Ask about the feeling of incomplete emptying, bladder pain (seen with interstitial cystitis), dysuria, haematuria, and recurrent UTI. Are there any symptoms of prolapse or bowel symptoms? It is important to check PMH, and record current drug treatment. How is the urinary incontinence affecting her quality of life (QOL)? Does it affect her relationship? *Frequency/volume charts* are a simple, objective way of obtaining information about fluid intake and voiding problems and should be filled in for 72h.

Examination Check weight, BMI, BP, and signs of systemic disease. Note manual dexterity and mobility as this can affect which treatment options are available to the woman. If symptoms suggest a neurological cause, perform a neurological examination (the most common cause of a neurogenic bladder in a woman is MS). Exclude an abdominal or pelvic mass, including a full bladder. Is the vulval/vaginal skin atrophic? Record any prolapse. Is there any urinary leakage on coughing?

Investigations

- *Urinalysis* and MSU for MC&S to exclude UTI; OGTT if diabetes is suspected.
- Check residual volume post micturition to exclude incomplete emptying.
- *Imaging* is not routinely used but may include US to exclude incomplete bladder emptying and define any pelvic mass.
- *Cystoscopy* is used to visualize the urethra, bladder mucosa, trigone, and ureteric orifices. Biopsies can be taken. Indicated if recurrent UTI, haematuria, bladder pain, suspected fistula, tumour, or interstitial cystitis.
- *Urodynamics* are a combination of tests which look at the ability of the bladder to store and void urine. Uroflowmetry screens for voiding difficulties and the patient voids in private onto a commode with a urinary flow meter, measuring voided volume over time and plotting it on a graph. Cystometry is more invasive and involves measuring pressure and volume within the bladder during filling and voiding, and is a test of bladder function. The bladder is filled with saline via a catheter, and an intravesical and rectal probe measure differences in pressure, to give the detrusor pressure. The patient is asked for first desire to void, strong desire to void, and to cough. The results are printed onto a graph and any detrusor contractions and/or leakage noted.

Classification *Stress urinary incontinence* is the involuntary leakage of urine on effort or exertion, or on sneezing or coughing. Commonly due to urethral sphincter weakness. *Urge urinary incontinence* is the involuntary leakage of urine with a strong desire to pass urine. Commonly coexists with frequency and nocturia and forms overactive bladder syndrome. *Mixed urinary incontinence* is the combination of stress and urge incontinence and usually one symptom will predominate (treat that first). *Overflow incontinence* is usually due to injury or insult eg postpartum. Treat with catheter.

Further reading

NICE (2013). *Urinary Incontinence in Women: Management* (CG171). London: NICE. https://www.nice.org.uk/guidance/cg171

Stress urinary incontinence (SUI) This is the most common urinary reason for which a woman will seek help. It affects up to 1 in 10, and in 50% will be pure stress incontinence. It occurs when detrusor pressure exceeds the closing pressure of the urethra. Pregnancy itself is a risk factor (mode of delivery much less so). At the menopause, oestrogen deficiency leads to weakening of pelvic support and thinning of the urothelium. Other causes include radiotherapy, congenital weakness, and trauma from radical pelvic surgery (eg for gynaecological cancer).

Investigations: Exclude UTI (this will worsen symptoms). A frequency/volume chart shows normal frequency and functional bladder capacity. Urodynamics are indicated when surgery is being considered, in order to confirm the diagnosis, check for detrusor overactivity (which can be worsened irreversibly by surgical procedures), and check for voiding dysfunction (a woman with a poor flow rate is at risk of long-term urinary retention).

Management:
- *Conservative measures* should be tried first. These include optimizing control of other medical problems, eg diabetes, weight loss, smoking cessation, treatment of chronic cough, and constipation. *Pelvic floor exercises* for at least 3 months and continued long-term (refer to a pelvic floor physiotherapist). Biofeedback uses a device to convert the effect of pelvic floor contraction into a visual or auditory signal.
- *Pharmacological agents* are not recommended as 1st-line treatment by NICE. Duloxetine is the only licensed drug for this but it is rarely used.
- *Surgery* is considered after other measures have failed. *Peri-urethral injections* of bulking agents are successful in 20–40% and have lower morbidity than other procedures. The *tension-free vaginal tape* (TVT) was the most common surgical procedure for SUI in the UK until 2018 when all vaginal mesh was temporarily banned due to problems with long-term outcomes—especially mesh erosion. A polypropylene mesh tape is placed under the mid-urethra via a small vaginal incision with a mean cure rate of 94%. Other risks of TVT include bladder injury and voiding difficulty. At present it is unclear how long the ban will be in place for. The laparoscopic colposuspension (insertion of non-absorbable sutures to elevate the bladder neck) is gaining in popularity with around an 80% success rate, but requires advanced laparoscopic skills and further training to make it more widely available.

Overactive bladder syndrome (OAB) OAB is a chronic condition affecting up to 1 in 6 women, and implies underlying detrusor overactivity (DO). DO is a diagnosis made on urodynamic testing. Incidence increases with age. It is mostly idiopathic, but may be found with MS, spina bifida, or secondary to pelvic or incontinence surgery. Symptoms may be provoked by cold weather, opening the front door, or by coughing or sneezing leading to confusion with symptoms of stress incontinence. It is unpredictable and the urine leakage may be significant, having a huge impact on the woman's QOL. *Investigations:* Exclude UTI. A frequency/volume chart typically shows ↑ diurnal frequency and nocturia. Urodynamics show involuntary detrusor contractions during filling and should be performed if there is doubt about the diagnosis, complex symptoms, or drug treatment has failed. *Management:* Avoid excessive fluid intake, caffeinated and carbonated drinks, and alcohol. Bladder retraining aims to suppress the urinary urge and extend the intervals between voiding. *Anticholinergics* are the mainstay of pharmacological therapy, blocking the parasympathetic nerves and relaxing detrusor. Try **oxybutynin** 2.5–5mg 1–4 times/day. Alternatives are **solifenacin** 5–10mg daily, or **mirabegron** 50mg daily (specialist advice only). SE include dry mouth, constipation, and nausea. *Intravaginal oestrogen cream* can help in those with vaginal atrophy. Other measures include *botulinum toxin* injected cystoscopically into detrusor (90% effective). Neuromodulation can help. Surgery is a last resort.

2 Gynaecology

A prolapse occurs when weakness of the supporting structures allows the pelvic organs to protrude within the vagina (fig 2.15). The weakness may be congenital, and is associated with prolonged labour, trauma from instrumental delivery, lack of postnatal pelvic floor exercise, obesity, chronic cough, and constipation. Poor perineal repair reduces support. Prolapse is exacerbated by the menopause and is not a danger to health—except for 3rd-degree uterine prolapse with cystocele when ureteric obstruction can occur.

Types of prolapse (fig 2.16) Named according to structure affected. Several types may coexist in the same patient. *Cystocele:* The anterior wall of the vagina, and the bladder attached to it, bulge. Residual urine within the cystocele may cause frequency and dysuria. It is associated with urethral prolapse (cystourethrocele). *Rectocele:* The lower posterior wall, which is attached to rectum, may bulge through weak levator ani. It is often symptomless, but she may have to reduce herniation prior to defecation by putting a finger in the vagina, or pressing on the perineum. *Enterocele:* Bulges of the upper posterior vaginal wall may contain loops of intestine from the pouch of Douglas. *Uterine prolapse:* Protrusion of the uterus downwards into the vagina, taking with it the cervix and upper vagina. If the woman has had a total hysterectomy, the vaginal vault is left and may also prolapse (15–20% risk after hysterectomy).

Grading of prolapse *1st degree:* The lowest part of the prolapse descends halfway down the vaginal axis to the introitus. *2nd degree:* The lowest part of the prolapse extends to the level of the introitus, and through the introitus on straining. *3rd degree:* The lowest part of the prolapse extends through the introitus and outside the vagina. *Procidentia:* Refers to 4th-degree uterine prolapse—the uterus lies outside the vagina.

Symptoms May be asymptomatic. Dragging sensation, discomfort, feeling of a lump 'coming down,' dyspareunia, backache. With cystocele, urinary urgency and frequency, incomplete bladder emptying, urinary retention if the urethra is kinked. With rectocele, constipation and difficulty with defecation. How do the symptoms affect her QOL? *Prevention:* Lower parity; better obstetric practices; pelvic floor exercises.

Examination Bimanual to exclude pelvic masses. Examine for prolapse with the woman in left lateral position using a Sims speculum or standing. Inspect anterior and posterior walls for atrophy and descent. If no obvious prolapse, ask the woman to strain. Arrange urodynamic studies if urinary incontinence.

Management *Conservative:* Mild disease may improve with reduction in intra-abdominal pressure, so encourage her to lose weight, stop smoking, and stop straining. Improve muscle tone with exercises or physiotherapy. *Pessaries:* Useful in those who decline surgery, are unfit for surgery, or if surgery is contraindicated. They affect sexual function. They should be changed every 6 months and if the woman is postmenopausal, topical oestrogen is useful to prevent vaginal erosion. Ring pessaries are the most common and come in many different sizes. It is placed between the posterior aspect of the symphysis pubis and posterior fornix of the vagina. The Gelhorn* pessary is similar in principle but is shaped like a mushroom. Shelves, cubes, and doughnuts are less commonly used. *Surgery:* Useful if symptoms are severe, the woman is sexually active, and pessaries have failed. The type of prolapse repair depends on type of prolapse. Repair operations (p. 177) excise redundant tissue and strengthen supports, but may reduce vaginal width. Marked uterine prolapse is treated by hysterectomy with or without sacrospinous fixation, or by laparoscopic sacrohysteropexy. Post-hysterectomy vault prolapse may be treated by sacrocolpopexy (eg with mesh). Anterior or posterior pelvic floor repair does not use mesh—it has been banned for prolapse repair due to the high complication rate.

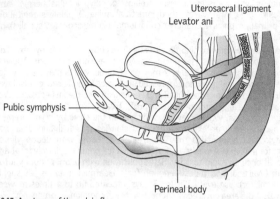

Fig 2.15 Anatomy of the pelvic floor.
Reproduced with permission from Impey L. (1999) *Obstetrics and Gynaecology*. Oxford: Wiley-Blackwell Publishing.

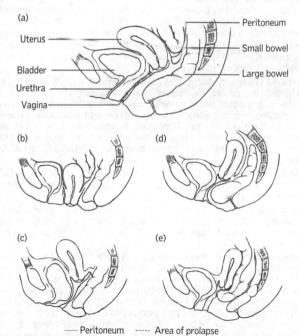

Fig 2.16 Types of prolapse. (a) Normal pelvis, (b) uterine prolapse, (c) cystocele, (d) rectocele, (e) enterocele.
Reproduced with permission from Impey L. (1999) *Obstetrics and Gynaecology*. Oxford: Wiley-Blackwell Publishing.

2 Gynaecology

Causes of vulval lumps Local varicose veins; boils; sebaceous cysts; Bartholin's cyst or abscess; uterine prolapse or polyp; inguinal hernia; varicocele; carcinoma; viral warts (condylomata acuminata); painless genital ulcer from primary syphilis (a chancre); condylomata lata (secondary syphilis); molluscum contagiosum.

Vulval warts Human papilloma virus (HPV)—is usually spread by sexual contact. *Incubation:* weeks. Her partner may not have obvious warts. The vulva, perineum, anus, vagina, or cervix may be affected. Warts may be very florid in the pregnant and immunosuppressed. HPV types 6 and 11 cause vulval warts and 16, 18, and 33 can cause vulval and cervical intraepithelial neoplasia. Warts may also cause anal carcinoma (*OHCM* p631). Treat both partners. Exclude other genital infections. Warts may be destroyed in the clinic by cryotherapy, trichloroacetic acid, or electrocautery/excision/laser. Vulval and anal warts (condylomata acuminata) may be treated at home with podophyllotoxin cream for 4–6 weeks, washed off after 30min (CI: pregnancy). Only treat a few warts at once, to avoid toxicity. Self-application with 0.15% **podophyllotoxin cream** (Warticon® 5g tubes—enough for 4 treatment courses—is supplied with a mirror): use every 12h for 3 days, repeated up to 4 times at weekly intervals if the area covered is <4cm². Relapse is common. In pregnancy, warts may grow rapidly and usually regress after delivery. Problematic warts can be treated with cryotherapy. It is not an indication for delivery by CS. *HPV immunization and cervical cancer:* See p. 166. NB: HPV types 6 and 11 may cause laryngeal or respiratory papillomas in the offspring of affected mothers (risk 1:50–1:1500; 50% present at <5yrs old). Any warty lesion in a postmenopausal woman should be biopsied to exclude vulval cancer.[41]RCOG

Urethral caruncle This is a small red swelling at the urethral orifice. It is caused by meatal prolapse. It may be tender and give pain on micturition. *Treatment:* Excision or diathermy.

Bartholin's cyst and abscess (fig 2.18) The Bartholin's glands and ducts lie under the labia minora. They secrete thin lubricating mucus during sexual excitation. If the duct blocks, a painless cyst forms; if this becomes infected the resulting abscess is extremely painful (she cannot sit down) and a hugely swollen, hot red labium is seen. *Treatment:* The abscess should be incised, and permanent drainage ensured by marsupialization, ie inner cyst wall is folded back and stitched to the skin, or by balloon catheter insertion.[42]NICE *Tests:* Exclude gonococcus.

Vulvitis Vulval inflammation may be due to infections, eg candida (p. 132), herpes simplex; chemicals (bubble-baths, detergents). It is often associated with, or may be due to, vaginal discharge.

Vulval ulcers (fig 2.19) *Causes:* Always consider syphilis. Herpes simplex is common in the young. Others: carcinoma; chancroid; lymphogranuloma venereum; granuloma inguinale; TB; Behçet syndrome; aphthous ulcers; Crohn's disease.

Herpes simplex (fig 2.17) Herpes type II classically causes genital infection, but either type can be the cause (30% type I). It is the third most common STI in the UK. The primary infection is usually the most severe, starting with the prodrome (itching/tingling of affected skin) and flu-like illness, progressing to vulvitis, pain, and small vesicles on the vulva. Urinary retention may occur due to autonomic nerve dysfunction. Recurrent attacks are usually less severe and may be triggered by illness, stress, sexual intercourse, and menstruation. *Treatment:* Strong analgesia, **lidocaine gel** 2%, salt baths (and micturating in the bath) help. Exclude coexistent infections. Aciclovir orally shortens symptoms. Oral dose: 200mg 5 times daily or 400mg/8h for 5 days (longer if new lesions appear during treatment or if healing is incomplete).

If immunocompromised/HIV+ve: 400mg 5 times daily for 7–10 days during 1st episode or 400mg/8h for 5–10 days during recurrent infection. If >6 outbreaks/year consider suppressive aciclovir for 6–12 months. Topical aciclovir is not beneficial. HSV can be transmitted during asymptomatic phases of viral shedding, and from areas of the genitals not protected by barrier contraception. Men are usually less symptomatic and may never have been aware of the infection, thereby unknowingly infecting their partners months or even years later, so don't assume infidelity.

For herpes in pregnancy, see p. 40.

Carcinoma of the vulva ►Refer unexplained vulval lumps urgently. 90% are squamous. Others are melanoma, basal cell carcinomas or carcinoma of Bartholin's glands. They are rare and usually occur in the elderly (age 70–80).

Presentation may be as a lump; as an indurated ulcer which may not be noticed unless it causes pain and bleeding hence often presenting late (50% already have inguinal lymph node involvement). There may be a preinvasive phase as VIN (for explanation and treatment see p. 131). *Treatment:*[41,RCOL] If tumour <2cm width and <1mm deep, lymph node excision is not needed. If >1mm deep do 'triple incision surgery' =wide (>15mm margin) local excision + ipsilateral groin node biopsy (and, if affected, sample contralateral side too). More advanced disease may need radical vulvectomy (wide excision of the vulva + removal of inguinal glands). Skin grafts may be needed. Radiotherapy may be used preoperatively to shrink tumours if sphincters may be affected. Chemoradiation is used if unsuitable for surgery, to shrink large tumours preoperatively, and for relapses. 5yr survival is >80% for lesions <2cm with no node involvement; otherwise <50%.

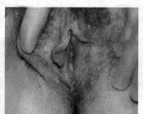

Fig 2.17 Herpes simplex.
Reproduced from Mitchell *et al.*, *Oxford Handbook of Genitourinary Medicine, HIV and Sexual Health* (2019), with permission from OUP.

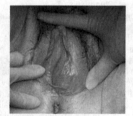

Fig 2.18 Bartholin's abscess.
Reproduced from Sarris *et al.*, *Training in Obstetrics and Gynaecology* (2009) with permission from OUP.

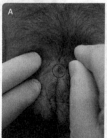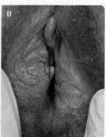

Fig 2.19 Vulval cancer.
Reproduced with permission from Simons, M. *et al.* (2010). A patient with lichen sclerosus, Langerhans cell histiocytosis, and invasive squamous cell carcinoma of the vulva. *American Journal of Obstetrics and Gynecology*, 203(2):e7–e10. doi: https://doi.org/10.1016/j.ajog.2010.04.023. Copyright © 2010 Mosby, Inc. All rights reserved.

This is the part of the uterus below the internal os. The endocervical canal is lined with mucous columnar epithelium, the vaginal cervix with squamous epithelium. The transitional zone between them—the squamocolumnar junction—is the area which is predisposed to malignant change.

Cervical ectropion/erosion (fig 2.20)
There is a red ring around the os because the endocervical epithelium has extended its territory over the paler epithelium of the ectocervix. Ectropions extend temporarily under hormonal influence during puberty, with the combined pill, and during pregnancy. As columnar epithelium is soft and glandular, ectropion is prone to bleeding, to excess mucus production, and to infection. *Treatment:* No treatment if asymptomatic, pregnant, or pubertal. If taking hormonal contraception consider changing to non-hormonal methods; cautery with diathermy as an out-patient if the woman wishes.

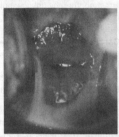
Fig 2.20 Cervical ectropion.
Courtesy of Mike Hughey.

Nabothian cysts These mucus retention cysts found on the cervix are harmless. **Cervical polyps** These pedunculated benign tumours of endocervical epithelium may cause increased mucus discharge or postcoital bleeding. *Treatment:* They may be simply avulsed in the outpatient clinic, but full assessment includes TVS ± hysteroscopy to exclude intrauterine polyps.

Cervicitis This may be follicular or mucopurulent, presenting with discharge. *Causes:* Chlamydia (up to 50%), gonococci, or herpes (look for vesicles). Chronic cervicitis (see fig 2.21) is usually a mixed infection. Cervicitis may mask neoplasia on a smear.

Cervical screening Persistent infection with HR–HPV is the key factor in the vast majority of cases of cervical cancer. Multiple subtypes have been linked to its pathogenesis (p. 166) and 80% of women become infected with HPV within 18 months of becoming sexually active. HR–HPV infection is asymptomatic, and usually cleared within 18 months. In persistent infection, the epithelium starts to become dysplastic and eventually (in about 10 years) invasive squamous cell carcinoma of the cervix.

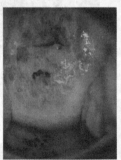
Fig 2.21 Chronic cervicitis.
Courtesy of Mike Hughey.

Cervical cells are collected (p. 165) and the sample is analysed for high-risk HPV (subtypes 16 and 18). Primary HPV screening has a lower false-negative rate than cytology alone (important because UK-wide vaccination of teenagers for subtypes 16 and 18 will lead to a reduction in CIN). If the sample is HR–HPV negative, no cytology is carried out and the woman goes back to routine recall. If HR–HPV is detected, the smear is then analysed for cytology and if this is abnormal (borderline, mild, moderate, or severe dyskaryosis), a colposcopy referral is automatically generated. Colposcopy correlates degree of cytology abnormality with histological diagnosis of CIN I–III. The higher the grade of CIN, the higher the risk of progression to carcinoma. Treatment is with LLETZ (p. 166).

About 72% of the total eligible UK population is now screened (the lowest since Jade Goody, a celebrity, died from cervical cancer in 2009), and mortality is 50% that of 1988 (the year screening started).

Risk factors for CIN:
- Persistent high-risk HPV (HR-HPV) infection.
- Exposure to HPV is increased by multiple partners.
- Smoking.
- Immunocompromise (HIV, transplant patients, immunosuppressants).
- The oral contraceptive pill is associated with CIN but probably due to reduced use of barrier contraception, thereby increasing exposure to HPV.

English cervical screening criteria:
- Sexually active women aged 25–64yrs.
- 3-yearly for woman 25–50 years, and 5-yearly until 64 (if normal).
- Yearly in HIV +ve women.
- 95% of abnormalities are identified by 3-yearly screening.
- In Scotland, screening begins at 20 years, and worldwide screening intervals vary considerably.

Taking a smear

- Explain the nature and purpose of the test, and how results will be conveyed. Warn that results are not always unequivocal.
- The cervix is visualized with a speculum (p. 106). Are there any suspicious areas? If so, carry on with the smear and indicate this on the referral form, and refer immediately for colposcopy under the 2-week rule.
- Cells are scraped from the squamocolumnar transformation zone with a special brush which is agitated in a liquid, ready for analysis (HR–HPV and liquid-based cytology).
- Suspensions can also be tested for *Chlamydia*.
- Ensure regular training and supervision, and audit of numbers of 'inadequate sample' reports. Don't do smears on a one-off basis (in the UK NHS, professionalism mandates formal methods of quality control, and specifies an acceptable number of smears per year, etc.).

Table 2.4 Management of abnormal smears

HR–HPV	Cytology	Management
Negative	Not analysed	Routine recall (3-5 years)
Detected	Normal	Repeat smear in 12 months; if HR–HPV negative, normal recall; if positive, colposcopy
Detected	Borderline, mild, moderate, or severe	Colposcopy referral; management depending on grade of CIN. Negative colposcopy: normal recall. CIN I: repeat smear in 12 months. CIN II–III: LLETZ
Moderate dyskaryosis	Treated CIN	Repeat smear at 6 months (test of cure)
Detected	Suspected invasion	50% invasion: 2 week rule referral to colposcopy

Further reading

Public Health England (2019). Cervical Screening: Implementation Guide for Primary HPV Screening. PHE, London. https://www.gov.uk/government/publications/cervical-screening-primary-hpv-screening-implementation/cervical-screening-implementation-guide-for-primary-hpv-screening#protocols

Aim to detect preinvasive disease by attendance at cervical screening. ~1900 women die yearly of cervical cancer in the UK. The main cause is human papilloma virus (eg HPV 16, 18, 31, 33, 35, 39, 45, 51, 52, 56, 58, 59, 68). Vaccines work only against a subset, eg Gardasil® covers HPV 6, 11, 16 & 18, the cause in 70% of cases. 99.7% of cervical cancers contain HPV DNA.

Dyskaryosis is a cytological term used to describe cervical smears. There are high false-positive (10–15%) and false-negative rates (5–15%), hence the need for further assessment by colposcopy.

Colposcopy This is the examination of the cervix by a colposcope—a binocular microscope which magnifies by 6–40×. The woman is in the lithotomy position and a bivalve speculum is inserted into the vagina. Once the cervix is visualized, the transformation zone is identified and painted with 5% acetic acid. This is preferentially taken up by neoplastic cells (fig 2.22 on p. 169). Lugol's iodine is also used, which is not taken up by neoplastic cells. Aceto-white areas identify abnormal areas and this enables a punch biopsy to be taken in order to gain a histological diagnosis (CIN or malignancy). If there is strong uptake of acetic acid (termed high-grade colposcopy), CIN II–III is more likely and the option is to 'see and treat'—perform definitive treatment in the same appointment without waiting for a biopsy result. CIN is also associated with vascular abnormalities. Very abnormal-looking vessels are associated with micro-invasive carcinoma. Colposcopy does not detect adenocarcinoma (it usually lies within endocervical canal). A pregnant woman can have colposcopy but not a LLETZ, and should wait until she is 12 weeks postpartum for definitive treatment.

Large loop excision of the transformation zone (LLETZ) CIN is managed according to grade of abnormality and patient preference, either conservatively or by excision. A LLETZ is usually performed in the colposcopy clinic under local anaesthesia, using loop diathermy. It is safe, easy to perform (all those treating CIN should be qualified to do so), and tissue is available for histology and confirmation of clear excision margins. It gives ~90% cure rates with one treatment.

Low-grade CIN (CIN I): Regresses spontaneously in 60% with no treatment. Repeat smear at 12 months; if HR–HPV negative, discharge to normal recall. May need LLETZ if persistent.

High-grade CIN (>CIN I): Progresses to cervical cancer in 3–5% of those with CIN II and 20–30% with CIN III within 10 years if left untreated. Spontaneous regression is possible but much less likely. It is therefore recommended for excision with LLETZ.

After LLETZ, the woman should have a test of cure smear at 6 months with high-risk HPV testing. If negative, she can return to 3-yearly smears. A positive HR-HPV test requires repeat assessment with colposcopy.

Complications of LLETZ: Include haemorrhage, infection, vaso-vagal symptoms and signs, anxiety, cervical stenosis, and a small risk of cervical incompetence and premature delivery (risk is thought to be increased with repeated LLETZ or biopsy depth >1cm).

CGIN This is cervical glandular intraepithelial neoplasia, and it can coexist with CIN or be a sole finding. It is also associated with high-risk HPV and can be difficult to manage, because the endocervical epithelium extends into the cervical canal and is therefore not completely visible at colposcopy, has no specific colposcopic appearances, and is associated with higher 'skip lesions'. It is managed with a cylindrical LLETZ or cone biopsy, or if family is complete, hysterectomy.

HPV vaccination HPV is a key player in the development of cervical cancer, and schoolchildren in the UK (girls and boys) are offered the HPV vaccine at 12 years, before their sexual debut. They offer no protection once HPV infection has occurred and are therefore not recommended in the management of CIN. The vaccines are primarily against HPV subtypes 6 and 11 (anogenital warts) and 16 and 18 (HR-HPV). They do not prevent all cancers (there are 15 HR-HPVS) and the long-term antibody response is at present unknown.

2 Gynaecology

83% of cervical cancer occurs in developing countries and is the 2nd most common cancer in women worldwide. Incidence has 2 peaks: the 1st at 30–39 years and the 2nd in the over 70s. Screening in the UK has increased the proportion of micro-invasive disease and adenocarcinomas (most are squamous carcinomas). High-risk HPV is strongly associated with cervical cancer. Risk factors are the same as for CIN (pp. 164–5). See fig 2.23 on p. 169.

Symptoms and signs
- Cervical smear showing ?invasion (unreliable).
- Incidental finding on treatment of CIN.
- Postcoital and/or postmenopausal bleeding; watery vaginal discharge.
- Features of advanced disease include heavy vaginal bleeding, ureteric obstruction, weight loss, bowel disturbance, vesicovaginal fistula, and pain.

Examination Colposcopy shows an irregular cervical surface, abnormal vessels, and dense uptake of acetic acid. On bimanual examination, the cervix feels roughened and hard, and if disease is advanced, there is loss of the fornices and the cervix is fixed. Speculum examination shows an irregular mass that often will bleed on contact.

Investigations Should include FBC, U&E, LFTS, punch biopsy for histology (LLETZ is contraindicated as it will bleed heavily and is not definitive treatment), CT abdomen and pelvis (staging), MRI pelvis (very accurate for staging and identifying suspicious lymph nodes). Examination under anaesthetic helps staging, and includes cystoscopy, hysteroscopy, PV/PR examination and sometimes sigmoidoscopy. MRI is so accurate that EUA is now performed less often. *Stage I* tumours are confined to the cervix; *Ia* microscopic; *Ib* macroscopic. *Stage II* have extended locally to upper ⅔ of the vagina; *IIb* if to parametria. *Stage III* have spread to lower ⅓ of vagina *IIIa;* or pelvic wall *IIIb*. *Stage IV* have spread to bladder or rectum. *IVb* if spread to distant organs. Most present in stages I or II. Up to stage Ib, 5 year survival is 90–95%.

Treatment Depends on stage and functional status:
- *Stage Ia1* (<3mm depth): local excision (fertility-sparing) or hysterectomy.
- *Stage Ia2* (<5mm depth) and *Ib1* (<4cm diameter): lymphadenectomy and if node negative, proceed to Wertheim's hysterectomy.
- *Stage Ib2* (>4cm diameter) and early *IIa:* chemoradiotherapy. If negative lymph nodes, consider Wertheim's hysterectomy.
- *>Stage IIb* : combination chemoradiotherapy.
- *Stage IVb* : chemoradiotherapy; palliative radiotherapy to control bleeding.

Laparoscopic lymphadenectomy is being used increasingly prior to hysterectomy; some units are now doing Wertheim's hysterectomy laparoscopically. Cisplatin is the main chemotherapy agent used.

Complications of treatment for Wertheim's (radical) hysterectomy and lymphadenectomy include bleeding, infection, VTE, ureteric fistula, bladder dysfunction, and lymphoedema. Radiotherapy can cause acute bladder and bowel dysfunction with tenesmus, mucositis, bleeding, ulceration, strictures and fistula formation, vaginal stenosis, shortening, and dryness.

2 Gynaecology

Primary vaginal cancers are extremely rare, accounting for <1% gynaecological malignancies. Vaginal tumours are most commonly due to metastatic spread from cervical, uterine, or vulval cancers. Of the true primary vaginal cancers, most are squamous in origin and present on older women. There is an association with previous CIN, pelvic radiotherapy, and long-term vaginal inflammation from pessaries or a procidentia (complete uterine prolapse). It is commonly HPV-related.

They are commonest in the upper third of the vagina. Presentation is usually with bleeding. Clear cell adenocarcinoma is associated with intrauterine exposure to diethylstilboestrol before 18 weeks' gestation but risk is low (0.1–1:1000). (Note: risk of invasive cervical carcinoma is also increased 3-fold, and structural abnormalities of the genital tract—uterine 69% and cervical 44%—are problems following past exposure).[43, RCOG] Spread is local and by lymphatics. Treatment is usually radiotherapy. Prognosis is poor eg 58% 5yr survival for squamous vaginal carcinoma; 34% for adenocarcinoma.

A note on cancer research, survival, and alternative medicine in the UK
Medical research in the UK is funded from 3 sources: government by allocation of funds from taxes (£2.5 billion), medical research charities (who distribute donor funds) (£1 billion), and private industry. How these funds are then allocated does not seem to be according to disease burden: great inequalities exist within the funding of research into cancer. It has been long-documented that some cancers have more 'funding appeal' than others—breast cancer received 13% of the total funding available in 2013 compared with 1% for ovarian cancer and 0.6% for cervical.[44] When funding is analysed against mortality (see table 2.5), the discrepancy increases even further—breast cancer again receives millions more despite having a relatively good prognosis compared with ovarian, lung, or pancreatic cancer.

Whilst the UK is one of the leaders in research investment, it lags behind Europe in terms of cancer mortality for lung, ovarian, and colorectal cancers. This is thought to be due to delayed diagnosis, lower use of successful treatments, and reduced access to these treatments, especially by the elderly.[45] However, rather than solely blame cancer care in the UK, it would be prudent to note that difference in lifestyle, smoking, alcohol use, and poor diet have not been accounted for.

When it comes to the use of complementary therapies, there is little evidence of benefit and potentially even evidence of harm. The problem seems to come from patients choosing alternative medicine instead of conventional cancer treatments with a resulting negative impact on survival.[46] Young women seem particularly at risk of choosing the alternative medicine path. However, when used alongside conventional treatment it appears safe, with benefits especially for psychosocial well-being, pain, and anxiety.[47] Beware herbal medicines—these potentially interact with chemotherapy. A low-fat diet with avoidance of processed food may be beneficial to survival but there is limited evidence for this at present.

Sources of support for women with gynaecological malignancy:
General: Macmillan (www.macmillan.org).
Ovarian: Ovacome (www.ovacome.org) and Target (www.targetovariancancer.org.uk).
Endometrial: Maggie's centres (www.maggiescentres.org).
Cervical: Jo's Trust (www.jostrust.org).

2 Gynaecology

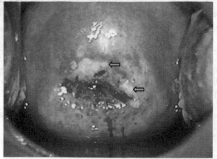

Fig 2.22 Colposcopic view of CIN III.
Reproduced from Sarris *et al. Training in Obstetrics and Gynaecology*
(2009) with permission from OUP.

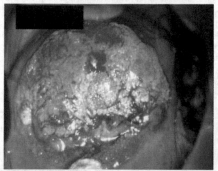

Fig 2.23 Exophytic cervical carcinoma.
Reproduced from Sarris *et al. Training in Obstetrics and Gynaecology*
(2009) with permission from OUP.

Table 2.5 Cancer in women by incidence with 1- and 5-year survival rates

	Registrations	1yr survival (%)	5yr survival (%)
Breast	45,656	96	86
Lung	17,821	40	16
Colorectal	15,371	75	57
Uterus	7,958	91	78
Melanoma	6,987	98	93
Ovary	6,430	77	50
Non-Hodgkin lymphoma	5,388	82	71
Pancreas	4,091	23	6
Kidney	3,392	78	63
Leukaemia	3,268	67	50
Cervix	2,594	85	67
Source: data from Cancer registration and survival statistics, England 2016 (Office for National Statistics) www.ons.gov.uk			

▶*Investigate postmenopausal vaginal bleeding **promptly** as the cause may be endometrial cancer.* Cancer of the endometrium is more common than cancer of the cervix. 91% of cases occur in postmenopausal women. Most are adenocarcinomas, and are related to excessive exposure to oestrogen unopposed by progesterone. There is marked geographical variation: North American:Chinese ratio ≈7:1, reflecting differences in risk factors, which are as follows:

• Obesity, type 2 diabetes, hypertension (increased peripheral oestrogens).
• Nulliparity (pregnancy associated with high progesterone levels).
• Anovulatory cycles, such as PCOS (absence of corpus luteum and therefore progesterone).
• Early/late menopause.
• Genetic predisposition: HNPCC (Lynch II syndrome) confers a high risk of colorectal, endometrial, and ovarian cancers.
• Breast cancer (similar lifestyle factors, and tamoxifen use).
• Oestrogen-only HRT.
• Protective factors are parity, and the combined oral contraceptive pill.

Presentation
Usually postmenopausal bleeding (PMB). A woman with PMB has a 10% risk of gynaecological cancer. Premenopausal women have heavy or irregular periods, and 1% are detected on routine smear. PV discharge and pyometra can also occur—50% with pyometra have underlying cancer.

Diagnosis
PMB is an early sign, and generally leads a woman to see her doctor, but examination is usually normal. TVS shows endometrial thickness >4mm. ET <4mm on scan has 96% negative predictive value with no requirement for biopsy, unless symptoms are recurrent. Biopsy can be performed either in out-patients (p. 171) or with hysteroscopy. Hysteroscopy enables visualization of abnormal endometrium to improve accuracy of sampling. Once diagnosis has been made, CT/MRI are used to help preoperatively stage.

Histology
Major prognostic indicators are grade of differentiation and FIGO stage of disease. It may metastasize to the vagina (5%), ovary (5%), or any of the pelvic lymph nodes (7%).

Staging
(See fig 2.24.) The tumour is …
I in the body of the uterus only.
II in the body and cervix only.
III advancing beyond the uterus, but not beyond the pelvis.
IV extending outside the pelvis (eg to bowel and bladder).

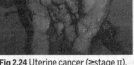
Fig 2.24 Uterine cancer (≥stage II).
Courtesy of Prof. J. Carter.

Treatment
Depends on stage and functional status of the patient.

Total hysterectomy with bilateral salpingo-oophorectomy preferably laparoscopically. Pelvic lymphadenectomy is controversial in early stage disease with Cochrane suggesting no survival benefit. Adjuvant radiotherapy is used in low-grade disease with deep myometrial invasion, and high-grade disease with superficial invasion. Radiotherapy has been shown to reduce pelvic recurrences but confers no survival benefit to late stage I disease, because those recurrences are responsive to radiotherapy if it has not previously been used. In advanced disease, high-dose progesterone helps with palliation of symptoms, and external beam radiotherapy can be used to control bleeding. Stage I disease has 85% 5-year survival, dropping to 25% by stage IV.

Endometrial sampling in outpatients

This bedside investigation is used primarily for the investigation of postmenopausal bleeding (investigation of menorrhagia should now be by out-patient hysteroscopy). It is cheap, reliable, and gives quick results without the need for anaesthesia. If transvaginal uterine us precedes the procedure, sample if endometrium >4mm thick. It is less useful in menorrhagia in women <45 years with regular cycles, as pathology is less common.

A sample is obtained using a side-opening plastic cannula in which a vacuum is created by withdrawal of a stopped central plunger mechanism. As the cannula is withdrawn and rotated in each quadrant of the uterine cavity, endometrial tissue is sucked into its interior, through the hole in its side (fig 2.25). Successful insertion is possible in 90–99% of women (hysteroscopy and biopsy possible in 99%). Adequate samples will be obtained in 91% of these, and in 84% of those for whom PMB was the indication. Abandon the procedure if it is impossible to enter the uterus, or if it causes too much pain.

Technique
1 Bimanual examination to assess size and position of uterus (p. 106).
2 Bend cervical cannula to follow the curve of the uterus.
3 Insert device, watching the centimetre scale on the side; observe resistance on entering the internal os (at 3–4cm) and then as the tip reaches the fundus.
4 When the tip is in the fundus, create a vacuum by withdrawing plunger until the stopper prevents further withdrawal. Then move sampler up and down in the uterus, rotate and repeat to sample whole cavity.
5 Remove cannula, and expel tissue into formalin. Send for histology. Vabra vacuum aspiration samples a greater area of tissue, and has higher cancer detection rates, but is more uncomfortable.[48]

Management
Reassure those in whom the results show normal or atrophic endometrium and those in whom tissue was sufficient for diagnosis. If those with PMB re-bleed, refer for hysteroscopy (polyps or a fibroid will be present in 20%). Those with simple hyperplasia on histology can be treated with progesterones. Refer those with polyps or necrotic tissue on histology for hysteroscopy and biopsy, and those with atypical hyperplasia or carcinoma for hysterectomy and bilateral salpingo-oophorectomy. If transvaginal us is not already done, perform in those on whom the procedure was impossible or abandoned to establish endometrial thickness (<4mm normal in the postmenopausal; refer if >4mm thick or if polyps seen, for hysteroscopy, biopsy, and polypectomy).

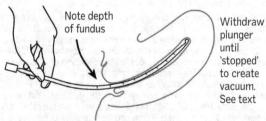

Note depth of fundus

Withdraw plunger until 'stopped' to create vacuum. See text

Fig 2.25 Endometrial sampling.

Redrawn from information supplied by Genesis Medical.

2 Gynaecology

Ovarian cysts are extremely common, and most often physiological due to either follicular cysts or corpus luteal cysts. In a woman of reproductive age, cysts <5cm should not cause concern unless imaging shows complex or suspicious features, or if she is symptomatic (most frequently pain). While most ovarian cysts are benign, one of the cornerstones of management is to identify cysts with a high risk of cancer so that the woman can be treated in a cancer centre.

Presentation
- Asymptomatic; an incidental finding on imaging for a different indication.
- Chronic pain with dull ache, dyspareunia, cyclical pain, or pressure effects.
- Acute pain due to bleeding into the cyst, ovarian torsion (the ovary does not tort unless a mass disturbs the balance), or rupture.
- Irregular vaginal bleeding.
- Hormonal effects eg sudden development of androgenic features.
- Abdominal swelling or mass; ascites suggests malignancy.

Cyclical pain and deep dyspareunia are features of endometriosis, which may be evident as an endometrioma on TVS (small deposits are poorly identified by US). *Ovarian torsion* is uncommon, classically presenting with severe lower abdominal pain and vomiting. The pain may then start to improve after 24h after the ovary starts to die. During torsion, the venous return from the ovary is occluded, causing the ovary to become oedematous, eventually leading to interruption of arterial blood supply. WBC and CRP may be normal or raised. Cyst rupture presents similarly to ovarian torsion but the woman may have additional features of haemorrhagic shock.

Examination May be normal if the cyst is small or the woman obese. If this is an acute presentation, be systematic and check observations and treat signs of shock first. Abdominal examination may reveal a mass arising from the pelvis, tenderness, peritonism, or ascites. Vaginal examination may show vaginal discharge or bleeding, cervical excitation, adnexal mass, or tenderness. Nodular uterosacral ligaments and a fixed retroverted uterus are features of endometriosis.

Investigations Check FBC; tumour markers depend on the age of the patient. Ca125 is less sensitive in women <40 years but should be checked in anyone >40. In women <40 years with complex cysts: AFP, Ca19-9, LDH, hCG, and CEA.

Imaging TVS is the most appropriate modality to start with. It is useful in distinguishing benign from malignant masses (concerning features: multilocular cyst, large papillary cyst wall projections, solid areas, metastases, ascites, and bilateral lesions). A cyst extending out of the pelvis will need transabdominal imaging with US, and in cysts >7cm consider MRI (superior for distinguishing benign from malignant disease; endometriomas and dermoid cysts have particular features on MRI). MRI and CT are used in staging malignancy.

Management Acute onset of symptoms with severe pain requires admission to hospital. If she is stable, arrange urgent TVS. If she is unstable, arrange urgent laparoscopy. *Premenausal women:* Aim to preserve fertility and exclude malignancy. If asymptomatic with simple cyst <5cm: no follow-up or 5–7cm: yearly scan. The COCP does not lead to resolution of a functional cyst. If the cyst is >7cm, she is symptomatic, or it is complex, arrange laparoscopic ovarian cystectomy. Avoid spilling cyst contents (if dermoid can lead to chemical peritonitis and if malignant can up-stage the disease). *Postmenopausal women:* Calculate Risk of Malignancy Index (uses menopausal status, Ca125 and US features). Low-risk cysts <5cm can be managed conservatively with repeat TVS and Ca125 every 4 months and the woman discharged if there is no change after 1 year. Moderate-risk cysts require (usually) bilateral oophorectomy; high-risk cysts require referral to a cancer centre for staging laparotomy (see BOX 'Calculating Risk of Malignancy Index (RMI)').

Ovarian tumours: pathology

Functional cysts These are enlarged or persistent follicular or corpus luteum cysts. They are so common that they may be considered normal if they are small (<5cm). They may cause pain by rupture, failing to rupture at ovulation, or bleeding. If <5cm they usually resolve over 2–3 cycles.

Endometriomas Ovarian cysts filled with old blood; also known as chocolate cyst (see pp. 140–1).

Serous cystadenomas These develop papillary growths that may be so prolific that the cyst appears solid. They are commonest in women aged 30–40 years. About 30% are bilateral and about 30% are malignant.

Mucinous cystadenomas The commonest large ovarian tumours; these may become enormous. They are filled with mucinous material and rupture may rarely cause pseudomyxoma peritonei (p. 175). They may be multilocular. They are commonest in the 30–50yrs age group. About 5% will be malignant. Remove the appendix at operation in those with suspected mucinous cystadenoma and send for histology. (Interestingly men can get pseudomyxoma from intestinal or appendicular neoplasms; most women with pseudomyxoma peritonei do not have overt rupture of ovarian tumours and 90% have concurrent intestinal or appendicular tumours and it is now thought that the ovarian tumours may be secondary to GI tumours.)

Fibromas These are small, solid, benign, fibrous tissue tumours. They are associated with *Meigs syndrome:* pleural effusion, often right sided + benign ovarian fibroma (or thecoma, cystadenoma, granulosa cell tumour) + ascites.

Teratomas These arise from primitive germ cells. A benign mature teratoma (dermoid cyst) may contain well-differentiated tissue eg hair, teeth. 20% are bilateral. They are most common in young women. Poorly differentiated malignant teratomas are rare.

Other germ cell tumours (All malignant and all rare.) Non-gestational choriocarcinomas (secrete hCG); ectodermal sinus tumours (yolk sac tumours—secrete α-fetoprotein); dysgerminomas.

Sex-cord tumours (Rare; usually of low-grade malignancy.) These arise from cortical mesenchyme. Granulosa cell and theca cell tumours produce oestrogen and may present with precocious puberty, menstrual problems, or postmenopausal bleeding. Arrhenoblastomas secrete androgens.

Calculating Risk of Malignancy Index (RMI)

RMI = U × M × Ca125

- U = US score (0, 1 or 3).
- M = menopausal status (1 = premenopausal, 3 = postmenopausal).
- Ca125 = serum Ca125 level (U/L).

US scoring system: 1 point for each of the following:
- Multilocularity
- Solid areas
- Metastases
- Ascites
- Bilaterality of lesions.

Score 0 for no features, 1 if 1 feature and 2 if there are 3 or more present.

Overall risk
- Low; RMI <25 with <3% risk of cancer.
- Moderate; RMI 25–250 with 20% risk of cancer.
- High; RMI >250 with 75% risk of cancer.

Further reading

RCOG (2016 & 2011). *The Management of Ovarian Masses in Pre- and Post-Menopausal Women* (Green-top Guidelines No. 34 & 62) London: RCOG.

2 Gynaecology

Ovarian cancer is the leading cause of death from gynaecological malignancy in the UK, and the majority are epithelial in origin. The peak incidence is in women aged 75–84 years. It causes more deaths than endometrial or cervical cancer because it often presents late, due to vague symptoms with an insidious onset.

Aetiology Originally thought to be related to irritation of the ovarian surface from ovulation. However, recent evidence suggests a role for the fallopian tubes in the development of ovarian cancer. It was found that in women with BRCA mutations, more had microscopic evidence of fallopian tube cancer than ovarian cancer at the time of salpingo-oophorectomy.

- Nulliparity increases risk.
- Early menarche and/or late menopause increases risk.
- Gene mutations in BRCA 1 and 2 increase risk of ovarian and breast cancer:
  - BRCA 1 has risk of 46% by age 70.
  - BRCA 2 has risk of 12% by age 70.
- HNPCC (Lynch II syndrome) gives a lifetime risk of ovarian cancer of 11%.
- Pregnancy, breastfeeding, and COCP are protective.
- Tubal ligation (female sterilization) is protective.

Refer for clinical genetics counselling and testing if there are two primary cancers in one 1st or 2nd degree relative; three 1st- or 2nd-degree relatives with breast, ovary, colorectal, stomach, or endometrial cancers; two 1st- or 2nd-degree relatives, one of whom has ovarian cancer at any age, and the other with breast cancer <50 years; two 1st- or 2nd-degree relatives with ovarian cancer at any age.

The role for screening Screening for ovarian cancer at present is not effective. If a gene mutation is identified, consider yearly TVS with CA125. If BRCA +ve offer BSO and warn of risk of finding incidental disease during surgery.

Presentation

- Often vague symptoms which may be misinterpreted as irritable bowel syndrome or diverticular disease and 50% present to a non-gynaecological specialty; 75% present once disease has reached FIGO stage III (see table 2.6).
- Bloating.
- Unexplained weight loss; loss of appetite; early satiety.
- Fatigue.
- Urinary symptoms eg frequency or urgency.
- Change in bowel habit.
- Abdominal or pelvic pain.
- Vaginal bleeding.
- Pelvic mass palpable by the woman or her GP.

Examination May reveal a fixed abdominal/pelvic mass, ascites, omental mass, pleural effusion, and/or supraclavicular lymph node enlargement.

Investigations

- FBC, U&E, LFTs.
- Tumour markers: Ca125 (raised in 80% of epithelial cancers and used to work out RMI, see BOX 'Calculating Risk of Malignancy Index (RMI)' p. 173). CEA is raised in colorectal cancers and normal in ovarian cancer. Ca19.9 may be raised in mucinous tumours. If the woman is <40 years, check AFP, LDH and hCG.
- TVS.
- CXR (looking for pleural effusion or lung metastases; needed for staging).
- CT abdomen/pelvis (to detect peritoneal disease, omental metastases, liver metastases and para-aortic lymph nodes).
- MRI is useful to further evaluate the ovarian mass and help distinguish benign from malignant disease.
- Ascites or pleural effusion can be sampled and sent for cytology.

Table 2.6 FIGO staging for ovarian cancer

Stage	Extent of disease	5yr survival
I	Limited to one or both ovaries; IC if the capsule is breached, tumour is present on the ovarian surface, or peritoneal washings are positive. Rupture of the cyst at time of surgery is IC.	75–90%
II	Limited to the pelvis	45–60%
III	Limited to the abdomen, including regional lymph node metastases	30–40%
IV	Distant metastases outside abdominal cavity	<20%

Treatment Best carried out in specialist centres; this depends on tumour stage.

Surgery: Consists of a full staging laparotomy through a midline incision by a cancer specialist (improves prognosis). As much tumour as possible should be removed. Stage III or IV cancers may benefit from neoadjuvant chemotherapy (chemotherapy prior to debulking surgery). A full staging laparotomy involves the following:
• Midline laparotomy.
• Hysterectomy.
• Bilateral salpingo-oophorectomy.
• Omentectomy.
• Para-aortic and pelvic lymph node sampling.
• Peritoneal washings and biopsies.

In a young woman with early disease, the uterus and other ovary may be left for fertility. Ensure optimal surgical staging (table 2.6). NICE says low-risk stage Ia or Ib disease may not need chemotherapy.[49]NICE

Chemotherapy: Recommended in everyone following surgery, unless disease is low-grade and stage Ia or Ib. Platinum agents are superior—carboplatin with paclitaxel (from Pacific yew trees) produces higher response rates and longer survival both when used for initial treatment and for treatment of recurrences compared to use of carboplatin alone. Advanced or relapsed ovarian cancer: see NICE guidance. Options include paclitaxel, pegylated liposomal doxorubicin, and topotecan. Palliative care involves relief of symptoms, which are generally due to extensive peritoneal disease.

Borderline ovarian tumours Epithelial in origin and not benign. They are more common in younger women and are staged as for ovarian cancer. Characteristics include confinement to one ovary, premenopausal age group, metastatic implants, difficulty in diagnosing histologically, and with a much better prognosis than ovarian cancer. In young women, conservative surgery is appropriate with unilateral oophorectomy and staging biopsies. Relapse can occur any time up to 25 years after initial diagnosis.

Pseudomyxoma peritonei Extremely rare and can arise from primary tumour of the appendix, but may be associated with mucinous cystadenoma (p. 173). There are thick, jelly-like deposits throughout the abdomen. Two specialist centres exist in the UK (Basingstoke and Manchester) and treatment involves cytoreductive surgery and hyperthermic intraperitoneal chemotherapy. In the past, this disease used to be treated palliatively but now, 5-year survival is between 53% and 88% depending on the type of tumour.

Hysterectomy

Performed less commonly now due to the success of the Mirena® IUS in treating menorrhagia and ablative procedures of the endometrium. It may be:

- *Total* (including the cervix) or *subtotal* (leaving the cervix behind; she will continue to need smears).
- *Approach* may be open, robotic, laparoscopic, laparoscopic-assisted or vaginal.
- *Removal of the tubes and ovaries* may be carried out at the same time and this depends on the woman's wishes, her menopausal status, and why she needs a hysterectomy. Due to the recent research suggesting that some ovarian cancer originates from the fallopian tubes, it is increasingly common to perform a salpingectomy if the woman wants to keep her ovaries.

A subtotal hysterectomy is an option if all smears have been normal or if pelvic adhesions make it impossible to remove the cervix. Women with endometriosis should have a laparoscopic total hysterectomy (with or without oophorectomy) plus excision of all visible disease in order to prevent recurrence. There is no link between better sexual function with or without a cervix, and a woman's sex life often improves after hysterectomy due to cessation of pain and heavy bleeding. 10% of women continue to have cyclical bleeding after a subtotal hysterectomy and should be warned of this. A *Wertheim's* (extended to include local lymph nodes and a cuff of vagina) is used for malignancy and has a higher rate of complications (particularly ureteric injury) due to the more extensive nature of the surgery. Patients who have had laparoscopic or vaginal hysterectomy have less postoperative pain and shorter recovery time. *Risks* include bleeding, infection, injury to bladder, bowel, vessels, or ureters, scarring (low transverse, midline, or laparoscopic scars), VTE, earlier menopause if ovaries retained (due to sharing of blood supply with uterine arteries). In a laparoscopic or vaginal procedure, there is a risk of converting to an open operation.

Hysteroscopy

One of the most common gynaecological procedures and can be carried out with simple analgesia, local, or general anaesthesia.[50] A fine scope (3–12mm) is inserted through the cervix into the uterus to visualize the endometrium. Visualization of both ostia (where the fallopian tubes join the uterus) confirms that the hysteroscope is in the correct cavity. It is mainly used in the diagnosis of abnormal uterine bleeding. A curette is used after removal of the hysteroscope to take endometrial biopsies. Depending on the findings, the surgeon may then proceed to transcervical removal of fibroid (TCRF), which uses an operating hysteroscope and monopolar or bipolar diathermy to shave off submucosal fibroids or polyps, or the endometrium (TCRE).

Risks of hysteroscopy: Risks include bleeding (usually spotting), infection, perforation of the uterus, or damage to the cervix, and if hysteroscopic surgery is being carried out and a perforation occurs, injury to surrounding organs. If the cervix is stenosed, it may be impossible to gain access to the uterus.

Out-patient hysteroscopy: Used for the investigation of postmenopausal or abnormal uterine bleeding, as well as: endometrial polypectomy, removal of small submucosal fibroids, endometrial ablation, removal of lost IUCDs, and transcervical sterilization. Miniature scopes (2.7–3.5mm diameter) are used with saline or CO_2 to give good views, reduced vasovagal episodes, reduced procedure time, and the ability to use cautery. Patients tolerate the procedure very well and satisfaction scores are high. Women are advised to take standard simple analgesia 1 hour prior to the procedure to reduce intra-and postoperative pain. Many units use these as 'see and treat' clinics to complete the patient episode in 1 visit. IUCDs/IUS can be fitted following hysteroscopy.

Endometrial ablation

By diathermy, microwave, electrical impedance (Novasure®), or thermal balloon (under GA or spinal ± paracervical block) reduces bleeding by destruction of the endometrium down to the basalis layer. It is most commonly performed with hysteroscopy immediately prior to the ablation. It is less effective if the endometrial cavity is >10cm. 90% of women have a reduction in bleeding by 9 months and 30% are amenorrhoeic. It has no effect on pain and should not be offered if dysmenorrhoea is significant. The woman should have completed her family and have reliable contraception. A Mirena® IUS can be fitted post procedure. *Risks:* Include bleeding, infection, uterine perforation with or without surrounding organ damage, failed procedure (eg if cavity too large or the ablative system used fails its safety checks), haematometra. Some endometrium remains in most (so give progesterone-containing HRT later, if needed).

Laparoscopy

May be diagnostic or operative and allows direct visualization of the pelvic organs. Minimal access surgery has the advantage of shorter hospital stays with minimal abdominal scarring. Many gynaecological procedures are carried out using this approach, including ovarian cystectomy, salpingectomy (for ectopic pregnancy), diathermy or excision of endometriosis, myomectomy, hysterectomy (total or subtotal), and some prolapse and urinary incontinence surgery. The abdomen is insufflated via a Verres needle in the umbilicus with carbon dioxide gas to create a pneumoperitoneum. Ports are introduced and instruments are inserted through the ports in the iliac fossae or suprapubically. *Risks:* Include bleeding (potential for large vessel injury on laparoscopic entry which is thankfully rare, and reduced with safe technique), infection, injury to bladder, bowel, vessels and ureters, failed entry, scarring, VTE, laparotomy, and any risks specific to the operation being performed.

Anterior and posterior vaginal repair (see p. 160)

The lack of support from the anterior or posterior vaginal wall in cases of prolapse is rectified by excising redundant mucosa and doing a fascial repair. It is *not* an operation to correct urinary incontinence. The operation may be combined with a vaginal hysterectomy. The more mucosa is removed, the narrower the vagina. Enquire before surgery if she is sexually active. An anterior repair may be performed as a day-case procedure, but posterior repairs are at higher risk of haematoma formation and many surgeons insert a vaginal pack and catheter overnight. It is approximately 90% curative. Vaginal mesh for prolapse is not used in the UK unless as part of a research setting due to the unacceptably high complication rates. *Risks:* Bleeding, infection, injury to bladder, bowel or ureters, dyspareunia, recurrence (10–20%), and VTE.

Surgical management of miscarriage (see p. 124–5)

Used to be known as 'evacuation of retained products of conception'. It is a day-case procedure that can be carried out under local, or most commonly, general anaesthetic. For miscarriage, gestational age should be <13 weeks (otherwise higher risk of complications, and medical management is safer). Prostaglandin administered PV prior to the procedure reduces the risk of uterine and cervical trauma especially in women who have never had a vaginal delivery. Once the woman is anaesthetized, the cervix is grasped and dilated to between 1 and 2cm. A rigid or flexible curette in the appropriate size is used to remove the products of conception under suction. *Risks:* Bleeding, infection, uterine perforation (rarely intraperitoneal injury), retained products of conception, intrauterine adhesions, and cervical tears.

Enhanced recovery

This looks at patient pathways with a view to optimizing preoperative and postoperative care, to minimize inpatient length of stay. Measures adopted include admission on the day of operation, early removal of drips and catheters, and early postoperative feeding. Daily ward rounds and good pain management are an integral part of care.

With many thanks to Dr Hugh Lemonde, our specialist reader, and junior readers Fraser Brown and Paul Hanna, for their contribution to this chapter.

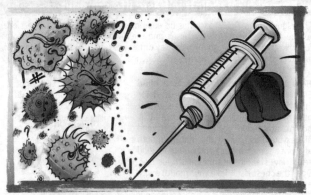

Fig 3.1 Vaccines are responsible for saving more lives worldwide than any other medical product or procedure. Edward Jenner was the first to develop and publish evidence that his smallpox vaccine was effective in the late 18th century; however, the Greek historian Thucydides first observed in 429 BC that those who survived smallpox did not become re-infected. From 900 AD the Chinese used a primitive form of vaccination called variolation by placing powdered scabs from people infected with smallpox under the skin or into the nose to provide immunity. Smallpox was a highly contagious and deadly disease killing up to 20% of those infected. Jenner, noting the common observation that those infected with the less virulent cowpox virus were immune to smallpox, used material from a cowpox vesicle on a milkmaid to inoculate an 8-year-old boy, proving by later challenges that the boy was immune. Use of this technique soon spread around Europe. In 1980 the WHO declared smallpox as being eradicated across the world—a miracle of modern medicine.

Pasteur developed and refined the use of attenuated vaccines by reducing the virulence of pathogens which stimulated an immune response, but which did not cause disease. Live attenuated vaccines continue to be widely used eg MMR, nasal flu, rotavirus, and shingles, as well as BCG and chickenpox.

Thousands of scientists have devoted their entire career to vaccine development, yet Maurice Hilleman is credited with saving more lives than any other medical scientist. Hilleman developed over 40 vaccines including those for measles, mumps, rubella, hepatitis A and B, chickenpox, meningitis, pneumococcus, and Haemophilus influenzae. When Hilleman's daughter contracted mumps, he cultivated a throat swab to develop the first mumps vaccine. The Jeryl Lynn strain (named in her honour) is still used in the MMR vaccine today.

Other vaccines—apart from live attenuated strains—include inactivated ('whole killed' vaccines eg Hep A) and subunit/acellular vaccines, which contain polysaccharides or proteins from the surface of bacteria or viruses which are recognized as foreign eg toxoid (diphtheria, tetanus, and pertussis), conjugate (eg Hib, Men C), and recombinant (eg Men B and HPV).

Future vaccines are likely to prolong immune memory, generate higher immune responses (via stronger adjuvants), as well as account for genetic variability.

▶Use your learning and knowledge to ensure the benefit of vaccination is shared with all parents and patients. Give time to counter the false myths peddled by anti-vaccine campaigners. Advances in immunology, molecular biology, and public health mean that vaccines will continue to have a massive impact by improving human health and longevity.

For the current UK immunization schedule see p. 257. For comment on the MMR vaccine scare see p. 256.

Artwork by Gillian Turner.

The algorithm in fig 3.2 assumes no equipment and that only 1 professional rescuer is present. Remove yourself and the child from danger. Perform CPR for 1min then phone or go for help. Key differences with adult BLS: respiratory arrest is more likely in paediatric arrest hence, 5 rescue breaths and ratio 15:2 rather than 30:2.

How to give rescue breaths to a child Ensure correct head position (neutral for infant, 'sniffing' for child).[1] Pinch the soft part of the nose. Open the mouth a little, but maintain chin up. Take a breath, and place your lips around the mouth (mouth and nose for an infant) and create a good seal. Blow steadily into the mouth for 1sec. Does the chest rise? Take your mouth away, and watch for the chest to fall. Give 5 successful rescue breaths. If the chest does not move, check position and retry. If the chest still does not move, respiratory obstruction may exist, open the mouth and look for any obvious obstruction. If one is seen, attempt removal but do not attempt blind or perform repeated finger sweeps.

How to give chest compressions Compress lower ½ of sternum to ⅓ of the chest's depth •For infants, 2 fingers are sufficient, or place both thumbs on sternum and encircle the entire thorax with your hands •For smaller children, use the heel of 1 hand in the middle of a line joining the nipples •For larger children (>8yrs) use adult 2-handed method.

Recovery position When breathing, place in the recovery position—as near to the true lateral position as possible, with mouth dependent to aid draining of secretions. The position must be stable (eg use pillows placed behind back). The degree of movement is determined by risk of spinal injury.

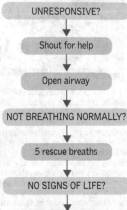

Paediatric Basic Life Support
(Healthcare professionals
with a duty to respond)

UNRESPONSIVE?

Shout for help

Open airway

NOT BREATHING NORMALLY?

5 rescue breaths

NO SIGNS OF LIFE?

15 chest compressions

2 rescue breaths
15 compressions

Fig 3.2 Paediatric basic life support (BLS), applicable only to healthcare professionals with a duty to respond.

Reproduced with the kind permission of the Resuscitation Council (UK).

Choking algorithm
- If coughing effectively, encourage cough.
- If ineffective cough and conscious: give 5 back blows then 5 thrusts (chest for infant, abdo for child) to increase intrathoracic pressure and dislodge obstruction. Reassess and repeat until improvement or child becomes unconscious. Deliver back blows with child in rescuer's lap head-downwards, prone position with the heel of the hand between the scapulae. Support the head without compressing the soft tissues of the neck. Chest thrusts are given to infant in head-downwards supine position, similar to compressions but sharper and more slowly. Abdominal thrusts for child >1yr performed from behind with clenched fist placed between umbilicus and xiphoid process and a sharp movement directed towards diaphragm.
- If child is unconscious, open airway, check for obstructions as previously described, give 5 rescue breaths and start CPR.

Paediatric advanced life support

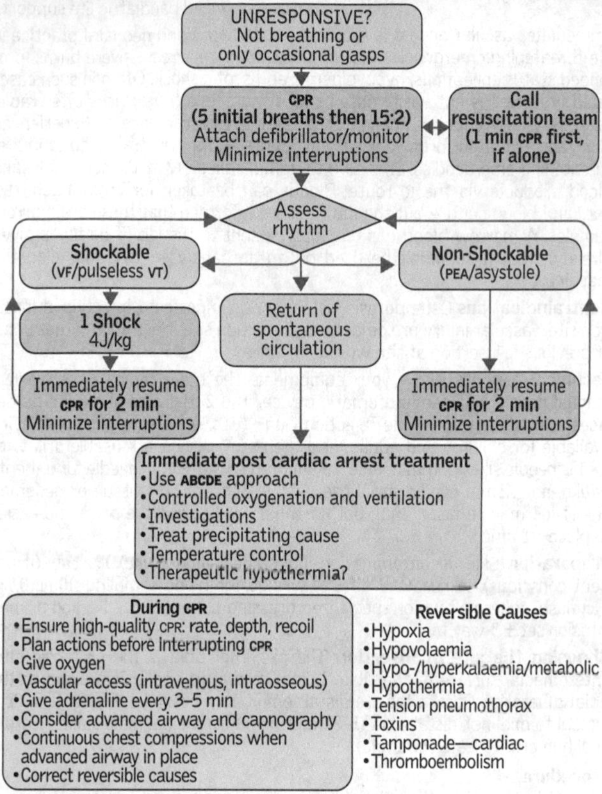

Fig 3.3 Paediatric advanced life support.

Reproduced with the kind permission of the Resuscitation Council (UK).

Fig 3.3 shows the paediatric advanced life support algorithm.[1] Order of assessment and intervention for any seriously ill or injured child follows the ABCDE principles: Airway (AC for airway and cervical spine stabilization for the injured child); Breathing; Circulation; Disability (level of consciousness and neurological status); Exposure to ensure full examination (while respecting dignity and temperature conservation). *Note:* 15:2 means 15 compressions (rate=100–120/min) to 2 ventilations. For neonates, see p. 185.

Non-shockable rhythm ▶▶Give adrenaline dose as soon as you have IV/IO access, and repeat on alternate cycles until spontaneous circulation returns.

Shockable VF/VT (Uncommon in children) ▶▶After 3rd shock, give **adrenaline** (epinephrine) 10mcg/kg IV/IO and repeat on alternate cycles. ▶▶ After 3rd shock also give **amiodarone** bolus 5mg/kg IV/IO. Repeat **amiodarone** 5mg/kg bolus one further time after 5th shock if still in VF/VT or at later stage if relapses into VF/VT. **At all times** Minimize interruptions to good-quality chest compressions, consider and correct reversible causes (4Hs and 4Ts), once intubated give continuous chest compressions and ventilate at rate of 10–12/min.

1 PEA = pulseless electrical activity.

(APLS=advanced paediatric life support.)

Immediate vascular access is required in paediatric and neonatal practice in life-threatening emergencies incl. cardiopulmonary arrest, severe burns, prolonged status epilepticus, hypovolaemic and septic shock. Often in such cases rapid IV access is not easily obtained. Intraosseous (IO) devices offer rapid, safe, easy, and effective means of obtaining vascular access.[2] Experienced clinicians will often forgo IV access attempts and move straight to IO in life-threatening emergencies. It is safe to administer all IV medicines, fluids, and blood products via the IO route. Bloods can be taken for crossmatch, FBC, U&E,[3] and blood culture but the lab must be informed that these are marrow samples. A marrow blood gas can also be sent to the lab (if no fluids given already)—but it shouldn't be used on an autoanalyser as it may clog the machine.

Contraindications Osteoporosis, osteogenesis imperfecta, infection at insertion site, vascular injury proximal to the insertion site, fracture in target bone, or previous IO insertion at site within 48 hours.

Technical aspects Know your equipment. The main choice is between a manual needle or a semi-automatic device. The 2 major semi-automatic devices available are the Bone Injection Gun® (B.I.G.®)—a spring-loaded device available for children and adults, and the EZ-IO® device, a reusable drill with 3 × 15G needle sizes (15mm needle for children <39kg, 25mm needle for patients >40kg, and 45mm needle for those with significant soft tissue or oedema). The EZ-IO® may be faster than both manual needles and the B.I.G.® and easier to place 1st time.[4]

Preparation Skin decontamination, **lidocaine** (=lignocaine) 1% 5mL (if patient conscious), IO needle ± device, syringe for blood sampling, 10mL 0.9% NaCl flush, adhesive tape or specialized dressing to secure needle, and primed infusion set ± 3-way tap.

Choosing the site of insertion The proximal tibia is the preferred site; anteromedial surface of the tibia, 1–2cm medial to and 1–2cm distal to the tibial tuberosity. Other sites are distal femur (1cm proximal to patella, 1–2cm medial to midline), distal tibia (1–2cm proximal to medial malleolus), or proximal humerus (greater tubercle).[5]

Procedure
- Clean the skin with antiseptic, infiltrate with lidocaine if patient conscious.
- Insert the IO needle at an angle of 90° to the skin; advance with a boring or screwing motion into the marrow cavity. Correct location of the needle is signified by a decrease in resistance on entering the marrow cavity.
- To prevent necrosis the needle flange should not be in contact with the skin.
- Verify the position by aspirating marrow (and taking blood samples), or by the easy flushing of 5–10mL of 0.9% NaCl, without any infiltration of surrounding tissue.
- The needle should stand upright without support, but should be secured with tape or specialized dressing.
- Connect to IV infusion via an extension ± 3-way tap: better flow rates are achieved by syringing in fluid boluses or using a pressure bag.

Complications (Infrequent.) Failure to enter bone marrow (extravasation), dislodgement, local infection (cellulitis, osteomyelitis), skin necrosis, fracture, pain, compartment syndrome, and fat or bone microemboli. These are more common with prolonged use—IO infusion should be discontinued as soon as adequate conventional IV access is attained (should be <24h).

NB IO delivery may also be used in adults.[6] The position on the tibia in adults is 2cm medial to tibial tuberosity and 1cm above it (as opposed to below it in children).

Never blame yourself for forgetting anything, except your humanity and the dose of adrenaline. See www.resus.org.uk.

Diagnostic criteria Sudden onset, life-threatening problems involving A, B, or C, and in ≈80%, associated skin changes.[7]

▶▶ Call the resuscitation/cardiac arrest team (paramedics if in the community).

▶▶ Remove the trigger eg bee sting; stop any drug or colloid IV infusion.

▶▶ ABCDE:[8] Airway (any swelling, hoarseness, stridor?); Breathing (rate↑, wheeze, fatigue, cyanosis, spo₂ <92%?); Circulation (pale, clammy, BP↓, faints?); Disability (confusion, conscious level eg drowsy/coma?); Exposure of skin (erythema/urticaria/angio-oedema?).

▶▶ Ideally place patient on back with legs raised. If they have significant respiratory distress, allow the patient to put themselves in a position of comfort. Do not let them stand or sit up rapidly. If comatose, use left-lateral position (to prevent caval compression).

▶▶ *The chief drug priority is adrenaline:* (table 3.1) Give intramuscularly (IM). Use a suitable syringe for measuring small volumes; absolute accuracy isn't essential.[9] Note strength! (1:1000 not 1:10,000.)

Table 3.1 IM dose of 3 drugs

IM dose of 3 drugs	Adrenaline 1:1000	Chlorphenamine	Hydrocortisone
If aged <6 months	0.15mL (150mcg)*	25mcg/kg	25mg
If aged 6 months–6yrs	0.15mL (150mcg)	2.5mg	50mg
If aged 6–12yrs	0.3mL (300mcg)	5mg	100mg
Adolescent/adult dose	0.5mL (500mcg)	10mg	200mg
* Drug dose not in *BNF*.			

▶▶ Repeat adrenaline dose after 5min if no improvement.
- Hydrocortisone and chlorphenamine can be given IM or slow IV, although there is little evidence these help much.
- Don't use the IV route for adrenaline (unless on ITU with experienced user; different doses apply).
- Also give: high-flow o₂ (± IPPV) & crystalloid (20mL/kg IV).
- *If bronchospasm is a feature:* Give IM adrenaline and also give bronchodilators as for asthma (see p. 213) but remember MgSO₄ may cause hypotension.
- *Continuously monitor:* Pulse , BP, spo₂, and ECG. If cardiac arrest, start CPR.
- *Differential diagnosis:* Asthma ; septic shock; breath-holding or panic attack.
- *Weight estimation:* APLS formulae weight (kg) ≈
    Age (in months)/2+4 for age <12 months.
    Age (in years) × 2+8 for age 1–5 years.
    Age (in years) × 3+7 for age 6–10 years.
- *After the emergency:* Try and identify the cause of the reaction; admit as an in-patient; offer referral to a paediatric allergist; provide education and training (recognition, trigger avoidance, biphasic reactions); consider a 3-day course of antihistamine or oral steroid—this may decrease chance of further reactions;[4] offer an adrenaline auto-injector with appropriate training.[7] There are several brands of auto-injectors.
- *Mast cell tryptase:* There is limited evidence for its use in children to confirm anaphylaxis, it is more useful if the suspected cause is drug related, idiopathic, or venom related. If considering, take 1st sample (>0.5mL in LFT bottle, ask lab to freeze) as soon as possible after emergency treatment and a 2nd sample ideally 1–2h after symptoms start but definitely within 4h. A 3rd sample after 24h may also be needed. Results should be interpreted by an allergy specialist.

Normal transition Most newborns are perfectly healthy and will make the transition to life outside the womb with little or no help. If baby is well at birth, cord clamping is delayed for 1 minute after complete delivery, the baby is dried and returned to mother. Mother-and-baby skin-to-skin contact (with baby's exposed surface covered by a dry towel) is the best way to maintain temperature and improves bonding and milk production.

Physiology of perinatal hypoxia Neonates who experience sufficient hypoxia pre delivery will attempt to breathe. If hypoxia continues the fetus will fall unconscious and enter primary apnoea. At this point the HR will decrease to approximately ½ the normal rate. If hypoxia continues, shuddering agonal gasps initiated by primitive spinal reflexes occur at a rate ≈12/min. If these fail to aerate the lungs the fetus enters secondary or terminal apnoea. The heart, until now resilient in the face of hypoxia, will slow and fail. *The key intervention in neonatal resuscitation is aeration of the lungs.* In the majority of resuscitations this will lead to a prompt increase in HR and restoration of adequate circulation.[10]

High-risk deliveries A paediatrician or nurse trained in advanced neonatal resuscitation should attend whenever there is concern about the fetus, including: emergency caesareans, breeches, twins/triplets, instrumental deliveries, prematurity, eclampsia, and thick meconium-stained liquor.

Preparation: Check and warm the resuscitaire and check other equipment (appropriately sized masks, BVM or Neopuff™, suction, laryngoscope, ET tubes, O_2 and air supplies). Have at least 2 towels available. Ascertain gestation, antenatal history, and any antenatal concerns. Do not hesitate to call for additional help at this or any time.

At birth:
- Assess colour, tone, breathing, if baby pink and crying: return to mother.
- If not, rub vigorously while drying baby (if <32 weeks' gestation, do not dry, place in plastic wrapping under radiant heater).
- Assess breathing *and* HR (use a stethoscope not peripheral pulses).
- If no spontaneous breathing, open airway and give 5 *inflation breaths* using *air* (via Neopuff™ or BVM). Apply pressure of 30cmH₂O in term infants (20–25cmH₂O in preterm infants) for 2–3sec to inflate the newborn's fluid filled lungs.
- Ensure the chest is expanding; if not, readjust the head position and consider airway adjuncts or a 2nd person to ensure an adequate technique. Consider direct inspection of oropharynx and suction.
- Look for chest expansion but the *key indicator of response is improvement in baby's HR.* Check HR and breathing every 30sec and after interventions. Ideally establish SpO_2 monitoring for continuous HR readout. If the HR is increasing it is safe to assume you have successfully aerated the lungs.
- Once 5 inflation breaths have caused adequate chest expansion, if the baby is still not making any respiratory effort, continue ventilation breaths 30–40 breaths/min using 4–5cmH₂O of PEEP if available until the baby is spontaneously breathing.
- If not pinking up, add oxygen stepwise (see acceptable *pre-ductal* (ie right arm) SpO_2 in fig 3.4).
- In the rare cases where HR <60/min after 30sec of adequate ventilation, start chest compressions at a ratio of 3:1 (⅓ depth of AP diameter, rate of 100–120/min), increase O_2 and call for neonatal arrest team if not already done, endotracheal intubation is likely to be needed.
- In exceptional cases drugs may be needed: adrenaline, glucose, crystalloid, blood, sodium bicarbonate. They may be given IV or IO but usually a UVC (umbilical venous catheter) is placed.
- **Adrenaline** 10mcg/kg (0.1mL/kg 1:10,000); if no response repeat with 30mcg/kg. 10% glucose is given as 2.5mL/kg bolus. If hypovolaemia is suspected (usually a clear history of peripartum haemorrhage), give 10mL/kg 0.9% NaCl over 10–20sec or o-negative blood and repeat as necessary.
- In prolonged resuscitation, **sodium bicarbonate** 1–2 mmol/kg (2–4 mL/kg of 4.2% solution) should be considered.

▶▶Newborn life support algorithm (2015)

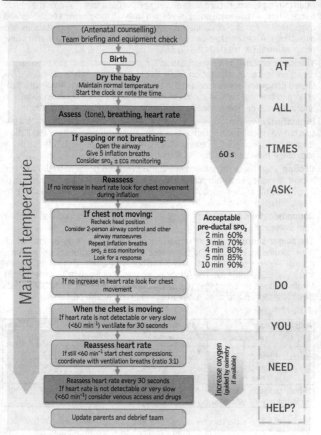

Fig 3.4 Newborn life support algorithm; 2015 guidelines.
Reproduced with the kind permission of the Resuscitation Council (UK).

Maintaining temperature Naked, wet, newborns cannot maintain their body temperature. Active measures are needed to avoid hypothermia (<36.5°c) and cold stress which is associated with *increased mortality* in all gestations and all settings. A resuscitaire can be used to help keep a newborn warm while being examined or treated (see fig 3.5).

Thick meconium The only indication for rapidly visualizing the oropharynx ± suctioning *before* stimulation and inflation breaths is in babies who are delivered floppy and apnoeic covered in thick viscous meconium. Tracheal intubation and tracheal suction should not be routine as it has not been shown to improve outcome. The emphasis remains on quickly initiating ventilation.

Prematurity Preterm infants <32 weeks' gestation may not require resuscitation but will require stabilization and assistance with temperature regulation, feeding, and respiration. The neonatal team should be present at the delivery to arrange transfer to the neonatal unit.

Cooling Therapeutic hypothermia initiated within 6 hours of birth has been shown to improve neurological outcome in evolving moderate to severe hypoxic ischaemic encephalopathy (HIE). The decision to cool should be made by an experienced senior clinician.

Communication As soon as feasible parents should be updated of their baby's progress.

The Apgar score A measure of physiological condition of a newborn which is performed at 1 minute and 5 minutes after birth. Scores ≥7 or more are normal. A score of 4–6 is low and ≤3 critically low, requiring immediate resuscitation. See table 3.2. The Apgar score was developed by us anaesthetist Virginia Apgar. Its purpose is to quickly determine whether a newborn needs medical attention and does not predict long-term health problems.

Table 3.2 Apgar score

Apgar*	Colour	Pulse	On stimulation	Muscle tone	Respirations
	Appearance	Pulse	Grimace	Activity	Respiration
2	Pink	>100	Cries	Active	Strong cry
1	Blue limbs	<100	Grimaces	Limb flexion	Slow, irregular
0	All blue or white	0	No response	Absent	Nil
*Apgar score: a score is given for each vital sign at 1, 5, and 10 minutes of age using the scoring system shown.					

Resources: The smartphone app 'Neomate', based on London's Neonatal Transport Service guidelines, is an excellent free resource full of useful calculators, references, and checklists for dealing with resuscitations and sick neonates.

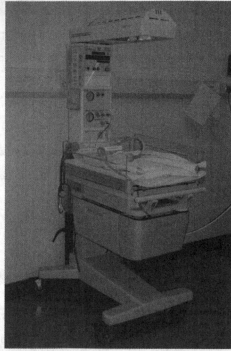

Fig 3.5 A resuscitaire. You may have noticed neonatal resuscitaires on the labour ward or SCBU. They are a workspace with integrated components for respiratory support, suction, and warming, as well as storing vital equipment needed for neonatal resuscitation.

There are 3 aims when taking a paediatric history:

1 Establish rapport with the child and their (extended) family. This builds trust and is critical to subsequent communication.

2 Formulate a differential diagnosis and ask questions to refute/support this.

3 Consider the history/diagnosis in the context of the child and family.

To facilitate this, remember to:

• Introduce yourself and explain what is going to happen.
• Talk first to the child, then to the carers, then to any relevant others.
• Smile!
• Get down to the child's level (sometimes physically).
• Use non-medical language with no jargon.

Always record the date and time when you undertook the consultation, who was present, and who gave the history. See table 3.3.

Presenting complaints Record the child's, parents', and GP's own words.

The present illness

• When and how did it start?
• Was he/she well before?
• How did it develop?
• What aggravates or alleviates it?
• Has there been contact with infections?
• Has the child been overseas recently?
• Have the carers sought medical attention before now?
• Which treatments have been tried?
• Especially in infants, enquire about feeding, wet and dirty nappies, alertness, and weight gain.
• After ascertaining the presenting complaint, use further questioning to test the various hypotheses of the differential diagnosis.

Past medical history *In utero:* Any problems (eg abnormal bleeding, infections, Rh disease); medication, alcohol, or recreational drug exposure? Were pregnancy US scans normal?

At birth: Gestation, mode of delivery, birthweight, resuscitation required? Birth injuries? Malformations?

As a neonate: Any jaundice, fits, fevers, bleeding, feeding problems? Did the baby receive vitamin K? Was the SCBU needed—if so, why and how long? Ask about later illnesses, operations, accidents, newborn screening tests, drugs, allergies, immunization and travel. Check the Red Book (UK only).[2]

Development (pp. 260–1) Ask about the age the child learned to sit, crawl, walk, and talk. Can they feed themselves, dress themselves, are they potty trained?

Drugs Prescribed, recreational, *in utero*, and over the counter. Drug intolerances, adverse drug reactions, and true allergies (ie rashes, anaphylaxis).

Family history Are there any medical problems that run in the family? Is there anyone in the wider family with medical, psychiatric, or learning difficulties? Has anyone had a child die? Consanguinity is common in some cultures and may be relevant to disease.

Social history Who is at home? Note ages of siblings. Do they all have the same father? Ask about play, eating, sleeping, schooling, and pets. Who looks after the child if the parents work? What work do they do? Ask about their hopes, fears, and expectations about the child's illness and hospital stay.

Ensure privacy whenever discussing sensitive issues.

▶If the family does not speak your language, find an interpreter.

2 The Red Book (and e-book) is a personal child health record given to parents in the UK at birth.

Table 3.3 Eliciting the history—systems review

	Neonate	Toddler	Older child
General condition	Weight gain, appetite, sleep	Weight gain, appetite, sleep, milestones, is the child their normal self?	Do they feel unwell, tired, or fatigued? How is school?
Cardiorespiratory	Tachypnoea, grunting, wheeze, cyanosis, cold sweats (heart failure), exposure to TB, smokers in the family? Is there a family history of heart murmur?	Cough, exertional dyspnoea, sputum, haemoptysis, exposure to TB, smokers in the family? Family history of heart murmur or rheumatic fever?	Exercise limitation? Cough, wheeze, sputum, haemoptysis, chest pain, exposure to TB, smokers in the family? Family history of heart murmur or rheumatic fever?
Gut	Appetite, D&V, feeding problems, jaundice, bleeding, appropriate weight gain?	Appetite, D&V, stool frequency, rectal bleeding, weight gain?	Appetite, D&V, abdominal pain, stool frequency, rectal bleeding, weight loss?
Genitourinary	Wet nappies (how often?)	Wet nappies (how often?) Is there a history of infection? Any haematuria?	Haematuria, dysuria, discharge, sexual development? History of infection? Any history of bedwetting? Menarche? Polydipsia/polyuria?
Neuromuscular	Seizures, attacks, jitters	Seizures, drowsy, hyperactive, hearing ↓, vision ↓, gait	Headaches, fits, odd sensations, drowsy, schooling, vision, hearing, coordination?
ENT, teeth	Noisy breathing. Did the baby have a newborn hearing test?	Are there problems with hearing or balance? Problems with ear infections or discharge? Any difficulty breathing? Nasal discharge, snoring, or bleeding? Any lumps or glands?	Earache, discharge, recurrent infections? Problems with hearing or balance? Difficulty breathing? Nasal discharge, snoring, or bleeding? Lumps or glands? Sore throat, dental problems, or mouth ulcers?
Skin	Is there a rash? Birthmarks or other marks on the skin?	Is there a rash? Is it itchy? Birthmarks or other marks on the skin?	Is there a rash? Is it itchy? Birthmarks or other marks on the skin?

3 Paediatrics

This is where you can make or break your relationship with the child and family. The child will observe your interaction with their carers. Investing a little time in establishing rapport with the child during history taking will usually pay dividends. Smile, talk to the child, ask about their toys, their friends, compliment them on their t-shirt. Explain what you are doing as you go along. It may help to examine their toy first if they are particularly nervous. Don't separate a young child from their family, examine on mum or dad's lap. Older children with whom you have established rapport and co-operation can be examined as adults.

A single routine will not work for all children. There is no correct order although *always* start with observation—you can't assess work of breathing when a child is crying. *Be opportunistic,* eg start with listening to a baby's heart and breathing while calm and settled in mum's arms as undressing and handling will likely make them cry. You may not need to examine each system each time but must if the source of infection is not clear. If the child is very ill, it is even more important that examination be thorough. Examine a painful area carefully but thoroughly, you don't want to have to do it twice, use analgesia beforehand if necessary. Sometimes if a child is really distressed (and not critically ill) it may be better to take a break, involve a play specialist, write some notes and return a little later to examine afresh.

1 Wash and warm your hands.

2 *Observation and general health.* Is the child ill or well? Alert, lethargic, in pain? If crying, is it high pitched or normal? Behaving normally and interacting with the parents and surroundings? Playing is obviously a good sign. Any jaundice, cyanosis, pallor, rashes? Nutritional status? Any dysmorphism (compare with parents' appearances)?

3 *Vital signs.* Temperature, heart rate, respiratory rate, SPO_2, BP. Review these beforehand if possible to give clues to focus your examination.

4 *Cardiovascular system.* Feel the hands, check peripheral ± central capillary refill (CRT) time (press for 5sec; CRT should be <2sec). Check pulse rate, rhythm, and volume, compare brachial and femoral for infants, radial is usually sufficient for older children. Check position of apex beat and for heaves and thrills. Auscultate the heart for s1, s2, and any added sounds. Note site, timing, grade, character, and radiation of any murmurs. Check for hepatomegaly and sacral or pedal oedema. Consider examining JVP in older children.

5 *Respiratory system.* Observation is absolutely key. What is the work of breathing (WOB)? Nasal flaring, head bobbing, abdominal breathing, tracheal tug, sub- or intercostal or sternal recessions, accessory muscle use, tripoding. Are there added sounds? Grunting, stridor, wheeze, cough. Can the child talk in full sentences, is the voice hoarse? Chest shape and movement; rate, depth, symmetry, regularity, inspiratory vs expiratory phases. Auscultate for breath sounds; normal, reduced, absent, bronchial, and added sounds; stridor (inspiratory, expiratory, biphasic), wheeze, coarse or fine crackles, pleural rub.[11] Percuss the chest for dullness or hyperresonance if appropriate. Do peak flow for obstructive airway disease.

6 *Gastrointestinal system.* Ideally examine supine and relaxed, with the knees bent. Look for distension, visible peristalsis, and hernias. Palpate for tenderness, rigidity, guarding, organomegaly and masses (describe size, shape, surface, edge, tenderness, movement with respiration and percussion note). Examine for shifting dullness if suspicion of ascites. Listen for bowel sounds. Always examine testicles as pain can be referred to abdomen. Don't perform a PR—this should be done once only and by a senior. If relevant check for anal patency, fissures, thread worms and prolapse. Check mouth for ulcers, stomatitis.

7 *Genitourinary system.* If relevant, examine external genitalia sensitively for evidence of ambiguity, congenital abnormality, and size. Note Tanner stage (p. 255, p. 255, p. 255). Examine once only using a chaperone for older children and maintain the child's dignity and privacy.

8 *Neurological system.* Observe muscle bulk, movements, symmetry, whether purposeful, involuntary. Check power, tone, reflexes, sensation, coordination, gait, cranial nerves. Often tricky with younger children, keep instructions simple, ask them to copy your movements or push against you, try and make it a game for them.

9 *Musculoskeletal system.* Watch the child walk and play. Examine limbs and joints, look, move, feel. Are there symmetrical skin creases on both thighs? If <6m check for congenital hip dislocation. Inspect the spine looking for dimples, hair tufts, skin changes, or absent spinous processes at the base. Is there any abnormal curvature or posture?

10 *Skin.* Don't forget to expose the skin fully to look for rashes, bruises, birthmarks, scars particularly if any suspicion of NAI.

11 *Other.* Check hydration status, sunken eyes, skin turgor, mucous membranes, fontanelle. Check Kernig's, Brudzinski's, and neck stiffness if appropriate (see 'Meningitis', pp. 198-9).

12 Is there anything else the parents would like you to see or check?

13 *Ears, nose, and throat.* Always best to leave until the end with young children. Position in the carer's lap is crucial. Examine around the ear; otitis externa, mastoiditis? Examine the tympanic membrane, note colour, lucency, bulging, effusion, perforation, foreign body. Use a spatula to check the tonsils, as well as inspect the teeth and oral and buccal mucosa. Can the child breathe through both nostrils? Is there rhinorrhoea? Check for neck lumps and lymphadenopathy.

14 *Height, weight, and head circumference.* Plot on centile charts. See also examination of the newborn pp. 282-3.

Is this child seriously ill? Prompt recognition of the seriously ill child is a central skill of paediatrics (see also APLS on p. 181).

Assessment *Airway, breathing, circulation:* then 'traffic light' assessment.[12]

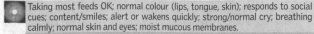

Taking most feeds OK; normal colour (lips, tongue, skin); responds to social cues; content/smiles; alert or wakens quickly; strong/normal cry; breathing calmly; normal skin and eyes; moist mucous membranes.

Taking ≤50% of feeds; pale; not responding to social cues; hard to wake; ↓ activity; no smile; nasal flaring; tachypnoea; SaO₂ <95%; crepitations; tachycardia; CRT>3sec; reduced urine output; dry mucous membranes; rigors; fever >5 days; limb or joint swelling, non-weight bearing/not using extremity; temp ≥39°c if 3–6 months.

Pale; mottled; ashen; blue. No response to social cues; appears ill to health professional; unrousable or doesn't stay awake when roused; weak, high-pitched, or continuous cry; grunting, RR>60, moderate to severe chest indrawing; ↓ skin turgor; non-blanching rash; bulging fontanelle; neck stiffness; status epilepticus; focal seizures; focal neurological signs; temp ≥38°c if <3 months.

Vital signs are a crucial part of your assessment. Sometimes the only clue to serious illness may be an abnormally high HR or RR. Carry a table of age-related normal ranges as it is impractical to try and learn them (table 3.4). Beware an inappropriately normal heart rate or respiratory rate in a tiring and peri-arrest child though this child is likely to appear obviously ill.

Table 3.4 Age-related normal ranges of vital signs

Age (yrs)[1]	Respiratory rate (breaths/min)	HR (beats/min)	Systolic BP (mmHg; 5th–50th centile)
<1	30–40	110–160	65–90
1–2	25–35	100–150	70–95
2–5	25–30	95–140	70–100
5–12	20–25	80–120	80–110
>12	15–20	60–100	90–120

Management of a critically ill child ▸▸ Manage A, then B, before moving on to C.

• ▸▸ *Get help early.*

• Establish an airway; use 100% O₂. Use jaw lift if necessary; suction nasopharynx and mouth as needed. Provide oral or nasopharyngeal airway. Do not force a distressed patient to lie down.

• Assess level of respiratory distress and if urgent treatment is needed eg bronchodilators for acute severe asthma; thoracocentesis for tension pneumothorax. Consider non-invasive ventilatory support.

• Start pulse oximetry and cardiac monitoring. Establish IV access. Have a low threshold for IO ac-

Causes
• Sepsis
• Meningitis
• Seizures
• DKA (p. 248)
• Intussusception (p. 220)
• Haemolytic uraemic syn.
• Epiglottitis
• Obstruction eg volvulus
• Myocarditis

cess if IV access is difficult (p.182). Take relevant bloods. Give IV fluid bolus (20mL/kg normal 0.9% NaCl) if volume depleted. Review and repeat until clinical improvement occurs. If no response to initial fluid bolus get senior help—inotropes may be required. See p. 201 meningococcal disease for additional R̠ of sepsis.

• Identify and treat the cause.

• Discuss with your seniors and the local PICU/retrieval service.

Fever Most emergency presentations to GPs and the ER are due to fever (≥38°c) and most children will have a self-limiting viral illness requiring no intervention. However, every parent and doctor's nightmare is the child with sepsis or meningitis. These children may be difficult to recognize in early stages and can deteriorate rapidly. If in doubt, do not hesitate to get a 2nd/senior opinion. A thorough history and examination are required to determine the source of the fever and extra caution is required if the source is not found. The younger the child, the more thorough the assessment needs to be. An infant <3 months with fever without obvious cause will require a full septic screen including lumbar puncture (LP).

Management of a child with fever This is according to the traffic light system and your clinical judgement. If you think the child is sick get help early. Have a lower threshold for investigation in children with comorbidities (cerebral palsy, learning difficulties, cardiac disease, immunosuppression, etc.). If a source of infection is found, treat accordingly.

Children <3 months:
- Children <3 months with fever should have the following investigations: urine, FBC, CRP, blood culture; ± CXR if any respiratory signs; ± stool culture if diarrhoea; nasopharyngeal aspirate (NPA); ± throat swab.
- LP should be performed on all <1 month, 1–3 months AND unwell-looking, OR 1–3 months AND WCC <5 or >15×10⁹/L.
- Exceptions may be made by experienced paediatricians for patients with a clear cause of the fever such as bronchiolitis or Men B vaccine.

Green features:
- A child with no 'amber' or 'red' signs may be managed at home even if the source of infection is not clear (but consider social and family circumstances). Urine should always be tested in young children. Oral antibiotics should not be prescribed to a child with fever and no clear source.
- Parents should be instructed to offer regular drinks or breastfeeding, to look for signs of dehydration (dry mouth, no tears, sunken eyes or fontanelle), look for a non-blanching rash, and check on their child during the night. Parents should not tepid-sponge or undress their child to control fever and only use antipyretics if the child appears distressed. The child should be kept off school or nursery while febrile.
- Parents should be given advice as to when to seek further help; if the child becomes more unwell, dehydrated, has a fit, or the fever lasts >5 days. If the child develops a non-blanching rash they should seek immediate help.

Amber features:
- Children with 1 or more 'amber' signs and no apparent source of fever should have the following tests done unless deemed unnecessary by an experienced paediatrician: urine, FBC, CRP, blood culture; ± LP if <1yr; ± CXR (particularly if fever >39°C or WCC >20×10⁹/L).

Red features:
- Red features indicate life-threatening illness, this child needs urgent treatment.
- Children with 1 or more 'red' signs and no apparent source of fever should have the following tests done; urine, FBC, CRP, blood culture; ± LP; ± CXR; ± blood gas and U&E; ± NPA; ± throat swab.
- Fluid bolus: if in shock give 20mL/kg IV 0.9%NaCl bolus.
- Antibiotics: maximum dose 3rd-generation cephalosporins (eg cefotaxime or ceftriaxone, use local guidelines) should be given to children with fever and signs of shock or unrousable, or signs of meningococcal disease. Common causes of serious infection: *Neisseria meningitidis, Streptococcus pneumoniae, Escherichia coli, Staphylococcus aureus,* or *Haemophilus influenzae* type B. If <3 months also cover for *Listeria* (eg ampicillin or amoxicillin).

Other points:
- If herpes simplex encephalitis is suspected, give IV aciclovir.
- If >3 months, and bacterial meningitis confirmed, give IV corticosteroid.[14]
- Children with fever of 5 days or more should be assessed by a paediatrician for Kawasaki disease (p. 850).
- Consider recent overseas travel or contact with serious infectious diseases.
- A period of observation in hospital may be useful for children with fever and no apparent source.
- If a child with any red or amber features was not admitted, parents should be provided with a 'safety net'—1 or more of: verbal or written advice as in 'Green features'; a follow-up appointment; or direct access for further assessment if required.

Further reading

NICE (2013). *Fever in Under 5s: Assessment and Initial Management* (cg160). London: NICE. http://www.nice.org.uk/guidance/cg160

'Children are not small adults' as paediatricians like to say. They experience a completely different range of illnesses and the age at which they present is often key to the ∆∆. Broadly speaking, the younger the child, the higher the likelihood of serious illness. To confound the problem the young child will most likely not be able to describe or localize symptoms. In contrast to adults, infectious diseases are much more common, particularly in under 5s and the unimmunized. Children with multiple comorbidities and complex needs are increasingly common as medical advances allow children to survive previously incurable conditions. **Terminology** A *neonate* is <28 days of age; an *infant* is <1yr; '*toddler*' is not well defined, '*pre-school*' or simply '*under 5*' is preferred; the legal definition of a *child* is <18yrs in most jurisdictions but many health services define a *child* as <16yrs.

This section lists common presenting complaints (PC) and their most common or important causes to signpost you to the relevant sections of the book and help you arrive at an effective working diagnosis or differential diagnosis.

▶▶**Seriously ill child** Children have less physiological reserve and may compensate for a period of time before rapidly deteriorating. See pp. 192–3 for initial recognition and management of sepsis, p. 183 for anaphylaxis, p. 201 for meningococcal disease, and pp. 234–5 for status epilepticus. For cardiac arrest see BLS (p. 180), APLS (p. 181), and NLS (p. 185) algorithms.

▶▶**Reduced consciousness** See p. 200 for assessment with AVPU and paediatric Glasgow Coma Scale. Consider: •Sepsis (pp. 192–3) •Meningitis (p. 198–9) •Encephalitis (p. 198) •Diabetic ketoacidosis (DKA, p. 248) •Seizure or post-ictal (pp. 232–3) •Raised intracranial pressure (p. 200) •Hypertensive crisis (p. 231) •Metabolic crisis (p. 252) •Drug or alcohol intoxication •Poisoning and overdose (pp. 276–7), and never forget to consider •Non-accidental injury (NAI, pp. 196–7).

▶▶**Faltering growth** (Previously known as 'failure to thrive'.) Any serious chronic disease can cause faltering growth; however, most cases are due to feeding problems. See pp. 264–5 for clues to pathological causes which include: •Coeliac disease (p. 217) •Cow's milk protein allergy (CMPA, p. 293) •Cystic fibrosis (pp. 214–15). Abuse and neglect must also be considered (pp. 196–7).

Fever Probably the most common PC, with parents presenting earlier and earlier, often before any localizing signs or symptoms of any infection evolve. NICE guideline: 'Fever in Under 5s' (p106) provides a useful traffic light framework for managing such children. ▶Fever in infants <3 months should always be assessed by a senior clinician. As well as viral and bacterial infections, also consider non-infectious causes: autoimmune—Kawasaki's (p. 850); malignancy—leukaemia (p. 242–3); endocrine—hyperthyroidism (p. 251).

Abdominal pain (p. 216) Another common, surprisingly non-specific PC in children, often no clear cause is found. Consider: ▶Appendicitis (tenderness, guarding, p. 220) •Functional abdominal pain (otherwise well, p. 216) •Mesenteric adenitis (associated with viral URTI, p. 216) •Gastroenteritis (p. 218) •Constipation (history is key, pp. 268–9) •Urinary tract infection (particularly in younger children, UTI, pp. 224–5) •Lower lobe pneumonia (cough, fever, pp. 210–11) •Parasitic (worm) infection (eosinophilia, anaemia) •CMPA (p. 293) •Inflammatory bowel disease (blood in stool) •Coeliac disease (faltering growth, p. 217) •Irritable bowel syndrome ▶Intussusception (unwell, obstruction, redcurrant jelly stools, p. 220) ▶Volvulus (obstruction, biliary vomiting, p. 223) •Meckel's diverticulum (melaena) •Pancreatitis •Diabetes (pp. 246–7) •HSP (purpuric rash, p. 241) •Peptic ulcer disease/*Helicobacter pylori* (epigastric) •Renal stones •Gallstones •Cholecystitis. *Consider:* ▶Testicular torsion in boys. Consider: •Menstruation/ovulation •Ovarian cyst •Ovarian torsion •Pelvic inflammatory disease, or ▶Ectopic pregnancy in older girls •Abdominal crisis in those with sickle-cell disease (p. 240).

▶Denotes *red flag* diagnoses not to miss.

3 Paediatrics

Abdominal mass Most commonly constipation but don't miss •Wilms' tumour (p. 229) •Neuroblastoma (p. 217) •Cysts •Hepatomegaly, or •Splenomegaly.

Respiratory disease See pp. 208-9 for causes of stridor: croup; epiglottis; bacterial tracheitis. Bronchiolitis, pneumonia, TB and pertussis are covered on pp. 210-11. Asthma, p. 212. Wheeze in <2yrs see p. 211. Cystic Fibrosis, pp. 214-15.

Rashes A transient maculopapular rash is a feature of many trivial viral illnesses. See pp. 204-5, p. 206 for specific viral illnesses presenting with rash: •Hand, foot, & mouth disease •Roseola infantum •Measles •Mumps •Rubella •Chickenpox. A *purpuric rash* may herald a more serious illness: ►Meningococcaemia (p. 201; Fig 3.6, p. 203) •Henoch–Schönlein purpura (HSP, p. 241) •Idiopathic thrombocytopenic purpura (ITP, p. 241) ►Leukaemia (pp. 242-3). See also •Scarlet fever (p. 414-15) •Eczema (p. 446) •Urticaria (p. 453) •Psoriasis (p. 444) •Pityriasis rosea (p. 452).

Headache p. 236 covers •Migraine •Tension-type •Cluster headaches and ►Red flags to consider for •CNS infection •Intracranial haemorrhage •CNS malignancy •Hydrocephalus, or •Other causes of raised ICP (p. 200). Consider also •Idiopathic intracranial hypertension (classically overweight, visual disturbance).

Seizures •Epilepsy •Febrile convulsions and conditions which can mimic seizures (cardiac arrhythmias; reflex anoxic seizures; Sandifer syndrome; non-epileptic seizures) are covered on p. 232-3.

Enuresis See pp. 268-9 covering primary enuresis and constipation but also consider UTI (pp. 224-5); new-onset diabetes if previously continent child (pp. 246-7); diabetes insipidus; psychosocial stressors and NAI/child sexual abuse (pp. 196-7).

Haematuria Differentiate microscopic, macroscopic, and myoglobinuria. Consider UTI (pp. 224-5); post-catheter insertion/trauma; acute glomerulo-nephritis (p. 227); menstruation; vasculitis (eg HSP, p. 241); rhabdomyolysis (eg from infection) or rarer causes: renal calculi; bladder/renal tumour; haemolytic uraemic syndrome (HUS, pp. 230-1).

Neonatal conditions and problems associated with prematurity These are covered from pp. 280-1 onwards.

►Involve colleagues/seniors and social services immediately when issues of abuse arise. Read what follows with local child safeguarding and NICE guidelines,[15] and relevant legislation in your country eg in England, the *Children's Act* (which states that *the child's welfare is* **always** *paramount*). *Child abuse* is defined as deliberate infliction of harm to a child or failure to prevent harm, and may be physical, sexual, emotional, neglect, or fabricated or induced illness (FII). *Neglect* is a persistent failure to meet a child's basic physical or psychological needs that is likely to result in serious impairment of the child's health and development and is the most common form of child abuse. FII (also known as *Munchausen's by proxy*) is a rare type of abuse where a carer fabricates or induces symptoms in the child for attention or other secondary gain. Prevalence of NAI: 1% of ED work.[16]

Risk factors for NAI Birthweight <2500g; mother <30yrs; unwanted pregnancy; stress; poverty;[17] prematurity; multiple medical conditions; child <2yrs; domestic abuse. Parental factors: substance and alcohol misuse; intellectual disability; history of childhood abuse; and mental health problems.[18]

History Child abuse may present following a disclosure by the child but all clinicians should consider it as a possible ΔΔ particularly if:
• History, inconsistent with injuries; odd mode of injury; odd set of signs.
• History inconsistent with the child's development eg bruising in children who aren't independently mobile.
• Significant unexplained injury; multiple injuries.
• Multiple or varying explanations from same or different carers.
• Delayed presentation to doctor, or taken by someone who is not a parent.
• Inappropriate responses from carer or child (evasive, unconcerned, aggressive) or unusual child–carer interaction.
• Multiple attendances particularly to several different services.

Examination If there is *any* suspicion of NAI, always examine the child thoroughly exposing the skin fully. This few-minute examination could save a child's life. Inspect external genitalia only, leave full examination to appropriate professional if necessary. Some patterns of injury may be highly suggestive of abuse:

Bruising: The most common injury in physical abuse. Research shows it is not possible to age a bruise by visual inspection.[18]
• Bruising on face, buttocks, abdomen, ears, neck, hands, arms.
• Bruising away from bony prominences.
• Bruises with uniform shape, the shape of an implement or finger marks, or in clusters.
• Bruising with petechiae not explained by medical cause.

Burns and scalds: Common accidental injuries particularly in toddlers. ~10% are related to abuse, predominantly neglect but sometimes intentional harm.[19]
• Immersion injury with glove and stocking distribution and clearly demarcated edges.
• Other bilateral, symmetrical scalds, particularly involving legs, buttocks.
• Contact burns not involving finger tips or palm, particularly if multiple.
• Multiple similar burns of same size and shape eg cigarette burns.

Other:
• Bite marks (not caused by small child); ligature marks.
• Oral injuries (torn lingual frenulum, perforated or lacerated pharynx) in the absence of clear explanation.
• Is the child clean, well kempt, well nourished? Is there poor school attendance?

Abusive head trauma (AHT): Predominantly seen in children <2yrs, may be very difficult to detect and has a high mortality. There may be an absence of history or external signs of injury. Symptoms may be vague, poor feeding, lethargy, or severe fits, apnoeas.

Fractures: Site or type of fracture cannot diagnose NAI, features associated with NAI are:[19]
- Rib # in very young children, particularly posterior, multiple, or same location on adjacent ribs.
- Humeral # in non-mobile child or spiral # of humerus any age.
- Femoral # in non-mobile child, once walking spiral # of femur can occur accidentally.
- Spinal # any age.

Investigation If physical abuse is suspected, children <2yrs should have a skeletal survey and an ophthalmology review (retinal haemorrhages indicate 71% chance of AHT in <3yrs[19]) to rule out occult injuries in this high-risk group. A head CT should be performed if <1yr and considered >1yr. Coagulation screen, FBC, and film in patients with unusual bruising, bone profile, vit D, and PTH in patients with #. Consider urine toxicology if poisoning is possible and medical photography to document injuries.

Information sharing: Children suffering abuse may present to several different services and combining information from different sources may lead to a very different view of the situation. It is routine procedure if the issue of abuse is just a possibility to contact social services and inquire if the child or family are known. If suspicion is high, GP practice, health visitor, school, and other services should be called. The need to share information usually overrides concerns about confidentiality but should be proportionate and considered.

ΔΔ Osteogenesis imperfecta; ITP; leukaemia; HSP; coagulation disorder; scurvy; blue spots (congenital dermal melanocytosis); osteoporosis eg from propionic acidaemia.[20][21]

Management You are not alone, remember that often your duty is not to diagnose child abuse, but to recognize possible abuse, and then to get help. All NHS organizations have a designated professional for safeguarding. A senior community paediatrician is often available by phone to discuss cases and give advice. The child's welfare is paramount—removal from danger may mean immediate admission to hospital or foster care. Always think about siblings/other children who may also be at risk. Never make assumptions, leave judgements to the courts. Be as open with the carers as possible if not endangering the child or others. In rare cases, the police may need to be contacted for an emergency protection order.

Other issues Talk to the child, let them tell their story. Don't delay, act quickly. Document contemporaneously and differentiate clearly what is fact and what is opinion. Don't forget children can be abusers too. Be aware of 'stress positions' which cause pain but leave no mark. Always be clear of who exactly is accompanying the child, be wary of private fostering arrangements.

Sexual abuse (CSA) or exploitation Know your local guidelines. Follow them. Inform social services and get help. Sexual activity <13yrs is illegal in the UK whether or not the child 'consented'. Suspect CSA if: genital, anal, or perianal injuries; persistent or recurrent anal or genital symptoms particularly if associated with behavioural change; STIs <13yrs. Consider CSA if: foreign bodies in vagina or anus; STIs <17yrs.[22] Consider exploitation or abuse where there is a clear difference in the power or mental capacity of the young person and the sexual partner. Conversion disorder is associated with CSA and other abuse.[23] Intimate examination and forensic specimens should only be done once by an expert in appropriate surroundings maintaining dignity and sensitivity. Forensic evidence may be obtained up to 7 days from vaginal intercourse. While vaginal discharge/vulvo vaginitis is more common in victims of CSA, it is common in girls generally and in most it is culture negative and not significant. Careful history and examination is important. STI screening is indicated where there is recurrent vaginal discharge or any clinical suspicion of CSA. Does abuse cause psychological harm? Yes, almost always. See p. 693. Psychological sequelae (stress; depression) can be a sign of sexual or emotional abuse.[3]

3 Hulme K (1984). *Bone People*. Auckland: Spiral/Hodder & Stoughton. This novel tests Samuel Johnson's aphorism that `it is better that a man should be abused than be forgotten'. Read it before making quick judgements about families.

Signs Altered behaviour, cognition, or consciousness; fever or recent febrile illness; fits; focal neurological signs; vomiting; meningism. High index of suspicion is needed—consider in children presenting with odd behaviour.

Causes *Infective:* HSV; mumps (ask about parotitis/testicular pain); varicella zoster (recent chickenpox?); rabies (dog-bite abroad); parvovirus (slapped cheek syndrome), immunocompromise (CMV, EBV, HHV-6); influenza; toxoplasmosis; TB; mycoplasma; malaria (if recent travel, see *OHCM* p416); dengue; Rickettsia; Lyme disease. *Non-infective:* acute disseminated encephalomyelitis (ADEM)—an acute demyelinating process which usually follows a non-CNS infection, antibody-mediated encephalitis (usually para-neoplastic).

ΔΔ Encephalopathies: metabolic (hypoglycaemia; DKA, ↑ ammonia), toxic, hypertensive, autoimmune, sepsis; Other CNS infection (meningitis, abscess), psychosis, lead or other poisoning, subarachnoid haemorrhage, malignancy, lupus.[24]

Investigations LP CSF opening pressure, protein, lactate, glucose, MC&S, and PCR (HSV, VZV, enteroviruses ±EBV and others); bloods incl. ammonia, serology; HIV; stool (enteroviruses); nose/throat swab (respiratory virus PCR); urine (mumps), MRI or CT.[25] EEG can be helpful in cases with subtle symptoms to differentiate psychiatric or organic cause.

Management Treat for bacterial meningitis, as signs and symptoms overlap. Empirically start treatment for mycoplasma, HSV, and any other causes suggested by clinical or epidemiological clues. A common practice in UK is 'triple therapy' with ceftriaxone, clarithromycin, and aciclovir.

HSV encephalitis The most treatable viral encephalitis. Nasolabial herpes or raised LFTs *may* be present. IV aciclovir 14–21 days, then repeat LP to confirm CSF is HSV negative. Corticosteroids are not routinely used. Mortality ~7%, 60% intact survival, neurological sequelae common.

▶▶Meningitis

Be clear on the difference between meningitis and meningococcal disease (p. 201): *meningitis* is an inflammatory disease of the meninges, causes may be bacterial, viral, fungal, or protozoal (see table 3.5); the relative frequency of causative pathogens depends on the child's age, immunization status, and immunocompetence (pp. 202–3). *Bacterial meningitis* is a *medical emergency* with high morbidity and mortality. **Presentation** Children with meningitis often present with non-specific signs and symptoms: poor feeding, fever, lethargy, irritability, vomiting, headache, myalgia, arthralgia. **Meningeal signs** Comparatively late, and much less common in young children, they are neither sensitive nor specific:[28] neck stiffness ('unable to kiss knee'), Kernig's sign (resistance to extending knee when hip flexed); Brudzinski's sign (hips flex on neck flexion); photophobia; opisthotonos. **Other signs** May be more specific but are late: bulging fontanelle; altered consciousness; seizures; focal neurological deficit; abnormal pupils; non-blanching rash (p. 201). **Other causes of stiff neck** Tonsillitis, lymphadenitis, subarachnoid bleed.

Investigations FBC, CRP, electrolytes, clotting, culture, meningococcal PCR, glucose, blood gas. LP if no contraindication. Also consider urine, nose/throat swab, stool virology, CXR.

Contraindications to LP Signs of raised ICP (p. 200); shock; respiratory insufficiency; spreading purpura; coagulopathy; ↓ platelets; local infection at LP site; during or after seizures until stable.[14] CT *cannot* show if LP will be safe. If in doubt give antibiotics. **Performing LP** Don't delay IV antibiotics to do LP. LP up to 96 hours after admission may still be useful.[14] *Technique:* (*OHCM* p768) Learn from an expert. • Explain everything to carers • Get IV access (if you are doing a procedure bigger than a cannula, you need a cannula first): acute deterioration is possible, consider monitoring options. Ask an experienced nurse to position child fully flexed (knees to chin) on the side of a bed, with back exactly at right angles with it • Mark a point just above (cranial to) a line joining the spinous processes between the iliac crests • Drape & sterilize the area; put on gloves • Infiltrate 1mL of 1% **lidocaine** superficially in the older child • Insert LP needle aiming towards umbilicus. Keep the needle perpendicular to the back at all times • Catch 5–10 CSF drops in each of 4 bottles for: urgent MC&S, virology, glucose, & protein (do simultaneous paired blood glucose too).

Treating pyogenic meningitis before the organism is known
▸▸ Manage ABC, high-flow O_2.
▸▸ Do not delay antibiotics for blood/CSF cultures, give immediate IV ceftriaxone if >3 months, cefotaxime plus amoxicillin/ampicillin if <3 months or IV/IM benzylpenicillin in pre-hospital settings (see BOX 'Giving IM benzylpenicillin before hospital admission' p. 203).[14]
▸▸ **Dexamethasone** (0.15mg/kg/6h IV eg for 4 days) with 1st antibiotic dose if child >3 months and not meningococcal septicaemia or TB (reduces hearing loss in pneumococcal meningitis but otherwise not clearly beneficial).
▸▸ Assess for signs of raised ICP (p. 200) and treat with **hypertonic saline** (3mL/kg of 2.7% or 3% NaCl) or **mannitol** (0.25g/kg of 20%) over 5min and discuss with senior and paediatric intensivist.
▸▸ Do not restrict fluids unless there are signs of SIADH p. 313 or ↑ICP.[14]
▸▸ Treat for *Cryptococcus* if HIV+ve.
▸▸ Add aciclovir if HSV encephalitis is suspected (p. 198).

Complications *Acute:* Seizures, ↑ICP, abscesses, infected subdural effusion. *Chronic:* Hydrocephalus , ataxia, paralysis, deafness (steroids reduce this), IQ↓, epilepsy.

Table 3.5 CSF in meningitis

	Bacterial/ pyogenic	Tubercular	Aseptic, viral	Normal range
Appearance [25,27,28]	Cloudy/turbid	Cloudy/yellow	Usually clear	Clear
Predominant cell	Polymorphs eg 1000/mm³	Mononuclear 10–350/mm³	Mononuclear 50–1500/mm³	≤5 lymphocytes; ~0 neutrophils (≤20 lymphocytes if <1 month old)
Glucose level	↓ (<⅔ of serum glucose)	↓ (<⅔ of serum glucose)	>⅔ of serum glucose	>⅔ of serum glucose
Protein (g/dL)	↑ (mean ≈3)	↑ >0.4 (mean ≈2)	≥0.4 and <1.5	<0.4

AVPU is a very quick and simple measure: Alert; responds to Voice; responds to Pain; Unresponsive.

Glasgow Coma Scale (GCS) GCS as modified for children[29,30] provides a more objective record of coma level to help monitor progress ± prognosticate. Use if <5yrs; if >5yrs, use adult GCS, p. 245.

Eye opening: E4: spontaneous. E3: to voice. E2: to pain. E1: none. C: eyes closed due to swelling/other local cause.

Verbal response: V5: alert, babbles, coos, words or sentences to usual ability (ie normal). V4: less than usual ability, irritable cry. V3: cries to pain. V2: moans to pain. V1: no response to pain. T: intubated.

Best motor response: M6: normal spontaneous movements. M5: localizes to pain (>9 months) or withdraws to touch. M4: withdraws from nailbed pain. M3: abnormal flexion to pain (decorticate—indicative of damage to cerebral hemispheres, thalamus, internal capsule, or midbrain). M2: extension to pain (adduction, internal rotation of shoulder, forearm pronation; decerebrate posture from brainstem damage). M1: no response to pain. NT: paralysed or other limiting factor. Painful stimuli: nailbed pressure, trapezius pinch, or supraorbital notch.

Total score ranges from 3 to 15, even if you are dead you score 3! eg no eye opening + no verbalization + no motor response to pain = 3. Although developed and validated for traumatic brain injury the GCS is widely used in other settings. As a rule of thumb, <8 ≈ intubation needed; 4–8 ≈ intermediate prognosis; 3 ≈ bad prognosis.

GCS-P The GCS Pupil Score published in 2018[29] recognizes the importance of pupil reaction. The pupil reactivity score (2: both pupils unreactive to light, 1: one pupil unreactive, 0: neither pupil unreactive) is *subtracted* from the GCS score to give a range from 1–15. Another alternative is the Blantyre Coma Scale which has been used in cerebral malaria research.[31]

▶▶Raised intracranial pressure (ICP)

Signs Drowsy; seizures; papilloedema; pupil changes (ipsilateral dilatation); abnormal posturing (decorticate/decerebrate); Cushing's triad (bradycardia, ↑BP, and irregular breathing) warns of imminent coning.

Management ABC is the initial priority. Maintain cerebral perfusion pressure (CPP = mean arterial pressure minus ICP; if CPP <40mmHg cerebral ischaemia is likely).

▶▶ Manage in ICU with neuroprotective measures: intubate and ventilate.

▶▶ Help venous drainage by keeping head in the midline, elevated at ~30°.

▶▶ Reduce metabolic demand: maintain normothermia (36–37°C) and oxygenation and muscle relax; prevent seizures (prophylaxis) and hypoglycaemia.

▶▶ Optimize CPP: low–normal pco_2, high–normal BP.

▶▶ Give **hypertonic saline** (3mL/kg of 2.7% or 3% NaCl) or **mannitol** (0.25g/kg of 20%) over 10–20min.[32]

▶▶ Fluid restriction & diuresis, avoiding hypovolaemia (keep Na+ 145–150mmol/L, and CVP to 2–5cmH₂O).

▶▶ Emergent neurosurgical transfer if intervention possible.

▶▶ Steroids may be useful: dexamethasone: if <35kg, 16.7mg IV (20.8mg if >35kg) then as per *BNFC*.

▶▶ *Don't do* LP (except in chronic stable ↑ICP).

Meningococcal disease (comprising *Neisseria meningitidis* meningitis or sepsis or both) progresses rapidly and there is a narrow window for diagnosis. Early signs may be subtle, 'classic' signs are often absent, particularly in young children. Consider in any seriously ill baby or child. ▶Get expert help from your senior. If there is any hint of meningococcal sepsis: ▶▶*Do not delay antibiotics* for blood/CSF cultures, give immediate IV ceftriaxone if >3 months, give cefotaxime plus amoxicillin/ampicillin if <3 months or give IV/IM benzylpenicillin in pre-hospital settings (see BOX 'Giving IM benzylpenicillin before hospital admission' p. 203).[14] **Early features** Last 4–8h are non-specific and common to many simple viral illnesses: T°↑; headache; misery; anorexia; vomiting; sore throat; coryza.[33] **Septic features** These occur next; cold hands/feet; limb pain; abnormal colour (pale/mottled); thirst; respiratory distress in younger children; and sometimes diarrhoea; DIC; pulse↑; BP↓; RR↑. **Non-blanching rash** (fig 3.6, p. 203) The classic sign is a late sign only seen in 40–70% of cases and after median 8–19h depending on age.[33] It evolves over hours from non-specific→petechial→purpuric/haemorrhagic. **Meningeal signs** Neck stiffness, photophobia, bulging fontanelle occur comparatively late (after 12–15 hours), and less common in young children. Unconsciousness, delirium, and seizures are very late signs.

Preventing deaths from meningococcal disease

Most children survive with prompt treatment:

▶▶ Get help early! This child is likely to need transfer to ICU.

▶▶ Manage ABC, high-flow O₂, give IV **ceftriaxone** 80–100mg/kg without delay.

▶▶ Access: 2 large IV cannulae or IO. Take blood gas (incl. lactate, glucose), electrolytes, FBC, clotting, culture, x-match, CRP, Men PCR, throat swab.

▶▶ Assess for signs of shock and treat immediately with 20mL/kg bolus over 5–10min and reassess. Repeat if necessary.

▶▶ If still in shock after 40mL/kg, child will require urgent intubation and ventilation (I&V) and inotropes: peripheral **dopamine** (10–20mcg/kg/min) or **adrenaline** 0.1mcg/kg/min if central or IO access.

▶▶ Assess for signs of raised ICP (p. 200) and treat as for meningitis (pp. 198–9).

▶▶ I&V to control CO₂ and institute other neuroprotective measures (p. 200).

▶▶ Do not perform LP if signs of shock or raised ICP or other contraindications (p. 199).

▶▶ Anticipate, monitor, and treat hypoglycaemia (glucose <3, give 10% **glucose** 2mL/kg as a bolus), anaemia, ↓K⁺, ↓Ca²⁺, ↓Mg²⁺, acidosis, coagulopathy. Alert haematology that blood and blood products may be required.

▶▶ Monitor pulse, respiratory rate, BP, ECG, pupil size/reactivity, level of consciousness, urine output (catheterize).

▶▶ Urgent discussion with and transfer to paediatric intensive care unit (PICU).

Heroic, non-standard ideas: Extracorporeal membrane oxygenation; terminal fragment of human bactericidal/permeability-increasing protein (rBPI21) to ↓ cytokines; heparin with protein C concentrate to reverse coagulopathy; plasmapheresis to remove cytokines, and thrombolysis (rTPA) for limb reperfusion.[34]

Other issues Inform your local health protection team early. Meningococcal prophylaxis for contacts ± vaccination may be advised, single-dose ciprofloxacin is now preferred to rifampicin.[35] Prevention is key, ensure immunization. 10 years after introduction of Men C vaccine in the UK in 1999, lab-confirmed cases of Men C fell by >90% in immunized age group and >⅔ in other age groups (due to reduced carriage).[35] A quadrivalent Men B protein vaccine was introduced to the UK schedule in 2015 but effectiveness is not yet established. ▶Stop parents smoking! 37% of cases are put down to aerosolized spread via smoker's coughs.[38]

The meningococcus, the pneumococcus, and, in the unvaccinated, *Haemophilus influenzae*, are the great killers. In the former, the interval between seeming well and coma is counted in hours. Antibiotic choice should be guided by culture and sensitivities.

Neisseria meningitidis Abrupt onset ± non-blanching rash (figs 3.6 & 3.8) (starts as non-specific rash); septicaemia may occur with no meningitis (Waterhouse–Friderichsen, OHCM p714), so early LPs may be normal, giving false reassurance. *Typical age:* Any. *Film:* Gram –ve cocci in pairs (long axes parallel), often within polymorphs. Drug of choice: **cefotaxime/ceftriaxone** or **benzylpenicillin** 50mg/kg/4h IV. If clear history penicillin and cephalosporin-induced anaphylaxis, give chloramphenicol (see later) or meropenem.[37] *Prevention:* p. 201.

Haemophilus influenzae (Rare if immunized). *Typical age:* <4yrs. CSF: Gram –ve rods. The lower the CSF glucose, the worse the infection. *Drugs:* Ceftriaxone or, where there is no resistance, **chloramphenicol** 12–25mg/kg/6h IVI (neonates: see BNF) + IV **ampicillin**—if ≤1wk old, 30–60mg/kg/12h (/8h if 1–3wks old;/6h if 3–4wks old). If >4wks old 25mg/kg/6h (max. 1g), doubled in severe infections. Rifampicin (see later) may also be needed. With chloramphenicol, monitor peak levels; aim for 20–25mcg/mL; usual doses may be far exceeded to achieve this. (Trough level: <15mcg/mL.) As soon as you can, switch to PO (more effective). Steroids (p.199) reduce hearing loss.

Strep pneumoniae *Typical age:* Any. *Risk factors:* Respiratory infections, HIV.[38] *Film:* Gram +ve diplococci. ℞: **Ceftriaxone**, or benzylpenicillin 50mg/kg/4h slow IV—or, if resistance likely (eg parts of Europe and USA) ± rifampicin. As an add-in or an alternative, consider **vancomycin**, if >1 month old: 15mg/kg/8h (max. 2g/24h) IVI over 1h, but CSF penetration is unreliable.[39] Monitor U&E.

Group B haemolytic streptococci Usually acquired via birth canal (so swab mothers whose infants suddenly fall ill at ~24h old). Infection onset may be delayed a month. Drug of choice: **benzylpenicillin** 25–50mg/kg/8–12h slow IV.

Escherichia coli This is a major cause of meningitis in neonates (in whom signs may consist of poor feeding, lethargy→apnoea, seizures, and shock). Drug of choice: cefotaxime + gentamicin.

Listeria monocytogenes Presents soon after birth with meningitis or septicaemia (± pneumonia). It is rare outside neonatal period unless immunocompromised. Microabscesses form in many organs (granulomatosis infantiseptica). Δ: Culture blood, CSF, placenta, amniotic fluid. ℞: IV ampicillin (see earlier) + gentamicin.[40]

TB meningitis has very high mortality, outcome depends on the stage at which treatment is started so early recognition is crucial. Consider in any child with ↓ glucose, ↑ protein, and lymphocytosis in CSF. Clinically divided into phases: 'prodromal' phase with gradual onset, malaise, headache, anorexia, and low-grade fever (can vary days to months with average around 2–3 weeks); 'meningitic' phase headache, vomiting, lethargy, confusion, meningism, and neurological signs; and 'paralytic' phase with coma, seizures, and paresis. Stage is based on level of consciousness and neurological signs: 1 Conscious with no neurological signs 2 Disturbed consciousness ± focal neurology 3 Comatose ± significant neurological deficit. *Complications:* communicating hydrocephalus, stroke, raised ICP. TB can also cause CNS tuberculomas (fig 3.7). *Investigations:* The 1st few CSFs may be normal, or show visible fibrin webs and widely varying cell counts. ℞ *example:* Isoniazid (± pyridoxine (vit B_6)) + rifampicin for 1yr + (for 2 months) pyrazinamide with eg streptomycin if >4wks old; alternative: ethambutol if old enough to report visual problems.[41,42] Adding dexamethasone improves survival (at least in those >14yrs old) but probably does not prevent disability.[43] Children <14 should be given **prednisolone** 4mg/kg/24h for 4 weeks then follow a reducing course.[44]

Other bacteria Leptospiral species (canicola); *Brucella; Salmonella, Staph. aureus*/CONS (in associated with ventricular drains/other foreign body).

Causes of 'aseptic' meningitis Viruses (eg measles, mumps, parecho, herpes, enteroviruses, arboviruses, polio), partially treated bacterial infections, *Cryptococcus* (in immunosuppressed, use India ink stain).

Giving IM benzylpenicillin before hospital admission

- 300mg IM up to 1 year old.
- 600mg if 1–9yrs.
- 1.2g if >10yrs.
- When in doubt, give it: it may be negligent not to do so.
- If penicillin-allergic, **cefotaxime** may be used (50mg/kg IM stat; if >12yrs 1g).[4]

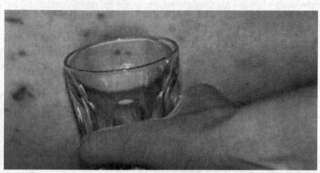

Fig 3.6 Image of glass test in purpuric rashes (seen in meningococcal disease). The rash does not blanch. © Dr Petter Brandtzaeg, and the Meningitis Trust.

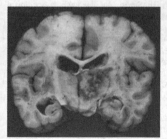

Fig 3.7 Tuberculoma. Caseous (cheese-like) necrotic material is surrounded by epithelioid cell granulomas. Rupture releases mycobacteria into the subarachnoid space, hence causing TB meningitis. © Prof. Dimitri Agamanolis.

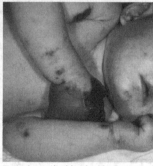

Fig 3.8 4-month-old girl with gangrene of hands due to meningococcaemia. Courtesy of the U.S. Centers for Disease Control and Prevention.

Measles⁰ (ND=notifiable disease) (RNA paramyxovirus)
↑ following 1998 MMR scandal. Epidemic in Europe
in 2018. *Spread:* Aerosol. *Incubation:* 6–19 days;⁴⁵ infective from prodrome (the 4Cs: cough, coryza, conjunctivitis, cranky), T°↑, until 5 days after rash starts.
Koplik spots on palate or buccal mucosa (fig 3.9) are
pathognomonic. They are often fading as the characteristic morbilliform rash appears (eg behind ears, on
days 3–5, spreading down the body, becoming confluent). Δ: IgM ± IgG +ve; PCR. *Complications:* Diarrhoea,

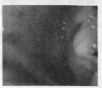

Fig 3.9 Koplik spots.
Courtesy of the U.S. Centers
for Disease Control.

stomatitis, otitis media, pneumonitis, meningitis,
encephalitis, myocarditis, acute disseminated encephalomyelitis (ADEM). More
common if <5yrs or >20yrs. Measles suppresses the immune system causing 2nd
infections: croup and tracheitis; pneumonia (the most common cause of death).
Encephalitis has 15% mortality and 25% neurological sequelae (fits, deafness, or
↓ cognition). *Subacute sclerosing panencephalitis (SSPE)* is a chronic complication of measles which develops 7–13yrs after primary infection (incidence: 4–11
cases per 100,000 cases of measles): progressive changes in behaviour, myoclonus, choreoathetosis, dystonia, dementia, coma, and death. R: Supportive.
Isolate—in hospital if the patient is ill or immunocompromised or malnourished,
or has pneumonitis, CNS signs, or dehydration, then:
- Ensure adequate nutrition (catabolism is very high). Continue breastfeeding,
  even during diarrhoea. Pass a nasogastric feeding tube if intake is poor.
- Give vitamin A in developing world or hospitalized patients: 2 doses, + 1 more at
  6 weeks later (pp. 374-5). CI: pregnancy; known not to be deficient.
- Treat secondary bacterial infection; antibiotics such as amoxicillin for otitis
  media or pneumonia. Prophylactic antibiotics are not indicated.⁴⁶

Immunization: (table 3.11, p. 257) 80% effective.⁴⁷ *Prognosis:* Good in rich countries; in poor areas death rate is up to 10%⁴⁸ (>1 million/yr, mostly in Africa).⁴⁶

Rubella⁰ (RNA virus.) *Spread:* Droplets. *Incubation:* 2–3wks. *Infectivity:*
5 days before to 5 days after start of rash. *Signs:* Macular rash; suboccipital
lymphadenopathy. R: Supportive. *Immunization:* Live virus, table 3.11, p. 257.⁴⁹
Complications: Small joint arthritis. Malformations *in utero* (p. 38). Infection
during the 1st 4 weeks of fetal development: eye anomaly (70%); wks 4–8: cardiac abnormalities (40%); wks 8–12: deafness (30%).

Mumps⁰ (RNA paramyxovirus.) *Spread:* Droplets/saliva. *Incubation:* 14–
21 days. *Immunity:* Lifelong, once infected. *Infectivity:* 7 days before and
5 days after onset of parotitis. *Signs:* Prodromal malaise; T°↑; painful parotid swelling, becoming bilateral in 70% (ΔΔ: Sjögren's; leukaemia; dengue;
herpes virus; EBV; HIV; sarcoid; pneumococci; *Haemophilus*; staphs; anaphylaxis; blowing glass or trumpets; drugs; fig 3.10). *Complications:* Usually none;
orchitis (infertility rare), arthritis, meningitis, **pancreatitis, myocarditis,
deafness, myelitis.** R: Supportive. *Immunization:* Table 3.11, p. 257, for *any*
non-immune adult or child (SE: rare parotitis/pancreatitis).

Erythrovirus ('Fifth disease', erythema infectiosum; parvovirus B19.). *Spread:*
Droplets. *Incubation:* 2–3wks. *Infectivity:* Not known but wholly before onset
of clinical disease. *Signs:* Usually a mild, acute infection, with malar erythema
('slapped cheek' fig 3.11), peri-oral pallor and a rash mainly on the limbs (gloves
and socks syndrome, in adults).⁵⁰ Arthralgia/arthritis are commoner in adults. It
can also suppress erythropoiesis (aplastic crisis)—serious if RBC lifespan is already short (eg sickle-cell disease, thalassaemia, spherocytosis, HIV). Δ: IgM (PCR if
immunocompromised). R: Symptomatic: transfusions and IVIg are rarely needed.⁵⁰
Pregnancy: Risk of fetal death is ~10% (esp. mid-trimester).⁵¹ If pregnant woman
exposed, check serum IgM/IgG for previous immunity. *Fetal infection:* anaemia
→hydrops fetalis (in ~3%; treat by intrauterine transfusion if severe); myocarditis
due to direct infection of myocytes; and in rare cases brain anomalies.⁵²

Hand, foot, & mouth disease *Cause:* RNA viruses—Coxsackievirus A16 or enterovirus 71 (suspect in outbreaks with herpangina, meningitis, flaccid paralysis ± pulmonary oedema). This has nothing to do with the bovine form. *Spread:* Droplets , faeco-oral, and vesicle fluid. *Incubation:* 5–7 days. *Presentation:* Low -grade fever, child is mildly unwell; develops vesicles on palms, soles, and mouth. They may cause discomfort until they heal, without crusting. *Treatment:* Symptomatic. *Herpangina* (also caused by Coxsackieviruses) entails high fever + sore throat + vesicles or macerated ulcers (on fauces, soft palate, or uvula, which heal over 2 days) ± abdominal pain and nausea.

Herpes infections See *онсм* p. 404. Varicella zoster/chickenpox: p. 206.

Roseola infantum *Cause:* Herpes virus 6 (HHV6; double-stranded DNA). *Synonyms:* Exanthem subitum, fourth disease, 3-day fever. *Presentation:* A common, mild, self-limiting illness in infants. A maculopapular rash appears as fever abruptly resolves after 3–5 days. Uvulo-palatoglossal junctional ulcers (Nagayama spots) may be a useful early sign.[53] It is neurotropic (a rare cause of encephalitis/focal gliosis on MRI, maybe accounting for why the not uncommon roseola 'febrile fits' tend to occur *after* the fever).[54]

Other causes of rashes in children See also skin diseases section (pp. 432–61).
• A transient maculopapular rash is a feature of many trivial viral illnesses (but a few macules may be a sign of early meningococcaemia).
• Purpuric rashes: meningococcaemia (p. 201); HSP (p. 241); ITP, ALL (check FBC and film).
• Drug rashes (maculopapular) from eg amoxicillin in glandular fever common.
• Scabies (p. 458); insect bites; scarlet fever (pp. 414–15).
• Eczema (p. 446); urticaria (p. 453); psoriasis—guttate psoriasis may follow a respiratory tract infection in children (p. 444); pityriasis rosea (p. 452).
• Still disease (JIA): transient maculopapular rash, fever, and polyarthritis.

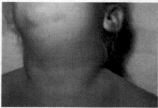

Fig 3.10 Mumps: generalized salivary swelling.
Courtesy of the U.S. Centers for Disease Control and Prevention.

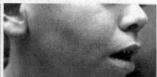

Fig 3.11 Slapped cheeks (parvovirus B19).
Courtesy of the U.S. Centers for Disease Control and Prevention.

Managing distressing fever in viral illnesses

►Unwrap ►Rehydrate ►Antipyretics. Antipyretics aren't always needed[55] (↑ mortality if used in severe sepsis).[56] Keep records of quantity used.

Ibuprofen 5mg/kg/8h if 1–2 months; 50mg/8h if 3–11 months; 100mg/8h if 1–3yrs old; 150mg/8h if 4–6yrs; 200mg/8h if 7–9yrs; 300mg/8h if 10–11yrs (max. 10mg/kg/8h) is better than paracetamol at 15mg/kg/6h, so try it first.

Oral paracetamol doses 30–60mg/8h (max. 60mg/kg/day) if 1–2 months; 60mg/4–6h if 3–5 months; 120mg/4–6h if 6–23 months; 180mg/4–6h if 2–3yrs; 240mg/4–6h if 4–5yrs; 240–250mg/4–6h if 6–7yrs; 360–375mg/4–6h if 8–9yrs; 480–500mg/4–6h if 10–11yrs; 480–750mg/4–6h if 12–15yrs; 0.5–1g/4–6h if 16yrs+. Maximum of 4 doses in 24h.

Paracetamol suppositories Are available (60, 120, 125, 240, 250, 500mg, or 1g).

Continue only as long as child is in discomfort, consider alternating antipyretics if discomfort persists, avoid giving simultaneously. Antipyretics *do not* prevent febrile convulsions.

3 Paediatrics

Chickenpox is a primary infection with vzv. Shingles (aka herpes zoster) (*OHCM* p404) is a reactivation of dormant virus in posterior root ganglia.

Chickenpox *Spread:* Droplets/vesicle fluid. It is one of the most infectious diseases known. 95% of adults have been infected; immunity is lifelong. Incubation: 11–21 days. *Infectivity:* 4 days before the rash, until all lesions have crusted (≈5 days). *Signs:* Crops of skin vesicles of different ages, often starting on face, scalp, or trunk. The rash is more concentrated on the torso than the extremities. *Δ:* Clinical, PCR useful in immunocompromised or atypical presentations. *ΔΔ:* Hand, foot, & mouth disease (p. 205); impetigo (p. 448); insect bites; scabies; eczema herpeticum; herpes simplex; dermatitis herpetiformis; rickettsia. *Course:* T°↑; rash starts 2 days later, often starting on the back: macule→papule→vesicle with a red surround→ulcers (eg oral, vaginal) →crusting. 2–4 crops of lesions occur during the illness. Lesions cluster around areas of pressure or hyperaemia. *Complications:* Cellulitis: vzv is associated with invasive group A strep cellulitis, necrotizing fasciitis, and toxic shock syndrome, if spots are blackish or coalescing and bluish, get urgent help on ITU; avoid ibuprofen. Be alert to pneumonia, encephalitis, myelitis, CNS thrombi, DIC, LFT↑, Guillain–Barré, Henoch–Schönlein, nephritis, pancreatitis, myositis, myocarditis, orchitis, cerebellar ataxia. If non-immune, *live attenuated vaccine* pre-cytotoxics/steroids may be wise. *Immunization:* Occurs in the USA/Japan/ Australia and other countries, but is not routine in the UK. Reasons not to vaccinate include paradoxically increasing shingles/chickenpox in adults[57] and lack of cost-effectiveness.[58] *Dangerous contexts:* Immunosuppression; cystic fibrosis; severe eczema; neonates; pregnancy. Keeping cool may reduce lesion numbers. Calamine lotion soothes. Trim nails to lessen damage from scratching. Consider daily antiseptic for spots (chlorhexidine). Flucloxacillin if bacterial superinfection—treat for septicaemia if worsening. If immunosuppressed or on steroids give aciclovir (5–7 days); begin within 24h of the rash. There is *no* clear evidence that aciclovir ↓ complications if immunocompetent, but it may help severe symptoms eg in adolescents, or 2nd- or 3rd-family contacts. If used, use at the 1st sign of infection, or as a 7-day *attenuating dose* of 10mg/kg/6h starting 1wk post-exposure. Famciclovir is less well-studied.[59]

Shingles *R̞:* Oral analgesia. Ophthalmic shingles: p. 335. Aciclovir may reduce pain, but also progression of zoster in the immunocompromised (may be rampant, with pneumonitis, hepatitis, and meningoencephalitis). **Aciclovir** IVI dose: 10mg/kg/8h (over 1h), with concentration <5mg/mL, over >1h.

Varicella in pregnancy Pneumonitis and encephalitis are no commoner in pregnancy, despite pregnancy being an immunocompromised state (1 in 400 and 1 in 1000, respectively). Infection in the 1st 20 weeks (esp. 13–20 weeks) may cause fetal varicella syndrome (FVS) in 2%.[60] *Signs of FVS* are variable eg cerebral cortical atrophy and cerebellar hypoplasia, manifested by microcephaly, convulsions, and IQ↓; limb hypoplasia; rudimentary digits ± pigmented scars. Maternal shingles is *not* a cause. If the mother develops chickenpox from 1 week before to 4 weeks after birth, newborn may suffer severe chickenpox with mortality up to 20%.[61] Give baby **antivaricella-zoster immunoglobulin** (VZIg) 250mg IM at birth[62] ± aciclovir;[63] isolate, and monitor closely for any clinical signs of varicella. Breastfeeding or expressed milk is recommended in babies receiving treatment.[63] Infection is preventable by pre-pregnancy vaccination with live varicella vaccine,[64] but testing for antibodies pre-conceptually is expensive, and cost-effectiveness depends on local rates of seronegativity. ~80% of those who cannot recall any previous chickenpox are, in fact, immune.[65]

vzv exposure in high-risk groups Postexposure VZIg prophylaxis may be indicated for the immunosuppressed, neonates, and pregnant women, algorithms are complex, see Green Book.[52] VZIg prevents infection in 50% of susceptible contacts.

In many sub-Saharan countries, ~40% of all under-5 mortality is a result of AIDS. If an HIV +ve mother breastfeeds, this ↑ risk of vertical transmission by ~50%. Mothers with HIV should formula feed in the UK, but in countries without reliable clean water, breastfeeding is less risky.[66,67] Infection can occur from the 1st trimester; ⅔ of infections occur at the time of delivery, and are more likely if mothers have symptomatic HIV infection or a high viral load. Full PMTCT intervention (prevention of mother-to-child transmission) reduces the rate of transmission from ≈25% to ≤1%[68] eg maternal and neonatal anti-retroviral therapy (ART), appropriate delivery, no breastfeeding. HIV infection in pregnancy/labour: p. 24; adult HIV: *OHCM*, p398.

Neonatal management
- PEP for 4 weeks starting <4h from birth: zidovudine monotherapy if maternal viral load <50 RNA copies/mL. 3-drug ART recommended for all other situations.[68]
- Exclusive formula feeding from birth regardless of maternal ART or neonatal PEP.
- Initiate PCP prophylaxis with co-trimoxazole from 4 weeks if tests +ve or equivocal.
- Delay BCG until confirmed HIV –ve unless high risk of TB exposure. Give other vaccines per routine schedule.

Neonatal testing HIV DNA PCR ± RNA PCR at birth, 6, and 12 weeks and HIV antibody at 18 months of age (+ additional monthly testing if infant is breastfed).[68] Sensitivity of PCR tests increases to near 100% at 3 months of age but results should be interpreted with caution by an expert. The all clear can only be given if all tests are negative at 18 months but infection unlikely if tests negative and the baby is well at 6 months.

Consider HIV in children with PUO; lymphadenopathy; hepatosplenomegaly; persistent diarrhoea; parotid enlargement; shingles; extensive molluscum; platelets ↓; recurrent slow-to-clear infections; faltering growth; clubbing, unexplained organ disease;[69] TB; pneumocystosis; toxoplasmosis; cryptococcosis; histoplasmosis; CMV; LIP (see later). **Suspect non-vertical seroconversion illness if:** T°↑, fatigue, rash, pharyngitis, lymphadenopathy, oral ulcers, D&V, headache, myalgia, arthralgia, meningism, peripheral neuropathy, thrush, weight ↓, night sweats, genital ulcers, WCC↓, platelets ↓, transaminases ↑.[70]

HIV & the lung: TB, lymphocytic interstitial pneumonia (LIP), immune reconstitution inflammatory syndrome, malignancy, bronchiectasis.[71] LIP: tachypnoea; hypoxia; clubbing; diffuse reticulonodular infiltrates on CXR; bilateral hilar lymphadenopathy. It is not AIDS-defining. It is less serious than pneumocystosis.

Prognosis By 3yrs old, up to half with early-onset opportunistic infection have died vs 3% of those with no such infection. Children with slow progression of HIV have persistent neutralizing antibodies. Transplacental passage of maternal neutralizing antibody may also have a role.

Ensure full course of vaccines (+ *Pneumococcus* + *annual influenza*; avoid live vaccines if very immunocompromised).[72,73]

Antiretroviral therapy (ART) All children with HIV should start ART *regardless* of CD4 count.[74] Use PENTA regimen (*OHCM* p403). *Obstacles:* Poor adherence (unpleasant tasting medicine); SE (lipids ↑, glucose ↑, bone metabolism ↓); lack of family routines.[75] Diarrhoea-related morbidity:[76] micronutrient (eg zn) zinc supplementation helps.[77]

▶Teach HIV+ve children about safe sex and other HIV issues before puberty.

90-90-90 BY 20 In 2015, new ambitious global targets for HIV control were adopted: By 2020, 90% of all people with HIV to know their status; 90% of those to receive sustained ART; 90% of those to have undetectable viral load.

Further reading

Pediatric European Network for the Treatment of AIDS: http://penta-id.org

For sore throat, see pp. 414-15.

Stridor ▸▸ Acute stridor may be a terrifying experience for children; this fear may lead to hyperventilation, which worsens symptoms. *Causes:* p. 416. The main concern is distinguishing viral croup from bacterial tracheitis or epiglottitis (rare in the UK since *Haemophilus* vaccination): see table 3.6. Don't forget to consider inhaled foreign body or laryngomalacia in babies if history doesn't seem right. Consider subglottic stenosis in ex-preterms.

Croup (Acute laryngotracheobronchitis.) *Causes:* Parainfluenza virus (1, 2, 3), respiratory syncytial virus, measles, and other viruses. *Age:* <6yrs (but can be recurrent in older, atopic children). *Epidemics:* Autumn. *Pathology:* Subglottic oedema, inflammation, and exudate. *Signs:* Stridor, barking cough, hoarseness from inflammation of the larynx. Croup is classified into mild/moderate, and severe disease (see table 3.7). Δ This is a clinical diagnosis. CXR or lateral neck x-ray may show 'steeple sign' or an enlarged epiglottis, but should be avoided. ℞ Mild illness may be sent home if settles—eg with **dexamethasone**, 0.15mg/kg PO stat (some give up to 0.6mg/kg[78]) *or* **prednisolone** 1-2mg/kg stat. *Moderate illness:* Observe for 3-4 hours, may be discharged if good response to treatment. *Severe:* Keep child calm and with parent, minimal interference, and close observation (T°, pulse, RR, SAO₂) by experienced nurses. *Watch for severe signs:* Restlessness; cyanosis (give O₂); recession; stridor at rest; rising HR/RR; tiredness, altered conscious level. Use nebulized **adrenaline**[79] 1:1000 (400mcg/kg up to 5mL) but remember duration of action is relatively short (2-3h); if poor response, repeat, and take to ITU. Nebulized **budesonide** (2mg) is another option. *Remember:* volume of stridor is a factor of flow; in severe disease, stridor will be very soft. Involve your senior colleagues, anaesthetist, and ENT team if requiring repeated nebulized adrenaline. Failure to improve with steroids/nebulized adrenaline should prompt the consideration of bacterial tracheitis.

Epiglottitis ▸▸ For signs, see table 3.6. *Avoid approaching the child and do not examine the throat.* This may precipitate obstruction. Do not cannulate the patient or upset them. Ask for senior help from an anaesthetist and ENT surgeon. Take the child to theatre for inhalation induction of anaesthesia and EUA if necessary. A smaller diameter endotracheal tube than normal for that age may be needed. A tracheostomy may be required if complete obstruction occurs. The cause is usually *Haemophilus influenzae* type B, treat with cefotaxime or ceftriaxone.

Bacterial tracheitis Defined by the presence of thick mucopurulent exudate and tracheal mucosal sloughing that is not cleared by coughing, and risks occluding the airway. There is often a history of a viral infection (such as croup) with an acute deterioration. Pronounced tracheal tenderness may be present. For signs, see table 3.6. Benefits from early intubation if severe, allowing suctioning of respiratory secretions and improved ventilation. Treat with cefotaxime + flucloxacillin. Hydrocortisone may be given, but isn't of proven value.

Diphtheria Caused by the toxin of *Corynebacterium diphtheriae*, exceedingly rare due to routine immunization. It usually starts with tonsillitis ± a pseudomembrane over the fauces. The toxin may cause polyneuritis, often starting with cranial nerves. Shock may occur from myocarditis, toxaemia, or cardiac conducting system involvement. *Other signs:* Dysphagia; muffled voice; bronchopneumonia; airway obstruction preceded by a brassy cough (laryngotracheal diphtheria); nasal discharge with an excoriated upper lip (nasal diphtheria). If there is tachycardia out of proportion to fever, suspect toxin-induced myocarditis (do frequent ECGs). Motor palatal paralysis also occurs causing fluids to escape from the nose on swallowing.

Δ: Swab culture of material below pseudomembrane; PCR.[80]

℞: ►►Diphtheria antitoxin: 10,000–30,000u IM (any age; more if severe, see *BNF*) and erythromycin; give contacts 7 days' **erythromycin oral suspension**: <2yrs old 125mg/6h PO (500mg per 6h if >8yrs) *before swab results are known*.

Risk ↑ if: Homeless/refugee; unimmunized; aged 3–6yrs old; in 'asocial' families. *Prevention:* Isolate until 3 −ve cultures separated by 48h. Vaccination: Table 3.11, p. 257.

Table 3.6 Distinguishing viral croup from bacterial tracheitis or epiglottitis

Mild croup	Bacterial tracheitis	Epiglottitis
Common	Uncommon	Rare
6 months–6 years	6 months–14 years	2–7 years
Onset over a few days	Viral prodrome for 2–5 days, then rapid deterioration	►►Sudden onset
Stridor variable	Continuous stridor	►►Continuous stridor
Stridor sounds harsh	Stridor may be biphasic	►►Stridor softer, snoring
Swallows oral secretions	Swallows oral secretions	►►Drooling of secretions
Voice hoarse	Very hoarse	►►Voice muffled
Apyrexial or low-grade fever	Moderate–high fever, appears toxic	►►Toxic and feverish (eg T° >39°C)
Barking cough	Barking cough	Cough not prominent

Table 3.7 Westley Croup Score[81]

Score	Stridor	Recessions	Air entry	SPO₂ <92%	Level of consciousness
0	None	None	Normal	Normal	Normal
1	With agitation	Mild	Mild decrease		
2	At rest	Moderate	Marked decrease		
3		Severe			
4				With agitation	
5				At rest	Decreased
Interpretation					
≤2	Mild	Alert, barking cough, no stridor at rest, mild or no recessions			
3–7	Moderate	Alert, barking cough, stridor at rest, mild to moderate recessions, no agitation			
8–11	Severe	Worsening stridor, moderate to severe recessions, reduced air entry, cyanosis, agitation			
≥12	Impending respiratory failure	Decreased consciousness, fatigue, cyanosis, chest movements may diminish or asynchronous chest and abdominal movements may be present			

►If severely ill, think of staphs, streps, TB, and *Pneumocystis* (HIV) (*OHCM* p166). *In chronic cough think of:* • Pertussis • TB • Foreign body • Asthma.

Bronchiolitis

The commonest lung infection in infants.[82] *Cause:* Most commonly respiratory syncytial virus (RSV), also rhinovirus, parainfluenza, adenoviruses, and many others. *Age:* <2yrs, peak 3–6 months. *Signs:* Coryza precedes cough, tachypnoea, wheeze, inspiratory crackles, poor feeding, intercostal recession, ± apnoea, ± cyanosis, ± fever (usually low grade). Illness peaks in 3–5 days then resolves, cough may last >3 weeks. *Risk factors for severe disease:* Preterm (esp. <32 weeks); age <3 months; congenital heart disease; chronic lung disease; immunodeficiency; other underlying medical conditions. *Admission criteria:* inadequate feeding (≤50%); dehydration; RR>60/min; severe respiratory distress; spO$_2$ <92%; apnoea. Δ: Clinical. Nasopharyngeal aspirate (NPA) for respiratory virus PCR or RSV rapid antigen may be useful for cohorting. If severe: CXR to exclude pneumothorax or lobar collapse; blood gases; FBC, U&E. ΔΔ: Pneumonia (if focal chest signs); heart failure (hepatomegaly); myocarditis (↑HR); *mycoplasma* or *pertussis* LRTI. R: Supportive, many things have been tried and don't work (nebulized hypertonic saline, adrenaline, salbutamol, ipratropium; systemic or inhaled steroids; montelukast). Give o$_2$ (when spO$_2$<92%); NG feeds or IV fluids (⅔ maintenance). Antibiotics are no benefit unless there is secondary bacterial infection. Consider in infants requiring respiratory support. ≈5% of admissions need respiratory support (CPAP or heated, humidified high-flow oxygen), a small proportion of those need ventilation and ICU. Mortality <1%; 33% if symptomatic congenital heart disease. *Prevention:* Palivizumab, a humanized monoclonal antibody to RSV is used prophylactically in very limited indications, ●✻ due to high cost and low impact.

Pneumonia

Causes: Pneumococcus, viruses, *Mycoplasma, Haemophilus, Staphylococcus*, TB.[83,84] *Signs:* T°↑, malaise, poor feeding. Respiratory distress: tachypnoea, cyanosis, grunting, recessions, use of accessory muscles. Older children may have typical lobar signs (pleural pain, crackles, bronchial breathing). *Admit:* If spO$_2$ <92%; signs of respiratory distress. *Tests:* Consider CXR/FBC/blood and sputum cultures if severe pneumonia. Investigations are not required in community acquired pneumonia in a child going home. Viral LRTI is more common than bacterial infection in children <2, so those with mild symptoms can typically be discharged without antibiotics (ensure follow-up if symptoms persist). *Oral R:* Amoxicillin is 1st-line; alternatives: co-amoxiclav, azithromycin, clarithromycin.[83] *Monitor:* TPR; spO$_2$.[85]

TB

Suspect if: overseas contacts, HIV+ve; odd CXR. *Signs:* Anorexia, low fever, faltering growth, malaise. Cough is common (may be absent). Prolonged course, not responding to antibiotics. *Diagnosis:* Difficult. Tuberculin skin test (*OHCM* p394); interferon-gamma release assays: culture + Ziehl–Neelsen stain of sputa (×3). CXR: consolidation, cavities. Miliary spread (fine white dots on CXR) is rare but grave. R: Get expert help. 6-month supervised plan:[86] isoniazid 3× a week + rifampicin 3× a week + pyrazinamide (1st 2 months only) 3× a week. Monitor U&E & LFT before and during treatment. Stop rifampicin if bilirubin ↑ (hepatitis). Isoniazid may cause neuropathy →give concurrent pyridoxine (vit B$_6$). ►Explain the need for prolonged treatment. Multiple drug resistance: *OHCM* p395. *Prophylaxis:* If TB with HIV, co-trimoxazole prophylaxis is likely to be needed.[86]

Whooping cough

(*Bordetella pertussis.*) *Signs:* Apnoea; bouts of coughing followed by whoop or vomiting (± cyanosis) worse at night or after feeds. Whoops (not always heard, particularly in young infants) are caused by inspiration against a closed glottis. Co-infection with RSV (see 'Bronchiolitis') is common. *Peak age:* Infants, with a 2nd peak in those >14yrs.[87] In the UK, the illness is often mild, with 1% needing admission (eg with secondary pneumonia); but may be fatal in the very young.[88] Δ: PCR via *pernasal swab*; or if symptoms >2 weeks, anti-pertussis toxin IgG in oral fluid swab. Culture is unsatisfactory. Absolute lymphocytosis is common (may be very high requiring leukapheresis). *Incubation:* 10–14 days. *Complications:* Prolonged illness (the '100-day cough'). Coughing bouts may cause petechiae (eg on cheek), conjunctival, retinal, & CNS bleeds (rare), apnoea, inguinal hernias± lingual frenulum tears. Bronchiectasis. ℞: A macrolide such as clarithromycin is often used in those likely to expose infants to the disease (benefit unproven). Admit if <6 months old (risk of apnoea). May need ventilating and even ECMO (p. 305). *Vaccine:* p. 257, not always effective. 30% of severe infections are via a fully vaccinated sibling. Vaccinating the mother during pregnancy reduces risk in babies. Immunity wanes steadily throughout childhood.

'Chesty' infants and viral-induced lower airways disease

Many children with cough and wheeze do not fit into the categories on pp. 210-11, and are too young for a diagnosis of asthma to be made with confidence. These infants often end up being treated with escalating bronchodilator therapy ± frequent courses of antibiotics against uncultured organisms. While it is true that asthma can begin in infancy, most of these chesty infants do not have asthma and symptoms diminish as they grow. NB: *viral-induced wheeze (VIW)/virally induced respiratory distress or virally induced lower airways disease* may be the appropriate label here: it is a non-atopic disorder; *respiratory syncytial virus* is more often the culprit rather than *Haemophilus*. When viruses are looked for (found in 80%), it turns out that together rhinoviruses, coronaviruses, human metapneumovirus, and human bocavirus account for 60% of viruses.[89] Although symptom scores and need for GP consultations are highest in infants with RSV, they are similar in infants infected with other viruses.[89]

Passive smoking does not trigger illness but does prolong symptoms. If the mother smoked during pregnancy, it significantly increases the risk of viral-induced wheeze in the child. 'Happy wheezers' (ie undistressed) probably need no treatment, but if chest symptoms start very early in life, a sweat test should be considered to rule out cystic fibrosis, especially if there is faltering growth and loose stools. Between these ends of the spectrum of 'chestiness' lie those who clearly need some help. These may benefit from inhaled β₂-agonists (via a spacer) ± inhaled steroids, given for ~8 weeks in the lowest effective dose. Assess benefit by ↓ in sleep disturbance. If ill enough to consider admission, 3 days' oral **prednisolone** 2mg/kg/day can ↓ duration of symptoms in children 6–35 months old with VIW.[90] Other randomized trials disagree, so some reserve steroids for the atopic.[91]

Aim to engage in a constructive dialogue with parents so that they understand that treatment is often unsuccessful, but that their child is unlikely to come to harm, while he or she is 'growing out of it'.

If cough is a chronic problem, exclude serious causes (eg TB; foreign body; asthma) and reassure. There is no good evidence that OTC cough medicines are effective for acute cough.[92]

(See BTS[93] & NICE[94] guidelines.) In the developed world, asthma is *the* leading chronic illness in children.[95] It implies reversible airway obstruction ± expiratory polyphonic wheeze, dyspnoea, or cough. 10% of the population is affected. **Prevalence** ↑ if Birthweight ↓; family history; bottle fed; atopy; ♂; pollution;[96] past lung disease.[97] *Genetics:* Asthma susceptibility genes are described (eg ADAM33). *Triggers:* Pollen; house dust mite; feathers; fur; exercise; viruses; cold air; chemicals; smoke; air pollution.

Diagnosis
No gold standard but use objective tests wherever possible (from age ≈5) to inform your clinical diagnosis: spirometry (FEV₁/FVC <70% demonstrates obstruction) and bronchodilator reversibility test (↑FEV₁ ≥12% is +ve). ΔΔ: Foreign body; pertussis; croup; pneumonia/TB;[98] hyperventilation; cystic fibrosis; VIW; heart failure; GORD + aspiration.

Treatment
Aims: Minimize symptoms and impact on life; reduce airway remodelling; reduce mortality. Use stepwise approach, achieve control, and then consider step-down. Most recent UK advice recommends more aggressive, *earlier use of inhaled corticosteroids* (ICS).

Stepwise management
Increase step if using reliever therapy ≥3×/week, consider step-down when asthma has been completely controlled for at least 3 months (no daytime symptoms, night-time waking, attacks, or reliever use).

Reliever therapy: Short-acting β-agonists (SABA) via pMDI[4] eg **salbutamol** 100mcg. • Step 1. ICS eg beclometasone: specify brand[99] as potencies vary: eg 50mcg **Clenil**® 2 puffs/12h[100] (or leukotriene receptor antagonist (LTRA) **montelukast** 4mg if <5yrs—can cause hyperkinesia and behavioural problems) • Step 2. ICS and inhaled long-acting β-agonist (LABA) in combined inhaler eg **Seretide**® (or ICS and LRTA if <5yrs) • Step 3. If no response to LABA, stop, and increase ICS eg 100mcg **Clenil**® 2 puffs/12h. Otherwise continue LABA and increase ICS or trial other therapy (LRTA) • Step 4. Increase ICS eg 200mcg **Clenil**® 2 puffs/12h, consider 4th drug (**theophylline** eg Slo-Phyllin® 125–250mg/12h PO if 6–11yrs) and referral to specialist • Step 5. Use daily oral steroid in lowest dose that controls asthma, continue ICS, refer to specialist. All steps: review diagnosis; check inhaler and spacer use/adherence; eliminate triggers. Use combination inhalers to aid adherence.

Exacerbations: Treat *early* (rescue **prednisolone** 30–40mg/day if >5yrs or 20mg/day if 2–5yrs for 5 days). In most cases antibiotics are not needed.

General management: Annual review of symptoms, exacerbations, oral steroid use, and time off school or nursery; check inhaler technique and medication concordance (always use a spacer[5]); make a personalized self-management action plan; advice regarding tobacco smoke exposure; monitor height and weight on centile charts.

Inhaler and nebulizer questions

• If <8yrs old, pressurized metered dose inhalers (pMDIs)[4] with a spacer[5] are best for routine use in stable asthma for both steroids and bronchodilators.
• In acute asthma, pMDIs with a spacer are at least as good as nebulizers (if not better) in mild to moderate attacks.[93]
• Fixed-dose combination ICS and LABA inhalers improve adherence.
• Maintenance and reliever therapy ('MART') combines ICS with 'fast-acting' LABA and is used both for daily maintenance and relief therapy. The SMART study showed real benefit, doctor dependency was less, and there were fewer asthma exacerbations.[101]

►Treating severe acute asthma

►►This is an emergency. Calmness helps. Give these treatments if life-threatening signs are present (table 3.8), or if not improving 15–30min after R_x starts.

1 Sit up; high-flow O_2 to maintain spO_2 94–98%.

2 Salbutamol 5mg (2.5mg if <5yrs) + ipratropium bromide 250mcg ± 150mg neb magnesium sulfate all O_2-nebulized every 20min for 1h.

3 Hydrocortisone 4mg/kg/6h (max. 100mg) IV; or prednisolone 2mg/kg to max 40mg (60mg if already on steroids & <12yrs), 50mg >12yrs for 3 days.

4 Consider one IV dose of magnesium sulfate 40mg/kg over 20min (≤2g) as 1st-line IV therapy if poor response to nebulizers.

5 Consider IV salbutamol bolus 15mcg/kg over 10min ± infusion (1–2mcg/kg/min) or aminophylline 5mg/kg IV over 20min (not if already on a xanthine); then infusion.

6 Salbutamol nebulizers continuously until improving, then eg 30min intervals, reducing frequency once improving. Give ipratropium 8hrly if needed.

7 Consider starting CPAP in the ED. Discuss with PICU, anaesthetist, and seniors if confused, tiring, silent chest, spO_2 remains <92% after R_x, high CO_2 (sign of tiring).

Before discharge *Ensure:* • Stable on 3–4hrly inhaled bronchodilators • Peak flow >75% of best or predicted • Good inhaler technique • Written management plan • Follow-up: GP in 2 days; in paeds asthma clinic in 1–2 months; by paeds respiratory specialist if life-threatening episode.

Table 3.8 Severity of acute asthma exacerbation

Near-fatal/ life-threatening	Respiratory acidosis and/or requiring mechanical ventilation with increased ventilation pressures
	Any one of the following: PEFR <33% best or predicted; sats <92%; silent chest; cyanosis; feeble respiratory effort; bradycardia; dysrhythmia; hypotension; exhaustion; confusion
Acute severe	Any one of: PEFR 33–50% predicted; RR 2–5yrs >40/min, 5–12yrs >30/min, >12yrs >25/min; pulse 2–5yrs >140bpm, 5–12yrs >125bpm, >12yrs >110bpm; inability to complete sentences
Moderate exacerbation	Increasing symptoms; PEFR 50–70% best or predicted; no features of severe asthma
Brittle asthma ♦✹	Type 1: wide variability in PEFR despite intensive therapy; type 2: sudden severe attacks despite apparently well-controlled asthma

Pitfalls in managing asthma

• Being satisfied with less than total symptom control.
• Inadequate perception of, and planning for, the severe attack.
• Faulty inhaler technique. Watch the patient operate the device. Always use a spacer.
• Unnoticed, marked diurnal variation in airways obstruction (consider peak flow diary). Always ask about nocturnal waking; it is a sign of dangerous asthma.

Further reading

Asthma UK (patient information and support): www.asthma.org.uk
BTS/SIGN (2014). *British Guideline on the Management of Asthma*. Edinburgh: BTS/SIGN.
NICE (2019). *Asthma*. http://cks.nice.org.uk/asthma

4 pMDI=press-and-breathe pressurized meter dose inhaler—as recommended by NICE.

5 *Spacers*: eg AeroChamber®—a responsive inspiratory valve allows opening on minimal effort to aid inhalation; it closes before exhalation disturbs retained aerosol. Static charge is a problem. Clean monthly. Wash in detergent. Dry in air. Wipe mouthpiece clean of detergent before use. Replace yearly.

Cystic fibrosis (CF) is one of the commonest autosomal recessive diseases (incidence at birth ~1:2500; ~1:25 of UK population are carriers[102]); it reflects mutations in the cystic fibrosis transmembrane conductance regulator gene (CFTR) on chromosome 7, which codes for a cyclic AMP-regulated sodium/chloride channel. There is a variety in severity of lung disease akin to bronchiectasis, exocrine gland dysfunction, meconium ileus in neonates (and its equivalent, distal intestinal obstruction syndrome, in children), pancreatic exocrine insufficiency, and a raised Na⁺ sweat level—depending in part on the type of mutation (85% from 5 mutations, the commonest of which is ΔF508) but other mutations, eg in intron 19 of CFTR, cause lung disease but no increased sweat Na⁺.

Antenatal (pp. 274-5) carrier-status testing is possible, as is preimplantation genetic diagnosis after *in vitro* fertilization.

Diagnosis ►In the UK since October 2007, all newborns are screened for raised immunoreactive trypsinogen (IRT) ± 2-stage genetic testing (commonest 4 ± 29 other CFTR mutations) on the newborn blood spot test (Guthrie card) with estimated 97% sensitivity.[102] Symptomatic presentations include:
- Neonatal meconium ileus (~1 in 7).
- Recurrent/chronic pulmonary disease (LRTIs, productive cough, CXR changes, ±clubbing).
- Faltering growth.
- Malabsorption: fatty, oily stools (steatorrhoea).

Sweat test: Sweat CL- <40mmol/L is normal (CF probability is low); >60mmol/L supports the diagnosis. Intermediate results are suggestive but not diagnostic of cystic fibrosis.[103] The test is technically challenging, so find an experienced centre.

Pitfalls of the sweat test:[104] *False-positive sweat test:* may be seen in atopic eczema, adrenal insufficiency, ectodermal dysplasia, some types of glycogen storage diseases, hypothyroidism, dehydration, malnutrition. On the first day of life, up to 25% of normal newborns show a sweat sodium concentration >65mmol/L, but this rapidly declines on the second day after birth. *False-negative sweat test:* Oedema is the most important cause. Poor technique can also give false-negative results.

Other tests: IRT; genetics; CXR: hyperinflation, increased anteroposterior diameter, bronchial dilatation, cysts, linear shadows, and infiltrates; malabsorption screen; random glucose; spirometry (obstructive pattern with decreased FVC and increased lung volumes); sputum culture. Mycobacterial colonization affects up to 20%; consider if rapid deterioration.

►*Genetic counselling* (pp. 274-5). Long-term survival depends on good MDT care from specialist centres, antibiotics, and good nutrition.

Respiratory problems (neutrophilic airway inflammation): Start physiotherapy (×3/day) at diagnosis. Teach parents percussion + postural drainage. Older children learn forced expiration techniques. Organisms are usually *Staph. aureus*, *H. influenzae* (rarer), and *Strep. pneumoniae* in younger children. Eventually >90% are chronically infected with *Pseudomonas aeruginosa*. In adolescence, aspergillosis and non-tuberculous mycobacteria can occur. *Burkholderia cepacia* (*Ps. cepacia*) is associated with rapid progression of lung disease (prompt diagnosis using PCR may be available: isolate the patient). Treat acute infection after sputum culture using higher than or double standard doses, and for weeks if necessary. If very ill, respiratory support becomes of utmost importance. Treat with **ticarcillin**, 80mg/kg (max 3.2g)/6–8h IV (if aged >1 month) + gentamicin, or **ceftazidime** (50mg/kg/8h IV) alone may be needed 'blind'. Nebulizing ticarcillin and tobramycin at home *does* prevent admissions.

Gastrointestinal problems & nutrition:
Energy needs rise by ~130% (∵ malabsorption and chronic lung inflammation). Most have steatorrhoea from pancreatic exocrine insufficiency and need replacement enzymes (eg Pancrex v® powder mixed with food for infants, and Pancrex v Forte® for older children, or Creon® which has enzymes in microspheres) to give regular, formed, non-greasy bowel actions. High-dose enzyme use can cause fibrosing colonopathy. Omeprazole (or cimetidine, or ranitidine) helps absorption by ↑ duodenal pH.[105]

Complications of CF
- Faltering growth
- DIOS
- Diabetes mellitus
- CLD/cirrhosis
- Male infertility
- ↓ female fertility
- Nasal polyps/sinusitis
- Rectal prolapse
- Osteoporosis
- Haemoptysis
- Pneumothorax
- Cholelithiasis (gallstones)

If all this controls steatorrhoea, a low-fat diet is not needed, but supplements for fat-soluble vitamins (A, D, E, and K) are still needed (eg **Abidec**® 0.6mL/24h PO (contains A & D) for infants or as multivitamin capsules for older children). Diet should be both high calorie & high protein. Fine-bore nasogastric or PEG feeding is needed only if growth cannot otherwise be maintained.

Distal intestinal obstruction syndrome (DIOS): Cause not fully understood, insufficient pancreatic enzymes, dehydration, and gut dysmotility are likely factors. Admit urgently to a specialist centre for medical treatment (eg with Gastrografin®); seek advice from the CF team (avoid laparotomy unless perforation has occurred). ∆∆: constipation (gradual onset), appendicitis, cholecystitis, intussusception.

Impaired glucose tolerance: Risk rises with age and is higher if homozygous for ΔF508 mutations. Screen yearly with OGTT from 12yrs. Insulin may be needed; optimize diet, then optimize dose, not vice versa. Only try oral hypoglycaemics if nutrition is satisfactory.[106]

Psychological help: Parents and children need expert counselling—and transitional clinics with multidisciplinary teams when transferring from paediatric to adult services. The Cystic Fibrosis Research Trust can help here. Online resources can provide contact between other CF patients without the risk of cross-infection.

Meconium ileus Abdominal distension, failure to pass stool in 1st 2 days of life ± vomiting. 'Inspissated' meconium obstructs the terminal ileus. ℞: Stabilize with NGT drainage and fluid management, hyperosmolar enemas, surgery (enterotomy and lavage, excision of the gut is last resort).

Prognosis Death may be from pneumonia or cor pulmonale. Most survive to adulthood (UK median survival is 47yrs, but babies born today are expected to live longer).[107] 5-year survivorship models take account of forced expiratory volume in 1sec (% of expected), gender, weight-for-age z score, pancreatic function, plasma glucose, *Staph. aureus* and *Burkholderia cepacia* infection, and number of acute lung exacerbations/yr.[108]

Newer options

Dornase alfa (Recombinant human deoxyribonuclease) (rhDNASE) (nebulized mucoactive agent) has been shown to improve lung function and reduce the number of pulmonary exacerbations. *Ivacaftor* (CFTR potentiator) improves lung function in those with G551D mutation.

Lung transplantation (heart + lung, or double lung) is getting safer; consider in those who are deteriorating (FEV₁ <30% of expected) despite maximum therapy, provided nutrition is good, and in whom there is no TB or aspergillus. Good results are limited by donor availability (avoid raising hopes).

Gene therapy aims to deliver normal copies of the cystic fibrosis gene into patients, so allowing them to make CFTR protein. A phase 2b clinical trial of the first gene therapy showed modest but significant benefit in FEV₁.[109]

3 Paediatrics

Acute abdominal pain One of the *most common* paediatric presentations and often no clear cause is found. The differential diagnosis is *wide* and varies significantly with age. The key is to address the carers' concerns, pick up the small number of children with potentially serious conditions, and give appropriate safety-netting advice. Children ≤8yrs old often have difficulty in localizing pain; other factors in the history may be more important.[110]

ΔΔ (acute)
- Appendicitis, most parents' main concern, don't let it be the elephant in the room, tackle it head on (p. 220).
- Viral illness (eg URTI) associated with mesenteric adenitis.
- Gastroenteritis.
- Constipation (history is key) (pp. 268–9).
- UTI (p226).
- ►Intussusception (p. 220).
- ►In boys always check for a torted testis.
- Consider menstruation, ovarian cyst, ovarian torsion, pelvic inflammatory disease, or ectopic pregnancy in older girls.
- Lower lobe pneumonia can present with pain referred to abdomen.
- Parasitic infection.
- Consider abdominal crisis in those with sickle-cell disease.

ΔΔ (recurrent) Very common presentation, ≥10% of children >5yrs suffer recurrent abdominal pains interfering with normal activity. No 'organic' cause in ~90%. NB: long-term follow-up indicates a 4-fold ↑risk of psychological problems manifesting in adult life.
- Functional abdominal pain: episodic or continuous pain at least ×1/week for ≥2 months + no evidence of organic disorder.
- Coeliac disease; GORD; IBS; lactose intolerance.
- In children with pica (p. 268), do FBC, iron, ferritin, and lead levels.
- Stress; depression; bullying; difficult family dynamics; NAI (pp. 196–7).

ΔΔ (rare) Volvulus; Meckel's diverticulum; pancreatitis; diabetes; peptic ulcer disease/*H. pylori*; inflammatory bowel disease (IBD); abdominal TB; renal stones; gall stones; cholecystitis; Henoch–Schönlein purpura.

►Red flags Weight loss; faltering growth; fever; bilious vomiting; significant vomiting; GI bleeding; chronic severe diarrhoea; gross abdo distension; palpable mass/organomegaly; specific tender area; oral ulcers; perianal fistulas; back pain; FH IBD. Be suspicious if pain is unusual in terms of site, character, frequency, or severity.

Investigations Difficult balance between excluding organic disorder and over-investigating functional abdominal pain. ►Always dip the urine. If any red flags are present, investigate as appropriate ± stool for occult blood; US; FBC; CRP/ESR; tTG (+ IgA level); amylase/lipase; TFTs (if constipation); barium studies and consider referral to a specialist.

R: Trials of laxatives or antacids may be appropriate if constipation or GORD are suspected. Simple analgesia and antispasmodics. Avoid dietary interventions unless there is positive history.

Abdominal distension

Causes Always remember acute GI obstruction as a cause; also consider:

Air:	Ascites:	Solid masses:	Cysts:
Faecal impaction	Nephrotic syn.	Wilms' tumour	Polycystic kidney
Air swallowing	Hypoproteinaemia	Neuroblastoma	Hepatic
Malabsorption	Cirrhosis; CCF	Adrenal tumour	Dermoid

Hepatomegaly *Infections:* Many, eg infectious mononucleosis, CMV, malaria.

Malignancy: Leukaemia, lymphoma, neuroblastoma.

Metabolic: Gaucher and Hurler diseases, cystinosis, galactosaemia.

Others: Sickle-cell disease and other haemolytic anaemias, porphyria.

Splenomegaly All the above-listed causes of hepatomegaly (not neuroblastoma).

Neuroblastoma This may be thought of as an embryonal neoplasm, derived from sympathetic neuroblasts. Presenting with decreasing frequency from birth to 5yrs of age. Some forms regress, while others present after 18 months old (eg with metastases ± DVT) and are highly malignant. Outlook depends on stage and has not improved over the last 25yrs. *Prevalence:* 1:6000–1:10,000— the most common solid tumour in the under 5s. *Signs:* Abdominal swelling. *Metastatic sites:* Lymph nodes, scalp, bone (causing pancytopenia ± osteo-lytic lesions). In 92%, urinary excretion of catecholamines (vanillylmandelic & homovanillic acids) are raised. *Treatment:* Refer to special centre. Excision (if possible) and chemotherapy (eg cyclophosphamide + doxorubicin). *Prognosis:* Worse if certain genotypes (pseudodiploid karyotypes, chromosome 1p deletions, N-myc gene amplifications), less mature catecholamine synthesis, and if >12 months old. Those <1yr do best. *Surveillance:* Pre-morbid screening by looking for excretion of catecholamines in the urine detects disease early, but may not save lives.[111] Uncertainty is added by a 2008 study which appeared to record lower mortality in a screened group (although it was a very large study, it is dubious, being retrospective).[112]

Coeliac disease: an example of malabsorption

Cause Enteropathy induced by gluten (in wheat, barley, and rye).

Signs Classically presents between 6 & 24 months, after introduction of gluten to diet, with diarrhoea, anorexia, abdo distension, pain, faltering growth ± anaemia (folate ↓; ferritin ↓). However, patients may present at *any* age. Signs may be less obvious in older children so investigate any faltering growth, unexplained anaemia, prolonged fatigue, persistent 'irritable bowel' symptoms, weight ↓, and short stature. See fig 3.12. Coeliac disease is associated with other autoimmune disorders (T1DM, thyroid disease, JIA), and Down and Turner syndromes. There is ↑ risk in 1st-degree relatives.

Δ: Serological tests show raised IgA anti-tissue transglutaminase (IgA-tTG), and endomysial antibodies (EMA) but *only* if the child is currently eating gluten. Also measure total IgA—if deficient measure IgG anti-gliadin antibodies.[113] Serology is less reliable if <18 months—IgA-AGA may be most useful in this age group.[114] Confirm by finding villous atrophy on small bowel biopsy via endoscopy. Villi return to normal on gluten-free diet; child should eat gluten ≥×2/day for at least 6 weeks before biopsy.[115]

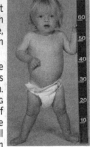

Fig 3.12 Coeliac disease.

℞: Dietician input to achieve gluten-free diet: no wheat, barley, rye (no bread, cake, pasta, pizza, pies). Rice, maize, soya, potato are OK as are oats produced in gluten-free environments.[116] Gluten-free biscuits, flour, bread, and pasta are prescribable. Minor dietary lapses may matter.

Other causes of malabsorption Cystic fibrosis; post-enteritis enteropathy; giardia; rotaviruses; bacterial overgrowth; worms; IBD; eosinophilic gastroenteritis.

3 Paediatrics

Diarrhoea may be an early sign of *any* septic illness. Faeces are sometimes so liquid they are mistaken for urine. NB: it is *normal* for breastfed babies to have loose, pasty stools. Under 5 mortality ≈525,000/yr worldwide.[117]

Gastroenteritis Rotavirus is the most common cause of gastroenteritis in infants and children. It causes ~215,000 <5yr deaths/yr (a rotavirus vaccine is part of the UK immunization schedule, p. 257).[118] *Other enteric viruses:* norovirus (most common cause in adults), astrovirus, adenovirus. *Treatment:* [119] Weigh, to monitor progress and quantify dehydration, if a recent previous weight is known. Start oral rehydration salts (ORS), eg **Dioralyte®**, at 50mL/kg over 4h (≈1mL/kg every 5min). Continue breastfeeding. If child refuses ORS, offer other fluids (eg bottle milk/water) or consider ORS via a NGT. Fruit juice can exacerbate diarrhoea but a 2016 study showed less treatment failure with diluted apple juice than ORS.[120] IV therapy is reserved for those who are persistently vomiting ORS, deteriorate on ORS or are in shock. Reintroduce milk after 4h of rehydration with ORS (even if <6 months), or sooner if improving or hungry (starving harms).[121] Use of antiemetics (**ondansetron** 0.1–0.15mg/kg) has been shown to decrease vomiting[122] and reduce need for IV fluids, hospital admission,[123] and overall costs,[124] but isn't officially recommended. *Complications:* Dehydration; malnutrition; temporary sugar intolerance after D&V with explosive watery acid stools. (Rare; manage with a temporary lactose-free diet.) Post-enteritis enteropathy resolves spontaneously after ~7wks. *Tests:* Stool: look for viruses, bacteria, ova, cysts, parasites. *Prevention:* Hygiene, good water & food, education, fly control.

Classification of diarrhoea by mechanism *Secretory:* (↓ absorption or ↑ secretion.) Stool is watery even if fasting, eg cholera, *c. difficile*, *E. coli*, carcinoid. *Osmotic:* (↑osmotic load in gut lumen). Stool is watery, acidic, and +ve for reducing substances. *Motility disorders: Increased:* thyrotoxicosis, irritable bowel syndrome. *Decreased:* pseudo-obstruction, intussusception (eg <4yrs old). *Inflammatory:* (eg bloody diarrhoea.) *Salmonella, Shigella, Campylobacter*, rotavirus, amoebiasis, NEC (p. 284), Crohn's/UC (look for weight ↓; anaemia; WBC↑; platelets ↑; ESR↑), coeliac disease, haemolytic uraemic syndrome (p232).

Malnutrition

:.: Rising food prices+global warming+political corruption + war. ►Being a major cause of death and misery, this is a global issue for us all. Undernutrition is associated with 45% of <5yrs deaths worldwide[125] and can be acute (low weight-for-height (W/H p. 319) or MUAC—mid upper arm circumference) or chronic (low height for age—stunting). Acute malnutrition manifests as 2 clinical syndromes: marasmus and kwashiorkor although there can be overlap. *Marasmus* is far more common. *Signs:* 'old man' appearance; emaciated; thin flaccid skin; prominent bones; alert; irritable; distended abdomen. *Kwashiorkor* has even higher mortality. *Signs:* bilateral pitting oedema; apathy; anorexia; skin/hair depigmentation and fragility; distended abdomen. Both forms are associated with failure of physiological and metabolic processes, reduced immunity, reduced gut absorption, and a vicious cycle leading to death. *R̥:* re-educate child, family, and politicians. Offer a gradually increasing, high-protein diet + vitamins. Most can be treated at home with fortified ready-to-use foods if >6 months, no serious medical complications, and able to eat. Those with complications or too weak to eat need a period of stabilization to restore physiological and metabolic processes while avoiding refeeding syndrome (↓K⁺; ↓Mg²⁺; ↓PO₄²⁻; oedema, seizures) before continuing treatment at home. Despite treatment, stature and head circumference may remain poor. *Prevention:* ►Give to charity eg. other charities are available... www.oxfam.org (to pay for fertilizers, high-yield seeds, and simple irrigation schemes). Medically, we often target the malnourished at aged ½–5yrs, found by screening, but better results are achieved by giving universal help at ½–2yrs in at-risk places.[126]

How does poverty impinge on childhood mortality & morbidity?

Worldwide, poor mothers are at ↑ risk of death: there is no worse start to life than the death of one's mother (100% fatal to her babies in some places).

Poverty-associated short stature, BMI <18.5 (p. 815), and iron deficiency in mothers accounts for 20% of maternal mortality.

Malnutrition causing stunting causes ~2.2 million deaths/yr and 21% of disability-adjusted life years (DALYs) in children <5yrs old.[127]

Deficiencies in vitamin A and zinc cause 1 million deaths/yr. Zinc supplementation cannot always be relied on to ↓ morbidity in children recovering from diarrhoea and respiratory illness in developing countries.[128] Prevention of the poverty which caused the diarrhoea is more important.

Not breastfeeding for the 1st 6 months of life (especially non-exclusive breastfeeding) causes 1.4 million deaths/yr in children <5yrs old.[129] NB: the position is further complicated by the fact that proteins, fat concentrations, and caloric value in breast milk from undernourished mothers are lower than in breast milk from well-nourished mothers.

These points account for 35% of child deaths and total global disease burden. In many other conditions (eg diarrhoeal diseases, HIV, asthma, obesity), poverty plays a leading role. But the main health issue is that it's harder to educate yourself if you live in a slum.

3 Paediatrics

Appendicitis

(*OHCM* p608) Uncommon <5yrs and diagnosis is often delayed leading to high rates of perforation and other complications in this group (up to 73%).[130]

Signs: Classic presentation of central abdo pain moving to right iliac fossa (RIF) with tenderness and guarding and fever can be seen in older children. Younger children may have anorexia, vomiting, abdo distension, mild diarrhoea, irritability, or even right hip pain/limp. Abdominal examination is key for which you will need the child's trust. Localized tenderness or signs of peritonism in RIF are very suggestive but difficult to elicit in younger children. Rovsing's (palpation of LIF → pain ↑ in RIF), obturator, and psoas signs are of limited help.[131] If the child appears well and can sit forward unsupported, and hop, appendicitis is unlikely.

Diagnosis: Primarily clinical and particularly difficult in young children. Tests have very low positive and negative predictive values as evidenced by the existence of multiple clinical scoring systems. WCC and CRP are routinely done. The use of imaging is controversial. In the UK, a period of 'active observation' in hospital with serial examination by a paediatric surgeon ± US is indicated for equivocal cases whereas in the US CT abdo is increasingly being used to aid Δ.

R: Appendicectomy with preoperative antibiotics, fluids, and analgesia. Interest in non-operative treatment (ie antibiotics only) is increasing and trials are ongoing.[132]

Intussusception

The most common cause of intestinal obstruction in children. The small bowel telescopes, as if it were swallowing itself by invagination. The vast majority are ileo-colic. Patients may be any age (typically 5–12 months; ♂:♀ ≈ 3:1) presenting with *episodic* intermittent inconsolable crying (every ~30min), with drawing the legs up (colic) ± vomiting ± blood PR (like red-currant jam or merely flecks—a late sign). A sausage-shaped abdominal mass may be felt. Child may be shocked and moribund. In between pains there may be no signs whatsoever. Older children may present differently: rectal bleeding is less common, and they may have a longer history ± contributing pathology acting as a lead point for the intussusception (Meckel's diverticulum; HSP; cystic fibrosis; Peutz–Jeghers syndrome; ascariasis: HUS; nephrotic syndrome or tumours such as lymphomas).

Tests: US is the preferred diagnostic modality (target sign). Abdominal x-ray may show a right lower quadrant opacity but is often unremarkable.

Management: The least invasive approach is US or fluoroscopic guided reduction by air enema (preferred to contrast). If reduction by enema fails, reduction at laparoscopy or laparotomy is needed ± resection of necrotic bowel.

Pre-op care: ►►Resuscitate, crossmatch blood, pass NGT. Recurrence rate: ~5–15% in infants.[133]

Infantile hypertrophic pyloric stenosis

Presents at 3–8 weeks (♂:♀ ≈ 4:1) with vomiting which occurs after feeds, and becomes projectile (eg vomiting over far end of cot). Pyloric stenosis is distinguished from other causes of vomiting by the following:
- The vomit does not contain bile, as the obstruction is so high.
- No diarrhoea: constipation is likely (occasionally 'starvation stools').
- Even though the patient is ill, baby is rarely obtunded: baby is alert, anxious, and always hungry—and possibly malnourished, dehydrated.
- The vomiting is large volume and within minutes of a feed.

Observe left-to-right LUQ (left upper quadrant) peristalsis during a feed (seen in late-presenting babies). Try to palpate the olive-sized pyloric mass: stand on the baby's left side, palpating with the *left* hand at the lateral border of the right rectus in the RUQ, during a feed from a bottle or the left breast. There may be *severe* water & NaCl deficit, making urine output & plasma Cl⁻ (also K⁺ & Ph) vital tests to guide resuscitation and determine when surgery is safe (CL⁻ should be >90mmol/L). The picture is of *hypochloraemic, hypokalaemic metabolic alkalosis*, sodium may be high or low.

Imaging: US imaging is used to confirm diagnosis. Barium studies are 'never' needed.

Management: Pass a wide-bore NGT and correct electrolyte and metabolic disturbances *before* surgery (Ramstedt's pyloromyotomy/endoscopic surgery).

Phimosis

The inability to retract the foreskin is usually physiological, in young boys. *It is normal to have a simple non-retractile foreskin up to the age of 4yrs.* By 11yrs or older, prevalence is <8%.[134] *Pathological phimosis:* The foreskin is too tight due to circumferential scarring. *Causes:* Recurrent balanoposthitis; repeated forced retraction. Time or a wait-and-see policy will usually obviate the need for circumcision. Topical corticosteroids are effective (esp. before 8yrs). Use twice-daily with stretching exercises for 15 days, then daily for 15 days.[135]

Other surgical problems: hernias, volvulus, torsion of the testis, acute abdomen: p. 194, *OHCM* p652 & p606.

▶Bilious (green) vomiting in neonates always needs urgent help (paediatric surgeon + neonatology team) for prompt investigation and management.

Hirschsprung disease Occurs in 1 in 5000 births.[136] Congenital absence of ganglia in distal colon ('long-segment' can involve whole colon or rarely even small bowel) leading to functional GI obstruction, constipation, and megacolon. *Signs:* Delayed passage of meconium (>48h) is common; abdominal distension; PR exam may reveal tight anal sphincter and explosive discharge of stool and gas. ♂:♀ ≈ 3:1. *Complications:* GI perforation, bleeding, ulcers, enterocolitis (may be life-threatening). Short-gut syndrome after surgery. *Tests:* Diagnosis through rectal suction biopsy of the aganglionic section, staining for acetylcholinesterase-positive nerve excess, is most accurate.[137] Excision of the aganglionic segment is needed ± colostomy.

Oesophageal atresia (OA) + tracheo-oesophageal fistula (TOF) A spectrum of abnormalities with OA plus a distal TOF being the most common (86%). Isolated OA (7%) and TOF without OA (4%) can also occur.[138] *Prenatal signs:* Polyhydramnios; small/absent stomach bubble. *Postnatal:* Respiratory distress, ↑ secretions, aspirating feeds. Severity of symptoms depends on anatomy, 'H-type' TOF may present much later. *Δ:* Inability to pass NG (Ryles) tube; x-rays show it coiled in the oesophagus. Avoid contrast imaging. *R:* NBM, continuous oesophageal pouch suction (Replogle tube). Primary surgical repair is possible in the majority of cases.[139] 50% have other anomalies.

Congenital diaphragmatic hernia (CDH) Defect in the diaphragm allowing herniation of abdominal contents into the chest. Leads to impaired lung development (pulmonary hypoplasia and pulmonary hypertension). *Incidence:* 1:2400. *Diagnosis:* Prenatal: US; postnatal: CXR. *Signs:* Difficult resuscitation at birth; respiratory distress; bowel sounds in one hemithorax (usually left so heart is best heard on the right). PH <7.3 and cyanosis augur badly (∵ lung hypoplasia).[140] *Associations:* 61% have a wide range of other malformations so actively look for them.[141] *R:* • *Prenatal:* fetal tracheal obstruction by balloon (encourages lung growth, pushing out other viscera) remains a controversial investigational therapy. • *Postnatal:* if prenatal diagnosis, at birth intubate, ventilate, and paralyse, with minimal pressures. Facemask ventilation is contraindicated (aim to keep any air out of the gut). Surgery in an appropriate centre.

Inguinal hernias These are due to a patent processus vaginalis (the passage which ushers the descending testicle into the scrotum). They present as a bulge lateral to the pubic tubercle eg during crying. In one series (n=6361), ♂: ♀≈5:1; there were 59% right, 29% left, and 12% bilateral hernias (almost all indirect), with a hydrocele in 19%.[142] 12% were incarcerated (irreducible by manipulation). *R:* Most surgeons aim to repair these promptly (laparoscopic repair is possible)[143] to avoid incarceration. Six/two rule: baby <6 weeks, operate within 2 days; <6 months, operate within 2 weeks; <6 years, within 2 months. Hydroceles are hard to distinguish from incarceration.

Hydroceles in infancy A processus vaginalis patent at birth, and allowing *only fluid* from the peritoneal cavity to pass down it, generally closes during the first year of life. If it persists until the age of 2 it may need surgical correction.[144] *Examination:* transillumination suggests hydrocele but does not fully exclude hernia. Absence of any palpable mass over the internal inguinal ring also suggests hydrocele. Communicating hydroceles are reducible, non-communicating are not.

Imperforate anus Covers a variety of anorectal abnormalities; muscle, nerves, GU tract, and spine may also be involved. Many girls have a posterior fourchette fistula; boys have a posterior urethral fistula (may pass meconium in urine). Do GU imaging to show commonly associated GU abnormalities. Posterior sagittal anorectoplasty is possible.[145] Babies with trisomy 21 commonly have imperforate anus without fistula.

Mid-gut malrotations ▶Bilious neonatal vomiting merits immediate surgical referral (pass NGT).[146] Absent attachment of the small intestine mesentery can cause mid-gut volvulus or obstruction of the 3rd part of the duodenum by fibrotic bands. Usually presents with obstruction in infancy but older children can have insidious onset or intermittent symptoms. Blood per rectum heralds mid-gut necrosis → emergency surgical decompression. *R*: Ladd procedure.
Acute gastric volvulus: Causes non-bilious vomiting, epigastric distention, and signs of pain, and is often associated with abnormalities of adjacent organs. There may also be feeding difficulty. Anterior fixation of the stomach to the anterior abdominal wall may be needed after upper GI imaging.

Anterior abdominal wall defects

Gastroschisis: (figs 3.13 & 3.14) A paraumbilical defect with evisceration (extrusion of viscera) of abdominal contents. Most are diagnosed antenatally on US. *Incidence:* ~1:3000; rising (especially in babies of young parents—or, in multips, if there has been a new father for this pregnancy (hence the idea that maternal immune factors play a role)).[147] Corrective surgery has

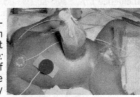
Fig 3.13 Gastroschisis.

a good outcome in 90%, plan delivery at centre with paediatric surgical facilities. At delivery, cover exposed bowel in cling film, avoid heat and fluid loss, and close the defect surgically as soon as possible. This may involve a staged procedure using a silo, because the abdomen at birth is too small to accommodate the gut. Intestinal function is slow to resume and the baby may require TPN for several weeks.

Exomphalos (omphalocele): (fig 3.14) Defect of the umbilical ring with herniation of abdominal viscera. Unlike gastroschisis, the viscera are covered by peritoneum and amniotic membrane. In exomphalos 'minor' the defect is <4cm and only contains bowel, if >4cm or the liver has herniated = exomphalos 'major'. The growth of viscera outside the abdominal cavity may lead the abdomen to be proportionately small making reduction more difficult. 72% of infants with exomphalos have other malformations: chromosomal, cardiac, or genitourinary.[148] Δ mostly by routine antenatal US (AFP↑ too).[149] *Postnatal management:* protect herniated viscera to prevent heat and fluid loss; NGT to decompress stomach; maintain fluids and electrolytes; broad-spectrum antibiotics. • Primary or staged closure may be used to repair the defect. Staged reduction may be over weeks or months with delayed closure as with big defects, closure can cause respiratory insufficiency, haemodynamic compromise, dehiscence, and death.[149,150]

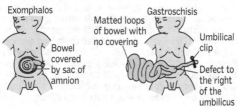

Exomphalos

Bowel
covered
by sac of
amnion

Gastroschisis

Matted loops
of bowel with
no covering

Umbilical
clip

Defect to
the right
of the
umbilicus

Fig 3.14 Exomphalos and gastroschisis.

3 Paediatrics

Definitions *Bacteriuria:* Bacteria in urine uncontaminated by urethral flora. Asymptomatic bacteriuria should not be treated with antibiotics[151] so don't test if asymptomatic! UTI denotes symptomatic bacteriuria that may involve the upper (pyelonephritis) or lower (cystitis) urinary tract. *Vesicoureteric reflux (VUR):* During micturition, urine may reflux up ureters, seen on a micturating cystourethrogram (MCUG) which requires catheterization and contrast. Grades: *I.* Incomplete filling of upper urinary tract, without dilatation. *II.* Complete filling ± slight dilatation. *III.* Ballooned calyces. *IV.* Megaureter. *V.* Megaureter + hydronephrosis. *Reflux nephropathy:* VUR is important as when associated with UTIs it is believed to cause progressive renal scarring which can cause hypertension and lead to end-stage renal disease (ESRD).

Incidence *UTIs:* Boys: ≤0.23%/yr; girls: 0.31–1%; ratios are reversed in neonates. UTIs are more common in uncircumcised boys. *Recurrence:* 35% if >2yrs old. *Prevalence of covert bacteriuria:* In schoolgirls: ~3%. *Prevalence of associated GU anomalies:* up to 40% (½ have reflux; others: malpositions, duplications, megaureter, hydronephrosis). *Renal scarring:* We used to concentrate on treating babies early, thinking new scars were rare after 4yrs old, but prospective ^{99m}Tc dimercaptosuccinic acid (DMSA) scintigraphy (the best test for scarring) shows new scars appearing on repeat scans in 43% of those <1yr old, 84% of those aged 1–5yrs, and 80% of those >5yrs old. VUR is more common in those with family history of VUR (consider screening siblings).

Presentation ▶Often the child may be *non-specifically* ill. Infants may present with fever without focus; vomiting; lethargy; poor feeding; faltering growth; prolonged jaundice or with collapse and sepsis. Toddlers as fever; frequency; dysuria; abdo pain; new incontinence; vomiting; offensive urine. Many with dysuria and frequency have *no* identifiable UTI, and often have vulvitis.

Tests Obtaining a clean sample is key due to the high rates of false negatives and positives from bag samples or cotton wool or pads in nappies. A 'clean catch' is best, wash the genitals gently with water, and tap repeatedly in cycles of 1min with 2 fingers just above the pubis (cold hands help), 1h after a feed, and wait for a clean voided urine (CVU) sample, avoiding the stream's 1st part. A catheter sample or suprapubic aspirate may be needed in a septic child. If >3 months, use dipstick test, if nitrites or WCC +ve, start ABx and send sample for MC&S (although if >3yrs and only WCC+ve use clinical judgement as UTI unlikely). In <3 months refer for urgent microscopy and specialist assessment.[6] Culture: >10^8 organisms/L of a pure growth signifies UTI.

▶*Upper vs lower UTI:* All infants and children with bacteriuria *and* either fever >38°C *or* loin pain/tenderness should be treated as upper UTI/acute pyelonephritis. Others with bacteriuria but no systemic signs or symptoms should be treated as lower UTI/cystitis. *Infants <3 months* should be referred for IV antibiotics (amoxicillin + gentamicin or cephalosporin and ampicillin (to cover *Listeria*) (p. 281)). *Children >3 months with upper UTI:* 7–10 days of oral cephalosporin or co-amoxiclav or refer for 2–4 days of IV cephalosporin followed by oral ABx. *Children >3 months with lower UTI:* 3 days of oral ABx guided by local micro guidance (eg trimethoprim, nitrofurantoin, cefalexin, amoxicillin/co-amoxiclav). Resistance to trimethoprim and ampicillin renders monotherapy insufficient in some places.[152] *All:* Treat constipation if necessary; ↑ oral fluids; encourage full or double voiding; clean the perineum from front to back; wear loose cotton underwear; avoid bubble bath. ▶Have low threshold for IV antibiotics in those with pre-existing renal disease. If on prophylaxis, use a different antibiotic ± consider previous culture sensitivities.

---

6 Microscopy is more reliable than dipstick tests for nitrites & leucocytes: *Effective Health Care* 2004: 8.6. https://www.york.ac.uk/media/crd/ehc86.pdf

Imaging The role of imaging in UTI is a complex and controversial issue. The urinary tract is normal in most, but up to 35% have VUR, ~14% have renal scars, ~5% have stones, ~3% develop hypertension. Each year in the UK, 10–20 children enter ESRD programmes. NICE recommend the following: children with atypical features (see BOX 'Atypical features') should have an *acute* US to identify any structural abnormalities.

- All infants <6 months should have US in <6 weeks.
- Infants <6 months with atypical or recurrent UTI should also have a DMSA scan and an MCUG.
- Those 6 months to 3yrs with atypical or recurrent UTI should have a DMSA scan.
- Those >3yrs with recurrent UTI should also have a DMSA scan.

The DMSA scan should be performed 4–6 months after the UTI for optimal detection of scarring. The MCUG can be performed earlier with a 3-day course of prophylactic antibiotics starting the day before the procedure. Children >6 months who respond well to treatment <48h do not require any imaging.

Atypical features
• Seriously ill/septicaemia.
• Poor urine stream.
• Abdominal or bladder mass.
• ↑ creatinine.
• Non-*E. coli* UTI.
• Failure to respond <48h.
Recurrent UTI:
• ≥2 upper UTIs.
• 1 upper UTI & ≥1 lower UTI.
• ≥3 lower UTIs.

Some believe the NICE guidelines lead to under-investigation. Clinicians must weigh-up the likelihood of disease vs burden on the family and NHS of unpleasant, invasive testing.

Prophylactic antibiotics May be considered on a case-by-case basis for children with recurrent UTI especially if the child has significant comorbidities. Prophylaxis is used if there is significant GU anomaly or renal damage and the child should be referred to a specialist. The role of prophylactic antibiotics for prevention of reflux nephropathy in VUR is controversial but antibiotics are shown to reduce the risk of recurrent UTIs in those with high-grade VUR. Some clinicians start prophylaxis while awaiting imaging results and stop when reflux has been ruled out if there is no scarring.

Surgical ℞ Surgical correction (ureteric reimplantation) of moderate reflux is 'unlikely to be beneficial', and in minor reflux is 'likely to be harmful' (carefully made EBM phrases!) and is unlikely to improve renal function.[153]

3 Paediatrics

Further reading
NICE (2007, updated 2017). *Urinary Tract Infection in Under 16s: Diagnosis and Management* (CG54). London: NICE. https://www.nice.org.uk/guidance/cg54

3 Paediatrics

Nephrotic syndrome (NS) This is the triad of oedema, proteinuria, and hypoalbuminaemia (± hypercholesterolaemia). Protein leaks from blood to urine through glomeruli, causing hypoproteinaemia, including loss of immuno-globulins and clotting factors. Before cortico-steroids (and antibiotics), many died from infections, steroids reduce mortality to ~3%.[154]

Causes of nephritis
• Post-infections (β-haemolytic strep, viruses, and many others)
• Chronic infections: IE/SBE; syphilis
• Henoch–Schönlein purpura
• SLE
• Membranoproliferative GN
• IgA nephropathy (Berger dis. OHCM p694)
• Anti-GBM (Goodpasture syn.)

Cause: Idiopathic in 90%, with peak age of onset <6yrs, ♂:♀ ratio 2:1. 85% of children with idiopathic NS have 'minimal change' disease and 10–15% have focal segmental glomerulosclerosis but biopsy is rarely needed. If <1yr the cause is likely genetic and the outcome poor. Any of the causes of nephritis (see MINIBOX 'Causes of nephritis') can also cause NS and should be considered particularly in children presenting >10yrs.

Presentation: Well child with insidious onset of pitting oedema, initially periorbital, then generalized. Often history of recent URTI. May progress to anorexia, GI disturbance, irritability, ascites, oliguria, SOB. Risk of infection and thrombosis.

Urine: Frothy; protein ≥3+; PCR >200mg/mmol; Na⁺ <10mmol/L suggests hypovolaemia (secondary hyperaldosteronism) but test invalidated by diuretic use.

Blood: Albumin <25g/L (so total Ca²⁺↓); U&E; lipids; C3/C4 (normal in INS); Hb (may be raised due to hypovolaemia); VZV immunity status. Note: visible haematuria, hypertension, and significantly raised creatine are not typically features of NS—if present consider GN, renal biopsy.

R: 1st line is corticosteroids. NS is classified by treatment response as steroid sensitive (SSNS), steroid dependent (SDNS), or steroid resistant (SRNS). **Prednisolone** 60mg/m2/day (max. 80mg) for 4 weeks, then 40mg/m2 alternate days for 4 weeks then taper[BNFC]. 90% respond within 8 weeks. Low-salt diet is recommended, high-protein diet is not. The value of fluid restriction is debatable although it is generally practised. Prophylactic antibiotics (PenV) are commonly used until oedema has resolved although evidence on efficacy is lacking. Pneumococcal and flu vaccines should be given.[155] Live vaccines are contraindicated in children receiving >20mg/day or >1mg/kg/day of prednisolone.

Symptomatic treatment: In severe cases fluid management is critical: the child may be intravascularly depleted at the same time as being grossly oedematous. Strict fluid balance, OD or BD weights. Give diuretics if very oedematous and no evidence of hypovolaemia. Albumin infusion (20% **albumin** 5mL/kg (1g/kg) over 4–6h) is only recommended in symptomatic hypovolaemia or severe diuretic-resistant oedema—discuss with senior.

Complications: ↑ susceptibility to infection due to loss of immunoglobulins and steroid immunosuppression particularly pneumococcal peritonitis. Have a low threshold for septic screen and IV ABx. There is ↑ risk of VTE although prophylactic anticoagulation generally not given due to lack of evidence on efficacy and safety.

Relapses: Relapse is defined as ≥3+ proteinuria for 3 consecutive days. 90% of children respond to corticosteroids; however, families should be advised 90% will experience at least 1 relapse and 40% will experience frequent relapses.[156] The length of initial treatment course was in debate but recent systematic reviews show no benefit from prolonging initial course beyond 2 or 3 months.[156,157] A 7-day course of low-dose steroids at the start of a minor infection may reduce the risk of a relapse.[157,158] First relapses may be treated with further steroid courses. Frequently relapsing NS or SDNS may be treated with alternate-day low-dose steroids or steroid-sparing agents such as cyclophosphamide, (ciclosporin), tacrolimus, or mycophenolate mofetil (MMF).[158]

Acute glomerulonephritis *Essence:* Immune-mediated glomerular inflammation causing haematuria, salt and water retention ± proteinuria ± BP↑ ± AKI. Peak age: 7yrs.

Presentation: Haematuria; pitting oedema (initially periorbital); ± oliguria; BP↑ present in ~50%.

Complicated presentations:
• *Hypertensive encephalopathy:* restless; drowsy; severe headache; fits; vision ↓; vomiting; coma.
• *AKI:* acidosis, hyperkalaemia, seizures, stupor.
• *Fluid overload:* pulmonary oedema, cardiac failure.
• Mixed nephritic-nephrotic syndrome.

Urine: Blood; protein; casts, red cell casts are pathognomonic for GN but not always present.

Blood: FBC, U&E (creatinine, K, bicarbonate, calcium, phosphate, and albumin), blood gas, C3, C4, ASOT/antiDNAaseB. ANA, anti-DNA antibodies (if SLE suspected), ANCA (if vasculitis suspected), syphilis serology, blood cultures, virology (EBV, CMV, Hep B).

Other tests: Throat swabs; CXR if fluid overload suspected. Renal biopsy indicated in severe cases (rare).

Treatment: Is mainly supportive with treatment of underlying infection or secondary cause if present. Low-salt diet, daily weights. Careful attention to fluid balance, fluid restrict if oliguric, consider furosemide if fluid overloaded. Treat hypertension. Check BP often. If encephalopathy, give sodium nitroprusside (p. 231). Renal replacement therapy may be necessary in severe cases of AKI failing to respond to medical management (↑K⁺; metabolic acidosis; symptomatic uraemia; fluid overload; pulmonary oedema).

Poststreptococcal glomerulonephritis (PSGN) The most common cause of acute GN in children and presents 7–21 days after a streptococcal infection (pharyngitis, impetigo) with hypertension, haematuria (microscopic to gross cola-coloured urine) ± oedema, malaise, anorexia, fever, and abdominal pain.

Investigations: As for acute glomerulonephritis. C3 is low. Recent streptococcal infection should be confirmed (ASO titre, anti-DNAaseB, throat swab). Typically, renal biopsy is not needed.

R: General measures as for acute glomerulonephritis. Oral penicillin for 10 days is given to reduce spread of nephritogenic bacterial strains. Oedema usually resolves in 5–10 days; however, hypertension, haematuria, and proteinuria may last for several weeks or months. Prognosis is very good (95% full recovery).

Pre-auricular pits or tags alone are *not* markers of renal anomalies, however consider renal us if maternal DM, other dysmorphic features, or FH of deafness or renal abnormalities.

Undescended testis—cryptorchidism (2–3% of neonates, 15–30% of prems; bilateral in 25% of these). On cold days, retractile testes may hide in the inguinal pouch, eluding all but the most careful examination (eg while squatting, or with legs crossed, or in a warm bath they may be 'milked' down into position). These retractile testes do not need surgery. If truly undescended it will lie along the path of descent from the abdominal cavity. Early (eg at 1 year) fixing within the scrotum (orchidopexy) may prevent infertility and reduces later neoplasia (untreated, risk is ↑ >5-fold).

Posterior urethral valves Affect males and occur from folds of bladder mucosa blocking the bladder neck, causing outflow obstruction. Usually diagnosed antenatally with oligohydramnios and renal tract dilatation or postnatally with absent or feeble voiding (± uraemia and a palpable bladder). *Micturating cystogram:* posterior urethral dilatation. Prognosis guarded, often cystic malformation of kidneys.

Hypospadias Affects 1:350 male births. Characterized by abnormal position of external urethral meatus on the ventral penis. May occur anywhere from the glans to the scrotum or even perineum, appearing ambiguous (pp. 302-3). Usually noted at birth. Most commonly causes difficulty urinating while standing and cosmetic appearance that is different to other boys. Occasionally, ventral curvature of the penis occurs (chordee). Avoid circumcision: use foreskin for preschool repair in one or more procedures with good prognosis.

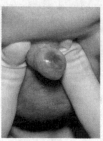

Epispadias (fig 3.15) (Meatus on dorsum of penis.) May occur with bladder exstrophy (see later).

Fig 3.15 Epispadias.

Some congenital/genetic disorders

Horseshoe kidney (crossed-fused kidney): Symptoms: silent or obstructive uropathy ± renal infections. us diagnosis: kidneys 'too medial'; lower pole 'too long'; anterior-rotated pelvis; poorly defined inferior border; isthmus often invisible.[159] Absence of 1 kidney or horseshoe kidney is associated with Mullerian anomalies in girls (such as unicornuate uterus).

Autosomal recessive polycystic kidney disease and congenital hepatic fibrosis (ARPKD-CHF): Characterized by cystic dilations of the collecting ducts associated with biliary dysgenesis and periportal fibrosis. PKHD1 is the responsible gene (on short arm of chromosome 6). Typically diagnosed by prenatal us (hyperechogenic, large kidneys ± oligohydramnios). Affects 1 in 40,000. Severe cases lead to pulmonary hypoplasia. 80% of those infants that survive the 1st month of life will live to 15. Affected children tend to develop hyponatraemia, hypertension, and renal failure. The histology of the liver is always abnormal. Survivors risk UTIs and portal hypertension with haematemesis.[160]

Ectopic kidney: May be seen on us (eg pelvic mass) or renal scintigraphy. Associations: anorectal abnormalities, UTIs; calculi.[161]

Renal agenesis: Causes oligohydramnios, Potter's facies, + death if bilateral. VACTERL association (vertebral, anal, cardiac, tracheo-esophageal, renal and limb anomalies). *Diagnosis:* prenatal us.[162]

Patent urachus: Urine leaks from the umbilicus. *Image:* excretory urogram.

Bladder exstrophy: Congenital anomaly which involves extrusion of the bladder through a defect in the abdominal wall. It is a spectrum of disease and can also involve the pelvic bones, ureters, bladder neck, and sphincters, and can be associated with other problems, such as inguinal and umbilical herniae, and undescended testes.[163]

Double ureter: Associations: ureterocele, UTI, pyelonephritis; may be symptomless.

Renal tubular defects: (eg renal glycosuria, cystinuria, or diabetes insipidus). In *renal tubular acidosis* conservation of fixed base is impaired, causing metabolic acidosis + alkaline urine. *Symptoms:* Faltering growth; polyuria; polydipsia.[164]

Wilms' tumour (nephroblastoma) The most common renal tumour of childhood (6–7% of all malignancies).[165] It is an undifferentiated mesodermal tumour of the intermediate cell mass. It is predominantly sporadic (~90%), but may be familial (~2%), or associated with Beckwith–Wiedemann syndrome (BWS, p. 842), WAGR (wilms', Aniridia, GU malformations, and intellectual disability (Retardation)) or other syndromes. One of the Wilms' tumour genes (WT1 on chromosome 11) encodes a protein which is a transcriptional repressor downregulating IGF2, an insulin-like growth factor.[166]

Median age at presentation: 3.5yrs. 95% are unilateral. *Staging:*

1 Tumour confined to the kidney.
2 Extrarenal spread, but resectable.
3 Extensive abdominal disease.
4 Distant metastases.
5 Bilateral disease.

The patient: 75% present <4yrs of age, mostly with a painless, palpable abdominal mass or swelling. Other features include fever, pain, and more rarely haematuria and hypertension. Metastases occur in 10%, most commonly in the lungs. us: renal pelvis distortion; hydronephrosis. *CT/MRI* provide the detailed anatomical information needed for surgical planning.[167]

Management: Surgery, chemotherapy ± radiotherapy. Avoid biopsy; nephrectomy + vincristine and actinomycin for 4 weeks pre-op can cure. Chemotherapy is used in all tumours. A 2-drug regimen is recommended for early Wilms' (without radiotherapy); more advanced stages need a 3-drug regimen + radiotherapy.[168] Genetic and biological factors guide risk categorization and help individualize care.[169,170] N=382

Prognosis: ~90% long-term survival.[171]

Acute kidney injury (AKI) A rapid fall in glomerular filtration rate (GFR) usually manifests as rising creatinine or development of oliguria/anuria.[172] *Causes: Pre-renal, intrinsic renal*, or *post-renal*. In developed nations: sepsis, cardiac surgery, bone marrow transplantation, and nephrotoxins (NSAIDs, aminoglycosides, vancomycin, aciclovir, and contrast);[173] in the tropics causes include: diarrhoea/dehydration (50%);[174] glomerulonephritis (34%); drug-induced haemolysis in G6PD deficiency (5%); snake bite (4%); haemolytic uraemic syndrome (2%); myoglobinuria and malaria (OHCM p298). *Acute tubular necrosis* (ATN) is a common form of intrinsic renal AKI caused by ischaemia (overlapping with pre-renal causes) or nephrotoxins. *Severity:* The paediatric RIFLE criteria grades AKI based on changes in eGFR or urine output (Risk, Injury, and Failure), and has 2 outcome measures (Loss of kidney function and End-stage renal disease).[175] Alternative criteria: AKIN[176] or KDIGO.[177] *Red flags:* Anuria; oedema/raised JVP/hepatomegaly/dyspnoea (fluid overload); headaches (BP↑↑); tremors/tetany (Ca²⁺↓); seizures.

Investigations: K⁺↑; creatinine ↑; urea ↑; PO₄³⁻↑ or ↔; Ca²⁺↓; Cl⁻↓. MSU: are there red cell casts (= GN, p. 227)? If no RBCs seen but dipstick +ve for RBCs, consider haemo/myoglobinuria (OHCM p319). Urine very concentrated in pre-renal (specific gravity >1.020, urine/plasma creatinine >40, Na⁺ <20) as opposed to intrinsic (<1.010, <20, >40 respectively). *Other tests:* serum and urine osmolality, ECG, blood gas, film, PCV, platelets, clotting studies (DIC), CK, LDH, C3/C4, ASOT, ANA, ANCA, anti-GBM antibodies. *Radiology:* ►Arrange urgent renal US if there is suspicion of post-renal or no clear cause.[178] Are the ureters dilated (eg stones: 90% radio-opaque)? If so, urgent surgery may be required.

Treatment: Remove or reduce the cause promptly. Involve paediatric nephrology team early. • Treat shock and dehydration (pp. 312-13)—then:
• Strict input/output and twice-daily weights.
• Maintain fluid balance and renal perfusion. Fluid resuscitate and use inotropes as necessary while avoiding overload. Replace losses + insensible loss (12–15mL/kg/day).
• Do *not* routinely use loop diuretics. Consider for fluid overload if renal function improving or while requiring renal replacement therapy.
• Monitor BP. If BP↑↑: sodium nitroprusside (see BOX 'Hypertensive emergencies').
• Minimize nephrotoxic drugs and adjust doses for renally cleared drugs.
• Treat ↑K⁺. Monitor ECG. Tall T-waves and QRS slurring prompt urgent lowering of K⁺ with nebulized salbutamol. Also give **calcium gluconate** (10%, 0.5mL/kg IV over 2–4min; monitor ECG: stop IVI if heart rate ↓) to stabilize myocardium; **sodium bicarbonate** (1mmol/kg IV over 20min) to correct acidosis; **calcium polystyrene sulfonate** (0.5–1g/kg max. 60g PO) to remove K⁺ from body. Insulin (+glucose) can be used to drive K⁺ into cells but must be used with extreme caution in AKI.
• Refer urgently for renal replacement therapy if the following fail to respond to medical management: ↑K⁺; metabolic acidosis; symptomatic uraemia; fluid overload; pulmonary oedema.[178] Many centres now prefer continuous haemofiltration to peritoneal dialysis.[173]

►► Significant polyuria may occur during recovery requiring further careful fluid management.

Haemolytic uraemic syndrome (HUS) An uncommon but important cause of AKI in children. *Essence:* Acute microangiopathic haemolytic anaemia (schistocytes, burr cells, OHCM fig 8.26 p333 & fig 8.12 p329), thrombocytopenia, renal failure (endothelial damage to glomerular capillaries). Typical HUS (95%) is associated with diarrhoea, atypical HUS (5%) is not.[179] *Typical:* HUS is more frequent in the summer months, and in children <3yrs. It is associated with Shiga toxin producing *E. coli* type O157:H7.[180] *Signs:* Abdo pain; diarrhoea (usually bloody); haemoglobinuria→; ± oliguria; pallor; bruising/petechiae; ↑BP; CNS signs→; encephalopathy. LDH↑. WCC↑. Coombs –ve. PCV↓. Hb↓. *Mortality:* 5–30% (<5% UK).

Treatment: Supportive. Liaise early with paediatric nephrology unit as early dialysis may be required. Antibiotics, fibrinolytics, and anticoagulation are *not* used.[181] ΔΔ: DIC, thrombotic thrombocytopenia purpura (TTP). TTP is rare in children and difficult to distinguish from HUS. It is associated with ADAMTS13 gene mutations and VWF deficiency.

Chronic kidney disease (CKD) *Causes:* Congenital dysplastic kidneys or renal tract abnormality, pyelonephritis, glomerulonephritis, recurrent infection, reflux nephropathy; AKI → cortical necrosis. ►Monitor growth, BP, U&E, Ca^{2+} (often ↓), Po_4^{3-} (often ↑). *The child:* Asymptomatic → faltering growth; poly/nocturia; lethargy; anorexia; vomiting; headache; BP↑; hypertensive retinopathy; anaemia; seizures. *Treatment:* (See BOX 'Chronic kidney disease: meta-

Chronic kidney disease: metabolic and other issues

Diet and growth Get help from a specialist dietician. Calorie needs may not be met if vomiting is a problem. Low-K^+ (±low Na^+), high-protein (100–140% of normal) diet is indicated. Vitamin drops may be needed. NGT or gastrostomy tube feeding has a role. Growth hormone therapy combined with optimal dialysis improves growth: see *BNF*.

Hypertension Strict BP control slows progression of CKD. Agents targeting the renin–angiotensin system such as ACE inhibitors or ARBs are preferred.

CKD mineral and bone disorder (CKD–MBD) is an umbrella term for the results of changes in Ca^{2+} and Po_4^{3-} metabolism and bone mineralization (osteoblast and osteoclast activity ↓): renal osteodystrophy (hyperparathyroidism, osteomalacia, and adynamic bone disease), extraskeletal (vascular) calcification. *Impact:* poor growth, muscle weakness, slipped epiphyses, bone pain, and bone deformity (±cranial nerve lesions).[182] As glomerular filtration falls, compensatory mechanisms to enhance phosphate excretion fail; resulting hyperphosphataemia promotes hypocalcaemia, so PTH rises, which enhances bone resorption to release Ca^{2+} in an attempt to correct hypocalcaemia. PTH↑ leads to marrow fibrosis (osteitis fibrosa). Also, the failing kidneys cannot convert enough 25-hydroxycholecalciferol to active 1,25-dihydroxycholecalciferol, so GI calcium absorption falls, worsening hypocalcaemia.

R: Complex due to changing normal values and requirements with age, sex, and puberty. Aims are to normalize calcium and ↓ associated hyperphosphataemia. Keep PTH within normal limits in predialysis children and 2–3× over upper normal limit in those on dialysis. Avoid aggressive use of calcium-based phosphate binders and vit D derivatives to prevent PTH oversuppression and development of adynamic bone disease.

Anaemia Common, and is the result of ↓ erythropoietin (EPO) ± poor iron and folic acid intake. A typical Hb is 60–90g/L. Do not transfuse, as this suppresses EPO production, give EPO (SC in pre-dialysis and peritoneal dialysis patients, and IV if on haemodialysis).

Acidosis Common, give oral bicarb if serum bicarb is <20mmol/L.[183]

►►Hypertensive emergencies

Rare.[184] ↑BP with severe symptoms or acute organ damage (headache, ↑ICP, encephalopathy, seizures, papilloedema, heart failure). Usually secondary to underlying disease. Get expert help. Aim to reduce BP slowly, by <25% over >8h. **Sodium nitroprusside** has rapid onset (seconds) and short half-life: 0.5mcg/kg/min IVI, ↑ slowly in 200-nanogram/kg/min increments as needed, up to 8mcg/kg/min (typical response ≈3mcg/kg/min). Photosensitive drug so protect from light. CI: severe hepatic impairment. Withdraw over ≥20min to prevent rebound hypertension. **Labetalol** is an easy-to-use alternative eg 0.25mg/kg/dose IV, doubled every 15min (as needed) up to 3mg/kg/h IV or as infusion (0.5mg/kg/h, ↑ to max. 3mg/kg/h); CI: asthma. Avoid short-acting nifedipine as it can cause severe complications due to sudden precipitous drop in BP.

Epilepsy This is a tendency to *recurrent, unprovoked* seizures (abnormal electrical brain activity).[185] 1% of children will have a seizure (not associated with fever) by the age of 14 years. ILAE *seizure type* classification[186] depends on whether onset is *generalized, focal,* or *unknown* and signs are *motor* or *non-motor*. Focal seizures originate within 1 hemisphere and may or may not have loss of awareness (previously 'simple partial' and 'complex partial'). *Generalized seizures:* Usually have loss of awareness and may be:

- **Generalized tonic/clonic** *(GTC or grand mal):* limbs stiffen (the tonic phase) and then jerk forcefully (clonic phase), with loss of consciousness.
- **Absences** *(petit mal):* brief (eg 10sec) pauses ('He stops in mid-sentence, and carries on where he left off'); eyes may roll up; he/she is *unaware of the attack*.
- **Infantile spasms** age: 3–9 months. Brief (<2sec) movements with flexion of trunk and extension of limbs ('Salaam attack').
- **Other** tonic (usually <1min sustained ↑ tone); atonic (abrupt loss of tone); clonic (rhythmic contractions); myoclonic (brief, usually single, sudden contractions).

Focal seizures: Can manifest with a wide variety of phenomena ranging from focal motor twitches to sensory or emotional disturbances to automatisms (eg lip smacking, rubbing face) or even fits of pure pleasure.[187,188] Todd paralysis, <48h weakness of affected muscles, may follow classic focal tonic–clonic seizures.

Diagnosis: Notoriously difficult and NICE recommends all children with a first afebrile seizure should be seen by a specialist. Identification of an *epilepsy syndrome* (a characteristic disorder based on age, seizure type, EEG, and other factors) is key for management and prognosis (examples on p. 233). If an epilepsy syndrome cannot be identified, the final level of diagnosis may be *epilepsy type:* generalized, focal, combined generalized and focal, or unknown. *Causes:* ILAE splits causes of epilepsy into structural (eg secondary to HIE, (p. 281), stroke, trauma), genetic (eg Dravet syndrome), infectious (eg neurocysticercosis TB, HIV), metabolic, immune (eg autoimmune encephalitides), and unknown (often no cause is found).

ΔΔ: There are many causes of seizures which are not epilepsy: acute infection (eg meningitis, encephalitis); glucose ↓, Ca^{2+}↓, Mg^{2+}↓; Na^+↑↓; ammonia; toxins; trauma; CNS tumour. There are also paroxysmal disorders that may mimic seizures: arrhythmias; migraine; narcolepsy; syncope (reflex anoxic seizures, p. 233); tics; Münchausen's by proxy (pp. 196-7) and non-epileptic seizures (NES).

Tests: If presenting acutely see pp. 234-5. Non-acute: EEG (±hyperventilation, photic simulation, and sleep) is important but difficult to interpret as EEG abnormalities are often seen in children without seizures and a normal EEG cannot rule out epilepsy. MRI is the imaging mode of choice but not required if epilepsy syndrome is clear. ECG if any possibility of syncope/arrhythmias.

Sudden unexpected death in epilepsy (SUDEP) A rare, catastrophic event which is poorly understood. The main risk factor is uncontrolled seizures.

Febrile seizures/convulsions (FS) A very common presentation to ED: a *single* tonic–clonic, symmetrical generalized seizure lasting <15min, occurring as temperature rises rapidly in a febrile illness in a normally developing child (½–6yrs old) and occurring no more than once in 24h. *Lifetime prevalence:* ~3% of children have at least 1 FS, positive family history is common. *Examination:* Find the source of infection, look for signs of meningitis. ℞: Give O_2, put in recovery position, check glucose; if fit lasting >5min treat as status epilepticus p. 234-5; antipyretics may reduce discomfort but do not treat nor prevent fits. *Tests:* As pp. 234-5 ± MSU, CXR, ENT swabs.[189] Your immediate concern is to differentiate from meningoencephalitis by careful history and examination although often by presentation the child is back to playing. *To LP or not LP?:* Risk of pyogenic meningitis is as low (<1.3%) as the risk in a febrile child with no seizures[190] if all the defining criteria listed are fulfilled. Avoid LP in the postictal period as a CNS assessment will be impossible. If doubt remains, then treat *now* for meningitis

Parental education: Allay fear (a child is *not* dying during a fit). A 1st FS is associated with a ≤3% risk of epilepsy, a modest ↑ over the general population.[191] The risk is higher if there is a +ve family history, complex features (see later), or developmental abnormality. Recurrence of FS is common (⅓ in <1yr).[192] If the seizure lasts >5min call an ambulance. *Prevention:* Evidence shows antipyretics do *not* prevent recurrence of FS.[192] Antiepileptic drugs (AEDs) have no role due to the benign nature of FS although benzodiazepines are recommended for prolonged FS. *Complex febrile seizures* have atypical features: focal onset, >15min duration, or >1 seizure in 24h, these are associated with an increased risk of epilepsy.

Are these paroxysmal/episodic 'spells' epilepsy?

This is a common and important dilemma, as epilepsy treatment can be toxic. Also, if it is harmful to label any child, it is doubly so to mislabel a child. Watching and waiting, repeat EEGs, and videos of attacks (eg on mobile phone), or video telemetry may be needed.[193] Neonates and infants commonly get benign neonatal sleep myoclonus. Toddlers may have breath-holding attacks and reflex-anoxic seizures (see later). In childhood, daydreaming can appear similar to an absence seizure. Syncope may be followed by tonic–clonic movements. Psychogenic non-epileptic seizures (NES) describe episodes of psychological origin; they may be triggered by specific situations, movements cannot be explained anatomically, and there is rapid return to normal. Injury and passing urine may occur. Psychogenic NES should be acknowledged by parents and the child that these attacks are non-epileptic and any gain from this behaviour should be removed. Psychological support is essential.

Reflex anoxic seizures (RAS) Paroxysmal, self-limited brief (eg 15sec) vagal-induced asystole triggered by pain, fear (eg at venepuncture) or anxiety. During this time the child is deathly pale ± hypotonia, rigidity, upward eye deviation, clonic movements, and urinary incontinence. Typical age: 6 months to 2yrs (but may be older). *Prevalence:* 0.8% of preschool children. ΔΔ· Accurate history is key. EEG is not indicated. ECG is indicated but has low yield. NB: tongue-biting is not described in RAS. *Management:* Education and reassurance. Drugs (atropine, β-blockers, SSRIs) have been tried but lack evidence of efficacy and are rarely needed. Pacemakers have been used in the US in extreme circumstances.[194] *What to tell parents:* Avoid the term 'seizure', as this is all that is likely to be remembered. *White breath-holding attacks* is a useful synonym. Emphasize its benign nature, and that the child usually grows out of it (but it may occur later in life, and in siblings).[195]

Some epilepsy syndromes

Benign epilepsy with centrotemporal spikes (BECTS/ 'rolandic' epilepsy.) 15% of all childhood epilepsy. Age 5–14yrs. Infrequent, focal seizures (often facial or oropharyngeal sensory-motor symptoms, speech arrest ± hypersalivation) ± secondary generalization usually occurring during sleep. Treatment is rarely needed.

Panayiotopoulos syndrome (6% of all epilepsies.) A benign focal epilepsy presenting in early childhood (4–7yrs). Autonomic symptoms predominate. It occurs mainly at night, with vomiting, sweating, eye deviation, impaired consciousness, and sometimes bilateral clonic activity. Many seizures last for 30min (some may last hours) but there is no brain damage. *EEG:* Shifting and/or multiple foci, often with occipital predominance. *Treatment:* Reassure as remission often occurs within 2yrs and medication is usually not needed.[196]

West syndrome/infantile spasms Peak age: 5 months. Clusters of infantile spasms lasting 3–30sec. IQ↓ in ~70%.[197] EEG is characteristic (hypsarrhythmia). ℞: Prednisolone, ACTH, or vigabatrin (SE: visual field defects). Prognosis is poor.[185]

Stepwise treatment of status epilepticus Call for help. ABC. See table 3.9.[198]NICE
(See also neonates: p. 284.)[185]

▶▶Table 3.9 Seizure control: proceed to the next step only if fits continue

0min	▶▶ABC. Secure airway. High-flow o_2. Check spo_2, pulse, glucose, BP, and temp. Secure IV/IO access. Estimate weight. Set a clock in motion
5min	▶▶Lorazepam 0.1mg/kg IV/IO; slow bolus; *or* buccal midazolam 0.5mg/kg (massage between lower gum and the cheek) *or* rectal diazepam 0.5mg/kg
15min	Repeat lorazepam. Call for senior help. Re-confirm epileptic seizure. Prepare phenytoin
25min	▶▶Phenytoin 20mg/kg IVI; over 20min (monitor ECG) *or* (if on regular phenytoin) ▶▶Phenobarbital 20mg/kg over 20min. *Call PICU & anaesthetist—prepare for intubation*, locate ET tube, etc. Optional 0.8mL/kg of paraldehyde 50:50 mixture may be given PR while preparing or infusing phenytoin/phenobarbital
45min	▶▶Rapid sequence induction with thiopental sodium 4mg/kg IV/IO. Transfer to PICU

▶These times refer to elapsed time on the clock from the start of the seizure, not gaps between each drug. ▶If hypoglycaemic, give 2–5mL/kg IV of **glucose 10%**, then repeat blood glucose. ▶For children with known epilepsy, check whether they have a patient 'passport' with personalized management plan. Other options include IV levetiracetam or sodium valproate. ▶Although convulsive status epilepticus (CSE) is defined as a continuous seizure, or multiple seizures without full recovery of consciousness, for 30min, treatment is started after 5min to break the cycle, 'time is brain'.

Tests For acute seizures: SaO_2; glucose; BP; and consider: electrolytes (Ca^{2+}↓, Mg^{2+}↓, Na^+↓↑); arterial gases; FBC; CRP; septic screen; anticonvulsant levels; toxicology screen; blood ammonia (requires special blood bottle); carbon monoxide; lead; and neurometabolic screen as appropriate. Serum prolactin is not recommended.[185] Perform CT if focal seizures or focal neurological signs.

Once the crisis is over Refer to a specialist: are further investigations (pp. 232–3), AEDs, or rescue medication needed? Drug choice is complex, side effects and interactions are many. Aim to use one drug only. Increase dose until seizures controlled, or toxic levels reached. Out of the context of status, choice of AED, if any, should be based on epilepsy syndrome or epilepsy type (pp. 232–3).

AED options by seizure type (See[198]NICE)
- *Generalized tonic–clonic:* 1st try sodium valproate in males. If female or unsuitable try lamotrigine (may exacerbate myoclonic seizures) or carbamazepine (may exacerbate myoclonic and absence seizures). Adjunctive treatment includes clobazam, levetiracetam, or topiramate.
- *Absences:* 1st choice, ethosuximide; 2nd, sodium valproate. If neither work, try lamotrigine, then try combinations. Avoid: carbamazepine, gabapentin, oxcarbazepine, phenytoin, pregabalin, tiagabine, and vigabatrin (may worsen seizures).
- *Myoclonic:* Sodium valproate, levetiracetam or topiramate are 1st line. Avoid: as for absences.
- *Tonic or atonic:* 1st line: sodium valproate, 2nd lamotrigine. Avoid carbamazepine, oxcarbazepine, gabapentin.
- *Focal:* 1st try carbamazepine or lamotrigine; then sodium valproate or oxcarbazepine or levetiracetam.
- *Prolonged seizures/CSE:* Buccal midazolam, rectal diazepam.

Other options *Ketogenic diet:* Consider under specialist supervision if 2 drugs fail to work (it can ↓ fits by ⅔).[199] SE: constipation, vomiting, ↓ energy, hunger. *Surgery:* Resective surgery can be used for refractory epilepsy with identifiable epileptogenic focus. *Vagus nerve stimulation:* An option for predominantly focal seizures refractory to medication and not amenable to epilepsy surgery.

Stopping anticonvulsants See *OHCM* p492. AEDs should never be stopped abruptly but the risk of seizure recurrence during the tapering down process is no greater if the tapering period is 6 weeks compared with 9 months. **Newer anticonvulsants** NICE reserves gabapentin, lamotrigine, oxcarbazepine, tiagabine, topiramate, and vigabatrin (as an adjunct for partial seizures) for children not benefiting from (or able to tolerate) older drugs or older drugs have contraindications/interactions (eg the OCP). Cannabidiols are an area of much media interest and have recently been approved by the US FDA for treatment of atonic seizures in 2 severe forms of epilepsy (LGS and Dravet) following +ve results in 2 RCTs.[200,201]

AED options by epilepsy syndrome See NICE CG137 table 2.[185]

Headache is a relatively common presentation to GPs or EDs and parents often assume the worst—if you don't address their concerns they will present somewhere else. **Causes** *Primary* (migraine, tension-type, or cluster) or *secondary* to an underlying cause. These are legion and include: meningitis (esp. viral); encephalitis; abscess; head injury; subdural/extradural bleeds (NAI? pp. 196–7); tumours; thrombosis;[7] Reye syndrome (p. 856); sinusitis; medication (overuse); substance abuse or withdrawal; menstruation; malignant hypertension (always check BP); idiopathic (previously benign) intracranial hypertension (IIH); stress; behavioural; infection. Consider a headache diary to aid diagnosis.

▶▶ **Red flags**[202] Fever; altered consciousness; sudden onset; worse in morning; varies with posture; worse with cough/Valsalva; wakes from sleep; unexplained vomiting (esp. early morning); recent head trauma; young age (<4yrs); bulging fontanelle; neurological signs; visual disturbance; rapidly increasing head circumference; cognitive decline; history of malignancy; immunosuppressed; early or late puberty; signs of raised intracranial pressure (p. 200).

Migraine In children we modify migraine criteria to include moderate to severe bifrontal or bitemporal as well as unilateral headache. Throbbing: lasting 1–72h; ± nausea/vomiting; ± photophobia: ± phonophobia (vertigo and abdo pain also occur); sometimes heralded by visual or sensory aura. The headache is aggravated by physical activity. If the headache occurs ≥15 days per month = chronic migraine. (See OHCM p458.) *Prevalence:* 5% (10% in adolescence). *Triggers:* Diet, dehydration, overtiredness, and stress. *Acute R:* (As early as possible in an attack); paracetamol (p. 205); ibuprofen (p. 205).[203] Consider an antiemetic. If this fails and >12yrs, add a triptan.[202,204] *Prophylaxis:* Avoid triggers and get enough sleep. If migraine is disrupting social activity or schooling on a regular basis, consider prophylaxis; topiramate, propranolol, or amitriptyline. **Riboflavin** (Vit B₂) 400mg OD may ↓ frequency and severity. Pizotifen is frequently used but evidence is lacking.[202] *Non-drug R:* Relaxation training, biofeedback, self-hypnosis, and guided imagery have a role.[205]

Tension-type headaches Diffuse, bilateral, pressing/tightening (non-pulsating), mild to moderate intensity (never severe), not exacerbated by activity, lasting 30min to 7 days with no nausea or vomiting.[206] There may be photophobia or phonophobia but not both together. Features may overlap with migraine, if so, diagnose and treat as migraine. If the headache occurs ≥15 days per month = chronic. *R:* Paracetamol; ibuprofen.

Cluster headaches Strictly unilateral headaches associated with ipsilateral parasympathetic autonomic features and occurring in clusters up to 8/day. The pain is severe to very severe and usually felt in orbital, supraorbital, and/or temporal areas, lasting 15min to 3h and causing agitation and restlessness. *Autonomic features:* Conjunctival injection; lacrimation; nasal congestion or rhinorrhoea; eyelid oedema; forehead and facial sweating; miosis (pupil constriction); ptosis (eyelid droop).[206] Rare, but does occur in children <10yrs, ♂>>♀. Δ: Clinical . Cluster headaches can occur secondary to structural brain lesions so discuss the need for neuroimaging with a specialist at the 1st presentation. *Acute R:* O₂ (100%, ≥12L/min via non-rebreathe mask) or SC or nasal triptan (in contralateral nostril). Do not use paracetamol, NSAIDs, opioids, ergots, or oral triptans for acute R.[202] *Prophylaxis:* Consider verapamil but get specialist advice. Other options include lithium, topiramate and steroids.

---

7 Venous sinus thrombosis risk ↑ if: infection; perinatal problems; blood dyscrasias. Signs: ↓ consciousness (50%), papilloedema (18%), cranial nerve palsy (33%), hemiparesis, hypotonia. Thrombolysis may be needed.[207]

Brain tumours May present with non-specific symptoms that overlap with common childhood illnesses so diagnosis is often delayed. Signs and symptoms are age and tumour location dependent. The *Children's Brain Tumour Research Centre* NICE accredited guidelines[208] identify discriminating features that are associated with increased incidence of tumours and therefore mandate urgent imaging (completed and reported <4wks if relatively low index of suspicion, faster if higher suspicion):

- *Headache:* Persistent (>2wks) headaches that wake child from sleep or occur on waking; persistent headaches in any child <4yrs; headache associated with confusion or disorientation; persistent headache + ≥1 sign/symptom suggestive of a tumour.
- *Vomiting:* Persistent (>2wks) vomiting on waking; persistent vomiting + ≥1 sign/symptom suggestive of a tumour.
- *Visual system:* Papilloedema ; optic atrophy; new-onset nystagmus; proptosis; new-onset paralytic squint/diplopia; reduced visual acuity or visual fields not due to ocular cause.
- *Motor system:* Motor skill regression (may be subtle—↓ handwriting, ↓ computer games); focal motor weakness; abnormal gait/ataxia, swallowing difficulties, or persistent head tilt without local cause; Bell's palsy (isolated lower motor CN VII palsy) with no improvement in 4 weeks.
- *Imaging is also recommended:* If there are 2 or more signs/symptoms suggestive of a tumour including those listed and: *Endocrine:* precocious, arrested, or delayed puberty; galactorrhoea; amenorrhoea; growth failure; diabetes insipidus (DI) (polyuria/polydipsia). *Other:* increasing head size/macrocephaly (the most common presenting symptom in <4yrs—you must measure head circumference); persisting lethargy; behavioural change (new mood disturbance, withdrawal, or disinhibition); dysphagia/dysphasia; new focal seizures.

▶▶**Referral** Discuss with specialist the same day if tumour suspected, child should be seen in <2wks, imaging reported <4wks. **Tests** MRI preferred, contrast CT if MRI unavailable. EEG is not useful.[209]

Types of tumour ⅔ are in the posterior fossa.

- *Medulloblastoma:* Midline cerebellar embryonal tumour (inferior vermis) causing ICP↑, speech difficulty, truncal ataxia ± falls. ♂:♀ ≈ 4:1. Peak age: 4yrs. Seeding is along CSF pathways.
- *Brainstem astrocytoma:* Most common brain tumour in children. Associated with neurofibromatosis 1 and prior radiation. Cranial nerve palsies; pyramidal tract signs (eg hemiparesis); cerebellar ataxia; signs of ICP↑ are rare.
- *Midbrain and 3rd ventricle tumours:* May be astrocytomas, pinealomas, or colloid cysts (cause posture-dependent drowsiness). *Signs:* behaviour change (early); pyramidal tract and cerebellar signs; upward gaze defect.
- *Suprasellar gliomas:* Visual field defects; optic atrophy; pituitary disorders (growth arrest, hypothyroidism, delayed puberty); DI. Cranial DI is caused by ADH↓, so that there is polyuria and low urine osmolality (always <800mosmol/L) despite dehydration.
- *Cerebral hemispheres:* Usually gliomas. Meningiomas are rare. Fits are common. Signs depend on the lobe involved (OHCM p499). *R:* manage seizures, ↑ICP (dexamethasone, CSF shunt), and endocrine abnormalities. Excision if possible; radiotherapy; chemotherapy.

Prognosis: Varies significantly with tumour type. Morbidity and complications are common and long-term follow-up is needed.

Other space-occupying lesions Aneurysms; haematomas; granulomas; tuberculomas; cysts (neurocysticercosis); ▶abscess: suspect if ICP↑; T°↑; WCC↑. Get help.

Spinal tumours Rare, consider in children presenting with back or neck pain, gait abnormalities, focal weakness, or scoliosis.

Incidence 8:1000 births (the most common type of birth defect).[210] 1 in 10 still-births have evidence of severe CHD. Many defects are identified antenatally during an anomaly scan or fetal echocardiography (pp. 12-3).

Symptoms Can present from minutes to days postnatally, to adulthood.

Presentation Can be cyanosis, circulatory collapse, heart failure, or incidental murmur. *Cyanotic lesions:* Have a R→L shunt or mixing: transposition of the great arteries (TGA), tetralogy of Fallot (ToF), truncus arteriosus, tricuspid atresia, or total anomalous pulmonary venous drainage (TAPVD), hypoplastic left heart (HLH). *Circulatory collapse:* Follows closure of the ductus arteriosus in the 1st days of life in duct-dependent (pulmonary or systemic) circulations: coarctation of aorta (CoA), some TGA, HLH, pulmonary or aortic atresia. *Heart failure (HF):* Presents with poor feeding, dyspnoea, tachycardia, gallop rhythm, sweating, hepatomegaly, cool peripheries, oedema, pulmonary venous congestion on CXR, faltering growth. Cardiac causes of HF: (large) L→R shunts (atrial septal defect (ASD), ventricular septal defect (VSD)); obstructive lesions (CoA, aortic stenosis); arrhythmias: cardio-myopathies. *Eisenmenger syndrome:* (p. 846) A L→R shunt causes ↑ pulmonary blood flow and, over time, damage to pulmonary vasculature and ↑ pulmonary vascular resistance. This eventually results in reversal of flow across the shunt and cyanosis. This is irreversible and heart–lung transplant is required.

Tests FBC, CXR, PaO_2 (air and 100% FiO_2), 4-limb BP, pre & post-ductal spO_2, ECG, echo, ± cardiac catheter/CT/cardiac MRI.

Initial ℞ *HF:* O_2, diuretics (**furosemide** 1mg/kg 1–3×/day ± spironolactone), cal-ories to promote growth. *Duct-dependent conditions:* Prostaglandin infusion (may cause apnoeas) to maintain duct patency, urgent transfer to cardiac centre.

VSD (30%) *Symptoms:* Usually mild. *Signs:* Harsh loud pansystolic blowing murmur ± thrill. ECG: Ventricular hypertrophy and strain. CXR: pulmonary en-gorgement, cardiomegaly. *Course:* Small or muscular defects close spontan-eously, 20% by 9 months. Larger defects often need surgery.

ASD (7%) *Symptoms:* Usually none. *Signs:* Widely split fixed s_2, systolic (pul-monary flow) murmur upper left sternal edge (ULSE).[211] ECG: RVH ± partial right bundle branch block, absence of sinus arrhythmia. CXR: cardiomegaly, globular heart. *Course:* Variable depending on site. ▶ Most require intervention.

Pulmonary stenosis (7%) Usually asymptomatic. *Signs:* Ejection systolic murmur (ESM) ULSE, thrill, soft s_2. See *OHCM* p148.

Patent ductus arteriosus (PDA) (12%) Failure of the duct to close postnatally (>1 month), very common in preterms. *Symptoms:* Rare unless large → HF. *Signs:* Continuous machinery murmur below left clavicle ± thrill, collapsing pulse/wide pulse pressure. ℞: Observation ± diuretics or closure. Closure in preterms may be achieved with oral or IV **ibuprofen** (10mg/kg then 5mg/kg at 24 and 48h).[212] Closure in term infants via catheter occlusion or surgical ligation.

Coarctation (5%) Usually no symptoms unless severe or interrupted arch type and so duct-dependent systemic circulation (see earlier). *Signs:* HTN (upper/lower limb difference in BP), ↓ femoral pulses, ejection systolic murmur at ULSE. CXR: rib notching (late), '3' sign. ECG: LVH may be seen. ℞: Stent or sur-gery by 5yrs to avoid HTN and HF.

TGA (5%) Systemic and pulmonary circulations are in parallel, survival is not possible without mixing/shunting (via PDA, VSD, or ASD). *Symptoms:* Cyanosis ± circulatory collapse. ℞: Maintain PDA (prostaglandin) ±balloon catheter atrial septal perforation to buy time for surgery (arterial switch).

Tetralogy of Fallot (5%) Large VSD, overriding aorta, (sub)pulmonary sten-osis, RVH. *Symptoms:* Cyanosis (↓ pulmonary blood flow with R→L shunt), 'spelling' (exacerbations of cyanosis with ↓↓ pulmonary blood flow during agi-tation). *Signs:* Harsh ESM LSE, clubbing. ℞: Corrective surgery at 6 months ± shunt formation as interim measure. Treat spells by bringing knees to chest, give O_2, ± morphine, β-blockers, and phenylephrine.

We hear innocent murmurs in ~80% of children, at some time (eg with fever, anxiety, exercise). A *flow murmur* is the most common: ejection systolic, low pitched, grade ≤III, ULSE caused by ↑ flow across the PV (hyperdynamic states: anaemia, fever, etc.) similar to an ASD murmur but without fixed splitting of s₂. A *venous hum* is heard above or below the clavicles, continuous, low pitched, grade ≤III, it is abolished by pressing the ipsilateral jugular or by lying down (PDA murmurs are similar, but don't change with posture). *Still's murmur* is heard at LLSE to apex, early systolic, vibratory, musical, grade ≤III, loudest on lying flat. Children with these murmurs are well with normal pulses and no red flags.

▶▶Red flags Signs of HF, faltering growth, chest pain, syncope, unexplained fever, cyanosis, clubbing, diastolic, thrills (grade ≥IV), heave. Have increased index of suspicion if: FH of CHD, dysmorphism or during neonatal period (check femoral pulses and pre- (right hand) and post- (either foot) ductal spo₂). When in doubt, refer to paediatrician with expertise in cardiology. CXR & ECG often mislead, skilled echocardiogram is the definitive investigation.[213]

Auscultation of murmurs If you have an ear for detail! Note timing, site, character, grade, and any radiation.
- *Ejection systolic* (innocent, or aortic or pulmonary stenosis).
- *Pansystolic* with no crescendo–decrescendo (VSD, PDA, COA, mitral incompetence).
- *Late systolic*, no crescendo–decrescendo (mitral prolapse, OHCM p144).
- *Early diastolic* decrescendo (aortic or pulmonary incompetence).
- *Mid-diastolic* crescendo–decrescendo (↑ atrioventricular valve flow, eg VSD, ASD; or tricuspid or mitral valve stenosis). An opening snap and presystolic accentuation suggest the latter.
- *Continuous murmurs* (PDA, venous shunt, or arteriovenous fistula).

Grade: The 6 grades for systolic murmurs (thrills mean pathology):

1 Just audible with a quiet child in a quiet room.	2 Quiet, but easily audible.
3 Loud, but no thrill.	4 Loud with thrill.

5 Audible even if the stethoscope only makes partial contact with skin.
6 Audible without a stethoscope.

Auscultation of heart sounds (s₁ and s₂) s₂ is more useful diagnostically than s₁: See fig 3.16.
- Is s₂ a double sound in inspiration, and single in expiration? (Normal.)
- Is s₂ split all the time? (ASD, VSD.)
- Is s₂ never split ie single? Fallot's; pulmonary atresia; severe pulmonary stenosis; common arterial trunk; transposition of the great arteries (the anterior aorta masks sounds from the posterior pulmonary trunk).
- Is the pulmonary component (2nd part) too loud? (Pulmonary hypertension.)

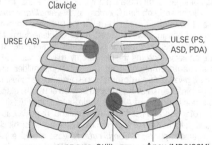

Fig 3.16 Auscultation of heart murmurs.

Normal HB levels vary dramatically with age, see reference ranges p. 314. When confronted by a child with pallor or an FBC showing anaemia, your 1st priority is: are there signs of serious illness? **▸▸ Red flags** Breathless; syncope; fever; lymphadenopathy; hepatosplenomegaly; bruising; jaundice; unexplained bone pain; haematuria; melaena; faltering growth; ↓ platelets, ↓WCC. ∆∆: Wide and depends on age. • ↓RBC production (diet, malabsorption, chronic disease, marrow disease, infections) or • ↑RBC loss (haemolysis, blood loss, haemoglobinopathies, hypersplenism, membranopathies).

Tests 1st line FBC, reticulocytes, & film; ferritin; CRP/ESR. *How should you proceed?*

1 Take a history (include travel, diet, ethnic origin); examine the child.

2 *Microcytic*: ?IDA (iron deficiency anaemia, ↓ferritin, see later); thalassaemia (Mediterranean/SE Asia areas, short stature, muddy complexion, icteric sclerae, distended abdomen ∴ hepatosplenomegaly; bossed skull, prominent maxillae, from marrow hyperplasia); G6PD deficiency; sideroblastic anaemia.

3 *Macrocytic*: ↓ folate (malabsorption; phenytoin), or ↓ vit B_{12} (breast milk from a vegetarian, ↓ intrinsic factor, malabsorption). Signs of vit B_{12}↓: poor feeding; late milestones; odd movements; microcephaly; faltering growth. Diamond–Blackfan (p. 844); Fanconi's anaemia (p. 848).

4 *Normocytic*: consider haemolysis, marrow failure (↓ reticulocytes, pancytopenia: malignancy; drugs; after infections (eg parvovirus B19); or thyroid, kidney, or liver failure) or anaemia of chronic disease (may also be microcytic).

5 *Eosinophilia* + tropics ≈ helminth infections (hookworm, roundworm, whipworm).

6 Severe tropical anaemias (eg Hb <50g/L): malaria; bacteraemia (eg non-typhoid salmonella[214]); worms; HIV; vit B_{12}↓; G6PD↓; malnutrition; sickle cell disease (SCD).

7 Next look at the ESR and CRP. This may indicate chronic disease.

8 *Film*: hypochromic, microcytic RBCs ≈ IDA; 'megaloblastic' (↑MCV and hypersegmented neutrophils) ≈ ↓ folate or ↓ vit B_{12}; target cells ≈ liver disease or thalassaemia; spherocytes ≈ hereditary spherocytosis or haemolysis; sickle cells ≈ SCD.

Iron deficiency anaemia (~26% of infants, worldwide;[215] peak age ~18 months.) This is despite fortification of formula, breakfast cereals, and noodles, etc.[216] Iron-deficient babies are less happy than others, with ↓ psychomotor development and poor cognition.[217] *Signs:* Pallor, lethargy, stomatitis, koilonychia, pica (p. 268). ∆∆: Poor diet (poverty, lack of education), malabsorption (coeliac disease, ↓vit C). In persistent IDA, suspect bleeding (menorrhagia, IBD, cow's milk protein allergy, Meckel's diverticulum). *R:* Trial of iron supplementation: ferrous fumarate syrup, or Sytron®. Aim for Hb rise of >10g/L/month (response confirms diagnosis). Warn of the dangers of overdosage, p. 277. In many places, the 1st step is deworming. *Prevention:* No cow's milk if <1yr; if formula-fed, use iron-fortified; wean at 4–6 months. Adequate vit C intake; iron supplements if premature.

Haemolysis Is malaria or SCD possible? Is the haemolysis intravascular haemolysis (haemoglobinuria) or extravascular (splenomegaly)? Is there an inborn error (haemoglobinopathy, membranopathy), or is the defect acquired (usually with +ve DAT—direct antiglobulin (Coombs) test)? *Hereditary spherocytosis* is the main cause of haemolysis in northern Europe (mainly autosomal dominant; spontaneous mutations in 25%). It is often mild. Splenectomy leads to ↑RBC survival and is sometimes indicated; gallstones may occur in the 1st decade, and if symptomatic cholecystectomy ± splenectomy may be needed.[218] *Hereditary elliptocytosis,* also autosomal dominant, is a similar but milder disease. *Sickle-cell disease (SCD):* OHCM p340. Autosomal recessive disorder causing production of abnormal β globin chains. HbS is produced instead of HbA (HbA₂ and HbF are still produced). Common in people of African origin, heterozygosity (sickle cell 'trait') confers some protection against falciparum malaria. Hypoxia causes polymerization of HbS and deformation of RBCs which can haemolyse or block small blood vessels. *Test:* Hb electrophoresis. *Complications:* Vaso-occlusive 'painful' crises, stroke, aplastic crises, sequestration crises. *R:* Antibiotic prophylaxis, pain control, hydration, hydroxycarbamide, transfusion programmes (+ iron chelation). Bone marrow transplant is curative but controversial.

Iron deficiency without anaemia

▶Don't think that if a child is not anaemic they are not iron deficient. CNS iron levels fall *before* RBC mass. If in doubt, check ferritin. Treating low ferritin may improve: • Memory • Lassitude • Developmental delay • Sleep • Mood • Cognition—in toddlers and adolescent girls, facing demands of puberty and menstruation. NB: pica (eating dirt, p. 268) is a sign of iron deficiency.

Non blanching rashes (NBR = petechiae or purpura)

▶**Key questions** Is the child well? Is there fever? Is the rash spreading rapidly?
- *If ill or rapidly spreading rash: Meningococcal septicaemia* (▶▶ceftriaxone, p. 201), *leukaemia*, or *disseminated intravascular coagulation* (check a visual non-automated blood film & WCC, discuss with lab); *haemolytic uraemic syndrome* (pp. 230–1).
- *If well looking + fever:* Do FBC, CRP, clotting, blood culture, glucose, and gas, whole blood PCR for meningococcus, and observe closely for signs of meningococcal sepsis.[14]
- *If well(ish) & platelets (plts)* ↔: Viruses eg measles; enteroviruses (95% petechial rashes will be viral);[219] HSP (see later); NAI (pp. 196–7); vigorous vomiting or coughing can cause petechiae in superior vena cava distribution; (rarely platelet function disorder).
- *If well & isolated ↓plts:* ITP (see later); hypersplenism; (rarely, Wiskott–Aldrich syndrome (p. 859) or Kasabach–Merritt syndrome—capillary haemangioma causing plt consumption).

Henoch–Schönlein purpura (HSP) An acute IgA complex-mediated vasculitis. Most patients have an antecedent URTI. The rash starts in dependent areas: ankles, backs of legs, buttocks. Δ· *Palpable* purpura (may be flat initially) plus 1 *or more of*: diffuse abdominal pain; acute arthritis or arthralgia (any joint); renal involvement (haematuria or proteinuria); IgA deposition on biopsy. ♂:♀ ≈ 1.3:1.[220] *Tests:* Urine dip—proteinuria (42%), BP, U&E, ESR↑ (57%), IgA↑ (37%), ASO titres ↑ (36%). C3, C4, ANCA. ℞: Simple analgesia. Most recover spontaneously in ≤2 months but monitor for haematuria, proteinuria, and ↑BP. Refer to nephrologist if abnormal renal function, ↑BP, >5 days' macroscopic haematuria, persistent proteinuria. Steroids may help resolve abdo pain,[221] but role in prevention of chronic kidney disease is less clear.[222] Recurrences, verified in 35%, correlate with ↑ESR. *Complications:* Intussusception; (massive) GI bleeds; and AKI (rare). Chronic kidney disease occurs in 5%.

Immune (idiopathic) thrombocytopenic purpura (ITP) The most common acquired bleeding disorder in childhood, autoantibodies destroy plts. *Presentation:* Well child with acute bruising, purpura, petechiae ± bleeding. Often a history of recent viral illness. *Tests:* Isolated ↓plts (<20×10⁹ in 80%); do a film to ensure no other abnormalities. Marrow is unnecessary, unless:[223]
- Unusual signs are present eg abnormal cells on a film, lymphadenopathy, significant mucosal bleeding, hepatosplenomegaly.
- Treatment is contemplated with steroids or immunoglobulin.

Intracranial haemorrhage occurs in <1% (mortality is 50%);[224] do CT if there is headache or CNS signs. *Acute ℞:* Mostly conservative, avoid contact sports, control menses, if severe bleeding: tranexamic acid, steroids, IVIg ± anti-D,[8] [211,212] (p. 11). Plt transfusions are reserved for life-threatening episodes as they are quickly consumed by the antibodies. 80% resolve over ~3 months with or without therapy. 20% become chronic (>6 months). *Chronic ℞:* Rituximab,[9] other immunosuppressants, and splenectomy are considered.

---

8 Anti-D: a single dose of 50mcg/kg IV ↑ platelet count to ≥20×10⁹/L in 70% of children within 3 days.

9 Rituximab can induce remission in ~30%. SE: T°↑, pruritus, throat tightness, serum sickness.

ALL is the commonest childhood cancer (~500 cases/yr[UK]); it is a malignant disorder of lymphoid progenitor cells. Other forms: OHCM pp354–59. Peak age is 2–6yrs, with a second peak >50yrs. Incidence is greater in white children than in black children. **Causes** Precise cause is unknown. There are genetic associations: ALL is concordant in ~25% of monozygotic twins; individuals with trisomy 21 have a 4-fold increased risk (also increased risk in Bloom syndrome, ataxia–telangiectasia). Chromosomal translocations such as t(12;21) resulting in the TEL-AML fusion gene are associated with 30% of cases (only present in 1% of the general population). t(9;22)—the Philadelphia chromosome—occurs in 15–30% (mostly adults) and is associated with a poor prognosis. Environmental risk factors which have been implicated include prenatal exposure to x-rays, *in utero* exposure to infection, delayed postnatal exposure to infection, and environmental radiation.[227, 228, 229]

Classification WHO classifies ALL into either b *lymphoblastic leukaemia* or t *lymphoblastic leukaemia*.[230] Prior to 2008 the term pre-B-cell ALL was used to distinguish B *lymphoblastic leukaemia* from mature B-cell ALL which is termed Burkitt lymphoma/leukaemia.

Presentation The period before diagnosis is often brief (2–4 weeks). Bone marrow infiltration → bone pain & pancytopenia: pallor; lethargy; (recurrent) infections; bruising, petechiae, bleeding. Reticuloendothelial infiltration → hepatomegaly; splenomegaly; painless, hard lymphadenopathy. Other organ infiltration → CNS: headache, vomiting, cranial nerve palsies; Testes: orchidomegaly ± general symptoms of fever, malaise, anorexia.

Tests *Bloods:* wcc↑, ↓, or ↔. Normochromic, normocytic anaemia ± platelets ↓, urate ↑, LDH↑. *Marrow:* 50–98% of nucleated cells will be blasts. *CSF:* Pleocytosis (with blast forms), protein ↑, glucose ↓. *Cytogenetic analysis:* 80% will have genetic abnormalities at diagnosis. CXR: May show mediastinal lymphadenopathy.

Prognosis Depends on clinical signs, biological features of lymphoblasts, and response to induction chemotherapy. Based on these features patients can be stratified into 4 risk categories. *Standard risk:* Patients are aged 1–9.9yrs, have wcc of <50×10⁹/L; lack unfavourable cytogenetic features, show a good response to initial chemotherapy, and have <5% bone marrow blasts by 14 days and <0.01% blasts by 28 days. *Low risk:* These patients meet the standard risk criteria and have favourable genetics, such as trisomy 4, 10, or 17. *High risk:* Patients do not meet standard criteria or have extramedullary involvement (eg brain/ testis). *Very high risk:* Have unfavourable genetics, such as the Philadelphia chromosome, hypodiploidy—or poor response to initial chemotherapy. *Eventfree survival:* At 5yrs is 95% in the low-risk group; 30% in the very high risk. Infant leukaemia has the worst outcome: 20%. Overall survival is 80%. Minimum residual disease (MRD) <0.01% at end of induction chemotherapy (seen in >40%) is associated with excellent prognosis (97% survival at 10yrs).

Treatment Typically has 3 phases: *Induction therapy:* 3-drug induction over 4 weeks (eg vincristine, dexamethasone,[231] asparaginase) + intrathecal (IT) therapy (methotrexate ± cytarabine + hydrocortisone) results in remission of >95%. High-risk patients may get a further agent eg daunorubicin.[230] ~2% die of infection. *Consolidation phase:* Cranial irradiation if known CNS disease. Further chemotherapy (eg cyclophosphamide; cytarabine; mercaptopurine). *Maintenance phase:* For ~2½yrs (daily mercaptopurine + weekly methotrexate ± vincristine/steroid pulses). 3-monthly intrathecal drugs.

Complications ►► *Neutropenic sepsis:* See BOX '►►Febrile neutropenia'. Cotrimoxazole prevents pneumocystosis. *Revaccinate* (1 dose of each type, p. 257) 6 months after chemotherapy (as vaccine-specific antibody ↓).[232] *Hyperuricaemia:* From massive cell death at induction: pre-treat with ↑ fluid intake + allopurinol. *Poor growth:* Monitor carefully.[233] *Cancer elsewhere:* Risk of CNS tumours or a 2nd leukaemia is 3%.

Pitfalls ►Ignoring quality of life; eg most cytotoxics may be given at home • Omitting to examine the testes (►a common site for recurrence) • Thiopurine methyltransferase deficiency may cause fatal myelosuppression (test prior to treating)[234] • Inappropriate transfusion (leucostasis, *OHCM* p354, if WCC >100×10⁹/L)[235] • SE of chemotherapy. NB: ondansetron is better than other antiemetics.

►►Febrile neutropenia

Children on anticancer treatment who are neutropenic (neutrophils ≤0.5×10⁹/L[236]) are at high risk for overwhelming sepsis. Emphasize to the parents and child the importance of urgent treatment. A recent FBC may not be available but any child on anticancer treatment with a fever >38°C is treated as *neutropenic sepsis* until deemed otherwise.

Initial management: Take cultures and start parenteral antibiotics ASAP (<60min): blood cultures (ideally peripheral and central); MSU; CXR if respiratory symptoms; swab all orifices and central line site; swab for respiratory viruses; FBC, U&E, LFTs, lactate, CRP, & serology. Follow local protocols for empiric antibiotic therapy. NICE recommends monotherapy with piperacillin–tazobactam, and to add gentamicin only if per patient specific or local protocol. Some units may use meropenem or imipenem ± teicoplanin. Central line infection should be considered but don't remove the line immediately. Liaise with child's oncology centre.

Further management: Child should be managed in hospital with care overseen by a clinician with experience in paediatric oncology until it is apparent whether this is a serious infection or not. If investigations and clinical course show likely viral or other low-risk infection, child may be discharged ± oral antibiotics. If blood culture is ve, other tests are inconclusive, and child has been afebrile for >24h, the antibiotics will often be continued empirically for 5 days. If blood culture does prove +ve, review antibiotic choice and duration with microbiological advice and oncology centre. If child continues to spike fevers, or becomes more unwell consider viral or fungal infections, line infection. Further investigations may be necessary, consider adding an antifungal (eg amphotericin) or aciclovir, liaise with the child's oncology centre.

Likely organisms: In one UK study, blood cultures were +ve in 30%. Grampositive organisms predominated (80%) and most were coagulase-negative staphs. 6% were Gram-negative isolates and <1% fungal.[237]

Primary immunodeficiencies (PIDs) are a group of disorders causing increased risk of infection and malignancy, many are X-linked or autosomal recessive and our understanding is rapidly evolving. The pattern and severity of clinical disease varies with the part of the immune system affected. They are important to recognize early as treatment can prevent life-threatening complications.

Presentation The neonate is usually protected by maternal antibodies so PIDs usually present after the first months of life with recurrent infections. Features to help differentiate PIDs from common multiple infections seen in infancy: faltering growth; family history of PID/consanguinity; unusual pathogens in unusual locations; persistent candidiasis; non-healing wounds; ≥2 episodes of pneumonia in a year; ≥2 episodes of meningitis or sepsis ever; complications with live vaccines; chronic sinusitis; chronic diarrhoea; absent tonsils.

Tests FBC, differential, and film; U&E; CRP/ESR; cultures; immunoglobulin levels (vary significantly with age); lymphocyte subsets (T and B-cells, monocytes, and natural killer cells); vaccine responses (measuring specific Igs); ± HIV. If tests are abnormal or there is strong suspicion of PID then refer to a paediatric immunologist.

ΔΔ Normal, a child with siblings or attending day care may have 12 self-limiting viral infections in a year; atopy, allergic rhinitis, or asthma may be misdiagnosed as infection; FII (pp. 196-7); chronic disease (eg CF, GORD with aspiration, congenital heart disease); acquired immunodeficiency (HIV, malignancy, drugs).

Management Treat infections promptly and aggressively. Prophylactic antibiotics may be considered. Issues around vaccination are complex and vary by disorder, avoid live vaccines. Caution with blood products as fatal graft vs host disease can occur in those with T-cell deficiency (use leucodepleted/irradiated blood products). Immunoglobulin replacement obviates most complications and is best delivered by an immunologist, after detailed assessment. The dose of immunoglobulin (IV or SC) is determined by the severity and frequency of infections, and the plasma level of IgG. SE: Headaches, abdominal pain, anaphylaxis. Have adrenaline, hydrocortisone, and an antihistamine at the ready.

Immune reconstitution *Haematopoietic stem cell transplantation (HSCT):* Provides a cure for certain PIDs including SCID (see later). Overall survival is 74% at 5yrs.[238] There is likely to be a limitation to initiation of normal thymopoiesis, HSCT at a younger age is associated with better outcomes. Absence of infection prior to or at time of HSCT is also associated with better outcomes. *Gene therapy:* Autologous (ie patient's own) haematopoietic stem cells transduced with the γc gene can restore immune system in children with SCID. A harmless retrovirus carries the replacement gene, and infects the stem cells *in vitro*. When these are replaced in the marrow an immune system develops within a few months.[10] It is an alternative to bone marrow transplants (eg if no HLA match can be found). Thymic transplant has been used with some success in infants with DiGeorge syndrome.

Complications *Chest:* Bronchiectasis, granulomas, lymphoma. *Gut:* Malabsorption, giardia, cholangitis, atrophic gastritis, colitis. *Liver:* Acquired hepatitis, chronic active hepatitis, biliary cirrhosis. *Blood:* Autoimmune haemolysis, ITP (p. 241), anaemia of chronic disease, aplasia. *Eyes/CNS:* Keratoconjunctivitis, uveitis, granulomas, encephalitis. *Others:* Septic arthropathy, arthralgia, splenomegaly.

Severe combined immunodeficiency (SCID) A syndrome of impaired cellular and humoral immunity caused by a heterogeneous group of inherited disorders. T-cell dysfunction usually causes combined immunodeficiency as T cells are necessary for B-cell differentiation. Perhaps the most important PID to recognize as, untreated, it is universally fatal in the 1st year of life. Presentation is in the 1st 6 months of life with faltering growth and severe, persistent, unusual infections. Newborn screening is possible and done in some US states but not the UK. *Treatment:* Stem cell transplant; gene therapy. *Prevalence:* ~1 in 50,000–75,000.[239]

3 Paediatrics

Other primary immunodeficiencies

IgA deficiency (IgA↓ + normal or ↑ levels of other immunoglobulins). It is the most common primary antibody deficiency. Many are asymptomatic. It may accompany CVID (see later). Patients tend to develop respiratory infections which may lead to bronchiectasis. Gastrointestinal infection (eg giardiasis) and disorders such as malabsorption, coeliac disease, ulcerative colitis are associated with IgA deficiency. Although rare, all blood products (incl. IVIg) can lead to severe, even fatal, anaphylaxis due to the presence of IgA. Ideally blood products if needed should be obtained from an IgA-deficient individual—or washed red cells given. Patients are recommended to wear a medical alert bracelet because of this.[240] *Prevalence:* Varies with ethnicity: 1 in 143 in Middle East; 1 in 875 in UK; 1 in 18,500 in Japan.[240]

Transient hypogammaglobulinaemia of infancy Temporary delay in antibody production. Onset: 3–6 months. It is more severe than normal antibody deficiency that happens at this age. Immunoglobulin levels become normal by 2–4yrs. *Prevalence:* ~1 in 10,000.[241]

Common variable immunodeficiency (CVID) (IgG↓, IgA↓, IgM variable). *Onset:* 2nd to 3rd decade of life. Enlarged tonsils, splenomegaly, gastrointestinal disease, liver dysfunction, and cancer (esp. lymphoma) may be present. *Prevalence:* ~1 in 10,000–50,000.[242]

Bruton x-linked agammaglobulinaemia Tyrosine kinase gene mutation (Xq21) causes ↓ mature B cells →↓ plasma cells →↓ immunoglobulins,[243] hence ↑ susceptibility to bacterial (but not viral) infections. *Onset:* 3 months–3yrs.[244] Also: arthropathy + absent Peyer's patches, tonsils, and appendix. *Prevalence:* ~1 in 250,000 males (the commonest inherited antibody deficiency).[243] *R:* HSCT or Immunoglobulin replacement therapy. Beware septicaemia and CNS infections (may require interferon alfa and high-dose IV immunoglobulin).[245] After marrow transplantation serum immunoglobulin rises to normal levels over ~3 months.[246]

IgG subclass deficiency There are ↓ levels of 1 or more of 4 subclasses of IgG. Total IgG levels may be normal. IgG₂↓ is the most common and often is associated with IgA↓, and ataxia–telangiectasia.

Chronic granulomatous disease A genetic defect of phagocytic cells (macrophages, neutrophils, and monocytes) leaving them unable to destroy certain bacteria and fungi. Life-threatening infections and granuloma formation occurs. *Test:* Neutrophil function tests (NBT reduction test—nitroblue tetrazolium). *R:* Antibiotic prophylaxis; HSCT; gene therapy.

Syndromes associated with immunodeficiency DiGeorge (22q deletion) p. 846; ataxia–telangiectasia; Wiskott–Aldrich p. 859; among many others.

---

10 T cells & repertoires of T-cell receptors were ~normal up to 2yrs post-op; thymopoiesis is shown by naive T cells. Antibody production is adequate.

3 Paediatrics

Type 1 DM The 3rd most common chronic disease in UK children (after asthma and cerebral palsy). It is an autoimmune disorder caused by T-cell-mediated destruction of pancreatic beta-cells, leading to insulin deficiency and hyperglycaemia. Genetic and environmental factors are implicated in its development, particularly the insulin-dependent diabetes mellitus (IDDM1) gene locus, part of the HLA DR/DQ locus on the major histocompatibility complex. Peak age of onset is 5–7yrs (but increasing in toddlers) and just before or at the onset of puberty, especially during winter. Good care of the child with diabetes requires involving the whole family unit *and* carers at school.

Presentation: Several weeks of polyuria, polydipsia, lethargy, and weight loss ± infection, poor growth; DKA (see p. 248). Secondary nocturnal enuresis is a classic presentation. *Diagnosis:* Based on WHO criteria:[247] symptomatic with ↑ venous blood glucose, ie ≥11.1mmol/L (random) or ≥7mmol/L (fasting), or raised venous blood glucose on 2 occasions without symptoms. Children with suspected DM should be referred **the same day** to a paediatric diabetes MDT. OGTT is rarely required and HbA1c should not be used for diagnosis in children. *ΔΔ:* Most children have T1DM. Consider T2DM in children with: obesity (p. 266), Asian (↑ risk ×13) or black ethnicity, no or very low insulin requirement after the 'honeymoon' period, strong FH T2DM or evidence of insulin resistance (eg acanthosis nigricans). C-peptide, islet cell autoantibody, anti-insulin antibody, anti-glutamic acid decarboxylase antibody, and anti-IA2 should not be used at presentation to distinguish T1 and T2DM. Consider monogenic or mitochondrial DM in children with: diagnosis in 1st year of life, absence of ketonaemia during hyperglycaemia, or syndromic features.

R: Complex and should be led by a multidisciplinary paediatric diabetes team providing 24h access to advice.[248, NICE] If not in DKA, children do not need IV fluids or hospitalization at diagnosis. All children should be supplied with blood glucose and ketone meters and test strips. Psychosocial aspects are important. Education of the child, family, and carers is key. Inform children and parents that they may experience a partial remission phase ('honeymoon period') with the start of insulin.

Insulin regimens:
• 'Basal bolus': a combination of regular daily longer-acting insulin with 'carb counting' and short- or rapid-acting insulin before meals. Most common/standard regimen.
• Continuous subcutaneous insulin infusion (CSII), an 'insulin pump'.
• 1–3 regular injections of mixed insulin (short- or rapid-acting insulin mixed in fixed ratio with intermediate-acting insulin).

Insulin requirements: 0.5–0.75 units/kg/24h is a sensible starting dose at diagnosis.[249] If using basal bolus regimen this total daily dose (TDD) should be split ½ as basal insulin and ½ as rapid-acting insulin in 3 divided doses before meals. If using mixed insulins usually ⅔ of the total daily dose is given pre breakfast, and ⅓ pre dinner. Insulin doses should be adjusted based on general trends.

Hypoglycaemia: Children, family members, and carers must know how to avoid, recognize, and manage hypoglycaemia. See BOX.

'Sick day rules': Illness generally increases blood glucose (BG) level (stress hormones) and the risk of ketosis.[250] There is usually relative insulin deficiency (never stop insulin) and intensive self-monitoring of BG and ketones with additional insulin doses during illness can avoid hospitalization. If negative blood ketones (<0.6mmol/L) and high BG take an insulin 'correction dose' in addition to normal insulin. If blood ketones are moderate (0.6–1.5mmol/L) take 10% of TDD or 0.1 units/kg fast-acting insulin. If ketones are high (>1.5mmol/L) take 20% of TDD or 0.2 units/kg fast-acting insulin. In all cases recheck BG and ketones in 2h and act on results. Keep well hydrated with sugar-free fluids. If not tolerating anything orally, hospitalization likely to be needed. D&V may cause hypoglycaemia or rarely 'starvation' ketones with normal BG. In D&V give sugar-containing fluids and fast-acting insulin may need to be decreased.

Targets: ≥5 capillary BG tests/day. Target 4–7mmol/L on waking and pre-meals, 5–9mmol/L 2h after meals. Measure HbA1c x4/y. Target ≤48mmol/mol (6.5%) while avoiding hypoglycaemia is ideal to minimize the risk of long-term complications but should be individualized to child/family circumstances.[251]

Real-time continuous glucose monitors with alarms are available and useful in neonates, infants, pre-schoolers and children with difficult BG control or inability to recognize or communicate hypoglycaemia symptoms.

Screening: Screen for coeliac and thyroid disease at diagnosis and annually thereafter.[251] Optician review every 2 years. From 12 years of age monitor annually for hypertension, albuminuria, and diabetic retinopathy. Be aware of rare complications; juvenile cataracts, necrobiosis lipoidica (a granulomatous skin disease), and Addison disease.

Hypoglycaemia

▶▶ *Signs and symptoms:* sympathetic—weakness, dizziness, shaking, palpitations, sweating, anxiety, hunger, vomiting. Neuroglycopenic—confusion, headache, blurred vision, lethargy, coma, convulsions. Also agitation, irritability, and other behavioural changes.

▶▶ *Mild or moderate episodes:* immediately give 10–20g of **fast-acting glucose** by mouth followed by (unless on CSII) a complex long-acting carbohydrate. If uncooperative or unable to eat, give oral glucose gel.

▶▶ *Sublingual 'kitchen' sugar* may be used as an immediate 'first aid' measure in managing hypoglycaemia. Place 1 level teaspoon of sugar moistened with water under the tongue every 10–12min until stable.

▶▶ *In hospital setting,* treat severe hypoglycaemia with 5mL/kg IV 10% **glucose**.

▶▶ *Severe hypoglycaemia out of hospital,* give GLUCAGON 1mg IM (500mcg if <8yrs or <25kg); Get help.

Expect quick return to consciousness. Recheck BG <15min; if low, repeat therapy, get help; if normal, ask yourself *is this is a post-ictal state after a hypoglycaemic fit?* Here, giving more glucose worsens cerebral oedema.

MODY: maturity-onset diabetes of the young

MODY is an autosomal dominant kind of non-ketotic diabetes, in childhood, or young adults.[252] The defect is one of pancreatic beta-cell dysfunction—leading to impaired insulin secretion.[253] MODY is caused by single gene defects, as opposed to T1 & T2DM which have polygenic and environmental causes. Classic MODY accounts for <5% of all diabetes in white children.[254]

MODY2 (GCK subtype) Caused by mutations in the glucokinase gene on chromosome 7. Glucokinase converts glucose to glucose-6-phosphate, which is needed to stimulate insulin secretion by the beta-cells. There is mild, asymptomatic, stable hyperglycaemia from birth. Complications are rare. Drugs are rarely needed.

MODY3 (HNF1A subtype) The most common type. It is caused by a defect on chromosome 12 leading to a progressive decrease in insulin production. It features severe hyperglycaemia after puberty, which often leads to a diagnosis of T1DM. Despite progressive hyperglycaemia, sensitivity to sulfonylureas is retained for years. Some children may be able to stop insulin (previously assumed to be lifelong treatment). Diabetic retinopathy and nephropathy often occur in MODY3. Frequency of cardiovascular disease is not increased. Owing to the pleiotropic character of transcription factors, most MODY subtypes are diseases with multiorgan involvement in addition to diabetes.

MODY5 (HNF-1B) More frequent than originally thought. It is associated with pancreatic atrophy, renal abnormalities, and genital tract malformations.

MODY1, 4, & 6 These subtypes of MODY are all rare.

Molecular diagnosis This matters because it has important consequences for prognosis, family screening, and management. Although MODY is dominantly inherited, expression varies, so a family history of DM is not always present.

Just 100 years ago, DKA was universally fatal. The 1st patient to receive insulin (on 11 January 1922), was Leonard Thompson—a 14yr-old boy, who went on to live a further 13 years. DKA results from a deficiency of insulin, often in combination with increased levels of counter-regulatory hormones (catecholamines, glucagon, cortisol, and growth hormone—eg due to sepsis). Children die from DKA, from cerebral oedema, hypokalaemia, or aspiration pneumonia.

The patient History of polyuria; polydipsia; weight loss; abdominal pain; vomiting; lethargy. *Look for:* Degree of dehydration; Kussmaul respiration (deep and rapid); ketotic (fruity-smelling) breath; signs of infection; shock. DKA is all too often the 1st presentation of diabetes.

Diagnosis Requires both •Acidosis (blood PH <7.3 or plasma bicarbonate <18mmol/L), and •Ketonaemia (>3 mmol/L, if blood ketones unavailable, urinary ketones can be used for diagnosis). Hyperglycaemia (≥11mmol/L) while expected may be absent in known diabetics with DKA.

▲▲ Hyperosmolar hyperglycaemic state, very high BG (>30 mmol/L), little or no acidosis or ketones. Requires different management—get help.

Management While DKA is an emergency, metabolic derangement has built up over time and the emphasis of management is slow correction of this derangement to avoid cerebral oedema. The trend is away from rapid fluid infusion.[11] Severity of DKA is categorized by degree of acidosis: mild or moderate—pH >7.1; severe—pH <7. 1 Follow local or national protocols and ask for senior help.

- *Resuscitate: ABC:* give 10mL/kg 0.9% NaCl bolus only if shocked. If still in shock after 1 bolus, consult with senior, consider sepsis, and consider inotropes or a 2nd 10mL/kg bolus.
- *Rapidly confirm diagnosis:* With history, BG, blood gas (incl. Na+, K+), blood ketones (urine dip if point-of-care testing unavailable, ≥2+ ketones).
- *Monitoring:* Frequent (<30min) GCS (p. 590; p. 200 if <4yrs), ECG monitoring (look for peaked T-waves of hyperkalaemia).
- *Use severity of acidosis to assess dehydration:* pH >7.1 assume 5% dehydration, pH <7.1 assume 10% dehydration.
- *Start IV fluids:* Requirement = fluid deficit + maintenance fluids. Fluid deficit should be corrected over 48h. Use lower fluid maintenance rates than APLS (see worked example). Start with 0.9% NaCl + 40mmol KCl/L.
- *Formal investigations:* Weight; FBC; U&E; lab glucose; Ca²⁺; consider infection screen.
- *Start IV insulin only after 1–2h of fluids:* Cerebral oedema may be more likely if insulin is started early. Do not give IV insulin bolus. Start infusion of fast-acting insulin at 0.05–0.1 units/kg/h. When venous glucose is <14mmol/L, do not stop insulin (it is still required to switch off ketogenesis), change IV fluids to use 0.9% NaCl + 5% glucose + 40mmol KCl/L.
- *Ongoing monitoring:* Hourly blood glucose, hourly fluid balance, 1–2 hourly blood ketones, U&E + lab glucose + blood gases 2h, then 4h. Weigh twice daily.
- *Stopping IV insulin:* When blood ketone levels are <1.0mmol/L, and patient is able to tolerate food. Give a dose of subcutaneous insulin; feed the patient. Stop infusion 30–60min after subcutaneous insulin injection.

Pitfalls in diabetic ketoacidosis

Cerebral oedema (see MINIBOX 'Cerebral oedema') is the big threat, and is almost exclusively a condition of childhood. It occurs in ~1% of childhood DKA and has a mortality of ~25%. Pathophysiology is poorly understood but more common in young age, new diagnosis, bicarbonate therapy, and with rapid fall in glucose or sodium. It usually occurs 4–12h from start of treatment, but it may be present at onset of DKA or up to 24h afterwards, presenting as a sudden CNS deterioration after initial improvement. *Aspiration pneumonia*—prevent using NGT if semi-conscious. *Potassium*—even if initial K⁺ is normal, child is whole body K⁺ deplete and K⁺ will drop when insulin is started so include 20mmol of K⁺ in every 500mL bag. *Persistent acidosis*—consider ↑ insulin dose, sepsis, hyperchloraemic acidosis, salicylate, or other poisoning. *Leucocytosis* may occur without any infection. *Infection* (there may be no fever)—do MSU, blood cultures, and

Cerebral oedema
Warning signs: headache, agitation, irritability, ↓ pulse, ↑BP (↑ICP), focal neurology (CN palsies), posturing, or falling consciousness:
▸▸ Call your senior.
▸▸ Exclude hypoglycaemia.
▸▸ Hypertonic saline 3–5 mL/kg of 2.7% NaCl over 10–15min.
▸▸ Mannitol (20% 0.5–1g/kg over 10–15min) if no 2.7% NaCl.
▸▸ Restrict IV maintenance fluids by ½ and replace deficit over 72h.
▸▸ Move to PICU and do CT.

CXR. Start broad-spectrum antibiotics if infection suspected. *Creatinine*—some assays for creatinine cross-react with ketone bodies, so plasma creatinine may not reflect true renal function. *Ketonuria* does not equate with ketoacidosis and drop in urine ketones may lag significantly behind blood ketones. Serum amylase is often raised (up to 10-fold), and non-specific abdominal pain is common even in the absence of pancreatitis.

Calculating fluid requirement in DKA

Hourly rate = (48h maintenance + deficit – boluses given in excess of 20mL/kg) ÷ 48

The BSPED suggests the following maintenance requirements based on weight (lower than APLS rates):

<10kg	2mL/kg/h
10–40kg	1mL/kg/h
>40kg	40mL/kg/h

A 20kg 6-year-old boy who is in severe DKA (pH <7.1 therefore 10% dehydrated), and who has already had 30mL/kg of 0.9% NaCl will require:

(48h maintenance + deficit – boluses in excess 20mL/kg) ÷ 48

$\approx$ 1mL/kg/h × 20kg × 48 (as 48h) + (100mL/kg × 20kg) – (10mL × 20kg) ÷ 48

$\approx$ (960mL + 2000mL – 200mL) ÷ 48

$\approx$ 2760mL ÷ 48 = 57.5mL/h

Hypothyroidism Virtually every cell in the body requires thyroid hormone, which controls cell metabolism and is necessary for growth and neurological development. Dysfunction may occur in the neonate, infant, or during childhood.

Congenital hypothyroidism 2 main groups:
- *Thyroid dysgenesis* (85%).
- *Dyshormonogenesis* (15%).

Also consider maternal antithyroid drugs (p. 28) and maternal iodine (I_2) deficiency (rare in the UK but common worldwide).

Signs: Mostly non-specific or develop late on, hence the crucial role of screening. Prolonged neonatal jaundice, widely opened posterior fontanelle, poor feeding, hypotonia, and dry skin are common. Inactivity, excessive sleepiness, slow feeding, hoarse cry, and constipation may occur.

Late signs: Coarse dry hair, a flat nasal bridge, a protruding tongue, hypotonia, umbilical hernia, slowly relaxing deep tendon reflexes (DTRs), pulse ↓. Untreated it leads to poor growth and cognitive disability. See fig 3.17.

Other later signs: IQ↓, delayed puberty (occasionally precocious), short stature, delayed dentition.[255]

Universal newborn screening: Day 5 dried blood spot. UK programme screens for elevated TSH so detects primary hypothyroidism but not the much rarer secondary or 'central' hypothyroidism.

Tests: ↓T_4, ↑TSH, thyroid imaging (US or radionucleotide scanning).

Acquired hypothyroidism Causes are divided into primary and secondary.
- *Primary:* prematurity; Hashimoto's thyroiditis (associated with: trisomy 21, T1DM, coeliac disease, Turner syndrome); I_2 deficiency; drugs (lithium, amiodarone): irradiation (haematopoietic stem cell transplantation—HSCT), post ablative (radioiodine, surgery).
- *Secondary:* hypopituitarism (intracranial tumours, cranial irradiation or surgery, developmental pituitary defects).

Signs: Insidious onset, weight gain, goitre, fatigue, constipation, bradycardia, cold intolerance, decreased height velocity, deteriorating school performance, dry skin, brittle hair, delayed relaxation of DTRs. High index of suspicion is needed.

Tests: T_4, TSH, thyroid antibody screen (anti-TPO, anti-thyroglobulin, blocking type TSH receptor Ab) ± pituitary function and imaging if secondary hypothyroidism.

Management Lifelong **levothyroxine** (LT_4): start neonates with ~15mcg/kg/day; adjust by 5mcg/kg every 2 weeks to a typical dose of 20–50mcg/day. <2yrs start with 5mcg/kg/day (max. 50mcg) adjust by 10–25mcg every 2–4 weeks; >2yrs start with 50mcg and adjust by 25mcg every 2–4 weeks.[256,257] Adjust according to growth and clinical state. Aim for high-normal T_4 and low-normal TSH levels.

Causes Graves disease; autoimmune thyroiditis (Hashimoto's); thyroid nodules, adenomas and carcinomas (rare).

Signs Hyperactivity, irritability, tachycardia, palpitations, tremor, anxiety, heat intolerance, diarrhoea, hyperreflexia, weight loss despite increased appetite, menstrual irregularity. *Specific to Graves disease:* exophthalmos/proptosis, lid lag, ophthalmoplegia.

Tests ↓TSH, ↑T_4. Radionucleotide thyroid scan.

Management 2 main strategies:
1 *Dose titration* with antithyroid drugs carbimazole or propylthiouracil.
2 *Block and replace*—induce complete thyroid suppression and replace with LT_4 to achieve euthyroidism.

Ablative treatment with radioiodine or thyroid surgery may also be considered particularly for multiple relapses.

Transient neonatal thyrotoxicosis Occurs in neonates born to mothers with Graves disease. TSH receptor-stimulating antibodies cross the placenta and cause transient thyrotoxicosis in the newborn.

Signs: Flushing, sweating, irritability, poor weight gain, tachycardia, and heart failure. Self-limiting but antithyroid drugs and supportive treatment may be required.

Other endocrine disorders Congenital adrenal hyperplasia, see p. 302; syndrome of inappropriate ADH secretion (SIADH), see p. 313.

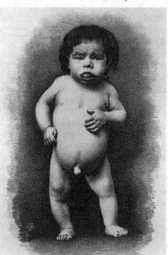

Fig 3.17 Cretinism was the term used to describe those affected by congenital hypothyroidism. The word is thought to originate from an Alpine dialect. Congenital hypothyroidism was common in mountainous regions due to a lack of dietary iodine. Iodine is needed to synthesize thyroxine and while found in many foods, the soil in mountainous regions is often iodine deficient. The resultant maternal hypothyroidism was a leading cause of congenital hypothyroidism. Typical features include short stature, coarse facial features, protruding tongue, and umbilical hernia.
Wellcome Collection.

3 Paediatrics

IMDs Involve a genetic defect (any mode of inheritance) that causes an enzyme in a cellular cycle to be dysfunctional or absent. This causes a 'block' in a metabolic pathway resulting in a lack of product from the pathway and/or a build-up of an intermediate compound that is toxic to the cell. Individually IMDs are rare diseases, but there are >1000 defined IMDs, a number that continues to increase. The most common IMDs, such as phenylketonuria (PKU) and medium-chain acyl-CoA dehydrogenase deficiency (MCADD) have an incidence of around 1 in 10,000. However, the incidence of combined IMDs is estimated at 1 in 800.

Presentation IMDs can present in almost any fashion, but it is most important to consider IMD in the acutely unwell child, as prompt diagnosis and treatment of IMD can drastically improve outcome. Common scenarios in which IMD should be considered include: the acutely unwell child, hyperammonaemia, and hypoglycaemia. Other considerations: see table 3.10.

The acutely unwell child Consider IMD in the ΔΔ of any acutely unwell child who does not have a clear diagnosis or is not responding to standard therapy. The acute presentation of IMDs is often non-specific and initially mistaken for sepsis. Types of IMD that can present in this manner include the organic acidaemias, urea cycle defects, and fat oxidation defects. *Red flags* that ↑ suspicion of IMD: neonatal presentation with short period (few days) of well-being/feeding prior to presentation; previous episodes triggered by illness/fasting (including cyclical vomiting); change in diet precipitating presentation (eg weaning); positive FH; consanguinity.

Tests Should include the following: blood gas; lactate; glucose; blood (or urine) ketones; ammonia; LFTs; CK. If an IMD is suspected, discuss urgently with an IMD centre, consider: plasma amino acids; acylcarnitine profile; urine organic acids. Consider sending DNA and skin biopsy if a child may not survive.

Management Includes stopping feeds containing potentially toxic substrate (protein, fat) while providing adequate energy to promote anabolism. Recognition and prompt treatment of hyperammonaemia and hypoglycaemia is also critical.

▸▸**Hyperammonaemia** is a medical emergency and should be discussed urgently with an IMD team. It causes cerebral oedema and ↑ICP. Outcome is dependent on degree and duration of hyperammonaemia. Unfortunately, delayed recognition is common and leads to severe neurodisability and death. Prompt measurement of blood ammonia level is crucial in all children presenting with unexplained drowsiness or encephalopathy. *Presentation:* Lethargy, vomiting, and altered conscious level that progresses to coma. Ammonia is a respiratory stimulant, so patients will often be tachypnoeic in early stages with a respiratory alkalosis. ΔΔ: Urea cycle defects; organic acidaemias; fat oxidation defects; and non-IMD (liver failure, poor sampling).

Hypoglycaemia Plasma glucose concentration low enough to cause signs and symptoms of impaired brain function. There are many causes of hypoglycaemia, IMD only representing a small portion. *Other causes:* Very ill child (sepsis, liver failure); fasting; hyperinsulinism; growth hormone deficiency; cortisol deficiency; hypothyroidism; ketotic hypoglycaemia; drugs; alcohol. Hypoglycaemia caused by an IMD is usually precipitated by fasting. Fasting tolerance can be as little as 90min (eg GSD1) or be relatively normal, only apparent when fasting is extended beyond normal, such as with intercurrent illness (eg fat oxidation defects). *Tests:* It is important to obtain samples at the time of ↓ glucose to aid Δ. However, this should not delay the emergency management (2–5mL/kg IV 10% **glucose** if ↓ consciousness). Lab glucose; 3βbetahydroxybutyrate (or bedside ketone measurement or ketones in 1st urine after episode); free fatty acids; lactate; LFTs; U&E; urine organic acids; acylcarnitine profile; plasma amino acids; insulin; c-peptide; ± cortisol; ± growth hormone; ± ammonia.

The glycogen storage disorders (GSDs) Result from defects in enzymes required for the synthesis and degradation of glycogen. Abnormal stores are deposited in liver, muscle, heart, or kidney. In some types there are CNS effects. Most types (there are >12) are autosomal recessive. There is considerable variability in severity and prognosis. Early diagnosis and treatment are important to minimize organ damage. Types include: von Gierke disease (type I, p. 859), Pompe disease (type II, p. 856), Cori disease (type III—hypoglycaemia, hepatomegaly, with faltering growth), Anderson disease (type IV), McArdle disease (type V), Hers disease (type VI), and Tauri disease (type VII). In McArdle's, (most common GSD in adolescents), the cause is myophosphorylase deficiency. Stiffness and myalgia follow exercise. Venous blood from exercised muscle shows ↓ levels of lactate & pyruvate. ↓ phosphorylase staining in muscle biopsy confirms diagnosis. There may be myoglobinuria. *Treatment:* Depends on type: specialized diets; enzyme replacement therapy; no extreme exercise; prevention of hypoglycaemia eg with bedtime meal of slowly digested complex carbohydrates (uncooked cornstarch).

Table 3.10 Signs which may indicate the presence of an IMD

Sign	Possible significance
Hepatosplenomegaly	Amino acid and organic acid disorders, lysosomal storage diseases (Anderson–Fabry disease)[11]
Coarse facies	Mucopolysaccharidoses, eg Hurler syndrome, p. 850, gangliosidoses, mannosidoses
Hypoglycaemia	Many diseases eg von Gierke syndrome; MCADD[12]
Faltering growth	Aminoacidurias, organic aciduria, cystinuria, lactic acidosis, storage diseases
Other	'Odd' body smells; developmental regression; consanguinity; multiple miscarriages or unexplained infant deaths

PKU (phenylalanine ketonuria)

Cause: Mutation of phenylalanine hydroxylase (PAH) gene (chromosome 1—autosomal recessive) leading to absent or reduced activity of phenylalanine hydroxylase. Classic PKU leads to gradual cognitive impairment. The defect leads to ↓CNS dopamine, reduced protein synthesis, and demyelination.[258] *Clinical features:* Fair hair, fits, eczema, musty urine. The chief manifestation is ↓IQ (eg dyscalculia ± poor spelling ± ↓cognition).[259] *Tests:* Detected in UK on newborn screening. Hyperphenylalaninaemia (reference interval: 50–120µmol/L). Treatment instigated in infants with levels >360µmol/L—to avoid ↓↓IQ which may start with levels of >394µmol/L.[260] *Treatment:* Dietary restriction with phenylalanine-free protein substitute enriched in tyrosine and <300mg–8g of natural protein/day (depending on age and severity of deficiency).[261] Aim to keep phenylalanine levels <360µmol/L.[262] Requires expert team and regular monitoring. Despite treatment, children are more prone to depression, anxiety, phobic tendencies, isolation, and a less 'masculine' self-image.[263] Adherence to the diet may be poor (it's unpalatable).[264]

Urine amino acids ↑ in:
- Alkaptonuria
- Canavan leucodystrophy
- Cystinosis
- Cystathioninuria
- Fructose intolerance
- Galactosaemia
- Hartnup disease
- Homocystinuria
- Hyperammonaemia

Maternal phenylketonuria: ▶Preconception counselling is vital. Effects on the baby: facial dysmorphism, microcephaly, growth retardation, IQ↓.

---

11 Anderson–Fabry disease may present with torturing, lancinating pains in the extremities (± abdomen) made worse by cold, heat, or exercise. It is a neuritis (vasculitis of the vasa nervorum). By adolescence, angiokeratomata appear (clusters of dark, non-blanching, petechiae) in the 'bathing trunk' area (esp. umbilicus & scrotum). Also: paraesthesiae, corneal opacities, hypohidrosis, proteinuria, and renal failure. It may respond to enzyme R (α-galactosidase is ↓). Carbamazepine may help the pain.

12 MCAD deficiency is screened for in neonates on the same sample as for PKU & hypothyroidism. It's an autosomal recessive (mutation of the medium-chain acyl-coa dehydrogenase gene; ACADM; 1p31). Signs: hypoketotic hypoglycaemic coma; metabolic acidosis; LFT↑; medium-chain dicarboxylic aciduria; 'SIDS'. ♀♂ ≈1:1. R: avoid fasting; diet to give more calories from carbohydrates & proteins, while minimizing lipids. It is the chief inherited disorder of mitochondrial fatty acid oxidation in N. Europe. Carrier rate: 1:65.

Puberty is a well-defined sequence of physical and physiological changes culminating in full physical and sexual maturity. Normal age of onset is earlier in females, (mean 10.5 (range 8.5–12.5) years, than males, 12 (10–13.5) years.[265]

Biology Hypothalamic–pituitary–gonadal (HPG) axis: increasing pulses of GnRH from the hypothalamus lead to increased secretion of LH and FSH from the pituitary. These stimulate 'gonadarche': growth of the gonads and secretion of sex steroids (primarily oestradiol and testosterone). This leads to the first physical signs of puberty; enlargement of the testes and the appearance of breast tissue. Pubic hair development and growth acceleration follow. Penis and breast enlargement continues in response to increasing sex steroids. Gynaecomastia may worry boys but is usually transient. Menarche occurs on average 2.5 years after the start of puberty. 'Adrenarche' is the maturation of adrenal androgen production (DHEA and DHEAS). This manifests as pubic hair development, acne, and adult body odour. Adrenarche is a temporally related but distinct process and is not controlled by the HPG axis.

Precocious puberty (PP) Signs of pubertal development before the age of ~8yrs in girls and ~9yrs in boys. This warrants referral to a paediatric endocrinologist. ♀:♂ ≈10:1.[266] Causes are divided into 'central' ('true' or 'gonadotrophin dependent') or 'peripheral' (gonadotrophin independent). *Central PP:* Occurs with early activation of the HPG axis and has a normal sequence of pubertal development. Causes: idiopathic (familial or non-familial), intracranial tumours (hypothalamic hamartoma, craniopharyngioma, astrocytoma, optic glioma), other CNS lesions (meningoencephalitis, hydrocephalus, trauma, irradiation) or secondary central PP (early maturation of the HPG axis due to long-term sex steroid exposure eg CAH or McCune–Albright syndrome (p. 854)). *Peripheral PP:* Usually has an abnormal sequence of pubertal development. Causes: gonadal (ovarian cysts or tumours, testicular tumours, or familial testitoxicosis), adrenal (see 'Premature pubarche'), HCG secreting tumours, profound untreated hypothyroidism or exogenous sex steroids. *'Premature pubarche':* The premature appearance of pubic hair ('pubarche'), axillary hair, acne, body odour, without other signs of puberty is independent of the HPG axis. Usually caused by premature adrenarche, a benign condition associated with obesity but needs to be differentiated from virilizing disorders; Cushing syndrome, CAH, exogenous androgen exposure, or virilizing tumours.

Assessment *Principles:* Central or peripheral PP or isolated androgen excess? Younger patient = higher suspicion and more urgency. *1st line:* History; growth charts; puberty staging (Tanner charts, figs 3.18-3.20); examination (skin lesions, abdominal or testicular masses, visual fields, fundoscopy); BP, electrolytes; T4; TSH; LH; FSH; oestradiol; testosterone; androgen levels (androstenedione, 17-OH progesterone, DHEAS); prolactin; HCG; AFP; GH; bone age (skeletal x-ray). *2nd line:* Adrenal, testis & pelvic US; brain MRI (if central PP), karyotype; GnRH stimulation test; ACTH stimulation test.

Management Detection and treatment of underlying pathological causes.[265] *Other aims:* Achievement of expected adult height; relief of psychosocial stress. *Central PP:* Continuous high levels of GnRH suppress secretion of pituitary gonadotrophins; GnRH analogues are given nasal, SC, or IM. There is a reversal of gonadal maturation and all the clinical correlates of puberty (except pubic hair, androgens secretion by adrenal cortex unaffected). There is deceleration in skeletal maturation.

Delayed puberty The commonest form of delayed puberty in males is constitutional delay.[265] Males over 14 years with no signs of puberty should be referred for assessment. A female with no signs of breast development by age 14 or absence of menarche by age 16 should be referred (see pp. 114–115).

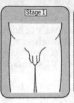

Fig 3.18 Tanner stages of puberty in males.

Reproduced from Butler *et al.*, *Paediatric Endocrinology and Diabetes* (2011), with permission from OUP.

Stage 1: Prepubertal with no pubic hair.
Stage 2: Scrotum and testes have enlarged and have more textured scrotal skin. Growth of slightly pigmented downy hair sparse.
Stage 3: The penis has grown, especially in length. Hair is darker and curlier.
Stage 4: Further penile growth, in length and breadth, has occured. Glans is larger and broader, and hair is adult in type.
Stage 5: The testes and scrotum are adult in size. Pubic hair is adult in quantity and pattern, and presents along the inner bordres of the thighs.

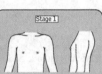

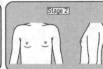

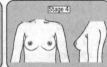

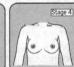

Fig 3.19 Tanner stages of breast development in females.

Reproduced from Butler *et al.*, *Paediatric Endocrinology and Diabetes* (2011), with permission from OUP.

Stage 1: Prepubertal.
Stage 2: Breast bud beneath the areolar enlargement.
Stage 3: Enlargement of the entire breast with no protrusion of papilla or of secondary mound.
Stage 4: Enlargement of the areola and papilla as a secondary mound.
Stage 5: Adult configuration of the breast with protrusion of the nipple.

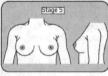

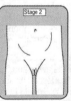

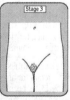

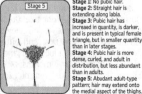

Fig 3.20 Tanner stages of pubic hair development in females.

Reproduced from Butler *et al.*, *Paediatric Endocrinology and Diabetes* (2011), with permission from OUP.

Stage 1: No pubic hair.
Stage 2: Straight hair is extending along labia.
Stage 3: Pubic hair has increaed in quantity, is darker, and is present in typical female triangle, but in smaller quantity than in later stages.
Stage 4: Pubic hair is more dense, curled, and adult in distribution, but less abundant than in adults.
Stage 5: Abudant adult-type pattern; hair may extend onto the medial aspect of the thighs.

3 Paediatrics

UK Healthy Child Programme This is the public health programme that offers every family a programme of screening tests, immunizations, developmental reviews, and information to support parenting and healthy choices.[267] It also provides an opportunity to identify families in need of additional support and children who are at risk of abuse/neglect.

Aims: To foster strong parent–child attachments and positive parenting (= better social and emotional well-being of children). To keep children healthy and safe by: • Promoting healthy eating & increased activity (= ↓ obesity) • Prevent serious/communicable diseases • Increase breastfeeding • Improve readiness for school & learning • To allow early detection of developmental delay, growth disorders, abnormalities, and ill health.

Summary of the screening schedule

- *Antenatal scans and other neonatal screening:* Assessment of the mother by 12 weeks of pregnancy + antenatal ultrasound scans and screening tests (see p. 10 & pp. 16–7).
- *Newborn:* Immediate physical external inspection after birth, followed by full physical examination by 72h (pp. 282–3).
- *Newborn Hearing Screening Programme:* (p. 398) Should be undertaken within 4–5 weeks of birth.
- *Bloodspot screening:* (Ideally day 5; up to day 8.) This is a heel-prick blood test to screen for hypothyroidism, CF, haemoglobinopathies and 6 IMDs: • PKU • MCADD • Maple syrup urine disease • Isovaleric acidaemia • Glutaric aciduria type 1 • Homocystinuria (pyridoxine unresponsive).
- *At 6–8 weeks:* Review + physical examination (usually undertaken by GP) to include general examination (including CVS, hips, eyes, testes) and to discuss any concerns.
- *By 5 years:* Pre-school hearing screen + screening for visual impairment.

Immunizations See table 3.11.

Health and development reviews These aim to • Assess family strengths, needs, and risks + any safeguarding concerns • Allow parents to discuss any concerns • Assess growth and development/detect abnormalities. 'Universal' service is for all families with enhanced services for families at higher risk.

- *Review by 14 days:* Face-to-face review with both parents to review feeding, assess maternal mental health, discuss home safety, SIDS risk, and promote sensitive parenting.
- *2–2.5-year health review:* Usually undertaken by health visitor: Review of the child's social, emotional, behavioural, and language development; review physical health, growth, development, hearing and vision, encourage positive parenting, promote language development (eg free books via Bookstart); and provide encouragement to take up early years education. It also allows review of immunizations, advice on diet, nutrition, and dental care, accident prevention, sleep management, and toilet training.

MMR scandal In 1998, *The Lancet* published a flawed and fraudulent[268] paper by Wakefield linking the MMR vaccine to autism. Despite its subsequent retraction by *The Lancet* and 11 of the 13 authors, and Wakefield being struck off by the GMC, the damage was done. The surrounding high-profile media coverage led to a drop in vaccine uptake across many countries and subsequent outbreaks of measles and mumps, including fatalities. Prior to 2006, the last death from acute measles in the UK was in 1992.[269] Large-scale reviews by Cochrane and WHO concluded there was no link between MMR and autism. In the UK, any non-immune adult is eligible for MMR (exclude pregnancy). If >18 months, the 2 doses of MMR should be separated by 3 months. MMR vaccine may also be offered to unimmunized, or measles-only immunized or seronegative postpartum women (avoid pregnancy for 1 month following immunization).

Immunization schedules

Immunization schedule (DOH^UK 2020) [270] (See also the *Green Book*) [271]

Table 3.11 UK immunization schedule

Stage	Vaccine
8weeks	3 vaccines: 1 DTaP/IPV/Hib/Hep B (6-in-1 diphtheria + tetanus + acellular pertussis + inactivated polio + haemophilus influenzae type B + hepatitis B): *Infanrix Hexa®* 2 Men B: (meningococcal group B) *Bexsero®*; note all doses of Men B should be given into *left* thigh, MenB can cause high fevers in infants and prophylactic paracetamol (3 doses of 60mg 4–6-hourly) is recommended [35] 3 Rotavirus oral vaccine: *Rotarix®L*
12weeks	3 vaccines: repeat 6-in-1 *Infanrix Hexa®* + oral *Rotarix®L* (note Men C no longer given at this age) and PCV (13-valent pneumococcal conjugate vaccine) *Prevenar 13®*
16weeks	2 vaccines: repeat 6-in-1 *Infanrix Hexa®* + *Bexsero®*
12months	4 vaccines: Hib/Men C (haemophilus influenzae type B & meningococcal group C): *Menitorix®* + MMR (measles, mumps, & rubella): MMR *VaxPRO®L* or *Priorix®L* + *Prevenar 13®* + *Bexsero®*
>3yrs 4 months	2 vaccines (known as the 'pre-school booster'): DTaP/IPV (diphtheria, tetanus, pertussis, & polio) *Repevax®* or *Boostrix-IPV®* + MMR: MMR *VaxPRO®L* or *Priorix®L*
12–13yrs	HPV (2 doses 6–24 months apart); protects against cervical cancer (p. 167) caused by human papillomavirus types 16 & 18 (and genital warts caused by types 6 & 11): *Gardasil®*
14yrs	2 vaccines: Td/IPV (low-dose diphtheria, tetanus, inactivated polio): *Revaxis®* + Men ACWY (meningococcal groups A, C, W, & Y): *Nimenrix®* or *Menveo®*
Flu	At-risk groups (asthma and other long-term health conditions or respiratory disease): aged 6 months–2yrs should have the inactivated injected quadrivalent influenza; aged 2–18yrs should have the annual live attenuated intranasal influenza vaccine *Fluenz Tetra®L* unless medical contraindications (severe asthma or immunosuppression) Other children: intranasal *Fluenz Tetra®L* should be offered annually to all children 2–9yrs (pre-school, reception, & school years 1–6)
BCG	Give BCG^L at birth if born in part of the country with high incidence or a parent or grandparent was born in a high-incidence country (>40,000/yr)
Hepatitis B	See OHCM p. 206. Babies born to HBsAg +ve mothers should receive vaccination (*Engerix B®* or *HBvaxPRO®*) at birth, 4wks & 12 months in addition to *Infanrix Hexa* at 8, 12, and 16 weeks. Hep B immunoglobulin should also be given at birth in some cases (mother is HBeAg+ve, or had high viral load during pregnancy or baby is ≤1500g); follow local protocol
Varicella	See p144. Routine in the USA, vaccination has greatly reduced incidence and hospitalizations/mortality [272]
Pregnancy	Give pertussis (as dTaP/IPV: *Boostrix-IPV®* or *Repevax®*) after 16 weeks' gestation and inactivated flu at any time

►L indicates live vaccines.
►An acute febrile illness is a contraindication to any vaccine.
►Give live vaccines either together, or separated by ≥3 weeks.
►Prematurity: give vaccines at chronological age, not corrected age. [273]

Immunocompromised See Royal College Guidelines [274] and *Green Book*. [273]
Don't give live vaccines if primary immunodeficiency (p. 244), or if on steroids (≥2mg/kg/day of prednisolone); or if HIV+ve (live vaccines except BCG can be given once immune reconstitution has been established with HAART).

3 Paediatrics

Speech develops in conjunction with hearing; therefore any impairment in hearing may delay language development. ►Always test the hearing. *Ensure the result is as reliable as possible.* Language is divided into expressive (speech) and receptive (comprehension) and should be assessed by a speech and language therapist. Delayed speech may also be part of global developmental delay or neurological problems or may occur in isolation. Check other developmental milestones, examine for neurological deficit, and consider autism, especially if there is regression of speech. *There is much variation in speech timing (first word between 11 and 20 months): what is 'clearly abnormal'?*

Speech and language development This dialogue portrays the mystery of language learning: *Daughter:* 'I don't want to eat my ice cream yet.' *Father:* 'Don't procrastinate!' 'Daddy, how can I understand you if you use words I don't understand? ' 'If I only ever used words you understood we could never have started talking.'

Early signs that the child is hearing and vocalizing normally:
- Newborn: quietens to voice and startles to loud noises.
- 6 weeks: responds to mother's voice.
- 12 weeks: begins to laugh, coo, and will vocalize when alone or spoken to.

Early language development:
- 6 months: uses consonant monosyllables eg ba and da.
- 8 months: non-specific 2-syllable babble eg mama, dada.
- 13 months: 2-syllable words become appropriate in their context; understands single words such as 'no'.
- 18 months: vocabulary of 10 words, can demonstrate 6 parts of the body; 2-word phrases eg 'Daddy come'.
- 24 months: subject–verb–object sentences appear eg 'I want ice cream!'

Conversation development:
- Sentence development becomes increasingly complex by the 2nd year.
- By age 3, the child knows their age, name, and several colours.
- At 3½yrs old … the child has mastered thought, language, abstraction, and the elements of reason, having a 1000-word vocabulary at his or her disposal, enabling sentences such as: 'I give her cake 'cos she's hungry'.

Words exist to give ideas currency, and so often that currency proves counterfeit—a process which so often starts with if eg 'If I hadn't thrown the cup on the ground, I might have got a pudding'. The uttering of 'If …', linked with an emotional response, is the most human of all constructions, opening up worlds divorced from reality, providing for the exercise of imagination, the validation of dreams, the understanding of motives, and the control of events. The rest of life holds nothing to match the intellectual and linguistic pace of these first years. Further linguistic development is devoted to seemingly conceptually minor tasks, such as expanding vocabulary.

Causes of delayed speech

- Hearing impairment: chronic otitis media is a common cause of delayed or poor clarity of speech in pre-school age children.
- Familial: family history of language delay; parents have been late in developing speech, or have had speech therapy.
- Environmental: deprivation; poor social interaction; neglect; other forms of abuse.
- Neuropsychological: global developmental delay; autism spectrum disorder (see p. 740); acquired epileptiform aphasia (Landau–Kleffner syndrome: epilepsy + progressive loss of language).

Vocabulary size: If <50 words at 3yrs old, suspect deafness—or:
- Expressive dysphasia or speech dyspraxia (eg if there is a telegraphic quality to speech, poor clarity, and deteriorating behaviour, eg frustration).
- Audio-premotor syndrome (APM). The child cannot reflect sounds correctly heard into motor control of larynx and respiration. Instead of babbling, the child is quiet, unable to hum or sing.
- Respiro-laryngeal (RL) dysfunction (dysphonia from incorrect vocal fold vibration/air flow regulation). The voice is loud and rough.
- Congenital aphonia (thin effortful voice; it's rare).

Speech clarity: By 2½yrs, parents should understand most speech. If not, suspect deafness—or:
- Articulatory dyspraxia (easy consonants are *b* and *m* with the lips, and *d* with the tongue—the phonetic components of babbling). ♂:♀ ≈ 3:1. Tongue-tie is a possible cause (∴ poor sounds needing tongue elevation—*d* and *s*)—surgery to the frenulum may be needed (+ speech therapy). Distinguish from phonological causes (disordered *sound for speech processing*—may present as *sound awareness problems* (difficulty in analysing sound structure of words)). Both are common.
- APM or RL dysfunction, as described above in 'Vocabulary size'.

Understanding: By 2½ years a child should understand 'Get your shoes', if not, suspect: • Deafness—if the hearing is impaired (eg 25–40dB loss) secretory otitis media is likely to be the cause. Worse hearing loss is probably sensorineural • Cognitive impairment • Deprivation.

Speech therapy Refer early, before school starts.

Global developmental delay Used to describe delay in ≥2 developmental domains; it may be more pronounced in fine motor, speech, and social skills. There are many causes although in some instances it remains unknown. The more severe the delay, the more likely a cause will be found (p272).
- *Genetic:* Chromosomal disorders eg Down syndrome, fragile x; Duchenne muscular dystrophy; metabolic eg PKU, MSUD.
- *Congenital brain abnormalities:* Hydrocephalus; microcephaly.
- *Prenatal cause:* Teratogens such as alcohol and drugs (including prescription), congenital infections (particularly rubella, CMV, or toxoplasmosis), hypothyroidism (rare in Westernized countries).
- *Perinatal cause:* Extreme prematurity leading to intraventricular haemorrhage or periventricular leukomalacia; birth asphyxia; metabolic disorders such as hyperbilirubinaemia (causing kernicterus) or hypoglycaemia.
- *Postnatal cause:* Brain injury from suffocation, drowning, head injury; CNS infection, particularly meningitis or encephalitis; hypoglycaemia; hypothyroidism.

Chronic childhood illness, and family support

Diseases such as asthma, CNS disease, and neoplasia may cause disintegration of even the most apparently secure families: ►*Consequent strife and marital breakdown may be more severe and have far-reaching consequences for the child and siblings.*

Remember that illness makes families poor, and movement down the social scale leads to unpredictable consequences in housing and (un)employment. Families experiencing housing instability and food insecurity (without homelessness or hunger) are known to miss out on healthcare.

Relationship disharmony may seem to be beyond the scope of paediatrics, but any holistic view of child health must put the family at the centre of all attempts to foster child health and well-being.

We see many families coping well with severe, prolonged illness in a child. But don't presume that because things are OK in clinic today, you can afford to neglect the fostering of family life. Given a certain amount of stress almost all families will show psychopathology, in time. Your job is to prevent this if possible. Counselling skills are frequently needed.

Developmental disorders are a group of conditions leading to impairment in at least 1 functional area—eg cognition, motor skills (gross or fine), social-emotional, or communication (speech, language, hearing, or vision). Around 20–25% of children have at least 1 developmental delay, and as many as 50% of these will not be detected before starting primary school.[275] Conditions falling under the umbrella of developmental disorders include autism spectrum disorder, speech-language impairment, learning disabilities, and psychosocial problems. *Biological risk factors* include: prematurity, low birthweight, birth asphyxia, chronic illness, and hearing/vision impairment. *Environmental risk factors* include: poverty, low parental education, parental mental illness and social isolation, maternal alcohol, or other drugs.[276]

Developmental surveillance Refers to an ongoing process of following a child's development over time. It involves discussing concerns with parents, eliciting a perinatal history, identifying risk factors, as well as observing the child attempting different skills at different times and referring the child when appropriate to other health professionals (eg health visitors, physiotherapists, speech and language therapists, or audiometrists). Developmental surveillance can be incorporated into well-child checks, general physical examination, and routine immunization visits. See table 3.12 for expected developmental milestones.

Developmental screening Refers to a standardized assessment aimed at identifying those children who require further investigation and assessment. It is typically carried out using a developmental screening tool. Screening should be carried out within the broader undertaking of developmental surveillance. Repeating screening at different ages increases the accuracy of the test. Parental concern about a child's development may in itself constitute a reliable screening test.[277] The first developmental screening tool *Denver Developmental Screening Test (DDST 1967)* and its successor the *Denver II (1992)* have largely been replaced with more sensitive tests. Screening may be based on parent report alone (parent-completed tests) or through direct observation together with parent report (directly administered tests). Some of the most commonly used tests are discussed as follows—all are copyrighted products:

The *Parents' Evaluation of Developmental Status (PEDS)* tool is a parent-completed test consisting of 10 questions (8 yes/no, 2 open ended). It can be given to parents to complete prior to attending health visits and takes less than 5 minutes to complete. It has a sensitivity of 74–80% and is suitable for children up to 8 years old.[275] It identifies children as low, moderate, or high risk for various disabilities and identifies an optimal course of action. www.pedstest.com.

The *Ages and Stages Questionnaire (ASQ)*, another parent completed test, consists of 21 age-specific questionnaires. It can be used to evaluate children aged 1 month to 5½ years old. It has a sensitivity of 85% and takes 10–20 minutes to complete.[275] It has a single cut-off score indicating which children need further referral. Available at: www.agesandstages.com.

The *Modified Checklist for Autism in Toddlers (M-chat)* is a 2nd-stage parent-completed test that is more specific for autism spectrum disorders. It has a sensitivity of 90%. Available free online at: www.firstsigns.org.

The *Schedule of Growing Skills (SOGS II)* is a directly administered test, eliciting skills from children. It covers all domains of development and cognition and can be used up to the age of 5 years. www.gl-assessment.co.uk

While the American Association of Pediatrics recommends both developmental surveillance and screening,[278] the National Screening Committee (UK) doesn't recommend developmental screening.[279]

Table 3.12 Developmental milestones

261

Average age	Milestone	Red flags
6 weeks	• *Smiles* • *Eyes follow an object past midline*	Strabismus (squint) persisting beyond 3 months
4–6 months	• *Sits with support* • *Rolls* • *Good head control* • *Reaches out for objects* • *Transfers objects from hand to hand* • *Starts babbling*	At 6 months if: • Lack of eye contact • No smile • No grasp • Not rolling • Poor head control
6–9 months	• *Crawls* • *Sits without support* • *Pulls to stand* • *Gives toy on request* • *Turns head to name* • *Responds to 'bye-bye'* • *Gestures with babbling* • *First tooth*	At 9 months if: • No response to words • No gestures • No passing of toys from hand to hand • Unable to roll or crawl or sit without support
7–12 months	• *Walks with support or using furniture ('cruising')* • *Develops pincer grasp* • *Plays 'peek-a-boo'* • *Waves goodbye*	At 12 months if: • Unable to pick up small items • Unable to crawl or bottom shuffle • Unable to stand holding on to furniture • No babbled phrases
12–15 months	• *Single words* • *Listens to stories* • *Drinks from cup*	
18 months	• *Speaks 6 words* • *Able to walk up steps* • *Names pictures* • *Walks independently* • *Scribbles* • *Builds with blocks*	At 18 months if: • Uninterested in playing with others • No clear words • Not walking without support • Not able to hold crayon • Unable to stack 2 blocks
1.5–2 years	• *Kicks/throws a ball* • *Runs* • *2-word sentences* • *Follows a 2-step command* • *Stacks 5–6 blocks* • *Turns pages* • *Uses a spoon* • *Helps with dressing*	At 2 years if: • Has <50 words • Difficulty handling small objects • Unable to climb stairs • No interest in feeding or dressing

3 Paediatrics

There is much individual variation but milestones should be achieved before red flag ages. ►If there is regression, or loss of a previously developed skill, this should be considered a red flag requiring immediate investigation. Other red flags at any age include poor interaction with others, difference in strength between right and left sides of body, emergence of hand preference before 12 months, abnormal tone, and strong parental concern.

Children usually learn to walk by 18 months of age. If this has not occurred, the child needs to be assessed: *History:* is development delayed in other areas? Is growth normal? Family history of late walking? *Examination:* dysmorphism; muscle tone; muscle weakness (Gower's sign=inability to get up from floor or squatting position without hands suggestive of muscular dystrophy); calf hypertrophy; plantar reflex; hepatosplenomegaly. *Causes:* the commonest causes reflect chronic illness, global developmental delay, cerebral palsy. Others: neglect; rickets; hypothyroidism; developmental coordination disorder; in boys consider Duchenne or Becker's muscular dystrophy. Delayed motor maturation (often familial) has no other features and is a diagnosis of exclusion. *Tests:* if history and examination normal check creatine kinase (CK). Consider referral to community or general paediatrician.

Cerebral palsy (CP) Comprises chronic disorders of central motor dysfunction caused by a non-progressive CNS insult sustained before 2yrs of age. As the brain is still evolving, motor manifestations also evolve. Non-motor symptoms *may* also be present (never assume): most commonly learning disability (35%), and epilepsy. *Causes:* (MINIBOX 'Typical causes'.) Most are due to antenatal events unrelated to birth asphyxia, however often no cause is found. *Prevalence:* 9% if gestation 23–27wks; 6% if 28–30wks; 0.1% if term.[280] ♀:♂ ≈ 1:1. *Signs:* Weakness; paralysis; increased tone; premature handedness (<12 months) or other motor asymmetry; delayed milestones; language/speech/swallowing problems.

Typical causes
Prenatal factors:
• APH (with hypoxia)
• Radiation
• Alcohol
• Intrauterine infection (CMV; rubella; HIV; toxoplasmosis)
• Rhesus disease
Perinatal factors:
• Prematurity
• Birth asphyxia (HIE p. 281)
• Hypoglycaemia
• Hyperbilirubinaemia (kernicterus)
Postnatal factors:
• Trauma/intraventricular haemorrhage
• Hypoxia
• Meningoencephalitis
• Cerebral vein thrombosis (from dehydration)

Classification: There are 4 main types: • Spastic • Dyskinetic • Ataxic • Mixed CP. Spasticity (velocity-dependent resistance to passive muscle stretch) suggests a pyramidal lesion. Most have either a spastic hemiplegia (arm>leg; delay in walking; increased deep reflexes of affected limb) or a spastic diplegia (both legs affected worse than the arms, so that the child looks normal until he or she is picked up, when the legs 'scissor'—hip adduction and internal rotation; with knee extension and feet plantar-flexed). Spastic quadriplegia is the most severe form and is associated with seizures and IQ↓.

• *Dyskinetic cerebral palsy:* uncoordinated, involuntary movements and postures suggest basal ganglia involvement. May be chorea (rapid, random contractions of small muscle groups), athetoid (slow writhing movements), or dystonic (sustained or repetitive muscle contractions). Association: kernicterus.

• *Ataxic CP:* rare and suggests cerebellar involvement. There may be hypo- or hypertonia and speech difficulties as well as incoordination and intention tremor.

Functional classification: The Gross Motor Function Classification System (GMFCS) is a more important classification in terms of the child's function and independence. It has 5 levels based on usual function: • Level 1: walks, runs, climbs stairs without rail, speed, balance and coordination limited • Level 2: uses rail for stairs, walks but may use handheld or wheeled device for long distance or uneven terrain, minimal ability to run or jump • Level 3: walks with handheld device in most indoor settings, uses wheeled device for longer distances • Level 4: Mobility requires physical assistance or powered mobility in most settings • Level 5: Children are transported in manual wheelchair in all settings, limited anti-gravity head, trunk, and limb control.

3 Paediatrics

Associations and complications: There are often other disorders of cerebral function and complications of CP: epilepsy; learning difficulties; hearing, vision, or speech impairments; swallowing difficulties (2° to retrobulbar palsy) may lead to recurrent aspiration, scoliosis causes restrictive lung disease, respiratory muscle weakness, and difficulty clearing secretions. These combine to make children with CP very high risk for respiratory infections; growth failure (use specific CP growth charts); constipation/intestinal paresis; osteopenia and fractures; joint subluxation and dislocation (particularly hips); fixed flexion deformities (contractures; should not occur with appropriate physiotherapy); neurogenic bladder; sleep disorders; and chronic pain (constipation, reflux, dystonia, joint subluxations) which may go unnoticed due to communication difficulties.

❖ **Management** Requires a multidisciplinary team. Children's views must be taken into account in all matters concerning them.[281] UN Convention on the Rights of the Child ▶*Assume that all disabled children are entitled to a 'full and decent life'.* The aim is quality of life and full integration into society. Because children have grown up hand-in-hand with disability and are often uncowed by it, they often score as high as anyone else on quality of life, if pain is treated.[281] Parents may find it a comfort to know this. Physio- and occupational therapists, orthopaedic surgeons, and orthoses experts aid holistic assessment: can they roll over (both ways)? Sit? Grasp? Transfer objects from hand to hand? Good head control? Ability to shift weight when prone with forearm support? Is continence possible? Can they hold a pen or a spoon? Muscle strengthening can help.[282] Splints may prevent deformity (equinovarus, equinovalgus, hip dislocation from excessive flexion/adduction). Attempts to show benefits of neurophysiotherapy (to help equilibrium and righting) don't show benefit over simple motor stimulation. Some parents try the Hungarian *Petö approach:* ☺Here the 'conductor' devotes herself to the child, using interaction with peers to reinforce successes: eg manipulation, art, writing, fine movement, and social skills.[283] Treat comorbidities such as epilepsy (p. 232). *Botulinum toxin* (p. 566) benefits many children with spasticity. *Epidural cord or deep brain electrostimulation & intrathecal or oral baclofen* (benefits uncertain).[271][272] **Prognosis** By 6yrs, 54% with quadriplegia (80% if hemiplegic or diplegic) gain urinary continence spontaneously. If IQ↓, 38% are dry at this age.[286] n=601

'Is growth normal?' is a *fundamental* question in determining a child's health. Normal growth = much reduced likelihood of a serious chronic condition. Take any opportunity to weigh and measure a child. A series of plots on centile charts (pp. 316-19) is infinitely more informative than one-off measurements. Birthweight (BW) is a reflection of *in utero* conditions whereas centile at 1 year of age is a better predictor of final adult height and is more genetically determined. Hence there is often a period of 'catch-up' or 'catch-down' growth in the 1st year. The growth rate in mid-childhood is 5–6cm/yr; this accelerates at puberty (peak height velocity) before epiphyses start to fuse. Be appropriately sceptical about reliability of data. Is the BW accurate? Was the child clothed during weighings? Length measurements are particularly error prone.

Faltering growth (Previously 'failure to thrive'.) Means inadequate weight gain outside of the neonatal period (p. 293). This means a fall across ≥2 centile lines on a WHO growth chart (or ≥1 if BW <9th centile, or ≥3 if BW >91st centile).[287] Head circumference is preserved relative to height, which is preserved relative to weight. If the head is not growing, a serious underlying disorder is likely. Check height/length centile

Features to note
• Signs of abuse (pp. 196-7)
• Feeding patterns
• Behaviour
• Activity level
• Family finances
• Health and happiness
• Parental mental health

and mid-parental height centile. If child is ≥2 centile spaces below the mid-parental centile, suspect chronic undernutrition or primary growth disorder. Check BMI if >2yrs:[13] BMI <2nd centile may indicate undernutrition or small build; BMI <0.4th centile is more likely to be undernutrition. *History: Breastfed* (p. 288): latching; swallowing; duration and frequency of feeds; urine passage; milk supply. *Formula fed*: appropriate volumes & frequency; mixing feed correctly; appropriate teat & technique. *Weaned*: age of weaning (beyond weaning, too much milk ↓ appetite for other foods); see MINIBOX 'Features to note'. *Causes:* In the vast majority of cases it is feeding related & the child is otherwise well. Worldwide, poverty is the big cause; in the UK it is difficulty at home; unskilled feeding; maternal interaction; delayed weaning; food aversion; unusual parental beliefs around nutrition; or, rarely, not enough breast milk. Neglect and abuse must be considered, does weight gain improve if the child is removed from the family? Is there evidence relevant to child safeguarding proceedings? *Tests:* Observation of feeding by a skilled professional. Other tests are rarely needed, in one study only 39 of 4880 tests were helpful.[288] NICE: consider MSU (or *clean catch* urine) & coeliac serology in all but consider other tests *only* if indicated. *Monitoring:* Repeat measurements not more frequently than: weekly if 1–6 months; fortnightly if 6–12 months; monthly if >12 months. ℞: Feeding support & education. Referral to breastfeeding specialist or paediatric dietician. Rarely supplementation with high-energy feeds. In non-organic faltering growth, studies favour weekly visits from trained lay visitors.[289] *Clues to pathological cause:* Stools (liquid, oily, mucousy, bloody); vomiting; polyuria & polydipsia; hyperhidrosis (↑ sweating); murmurs; clubbing; hepatosplenomegaly; abdominal mass; neurological signs; cleft palate; dysmorphism; FH of serious condition. Remember: ►*Any serious chronic disease can cause faltering growth.* Consider these which may have few other signs unless looked for: anorexia; bulimia; coeliac disease; IBD; CMPA (p. 293); HIV; TB; CF; helminth infection; metabolic disorders; malignancy. *Tests:* FBC; U&E: blood pH; glucose; LFTs; immunoglobulins; CRP/ESR; TFTs. ±: sweat test; urine organic acids, plasma amino acids & acylcarnitine profile; stools (MC&S, OCP, occult blood, reducing substances); HIV; CXR; renal or CNS US; skeletal survey for dwarfism and abuse; ECG; echo. ℞: Appropriate specialist referral.

13 https://www.nhs.uk/live-well/healthy-weight/bmi-calculator/

(side margin) 3 Paediatrics

Short stature = height <2nd centile (pp. 316-19). *Causes:* ▶*Any chronic disease can cause short stature* (see 'Causes of faltering growth'). However, familial short stature and constitutional delay of growth and puberty (CDGP) are by far the most common causes and are non-pathological. *Endocrine causes:* Usually have excessive weight for height: growth hormone deficiency (may be part of hypopituitarism); hypothyroidism; Cushing's. *Other causes:* Drugs (steroids, stimulants); syndromes (Turner's p. 859, Noonan's p. 854, Prader–Willi p. 856).

- *Familial short stature:* Use the method shown on growth charts to calculate mid-parental height centile. The further the child's centile from this, the less likely it is to be familial.
- *CDGP:* Birthweight normal but at 6–24 months drops to below 2nd centile, after 3yrs growth is below but parallel to 2nd centile, typically delayed puberty with catch up growth during puberty. x-ray shows delayed skeletal age. GH↓: If congenital, usually manifests by age of 2yrs: look for relative obesity, with low growth velocity. Acquired GH↓ may be secondary to a pituitary tumour (red flags: headache, vomiting, weight loss, bitemporal hemianopia) and hypopituitarism (always assess other pituitary hormones, OHCM p232). *Tests:* IGF-1 & IGFBP-3 then GH stimulation test (+ve if impaired rise in GH after a stimulus of arginine or hypoglycaemia, induced by IV insulin (OHCM p232)). *R:* SC synthetic GH, to be effective start early. Expect growth velocity to ↑ by ≥50% from baseline in year 1 of treatment. *Causes of height ↑:* familial tall stature; nutritional; hyperthyroidism; precocious puberty; GH↑; Klinefelter's; Marfan's; homocystinuria.[287]

Ethnospecific growth charts

It is clear that some populations are inherently shorter than others, and this poses problems when using UK90 growth charts (ie charts for children >4yrs); which are based on cohorts of UK children in the 1980s (see also p. 316).[290] Consider these facts:

- The Dutch are the tallest *nation* on earth (mean ♂ height 1.84m): the tallest *population group* is the Masai people (eg in Tanzania and Kenya).
- African and Afro-Caribbean 5–11yr-olds' height is ~0.6 standard deviations scores (SDs) greater than white children living in England.
- Gujarati children and those from the Indian subcontinent (except those from Urdu- or Punjabi-speaking homes) have heights ~0.5 SDs less than white children living in England. NB: Sikh children are taller and heavier than Caucasians.[291]
- Gujarati children's weight is ~1.5 SDs < for white children living in England.
- Published charts have centile lines 0.67 SDs apart; for height and weight so shift the centile lines up by 1 centile line division for African-Caribbeans.
- Body mass index centiles are said to be appropriate for African-Caribbeans, but need some adjustment for Indian subcontinent children as noted earlier.

Trends towards tallness with each generation occur at varying rates in all groups, so 3rd-generation immigrants are taller than expected using 2nd-generation data. Intermarriage adds further uncertainty.

Obesity in childhood has risen fast in the West, and appears now to be slowing. However, it remains a huge public health problem, not only in childhood, but also in the medium and long term: obese and overweight children are far more likely to become obese adults with the resultant effects on health.

Prevalence In the UK, in 2016/17 10% of reception class children were obese, rising to 20% by school year 6 (age 11).[292]

Causes Essentially an imbalance between energy intake and expenditure.

- *Dietary:* Fast and processed foods, especially those high in carbohydrates.
- *Exercise:* There has been an overall decline in physical activity of children in the UK, with reduced time playing sports at school, and an increase in sedentary activities at home (TV, computer games, social networking).
- *Sleep deprivation:* Leads to low leptin levels (a hormone which communicates adequate fat levels) and high ghrelin levels (released by the stomach to signal hunger); this increases appetite.
- *Socioeconomic background:* The more deprived areas have over double the prevalence of childhood obesity than the least deprived. Higher levels of parental education appear to be protective against childhood obesity.
- *Genetics:* Obese parents are more likely to have obese children; however, it is difficult to establish how much of this effect is due to genetics versus growing up in an obesogenic environment.
- *Medication:* Can increase weight gain eg steroids, sodium valproate, carbamazepine, mirtazapine. *Others:* High or low birthweight; intrauterine exposure to maternal gestational diabetes or maternal obesity.

Medical causes Extremely rare (except steroid use) but more common with short stature so check height (p. 265). Consider hypothyroidism, Cushing syndrome, growth hormone deficiency, and Prader–Willi syndrome.

Diagnosis Normal BMI varies with age, use UK-WHO charts for children <4; once >4 years old use UK 1990 BMI percentile charts. A BMI >91st centile is overweight, >98th centile obese, and >99.6th centile severely obese. This needs sensitive discussion with the child and their parents. Parents often do not have the correct perception of their child's weight. Emphasize the long-term problems associated with being overweight or obese and this being a good opportunity to improve their child's health in the future. Is the child having any physical or emotional problems resulting from being overweight? Talk about factors which may be contributing—diet, exercise, lifestyle, family circumstances, disability, other medical or family problems. *Screen:* For comorbidities eg hypertension, diabetes, non-alcoholic fatty liver disease (NAFLD), and hyperlipidaemia.

Management
- What has been tried before? It is important to involve the whole family.
- The primary treatment is dietary modification and exercise.
- Diet alone is not recommended.
- Referral to a dietician can be very helpful; aim to eat a healthy diet.
- Aim for moderate exercise of at least 60 minutes per day. Exercise not only increases energy expenditure but also increases self-esteem and helps sleep.
- The MEND programme (Mind, Exercise, Nutrition … Do it).
- Refer: BMI >98th centile; weight-related morbidity; suspicion of medical cause.

Medium-term consequences: Insulin resistance, type 2 diabetes, obstructive sleep apnoea, orthopaedic problems, NAFLD, psychosocial morbidity, polycystic ovarian syndrome, vitamin D deficiency. *Long-term problems:* Atherosclerosis, early-onset cardiovascular disease, many cancers, subfertility, hypertension.

Further reading

NICE (2013). *Managing Overweight and Obesity among Children and Young People: Lifestyle Weight Management Services* (PH47). London: NICE. https://www.nice.org.uk/guidance/ph47

Stage I hypertension in children is BP >95th centile of average systolic & diastolic BP adjusted for *age, height,* and *sex* (stage II is >99th centile +5mmHg). You *must* use the correct cuff size (the *bladder* must be long enough to encircle ≥80% of upper arm *circumference* and the bladder width ≥40% the circumference) and a manual sphygmomanometer. Take ≥3 BPs >1 week apart (in general) before diagnosing hypertension. Use the 1st and 5th Korotkoff sounds. Ambulatory BPs can show that white coat hypertension is about as common in children as in adults.[293,294]

Prevalence In the USA is 3–4% of 3–18-year-olds.

Risk factors • High salt intake; fast and processed foods are particularly to blame • Obesity • Low birthweight in those who go on to develop obesity.

Causes of raised blood pressure in children

Child <6yrs Renal parenchymal disease, renal vascular disease, coarctation of the aorta, endocrine causes, essential hypertension, drugs (steroids).

6–12yrs Renal parenchymal disease, essential hypertension, renal vascular disease, endocrine causes, coarctation, iatrogenic cause.

Adolescence Essential hypertension, iatrogenic illness, renal diseases, coarctation of the aorta, endocrine causes.

As a general rule, the younger the child, the higher the probability of identifying the cause. In 80% the cause is renal parenchymal disease (pp. 224–5, pp. 230–1).

History and examination Symptoms/signs are non-specific in a neonate. In older children. headaches, fatigue, blurred vision, epistaxis, Bell's palsy. Ask about prematurity, bronchopulmonary dysplasia, umbilical artery catheterization, head or abdominal trauma, family history of hypertension, neurofibromatosis, and multiple endocrine neoplasia; urinary tract infection, medication (especially steroids and drugs used to treat ADHD), sleep-disordered breathing and diet. *Examine* the child from head to toe; check height and weight against centile charts. Points of interest: goitre, signs of left ventricular hypertrophy, poor amplitude of peripheral pulses (aortic coarctation); abdominal mass (Wilms' tumour); virilization (congenital adrenal hyperplasia).

Investigations • Urine to check for protein & blood • U&E; creatinine; FBC; TFTs; glucose; fasting lipid profile (check extent of disease, comorbidities, anaemia from renal disease) ± plasma renin & aldosterone • Renal US to exclude structural abnormalities ± renal artery Doppler US • Screen for end-organ damage: ECG (LVH/strain), echocardiogram (hypertrophy); retinal screening.

Treatment *Lifestyle modification:* Weight loss if necessary; a healthy, low-salt diet, regular exercise; avoidance of smoking and alcohol. *Referral and treatment:* Required if the child is symptomatic, has secondary hypertension, diabetes, end-organ damage, or persistent hypertension despite lifestyle modification. This is with ACE-inhibitors, β-blockers, thiazide diuretics, and calcium channel blockers. ▶Hypertensive crisis, see p. 231.

3 Paediatrics

►*Only enter battles you can win.* If the child can win, be more subtle eg consistent rewards, not inconsistent punishments. Get a health visitor's advice; ensure everyone is encouraging the same response from the child.

Food refusal and *food fads* Are common. Reducing pressure on the child, discouraging parental over-reaction, and gradual enlarging of tiny portions of attractive food are usually all that is needed. Check ferritin and FBC. Keep a watchful eye on growth and weight gain.

Overeating: Eating comforts, and if the child is short on comfort, or if mother feels inadequate, the scene is set for overeating and lifelong patterns are begun (see 'Childhood obesity', p. 266). Medical causes of hyperphagia are very rare (consider Prader–Willi, p. 856).

Pica: Eating things which are not food, eg soil, plastic, cloth, string; if persistent >1 month, look for other disturbed behaviours, autism, or ↓IQ. *Causes:* Iron or other mineral deficiency; obsessive-compulsive disorder. *Complications:* Lead poisoning; worm infestations.[295] Treating iron deficiency helps; otherwise behaviour modification.[296]

Constipation Difficulty in defecation; it may comprise of <3 stools per week; large hard stool; 'rabbit dropping' stool; distress/straining/bleeding with passage of stool. It may lead to abdominal pain, abdominal masses, overflow soiling or diarrhoea ± 'lavatory-blocking' enormous stools (megarectum), and anorexia. *Causes:* Diet, poor fluid, or fibre intake—or fear eg as a result of a fissure. Rarely Hirschsprung disease (p. 222). Failure to pass meconium in first 48h? Meconium ileus is suggestive of cystic fibrosis pp. 214–15. Ask about onset of constipation and precipitants (fissure/change in diet/timing of potty training/fears and phobias/moving house/acute infections/family upheavals).

Red flags: Include:[297 NICE]

- 🚩 Constipation from birth or first few weeks.
- 🚩 Failure to pass meconium within 48h.
- 🚩 Faltering growth (consider coeliac disease/hypothyroid).
- 🚩 New weakness/abnormal reflexes in legs, delayed locomotion.
- 🚩 Abnormal appearance of anus/skin in sacral/gluteal region (look for sacral dimples/hairy patches/flattening of gluteal muscles/multiple fissures).
- 🚩 Gross abdominal distension with vomiting.

Action: •Find out about potty/toilet refusal •Does defecation hurt? •Is there parental coercion? Break the vicious cycle of: large faeces → pain/fissure → fear of the pot → rectum overstretched → call-to-stool sensation dulled → soiling → parental exasperation → coercion. ►Exonerate the child to boost confidence for the main task of obeying calls-to-stool to keep the rectum empty.

Treat: Faecal impaction with escalating dose 'disimpaction regimen' of **polyethylene glycol 3350 + electrolytes** eg 'Movicol® Paediatric Plain' as 1st-line intervention. NICE[297 NICE] suggests doses, which exceed those in the *BNFC*, as follows:

- If <1yrs then ½–1 sachet daily.
- 2–5yrs: 2 sachets on day 1; increase by 2 sachets every 2 days to max. of 8 sachets daily.
- 5–12yrs: start on 4 sachets and increase in steps of 2 to a maximum of 12 per day.
- If >12yrs use Movicol® or equivalent (lacks electrolytes and contains a higher dose of polyethylene glycol 3350) at 4 sachets on day 1, escalating by 2 sachets/day to a maximum of 8.

Follow this with maintenance 'Movicol® Paediatric Plain' (<12yrs)/Movicol® (>12yrs) or lactulose ± stimulant laxative (eg senna), adjusting dose to produce regular soft stools. Disimpaction is unpleasant for all involved and takes a concerted effort over many days. ERIC website (https://www.eric.org.uk/) has excellent resources and advice for families.

NB: behaviour therapy in combination with laxatives is effective,[298] but biofeedback methods are not.[299] Clinics run by nurse specialists can be more effective than those run by consultants.[300] Dietary modifications to ensure a balanced diet, with sufficient fluids and fibre are necessary but not sufficient by themselves. Encourage daily physical activity. Digital rectal examination and abdominal x-rays are rarely required. Do not use enemas until all attempts at oral medication have failed.

Faecal incontinence, encopresis, and soiling These are terms often used interchangeably and don't have clear definitions although in the UK, encopresis is used more often when in association with emotional or behavioural difficulties. Incontinence may be voluntary or non-voluntary. In 80% it is due to constipation and 'overflow' (retentive encopresis), but may occasionally be a behavioural response to abuse or emotional difficulties. Rarely there is a physical/anatomical lesion or neuromuscular cause (Hirschsprung disease, anal malformation, anal trauma, imperforate anus with fistula, meningomyelocele). Treat retentive encopresis with extra dietary fibre, laxatives, and 'mandatory' daily toilet sittings ~15–30min after eating. *Functional (non-retentive) faecal incontinence* is the repeated passage of normal stool in inappropriate places in those >4yrs old. ♂:♀ ≈ 5:1. Try behaviour therapy and referral to a child and adolescent psychiatrist—it is usually part of an emotional disorder.[301] NB: this demarcation is not absolute: behavioural techniques such as differential attention, contingency management, and contracting are relevant to both forms of encopresis.[302]

Enuresis Infrequent bedwetting (<2 nights/week) occurs in ~15% at 5yrs and 5% at 10yrs.[NICE][303] 1–2% of >15yrs continue to wet the bed, usually from delayed maturation of bladder control (family history often +ve). Girls are earlier to achieve bladder control than boys; enuresis is defined as continued wetting >5yrs in ♀ and >6yrs in ♂. Tests for diabetes, UTI, and GU abnormality (pp. 228–9) can occasionally yield surprises but are by no means compulsory unless there are clinical suspicions. The term 'secondary enuresis' implies bedwetting after >6 months' dryness, and raises concerns about worries, illness (diabetes), or abuse.

History: Ask about nights per week she/he wets the bed? Does it happen more than once per night? Severe bedwetting is less likely to resolve spontaneously. Are there any daytime symptoms? Frequency/urgency may indicate an overactive bladder; diurnal wetting may respond to oxybutynin. How much do they drink during the evening? Is there constipation/soiling; history of recurrent UTI (underlying urological abnormality)?

Treatment: Start with advice and reassure parents that many children continue to wet the bed after achieving day-time dryness. Ensure that caffeine-based drinks are avoided and the toilet is used regularly during the day (4–7 times is typical). Reassure that he is neither infantile nor dirty. A system of rewards for *agreed behaviours* (eg drinking recommended levels of fluid, using the toilet before bedtime, taking medicines, or helping change the sheets (*not for* dry nights which the child can't control)) may be effective. Alarms (± vibrations) triggered by urine in the bed can make 56% dry at 1yr; relapses are preventable by continuing use after dryness. They are cheap—eg Drinite®.[304] **Desmopressin** (synthetic vasopressin/ADH) sublingual dose (if >5yrs): 120mcg at bedtime (max. 240mcg); useful for sleepovers and school trips but relapse is common. Have 1wk every 3 months with no drugs. CI: D&V, cystic fibrosis, uraemia, BP↑.

Further reading

NICE (2014). *Clinical Knowledge Summaries: Bedwetting (Enuresis).* http://cks.nice.org.uk/bedwetting-enuresis#!scenariorecommendation:7.

WHO definitions *Disability* is an umbrella term covering: *impairment* (a pathological problem in body function or structure), *activity limitation* (difficulty experienced by an individual in performing a task), and *participation restriction* (problem with involvement in life situations) eg spina bifida, causing difficulty walking, resulting in eg inability to participate in all activities in school.[305]

Learning disability *The mother often makes the first diagnosis.* Learning (or intellectual) disability entails deficits in intellectual and adaptive skills and may be classified as mild, moderate, severe, or profound (IQ <70, <50, <35, and <20 respectively, see p. 742). ▶Beware equating IQ with intellect: the latter implies more than problem-solving and memory. Intellect entails the ability to speculate, to learn from mistakes, to have a view of oneself and others, to see relationships between events in different domains of experience—as well as the ability to use language either to map the world, or to weave ironic webs of truth and deceit (and, on a good day, to do both simultaneously). If a child is failing to meet milestones in multiple developmental domains, the term *Global Developmental Delay* (GDD) is used (p. 259). *Causes:* Severe mental impairment usually has a definable cause, whereas mild intellectual disability is often familial, with no well-defined cause. *Congenital disorders* are legion: chromosomal (eg Down's; fragile X, p. 852); metabolic (individually rare but many and varied, pp. 252-3). *Acquired:* perinatal infection pp. 38-9, pp. 40-1, birth injury, trauma, meningitis, fetal alcohol spectrum disorder.

Diagnosis and management: Refer to an expert, so that no treatable cause is missed. Recent evidence supports genetic and metabolic testing as *1st line* in all children with unexplained learning disability/GDD.[306] Would the family like help from a group, such as MENCAP? Other members of the family may need special support (eg normal siblings, who now feel neglected). If the IQ is >35, life in the community is the aim.

Learning disorders Or specific learning difficulties are recognized syndromes with impact on a particular area of learning: eg dyslexia, dysgraphia, dyscalculia.

Physical disability

• *Sensory:* Deafness, see pp. 398-9. Blindness: congenital defects, see p. 380. Principal acquired causes of blindness are: retinopathy of prematurity (p. 306), eye injuries, cataract (eg Down syndrome), and in developing countries: vitamin A deficiency, trachoma, onchocerciasis (p. 374).

• *CNS & musculoskeletal problems:* (Congenital or acquired.) *Causes:* accidents (eg road traffic accidents), cerebral palsy (pp. 262-3), spina bifida (p. 285), meningitis, polio, congenital infections, tumours, syndromes (pp. 842-59).

• *Wheelchairs:*[14] For indoors or outdoors? Patient-operated, motorized, or pushed? What sort of restraints/supports? Must it fit into the car? Are the sides removable to aid transfer from chair to bed? Can the child control the brakes? Are there adjustable elevated leg rests? Liaise with the physio and occupational therapist.

• *Knee–ankle–foot orthosis (KAFO):* (aka *Callipers.*) Will allow some patients to stand and walk. KAFOs with a knee-lock are used to prevent the knee bending when there is quadriceps weakness. The lock and foot section prevents foot drop. Modern KAFOs are lightweight, use moulded plastics, and fit into shoes. There are various designs, each determined by individual disability/ functionality.

14 Disabled Living Foundation: www.dlf.org.uk

Checklist to guide management of disability

In hospitals or the community, we should address each of these points:
• Screening and its documentation on local disability registers.
• Communication with parents.
• Referring to/liaising with district team & community paediatrician.
• Access to specialist services, including physiotherapy, orthopaedic surgery.
• Assessing special needs for schooling and housing.
• Coordinating neuropsychological/neurodevelopmental assessments.
• Coordinating measures of severity (eg electrophysiology ± CT/MRI).
• Liaison with dietician on nutrition.
• Promotion of long-term concordance with treatment/education programmes.
• Education about the consequences of the illness.
• Encourage contact with family support groups.
• Offering family planning *before* patients become unintentionally pregnant.
• Pre-conception counselling; referral to geneticist if appropriate.
• Coordinating prenatal diagnostic tests and fetal assessment.

Society, paediatrics in the community, and family-oriented care

Most paediatric care goes on in the community, provided by mothers, fathers, GPs, nurses, physios, community paediatricians, child-minders, special-needs teachers, and their assistants. Inevitably if you are studying paediatrics within hospital you will have a biased view of what paediatrics is like—nowhere more at odds with reality than in the spheres of impairment and disability. ►*If you really want to make a difference to children's lives, get out into the community.* Find out what is going on—and then start contributing.

Increasingly, this is being advocated by paediatric training programmes in the UK and abroad—eg the *Community Paediatrics Training Initiative.*[307]

Children's health and well-being are inextricably linked to their parents' physical, emotional, and social health, social circumstances, and parenting ability.[308] These cannot be appreciated or moulded to the child's advantage without at least one foot in the community.

No paediatrician can work well without understanding the demographics of the population from which their patients come. The proportion of children who live in poverty is ~5-fold greater for female-headed families than for married-couple families.[308] In the UK, 4.1 million children live in poverty, ⅔ of whom live in a family where at least one parent works.[309] This has a greater effect on children's health than all the goings on in paediatric wards and hospitals.

Most families with young children depend on child care, of varying quality with ↑ costs (only partly mitigated by government support).

More and more parents are devoting time once available to their children to the care of their own parents. They won't tell you of this in brief ward encounters, but these facts become clear when working in the community.[308]

Paediatricians have a key role in fostering interdisciplinary collaboration between schools, hospitals, and other child-related institutions, and they must feel able to refer parents for physical, emotional, or social problems, or health risk behaviours that can adversely affect the health or emotional or social well-being of their child.

3 Paediatrics

Genome sequencing This is sequencing a person's entire exome (coding regions) or genome (coding and non-coding regions). What to do with this wealth of information is the current dilemma, particularly variants of unknown significance. In the future, whole genome sequencing is likely to be common and the basis of 'personalized' or 'precision' medicine.

Single gene analysis This is used to identify mutations to a specific gene; a targeted test so only useful where there is high pre-test probability/clinical suspicion of a single gene disorder. Tests may be PCR for a specific mutation or a panel of PCRs for multiple disease causing mutations (eg cystic fibrosis) or sequencing of the whole gene.

Genotyping Identifies both alleles at a specific gene locus to determine whether the patient is homozygous, heterozygous, or compound heterozygous (carrying 2 disease-causing variants).

Gene panels Used for specific presentations and test for a number of genes that are known causes of that clinical syndrome (eg immunodeficiency).

Chromosomal studies Karyotyping uses visual examination to determine the number of each chromosome. Array comparative genomic hybridization (CGH) detects copy number variants which reveal aneuploidies or smaller duplications or deletions. Array CGH is quicker and does not require cultured cells so is now the 1st line for suspected chromosomal abnormalities. However, only karyotyping can detect translocations which is important for risk of recurrence.

Prenatal testing Non-invasive prenatal screening (NIPS) can now be performed on fetal DNA (cell-free DNA) circulating in maternal blood to detect chromosome aneuploidies. While this has high sensitivity (eg 99% for trisomy 21)[310] there are occasional false positives and it is still considered a screening test. The gold standard (using fetal DNA from amniotic fluid cells (amniocentesis) in the 2nd trimester, or from chorionic villus sampling in the 1st) is recommended for those who screen positive.

Non-disjunction After meiosis, 1 gamete contains 2 chromosome 21s (say)[15] and the other gamete has no chromosome 21. After union of the 1st gamete with a normal gamete, the conceptus has trisomy 21 (50% spontaneously miscarry). This is the cause in ≥88% of babies with trisomy 21, and increases significantly in mothers over 40 (p. 16).

Translocation Where 2 chromosomes have been broken and rejoined in the wrong combination. They can be balanced, entailing no net gain or loss of chromosomal material, or unbalanced with a change to the genetic material.

Robertsonian translocations (fig 3.21) Entail a translocation at the centromeres of 2 chromosomes with loss of the short arms. A chromosome with 2 long arms is formed, 1 derived from each chromosome. They involve any 2 of chromosomes 13, 14, 15, 21, & 22 (all acrocentric ie the centromere is close to one end). As the genetic material on the short arms is not significant this leads to a balanced karyotype with 45 chromosomes

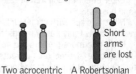

Two acrocentric   A Robertsonian
chromosomes   translocation

Short
arms
are lost

Fig 3.21 A chromosome with 2 long arms.

and a normal phenotype. The offspring, however, are at risk of monosomy or trisomy and this is how 4% of Down syndrome cases occur (unrelated to maternal age). If the father carries the translocation, risk of trisomy 21 is 10%; if it is the mother, the risk is 50%. 0.3% of mothers have this translocation.

Mosaicism A trisomy may develop during early divisions of a normal conceptus (∴ somatic, not germline). If the proportion of trisomy 21 cells is low (eg 4%) CNS development may be 'normal'. It accounts for ≤8% of Down syndrome babies.[311]

15 Chromosome 21 contains only 225 genes: most of its DNA is apparently meaningless.

Causes : See p. 272. *Recognition at birth:* Flat facial profile, abundant neck skin, dysplastic ears, muscle hypotonia, and x-ray evidence of a dysplastic pelvis are the most constant features. Other features: see BOX 'Features of trisomy 21'. Δ: It is best to ask an expert's review, rather than cause anxiety for the family by taking karyotype tests 'just in case it's Down's'.[16] Fluorescent *in situ* hybridization (FISH) can give rapid results, karyotyping is needed to determine whether the trisomy is as a result of a translocation (and therefore ↑ risk of recurrence) or not. Helping the mother accept her child may be aided by introducing her to a friendly mother of a baby with trisomy 21. *Prenatal diagnosis:* pp. 12-3, pp. 16-7.

Features of trisomy 21

Clinical features
- Hypotonia.
- Flat face and small round head (brachycephaly).
- Upward slanted palpebral fissures and epicanthic folds.
- Speckled irises (Brushfield spots).
- Protruding tongue (pseudo-macroglossia).
- High-arched palate.
- Single palmar crease.
- Short broad hands and fingers (brachydactyly).
- Hypoplasia of middle phalanx of (incurving) 5th finger (clinodactyly).
- Pelvic dysplasia.
- Wide space between 1st and 2nd toes (sandal gap).
- Cardiac malformations.
- Intestinal atresia (esp. duodenal), Hirschsprung's, and imperforate anus.
- Short stature.

Associations
- Intellectual impairment.
- Lung problems (lung capacity is reduced in almost all).
- Congenital heart disease (42%) AVSD, VSD, ASD, ToF, PDA.
- Digestive problems (6%).
- Hypothyroidism.
- Hearing loss (60%).
- Leukaemia (ALL and AML).
- Early-onset Alzheimer disease (50%).
- 44% survive to age 60 years.

The health needs approach to someone with trisomy 21 This approach starts by asking: 'How can I help?' Health maintenance for children with trisomy 21 is more important, not less, compared with the needs of other children—because their families are vulnerable, and many conditions are more likely in those with this condition. Examples are otitis media, refractive errors, congenital cataracts, coeliac disease, type 1 diabetes, leukaemoid reactions, dental problems, and feeding difficulties.[312]

The patient-centred approach Different approaches are needed at different times: a key skill in becoming a good doctor is to be able to move seamlessly from one approach to another—and knowing when to adopt which approach.

---

16 Even in good hands, accuracy of suspicion is only 64%, so at some stage karyotyping is needed.[313]

Chromosome terminology Autosomes (non-sex chromosomes) are numbered 1 to 22 roughly in order of size, 1 being the largest. The arms on each side of the centromere are named 'p' (petite) for the short arm, and 'q' for the long arm (remember, there's always a long Q for a short P). Thus 'the long arm of chromosome 6' is written '6q'.

Chromosomal disorders The most important chromosomal abnormalities are aneuploidies (abnormalities in chromosome number)—eg Down syndrome, (trisomy 21 (T21), p. 273). Many genes are involved when the defect is large enough to be seen microscopically and most spontaneously abort or are incompatible with life (Edward's (T18, p. 846), and Patau's (T13, p. 854)). Sex-chromosome aneuploidies are Turner (45,X0, p. 859) and Klinefelter (47,XXY, p. 850) syndromes. *Cri-du-chat* syndrome is an example of chromosome deletion. The short arm of chromosome 5 is missing, causing a high-pitched cry, CVS abnormalities, microcephaly, widely spaced eyes, and a 'moon' face.

Autosomal dominants Adult polycystic kidney (16p), Huntington's chorea, (4p). A single copy of a defective gene causes damage. Some people inheriting the defective gene are phenotypically normal (=*reduced penetrance*).

Autosomal recessives Infantile polycystic kidney; cystic fibrosis (7q), β-thalassaemia, sickle cell (11p), most metabolic conditions, and almost all which are fatal in childhood. In general, both genes must be defective before damage is seen, so carriers are common. Both parents must be carriers for offspring to be affected, so consanguinity (marrying blood relatives) increases risk.

x-linked Duchenne muscular dystrophy, p. 846; haemophilia A & B; fragile x (p. 852). In female (xx) carriers a normal gene on the 2nd x chromosome prevents manifestation of disorder. Males (xy) have no such protection.

Genetic counselling Aims to provide accurate, up-to-date information on genetic conditions to enable families and patients to make informed decisions.
►Genetic counselling is best done in regional centres to which you should refer.
Consider the consequences of doing any test on a child—but especially a genetic test. Discuss with a geneticist or senior doctor first—will the child be glad of the information when they are old enough to understand?

In order to receive most benefit from referral
- The affected person (proband) ideally comes with family (spouse, parents, children, siblings); individuals can of course be seen alone as well.
- The family should be informed that a detailed pedigree (family tree) will be constructed, and medical details of distant relatives may be asked for.
- Irrational emotions (guilt, blame, anger) are common. Deal with these sensitively, and do not ignore. *Remember:* you do not choose your ancestors, and you cannot control what you pass on to your descendants.
- Warn patients that most tests give no absolute 'yes' or 'no' but merely 'likely' or 'unlikely'. In gene tracking, where a molecular fragment near the gene is followed through successive family members, the degree of certainty of the answer will depend on the distance between the marker and the gene (as crossing-over in meiosis may separate them).
- Accept that some people will not want testing eg the offspring of a Huntington's patient—or a mother of a boy who might have fragile x syndrome, but who understandably does not want her offspring labelled (employment, insurance, and social reasons). Offer a genetic referral to ensure that her decision is fully informed (but remember: 'being fully informed' may itself be deleterious to health and well-being).

NB: being pregnant and unwilling to consider termination does *not* exclude one from undergoing useful genetic counselling.

'Couple screening' A big problem with counselling is the unnecessary anxiety caused by false +ve tests. In cystic fibrosis screening of prospective parents (analysis of cells in mouthwash samples), this is reducible by 97% (0.08% vs 3.2%) by screening mother and father together—there is no cause for concern unless *both* are screen-positive. Many forget that they will need future tests if they have a different partner, and those who do not are left with some lingering anxieties.

Genetic counselling to try to influence pregnancy outcome?

The increasing use of genomic tests around pregnancy can lead to difficult ethical decisions. There may be tensions between the interests of different individuals including people who don't yet exist or exist as embryos *in vitro* or fetuses *in vivo*. *Pre-implantation genetic diagnosis* for couples with known genetic mutations can provide reassurance but these techniques have been used in other ways: sex selection; HLA typing to provide a match for a sick sibling; selecting an embryo with the same disability as the parents, such as deafness. Genetic screening is increasingly available from commercial suppliers including preconception carrier screening for x-linked and autosomal recessive disorders and circulating cell-free DNA screening in pregnancy for fetal chromosomal abnormalities. This may result in information, such as copy number variants of uncertain significance, which may push people towards an 'unnecessary' termination.[314]

Couples should not undergo testing without sufficient pretest genetic counselling to fully inform their decision-making. They should be given balanced, up-to-date information and psychological support to help them weigh up the pros and cons of undergoing testing.[315] Non-directive counselling is something of a mantra among counsellors. We should explore the patient's world view and their expectations, and then use this knowledge to reframe the information in a way that makes sense to the individuals concerned, taking into account their cultures and systems of beliefs and allowing them to make truly informed decisions.

Most commonly seen between age 2 & 3yrs (accidental), in older children it is usually self-harm or a suicide attempt. Determine *how much, when,* and *what exactly* was ingested; the number of tablets dispensed is often on the pack—count what remains and calculate the maximum dose ingested. Ask if *other medicines/chemicals* are kept in the same place and could the child have taken more than one type? Was this child playing with any *others*? If so, they too may have shared some of the poison. If the tablets are from an unlabelled box, the dispenser may have records and be able to name the tablets; to help identify medication from loose tablets brought in by parents use sites such as www.drugs.com/pill_identification.html—this is usa based—your hospital may subscribe to an equivalent local system. Once the poison has been identified consult TOXBASE® (www.toxbase.org) or local equivalent.

▶Contact a National Poisons Information Service (NPIS, eg 0844 892 0111 in UK). **Examination** Look for signs of toxidromes (see 'Toxidromes'). Ensure complete set of vital signs are obtained. Note GCS and pupils.

Principles of management

- As always: ABC is your priority, but also DEFG, don't ever forget glucose.
- Consider intubation if GCS <8, or respiratory failure; if GCS 8–14 consider oral/nasopharyngeal airway (caution if vomiting) and put in recovery position.
- Maintain BP; correct hypoglycaemia; monitor urine output.
- Baseline studies may include: FBC, U&E; glucose; ECG.
- Do a blood gas: a metabolic acidosis with an increased anion gap can be due to drugs such as metformin; alcohol; ethylene; toluene; cyanide; isoniazid; iron; aspirin; paraldehyde; or other causes (DKA; lactic acidosis).
- Certain drugs can be measured in serum, so test for paracetamol; ethanol; methanol; ethylene glycol (in antifreeze); salicylates; iron; anticonvulsants; lithium; digoxin; theophylline; carboxyhaemoglobin if these are suspected.
- The mainstay of care is *supportive management.*
- Determine if a *specific antidote* is available (see 'Specific antidotes' and p. 278, p. 279).
- Haemofiltration may be required for extremely unwell children.
- Consider *gastric decontamination*—discuss with a toxicologist.
- *Activated charcoal* is controversial as there is no evidence it improves clinical outcome.[316] It is most effective if given within 1h of ingestion. Concerns exist about the risk of aspiration of charcoal if the patient vomits or becomes drowsy. Avoid with lithium, alcohol, cyanide, iron ingestions, or rapid acting ingestions.[316]
- *Ipecacuanha,* or any form of forced vomiting, is no longer recommended.[317] *Cathartics* (which accelerate defecation) and *gastric lavage* are virtually never indicated.[304,305,306] *Whole-bowel irrigation* should not be routinely used, but it may be of benefit in sustained released ingestions. Only use after consulting NPIS or if specifically recommended in TOXBASE®.[320]

Specific antidotes See also OHCM p842.
- *Opioids:* Use IV naloxone 100mcg/kg (max. 2mg); if no response, repeat at 1min intervals up to 2mg and review Δ. Half-life is short so repeated doses or infusion may be required. IM can be used.
- *Beta-blockers:* Cause hypotension, bradycardia, heart block, and heart failure. Monitor ECG; atropine 40mcg/kg IV for bradycardia, then glucagon (50–150mcg/kg IV + infusion of 50mcg/kg/h in 5% glucose). Consider adrenaline or dopamine infusions.
- *Carbon monoxide:* High-flow oxygen, treat raised ICP conventionally.
- *Digoxin:* Atropine is used if bradycardic. Digoxin-specific antibody (Digibind™) is used in those with severe dysrhythmias/hyperkalaemia.

3 Paediatrics

Toxidromes
- *Opioid:* eg morphine, codeine, tramadol, fentanyl, methadone, oxycodone, heroin; miosis (pin-point pupils), respiratory depression, ↓ consciousness, bradycardia, and hypotension.
- *Cholinergic:* eg organophosphates; pilocarpine: *DUMBBELLS:* *D*iarrhoea; *U*rination; *M*iosis; *B*ronchospasm (and secretions); *B*radycardia; *E*mesis; *L*acrimation; *L*ethargy; *S*alivation. Also muscle weakness, respiratory depression, ataxia, and seizures.
- *Anticholinergic:* eg antihistamines, tricyclic antidepressants, deadly nightshade, atropine—these patients are *Hot as a hare, Red as a beet, Dry as a bone, Blind as a bat,* and *Mad as a hatter*—with hyperthermia, facial flushing, dry skin, mydriasis (dilated pupils), and delirium. They also have tachycardia, arrhythmias, and urinary retention.
- *Sympathomimetic:* eg cocaine, amphetamines, pseudoephedrine—patient is tachycardic, hypertensive, hyperthermic, and has mydriasis. Risk of seizures and MI.

Iron poisoning

Iron is a common childhood poison. It is absorbed as Fe^{2+}, oxidized to Fe^{3+}, and bound to transferrin. Toxicity occurs when transferrin binding capacity is exceeded.

Identify the exact preparation As formulations contain different amounts of elemental iron (don't forget some multivitamins contain iron). A 300mg ferrous fumarate tablet may contain 100mg of iron (depends on brand), whereas a 300mg ferrous gluconate tablet may only contain 35mg iron. Expect mild toxicity at doses of >20mg/kg of elemental iron. Moderate–severe toxicity occurs with doses of >60mg/kg.[321,322] Doses of 200–250mg/kg are potentially fatal.

Presentation Nausea, vomiting, abdo pain, haematemesis, diarrhoea, altered mental status, or hypotension. Between 6 & 12 hours there may be a phase of apparent improvement. Between 12 & 24 hours cardiovascular collapse and massive GI bleeding can occur. Severe metabolic acidosis with raised anion gap may develop as each Fe^{3+} ion combines with water to produce $3H^+$ and $Fe(OH)_3$. Renal and hepatic failure may ensue. Hepatotoxicity is a marker of severity and is a common cause of death. Survivors may develop pyloric strictures after 4–6 weeks secondary to scarring. *Tests:* Blood gas, serum iron concentration, U&E, FBC, LFTs, clotting, glucose, ECG. Iron levels at 4–6h indicate severity. Levels of <3mg/L (~55μmol/L) are associated with minimal symptoms and >5mg/L (~90μmol/L) serious toxicity. An abdominal x-ray may show tablets within the gut and reveal a bezoar (a mass within the gastrointestinal system).

Management
► In severe toxicity do not wait for tests: start desferrioxamine.
- Obtain expert help as this is one of the few instances when gastric lavage/endoscopy to remove tablets in the stomach may be recommended.
- Activated charcoal is not given as it does not bind iron.
- Whole-bowel irrigation may help (esp. in slow-release preparations).[323]
- Supportive care—IV fluids and sodium bicarbonate to correct acidosis.
- Chelation with IV **desferrioxamine** (15mg/kg/h until 80mg/kg given then discuss with national poisons service). Therapy should be stopped when the acidosis improves. It is rarely required for >24h. Use of desferrioxamine leads to orangey-red urine which demonstrates that free iron has been bound to the desferrioxamine. It is also associated with hypotension, rashes, pulmonary oedema, and acute respiratory distress syndrome.
- Haemofiltration has been used in children, in combination with desferrioxamine to rapidly reduce iron levels.[324]

Refer to TOXBASE® (www.toxbase.org) and *BNFC*. The therapeutic dose is 15mg/kg. Hepatotoxicity can occur if ≥150mg/kg ingested but has been reported rarely with ingestion as low as 75mg/kg. Initial features are minimal (nausea and vomiting) and usually settle <24h. Hepatic enzymes rise after ~24h. Jaundice and an enlarged, tender liver occur after 48h. Maximal liver damage is 3–4 days post ingestion. Hypoglycaemia, hypotension, encephalopathy, coagulopathy, coma, and death from liver failure may also occur.

Management of single oral paracetamol overdoses

- If you are certain the ingested paracetamol is <75mg/kg in a child, then management may be safely done at home after addressing risk of self-harm.[325]
- Admit those ingesting >75mg/kg (or an unknown amount) and do a serum paracetamol concentration at ≥4h post ingestion, with venous gas, U&E, bicarbonate, FBC, LFTs and clotting. If presenting <1h, and >150mg/kg ingested, and no contraindication (eg vomiting; ↓GCS), give activated charcoal.*BNFC*
- Consult the nomogram in fig 3.22. If plasma paracetamol level is on or above the line, *or* the patient has an abnormal INR, ALT, or creatinine, treat with **acetylcysteine** (NAC).
- The initial dose of NAC is 150mg/kg in up to 200mL (depending on weight; see *BNFC*) of 5% glucose infused over 1h, followed by 50mg/kg IVI over the next 4h, and 100mg/kg IVI over the next 16h. It is very effective in preventing liver damage if started <8h after overdose.
- Patients who present 8–24h after ingestion, should have NAC started immediately if ingested dose is >150mg/kg, or dose is unknown. NAC can then be stopped if paracetamol level is below the treatment line on fig 3.22, patient is asymptomatic, and INR, LFTs, and creatinine are normal.
- Prognostic value of paracetamol levels >15h after ingestion is uncertain. Treat if above the line, contact the national poisons service if in doubt.
- There is generally no indication to start NAC before obtaining the paracetamol level if that can be obtained and acted on in <8h.
- In obese patients use actual weight for calculating toxic dose and NAC dose up to a maximum of 110kg.
- Consider the cause. All deliberate overdoses need psychiatric evaluation, preferably by child and adolescent mental health specialists. Causes may be extremely complex and deep-seated: although the patient may claim a seemingly superficial cause, this may be hiding deep social or psychiatric pathology.

Special circumstances

- Neonates with corrected gestational age of <45 weeks are at higher risk of liver damage, seek expert advice for all cases.
- Staggered overdoses or therapeutic excess (a potentially toxic dose taken over a period >1h): if >150mg/kg taken in any 24h period, start NAC and seek expert advice unless >24h have elapsed since last ingestion, patient is asymptomatic, paracetamol level is undetectable and blood results are normal.
- With IV paracetamol overdoses, the nomogram does not apply. Discuss all cases with national poisons service. Start NAC if >60mg/kg given.

Further reading

The Royal College of Emergency Medicine (2012). *Paracetamol Overdose in Adults and Children.* www.rcem.ac.uk/RCEM/Quality-Policy/Clinical_Standards_Guidance/RCEM_Guidance.aspx
Information relating to all poisonings: www.toxbase.org (will require an institutional login).

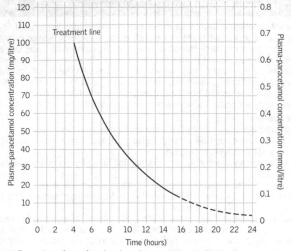

Fig 3.22 Paracetamol overdose treatment nomogram.

Reproduced from Drug Safety Update September 2012, vol 6, issue 2: A1 © Crown Copyright 2013. Contains public sector information licensed under the Open Government Licence v3.0. Available at https://www.gov.uk/drug-safety-update/treating-paracetamol-overdose-with-intravenous-acetylcysteine-new-guidance

Salicylate poisoning

The most common salicylate is acetylsalicylic acid ie aspirin, which is not recommended in children <16yrs due to its association with Reye syndrome (p. 856). Choline salicylate is found in Bonjela™ for adults. Since 2009, Bonjela teething gel™ in the UK has used lidocaine as its active ingredient, however Bonjela teething gel™ in other countries (eg Australasia) continues to contain choline salicylate (8.7%) and there are reports of toxicity in children.[326] Methyl salicylate is found in oil of wintergreen (98%). As little as 3mL can be fatal in children.[327] Methyl salicylate is also found in muscle rubs such as Bengay™, Deep Heat™, and Tiger Balm™ (~15–40%). **Presentation** Toxicity occurs at ~100mg/kg aspirin. Early signs include tinnitus and hearing loss. Stimulation of respiratory centres leads to tachypnoea and a respiratory alkalosis. Interference with aerobic metabolism leads to the metabolic (lactic) acidosis which is characteristic of salicylate poisoning. GI irritation (nausea, vomiting, abdominal pain is common). Central effects lead to agitation, delirium, and seizures. Rhabdomyolysis, pulmonary oedema, and electrolyte disturbances may also occur, particularly hypokalaemia. **Tests** Blood gas; FBC; U&E, clotting, glucose, ECG. Salicylate levels are best obtained at 6h (reflects a peak level); however, do an initial level to confirm diagnosis, and then levels every 2h to confirm levels are decreasing—enteric coated (EC) preparations can lead to delayed absorption. Large bezoars of EC aspirin may be seen on x-ray. **Management** Avoid intubation unless in respiratory failure, sudden loss of hyperventilatory drive can lead to decompensation and death. Resuscitate with boluses of 10–20mL/kg of 0.9% NaCl. Correct hypokalaemia. Severe toxicity is likely with levels >700mg/L (5.1mmol/L)—consider urinary alkalinization with IV sodium bicarbonate to enhance elimination (under expert guidance in ITU). Activated charcoal is effective in adsorbing aspirin, give via NGT. Repeat doses can be given. Haemodialysis is the definitive treatment: use when evidence of end-organ injury[328] (seizures, severe acidosis, rhabdomyolysis, renal failure, pulmonary oedema). *Seek expert help.*

Neonatal collapse Neonates can become unwell rapidly and present unresponsive, in shock, ± respiratory distress, ± DIC, ± seizures. Sepsis is by far the most common cause but ΔΔ is *wide*: cardiac (congenital heart disease, arrhythmia, myocarditis), metabolic disease (p. 252-3), undiagnosed congenital abnormality (congenital diaphragmatic hernia, oesophageal atresia, tracheo-oesophageal fistula), necrotizing enterocolitis (NEC, p. 284), MAS (pp. 284-5), PPHN (p. 305), RDS (p. 304), blood loss (placental haemorrhage; twin–twin transfusion; intraventricular haemorrhage; haemorrhagic disease of the newborn).

Management:
- Initially supportive, + antibiotics, ± prostin, then as directed by cause.
- ABC: high-flow O_2, ventilate as needed, give **crystalloid** 20mL/kg (caution if signs of heart failure), repeat as needed.
- Fluid refractory shock: inotropes eg **dopamine** 10mcg/kg per min and intubate and ventilate.
- Blood gas, lactate, glucose, FBC, CRP, U&E, clotting, ± ammonia, ± ECG.
- Blood culture, CXR, urine (if >72h old), LP (when stable enough), skin swab if signs, ± HSV PCR, ± stool virology, ± urine CMV PCR.
- Consider duct-dependent cardiac lesion (poor femoral pulses, cyanosis without respiratory distress and not responding to O_2, heart murmur, cardiomegaly, differential pre- and post-ductal O_2 saturations): start prostin (apnoeas common) and discuss with cardiology centre.

Neonatal sepsis More common in premature than term babies. Acquired transplacentally, via ascent from vagina, during birth, or from the environment. Mortality up to 15% (30% if low birthweight). Defined as early onset (<72h of birth) or late onset. *Presentation:* Variable, signs may be non-specific and subtle (poor feeding, vomiting/feed intolerance, abdo distension, lethargy, jaundice <24h of birth, temperature <36° or >38°c, ↑ or ↓ glucose, ↑RR, apnoeas, ↑HR) through to neonatal collapse.[329]

Risk factors for neonatal sepsis

Risk factors for early-onset neonatal sepsis
- Mother known carrier of group B *Streptococcus* (GBS) from vagina or urine, or previous infant affected by it (this is the most important risk factor but can be negated by intrapartum antibiotics: see p. 41).
- Intrapartum maternal pyrexia >38°c or suspected chorioamnionitis (pp. 88-9).
- Prolonged (>18h) or pre-labour rupture of membranes (ROM) (p. 57).
- Spontaneous preterm labour (<37wks).
- Suspected maternal invasive bacterial infection.

Causes: Organisms acquired from the mother—usually GBS, *E. coli* or *Listeria*. Other agents include herpes simplex (highest risk to neonate is from primary vulval herpes infection within 6 weeks of delivery), *Chlamydia trachomatis*, anaerobes, and *H. influenzae*.

Risk factors for late-onset neonatal sepsis
- Prematurity.
- Low birthweight.
- Central lines and catheters.
- Congenital malformations eg spina bifida.
- Parenteral nutrition.
- Immunodeficiency.

Causes: Tend to be environmental organisms, eg coagulase-negative staphylococci, *Staph. aureus*, *E. coli*, and GBS. Viral (HSV) or fungal sepsis (from *Candida* spp.) also occur.

Initiation of treatment:
- Treatment may be initiated on the basis of clinical findings or, in early-onset sepsis, on the basis of risk factors alone. Such decision-making inevitably leads to overtreatment to prevent a small number of devastating neonatal infections.
- Most institutions will have their own policy on when to 'screen and treat' based on risk factors alone (eg if term and ≥2 risk factors) or follow NICE CG149.[329]
- More advanced decision support tools (eg Kaiser Permanente Neonatal Early Onset Sepsis calculator: https://neonatalsepsiscalculator.kaiserpermanente.org/) are increasingly available with the potential to reduce unnecessary costs and harms.[330,331]

Investigation: FBC, CRP (may be normal; helpful if raised; bacterial sepsis unlikely if both CRP and repeat CRP 12h later are normal), glucose and blood cultures (results take 36–48h). Consider LP, CXR, catheter urine (not in early-onset sepsis), viral PCR.

Antibiotic choice in early-onset neonatal infection:
- Give broad-spectrum antibiotics eg benzylpenicillin + gentamicin until blood culture results are available.
- If meningitis is suspected, *add* cefotaxime ±aciclovir.
- If *Listeria* suspected (discoloured amniotic fluid, premature delivery, maternal infection), give ampicillin/amoxicillin + gentamicin.

Antibiotic choice in late-onset neonatal infection:
- Broad-spectrum antibiotics eg flucloxacillin + gentamicin.
- Add cefotaxime ± aciclovir if meningitis likely.
- Use amoxicillin, gentamicin, and metronidazole if abdominal source is suspected.
- Coagulase –ve staph sepsis is more likely in preterm infants with central lines— treat with vancomycin & discuss line use/removal with a senior.
- Consider empirical therapy for multidrug-resistant organisms in neonates who have been hospitalized since birth.
- Consider fungal or viral sepsis if failure to respond to standard treatment.

Duration of treatment:
- If baby clinically well, blood culture negative, ×2 CRP 'reassuring' (exact level controversial), and pretreatment level of suspicion low, stop antibiotics after 36h.[329]
- Otherwise, 5–10 days depending on pretreatment level of suspicion, results, and clinical course.
- 14–21 days if meningitis confirmed or highly suspected.

Hypoxic-ischaemic encephalopathy (HIE) A clinical syndrome of brain injury secondary to perinatal hypoxic-ischaemic insult in term babies. In developed countries, the incidence is 2–5/1000 live births, of which 1–2/1000 are moderate to severe. The cause may be antenatal, intrapartum, or postpartum eg cord prolapse, placental abruption, any cause of maternal hypoxia, or inadequate postnatal cardiopulmonary circulation. Presentation varies depending on the severity of cerebral hypoxia. The baby will be unwell at birth, usually requiring resuscitation. Encephalopathy develops within 24h of birth. *Management:* Resuscitation (NLS p. 184), supportive management, monitoring and treatment of seizures (eg using CFAM, p. 284), and assessment of suitability for cooling. Therapeutic hypothermia reduces death and disability. TOBY cooling criteria: ≥36wks' gestation with moderate to severe encephalopathy and either: APGAR score ≤5 or continued need for ventilation at 10min after birth or acidosis (pH <7.00 or base deficit ≥16 mmol/L).[332]

Disseminated intravascular coagulation (DIC) Newborns (particularly preterms) have low levels of coagulation factors and are vulnerable to DIC. *Signs:* Petechiae; bleeding (cutaneous, mucosal, umbilical, GI). *Causes:* Sepsis; NEC; HIE; RDS. *Tests:* Platelets ↓; schistocytes (fragmented RBCs); INR↑; APTT↑; fibrinogen↓.[333,334] *Treatment:* Get help; treat cause (eg NEC, sepsis, etc.); give vit K 1mg IV & blood products as required (platelets; FFP; cryoprecipitate; fibrinogen concentrate; antithrombin III; red cells).[335,336] In most severe cases, consider exchange transfusion.

This is a thorough examination to screen for abnormalities and should be performed within 72h of birth and again at 6–8wks of age (as specified by the NHS Newborn and Infant Physical Examination Screening Programme). Before the examination review: antenatal US scans and serology; gestation; birthweight; any problems during pregnancy or delivery; maternal illness; FH of CHD, jaundice, diabetes, SLE, Graves disease; maternal rhesus status; has baby passed urine/stool? Are they feeding? Does mum have any questions or difficulties? Are there risk factors for sepsis (p. 280)? Find a quiet, warm, well-lit room with stethoscope, tape measure, tongue depressor, and ophthalmoscope. Enlist the mother's help. Explain your aims. Listen if she talks. Examine systematically eg listen to the heart and lungs first when baby is calm then proceed head-to-toe but be opportunistic and check eyes when spontaneously opened. Wash your hands meticulously. Note observations (eg T°, RR, HR).[337,338]

Head Measure and document circumference (50th centiles, ♂=35cm, ♀=34cm, pp. 316–19), shape (odd shapes from a difficult labour soon resolve), fontanelles (tense if crying or intracranial pressure ↑; sunken if dehydrated), and any birth injuries: caput succedaneum, cephalhaematoma, chignon, & subgaleal bleed (pp. 82–3). *Complexion:* Cyanosed, pale, jaundiced, or plethoric (polycythaemia)? *Eyes:* Red reflex *must* be observed (absent in cataract & retinoblastoma); corneal opacities; conjunctivitis. *Ears:* Shape; position. Are they low set (ie below eyes)? Ensure oto-acoustic screening is done (p. 398). *Mouth:* The palate must be visualized *and* palpated to ensure it is intact. Breathing out of the nose (shut the mouth) tests for choanal atresia. Is suck good? *Face:* Facial nerve injury (if forceps delivery). Does the baby's face look normal? Dysmorphism can be difficult to detect soon after birth as the baby may have some puffiness in the face. Is there torticollis (wry neck)?

Arms & hands Number of digits (polydactyly is common). Single palmar creases (normal or trisomy 21). Brachydactyly and clinodactyly (trisomy 21, see p. 273). Waiter's tip sign of Erb's palsy of: C5 & C6 brachial plexus injury (p. 74 & pp. 210–11).

Thorax Watch respirations; note grunting and intercostal recession. Palpate the precordium, apex beat (dextrocardia), brachial and femoral pulses (coarctation). Listen to the heart and lungs. Any murmur or suspected cardiac abnormality needs prompt senior review. Palpate the clavicles. Inspect and palpate the vertebral column for neural tube defects.

Abdomen Expect to feel the liver edge. Any other masses? Inspect the umbilicus. Next, lift the skin to assess skin turgor. Inspect genitalia and anus. Are the orifices patent? Ensure the baby passes urine in the 1st 24h (consider posterior urethral valves in boys if not) and stool in the 1st 24h (consider Hirschsprung's, cystic fibrosis, hypothyroidism). Is the urinary meatus misplaced (hypospadias), and are both testes descended? The neonatal clitoris often looks rather large, but if very large, consider CAH, p. 302. Bleeding PV may be a normal variant following maternal oestrogen withdrawal.

Legs Test for developmental dysplasia of the hip (p. 492). Avoid repeated tests as it hurts, and may induce dislocation. Note talipes (pp. 492–3) and whether it is positional (self-resolving) or fixed (referral needed). *Toes:* Too many, too few, or too blue?

Buttocks/sacrum Is there a patent anus? Tufts of hair ± dimples suggest bifida occulta. If you can't see the bottom of a dimple, or is large and >2.5cm from anus, arrange US. Is there congenital dermal melanocytosis ('mongolian' or 'blue' spots—harmless, fades over years)?

cns Assess posture and handle the baby. Intuition can be most helpful in deciding if a baby is ill or well. There should be some control of the head. Do limbs move normally? Is the tone floppy or spastic? Are responses absent on one side (hemiplegia)? The Moro reflex should be symmetrical. It is checked by sitting the baby at 45°, supporting the head. On momentarily removing the support to the head the arms will abduct, the hands open and then the arms adduct. Touch the palm to elicit a grasp reflex.

Pulse oximetry screening Screening of pre and post-ductal o₂ saturations to detect congenital heart disease is currently being piloted in the UK.

The assessment should be recorded in the newborn's 'red book' in the UK.

▶If uncertain about your findings, get a senior review before unduly alarming the parents.

Minor neonatal problems

Most neonates have a few minor lesions; the more you examine neonates, the better you will become at reassuring mothers.

Strawberry naevus (fig 3.23) May not be present at birth, increases in size over first few months, then fades again. Some may ulcerate or bleed. If large or in critical area (over eye or joint), consider early propranolol to shrink the lesion.

Milia 1–2mm pearly white/cream papules caused by retention of keratin in dermis. Found on forehead, nose, cheeks. Will resolve spontaneously.

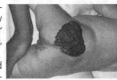
Fig 3.23 Strawberry naevus.

Erythema toxicum neonatorum These red blotches, usually with a central white pustule, often cause concern for parents but are harmless. Present at birth or <48h, appears more florid when warm and resolves spontaneously in 5–7 days.

Miliaria *Miliaria crystallina* develop due to transient sweat-pore disruption[339] or immaturity[340]—hence its characteristic 1–2mm retention vesicle.[341] Prevalence: ≤ 8%.[342] In *miliaria rubra* there is also a surrounding flush (a prickly-heat like-rash).

Stork bites These are areas of capillary dilatation on the eyelids, central forehead, and back of the neck—where the baby is deemed to have been held in the stork's beak. They blanch on pressure and fade with time.

Peeling skin/desquamation Common in postmature babies, it does not denote future skin problems.

Petechial haemorrhages, facial cyanosis, subconjunctival haemorrhages These temporary features generally reflect suffusion of the face during delivery.

Swollen breasts These occur in both sexes and occasionally lactate ('witch's milk'). They are due to maternal hormones and gradually subside if left alone, but if infected (mastitis or abscess) need antibiotics. Milk may persist until 2 months old.

The umbilicus It dries and separates around day 7 but may persist up to 3 weeks. Infection (omphalitis) is rare in developed settings. *Granuloma:* Don't cauterize with a silver nitrate stick, table salt applied BD for 2 days usually leads to complete resolution.[343]

Sticky eye Very common in neonates, usually not infected and responds to cleansing. If persists may be due to a blocked tear duct, p. 340. If copious, purulent discharge or conjunctivitis swab and treat as infection, see p. 41.

Red-stained nappy This is usually due to urinary urate crystals but may be blood from the cord or baby's vagina (oestrogen withdrawal bleed).

Harlequin colour change Transient, episodic, demarcated erythema on left or right, with simultaneous contralateral blanching, harmless, self-limiting.

Neonatal seizures (~4/1000 births) Most occur 12–48h after birth, and may be generalized or focal, and tonic, clonic, or myoclonic.

Causes:
• Hypoxic-ischaemic encephalopathy (p. 281).
• Infection (meningitis/encephalitis).
• Intracranial haemorrhage/infarction.
• Structural CNS lesions (focal cortical dysplasia/tuberous sclerosis).
• Metabolic disturbance (hypoglycaemia; ↓Ca²⁺; ↑ or ↓Na⁺; ↓Mg²⁺).
• Metabolic disorders (urea cycle disorders/amino acid metabolism).
• Neonatal withdrawal from maternal drugs or substance abuse.
• Kernicterus (pp. 294-5).
• Benign neonatal convulsions (AKA 5th day fits, a Δ of exclusion).

Diagnosis: Can be very difficult to diagnose as there may only be subtle clinical signs, eg lip-smacking, limb-cycling, eye deviation, apnoeas. CFAM (see later) or EEG can confirm seizure activity but only video EEG telemetry during episodes can exclude.

Management: ABC, check glucose. Turn on the side if any aspiration risk.
• A single short seizure does not need to be treated with anticonvulsants. If prolonged (>3–5min) or repeated seizures consider anticonvulsants. *1st line:* **phenobarbital**. Loading dose: 20mg/kg IV as slow injection. *2nd line:* **phenytoin** 18mg/kg IVI. Other agents: clonazepam; midazolam; paraldehyde, levetiracetam. If intractable seizures consider trials of pyridoxine (vit B₆), pyridoxal phosphate, or biotin supplements in case of pyridoxine or biotin deficiencies.[344]
• Consider starting empirical antibiotics.
• Insert IV access and take blood for FBC, culture, CRP, U&E, LFTs, Ca²⁺, Mg²⁺, glucose and blood gas. Consider LP.
• If available, commence cerebral function analysis monitoring (CFAM—a basic bedside EEG monitor).
• Radiological investigation may include cranial US, and MRI.
• Other tests include toxicology screening, ammonia, urine organic acids, serum amino acids, karyotype, and TORCH screen (pp. 38–9).
• Treat the cause where possible. *Hypoglycaemia:* 10% **glucose** 2–5mL/kg IV. *Hypocalcaemia:* IV **calcium gluconate** 10%, 1mL/kg (over 5–10min). Monitor ECG. Repeat once if necessary. *Hypomagnesaemia:* give 100mg/kg of **magnesium sulfate** 10% (=100mg/mL), IV over >10min.[346]

Necrotizing enterocolitis (NEC) An ischaemic, inflammatory bowel necrosis. Main risk factors: prematurity, ↓BW. If weight <1500g, 5–10% develop NEC. Other risk factors: non-human milk feeds, comorbidities affecting gut perfusion (eg congenital heart disease, IUGR, sepsis).[346] Probiotics ↓ risk (*Lactobacillus* ± *Bifidobacterium*).[347] *Signs:* If mild, just some abdominal distension, ↑ aspirates (esp. bilious), faecal occult blood. Temperature instability, lethargy, apnoea, blood/mucus PR. If severe, there is marked abdominal distension, discolouration, tenderness (± perforation), shock, DIC, & mucosal sloughing. *Tests:* Abdo x-ray (AXR), abdo US (pneumatosis intestinalis (gas in the gut) is pathognomonic); FBC + film; clotting; cross-match; CRP; U&E; blood gas + lactate. ℞: NBM; NGT on free drainage; IV antibiotics: eg amoxicillin, gentamicin, & metronidazole; barrier nurse; TPN; analgesia; low threshold for intubation.[348] Liaise early with surgeon; repeated AXR and girth measurement. Platelets mirror disease activity; <100×10⁹/L is 'severe'.[349] *Laparotomy indications:* Progressive distension, perforation (up to 50% die).

Meconium aspiration syndrome (MAS) Meconium-stained amniotic fluid (MSAF) occurs in ~8–25% of births when the faecal material that accumulates in the fetal colon is passed *in utero* due to fetal maturity or distress. MAS occurs in ~5% of these infants;[350] it is defined as respiratory distress in the infant born through MSAF which cannot otherwise be explained. Aspiration of meconium mostly occurs *in utero* with prolonged hypoxia.[351] Risk of MAS ↑ with ↑ gestational age >31wks. It may lead to airway obstruction, surfactant dysfunction, pulmonary vasoconstriction and persistent pulmonary hypertension of the newborn (PPHN, p. 305), infection, chemical pneumonitis, and pneumothorax. Intrapartum suctioning of the oro/nasopharynx wastes time and makes no difference.[352] Endotracheal suctioning is only needed for those infants who are flat at birth.[352] Cricoid and/or chest compression at birth to prevent aspiration have not been shown to be useful.[353] Surfactant, ventilation, inhaled nitric oxide, antibiotics, chest drains, and ECMO may be required.[338] Avoid CPAP (↑ risk of pneumothorax).

Transient tachypnoea of the newborn (TTN) Due to slow clearance of lung fluid. Features: starts <4h of age, ↑RR ± mild ↑ work of breathing. CXR shows features of pulmonary oedema. More common in caesarean delivery without labour. Usually resolves spontaneously within 24h.

Vitamin κ deficiency bleeding (VKDB=haemorrhagic disease of the newborn.) Usually occurs ~2–7 days postpartum but can be up to 6 months. *Cause:* Poor placental transfer of vit κ, immature liver, no enteric bacteria to make vit κ. *Signs:* The baby is usually well, apart from bruising/bleeding although intracranial haemorrhage does occur. Prothrombin & partial thromboplastin times (PT & PTT) ↑; platelets ↔. *R̶:* **vit κ** 1mg IV TDS ± FFP 15–20mL/kg if severe.[354] Prevention is very effective: vit κ 1mg IM at birth (0.4mg/kg if <2.5kg); or oral colloidal (mixed micelle) **phytomenadione** 2mg at birth, repeated at 4–7 days; if exclusively breastfed, give a 3rd oral dose at 1m old (infant formulas are fortified).

Neural tube defects (NTDs) Result from failure of the neural tube to close between the 3rd and 4th week of *in utero* development. *Terminology:* **Spina bifida:** incomplete vertebral arch. *Myelocele:* failure of cord fusion so that there is a flat neural plaque. *Meningocele:* herniation of dura & arachnoid mater through a bony defect. *Meningomyelocele:* herniation involving meninges and cord (fig 3.24). *Closed spinal dysraphism (spina bifida occulta):* vertebral arch defect ± spinal cord abnormality with intact overlying skin. 95% of major lesions are detected on antenatal US. Termination of pregnancy is offered at any stage of pregnancy in the UK if an NTD is discovered. *Neurological deficit* is variable, depending on level of the lesion and the degree to which the lower cord functions independently from the upper cord. Hydrocephalus is common as are urinary and faecal incontinence and sexual dysfunction. Those with lumbosacral myelomeningoceles usually learn to walk with callipers by the age of 3, but ≤20% with higher lesions ever walk. *R̶:* Surgical closure shortly after birth is indicated to prevent CNS infection. Further operations may be needed for spinal deformity (often severe and very hard to treat), cord untethering, and hydrocephalus (ventriculoperitoneal CSF shunts). *Prevention:* **Folic acid** 0.4mg daily for 3 months pre-conception until 13wks' gestation ↓ risk. In mothers who have had an affected baby, folic acid (5mg/day) reduces the risk of recurrence by 72%.

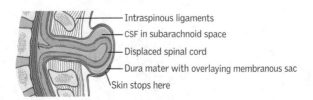

— Intraspinous ligaments
— CSF in subarachnoid space
— Displaced spinal cord
— Dura mater with overlaying membranous sac
Skin stops here

Fig 3.24 Meningomyelocele.

3 Paediatrics

Breastfeeding (± expressed breast milk, p. 288, p. 291) is the ideal way to feed term and pre-term babies. Small babies may remain small and this is not helped by overfeeding. Adequate incremental weight gain is more important than overall size—a good rule of thumb is 'an ounce (28g) a day with a day off on Sundays'.

Nasogastric tube feeding *Indications:* Any sick infant who is too ill or too young to feed normally (eg respiratory distress syndrome). Expressed breast milk or formula milk is fed via a naso- or orogastric tube either as a bolus or as a continuous infusion. If gastro-oesophageal reflux or aspiration is a problem, then a silastic naso-jejunal tube can be used. After entering the stomach, the tube enters the jejunum by peristalsis: confirm its position on x-ray. When the baby improves, start giving some feeds by mouth (PO) eg by increasing the ratio of oral to NG feeds, either in whole feeds, or by fractions of each feed. If during oral feeds, cyanosis, bradycardia, desaturation, apnoea, or vomiting supervene, you may be trying too soon.

Trophic feeding *Synonyms:* Minimal enteral or hypocaloric feeding; gut priming. *Rationale:* If prems go for weeks with no oral nutrition, normal GI structure and function are lost despite an anabolic body state. Villi shorten, mucosal DNA is lost, and enzyme activity is less. Early initiation of sub-nutritional enteral feeding may help by promoting gut motility and bile secretion, inducing lactase activity, and by reducing sepsis and cholestatic jaundice.[355] See fig 3.25. *Technique:* Typically, milk volumes of ~1mL/kg/h are given by tube starting on day 2–3. Use expressed breast milk (or a preterm formula eg Nutriprem®). *Effects:* Studies show that weight gain and head growth is better, and that there are fewer episodes of neonatal sepsis, fewer days of parenteral nutrition are needed, and time to full oral feeding is less. If too much is given, NEC (p. 284) may ensue.[356] *Eligibility:* Experience shows that almost all prems with non-surgical illness tolerate at least some milk as trophic feeds.[357]

Parenteral nutrition (PN, via a central vein.) *Indications:* preterm, low birth-weight; too unwell for enteral nutrition (eg high dose inotropes); and gut malfunction requiring gut 'rest' (eg necrotizing enterocolitis or septic ileus). ▶*Sterility is vital*; prepare using laminar flow units. Monitoring of electrolytes must be meticulous.[17] *Daily checks:* Weight; fluid balance; U&E; blood glucose; Ca^{2+}. Test for glycosuria. Change IVI sets/filters; culture filters, Vamin®, and Intralipid® samples. *Weekly:* Length; head circumference; skinfold thickness. Mg^{2+}; PO_4^{3-}; ALP; triglycerides; LFTs; direct and total bilirubin; FBC; CRP (helps determine if there is line sepsis). *Complications:* Electrolyte imbalances; thrombophlebitis; sepsis; PN associated liver disease; acidosis. *Stopping IV nutrition:* Grade onto enteral feed in stages to prevent hypoglycaemia.

Daily water and electrolyte requirements

Daily water requirements See pp. 312-13. After the first 4 days of life, an intake of 150mL/kg/day (range 120–200mL/kg/day) of human or formula milk meets the water needs of most term and preterm infants under normal circumstances. In infants with heart failure, water restriction is necessary (eg 100mL/kg/day).

Daily IV electrolytes Na⁺: 4–8mmol/kg/day. K⁺: 2–4mmol/kg/day. Ca²⁺ ~1.5mmol/kg/day. Phosphate ~1.5mmol/kg/day.

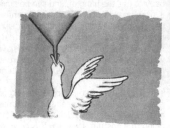

Fig 3.25 'Gavage' (from an old French word meaning 'to gorge') denotes a controversial farming and gastronomic method entailing insertion of a long funnel into a goose's throat. Down this funnel is pumped a slurry of ground corn and water, to produce obesity—and, to some palates, a delicious (if unnaturally fatty) pâté—*pâté de foie gras*. On the neonatal unit, gavage feeding should not be quite so enthusiastic. But French farmers were right about one thing: *bolus* gavage feeding is better than *continuous* tube feeds, at least with regard to trophic feeding.[358]

3 Paediatrics

It is better to talk to a breastfeeding mother while pregnant than to rely on simple encouragement and leaflets.[359]

Reflexes Rooting (searching, with wide-open mouth) → suckling (jaw goes up and down while the tongue compresses the areola against the palate) → swallowing reflex (as milk hits the oropharynx, the soft palate rises and shuts off the nasopharynx; the larynx rises, and the epiglottis falls, closing the trachea).

Skill Don't assume this comes naturally; it can be difficult for both mother and baby to get the hang of, and can be anxiety provoking. The best way to learn is from an experienced person in comfortable surroundings—eg sitting in an upright chair, rather than inadequately propped up in bed. Reassure that a few problematic feeds do not mean that the baby will starve, and that bottle feeding is needed. *Most term babies have plenty of fuel reserves*—and perseverance will almost always be rewarded. Furthermore, 'top-up' bottle feeds may undermine confidence, and, by altering the GI milieu, diminish the benefits of breastfeeding.

A good time to start breastfeeding is just after birth (good bonding; PPH risk ↓), but labour procedures may make this hard, eg intrapartum opiate analgesia ± operative delivery, T° and BP measurements, washing, weighing, going to a postnatal ward. ►*It is never too late to put to the breast.*

From the baby's viewpoint, breastfeeding entails taking a large mouthful of breast-with-nipple, which he or she gets to work on with tongue and jaw. Ensure the baby is close to the mother with the shoulders as well as the head facing the breast—which, if large, may need supporting (mother's fingers placed flat on the chest wall at the base of the breast: avoid the 'scissors' grip which stops the baby from drawing the lactiferous sinuses into the mouth).

- Avoid forcing the nipple into the mouth; so do not place a hand over the occiput and press forwards. Cradle the head in the crook of the arm.
- Explain the signs of correct attachment:
  - Mouth wide open, and chin touching the breast (nose hardly touching).
  - The baby should be seen to be drawing in breast, not just nipple.
  - Lower lip curled back, maximally gobbling the areola (so angle between lips >100°). (Don't worry about how much areola can be seen above the top lip: this gives little indication of where the tongue and lower jaw are.)
  - Slow, rhythmic, and deep jaw movements, as well as sucking movements. The 1st few sucks may be fast, shallow, and non-nutritive: here the baby is inducing the 'let-down' reflex, which promotes flow.
- When helping with placing, it is quite appropriate to 'tease' the baby by brushing the lip over the nipple, and then away. This may induce a nice big gape. With one movement bring to the breast, aiming the tongue and lower jaw as far as possible from the base of the nipple—so the tongue can scoop in the nipple and a good mouthful of breast.
- Keeping on the postnatal ward for a few days, and having the mother learn with an experienced, friendly midwife is very helpful, but this is rare in the UK, as cost and other pressures make admissions shorter. Most hospitals have a breast-feeding expert (usually a senior midwife) who can help troubleshoot if problems persist.

3 Paediatrics

How to express breast milk

It is good for every breastfeeding mother to learn this skill (access to teaching is *required* before the accolade of 'baby-friendly' can be granted to UK hospitals). There are at least 4 times when expressing is valuable:

• To relieve (sometimes very) painful breast engorgement between feeds.
• To keep milk production going when it is necessary to give nipples a rest owing to soreness—which is quite a common problem.
• To aid nutrition if sucking is reduced for any reason (eg prematurity or cleft lip).
• If the mother is going to be separated from her baby for a few feeds (eg going out to work).

The best way to learn is from a midwife, and by watching a mother who is already successfully expressing milk. Pumps are available from any chemist. If not, wash hands, and dry on a clean towel. Then, try to start flow by:

• Briefly rolling the nipple: this may induce a let-down reflex, especially if the baby is nearby.
• Stroke the breast gently towards the nipple.
• With circular movements, massage the breast gently with the 3 middle fingers.

Applying warm flannels, or expressing in the bath may aid flow eg while the mother is learning, and only a few drops are being expressed.

Teach the mother to find the 15 or so ampullae beneath the areola: they feel knotty once the milk comes in. Now with the thumb above the areola and the index finger below, and whole hand pressing the breast back on the chest wall, exert gentle pressure on the ampullae. With rhythmic pressure and release, milk should flow. Use a sterile container.

Take care that the fingers do not slip down on to the nipple, and damage the narrowing ducts. Fingers tire easily: practice is the key. Concentration is also needed to be sure to catch oddly angled jets.

If kept in a fridge, the milk lasts 5 days. Frozen milk should be used within 6 months. It is thawed by standing it in a jug of warm water. Any unused milk should be discarded after 24 hours, not refrozen. NB: it is known that the antioxidant level of stored breast milk falls, but it is not known if this matters. Refrigeration is better than freezing and thawing.[360]

Mastitis

This is a common reason to give up breastfeeding and is easily treatable.

Symptoms
• Tender, hot, reddened area of breast.
• Fever may be present or absent.

Treatment
• **Flucloxacillin** 500mg QDS PO for 7–10 days if not penicillin allergic (it is safe for her baby).
• Give analgesia and continue breastfeeding.
• If breastfeeding too painful, express the milk.
• Consider checking breastfeeding technique with a breastfeeding expert.
• If a breast abscess forms, discard the milk if it is pus-like, give flucloxacillin but drainage may be needed.
• Consider candidal infection particularly if infant has oral candidiasis.

3 Paediatrics

Factors which make starting breastfeeding harder • Family pressures, including partner's hostility (10% breastfeed vs ~70% if he approves).
• If mother and baby are separated at night in hospital.
• Unfriendly working environments.
• Cultural reframing of breasts as sex objects; no non-sexual role models.
• The commitment a breastfeeding mother makes is huge and sustained—24/7 for many months (WHO advises exclusive breastfeeding for 6 months).[18] ♂⚢

Breastfeeding advantages ▶Mutual gaze ↑ emotional input from mother.
• Sucking promotes uterine contractions, so avoiding some PPHs.
• Breastfeeding-induced oxytocin surges promote trust and diminish fear.[361,362]
• Less insulin resistance, BP↑, & obesity (growth is less rapid)[363] due to ↑ breast milk long-chain polyunsaturated fatty acids (LCPUFAs)[364] ▶LCPUFAs *may* also ↑IQ.[365]
• Breast milk is free and clean, and gives babies an attractive smell.
• Colostrum has endorphins: good for birth-associated stress?[366]
• IgA, macrophages, lymphocytes (with interferon), and lysozyme protect from infection. Acids in breast milk promote growth of friendly lactobacilli in the baby's bowel. Gastroenteritis may be less severe if the mother makes and transfers antibodies (an 'immune dialogue').
• Infant mortality, otitis media, pneumonia, & diarrhoea are less if breastfed.[367]
• Breast milk contains less Na^+, K^+, and Cl^- than other milk, so aiding homeostasis. If dehydration occurs, risk of fatal hypernatraemia is low.
• Exclusive breastfeeding may ↓ risk of: type 1 DM, rheumatoid arthritis, inflammatory bowel disease.[308]
• Breastfeeding helps mothers lose weight, and is contraceptive (unreliable!).
• Some protection in premenopausal years against maternal breast cancer.

Why is feeding on demand to be encouraged?
• It keeps the baby happy, and enhances milk production.
• Fewer breast problems (engorgement, abscesses).

NB: feeding by routine is possible with a structured plan (see *The New Contented Little Baby Book*),[369] which may help to promote a diurnal sleep cycle.

NB: although co-sleeping (a baby sleeping in the parental bed) can aid parental sleep, there is a risk of inadvertent smothering (pp. 310–11).

Contraindications to breastfeeding Are few. • An HIV +ve mother in developed countries • Amiodarone • Antimetabolites • Antithyroid drugs • Some drugs are relative contraindications: consult the online Drugs and Lactation database Lactmed or *BNF*.

Problems Treat *breast engorgement* by better breast technique and better latching-on; aim to keep breasts empty eg by hourly feeds or milk expression. Treat *sore nipples* by ensuring optimal attachment (p. 288), and moist wound healing (paraffin gauze dressing or glycerin gel)[370] ± nipple shield *not* by resting, except in emergency. For mastitis and breast abscess, see p. 289.

Prematurity Preterm breast milk is different and is the best food for prems. Give unheated, via a tube (p. 286). Preterm babies need multivitamins, folic acid, and iron. Phosphate supplements may be needed. Even term babies may (rarely) develop rickets ± hypocalcaemia (eg fits, recurrent 'colds', lethargy, or stridor) if exclusively breastfed, unless vitamin supplements are used.

---

18 However, evidence is insufficient to say confidently 'Breastfeed exclusively for 6 months' in developed countries, as breast milk may not meet full energy needs of some infants at 4–6 months old—and there may be risk of specific nutritional deficiencies. Further evidence is awaited.[371]

There are few contraindications to breastfeeding but many pressures not to. In many communities >50% mothers are breastfeeding at 2 weeks but this reduces to ≤40% at 6 weeks. Most change to bottle because of lack of knowledge or encouragement. Advertising also has a role. The WHO/UNICEF *International Code of Marketing of Breastmilk Substitutes* bans promotion of bottle feeding and sets out requirements for labelling and information on feeding.[371] The advantage of bottle feeding is that fathers and others can help. Knowing how much milk the baby is taking can be reassuring to mothers.

Teats Babies fed with a cross-cut teat (lets the baby determine rate) cry less and spend more time awake and content than babies fed with standard teats.

Standard infant formulas (Cow's milk 'humanized' by reducing the solute load and modifying fat, protein, and vitamin content.) As with breast milk, the protein component is whey-based. Brands are similar so shopping around for a brand which 'suits better' is unlikely to be an answer to feeding problems.

Follow-on formula milks These are like standard formulas, but the protein component is casein-based (∴ delays stomach emptying and allows less frequent feeds). These are marketed to satisfy hungrier babies before they start weaning. Typical age of use: 6–24 months.

Soya milks These are no longer recommended. They contain high levels of phyto-oestrogens which have oestrogen-like properties. This could affect immunity and thyroid function, as well as the more obvious hormonal disruption, especially in boys. Soya milks are still on sale in the supermarket: try to discourage parents from their use. Soya milk is *not* indicated in re-establishing feeding (regrading) after gastroenteritis.

Hydrolysed formula A cow's milk formula where protein is hydrolysed into short peptides (eg Nutramigen®). Indications: *cow's milk protein ullergy* (p. 293) or *soya allergy*. Cow's milk can be reintroduced eg at 1 year.

Specialist milks Many types exist (eg for gastro-oesophageal reflux, malabsorption, metabolic diseases, etc.). Get help from a paediatric dietician.

Preparing feeds Hands must be clean and boiled water used—infective gastroenteritis causes many deaths in poor countries and considerable morbidity in the UK. UK authorities advise sterilizing feeding equipment until baby is 12 months old but evidence is poor[372] and this is not done in the US. Powder must be accurately measured. Understrength feeds lead to poor growth and overstrength feeds have caused dangerous hypernatraemia, constipation, and obesity.

Feeding After the first few days, babies need ~150mL/kg/24h (1oz=28.4mL) over 4–6 feeds depending on age and temperament; be led by baby. If small-for-dates, up to 200mL/kg/day may be needed; if large-for-dates, <100mL/kg. Feeds are often warmed; there is no evidence that cold milk is bad. Flow should almost form a stream; check before each feed as teats silt up. The hole can be enlarged with a hot needle. Bottles are best angled so that air is not sucked in with milk.

Weaning Introduce solids at 4–6 months by offering a selection of finger foods with or without puree. Avoid adding salt or sugar. Encourage home cooking and eating together as a family. Do not delay introduction of highly allergenic foods, recent trials show reduced rates of allergy with early introduction.[373] Normal *full-fat* supermarket cow's milk can be used from 12 months of age. By then children should be getting the majority of their calories from solids and not be drinking large amounts of milk. It is recommended to maintain 2 servings (~350mL) of milk or dairy products per day for calcium intake. Semi-skimmed milk *not* be used until at least 2yrs and only if child has a good appetite and is growing well. Unsweetened, calcium fortified, soya, almond, or oat drinks can also be used from 12 months but avoid rice drinks due to high level of arsenic.

3 Paediatrics

Crying Up to 20% report problems with crying in the 1st 3 months of life; usually no cause is found. Crying peaks at 6–8 weeks old (~3h/day, worse in the evenings) and subsides by 4 months.[374] Cries of hunger and thirst are indistinguishable. The demand feeding vs routine feeding debate rages among parents, with each group convinced that they have the happier babies. Crying worsens 'postnatal blues' and may be the last straw for a parent with few reserves. Aim to offer help before this stage (www.purplecrying.info, www.crysis.org.uk). Don't make parents feel inadequate; encourage parents to take it in turns to sleep. Encourage *grandparent* involvement. Explain normal crying and sleeping. Remember: a crying baby may be a sign of major relationship problems.

- Baby-centred approach to help parents help the baby deal with discomfort.
- Take parents' concerns seriously.
- Help parents recognize when their baby is tired and hungry ('read-your-baby' lessons may be needed), and to apply a consistent approach to care.
- Involve the health visitor.
- Vocal (singing), vestibular (rocking, going for a drive), or tactile stimulation (hugs) may help. Encourage help from friends/family. Simplify daily living.
- If not coping, admit to a parenting centre or hospital;[375] don't over-medicalize!

Colic (Paroxysmal crying with pulling up of the legs, for >3h on ≥3days/wk.) There is an association with feeding difficulties.[376] ΔΔ: CMPA see p. 293. ℞: *Movement* (carry-cot on wheels) is often tried and may help.[377] Let the baby *finish the first breast first* [Fisher's rule] (hindmilk is easier to digest).[378] If breastfeeding, a low-allergen diet and probiotics are *unproven* interventions to try as a last resort. The key question is, is baby gaining weight? If so: *reassure strongly; reduce stress.*[379]

Nappy rash/diaper dermatitis 3 main types (may coexist):[380]

1 The common 'nappy rash' is a contact dermatitis—red desquamating rash, sparing skin folds (as opposed to seborrhoeic dermatitis, which doesn't), due to prolonged contact with moisture and waste products.[381] It responds to frequent nappy changes (cloth nappies retain more moisture than disposables), or nappy-free periods, careful drying, and emollient creams. Best treatment: leave nappy off. Use barrier cream: eg Sudocrem® (zinc oxide cream).

2 Candida/thrush is isolatable from ~½ of all nappy rashes. Its hallmark is satellite spots beyond the main rash. Mycology: see p. 448. Always check and treat for concurrent oral candidiasis. ℞: nystatin, + clotrimazole. Avoid oral antifungals (hepatotoxic), topical steroids (only temporary improvement and may thin skin) and gentian violet (staining is disliked).

3 Seborrhoeic dermatitis: a diffuse, red, shiny rash extends into skin folds, often occurs with other seborrhoeic areas, eg occiput (cradle cap), neck, axillae. ℞: as for 1.[382]

ΔΔ: Infantile psoriasis, scabies, Langerhans cell histiocytosis, eczema (usually spares nappy area)

Sleep problems See p. 739.

Vomiting

- Effortless regurgitation of milk is common during feeds, this is 'posseting'.
- Non-pathological vomiting between feeds is also common. As with colic, the key question is weight gain: if baby is gaining weight a pathological cause is unlikely.
- Gastro-oesophageal reflux, gastritis.
- Over-feeding (150mL/kg/day is normal, see p. 291).
- Pyloric stenosis presents at ~3–8 weeks old. Vomiting is projectile (eg over the end of the cot) and baby is very hungry, see p. 210.
- Almost any infection eg UTI.
- CMPA (see later).
- Adverse food reaction.
- Infective gastroenteritis.

Rarer causes
- Raised intracranial pressure (eg hydrocephalus).
- Pharyngeal pouch.
- Poisoning.
- Metabolic conditions eg galactosaemia, organic acidaemias.

Bilious (green) vomiting: Often a surgical emergency, get urgent help: consider malrotation with volvulus (p. 223), duodenal obstruction, or intussusception.

Feeding anxieties and weight loss Healthy term babies require little milk for the first few days and early poor feeding is not an indication for investigation or bottle top-ups. The exceptions are babies of diabetic mothers, LBW or preterm babies who are at risk of hypoglycaemia. It is normal for babies to lose weight in the first week of life and loss of up to 10% in an otherwise well baby is not cause for concern. Weight loss of >15% is concerning and requires investigation. Weight loss of 10–15% should be reviewed by a doctor or experienced midwife. New babies may have difficulty coordinating feeding and breathing, and briefly choke, gag, or turn blue. Exclude disease, check feeding technique (too much? too fast?) and reassure.

Cow's milk protein allergy (CMPA) This is either IgE or non-IgE-mediated. Prevalence: 2–3% of 1–3yr-olds in the UK.[383]
- *IgE mediated* is easier to Δ with onset of classic allergic symptoms (pruritus, urticaria, angio-oedema, rhinitis, conjunctivitis, ±GI symptoms) within minutes of exposure (rarely up to 2h).
- *Non-IgE mediated* is much more common and much more difficult to Δ, there are no tests. *Signs:* Mostly non-specific: colic, reflux, vomiting, food aversion, constipation (early onset), eczema not responding to treatment, blood/mucus in stools, and in severe cases, faltering growth. Δ: Usually several symptoms are present but not all. An exclusion trial is necessary (minimum 2 weeks) and the Δ is *only confirmed* if symptoms return on reintroduction of CMP to the child's diet (may take up to 1wk). R: Breastfed babies: mother to completely exclude cow's milk protein from her diet and take Ca²⁺ & vit D supplements. Formula-fed babies: change to an extensively hydrolysed or amino acid formula. Refer to dietician if allergy confirmed. If symptoms do not improve, refer to local paediatric allergy service. Multiple food exclusions are rarely necessary. Any food exclusion can have serious deleterious effects on the child's growth and health and should only be done with the support of a paediatric dietician. The prevalence of parental reported food allergy is much higher than the true prevalence and only around 25–40% are confirmed on food challenge.[384]

Further reading

Venter C *et al.* (2017). Better recognition, diagnosis and management of non-IgE-mediated cow's milk allergy in infancy: iMAP—an international interpretation of the MAP (Milk Allergy in Primary Care) guideline. https://ctajournal.biomedcentral.com/articles/10.1186/s13601-017-0162-y

Jaundice is caused by raised bilirubin levels, divided into conjugated (direct) and unconjugated (indirect) bilirubin. Neonatal jaundice is very common, occurring in 60% of term and 80% of preterm neonates[385] and is divided into 3 categories:

- *Early jaundice*—clinical jaundice <24h is nearly always pathological and needs urgent action.
- *Jaundice 24h to 14 days* is mostly physiological, however severe hyperbilirubinaemia is a risk and pathological causes still occur.
- *Prolonged jaundice* is visible jaundice >14 days (>21 days if preterm). Physiological jaundice is still the most common cause but there is increasing likelihood of underlying pathological cause.

Assessment Jaundice can be difficult to detect, especially in non-white skin. Check baby in bright, preferably natural light. Jaundice is best seen in the sclerae, gums, or on blanched skin of forehead, nose, or sternum. If jaundice is detected it must be measured:

- Transcutaneous bilirubinometers can be used in babies ≥35wks' gestation who are >24h old. They *are* validated for non-Caucasian babies.
- Serum bilirubin measurements should be used in all other situations or if the transcutaneous bilirubin measurement is >250μmol/L or > the relevant treatment threshold for a baby (also use serum bilirubin for all subsequent measurements in such babies).

Early jaundice *Causes:*

▶ Sepsis, (pp. 280–1); or:
- *Rhesus incompatibility*: +ve direct antiglobulin test (DAT, previously DCT or Coombs test) see p. 296.
- *ABO incompatibility*: (mother O; baby A or B, or mother A and baby B, or vice versa) DAT +ve in 4%; indirect antiglobulin test +ve in 8%. Maternal IgG anti-A or anti-B haemolysin is 'always' present.[386]
- *Red cell anomalies*: congenital spherocytosis (fragility tests/EMA binding, p. 240); or elliptocytosis; glucose-6-phosphate dehydrogenase deficiency (do enzyme test).[387]

Tests: Partial septic screen (FBC, CRP, blood culture); packed cell volume; blood film; group & save; DAT; maternal blood group; ±G6PD level.[388]

Hyperbilirubinaemia between 24h and 14 days Usually 'physiological':

1 Increased bilirubin production in neonates due to shorter RBC lifespan.
2 Decreased bilirubin conjugation due to hepatic immaturity.
3 Absence of gut flora impedes elimination of bile pigment.
4 Exclusive breastfeeding (esp. if there are feeding difficulties →↓ intake → dehydration →↓ bilirubin elimination + ↑ enterohepatic circulation of bilirubin—not a reason to stop[389]).

Physiological jaundice is unconjugated, the natural history is rising bilirubin levels in first 3–5 days then spontaneous resolution over 1–2wks. However, levels should be monitored to prevent kernicterus.

Remember *pathological causes* are still possible: all the causes of early jaundice above-mentioned, or polycythaemia; resorption of cephalohaematoma; parenteral nutrition associated liver disease (p. 286); hypothyroidism; haemoglobinopathies; TORCH infections (pp. 38–9); viral hepatitis.

Kernicterus Refers to the permanent neurological sequelae of severe hyperbilirubinaemia and acute bilirubin encephalopathy (ABE). Exact mechanism is poorly understood but risk ↑ with extremely high unconjugated bilirubin levels (>350μmol/L; lower in prems). ABE: lethargy/poor feeding/ hypotonia shrill cry progressing to irritability/hypertonicity/opisthotonos then apnoeas/seizures/coma/death. Long-term sequelae in survivors include choreoathetoid cerebral palsy, deafness, and ↓IQ. It is prevented by photo-therapy ± exchange transfusion ±IVIg.[390]

Treatment *Phototherapy:* Uses light (wavelength 460–490nm) energy to convert bilirubin to soluble products (lumirubin and other isomers) that can be excreted without conjugation. Efficacy depends on irradiance (measured in μw/cm²)—so exposing baby will lead to more rapid reduction in serum bilirubin, as will using light from above and below (ie a 'biliblanket'). Breastfeeds should be brief to maximize time under the lights. SE: T°↑, ↓; eye damage (baby will need eye protection); diarrhoea; separation from mother; fluid loss. *Intense phototherapy* is an adjunct to exchange transfusion.[391,392] The treatment threshold levels for phototherapy vary with gestational age, and postnatal age. Use NICE guidelines (www.nice.org.uk/cg98, also available on the handy BiliApp smartphone app), or your unit's protocol.

Exchange transfusion: Uses warmed blood (37°c), 170mL/kg (double volume), given ideally via umbilical vein IVI, with removal via umbilical artery. The aim is to remove bilirubin in those with severe or rapidly rising hyperbilirubinaemia.

IVIg: For babies with proven isoimmune haemolytic disease (Rh, ABO, or other incompatibility) and rapidly rising bilirubin, IVIg may obviate the need for exchange transfusion.

Prolonged jaundice The bane of the neonatal SHO's week is the prolonged jaundice clinic: most of these babies will have physiological or breastmilk jaundice but a small subset will have life-changing pathology that is treatable. *Red flags:* Pale stool; hepatosplenomegaly; ascites; bruising/bleeding; neurological signs. *1st-line screening tests:* Total & conjugated bilirubin; FBC; film & retics; group & DAT; TFTs; ± LFTs; ± G6PD (depending on ethnicity). NICE recommends MSU but false +ves are high so most units only do if there are other clinical signs. *Causes:* Split into conjugated and unconjugated: an abnormal conjugated fraction is conjugated bilirubin >25μmol/L and >25% of total bilirubin.
- *Unconjugated:* As above, plus: UTI; Crigler–Najjar p. 844 and Gilbert syndromes.
- *Conjugated:* These are legion but include several not to miss: hypothyroidism; biliary atresia; choledochal abnormalities; galactosaemia; tyrosinaemia; α1-antitrypsin deficiency; Alagille's; neonatal haemochromatosis; cystic fibrosis. 2nd- and 3rd-line tests as per BSPGHAN Guideline for the Investigation of Neonatal Conjugated Jaundice.[393] If baby is unwell, involve liver centre early.

Biliary atresia

Incidence 1:17,000. Rare but serious. Apparently healthy term babies have jaundice, dark urine, and pale stools due to biliary tree occlusion by progressive cholangiopathy. 20% have associated cardiac malformations; polysplenia; ± situs inversus. It can also occur in preterms. The spleen becomes palpable after the 3rd or 4th week—the liver may become hard and enlarged. Δ Babies suspected of biliary atresia should be urgently assessed in a liver unit. Percutaneous liver biopsy may show bile duct proliferation and bile plugs. ℞ Early surgery (Kasai procedure = hepatoportoenterostomy—the extrahepatic biliary tree is identified, a cholangiogram performed to check diagnosis, and an intestinal limb (Roux-en-Y) is attached to drain bile from the porta hepatis) has a good chance of restoring flow of bile to bowel (60% success if done <60 days of age) but if presenting for operation late (eg at 100 days) Kasai procedure is unlikely to be successful due to advanced liver damage and cirrhosis; and the baby will likely need liver transplant before 12 months.

Further reading

NICE (2010). *Neonatal Jaundice* (cg98). London: NICE. https://www.nice.org.uk/guidance/cg98

Incompatibility between maternal and fetal blood groups → production of IgG which crosses the placenta → haemolysis in the fetus and neonate → unconjugated *hyperbilirubinaemia* (pp. 294-5) and severe *anaemia*. Most important/severe disease seen in rhesus D incompatibility.

Physiology When a RhD−ve mother delivers a RhD+ve baby a leak of fetal red cells into her circulation may stimulate her to produce anti-D IgG antibodies (isoimmunization). In subsequent pregnancies, these can cross the placenta, causing worsening rhesus haemolytic disease (*erythroblastosis fetalis*) with each successive RhD+ve pregnancy. First pregnancies may be affected due to leaks prior to delivery eg: •Threatened miscarriage •APH •Mild trauma •Amniocentesis •Chorionic villous sampling •External cephalic version.

There is a wide clinical spectrum. A severely affected oedematous fetus (with stiff, oedematous lungs) is called a *hydrops fetalis*. Anaemia-associated CCF causes oedema, as does hypoalbuminaemia (the liver is preoccupied by producing new RBCs). ΔΔ: Thalassaemia; infection (eg toxoplasmosis, CMV, pp. 38-9); maternal diabetes.

Clinical Rh disease ►*Test for D antibodies in all RhD−ve mothers, at booking, 28 & 34 weeks' gestation* (p. 11). Anti-D titres <4u/mL (<1:16) are very unlikely to cause serious disease; it is wise to check maternal plasma every 2 weeks if positive. If >10u/mL, get the advice of a referral centre: fetal blood sampling ± intraperitoneal (or, with fetoscopy, intravascular via the cord) transfusion may be needed. Expect fetal Hb to be <70g/L in 10% of those with titres of 10–100u/mL (75% if titres >100u/mL).

Do regular US (+amniocentesis if anti-D titre >4u/mL). Timing is vital. Do it 10 weeks before a Rh-related event in the last pregnancy (eg if last baby needed delivery at 36 weeks, expect to do amniocentesis at 26 weeks). Fetuses tolerating a high bilirubin level may be saved risky transfusions (fatality 2–30%) if monitored by serial measurements of fetal Hb (by fetoscopy or non-invasive middle cerebral artery peak velocity) and daily US to detect oedema, cardiomegaly, pericardial effusion, hepatosplenomegaly, or ascites.[394]

Anti-D is the main rhesus antibody but there are others: Rh C, E, c, e, Kell, Kidd, Duffy (all are IgG). Low concentrations sometimes produce severe disease. Prognosis is improving. Mortality is <20% even for hydropic babies. Note that maternal antibodies persist for some months, and continue to cause haemolysis during early life.[395]

Presentation Ranges from mild to moderate self-limiting haemolysis (jaundice <24h; anaemia; lethargy; ↑HR) to life-threatening hydrops fetalis (p. 297).

Exchange transfusion *Indications/technique:* p. 295 If Hb <70g/L, give 1st volume of the exchange transfusion (80mL/kg) as warmed packed cells, and subsequent precise exchanges according to response. ►*Keep the baby warm.*

Phototherapy (p. 295) May be all that is needed in less severe disease.

Giving Rh−ve mothers anti-D immunoglobulin (p. 11) This strategy has markedly reduced need for exchange transfusion.[396,397]

ABO incompatibility 1 in 45 of group A or B babies born to group O mothers will have haemolysis from maternal antibodies. Disease is usually less severe with most neonates needing phototherapy only. Rarely, exchange transfusion is needed, even in firstborns (isoimmunization occurs as A & B antigens are present in food and bacteria). May manifest as late anaemia (7–21 days after birth) which is usually treated with iron and folic supplements and rarely transfusion.

Neonatal alloimmune thrombocytopenia (NAIT) Similar to haemolytic disease, mothers may develop antibodies to fetal platelet antigens causing NAIT (1:2000 births). It develops *in utero*. 50% are firstborn (it recurs in ~80% of later pregnancies with same or ↑ severity). If affected *in utero*, ~25% have intracranial haemorrhage. Platelets fall for 48h of life. Treat severe thrombocytopenia with compatible platelets (matched to mother's cells) or irradiated maternal platelets. IVIg 400mg/kg/day for 48h and steroids may help. Maternal steroids and IVIg from 12wks may be needed in later pregnancies. Diagnose by detecting maternal platelet alloantibody against father's platelets. Neonatal thrombocytopenia may also occur secondary to maternal autoimmune disease as autoantibodies may also cross the placenta (<10% of babies of women with ITP are affected (p. 99)).

Hydrops fetalis: management

Hydrops is a syndrome of excessive fluid accumulation in the fetus manifest as: oedema; ascites; pleural and pericardial effusions; ± circulatory collapse & shock. Causes are split into *immune* (alloimmune haemolytic disease, p. 296, 10%); and *non-immune* (90% of cases, wide range of causes from congenital infection, abnormalities, and genetic defects to fetomaternal or twin-to-twin transfusion).

• Get expert help, very high mortality.
• At birth, take blood for FBC & film, bilirubin (conjugated and unconjugated), blood group, direct and indirect antiglobulin test, LFT, TORCH screen (p. 38-9), array CGH, Hb electrophoresis, culture, viral and bacterial serology. Also CXR, abdominal x-ray, ECG, US head, abdo, chest, echo. Maternal blood for Kleihauer test and TORCH screen.
• Expect to need to ventilate with high peak inspiratory pressure (PIP) and positive end-expiratory pressure (PEEP). HFOV and inhaled NO may be needed, pp. 308-9.
• Drain ascites and pleural effusions If affecting ventilation.
• Inotropic support as needed.
• Restrict IV fluids to 60mL/kg/24h (crystalloid); if exchange transfusing, aim for a deficit of 10-20mL/kg. Monitor urine output. Give diuretics.
• Correct anaemia, have o-ve blood ready at delivery.
• Treat hyperbilirubinaemia (p. 295)
• Prognosis: 90% of those with non-immune hydrops die *in utero*; 50% die postnatally. Babies with non-immune hydrops not secondary to infection have a good neurological outcome.[398]

3 Paediatrics

Some definitions *Preterm:* A neonate whose calculated gestational age (GA) from the last menstrual period is <37 completed weeks—ie premature. *Low birthweight (LBW):* Birthweight of <2500g regardless of gestational age. Thus a LBW baby may not be small for gestational age (see later) if they are born preterm. 6% of UK infants are <2500g at birth, and 50% of these are preterm. 10% of pregnancies end in spontaneous preterm delivery, and 70% of all perinatal deaths occur in preterm infants.

Very low birthweight (VLBW): Birthweight of <1500g regardless of age. *Extremely low birthweight (ELBW):* Birthweight <1000g regardless of age. *Small for gestational age (SGA):* Typically SGA refers to a birthweight below the 10th percentile for gestational age (SGA). In *intrauterine growth restriction (IUGR)* there is a reduction of expected fetal growth *in utero*, which may or may not result in the baby being IUGR. *Asymmetric (disproportional)* IUGR: the most common type, weight centile is < length and head circumference (head sparing). It is usually due to IUGR and an insult later in pregnancy eg pre-eclampsia. These babies have a higher risk of complications than non-SGA babies. *Symmetric (proportional)* IUGR: all growth parameters are symmetrically small, suggesting that the fetus was affected from early pregnancy. This is seen in babies with chromosomal abnormalities and in the constitutionally small. *Chief causes:* ►Poverty/poor social support may account for 30% of variance in birthweights.[399] *Other causes:* constitutional factors; malformation; twins; congenital infection; placental insufficiency (maternal heart disease, BP↑, smoking, diabetes, sickle-cell disease, pre-eclampsia).[400] Gestational age (based on US) is more important for predicting survival than the birthweight alone. *Are SGA effects permanent?* 90% of SGA catch up growth in the first 2yrs, however as adults they are on average 1 standard deviation shorter than the mean adult height.[401] There may be an association between SGA and adult risk of coronary heart disease, hypertension, and obesity.[401] *Complications:* Increased risk of fetal death; risks from congenital infection or malformations if present, hypoglycaemia, hypothermia, polycythaemia (secondary to chronic intrauterine hypoxia), NEC (p. 284), meconium aspiration.

Causes of prematurity Mostly unknown (40%); smoking tobacco, poverty, and malnutrition play a part. Others: past history of prematurity; genitourinary infection/chorioamnionitis; systemic infection; pre-eclampsia; diabetes mellitus; polyhydramnios; closely spaced pregnancies; multiple pregnancy; uterine malformation; placenta praevia; abruption; premature rupture of the membranes; cervical insufficiency. Labour may be induced early on purpose or accidentally (p. 60).

Estimating the gestational age Check EDD on 12 week scan (later scans less accurate). If no scans in pregnancy or LMP available, a scoring system is used to estimate the GA. The New Ballard score[402] uses 6 physical and 6 neurological criteria and has largely replaced the more detailed Dubowitz score.

Management Delivery should take place in a centre capable of caring for preterm babies; arrange *in utero* transfer if possible (better outcomes than *ex utero*). Once born, ensure adequate resuscitation (p. 184) and take to NICU/SCBU (pp. 306-7). Preterm babies are likely to need support with thermoregulation; nutrition (p. 286), encourage mother to express from day 1; ± respiration (pp. 308-9) and other support. Parents also need support (eg www.bliss.org.uk).

Survival if very premature 40% of infants born before 23 weeks die on labour ward. Of those surviving labour ward, 75% died on the neonatal unit. 47% survive at 24 weeks and 67% at 25 weeks.[EPICure2] Mortality is associated with intracranial abnormalities seen ultrasonically.

Disability *As a percentage of live births:* if 23 weeks' gestation: 5% had no or minor subsequent disability (24 weeks ≈ 12%; 25 weeks ≈ 23%). Morbidity relates to cerebral palsy, squint, and retinopathy (p. 306).[403]n>150 Disability may be subtle but specific: one pattern is ↓ numeracy if gestation is <30/40, associated with ↓ grey matter in the left parietal lobe.[404] ADHD risk ↑ (p. 741).

Is this baby small for gestational age?

Use centile charts which take into account that firstborns are lighter than subsequent births: table 3.13 gives sample data.

Table 3.13 Sample data: 10th centile weights at different gestational ages

Weeks of gestation	10th centile weight (grams)			
	Firstborn		Subsequent births	
	Boy	Girl	Boy	Girl
32	1220	1260	1470	1340
33	1540	1540	1750	1620
34	1830	1790	2000	1880
35	2080	2020	2230	2100
36	2310	2210	2430	2310
37	2500	2380	2600	2480
38	2660	2530	2740	2620
39	2780	2640	2860	2730
40	2870	2730	2950	2810

Preventing neonatal deaths—worldwide

In 2016, of the ≈136 million babies who were born, ~2.6 million died in the 1st 4 weeks of life (the neonatal period)—most from preventable causes. ⅔ occur in India, China, Pakistan, Nigeria, Bangladesh, Ethiopia, DRC, Indonesia, Afghanistan, and Tanzania. Most of the deaths were caused by pre-term births, birth asphyxia and birth trauma, sepsis, congenital abnormalities, respiratory problems, and tetanus.[405] (Malaria and diarrhoeal diseases are less important in the neonatal period.) Prevention depends on:

• Vaccination, access to antibiotics and breastfeeding advice.
• Sanitary delivery rooms with basic emergency services (caesarean sections and blood transfusion; obstructed labour is a major problem).
• Preventing and managing low birthweight. Low birthweight affects 14% of births worldwide, but accounts for ~70% of neonatal deaths. Managing low birthweight babies need not require expensive technology. Much could be achieved by application of known primary care principles of warmth, feeding, and the prevention and early treatment of infection.
• Preventing maternal mortality (0.5 million maternal deaths/yr) is a prerequisite for preventing many neonatal deaths. In one small but harrowing study from Gambia, *all* the children born to mothers who died from pregnancy-related causes were themselves dead at 1 year.[406]

Non-pharmacological methods to reduce pain in neonates

Pain relief through non-nutritive sucking (NNS), rocking, massage, 20% sucrose (12mg may be enough),[407] distilled water, and expressed breast milk (EBM) have been studied in a randomized way—in the context of a heel-prick (for obtaining blood for testing). Duration of cry and pain score were used as objective measures of pain. Pain scores and duration of crying were lowest in the NNS and rocking groups compared with sucrose, distilled water, expressed breast milk, and massage.[408] Other trials show that for venepuncture, breastfeeding or glucose plus use of a pacifier provides good analgesia.[409,410] Other alternatives: kangaroo care (skin-to-skin with mum); morphine; fentanyl. Whenever you hear *siren cry* (sequence of almost identical cries with a period of 1sec) think: 'How can I help this baby? What is going wrong?'[411]

Orofacial clefts (cleft lip and palate)

This is the most common facial malformation. It results from failure of fusion of maxillary and premaxillary processes (during week 5). The defect runs from lip to nostril. It may be bilateral, when there is often a cleft in the palate as well, with the premaxillary process displaced anteriorly. Palate clefts may be large or small (eg of uvula alone). **Incidence** ~1:1000. ♂:♀ >1:1. **Causes** Genes, benzodiazepines, antiepileptics, rubella. Other malformations are common eg trisomy 18, 13–15, or Pierre–Robin short mandible (causing intermittent upper airway obstruction). **Prevention** Quit smoking pre-pregnancy.[412] **Folic acid** 5mg/day periconception ± multivitamins may help if the woman already has an affected child.[413,414] Avoidance of antiepileptics. **Interdisciplinary treatment** Orthodontist, plastic surgeon, oral surgeon, GP, paediatrician, speech therapist. Feeding with special teats may be needed before plastic surgery (usually, lip repair at 3 months, and palate at 6 months). Repair of unilateral complete or incomplete lesions often gives good cosmesis. Refer to expert centres. If bilateral, there is always some residual deformity. Surgery may involve iliac bone grafts + insertion of Gore-Tex® membranes.[415] **Complications** Otitis media, aspiration, post-op palatal fistulae, poor speech (speech therapy helps). Social adjustment ↓.[416] Avoid taking to NICU—may ↓ bonding—a big problem (also the dopaminergic 'high' a normal baby's smile induces in the mother's putamen may be subverted by the defect).[417]

Other head & neck malformations

Eyes Anophthalmos: there are no eyes; rare; part of trisomy 13–15. *Ectopia lentis:* Presents as glaucoma with poor vision. The lens margin is visible; seen in Marfan's (*OHCM* p706), Ehlers–Danlos (p. 846), homocystinuria; incidence: <1:5000; autosomal-dominant (AD) or recessive (AR). *Cataract:* Rubella, Down's. *Coloboma:* Notched iris with a displaced pupil; incidence: 2:10,000; (AR). *Microphthalmos:* Small eyes; 1:1000; due to rubella—or genetic (AD).

Ears *Accessory auricles:* Seen in front of the ear; incidence: 15:1000. *Deformed ears:* Treacher Collins syndrome (p. 859). *Low-set ears:* Associations—Down syndrome; congenital heart disease.

Nose/throat *Choanal atresia: Signs:* postnatal cyanotic attacks; nasal catheter doesn't go into the pharynx because of nasal malformation. *Incidence:* ≤1:5000. *Surgery:* consider a micro-endoscopic nasal approach.[418] *Branchial fistula:* These open at the front of sternomastoid (a remnant of the 2nd or 3rd branchial pouch). *Incidence:* <1:5000. Branchial and thyroglossal cysts: p. 426.

Skull & spine *Brachycephaly:* Short, broad skull from early closure (craniosynostosis) of the coronal suture; incidence: <1:1000; Down's-associated or AD. *Cleidocranial dysostosis:* No clavicles (so shoulders meet). Slow skull ossification, no sinuses, high-arched palate; incidence <1:5000; AD.

Craniofacial dysostosis: Tower skull, beaked nose, exophthalmos. Δ: CT. Klippel–Feil syndrome (p. 850): fused cervical vertebra (so the neck is short).

CNS *Hydrocephalus:* Incidence 0.3–2:1000. Ante- or neonatal injury, infection, or genes (sex-linked) may cause aqueduct stenosis. Dandy–Walker syndrome (p. 844); Arnold–Chiari malformation (*OHCM* p694). *Microcephaly: Causes:* genetic,[419] intrauterine viruses (eg rubella, Zika), hypoxia, x-rays, maternal alcohol. *Incidence:* 1:1000. Recurrence risk: 1:50. For spina bifida, see p. 285.

Fetal alcohol spectrum disorder Severity depends on how much alcohol the mother had in pregnancy. *Features:* Microcephaly, short palpebral fissures, hypoplastic upper lip, absent philtrum, small eyes, IQ↓, cardiac malformations.

Head words

To outsiders, it seems as if paediatricians are obsessed with measuring head circumference and head shape, and translating the latter into Latin—as if defining the *outside* could explain what is going on *inside*. To insiders, though, ▶*it is to diagnose and treat craniostenosis that we measure heads.* So ... always know where your patient is on his or her centile charts.

Plagiocephaly If fully expressed, synostosis affects coronal (rarely lambdoidal) sutures (± palpable bony ridge) with a flat forehead and elevation of the orbit on one side. Minor (unfused) plagiocephalic asymmetry is common in infants sleeping on their backs, improves with time, and is of no significance. Associations: scoliosis and pelvic obliquity (fig 3.26).

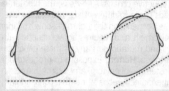
Fig 3.26 Plagiocephaly from positional flattening.
© The Royal Children's Hospital, Melbourne, Australia; Kids Health Info, www.rch.org.au/kidsinfo/fact_sheets/Plagiocephaly_misshapen_head/

Craniostenosis (=craniosynostosis=premature closure of one or more of the skull's fibrous sutures by ossification) It affects ~1:2000 of whom 2–11% have a family history. 15–40% have one of 180 recognized syndromes (with a family history it's 50%). Normal time for sutures to close is 3–9 months for the metopic (frontal) suture, 22–39 months for other sutures (sagittal, coronal, lambdoid). The skull compensates for closure by growing in the direction parallel to the closed suture. If the compensatory growth allows insufficient space for the growing brain there will be ↑ICP ± visual loss, sleep impairment (obstructive sleep apnoea), eating problems and ↓IQ. Babies with insufficient head growth (centile charts pp. 316-19) or skull deformity need assessment by a craniofacial surgeon. 4–20% of children with single suture closure have raised ICP, up to 60% if more than one suture involved. Look for papilloedema. Skull x-ray: single closed suture. CT: structural brain abnormalities and suture fusion and will diagnose deformational plagiocephaly (due to absent suture) and pansynostosis secondary to microcephaly. Subarachnoid spaces are larger in microcephaly. Surgery at 6–12 months aims to normalize the cranial vault and to allow for brain growth.

Dolichocephaly (Also scaphocephaly—boat shaped.) The head is elongated eg as in Marfan's, or El Greco portraits.

Holoprosencephaly (A whole, ie single-sphered, brain.) Hypotelorism with cleft palate ± premaxillary agenesis ± cyclopia ± cebocephaly (monkey-like)—follows failure of the lateral ventricles to separate (defective cleavage of the prosencephalon) eg with fusion of the basal ganglia.

Lissencephaly Smooth cortex with no convolutions (agyria).

Oxycephalic (=turricephaly=acrocephaly) The top of the head is pointed.

Wormian bones Supernumerary bones in the sutures of the skull.

3 Paediatrics

This is rare, but devastating for the parents (see BOX 'Assigning sex and gender'). It can be a life-threatening endocrinological emergency, CAH (see later) is the commonest cause of ambiguous genitalia,[420] so *investigate* and *refer promptly*. **Physiology** Early XX and XY fetuses have the same rudimentary reproductive organs. At ~7wks, the bipotential gonads begin to differentiate into testes driven by the SRY gene (on the Y chromosome); ovarian development also requires active genetic pathways and mutations in any of these genes can lead to DSD. **History** Exposure to progesterone, testosterone, phenytoin, aminoglutethimide; FH of unexplained neonatal deaths; consanguinity. **Examination** Note penis size and urethral position (fig 3.27). Are the labia fused? Is there a

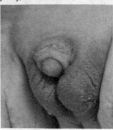

Fig 3.27 Ambiguous genitalia.

vaginal opening? Have the gonads descended? Is there dysmorphism? Preterm girls have prominent labia and clitorises; preterm boys have undescended testicles until 34wks' gestation. If sex is not clear from examination, investigation is indicated. There are also small but significant rates of chromosomal abnormality with: isolated bilateral cryptorchidism (at term), even if a penis is present; unilateral cryptorchidism with hypospadias; or isolated penoscrotal or perineoscrotal hypospadias. **Tests** Parents and relatives will be anxious to know the sex of their baby. However, any decision regarding the infant's sex must be delayed until a multidisciplinary team assessment has been carried out (see BOX 'Assigning sex and gender'); it is not the result of a single test. Tests are needed to rule out life-threatening complications, assess anatomy, and determine chromosomal sex: glucose; repeated serum electrolytes (may be normal until ~day 4 of life); serum 17OH-progesterone (may be normal <36h old); testosterone; other serum steroid metabolites; urine for steroid profile. Pelvic US, expert examination ± endoscopy are used to assess anatomy. FISH for X and Y chromosomes plus karyotype. If karyotype is normal, further testing (array CGH, targeted gene panels) is advised eg terminal deletion of 10q deletes genes essential for normal male genital development.[421]

Congenital adrenal hyperplasia (CAH) From deficiency of 21-hydroxylase, 11-hydroxylase, 17-α-hydroxylase or 3-β-hydroxysteroid dehydrogenase from a defect on the gene CYP21. Cortisol is inadequately produced, leading to a rise in adrenocorticotrophic hormone, adrenal hyperplasia, and overproduction of androgenic cortisol precursors (particularly 17OH-progesterone, →↑ testosterone production). Most affected infants are also salt losers, as 21-hydroxylase is needed for aldosterone biosynthesis. In boys this is usually the sole early manifestation (excess virilization may be early or in adulthood). Biochemical screening is carried out in some centres in boys, to diagnose before life-threatening adrenal hyperplasia. Girls are detected by finding virilization at newborn examination. Prenatal diagnosis is possible (eg after affected sibling) and treatable by giving the mother dexamethasone from early in pregnancy. The variation in time of onset and clinical presentation, despite identical CYP21 mutations, makes adrenal hyperplasia a continuum of disorders. *Incidence:* 1:14,000.[422] *Signs:* Vomiting , dehydration, and ambiguous genitalia. Girls may be masculinized. Boys may be normal at birth, but have precocious puberty, or ambiguous genitalia (↓ androgens in 17-hydroxylase deficiency), or incomplete masculinization (hypospadias with cryptorchidism from ↓3β-hydroxysteroid dehydrogenase). *Hyponatraemia* (with paradoxically ↑ urine Na⁺) and *hyperkalaemia* are common. ↑ plasma 17-hydroxyprogesterone in 90%; urinary 17-ketosteroids ↑ (not in 17-hydroxylase deficit). *Treatment:* Medical (glucocorticoid replacement in all; mineralocorticoid replacement (fludrocortisone) if salt-wasting form); and surgical (clitoral reduction and vaginoplasty). Growth and fertility are also impaired.[423]

Aromatase deficiency Rare. CYP19 genes are needed for normal oestrogenization: recessive mutations cause ambiguous genitalia in 46,XX individuals; at puberty there is hypergonadotropic hypogonadism, with no secondary sexual characteristics, except for progressive virilization. Boys have normal male sexual differentiation but are tall with brittle bones. Oestrogen receptor gene mutations are similar.[424]

▸▸Emergency treatment of adrenocortical crisis

Babies may present with an adrenocortical crisis (circulatory collapse) in early life (10–20 days). Presentation in older children may be brought on by stressors such as infection, trauma, and surgery. The adrenal gland is unable to respond to the stressor by increasing production/secretion of cortisol. Other presentations include hyponatraemic seizures in infancy (often misdiagnosed as a febrile convulsion).

Symptoms/signs
- Abdominal pain, nausea, vomiting.
- Hypoglycaemia.
- Lethargy.
- Hypotension, shock.

▸▸Urgent treatment is needed with
- 20mL/kg 0.9% NaCl IV bolus, repeat up to 3 times.
- Bolus of 10% **glucose** 2–5mL/kg, *repeat as necessary*.
- **Hydrocortisone**—neonate: 10mg slow IV stat, then 100mg/m² daily by IVI; child 1 month–1yrs: 2–4mg/kg/6h; >12yrs: 100mg/6–8h slow IV.
- Rarely insulin and glucose for hyperkalaemia.

Assigning sex and gender

▸There are 2 pieces of information every new parent is asked: the weight and the sex. It is traumatic for them not to be able to answer. However, you must tell parents that you do not know whether their baby is a boy or girl, and that tests must be done. This is unsatisfactory, but much better than having to reassign gender. This is why a neonate with ambiguous genitalia is an emergency for the parents and the well-being of the wider family. Choice of gender must take into account chromosomal and gonadal sex, the hormonal milieu during fetal life, surgical aspects, internal anatomy, fertility issues, psychosexual development, and adult sexual function. NB: ♀ karyotype does not guarantee absence of intra-abdominal testes—so future risks of malignancy have to be assessed too.[425]

The MDT: paediatric endocrinologist with psychological expertise, a neonatologist or general paediatrician, clinical psychologist, paediatric urologist, gynaecologist, geneticist, radiologist, psychologist, and clinical biochemist.

Prenatal preparation entails comparing prenatal karyotype with US genital scans to formulate a differential diagnosis—but US is unreliable in >50% of ♀ pseudohermaphroditism.[426,427] NB: it is common to assign ♀ gender when in doubt,[428] but while some favour a gender compatible with the chromosomal sex, if possible, others point out that this is a simplification as we don't fully understand determinants of gender role (social sex).[429,430] It is important not to think simply in terms of what promotes the greatest efficiency in the act of sexual intercourse.[431]

Advise against registering the birth until a definite treatment plan is in place. Once registered, legal sex cannot be changed in most countries; however, this is changing with ↑ rates of gender dysphoria (p. 725).

RDS is due to a deficiency of alveolar surfactant, which is common in premature babies. Insufficient surfactant leads to atelectasis; re-inflation with each breath exhausts the baby, and respiratory failure follows. Hypoxia leads to ↓cardiac output, hypotension, acidosis, and renal failure. It is the major cause of death from prematurity. *Infants at risk:* 91% if 23–25 weeks; 52% if 30–31 weeks.[432] In late preterms, ↑ risk with maternal diabetes, males, 2nd twin, caesareans.

Signs Increased work of breathing shortly after birth (1st 4h)—tachypnoea (>60/min), grunting, nasal flaring, intercostal recession, and cyanosis. CXR: diffuse granular patterns (ground-glass appearance) ± air bronchograms.

ΔΔ Sepsis (p. 280–1). TTN (p. 285); meconium aspiration syndrome (pp. 284–5); congenital pneumonia; tracheo-oesophageal fistula (rare; suspect if respiratory problems after feeds); congenital lung abnormality.

Prevention Glucocorticoids should be offered to all women at risk of preterm delivery from 24–34wks (consider if 23, or 35–36wks, p. 53); *in utero* transfer, if safe, to centres with experience in managing prematurity/RDS.

Treatment If neonate does not need immediate resuscitation (pp. 226–7) delay clamping of cord (p. 53) to promote placenta–fetal transfusion. Attach pulse oximeter: sats should reach 85% by 5min and 90% by 10min of life in healthy preterms.[432] If not, give oxygen via an oxygen–air blender, starting with 30%, and increase O_2 by 10% every min until improving. Further management depends on spontaneous respiratory effort and work of breathing (± blood gases), options are:
- CPAP (5–6cm H_2O).
- Nasal intermittent positive pressure ventilation (NIPPV).
- Intubation and mechanical ventilation (MV).

See pp. 308–9 for details of types of respiratory support. Caffeine is given as a respiratory stimulant to preterms with apnoeas. Some units give routine caffeine to all babies <30wks' gestation until about 32wks CGA. Inositol is an essential nutrient that has been shown to reduce adverse outcomes in preterms with RDS (↓ death; ↓ retinopathy of prematurity, p. 306; ↓IVH, p. 306; ↓ bronchopulmonary dysplasia (BPD).[433]

Surfactant In the era of prenatal steroid use, prophylactic surfactant has been replaced by 'early selective surfactant administration'. If gestation ≤26wks and FiO_2 >0.3, or >26wks and FiO_2 >0.4 intubate and give prophylactic surfactant via ET tube ±2 further doses if ongoing high O_2 demand/ventilation requirement.[434] Some centres give a dose of surfactant then immediately extubate to non-invasive CPAP ('INSURE' method—INtubate, SURfactant, Extubate); others keep the baby intubated and wean as tolerated. Monitor ventilatory pressures, tidal volumes, and O_2, as needs may suddenly ↓ after surfactant.[435] New minimally invasive surfactant delivery techniques are being developed with the aim of avoiding intubation and mechanical ventilation.
- *Traditional ventilator settings:* (pp. 308–9) On connecting the endotracheal tube, check chest movement is adequate and symmetrical. Auscultate for breath sounds. *Oxygenation:* paO_2 is increased by ↑ mean airway pressure (not too high). *Ventilation:* $paCO_2$ is decreased by ↑ minute volume (↑ breath frequency or ↑ tidal volume (↑PIP or ↑ inspiratory time)). Always use end-tidal CO_2 monitoring. Ask a senior colleague for advice.[436, 437]
- *Fluids:* Start with 10% glucose IV maintenance (p. 287). Full parenteral nutrition can be started on day 1 as can trophic feeding with expressed breast milk (p. 286).[432]

Bronchopulmonary dysplasia (BPD)

This complicates ventilation for RDS in 40% of babies of <1kg birthweight.[438] Defined as a persistent oxygen requirement after 28 postnatal days or 36wks CGA (whichever is later). 'Old' BPD is mainly from barotrauma and oxygen toxicity, whereas 'new' BPD (in babies receiving surfactant) is multi-factorial with airway infections triggering inflammatory cascades. Without surfactant, many would not survive to get BPD.[439] Oxidative processes may also play a key role, but antioxidants are unproven.[440]

Tests *CXR:* Hyperinflation, rounded, radiolucent areas, alternating with thin denser lines. *Histology:* Necrotizing bronchiolitis with alveolar fibrosis.

Mortality Variable, ∴ complex interaction with surfactant use.[439]

Early sequelae Ventilator dependence; pulmonary hypertension; subglottic stenosis, tracheobronchomalacia. Feeding problems. O_2 desaturation during feeds is not uncommon; severe RSV bronchiolitis; gastro-oesophageal reflux.

Late sequelae ↓IQ; cerebral palsy; by adolescence/early adulthood the main changes remaining are asthma and exercise limitation.

Prevention Steroids (antenatal & postnatal); surfactant and 'suitably high' calorie feeding.[441]

Pulmonary hypoplasia

This is very rare. Suspect this in all infants with persisting neonatal tachypnoea ± feeding difficulties, particularly if prenatal oligohydramnios. Hypoplasia may be a consequence of oligohydramnios eg in Potter syndrome or premature rupture of the membranes. In congenital diaphragmatic hernia and cystic adenomatoid malformations, it is a consequence of the 'space-occupying lesion'. They are often detected on the fetal anomaly US. CXR may be misleadingly reported as normal. The condition need not be fatal: postnatal catch-up growth can occur.

ΔΔ RDS, meconium aspiration, sepsis, or primary pulmonary hypertension.[442] Some degree of pulmonary hypoplasia is the price of adopting an early elective delivery for early spontaneous rupture of the membranes, but despite this, expectant management leads to fewer deaths.[443]

Persistent pulmonary hypertension (PPHN)

With our 1st breath, pulmonary vascular resistance (PVR) falls, and there is a rush of blood to our lungs. This is partly mediated by endogenous nitric oxide (NO). This breath initiates changes from fetal to adult circulation—a process which may be interrupted in various conditions eg meconium aspiration, pneumonia, respiratory distress syndrome, congenital lung disease, sepsis, and pulmonary hypoplasia. These adverse events cause abnormal persistence of elevated PVR. In rare cases, it may be due to hypertrophy of the muscular layer in the pulmonary arteries (=*primary pulmonary hypertension*). *Signs:* ↑RR; cyanosis despite intensive O_2 therapy; pre and post-ductal SpO_2 difference; systolic murmur; + signs of underlying cause (see earlier). *Test:* Echocardiography shows ↑RV pressure and right-to-left shunting at the ductus arteriosus in the absence of structural heart disease. R_x: Treat underlying cause; supportive care (ventilate, inotropes); correct reversible contributory factors (hypothermia, polycythaemia, hypocalcaemia, hypoglycaemia). Give surfactant as indicated. Inhaled NO is a potent pulmonary vasodilator; ECMO may be required until PVR falls.

Extracorporeal membrane oxygenation (ECMO) A complex procedure available in a limited number of tertiary units. In veno-venous ECMO, blood is removed, oxygenated, and returned to a central vein precluding the need for lung gas exchange. In veno-arterial ECMO, oxygenated blood is returned to the aorta thereby replacing or supporting the function of both the heart and the lungs.

Neonatal intensive care is a technological development of the basic creed of first aid— ABC; Airway, Breathing, and Circulation. There is also an E. Epithelial cells determine whether low birthweight babies survive outside the uterus. They manage all interactions with the *ex utero* world: • Lung mechanics/gas exchange • Renal tubular balance of fluid and electrolytes • Barrier functions of the gut and skin for keeping bacteria out and water in, plus enabling digestion • Intact neuroepithelium lining of the ventricles of the brain and retina.[444]

Monitor $T°$, HR, RR, SaO$_2$, BP (intra-arterial if critical), blood gases, U&E, bilirubin, FBC, weight, weekly head circumference.

Problems facing babies on NICU
- Hypothermia: incubators allow temperature to be controlled.
- Respiratory distress syndrome (p. 304).
- Hypoxia (respiratory support, pp. 308–9).
- Hypoglycaemia and nutrition (p. 286).
- Persistent ductus arteriosus (PDA).
- Infection (pp. 280–1).
- *Intraventricular haemorrhage:* Occurs in 25% if birthweight ≤1500g.[445] Preterm infants are at risk of IVH due to unsupported blood vessels in the subependymal germinal matrix and the instability of blood pressure associated with birth trauma and respiratory distress. Delayed cord clamping in prems may ↓ risk.[446] *Signs:* seizures, ↓Hb, bulging fontanelle, and cerebral irritability but many will have no clinical symptoms.[447] *Tests:* US; MRI. *Complications:* IQ↓, cerebral palsy, hydrocephalus. Many survive without any sequelae.
- *Apnoea:* Prevalence is 25% of neonates <2.5kg, higher with lower birthweights. Common causes are prematurity, infection, hypothermia, aspiration, congenital heart disease. Caffeine is used in babies <28 weeks. *Prevention:* maternal corticosteroids for fetal lung maturation to increase surfactant production in those at risk of preterm delivery (23–34^{+6} weeks' gestation, p. 53).
- *Anaemia:* ↓EPO production, blood loss from phlebotomy, ↓RBC life span.
- *Necrotizing enterocolitis:* See p. 284.
- *You* may become the problem: overzealous investigation/handling is damaging,[448] but so is under-intervention.[449]
- *Retinopathy of prematurity (ROP):* A disorder of the developing retina. Abnormal fibrovascular proliferation or retinal vessels may lead to retinal detachment and visual loss. Major risk factors are low birthweight and prematurity. Exposure to supplemental oxygen is a cause, in particular large fluctuations in paO$_2$, so careful titration of O$_2$ levels has led to a decrease in the incidence of ROP. *Prevalence (lower limits):* <750g: 62%, >1000g: 10%[450] *Classification:* there are 5 stages, depending on site involved, extent of vascularization, and the degree of retinal detachment. *Treatment:* laser photocoagulation causes less myopia than cryotherapy. Intravitreal anti-VEGF monoclonal antibodies are also used. Screening: see BOX 'Screening for retinopathy of prematurity'.
- *Oxygen saturations:* Target is a contentious issue. A Cochrane review with follow up to 18–24 months of age showed that lower target ranges (85–89%) are associated with ↑ death and ↑NEC, higher target ranges (91–95%) are associated with ↑ROP. However there was no difference in composite outcome of death or major disability.[451] Targeting 90–94% is recommended by a consensus group of European neonatologists.[434]

Screening for retinopathy of prematurity

Screening is performed by indirect ophthalmoscopy (a light attached to a headband with a small handheld lens, giving a better view of the fundus than direct fundoscopy), or wide field digital retinal screening.[452]

Screening criteria
- If ≤27 weeks, screen at 30–31 weeks postmenstrual age.
- If born at 27–32 weeks, screen at day 28–35 of life.
- Screening is repeated 1–2 weekly depending on severity of disease.

Communicating with parents

Take time to explain to parents exactly what is happening to their baby. Structured, tested interviews yield these guidelines:[453]
- Ask both parents to be present (plus a nurse whom they trust).
- Elicit what the parents now know. Clarify or repeat as needed.
- Hand your bleep to a colleague. Allow time. Call the parents by name.
- Look at the parents (mutual gaze promotes trust).
- Name the illness concerned with its complications. Write it down.
- Give support group details: www.bliss.org.uk or www.cafamily.org.uk.
- Answer any questions. Arrange follow-up (<50% may be remembered).

Doctors' decisions are increasingly being questioned by parents. If you and your team are sure your actions are in the child's best interests, and the parents take a different view, take any steps you can to resolve the issue in a non-confrontational way. Violent fights between doctors and parents endanger other children (some UK units have had to be evacuated while police are called). You should know emergency procedures for contacting the High Court to settle the issue (go through the on-call manager: your Trust can make applications day or night). Failure to get Court approval will leave you open to criticism from the European Court of Human Rights, which is likely to take the view that 'do not resuscitate' notices fail to guarantee respect for the child's 'physical and moral integrity'—guaranteed by Article 8 of the Convention on Human Rights—see *Glass* vs *United Kingdom*, 2004 (61827/00).[454]

Signs of a poor prognosis If, despite everything, the baby is still deteriorating, enlist senior help. In extreme prematurity or significant congenital abnormality, it may be appropriate to not escalate treatment any further, or even to withdraw treatment; this is a consultant/MDT decision. Explain what is happening to the parents. Encourage christening, or what is congruent with parents' beliefs. Relieve pain; keep the baby comfortable. In the light of dialogue with parents and nurses it may be appropriate to disconnect the tubes, so allowing the parents to hold the baby, and, in so doing, to aid their grief. NB: contact your Trust's head and defence organization if legal issues beckon.[455]

This is a skill to be learned at the cot side. Nurses and specialist respiratory therapists will help you. Needs of apparently similar babies vary, so what follows is only a guide to prepare your mind before teaching. Continuous refinement in the light of transcutaneous and blood gas analysis is needed. The aims are to improve gas exchange, decrease work of breathing, and enable ventilation for those with respiratory depression or apnoea.

Non-invasive ventilation

CPAP (continuous positive airways pressure): Pressure is delivered throughout the respiratory cycle, assisting spontaneous ventilation. It prevents airway collapse and loss of lung volume. Complications include pneumothorax, nasal trauma, feed intolerance, and reflux. It is used in RDS as respiratory support, particularly in preterm infants, post-extubation, and in upper airway obstruction (eg Pierre–Robin sequence). CPAP is delivered by nasal mask or binasal prongs, or rarely via face mask.

NIPPV (nasal intermittent positive pressure ventilation): Also called bi-level positive airway pressure (BiPAP). This combines nasal CPAP with superimposed ventilator breathing at a set pressure—it can be used as a bridge between invasive ventilation and CPAP.

HFNC (high-flow nasal cannula): A high-flow nasal cannula delivers a distending positive pressure to the airways similar to CPAP. Heating and humidifying the gas delivered reduces side effects of mucosal dryness. Use of HFNC may reduce the number of ventilated days compared to CPAP, but it is not yet considered to be standard practice.[456]

Nasal cannula: O_2 is delivered via soft prongs in the nares at up to 2L/min. The FiO_2 varies with several factors (RR, tidal volume, and degree of mouth breathing) as air is entrained along with the O_2. The oxygen should also be heated and humidified to avoid drying the airway mucosa.

Invasive ventilation Invasive ventilation is broadly composed of *conventional mechanical ventilation* (CMV) (AKA intermittent mandatory ventilation (IMV)) and *high-frequency ventilation* (HFV). Different ventilator models have a bewildering array of different acronyms for their modes which are neither descriptive nor intuitive (SIMV, SIPPV, Assist Control, Pressure Support). Basic terminology common to all: PIP—peak inspiratory pressure; PEEP—positive end-expiratory pressure; MAP—mean airway pressure; T_i—inspiratory time; T_e—expiratory time; TV—tidal volume.

Conventional ventilation: May be pressure targeted (the machine delivers a set PIP for a set T_i, the delivered TV is dependent on lung compliance) or volume targeted (the ventilator delivers a set TV, the PIP and T_i may vary from breath to breath within set limits).

- *TCPL (time-cycled pressure limited ventilation)* is the simplest mode of ventilation. The ventilator delivers PIP on a set time cycle, it does not synchronize with any spontaneous breathing so is rarely used (unless patient is muscle relaxed).
- *PTV (patient-triggered ventilation), including SIMV and SIPPV.* PTV uses a sensor which detects spontaneous breaths. The ventilator then delivers a breath which is synchronized with the infant's own inspiratory effort. In PTV, PIP, and PEEP or TV and is set by the operator, but the rate (within limits) set by the baby. PTV is associated with a shorter duration of ventilation.[457,458] Hiccups can cause problems if abdominal movement is used to detect inspiration.
- *Initial settings:* Set PIP to give good chest inflation and air entry on auscultation or set TV 5–7mL/kg (usually start at 5mL/kg) if using volume targeted. Set PEEP 4–6cmH₂O. Set FiO_2 to give adequate SaO_2. Typical T_i 0.35–0.4sec, and rate 40–60 cycles/min. Adjust in view of blood gas results.

High-frequency ventilation: Delivers small volumes of gas at very rapid rates. Its aim is to reduce ventilator-associated lung injuries for those babies requiring very high pressures to oxygenate. There are several different types—high-frequency positive pressure ventilation (HFPPV), jet ventilation, flow interruption, and oscillatory ventilation (HFOV). HFV may reduce incidence of air leak compared to CMV (see BOX 'Other factors').[459]

Sedation This is given prior to elective intubation with an opiate such as morphine or fentanyl, with a muscle relaxant (suxamethonium). Then **morphine infusion** at 5–20mcg/kg/h (rarely up to 40mcg/kg/h) for ongoing sedation. This is thought safe, and lowers catecholamine concentrations. Most babies do not need long-term paralysis. Nasotracheal ETT siting is best (fewer tube displacements and more comfortable).[460]

Factors associated with a good outcome from ventilation

Factors associated with a better outcome: antenatal corticosteroids, singleton pregnancy, ♀ sex, and higher birthweight.[461]

Complications of mechanical ventilation of neonates

Lung Pneumothorax; pulmonary haemorrhage; bronchopulmonary dysplasia (p. 305); interstitial pulmonary emphysema; pneumonia. Multidrug-resistant organisms may be the cause of late-onset ventilator-associated pneumonia (cefepime has a role here).[462] Post extubation atelectasis may be more frequent after nasal intubation (esp. in very low birthweight infants).[463]

Airways Upper airway obstruction (worse in inspiration and may cause stridor). Consider bronchoscopy (may show supraglottic lesions). Laryngomalacia and gastro-oesophageal reflux also occur, but more rarely.[464]

Others Patent ductus arteriosus; ↑ intracranial pressure ± intraventricular haemorrhage (p. 306); retinopathy of prematurity (p. 306); subcutaneous emphysema; pneumomediastinum; pneumopericardium; pneumoperitoneum.

Weaning from the ventilator

As the baby's condition improves, ventilatory support is weaned. Reduce oxygen to lowest level needed to maintain paO_2/SaO_2. This ↓ROP risk. Decrease the rate of CMV and ↓PIP by 2cmH₂O at a time; try extubating if blood gas OK with ~4cmH₂O PEEP and a PIP of 12–14 with consistent spontaneous breathing above the backup rate. Preterm infants benefit from starting nasal CPAP following extubation. If ventilation has been short term, extubation without CPAP may be appropriate.

Other factors

▶▶Acute deterioration while ventilated, check DOPES: Displaced ETT, Obstructed ETT (secretions, blood), Pneumothorax, Equipment failure (ventilator, tubing), Stomach (splinting diaphragm from BVM ventilation, CPAP, or feeds).

Air leak/pneumothorax Air ruptures alveoli, tracks along vessels and bronchioles (pulmonary interstitial emphysema), and may extend intrapleurally (pneumothorax ± lung collapse), or into the mediastinum or peritoneum. Associated with high PIP, it is less common with HFOV. *Signs:* Tachypnoea , cyanosis, chest asymmetry. Auscultate and transilluminate. The CXR (supine or lateral decubitus) is often diagnostic if you have time.

▶▶Prompt 'blind' needle aspiration of a pneumothorax (thoracocentesis) may be needed in an acute deterioration. Aspirate through the 2nd intercostal space in the midclavicular line with a 25G 'butterfly' needle and a 50mL syringe on a 3-way tap. Following this, insert a chest drain.

Definition *Sudden unexplained infant death (SUID)* is any infant death that is unexpected and initially unexplained. Sometimes, a cause of death is determined after a thorough investigation and autopsy. The deaths that remain unexplained are defined as *sudden infant death syndrome* (SIDS; AKA 'cot death'), the sudden death of an infant under 1 year of age, which remains unexplained after a thorough investigation including an autopsy, examination of the death scene, and review of the clinical history.

Putative causes
Obstructive apnoea:
• Inhalation of milk
• Airways oedema
• Passive smoking
Central apnoea:
• Faulty CO_2 drive
• Prematurity
• Brainstem gliosis
Others:
• Long QT interval
• Staph infection[19]
• Overheating
• ↑ vagal tone or Mg^{2+}↑
• Immature diaphragm
• Genetic & viral causes

Epidemiology Peak incidence: 1–4 months. Risk ↑ if: poor; parents are smokers; baby is male, twin, premature, or LBW; co-sleeping; winter; previous sibling affected by SIDS; coexisting minor upper respiratory infection is common. There are many causal theories (see MINIBOX 'Putative causes').

Prevention Sleeping position is the most important modifiable risk factor, always sleep supine.[465] Breastfeeding; room sharing (as opposed to co-sleeping); removing loose blankets or pillows; preventing overheating; and ↓ cigarette smoke exposure are the other chief preventive interventions: risk from passive smoking is dose dependent, and often at least doubles risk.[466] The face is an important platform for heat loss—and it is known that the incidence of SIDS is ~5–10-fold higher among infants usually sleeping prone (17-fold higher if sleeping in a room separated from parents). Studies have shown no benefit from cardiorespiratory monitors and they may have negative psychological effects on the parents.[467,468] However, these are used in the UK CONI programme (care of next infant for families who suffered SIDS). Advise as follows:

▶*Always* sleep supine ('back to sleep', even for short naps).
• Do not overheat the baby's bedroom. Aim for a temperature of 16–20°C.
• Do not use too much bedding, and avoid duvets if <1 year of age.
• If ill or feverish, consult a GP—do not increase the amount of bedding.
• Use a grow-bag; this is a modified sleeping bag for a baby, containing arm holes and prevents the baby migrating under the blanket.
• While sleeping, avoid heaters, hot water bottles, electric blankets, and hats. Do wrap up for trips out in winter, but unwrap once indoors, even if this means disturbing the baby. Never tuck in blankets higher than the armpit.[469]
• Babies >1 month do not need to be kept as warm as in hospital nurseries.
• Room share but avoid co-sleeping (even if very tired ie most new parents!), especially if parents are deep sleepers, or if they have had any alcohol or drugs.[470,471]

Autopsy This is unrevealing; minor changes are common; petechial haemorrhages over pleura, pericardium, or thymus, and vomit in the trachea may be agonal events. *Causes to exclude:* Sepsis, metabolic defects, and heart defects.

Action after failed resuscitation in the Emergency Department
• Document all interventions, venepuncture sites, and any marks on the baby. You don't have to keep all tubes *in situ*, but ensure that someone who did not intubate confirms endotracheal placement of the tube before extubation.
• Keep all clothing and the nappy.
• Explain clearly to parents that despite your best efforts, the baby has died.
• Unless the cause is obvious, be non-committal about cause of death. Explain the baby *must* have a postmortem (this is a coroner's case).
• Contact the consultant on call, the police, child protection team, and the coroner at once; also GP, health visitor, and any other involved professions.

19 Staphs in mattress foam are implicated (do not reuse).

How the GP can help the family on the first day

- A prompt visit to express sympathy emphasizing that no one is to blame.
- Explain the legal requirement for an autopsy and coroner's inquest. The parents may be called upon to identify the body.
- Bedding may be needed to help find the cause of death.

Subsequent help

Don't *automatically* suppress lactation, but if this becomes necessary **cabergoline** (250mcg/12h PO for 48h) is preferred to bromocriptine. NB: continued lactation may be an important way of grieving for some mothers.

Advise the parents of likely grief reactions (guilt, anger, loss of appetite, hearing the baby cry). Make sure that the coroner informs you of the autopsy result; a consultant paediatrician or GP should explain the findings to the parents. They should already have a routine appointment with a consultant paediatrician. This can provide an opportunity for the parents to ask questions. Programmes exist to prevent a future SID—eg the CONI programme and parents can contact them in future pregnancies. The parents may find an electronic apnoea alarm reassuring in caring for later infants despite the lack of efficacy.

3 Paediatrics

Further reading

Care of Next Infant: www.lullabytrust.org.uk/coni

Estimating dehydration This is difficult. In the West, dehydration >7.5% is rare, even with DKA. *Mild dehydration (0–5%):* Dry mucous membranes; thirsty child; may have decreased urine output. *Moderate dehydration (5–10%):* Dry mucous membranes; cold peripheries; oliguria; ↓ skin turgor; sunken eyes; sunken fontanelle; ↑HR; capillary refill time >2sec; irritable or lethargic. *Severe dehydration (>10%):* As moderate + weak, thready pulse; anuria; reduced consciousness; ↑RR; shock.

Ongoing losses Don't forget to estimate and account for ongoing losses in your fluid regimen eg diarrhoea, vomiting, or NG or drain losses in surgical patients. Ideally the replacement of these fluids should reflect the electrolyte composition of the losses. Beware hidden losses (oedema, ascites, GI pools), and shifts of fluid from the intravascular space to the interstitial space ('third-spacing').

Enteral fluid management Always use enteral fluids, if tolerated, as this is far safer. In dehydration use low-osmolality oral rehydration salts (ORS) with 240–250 mosm/L. Higher osmolalities can cause osmotic diarrhoea. ORS comes in sachets which contain glucose, Na⁺, and K⁺. Show the parent/guardian how to make it up (with the correct volume of water!). Fruit juices and carbonated drinks are not recommended due to high osmolality; however, 1 study showed dilute apple juice is as effective as ORS and more palatable.[472] If child is breast-feeding, continue and give ORS on top as necessary. Use of a NGT may overcome problems of vomiting and palatability but is often not tolerated by pre-school children who may pull the tube out. Antiemetics may be useful in gastroenteritis but evidence is lacking and they may ↑ diarrhoea so are rarely used. *Mild dehydration:* Best managed at home. Encourage parents to give little and often (ie 2.5–5mL every 5min by syringe). The child will not need further treatment unless they become more dehydrated. *Moderate dehydration:* May be managed at home if child is tolerating oral fluids, has improved following a period of observation and there are no longer any red flags.

IV fluid management in dehydration *Indications:* Failure of enteral therapy, severe dehydration, shock. *Fluid choice:* Depends on sodium status. However, for the vast majority of children, use 0.9% NaCl with 5% glucose (± KCL) for IV maintenance and deficit replacement. The glucose content contains few calories, but prevents ketosis. Remember glucose (dextrose) is rapidly metabolized by cells so does not remain in the intravascular space and makes *no contribution* to tonicity (0.9% NaCl and 0.9% NaCl with 5% glucose have the *same* tonicity). Add in KCL (10–20mmol/500mL) once the child has passed urine. *Fluid rate:* Give maintenance fluid requirement (table 3.14) and replace deficit over 48h if >5% dehydrated. Give additional fluid to replace ongoing losses as necessary. Most dehydration in children is *isonatraemic* and rehydration should be with isotonic NaCl as previously described.

Hypernatraemic dehydration: Fairly common, especially in younger children with increased insensible losses. The main danger is too rapid rehydration which can cause cerebral oedema and seizures if serum Na⁺ drops too quickly: ▶▶*correct slowly*. Aim for decrease in serum Na⁺ of <0.5 mmol/L/h. Generally, isotonic NaCl with glucose at rates as above-mentioned is safe and effective. Hypotonic solutions should *only* be used by experienced staff in renal or liver units or PICU with frequent monitoring.

Hyponatraemic dehydration: Rare, often iatrogenic (use of hypotonic IV fluids) or as a result of SIADH. If Na⁺ >125mmol/L use isotonic NaCl with glucose at rates as above-mentioned and this will correct hypovolaemia and hyponatraemia. Children with Na⁺ <120mmol/L are at increased risk of central pontine myelinolysis (osmotic demyelination syndrome) if the Na⁺ is raised too rapidly, seek help. ▶▶Symptomatic hyponatraemia with seizures requires emergency administration of hypertonic saline (3mL/kg of 3% NaCl) seek senior advice. *'Rapid rehydration':* An alternative strategy advocated by the WHO which, in stark contrast to traditional slow correction of fluid deficit over 24h, involves 4h of 10mL/kg/h 0.9% NaCl then maintenance after if needed.[473] Ensure the nurses are aware to drop the fluid rate after 4h. This is thought to be safe in acute gastroenteritis but should not be used in children with significant electrolyte abnormalities as above-mentioned. *Monitoring:* Clinical signs. U&E (± blood gas, osmolality) on admission, and *at least* daily for any child on IV fluids. Initial metabolic acidosis usually corrects itself (although prolonged infusion of NaCl may lead to hyperchloraemic metabolic acidosis). Strict fluid balance. Catheter may be needed to monitor urine output. OD or BD weights are useful in protracted cases. Urinary Na+ may be useful in unusual cases.

Maintenance requirements
See table 3.14. eg for a 23kg child, daily maintenance fluid requirement = 10kg × 100mL/kg + 10kg × 50mL/kg + 3kg × 20mL/kg = 1560mL/day = 65mL/h. This includes insensible water losses (via skin and respiratory system) which vary with body surface area ($\approx$300–400mL/m^2/day).

Table 3.14 Daily IV fluid maintenance needs

Weight (kg)	Water (mL/kg/day)
Neonates	150
First 10	100
10–20	50
>20	20
Maximum	2500mL/day

Calculating pre-existing deficit In mL $\approx$ % dehydration × weight (kg) × 10 (eg for a 10kg child who is 7.5% dehydrated = 750mL).

▶▶ **IV fluid management in hypovolaemic shock (APLS)** Treatment aims to restore any circulatory compromise, then to correct deficits over 48h. If IV access fails, use the intraosseous route (p. 182).
• Give 20mL/kg 0.9% NaCl bolus and reassess. If still in shock, repeat.
• If remains in shock after 40mL/kg consider other causes of shock. Further fluid boluses, inotropes, blood, and ventilation may be needed, discuss urgently with seniors and PICU.

Initial resuscitation should always be with isotonic crystalloids. Colloids are an option but have failed to show superiority over crystalloids in trials. Use blood in haemorrhagic shock.

SIADH Hyponatraemia in children is usually caused by the syndrome of inappropriate ADH secretion (ΔΔ: use of hypotonic IV fluids). SIADH occurs with several conditions: infections; surgery; medications; but probably most commonly with respiratory infections. R: Treat underlying cause, fluid restrict. Most units will give ⅔ IV maintenance fluids to children with respiratory infections to anticipate and prevent ↓Na from SIADH.

Special circumstances Neonates (p. 287); DKA (p. 248); nephrotic syndrome (p. 226); burns—greatly increased skin losses; cardiac disease—increased risk of fluid overload; diabetes insipidus; renal failure; severe acute malnutrition—increased risk of fluid overload.

Key points • First correct shock • If tolerated, always use *oral* rehydration • 0.9% NaCl with 5% glucose (± KCl) is the fluid of choice for the majority of children • Avoid rapid changes in Na+ (↑ or ↓) • Check U&E *at least* daily, more often if abnormal • *Keep it simple*, complex regimens cause errors.

Table 3.15 Reference ranges

	Age	Range		Age	Range
Haematology			**Coagulation screen**		
Haemoglobin	0–6d	145–220g/L	PT, term babies	0–3mths	8.5–14.1sec
	7d	140–186g/L	PT, preterm babies (born at 30–36wks)	0–3mths	8.5–17.0sec
	8d–3mths	95–125g/L	PT	Adult	10–12sec
	3mths–4yrs	110–140g/L	APTT, term babies	0–3mths	28.0–55.0sec
	5–12yrs	115–140g/L	APTT, preterm babies (30–36wks' gestation)	0–21d	27–75sec
	Adult ♂	130–175g/L		22d–3mths	26.9–62.5sec
	Adult ♀	115–165g/L	APTT, term & preterm	3mths–12yrs	28.0–45.0sec
Platelets		150–450×10⁹/L	APTT	Adult	22–41sec
	Adult	150–400×10⁹/L	**Electrolytes**		
MCH	0–3mths	31–37pg	Sodium		133–146mmol/L
	3–4mths	27–33pg	Potassium		3.5–5.5mmol/L
	4mths–12yrs	23–31pg	Chloride		95–106mmol/L
	Adult	27–33pg	Urea	0–12mths	0.8–5.5mmol/L
MCHC		32–35g/dL		1–16yrs	2.5–6.5mmol/L
MCV	0–3mths	100–130fL	Creatinine	Neonate	21–75µmol/L
	3–4mths	85–100fL		1mth–4yrs	13–39µmol/L
	4mths–4yrs	70–86fL		5–11yrs	29–53µmol/L
	4–12yrs	77–91fL		12yrs+	40–90µmol/L
	Adult	80–96fL	Calcium	<4wks	2.0–2.7mmol/L
WCC	0–6d	10.0–26.0×10⁹/L		4wks–16yrs	2.2–2.7mmol/L
	7d	5.0–21.0×10⁹/L	Magnesium		0.6–1.0mmol/L
	8d–6mths	6.0–15.0×10⁹/L	Phosphate	<1yr	1.3–2.6mmol/L
	7mths–5yrs	5.0–12.0×10⁹/L		1–16yrs	0.9–1.8mmol/L
	Adult	3.0–10.0×10⁹/L	Fasting glucose	Neonate	2.5–5.5mmol/L
Neutrophils	0–3d	5.0–13.0×10⁹/L		Child	3.0–6.0mmol/L
	4d	1.5–10.0×10⁹/L	**Liver function**		
	5d–6yrs	1.5–8.0×10⁹/L	Albumin	<4wks	25–45g/L
	7–11yrs	2.0–6.0×10⁹/L		4wks–1yr	30–45g/L
	Adult	2.0–7.5×10⁹/L		1yr–adult	35–50g/L
Lymphocytes	0–2d	2.0–4.5×10⁹/L	ALT	0–12mths	0–41IU/L
	3d	3.0–9.0×10⁹/L		1–2yrs	0–28IU/L
	4d–12mths	4.0–10.0×10⁹/L		3–6yrs	0–29IU/L
	1–6yrs	1.5–9.5×10⁹/L		7–12yrs	0–36IU/L
	7–10yrs	1.5–7.0×10⁹/L		13–17yrs	0–37IU/L
	Adult	1.5–4.0×10⁹/L	AST	Neonate	18–92IU/L
Monocytes	0–3d	0.5–1.5×10⁹/L		Child	8–60IU/L
	4d–6yrs	0.3–1.1×10⁹/L	Alkaline phosphatase	Neonate	73–391IU/L
	7–10yrs	0.2–1.2×10⁹/L		Infant	59–425IU/L
	Adult	0.2–1.0×10⁹/L		1–14yrs	76–308IU/L
Eosinophils	0–3d	0.1–2.0×10⁹/L		14–16yrs	49–242IU/L
	4d–6yrs	0.1–1.0×10⁹/L		Adult	25–115IU/L
	7–10yrs	0.1–0.8×10⁹/L	Bilirubin	14d–16yrs	<21µmol/L (conjugated <2µmol/L)
	Adult	0–0.4×10⁹/L	γGT		9–40IU/L
Basophils		0–0.1×10⁹/L	**Haematinics**		
ESR		<20mm/h	Serum vitamin B₁₂		160–925ng/L
			Serum folate		3–15mcg/L
			Ferritin		12–200mcg/L

3 Paediatrics

Table 3.15 Reference ranges (contd.)

	Age	Range		Age	Range
Endocrine			**Arterial blood gas**		
TSH	0–3d	5.2–14.6mU/L	pH		7.35–7.45
	4d–12mths	0.6–8.1mU/L	pao₂		11–15kPa
	Child	0.5–4.5mU/L	pao₂ preterm neonatal target		8–12kPa
	Adult	0.3–4.2mU/L			
Free T3		3.0–9.0pmol/L	paco₂		4.6–6.4 kPa
	Adult	4.0–7.2pmol/L			
Free T4	0–6d	11–32pmol/L	Bicarbonate	Neonate	14–28mmol/L
	7d–3mths	12–18pmol/L		Child	19–28mmol/L
	>3mths	12–24pmol/L		Adult	22–30mmol/L
	Adult	9–25pmol/L	Base excess		–2 to +2mmol/L
Cortisol (9am)		200–700nmol/L			

Adult reference ranges apply after the last listed upper age limit, where applicable. Check your haematology and biochemistry lab for local reference ranges which vary between populations and age groups

Source: data from RCPCH (2016) https://www.rcpch.ac.uk/sites/default/files/rcpch/HTWQv8.4/Normal%20ranges.pdf

3 Paediatrics

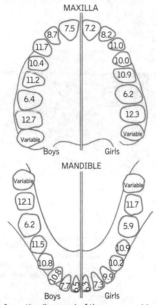

MAXILLA

Boys — Girls

MANDIBLE

Boys — Girls

Fig 3.28 Mean times of eruption (in years) of the permanent teeth.

Table 3.16 Mean age of eruption of deciduous 'baby' teeth

Deciduous teeth	Months		Months
Lower central incisors	5–9	1st molars	10–16
Upper central incisors	8–12	Canines	16–20
Upper lateral incisors	10–12	2nd molars	20–30
Lower lateral incisors	12–15		
A 1-year-old has ~6 teeth; 1½yrs ~12 teeth; 2yrs ~16 teeth; 2¼yrs ~20.			

3 Paediatrics

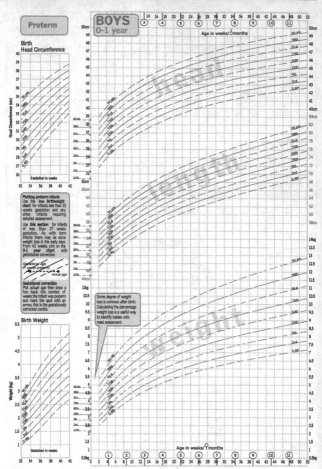

Fig 3.29 UK-WHO growth charts—boys aged 0–1yrs.
Source: RCPCH/WHO/Department of Health. © 2009 Department of Health. Reproduced with permission of Royal College of Paediatrics and Child Health.

In 2006, the WHO introduced new growth standards which were adopted in the UK in 2009 (2010 in Scotland) for children 0–4yrs (UK-WHO charts, figs 3.29 & 3.30). These growth standards were compiled from data from breastfed babies (in whom growth is slower than formula-fed infants)—from 6 different nations (the USA, Norway, Oman, Brazil, India, and Ghana). The linear growth patterns were similar between nations—so for this age group there aren't thought to be any ethnospecific differences in rate of growth. This rate of growth is taken to be an optimal growth rate for children, as opposed

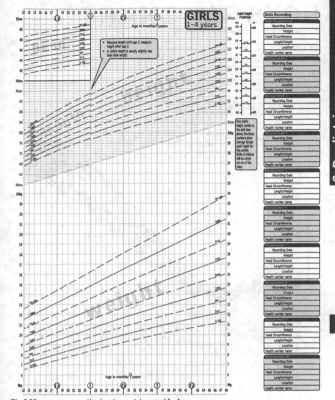

Fig 3.30 UK-WHO growth charts—girls aged 1–4yrs.
Source: RCPCH/WHO/Department of Health. © 2009 Department of Health. Reproduced with permission of Royal College of Paediatrics and Child Health.

to the previous growth charts (UK90) which described the prevailing growth patterns of UK children compiled from surveys done in the 1980s. As a result the UK-WHO charts have an increased number of overweight children and fewer underweight children, when compared with the UK90 charts. For <4yrs, the UK-WHO charts replace the UK90 charts. The UK90 charts are still used for children >4yrs (not reproduced here). Separate charts exist for children with Down syndrome, Turner syndrome, achondroplasia, and significant prematurity (<32wks).

BOYS BMI CHART

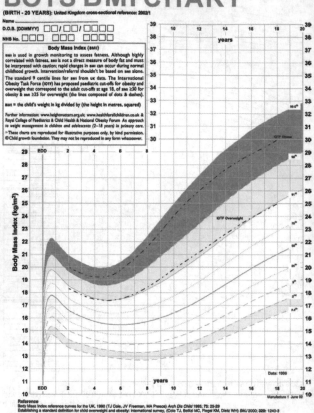

Fig 3.31 Boys' BMI chart.

© Child Growth Foundation reproduced with kind permission. www.childgrowthfoundation.org.

Risk factors for childhood obesity Changes in food availability and activity levels during the past 30 years are well known. Also: low socioeconomic status, maternal obesity, rapid infancy weight gain. *Obesity prevention programmes* have some success and show that changes in school and community environments can decrease childhood weight gain. In France, for example, children are weighed in school regularly, and regular exercise and healthy eating (not diets) are promoted in systematic ways. Input from a family healthy-eating coach has also been found to help.[474,475] Peer encouragement and feedback in the form of pedometer readings is one way of promoting more exercise.[476]

For methods of preventing adult consequences of childhood obesity by intervening in childhood, see p. 266.

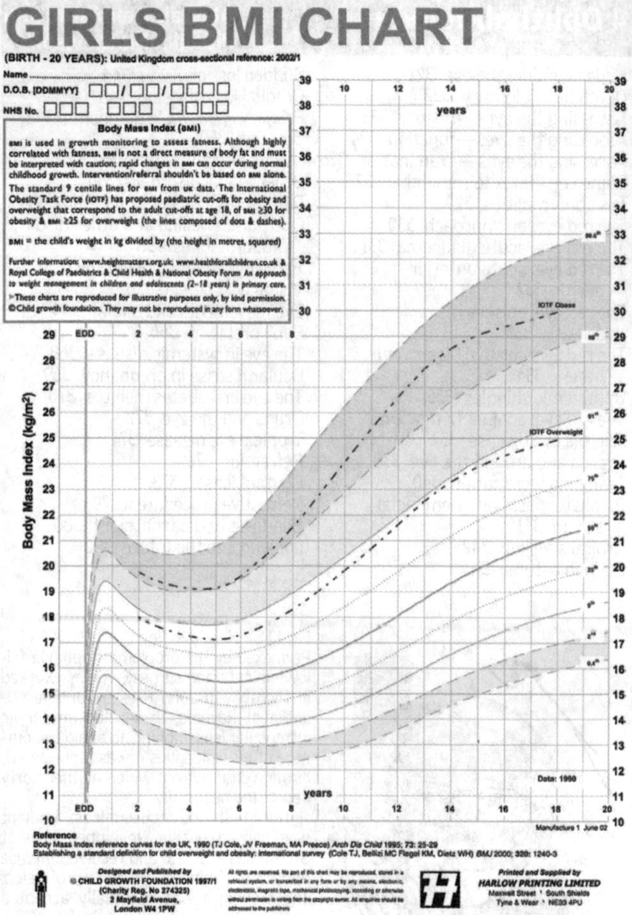

GIRLS BMI CHART

(BIRTH - 20 YEARS): United Kingdom cross-sectional reference: 2002/1

Name ....

D.O.B. [DDMMYY] ☐☐/☐☐/☐☐☐☐

NHS No. ☐☐☐ ☐☐☐ ☐☐☐☐

Body Mass Index (BMI)

BMI is used in growth monitoring to assess fatness. Although highly correlated with fatness, BMI is not a direct measure of body fat and must be interpreted with caution; rapid changes in BMI can occur during normal childhood growth. Intervention/referral shouldn't be based on BMI alone.

The standard 9 centile lines for BMI from our data. The International Obesity Task Force (IOTF) has proposed paediatric cut-offs for obesity and overweight that correspond to the adult cut-offs at age 18, of BMI ≥30 for obesity & BMI ≥25 for overweight (the lines composed of dots & dashes).

BMI = the child's weight in kg divided by (the height in metres, squared)

Further information: www.heightmatters.org.uk; www.healthforallchildren.co.uk & Royal College of Paediatrics & Child Health & National Obesity Forum An approach to weight management in children and adolescents (2–18 years) in primary care.

▷These charts are reproduced for illustrative purposes only, by kind permission. © Child growth foundation. They may not be reproduced in any form whatsoever.

Fig 3.32 Girls' BMI chart.

© Child Growth Foundation reproduced with kind permission. www.childgrowthfoundation.org.

Reference
Body Mass Index reference curves for the UK, 1990 (TJ Cole, JV Freeman, MA Preece) *Arch Dis Child* 1995; 73: 25-29
Establishing a standard definition for child overweight and obesity: international survey (Cole TJ, Bellizi MC Flegal KM, Dietz WH) *BMJ* 2000; 320: 1240-3

z-scores for weight, height, and BMI: what do they mean? A z score (for weight-for-age) of −1 indicates that weight is 1 standard deviation below the median for that age/sex group. This means mildly underweight. z −2 (minus 2 standard deviations) is moderate, and z−3 is severe. Ditto for height. In the care of children with chronic diseases eg HIV, monitoring and improving the BMI z-score is an important way of reducing morbidity and mortality.[477]

A BMI z-score of +2 to +2.5 counts as moderate obesity (severe if >2.5).[478,479] BMI z-score is a key determinant of metabolic syndrome in children;[480] a 1-point increase in BMI z-score yields a 2-fold increase in its prevalence (↑ from 27.6% to 60.7% if BMI z-score increases from 2.3 to 3.3). (See figs 3.31 & 3.32 for BMI charts.)

BMI z-scores also help monitoring weight-intervention programmes.[481]

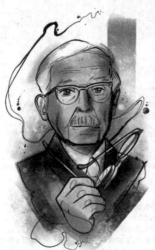

Fig 4.1 Sir Harold Ridley.
Perplexed by the problem of aphakia following cataract surgery, Ridley worked in secret with John Pike, an optical scientist at Rayners, to develop an acrylic intraocular lens implant. To avoid the outrage of his colleagues it was a purely scientific venture, from which neither party benefitted financially.

The first intraocular lens implant was carried out in November 1949 at St Thomas' hospital and received intense opposition from the medical profession. The technique was eventually accepted by the medical profession in the late 1970s. Intraocular lenses have since been used to restore eyesight in millions of patients worldwide. In the 1990s Ridley underwent bilateral intraocular lens implantation at St Thomas's hospital, himself benefitting from the surgery he had pioneered there decades earlier.[1]

Artwork by Gillian Turner.

With many thanks to our junior reader Nikhil Joshi for their contribution to this chapter.

Understanding the eye

If you understand the basic anatomy (fig 4.2) and function of the key parts of the eye, most of the rest—clinical presentation, pathology, and treatment—falls into place.

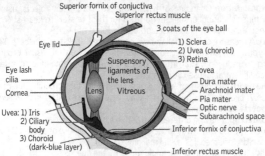

Fig 4.2 Anatomy of the eye. The average human eye has a length of 24 millimetres and weighs about 7.5g. It is composed of 6g of water.

Ocular surface

Conjunctiva: Anatomy: thin membrane covering most of the anterior surface of the eye, continuous from edge of cornea (limbus) to lid margin. *Function:* mucous membrane; contributes to tear film.

Episclera: Anatomy: thin connective tissue layer between conjunctiva and sclera. *Function:* connective tissue.

Sclera: Anatomy: the tough outer coat of the eyeball, continuous with the cornea anteriorly; the 'white' of the eye. *Function:* maintains eye shape (for refraction), barrier (vs infection), protective (vs trauma).

Cornea: Anatomy: thick collagen layer of remarkable transparency forming the most anterior part of the eyeball; continuous with the sclera. *Function:* the 'window' of the eye, allowing light transmission and responsible for ~⅔ of refraction; also structural/barrier function similar to sclera.

Structures in the eye

Lens: Anatomy: transparent biconvex structure suspended by lens zonules; naturally spherical but is held in tension and therefore more oval; mainly composed of proteins called crystallins. *Function:* light transmission; refraction, by contraction/relaxation of the ciliary muscle for changing focus ('accommodation'). Ciliary muscle contraction → zonules relax → lens ↑ spherical → focusing power ↑.

Iris: Anatomy: anterior part of the highly vascular layer known as the uvea; contains radial and circular muscle fibres working in opposition. *Function:* aperture of the eye controlling light entry.

Ciliary body: Anatomy: middle part of the uvea, continuous with iris anteriorly and choroid posteriorly; comprises ciliary epithelium and ciliary muscle. *Function:* ciliary epithelium produces aqueous humour; ciliary muscle causes accommodation.

Choroid: Anatomy: posterior uvea, continuous with the ciliary body anteriorly; highly vascular. *Function:* provides oxygen and nutrients to the outer layers of the retina.

Retina: Anatomy: transparent tissue containing the photoreceptors (rods and cones); lies anterior (ie on the inner aspect of) the choroid; within the retina, multiple neural layers overlie the photoreceptors, which overlie the retinal pigmented epithelium (RPE). *Function:* transduction of light into a neural signal; transparency through the neural layers to reach the photoreceptors.

Optic nerve: Anatomy: CN II; comprising 1.2 million axons of the retinal ganglion cells; about 5cm long running from the optic disc to the optic chiasm. *Fluids filling the eye: Aqueous humour:* transparent watery fluid filling the anterior chamber of the eye (the space in front of the lens); *Vitreous humour:* transparent gel filling the globe behind the lens.

Starting in another speciality can feel like moving to a different country with its own language and customs. Here is a short phrasebook to get you started.

Accommodation Changing of lens shape to focus near objects, using the ciliary muscle. Young lenses can go from furthest (a star) to nearest (7cm) in 0.35 seconds (approaching kisses go out of focus at ~7cm).

Acuity A measure of how well the eye sees a small or distant object (p. 324).

Amblyopia A common developmental defect of central visual processing leading to reduced vision in one or both eyes, occurring due to a lack of balanced bilateral focused visual stimulation.

Amsler grid Test chart of intersecting lines used for screening for macular disease. If present, lines may appear wavy and squares distorted or absent.

Anisocoria Unequal pupil size (p. 367).

Anisometropia Having different refractive errors in each eye.

Aphakia The state of having no lens (eg removed because of cataract).

Blepharitis Inflamed lids/eyelid margins (p. 338).

Canthus The medial or lateral angle made by the open lids.

Chemosis Oedema of the conjunctiva.

Cycloplegia Ciliary muscle paralysis preventing accommodation.

Dacryocystitis Inflammation of the lacrimal sac.

Dioptre Units for measuring refractive power of lenses.

Ectropion Abnormal eversion of the lid (commonly lower lid).

Endophthalmitis Inflammation of the internal eye, often secondary to infection following surgery.

Entropion Abnormal inversion of the lid (lashes may irritate the eyeball).

Epiphora Passive overflow of tears on to the cheek.

Fornix The fold of conjunctiva connecting the palpebral (lid) conjunctiva with the bulbar (eyeball) conjunctiva.

Fovea Cone-rich area of macula capable of highest acuity vision (p. 352). See also foveolar (p. 352).

Fundus That part of retina normally visible through the ophthalmoscope.

Gonioscopy The use of a goniolens (+slit lamp) to evaluate drainage of aqueous humour by examining the 'angle' of where the cornea and iris meet.

Hypermetropia 'Long-sighted.' Distant objects appear more clearly and near objects appear blurred, due to light focusing behind the retina (p. 376).

Keratoconus The pathological process whereby the cornea is shaped like a cone.

Limbus The annular border between clear cornea and opaque sclera.

Macula Central most posterior part of the retina, approximating to 550μm oval centred on the fovea (p. 352).

Miotic An agent causing pupil constriction (eg pilocarpine).

Mydriatic An agent causing pupil dilatation (eg tropicamide).

Myopia 'Short-sighted.' Close objects look clearer but distant objects are blurred due to a refractive error where light focuses in front of (instead of on) the retina (commonly due to long axial eye length) (p. 376).

Near point Where the eye is looking when maximally accommodated.

Optic cup The cup-like depression in the centre of the optic disc (p. 349).

Optic disc (Optic nerve head.) That part of optic nerve seen ophthalmoscopically in the fundus.

Papillitis Inflammation of the optic nerve head.

Photophobia Painful sensitivity to light.

Presbyopia The loss of accommodation resulting in failure to focus on near objects due to loss of elasticity of the lens; usually age related.

Pterygium Wing-shaped degenerative conjunctival triangular fibrovascular band of conjunctiva which spreads across the cornea (p. 338).

Ptosis Drooping lid(s).

Refraction Light ray deviation on passing through media of different density; or determining refractive errors and correcting them with lenses.

Retinal detachment The sensory retina separates from the pigmented epithelial layer of retina ; or an area of full thickness retina separates from the choroid.

Scotoma A 'blind-spot'; part of the field of view is missing.

Slit lamp A device which illuminates and magnifies structures in the eye (p328).

Strabismus (Squint.) Misalignment of the eyes such that the visual axis of each eye is not directed at the same point.

Tarsorrhaphy A surgical procedure for joining upper and lower lids.

Tonometer A device for measuring intraocular pressure.

Uvea Iris, ciliary body, and choroid.

Vitrectomy Surgical removal of the vitreous.

Assessing the eyes—history

If you allow the patient enough time to talk they may well give you the diagnosis. The history will focus your examination and narrow down likely diagnoses. Key presentations are listed in table 4.1.

Table 4.1 Presentation of eye symptoms

Presentation	Diagnostic pointer
Pain/redness/discharge/ photophobia	Front of the eye problem See 'The red eye', p. 330
Loss of vision	Usually back of the eye problem (especially if painless) See 'Loss of vision', pp. 344–5
Distortion of vision	Usually macula problem See 'Macula', p. 352
'Flashes and floaters'	Usually vitreous or retinal problem See pp. 356–7
Double vision	Usually a cranial nerve problem or a decompensating childhood squint, but may arise anywhere from brainstem to orbit See pp. 364–5

History

Symptoms (uni- vs bilateral):
• Pain (severity, character, duration, location, precipitants), discharge (purulent/ watery).
• Redness (duration, location).
• Photophobia.
• Loss of vision (onset, pattern, duration).
• Distortion.
• 'Flashes and floaters'.
• Double vision (onset, variability).

Specific questions are considered further under the specific presentations—see the relevant sections, eg 'The red eye', p. 330.

Past ophthalmic history: Contact lens (CL) wearer p. 378 (type of CL and CL hygiene); previous eye surgeries/injections; approximate refraction if known.

Social history: Employment; smoking; relevant specific exposures (eg sexual history).

Past medical history: Eye disease is a common presenting issue for inflammatory conditions.

Inside the eye hides a world of medical signs in miniature, providing clues to both ophthalmic and systemic pathology. Work systematically—assess function, then examine the eye from 'outside-in'.

Assessment of visual function *Visual acuity:* This is the clarity or sharpness of vision. Accurate assessment of visual acuity (VA) is the cornerstone of any ophthalmic examination. The distance at which the Snellen chart is read is the numerator (usually 6m); the smallest line which the patient can read is the denominator (fig 4.3). If a patient can read the 60m line at 4m then the visual acuity is 4/60. Distance glasses should be worn, and one eye should be tested at a time. The fellow eye must be occluded (ensure the patient doesn't peep with the better-seeing eye). If the patient sees less than 6/6 with or without glasses, examine with a pinhole in front of the eye. In simple refractive errors, acuity will improve through the pinhole. This test can estimate the extent to which a patient's reduced vision is due to refractive error. For acuities <6/60 patients can be brought forward to 5, 4, 3, 2, and 1m from the chart to read the top line. If vision is below 1/60 ask the patient to count fingers (CF) at 50cm distance; if this fails see whether they can detect your hand movements (HM), and then perception of light (PL). If all of this fails then the patient has no perception of light (NPL) ie the eye is completely blind.

4 Ophthalmology

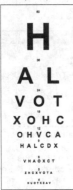
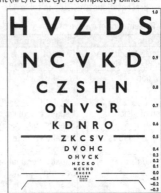

Fig 4.3 The familiar Snellen chart is known throughout the world, with comic variations appearing in memes and on mugs. The alternative LogMAR chart is less well known but commonly used in hospital eye services. It has a number of advantages, including having an equal number of letters on each line. The chart is normally used at 4m. Each correct line (worth 0.1u) and each correct letter (worth 0.02u) is subtracted from 1.0 to give the final score.

Reproduced from Denniston A. and Murray P.I.., *Oxford Handbook of Ophthalmology* (2018), with permission from OUP.

Visual acuity testing in children

Visual acuity can be tested in babies and young children by checking if they 'fix and follow' with each eye tested separately. To do this cover one eye and then see if they watch your face as you move from side to side. If the child cries when one eye is covered, then it raises the suspicion that vision in the fellow eye is poor.

Visual field The area seen without shifting gaze. See p. 362.

Extraocular movements (See pp. 364-5.) Always examine in those with diplopia. Ask the patient to watch a pen move into the 9 positions of gaze and ask which movement provokes most diplopia, and when looking in that direction, block each eye in turn and ask which one sees the *outer* image: that is the eye with pathology.

Pupil examination and reflexes See p. 366.

Colour vision and colour blindness

A disorder characterized by a deficiency in colour detection or processing. In order for light rays to make the images we see, the rays need to pass through the photoreceptors. We require all 3 cones, red, green, and blue, to perceive colour. If any are missing or not functioning, one can be colour blind in that spectrum of colour. There are at least 19 different chromosomes involved in colour vision deficiencies. However, the condition is mostly inherited on the x chromosome.[1] 8% ♂ and 0.5% ♀ affected—so those with Turner syndrome have ♂ incidence and those with Klinefelter's have ♀ incidence. **Diagnosis** This is by use of coloured pattern discrimination charts (eg Ishihara plates, see fig 4.4). Depressed colour vision may be a sensitive indicator of acquired macular or optic nerve disease (eg reduced red saturation in optic neuritis).[2]

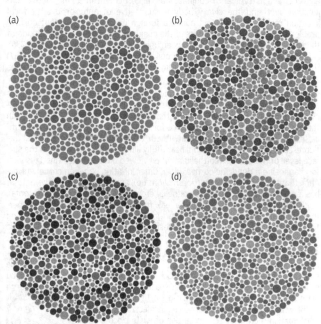

Fig 4.4 Ishihara Test for colour deficiency. (a) Demonstration plate: everyone should read '12'. (b) Normal vision read '3'; red–green deficiency read '5'. (c) Normal vision read '42'; in protanopia (blindness to red) and protanomalia (insensitivity to red) only '2' is read (or '2' is clearer than '4' in mild protanomalia); in deuteranopia and deuteranomalia (blindness/insensitivity to green) only '4' is read (or '4' is clearer than '2' in mild deuteranomalia). (d) Normal vision read '6'; the majority with colour vision deficiency cannot read a number or read it incorrectly.

NB: These plates should *not* be used for diagnostic purposes. Please note that the sample images reproduced here should not be used for the test of colour anomaly. The plates of 'Ishihara Test for Colour deficiency' reproduced with permission, The Public Interest Incorporated Foundation Isshinkai, Tokyo, Japan.

1 This is due to the fact that males have only one x chromosome. Females inherit 2 copies of the x chromosome. For the deficiency to be present, females need relevant mutations in both x chromosomes present which is highly unlikely.

Examining the front of the eye

If you have access to a 'slit lamp' (a biomicroscope) then use it. This instrument has a bright light source and a horizontally mounted microscope to examine the structures of the eye. The light source can be converted to a slit (hence the name). Attachments allow intraocular pressure measurement ('tonometry'). When you are working in the ED, ask someone to show you how to use it; the basics are within your grasp, you will be amazed by the beautiful detail you can see with a little focusing. In the absence of a slit lamp, use a good light source (eg a bright pen-torch or ophthalmoscope).

Conjunctiva Can be seen best by asking the patient to look up, down, left, and right. Look for engorgement ('injection') of the conjunctival vessels suggestive of inflammation, a common cause of 'the red eye'. Diffuse vascular engorgement is typical of conjunctivitis; engorgement in a ring of the conjunctiva overlying the ciliary body is suggestive of anterior uveitis; focal injection may be related to trauma, a foreign body, or an adjacent corneal problem (fig 4.7). Diffuse redness of the conjunctiva which extends outside of the vessels is probably due to a subconjunctival haemorrhage (fig 4.18 p. 336).

To examine the tarsal conjunctiva pull down the lower lid and evert ('flip') the upper lid to reveal retained foreign bodies, or allergic changes such as papillae.

Cornea Best examined with a sideways slit-lamp beam, which enables visualization of the anterior and posterior surfaces. This will enable you to appreciate the depth of a foreign body in the cornea, if it has penetrated through the posterior surface, and to examine for corneal scarring (fig 4.6). No examination of the cornea is complete without using fluorescein. This yellow dye fluoresces at the correct dilution, beautifully illuminating any defect in the surface layer of the cornea (epithelium) when viewed under a blue light. It is vital for diagnosing a dendritic corneal ulcer, differentiating between corneal ulceration (lights up) and scarring (doesn't light up), and showing you if the patient has a dry eye (lots of punctate epithelial erosions = diffuse tiny yellow spots). It is also valuable for diagnosing a leak from the cornea: if it has been perforated, fluorescein can highlight a bright yellow river of aqueous streaming from the front of the eye (= Seidel's test positive requiring urgent ophthalmic intervention to save the eye).

Anterior chamber Can be seen by using a sideways slit-lamp beam and examining the space between the cornea and the iris. This is done by focusing on the cornea and then gradually focusing backwards to the iris. In a normal eye you shouldn't be able to see anything in this space. Look for blood in the anterior chamber (hyphaema) (fig 4.5). In trauma, it can fill the whole anterior chamber if severe. In infection or severe inflammation there may be a collection of white blood cells at the bottom of the anterior chamber (hypopyon). Individual white blood cells can be seen in uveitis (with a narrow slit-lamp beam and on maximum magnification, use the black pupil as a backdrop to see the cells). There can also be 'flare' (like headlamps in the fog).

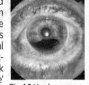

Fig 4.5 Hyphaema.
Courtesy of Prof J Trobe.

Pupil May be small and irregular in anterior uveitis (p. 332), and semi-dilated and fixed in acute glaucoma (p. 331). Pupil examination is covered in detail on p. 366.

Lens Normally transparent, but can become white or brown in cases of cataract (seen as a white pupil, 'leucocoria').

The ophthalmoscope can be used to detect pathology in the lens, vitreous, and retina. Start with high + numbers (often marked in colour on the dial). To examine the lens and the vitreous, focus the beam of the ophthalmoscope at the pupil at ~1m from the eye. In the normal eye there is a red glow from the choroid (the red reflex). Red reflexes are absent with dense cataract and intraocular bleeding. Any lens opacity (cataract) will be seen as a black pattern obstructing the red reflex.

Vitreous, retina, and choroid Blood or debris in the vitreous are seen by the patient as black floaters. When the retina is in focus, ask the patient to look ahead into the distance. This may bring the optic disc into view. It should have precise boundaries (p. 358) and a central cup (p. 349). Examine radiating vessels and lastly the macula (ask the patient to look at the light).

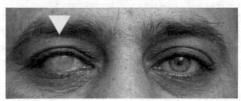

Fig 4.6 Corneal opacity in the right eye preventing view of the iris and pupil. The aetiology of corneal opacities include genetic, metabolic, and idiopathic. The most common cause of corneal opacity is scarring secondary to corneal infections. When looking for a cataract, only the lens (seen through the pupil) will look hazy.

Reproduced with permission from the article by Zahid H Sheikh, Wasif Hafeez. The Unknown Source of Communicable Disease. *Pak J Ophthalmol* © Oct 2001;17(4):110–4.

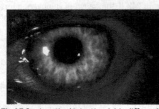 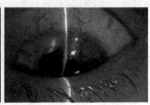

Fig 4.7 Conjunctival injection (a) is diffuse dilatation of peripheral conjunctival vessels caused by conjunctivitis (p. 336); it may cause discomfort but is not painful. Ciliary injection (b) is dilatation of deeper vessels around the limbus. It is associated with corneal injury, episcleritis, scleritis, anterior uveitis, infection, and acute glaucoma + moderate–severe pain.

Image (a) reproduced from Simon C *et al*, *Oxford Handbook of General Practice* 2014, with permission from OUP; image (b) reproduced from Sundaram V. *et al*, *Training in Ophthalmology* 2016, with permission from OUP.

Further reading

International Council of Ophthalmology (2009). *Handbook for Medical Students Learning Ophthalmology*. http://www.icoph.org/downloads/ICOMedicalStudentEnglish.pdf

4 Ophthalmology

4 Ophthalmology

1 *Always test visual acuity* in each eye separately and wearing glasses (if worn). A 1mm pinhole will improve acuity in refractive errors.

2 *More mistakes in medicine are made by not looking than not knowing.* Optimize illumination and magnification (slit lamp optimal) for examination of the fundus. Use g. tropicamide 1% (if no head injury and no shallow anterior chamber) to dilate the pupil.

3 *Examine the pupil reflexes* to determine if there is a problem with optic nerve function (p. 366).

4 *Visual field examination* can differentiate an ocular cause from central cause of vision loss. Peripheral defect in glaucoma, horizontal defect in branch retinal artery, or vein occlusion; bitemporal vertical defect in pituitary tumour; homonymous vertical defect in intracranial lesion or cerebrovascular accident (p. 362).

5 *No child is too young for an eye exam.* Check the red-reflex of every newborn and refer any suspected squint immediately.

6 *Sudden loss or blurring of vision is an emergency.* Always exclude temporal arteritis because of immediate risk to other eye. Other causes are retinal artery or vein occlusion (p. 345), vitreous and macular haemorrhage, retinal detachment (vision loss preceded by floaters and flashes), and optic nerve ischaemia. Distortion of vision may indicate macular disease (pp. 352-3).

7 *Never ignore new-onset diplopia.* Binocular diplopia can be the first sign of temporal arteritis or posterior communicating artery aneurysm.

8 *Orbital cellulitis* is a life-threatening infection; pain on eye movement is often the first sign of orbital involvement in a patient with lid swelling and redness (p. 342).

9 *Headaches are rarely due to a refractive cause.* Ocular causes include acute closed-angle glaucoma and anterior uveitis.

10 *Always irrigate chemical burns immediately.* Irrigate copiously with water for 15min (instil local anaesthetic eye drops to assist).

11 *A corneal abrasion* should improve in 24h if the cause is removed. Evert the eyelid to check all foreign bodies have been removed and check conjunctival fornices. Exclude corneal ulcer (p. 334).

12 *Irritable eyes* are often dry eyes if they burn and sting. Consider blepharitis (p. 338) if lids are red and raw, and allergy if itchy.

13 *Viral conjunctivitis* is almost always bilateral, usually self-limiting, and will resolve without antibiotics. It can last up to 2wks.

14 *Topical steroid drops* should only be initiated by an ophthalmologist due to the risk of promoting infection (HSV, fungal). They may also cause increased pressure in the eye and cataract.

15 *Blindness in diabetes mellitus* is largely preventable with tight glycaemic control, reducing lipid and blood pressure. Refer all patients with diabetes for retinopathy screening and concurrent management of hypertension. Refer as soon as diagnosed (pp. 370-1).

16 *Age-related macular degeneration* may be treatable. Suspect age-related macular degeneration if gradual vision loss and distortion on Amsler grid. Sudden changes need urgent assessment (pp. 352-3).

17 *Simple lifestyle advice can improve ophthalmic health.* Regular eye exam every 2 years. Use eye protection (sports, industry, and sunglasses). UV exposure is related to pterygium, cataract, macular health, and lid tumours (most are basal cell carcinomas). Eat fish and green vegetables (macular health). Smoking cessation (macular health, diabetic, cataract risk).

Adapted from Dr John Colvin's 'Golden eye rules', The Royal Victorian Eye and Ear Hospital. www.eyeandear.org.au

Iris abnormalities

Heterochromia See fig 4.8 **and** 4.9 **below**

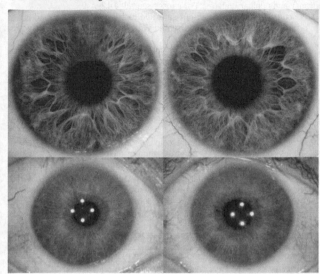

Fig 4.8 Heterochromia (sectoral above; central below). Both may be a normal variant; sectoral heterochromia may be a feature of Waardenburg syndrome (ws). Type 1 ws is an autosomal dominant disorder whose other signs are hearing loss, pigmental abnormalities of the hair and skin, and dystopia canthorum (wide nasal bridge due to sideways displacement of the inner angles of the eyes).

Courtesy of Jon Miles.

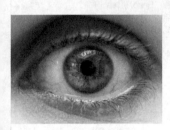

Fig 4.9 Sectoral iris heterochromia. Different coloured irises can look very striking.

© Heather Smyth, with thanks to
Megan Hale.

Carefully examine all red eyes to assess visual acuity, cornea (use fluorescein drops), and pupillary reflexes. For causes see table 4.2. Ask:

1 *Is acuity affected?* A quick but sensitive test is the ability to read newsprint with refractive errors corrected with glasses or a pin-hole. ↓ acuity suggests more serious pathology.

2 *Is the globe painful?* Actual pain is potentially sinister; foreign body sensation is of less concern.

3 *Is there photophobia?* Suggests more serious conditions such as anterior uveitis or significant corneal pathology.

Look:

1 *What is the distribution and depth of the redness?* (table 4.2)

2 *Is there discharge?* Discharge suggests ocular surface issues, most commonly conjunctivitis.

3 *Is the cornea intact?* Use fluorescein eye drops (p. 326). Staining demonstrates corneal damage eg due to trauma or ulcers.

4 *Does the pupil respond to light?* Absent or sluggish response is sinister.

Ask about trauma and discharge, general health and drugs; remember to check for raised pressure. Use of contact lenses? (Risk of bacterial infections and corneal ulcers.) Past history of eye disease? Any systemic features?

Immediately refer: suspected cases of acute glaucoma, anterior uveitis (iritis), keratitis/corneal ulcers, scleritis.

Causes of the red eye			
Common causes		Uncommon causes	
• Conjunctivitis	• Corneal ulcer	• Acute glaucoma	• Scleritis
• Foreign bodies	• Subconj. haem'ge	• Acute iritis	• Episcleritis

Table 4.2 Differential diagnosis of the red eye

	Conjunctivitis	Episcleritis	Scleritis	Anterior uveitis	Acute glaucoma
Hyperaemia	Diffuse	Sectoral superficial injection	Deep, often diffuse injection	++	++
Pain	Mild irritation	Mild irritation	++ Dull aching Painful movements	++	++ to +++
Photophobia	+	±	±	++	–
Visual acuity (VA)	Normal unless keratitis	Normal	Normal initially	Mild ↓	↓
Discharge	+	–	–	No discharge but lacrimation ++	–
Cornea	Normal	Normal	Normal	Normal/ keratitic precipitates	Steamy or hazy
Pupil	Normal	Normal	Normal	Usually small	Large Mid-dilated
IOP	Normal	Normal	Normal	↑ ↔ or ↓	↑
Referral?	No	Only if very painful	Within 24h	Within 24h	Immediately

4 Ophthalmology

The red eye: acute glaucoma

Acute closed-angle glaucoma

(figs 4.10 & 4.11) A form of glaucoma where the angle of anterior chamber narrows acutely causing a sudden rise in intraocular pressure (IOP) to ≥30mmHg (normal 12–21), the pupil becomes fixed and dilated, and axonal death occurs. ↑IOP may make the eye feel hard. *Primary angle-closure* occurs in patients with anatomical predisposition. *Secondary angle-closure* arises from pathological processes (eg traumatic haemorrhage pushing the posterior chamber forwards). Peak incidence in ages 40–60

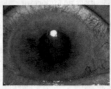

Fig 4.10 Acute closed-angle glaucoma.

Courtesy of Prof J Trobe.

and more common in Asia. *Presentation:* Patients are often generally unwell with nausea and vomiting; they can sometimes present to the acute medical team with no visual complaints. In 25%, acute uniocular attacks occur with headache and a painful red eye, often preceded by blurred vision or haloes around lights, at night. Onset is over hours–days. Ask about precipitating factors, eg has the patient been given dilating drops?[2] ▸▸Send to eye unit *now* for treatment. *R:* Treat according to local protocol which may include β-blockers to suppress aqueous humour production, eg **timolol 0.5%**, **pilocarpine 2–4% drops/2h** (miosis opens a blocked, 'closed' drainage angle, fig 4.11) + 500mg IV **acetazolamide** stat then 250mg/8h PO/IV (it ↓ aqueous formation). Analgesia and antiemetics may be used. Admit to monitor IOP. Peripheral iridotomy (laser or surgery) is done in both eyes once IOP is controlled (rarely as an emergency if IOP uncontrollable). The hole in the iris breaks the cycle, reducing pressure and allowing the drainage angle to open up again.[3] *Complications:* Include visual loss, central retinal artery or vein occlusions and repeated episodes in either eye.[4]

▸▸If you suspect acute closed-angle glaucoma, you should refer immediately to your local emergency eye unit.

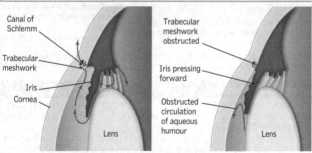

Fig 4.11 Normally, aqueous humour is produced by the ciliary body and flows through the pupil and empties out at the drainage angle through the canal of Schlemm. Any structural changes to this angle will block the flow and raise intraocular pressure. Predisposing factors include shallow anterior chamber, thick lens, thin iris or ciliary bodies (eg pupil dilation at night), and hypermetropic eye (short axial eye length).

Further reading

Denniston A and Murray PI (2018). *Oxford Handbook of Ophthalmology 4th edition*. Oxford: Oxford University Press.

Kent C (2013). Managing narrow angles and glaucoma. *Rev Ophthalmol* http://www.reviewofophthalmology.com/content/i/2417/c/41056/

2 Topical mydriatics will dilate the pupil and push the iris forwards.

Uveitis is an important cause of visual impairment in people of working age. The commonest form is acute anterior uveitis (iritis) which presents with an acute red eye. Provided it is treated promptly, it tends to have a good visual prognosis; other forms of uveitis affect the more posterior parts of the eye and can lead to significant visual impairment.[5]

Presentation Classically with pain, blurred vision, & photophobia. The red eye starts with conjunctival injection around the junction of the cornea and sclera and increased lacrimation (no sticky discharge, unlike in conjunctivitis). The pupil may be small, initially from iris spasm; later it may be irregular due to adhesions between lens and iris (synechiae) (fig 4.12). Onset is over hours/days. Ask about any features of systemic disease. *Diagnosis:* This is by slit lamp with a dilated pupil to visualize the location of inflammatory cells (in anterior uveitis you see leucocytes in the anterior chamber).[3]

R: ▶▶Urgent eye clinic referral. Use the slit lamp to monitor inflammation; it may relapse so regular eye clinic care and follow-up is vital. Drops: topical corticosteroids eg 0.5–1% prednisolone/2h or 0.1% dexamethasone, to ↓ inflammation. To prevent adhesions between lens and iris (synechiae) and to relieve spasm of ciliary body keep pupil dilated with cyclopentolate 1%/8h, unless very mild. Aim to prevent damage from prolonged inflammation (eg synechiae disrupts flow of aqueous→glaucoma ± adhesions between iris & lens).

▶▶Involve multidisciplinary care if systemic disease as controlling the underlying disease is key.[4]

Types & causes of uveitis
Anterior uveitis:[4]
• Ankylosing spondylitis; reactive arthritis, IBD
• Sarcoid; Behçet's, etc.
• Juvenile idiopathic arthritis
• Herpes simplex/zoster, TB, syphilis, HIV
• Tarantula hairs
Intermediate uveitis:
• MS; sarcoid; lymphoma
Posterior & panuveitis:
• Herpes simplex, herpes zoster; toxoplasmosis; TB; CMV; bacterial or fungal endophthalmitis
• Lymphoma; sarcoidosis
• Behçet's

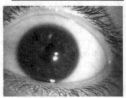

Fig 4.12 Posterior synechiae. The iris adheres to the lens and when inflamed causes an irregular pupillary border.

Courtesy of Alastair Denniston.

▶▶If you suspect acute anterior uveitis, you should refer immediately to your local emergency eye unit.

Other forms of uveitis

In anterior uveitis the primary site of inflammation is the iris + ciliary body; in intermediate uveitis it is the vitreous; in posterior uveitis it is the choroid (+ retina); and in panuveitis it is all of them.

Intermediate, posterior, and panuveitis forms of uveitis are much less common than anterior. They are usually painless and present with blurred vision or floaters. The eye is typically not red.

Ocular imaging such as fundus fluorescein and indocyanine green-angiography are used to further examine for retinal and choroidal disease.

Topical treatments do not penetrate sufficiently posteriorly for these forms of uveitis, necessitating systemic or intraocular therapies. NICE has approved both adalimumab and two intravitreal steroid implants (Ozurdex® and Iluvien®) for these forms of uveitis.[5]

Visual loss is common in uveitis due to: cystoid macular oedema, glaucoma, cataracts, chorioretinal scarring, choroidal neovascular membranes, retinal detachment, and vitreous opacities.[6]

The red eye: episcleritis and scleritis

Inflammation of the episclera and sclera Manifests as episcleritis and scleritis. The former is common, frequently self-limiting, and usually benign. In contrast, scleritis is much rarer, very painful with sight-threatening sequelae, and a strong association to systemic disease (see later).

▶ **Clinical distinction between scleritis and episcleritis** The episclera lies superficially and consequently the episcleral vessels will move when probed with a cotton bud and blanch with the application of 10% phenylephrine. The deeper scleral vessels will neither move nor blanch.

Episcleritis (fig 4.13) Inflammation below the conjunctiva in the episclera is common, 70% of patients are women. Bilateral in 30%. It may be focal or diffuse. Discomfort is usually minor. Acuity is normal. No cause is found in 70%,[7] but may occur in connective tissue diseases such as SLE. Rᵪ: Symptomatic relief is the mainstay with artificial tears and topical or systemic NSAIDs.

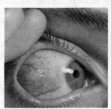
Fig 4.13 Episcleritis.

Scleritis (fig 4.14) Generalized inflammation of the sclera itself with oedema of the conjunctiva, scleral thinning, and vasculitic changes. Characterized by deep severe pain of the globe. Anatomically divided into: anterior (90%) and posterior (10%) scleritis. The necrotizing variety can cause globe perforation. 50% of patients have associated systemic disease (typically rheumatoid arthritis or granulomatosis with polyangiitis).[8] Patients describe a constant, severe dull ache which 'bores' into the eye and can wake them at night. Ocular movements are painful since the muscles insert into the sclera. May present with headache and photophobia. Rᵪ: ▶Urgent referral. Management is guided by subtype: non-necrotizing anterior scleritis may only require oral NSAIDs ± oral high-dose prednisolone. Posterior scleritis or any form of

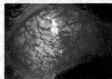
Fig 4.14 Scleritis.
Reprinted by permission from Macmillan Publishers Ltd: *Nature Reviews Rheumatology*, Artifoni *et al*, Ocular inflammatory diseases associated with rheumatoid arthritis, volume 10, issue 2, p.108–116, copyright (2013).

necrotizing scleritis requires more aggressive therapy. Systemic immunosuppression is influenced by underlying systemic disease; typically cyclophosphamide or rituximab and a course of methylprednisolone. Recalcitrant disease may benefit from infliximab.[8] Imminent globe perforation requires surgical intervention. Prognosis tends to follow that of the underlying systemic disorder. Visual loss is common in those with the necrotizing form.

▶▶If you suspect scleritis, you should refer immediately to your local emergency eye unit.

---

3 Talbot's test is +ve: pain increases on convergence (and pupils constrict) as patients watch a finger approach their nose.

4 In juvenile idiopathic arthritis (JIA), screening is important as the child often does not get symptoms until late in the disease.

Further reading

Denniston A and Murray PI (2018). *Oxford Handbook of Ophthalmology 4th edition*. Oxford: Oxford University Press; pp320–32.

Mahmood AR *et al*. (2008). Diagnosis and management of the acute red eye. *Emerg Med Clin North Am* 26:35–55.

NICE (2012). *Clinical Knowledge Summaries: Red Eye*. http://cks.nice.org.uk/red-eye

Wittenberg S (2008). 10 *Clinical Pearls for Treating Uveitis*. http://www.aao.org/young-ophthalmologists/yo-info/article/10-clinical-pearls-treating-uveitis

4 Ophthalmology

▶▶Accurate, rapid diagnosis is vital! **Corneal abrasion/erosion** An epithelial breach causing pain, photophobia, ± ↓ vision. 'Abrasions' result from trauma (scratches, contact lenses); 'erosions' from failure of local tissue health (previous corneal disease, chemical injury). Use fluorescein drops and the blue light on a slit lamp to aid diagnosis. Corneal lesions stain green (drops are orange and become more yellow on contact with the eye). Always evert the eye lid to look for foreign bodies. ℞: Chloramphenicol ointment ± cycloplegia. Simple abrasions usually heal quickly.

Keratitis Corneal inflammation (identified by a white area on the cornea—indicating a collection of white cells in corneal tissue). Keratoconjunctivitis refers to conjunctivitis with associated corneal involvement. Microbial keratitis is secondary to bacterial infection.

Corneal ulcers ▶▶If you suspect a corneal ulcer, you should refer immediately to your local emergency eye unit. May be bacterial (beware *Pseudomonas* which may progress rapidly), herpetic (see BOX 'Herpes simplex (dendritic) corneal ulcers (epithelial keratitis)'), fungal (*Candida*; *Aspergillus*), protozoal (*Acanthamoeba*), or from vasculitis, eg in rheumatoid arthritis. Ask contact wearers if they sleep with lenses in and how they are changed. Don't try treating corneal ulcers on your own: perforation, scarring, and visual loss may occur. ℞: Liaise with microbiologist. In early stages of ophthalmic shingles, use oral aciclovir (p. 335). Cycloplegics ease photophobia. *Management of corneal ulcers:* Urgent eye clinic referral with review today by an eye specialist for urgent diagnostic smear/Gram stain and scrape, and initiation of empirical treatment. Remove contact lenses. Test cranial nerve V. HIV +ve? Until cultures are known, Gram +ve and –ve cover is required with either topical fluoroquinolone (eg ofloxacin) or alternating cefuroxime 5% and gentamicin 1.5% (check local protocol). Adapt in the light of cultures. Admit if diabetes, immunosuppression, or if the patient won't manage the drops. Steroid drops can be added once recovery starts. ▶See BOX 'Steroid eye drops', p. 373 for the dangers of steroid drops.

Herpes simplex (dendritic) corneal ulcers (epithelial keratitis)

Herpes simplex virus (HSV) type 1 has multiple ocular manifestations. Keratitis is the most common and is a major cause of corneal blindness through corneal scarring. Acute presentation with pain, photophobia, and watering. Ask about past eye, mouth, or genital ulcers. Use a slit lamp and apply fluorescein 1% staining to look for dendritic ulcers which suggest active virus replication (fig 4.15). If steroid drops are used without aciclovir cover, corneal invasion and scarring may occur, risking blindness. ℞: aciclovir 3% eye ointment 5× daily. Corneal transplants are considered for those with significant visual impairment due to scarring.[9]

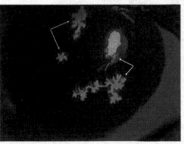

Fig 4.15 Dendritic ulcers (short arrows) are classic for HSV keratitis. Read about this patient's case study here: http://qjmed.oxfordjournals.org/content/early/2014/12/22/qjmed.hcu250

Reproduced from J. Mare Njoya, *et al.* Herpetic epithelial keratitis. *QJM: An International Journal of Medicine* (2015) 108 (7): 595, by permission of OUP.

Further reading
See online references.[10,11]

Herpes zoster ophthalmicus (HZO) (Also see BOX 'Common viral infections', p. 449.) Varicella zoster infection has 2 distinct forms: it tends to first occur in childhood as chickenpox (varicella), it then lies dormant within the sensory ganglia for years until in 20–30% of individuals it reactivates and spreads across a dermatome as shingles (zoster). The most common site of shingles (55%) is the thoracic nerves, followed by the 1st (ophthalmic) branch of the trigeminal nerve (10–20%).[12] *Risk factors:* While the rate of HZO increases with age, more than half of cases occur in people under age 60. HZO is more common and severe in people with immunocompromise; however, the majority of cases occur in people who are immunocompetent. Young healthy patients can develop neurological sequelae from HZO.

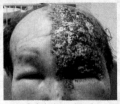

Fig 4.16 Ophthalmic shingles.
From *The New England Journal of Medicine*, Wills C *et al.* 362(12), 1128. Copyright © (2010) Massachusetts Medical Society. Reprinted with permission from Massachusetts Medical Society.

4 Ophthalmology

Presentation Pain and neuralgia in the distribution of cranial nerve VI dermatome (p. 552) precedes a blistering inflamed rash (fig 4.16). *Predictors of ocular involvement:* In up to 65% of those with HZO the globe is affected (corneal signs ± iritis). Nose-tip involvement (Hutchinson's sign) makes it likely that the eye will be affected (since it indicates involvement of the nasociliary branch of the 1st (ophthalmic) branch of the trigeminal nerve, which also supplies the globe). The eye can be seriously affected with little rash elsewhere; so age and severity of rash are not reliable predictors.[12] Beware dissemination if immunocompromised. Varicella zoster virus (VZV) may persist in the eye.

Assessment Good visual acuity and normal corneal appearance is reassuring. Refer for more detailed examination if pain, redness, or altered vision is reported. Look carefully for Hutchinson's sign.

R: Commence 7-day course of oral antivirals within 72h of rash to reduce ocular complications from 50% to 30%; does not prevent post-herpetic neuralgia. **Famciclovir** (750mg 1–2×/day or 500mg 3×/day for 7 days; SE vomiting; headache)[13] or **aciclovir** (800mg 5×/day for 7 days; SE hepatitis and renal failure)[13] or **valaciclovir** 1000mg TDS for 7 days (SE hepatitis and renal failure).[13] Prolonged steroid eye drops may be needed for stromal keratitis/anterior uveitis and should be prescribed by an ophthalmologist. Acute retinal necrosis and progressive outer retinal necrosis are rare complications of HSV or VZV and are ophthalmic emergencies. Advise isolation from pregnant women with no immunity to chickenpox until several days after the vesicles dry up.

HZO complications • Conjunctivitis • Keratitis • Glaucoma • Anterior uveitis (±atrophy) • Necrotizing retinitis (acute retinal necrosis/progressive outer retinal necrosis) ▸▸ophthalmic emergency • Episcleritis/scleritis • Optic neuritis • Cranial nerve palsy • Stroke (rare, secondary to cerebral vasculitis) • Post-herpetic neuralgia (common and debilitating).

Post-herpetic neuralgia: (9–45% of all cases.) Can persist from months to years. It is associated with older age, ocular involvement, and severe rashes. Treatment involves early commencement of antivirals and neuropathic analgesics (eg tricyclic antidepressants, gabapentin/pregabalin) to decrease the pain. Post-herpetic neuralgia has been cited as the commonest cause of suicide in patients with chronic pain who are >70 years of age.[14]

Ramsay Hunt syndrome See p. 856.

Further reading
See online references.[15-19]

Conjunctivitis[20] The conjunctiva is inflamed with injection of the superficial vessels. It can only be diagnosed by ruling out sight-threatening features: acuity, pupillary responses, and corneal lustre are unaffected. Eyes itch, burn, and lacrimate. It is often bilateral with discharge sticking lids together.

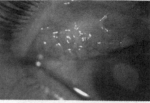

Non-infectious causes: Allergic conjunctivitis (p. 337) is the most frequent cause of all cases, affecting 15–40% of the population. Few seek medical attention.[21]

Other causes: Toxic, autoimmune, neoplastic. Contact lens wearers may develop a reaction to lens presence (fig 4.17). ►Be aware of conjunctivitis may include abnormal conjunctival adhesions (symblephara), due to a chronic cicatrising (scarring) conjunc-

Fig 4.17 Giant papillary conjunctivitis is characterized by the formation of papillae (>1mm) on the inner aspect of the upper eye lid. Note the grey, oval corneal ulcer ('shield' ulcer) due to corneal erosion. *Symptoms:* intense itch + mucoid discharge. *Cause:* contact lenses, foreign bodies. *Treatment:* abstain from wearing lenses for 1wk, reduce time wearing lenses + replace frequently. Ensure correct lens hygiene.[22]

Courtesy of Mr D Tole FRCO.

tivitis, such as *ocular mucous membrane pemphigoid*. Scarring of the lids and secondary damage to the cornea can progress quickly, with rapid bilateral loss of vision. Urgent specialist input is needed.

Infectious causes: Non-herpetic viral (usually a 'watery' serous discharge) is the most common infectious cause; ~80% are adenoviruses (small lymphoid aggregates appear as follicles on conjunctiva) and can cause intense itching. Bacterial (purulent discharge more prominent, especially in gonococcal infection).

Investigations: Conjunctival cultures are only needed if you suspect gonococcal/chlamydial infection, neonatal conjunctivitis, or in recurrent disease not responding to therapy.

Treatment: Most cases are viral and only need symptomatic relief with artificial tears and cold compresses. Topical antiviral treatment does not help. Topical antibiotics supposedly prevent 2° bacterial infection. Viral conjunctivitis is highly contagious so educate patients on hand and face washing. Bacterial conjunctivitis also tends to be self-limiting (60%) within 1–2 weeks; topical antibiotics can ↓ duration of symptoms and transmission risk. Antibiotic drops are especially useful in culture-proven bacterial conjunctivitis. Start antibiotics immediately if sexual disease is suspected, contact lens wearers, or immunocompromised. **Chloramphenicol** 0.5% drops/4–6h are often used (or fusidic acid). Staphylococci are common causes. In prolonged conjunctivitis, esp. in young adults, consider chlamydial infection (get expert help; see 'Ophthalmia neonatorum', p. 330). For allergic conjunctivitis: try antihistamine drops eg **azelastine** 0.05% 2–4×/day for 6wks max or **olopadine** 1mg/mL 2×/day for 4 months, refer if not settling. Steroid drops (after advice from an ophthalmologist) may help.

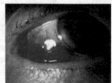

Fig 4.18 Subconjunctival haemorrhage.

Reprinted by permission from Wells, A. et al (2004). Spontaneous inferior subconjunctival haemorrhages in association with circumferential drainage blebs. *Eye*, 19:269–272. doi: https://doi.org/10.1038/sj.eye.6701496. Copyright © 2004, Springer Nature.

Subconjunctival haemorrhage (fig 4.18) This harmless but alarming pool of blood behind the conjunctiva is from a small bleed; check BP and history of anticoagulants. It often occurs in the elderly. If there is a history of trauma ensure there is no globe rupture.

Allergic eye disease affects ~20% of the population and incidence is increasing. Peak age of onset is 20yrs.[24] Acute allergic conjunctivitis is caused by IgE-mediated type 1 hypersensitivity, triggering release of inflammatory mediators by mast cells. Most have a history or family history of atopy.

Chronic allergic disorders are characterized by an increase in the number of local conjunctival τ-cells, with a mixed cellular infiltrate of mast cells, eosinophils, neutrophils, and macrophages.

Seasonal allergic conjunctivitis Up to 50% of allergic eye disease. Allergens include grass, tree, and weed pollens. Symptoms are seasonal and mild—but may continue long after allergen exposure. Examination shows small papillae on the tarsal conjunctiva. It is self-limiting and not sight-threatening. R: Lubricating eye drops if mild. If moderate antihistamine drops (**azelastine** 0.05% 2–4×/day for 6wks maximum, **olopatadine** 1mg/mL 2×/day for 4months). Mast cell stabilizers (**sodium cromoglicate** 2% 4×/day or **lodoxamide** 0.1% 4×/day) may be used prophylactically. If severe, referral to an ophthalmologist for consideration of topical steroids, ± referral to an immunologist for desensitization therapy.

Perennial allergic conjunctivitis Symptoms are mild and may persist all year with seasonal exacerbations. Allergens include animal dander and house dust mite. Small papillae are found on the tarsal conjunctiva. *Management:* As for seasonal allergic conjunctivitis.

Vernal keratoconjunctivitis[25] Comprises only 0.5% of allergic eye disease. It can lead to corneal scarring and blindness in its severest form so needs to be managed in a specialist clinic. The typical patient is an atopic boy living in a warm, dry climate with severe bilateral symptoms of itchy eyes, foreign body sensation, photophobia, and giant cobble-stone papillae under the upper eye lid (fig 4.17 p. 336). Lid skin is spared, unlike atopic keratoconjunctivitis (see later). R: Topical lubricants (preservative free), topical antihistamines eg olopatadine or lodoxamide (BOX '3 principles'). If uncontrolled or if corneal disease, steroid drops are needed (eg 1% prednisolone acetate/2h; taper rapidly). Ciclosporin drops 0.1% also help. Corneal involvement needs careful eye clinic review and coverage with steroids, antibiotic drops, and lid hygiene to limit staphylococcal colonization. If severe blepharitis, oral erythromycin or doxycycline (in adults) can help.

Atopic keratoconjunctivitis Affects 1.5% of the population. Symptoms are severe with pain, redness, and reduced vision. Associated with atopic dermatitis, including eczema of the eyelids, and staphylococcal lid disease. Signs include conjunctival papillae and eventual conjunctival scarring which can lead to corneal opacification and neovascularization. *Management:* Combination of mast cell stabilizer, topical steroids, topical ciclosporin ± unlicensed use of topical tacrolimus.

Giant papillary conjunctivitis (fig 4.17 p. 336) An iatrogenic condition related to foreign bodies eg contact lenses, ocular prosthesis, and sutures. *Management:*Involves removal of the foreign body and treatment with topical mast cell stabilizers or steroids.

Differential diagnoses Dry eyes, blepharitis, any causes of red eye (p. 330).

3 principles for successfully managing allergic eye disorders

1 Remove the allergen responsible where possible ('don't travel to places which make your symptoms worse').[26] Consider referral to an immunologist if severe.

2 General measures: • Cold compresses • Artificial tears to wash out allergens and ↓ itch (preservative free) • Oral antihistamines for symptom relief, eg **loratadine** 10mg/day PO • Nasal steroid sprays may help even if no nasal symptoms.[27]

3 Eye-drop specifics (rapid action + fewer SE, being topical)—eg antihistamines (eg azelastine), drugs inhibiting mast cell degranulation (cromoglicate; lodoxamide), and accessory drugs, eg steroids (specialist use only), ±NSAIDs (eg ibuprofen), immunosuppressants (ciclosporin, specialist use only).

Further reading

See online references.[23]

Blepharitis

Common inflammation of the eyelid margin secondary to blockage of the Meibomian glands and infection with *Staph. aureus*. Suspect in rosacea and seborrheic dermatitis. It causes redness/irritation of the lid and eye ± marginal keratitis (sterile inflammation of the cornea). *Treatment:* Meticulous lid hygiene; warm compress with bean bag 10min, lid massage, lid cleaning wipes. Consider oral doxycycline in adults or erythromycin in children.

Stye/hordeolum

Bacterial infection of an eyelash follicle and adjacent glands of Zeiss or Moll, causing small, red, tender spot (fig 4.25). Often associated with blepharitis. Can develop into cellulitis. *Treatment:* Warm compresses + lid hygiene. Topical antibiotics may occasionally be needed (eg **chloramphenicol** 1% 4×/day). Removal of the associated lash can also help.

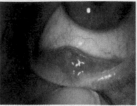

Fig 4.19 Chalazion (meaning hailstone in Greek). A granular mass to palpation.

Courtesy of Mr Murray and University Hospitals Birmingham NHSFT, with thanks to Mark Lane for image collection.

Chalazion

(fig 4.19) Focal inflammation of Meibomian gland. It can present as a tender or non-tender round eyelid swelling/lump. Also associated with blepharitis. *Treatment:* Warm compresses + massage. May require incision and curettage if persistent but most resolve within a few months.

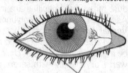

Pinguecula

Fig 4.20 Diagrammatic representation of pinguecula either side of the cornea.

Pinguecula

(fig 4.20) Degenerative vascular yellow-grey nodules on the conjunctiva either side of the cornea (esp. nasal side). *Typical patient:* Adult male. *Associations:* ↑ hair and skin pigment; sun-related skin damage. If inflamed (pingueculitis) topical steroids are tried.

Pterygium

Similar process as pinguecula but invading the surface of the cornea; associated with dry, dusty conditions and high UV exposure (fig 4.21); surgery may be needed if encroaching on the visual axis or causing astigmatism.

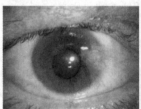

Fig 4.21 Pterygium encroaching on the cornea.

Courtesy of Mr Murray and University Hospitals Birmingham NHSFT, with thanks to Mark Lane for image collection.

Entropion

(fig 4.22) Lid turns in and eyelashes rub on the cornea. Typically due to lower lid laxity. Taping the (lower) eyelids to the cheek can give temporary relief, with regular lubricating eye ointment. Surgery is usually indicated.

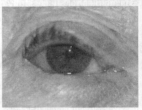

Fig 4.22 Lower lid entropion.

Courtesy of Bristol Eye Hospital.

4 Ophthalmology

Ectropion (fig 4.23) Lower lid rolls out leading to irritation, watering (drainage punctum malaligned) ± exposure keratitis. *Associations:* Lid laxity; facial nerve palsy. Surgically corrected.

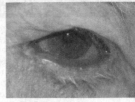

Fig 4.23 Ectropion.
Courtesy of Bristol Eye Hospital.

Ptosis

Upper lid is abnormally low when patient looks forward. Causes include: • Congenital (absent nerve to levator muscle; poorly developed levator) • Mechanical (oedema, xanthelasma, or upper lid tumour) • Myogenic (muscular dystrophy, myasthenia) • CNS (III nerve palsy, p. 364–5; Horner's, p. 366). Congenital ptosis is corrected surgically early if the pupil (visual axis) is covered (risk of amblyopia, p. 364). Pseudoptosis may occur due to abnormal position or size of the globe itself. Dermatochalasis denotes excess eyelid skin hanging over the upper lid (may obstruct sight).

Lagophthalmos

The inability to close the eyelids. *Causes:* Exophthalmos (eg thyroid eye disease); mechanical impairment of lid movement (eg injury or lid burns); leprosy; paralysed orbicularis oculi (eg VII nerve palsy). Exposure keratopathy and corneal ulcers may follow. ℞: Lubricate eyes with regular lubricants throughout the day and liquid paraffin ointment, especially at night. If corneal ulcers develop, temporary tarsorrhaphy (stitching lids together) may be needed.

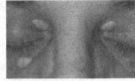

Xanthelasma

(fig 4.24) Lipid depositions under the skin, often around the eyelids, seen in hyperlipidaemia.

Fig 4.24 Xanthelasma.
Courtesy of Jon Miles.

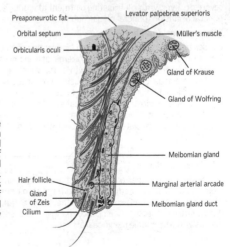

Fig 4.25 Anatomy of the eyelid. Styes occur on the eyelid margin and are due to infection of the eyelash follicle and glands of Moll or Zeiss. Chalazions are cysts due to inflammation of the Meibomian gland and can occur away from the eyelid margin.

Preaponeurotic fat — Levator palpebrae superioris — Orbital septum — Müller's muscle — Orbicularis oculi — Gland of Krause — Gland of Wolfring — Meibomian gland — Marginal arterial arcade — Hair follicle — Gland of Zeis — Meibomian gland duct — Cilium

4 Ophthalmology

4 Ophthalmology

Tears play an essential role in refraction. A poor tear film causes blurring of vision. The anatomy of the tear drainage system is outlined in fig 4.26. Tears consist of a lipid layer, an aqueous layer, and a mucin layer. The volume of tears normally in the eye is 6µL, the turnover rate being 1.2µL/min. Tears are similar in electrolyte concentration to plasma, but rich in proteins, especially IgA. They also contain lysozyme and beta-lysin which have antibacterial properties. Meibomian glands, conjunctival glands, goblet cells, and lacrimal glands produce tear fluid. Reflex secretion is from the lacrimal gland alone via parasympathetic fibres of the trigeminal nerve.[28,29]

Dry eyes (*keratoconjunctivitis sicca*)

Can have an immense impact on quality of life causing a gritty burning sensation and ↓ vision. Watering can occur if the quality of the tear film is poor, as reflex lacrimation occurs. Risk of corneal ulceration and perforation if severe.

Causes of dry eye: ↓ tear production by lacrimal glands in old age, or rarely in: • Sjögren syndrome (associated with connective tissue disorders, esp. RA); • Mumps • Sarcoidosis • Amyloidosis • Lymphoma • Leukaemia • Haemochromatosis. *Other causes:* • excess evaporation of tears can occur when the eyelids do not close properly (lagophthalmos) such as in a CN VII palsy, entropion, or ectropion • Mucin deficiency • Avitaminosis A • Stevens–Johnson syndrome • Pemphigoid • Chemical burns. ▶▶Consider blepharitis and chronic allergy (p. 338).

Examination: Evaluate whether the cornea is at risk by examining for *entropion, ectropion,* and *lagophthalmos.* The upper lid should act as a windscreen wiper and smooth the tears over the cornea each time the patient blinks. Check corneal sensation: ↓ sensation → risk of ulceration esp. if risk of exposure eg CN VII palsy. Examine with fluorescein for corneal punctate epithelial erosions. *Schirmer's test* (strip of filter paper put overlapping lower lid; tears should soak >15mm in 5min) reveals ↓ tear production.

Management: Artificial tears ↓ symptoms and can be given up to hourly in severe dry eyes, with a lubricating ointment at night. Tear drainage can be ↓ by punctal occlusion (punctal plugs/cautery).

'Watery eyes' (epiphora)

Causes of 'watery eyes' or increased lacrimation can be 2° to:
• ↑ tear production: in corneal injury/allergic conjunctivitis/meibomian gland dysfunction (tears contain ↑nerve growth factor, which aids healing), or
• ↓ tear drainage: punctal stenosis/obstruction of the canaliculus (can be 2° to herpetic infection), nasolacrimal duct obstruction, or pump failure. On blinking, positive and negative pressure is created in the lacrimal sac which accordingly sucks tears into it. This is the tear pump. Gravity helps keep the sac empty. Pump failure may be associated with entropion, ectropion, or CNS causes (myasthenia, CN VII palsy).

The lacrimal glands

These are in the upper outer area of the orbit (lacrimal fossa of the frontal bone) and have autonomic innervation. Parasympathetics start in the lacrimal nucleus of the facial nerve in the pons. Sympathetic postganglionic fibres start in the superior cervical ganglion and travel as a periarteriolar plexus with the middle meningeal artery.

Blepharospasm and hemifacial spasm

Essential blepharospasm is an *involuntary* bilateral contraction of orbicularis oculi and is a form of *focal dystonia* (OHCM p. 469). Exacerbated by stress, in its most severe form this forceful prolonged blinking can lead to functional blindness. Quality of life can be significantly impaired with difficulty reading, writing, and driving.[30]

Presentation

♀:♂ ≈ 3:1. Blepharospasm is often preceded by exaggerated blinking. Other dystonias may be present (eg oro-mandibular). It can start unilaterally, becoming bilateral. Patients may develop tricks to reduce it, such as touching or pulling the eyelids—a variation of '*geste antagoniste*' seen in other forms of dystonia. *Causes:* (Mostly unknown.) Neuroleptic drugs, Parkinson disease, progressive supranuclear palsy, paraneoplastic (eg from lung cancer).

Treatment

Drugs—botulinum neurotoxin: Causes of secondary blepharospasm (trichiasis, dry eye, corneal and external eye disease) should be excluded. Palliation is achieved with small doses injected to orbicularis oculi; here it produces a temporary flaccid paralysis. It can help some people recover effective vision. It binds to peripheral nerve terminals and inhibits release of acetylcholine. Regular treatments are needed. Oral agents provide only short-term relief and unwanted side effects so are reserved as 2nd line treatment.[31] *Supportive treatment:* If the cause is apraxia of lid opening, wearing goggles may help.[32]

Hemifacial spasm

A form of segmental myoclonus characterized by unilateral contractions of the face. It is most common in women (2:1) in the 5th and 6th decades. The majority of cases are sporadic. While neurosurgical intervention is possible, if there is MRI evidence of facial nerve root irritation complication rates are high, so as for blepharospasm, botulinum neurotoxin forms the mainstay of treatment.

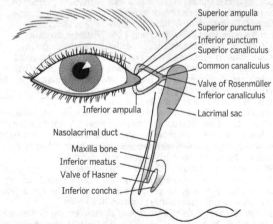

Superior ampulla
Superior punctum
Inferior punctum
Superior canaliculus
Common canaliculus
Valve of Rosenmüller
Inferior canaliculus
Inferior ampulla
Lacrimal sac
Nasolacrimal duct
Maxilla bone
Inferior meatus
Valve of Hasner
Inferior concha

Fig 4.26 Anatomy of nasolacrimal system. © D P Austin.

Further reading

Defazio G *et al.* (2013). Development and validation of a clinical guideline for diagnosing blepharospasm. *Neurology* 81:236–40.

Reimer J *et al.* (2005). Health-related quality of life in blepharospasm or hemifacial spasm. *Acta Neurol Scand* 2005;111:64–70.

The Dystonia Society: www.dystonia.org.uk

The bony orbit is a confined space; any ↑ volume will cause the eyes to move forwards (proptosis) and the lids to become tight. Compression of the optic nerve and loss of vision can ensue. If pressure is eccentric there will be deviation of the eyeball ± diplopia. *Causes*: infection (orbital cellulitis), inflammation (thyroid eye disease, see pp. 342-3), primary malignancy/metastatic deposits, or vascular distension (carotid-cavernous fistula). Be sure to examine optic nerve function (visual acuity, RAPD, colour vision) and promptly refer to an ophthalmologist.

Preseptal cellulitis[33] Strictly not an orbital pathology since infection is anterior to the orbital septum (fig 4.27a; see also table 4.3). Commonly caused by infection of adjacent structures; dacryocystitis (infected swelling of the lacrimal sac), insect bites, hordeolum, trauma, etc. Characterized by inflamed eyelids but white eyes and normal VA, painless eye movements with no diplopia. If in doubt, treat as for orbital cellulitis. ℞: Based on empirical treatment for cellulitis eg **flucloxacillin 500mg** QDS 7 days. Compared to orbital cellulitis, it is much more common, has a better response to treatment, and a minimal risk of recurrence. ▶▶Be cautious in very young children who have not yet developed an orbital septum and are at risk of orbital cellulitis developing quickly.

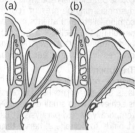

Fig 4.27 Patterns of infection within the orbit: (a) preseptal, (b) postseptal.

Orbital cellulitis ▶▶Severe sight- and life-threatening emergency. Infection of soft tissues posterior to the orbital septum (fig 4.27b; see also table 4.3) most commonly with *Strep. pneumoniae, Staph. aureus, Strep. pyogenes*, and *Haemophilus influenzae*.[35] Spread is typically via paranasal sinus infection (or eyelid, dental infection, or recent lacrimal surgery). *Typical patient:* A child with inflammation in the orbit, fever, lid swelling, and ↓ eye mobility ± diplopia; eye movements will be painful. Conjunctival swelling (chemosis) and proptosis may be present. *Complications:* Subperiosteal and orbital abscesses (confirmed by CT). Extraorbital extension is rare but devastating. Visual loss 2° to optic nerve inflammation or central retinal vein or

Indications for CT of orbits[34]
• Neurological symptoms 2° to infection
• Central signs
• Inability to accurately assess patient's vision
• Gross proptosis
• Bilateral oedema
• Ophthalmoplegia
• Deteriorating visual acuity or colour vision
• No improvement at 24h/ pyrexic at 36h

artery occlusion (see p. 344). Intracranial involvement can result in meningitis, brain abscesses and thrombosis in the dural or cavernous sinuses. ℞: Admit for prompt ENT and ophthalmic opinion + IV antibiotics (eg either **cefuroxime 750mg–1.5g** 3×/day or **ceftriaxone** 1–2g once daily with **metronidazole 500mg** 3×/day if history of chronic sinus disease). Abscesses ± sinuses may require surgical drainage.

Carotid-cavernous fistula *Causes:* Spontaneous; trauma; post-septorhinoplasty. There is engorgement of eye vessels + lid & conjunctival oedema. Exophthalmos may be pulsatile, ± bruit over the eye ± tinnitus. Arterial ligation or embolization may occasionally be tried.

Thyroid eye disease Autoimmune thyroid dysfunction (eg Graves) leading to enlargement of the extraocular muscles and orbital fat causing proptosis ± optic nerve compression, and loss of vision. Associated with lid retraction, lid lag, chemosis, conjunctival injection, and ↓ extraocular movements. *Management:* Treat thyroid dysfunction. Urgent orbital decompression if severe.

Further reading

Denniston A and Murray PI (2018). *Oxford Handbook of Ophthalmology 4th edition.* Oxford: Oxford University Press; pp666–7, 670–80.

NICE (2015). *Clinical Knowledge Summaries: Cellulitis—Acute.* http://cks.nice.org.uk/cellulitis-acute

4 Ophthalmology

Table 4.3 Orbital vs preseptal cellulitis

	Orbital	Preseptal
Proptosis	Present	Absent
Ocular motility	Painful + restricted	Normal
VA	↓ (in severe cases)	Normal
Colour vision	↓ (in severe cases)	Normal
RAPD	Present (in severe cases)	Absent (ie normal)

Reproduced from Denniston A. and Murray P.I., *Oxford Handbook of Ophthalmology* (2018), with permission from OUP.

Retinoblastoma

Commonest primary intraocular tumour of childhood.

Signs Strabismus and leucocoria (ie a white pupil). Always suspect retinoblastoma when the red reflex is absent (fig 4.28; eg absent red reflex during flash photography). NB: multiple tumours may be present.

Inheritance Retinoblastomas highlight the genetic component aetiology of cancer. The Rb gene is a tumour suppressor gene, its product is a nuclear phosphoprotein which helps regulate DNA synthesis. In hereditary retinoblastoma every cell in the body is missing one copy of the Rb gene. In somatic cases a single developing retinal cell has lost the gene. When a 2nd copy of the gene is lost the patient develops retinoblastoma (Knudson's two-hit hypothesis). Hereditary cases can be bilateral. Mean age of presentation: <12months (hereditary) and ~24months (sporadic).

Associations 5% occur with a pineal or other tumour (=trilateral retinoblastoma). Secondary malignancies such as osteosarcoma and rhabdomyosarcoma are more frequent and are the main cause of death.

Treatment Is in highly specialist centres. There is a trend away from enucleation (eye removal) towards focal procedures to preserve eye and sight, if possible:
• *Chemotherapy:* Useful if bilateral. Includes carboplatin, etoposide, and vincristine.
• *Enucleation:* May be needed with large tumours, long-standing retinal detachments, and optic nerve invasion or extrascleral extension.
• *Laser treatment (transpupillary thermotherapy):* Can be used to treat small tumours or larger tumours after they have been shrunk by chemotherapy.
• *Cryotherapy:* Can be given to treat tumours in the peripheral retina.
• *External beam radiotherapy:* Reserved for diffuse disease in the only remaining eye, or recurrent non-responsive disease. It may cause 2° non-ocular cancers in the radiation field (esp. if carrying the Rb-1 germline mutation).
• *Plaque brachytherapy:* Involves suturing a radioactive plaque to the sclera. This has a more focal and shielded radiation field and carries less risk of 2° tumours.

Screening parents and siblings This is needed for accurate genetic counselling and to allow presymptomatic detection and treatment.

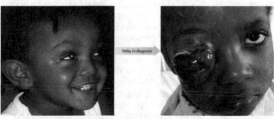

Fig 4.28 Absent red reflex during flash photography is a worrying sign; if untreated, retinoblastomas have a high risk of local metastasis and death within 2 years. Early recognition and treatment can be life- and vision-saving.

Reprinted with permission from Elsevier (*The Lancet*, 2012, Volume 379(9824), pp. 1436–1446).

▶▶All episodes of sudden visual loss need to be immediately referred to an eye specialist for same-day review. Most are painless and are often vascular—effectively 'strokes' to the optic nerve (AION, see later) or retina (arterial/venous occlusions). Consider also retinal detachment or vitreous haemorrhage.

Causes of sudden/rapid onset sustained vision loss

Painless
- Anterior ischaemic optic neuropathy (AION)
- Retinal artery occlusion
- Retinal vein occlusion
- Macular degeneration (wet)*
- Retinal detachment
- Vitreous haemorrhage
- Severe uveitis* (intermediate, posterior)

Painful
- Acute glaucoma
- Severe corneal pathology*
- Severe uveitis* (anterior, panuveitis)
- Endophthalmitis*
- Optic neuritis*

*These conditions tend to cause progressive visual loss over days/weeks, whereas the others can be minutes/hours.

Causes of transient vision loss

▶Always think of vascular causes, such as microemboli from atherosclerotic plaques in the carotid arteries (any stenosis or bruit?).

Typical causes
- Amaurosis fugax/TIA.
- Migraine.
- Papilloedema causing transient visual obscuration (ask about pulsatile tinnitus and other symptoms of raised intracranial pressure).

Anterior ischaemic optic neuropathy (AION) The most common cause of optic neuropathy in older patients. The optic nerve is damaged if posterior vascular supply is blocked by inflammation or atheroma. There are 2 main types: *non-arteritic* AION (90–95%) and *arteritic* AION (5–10%). Despite the differing pathophysiology between the types of AION, both result in ischaemic loss of vision. *Fundoscopy:* Pale/swollen optic disc.

Arteritic AION and giant cell arteritis (GCA; temporal arteritis) *(OHCM p556)* GCA is the most common cause of arteritic AION. It is described as a medium to large vessel systemic vasculitis. Typically seen in patients >70yrs old; rarely occurring before the age of 50. Lifetime risk is 1% in women and 0.5% in men.[36] *Symptoms:* New-onset headache, malaise, jaw/tongue claudication (chewing pain) ± tender scalp and temporal arteries (thickened ± absent pulses), neck pain. Visual loss is typically monocular (rarely bilateral, this is a more worrying sign). Permanent vision loss can be preceded by multiple episodes of amaurosis fugax or can occur at first presentation.[37] There is a strong association with polymyalgia rheumatica, hip and shoulder girdle aching, and morning stiffness. Onset of symptoms tends to be subacute, but in some the onset can be sudden. Not all patients experience this constellation of symptoms so retain a high index of suspicion and request the following: *Immediate:* ↑ESR, ↑CRP, FBC (↑ platelets) are supportive of GCA; temporal artery biopsy within 1wk of starting prednisolone; may miss affected sections of artery (skip lesions). Temporal artery ultrasound. *R:* ▶▶The other eye is at risk so give steroids urgently. **Prednisolone** 60mg/24h PO (consider higher IV doses if vision is involved)[38] with a proton pump inhibitor ± low-dose aspirin if no contraindication.[38] Tailing off steroids as ESR and symptoms settle may take >1yr.[38] Despite this, ~20% of patients are left with partial or complete visual loss.[37]

Non-arteritic AION (NAION) Commonest acute optic neuropathy in patients >50yrs old; visual loss is usually painless and field loss is usually altitudinal. Associations: ↑BP; ↑ lipids; DM, smoking. The role of low-dose aspirin is uncertain in protecting other eye.[39]

Central retinal artery occlusion This is an emergency. Dramatic loss of vision occurs within seconds of occlusion (in 90%, acuity is finger counting or worse). ►►This is considered a form of stroke and should be managed according to local stroke protocols. Occlusion is often thromboembolic (eg carotid artery atherosclerosis in the elderly) but consider all causes of stroke (*OHCM* p470). Look for signs of atherosclerosis (bruits; ↑BP), atrial fibrillation, heart valve disease, diabetes, smoking, or ↑lipids. An afferent pupil defect (p. 366) appears within seconds and may precede retinal changes by 1h. The retina appears white, with a cherry red spot at the macula (figs 4.29 & 4.30). Exclude temporal arteritis (*OHCM* p556). *Management:* ►►If seen within 100min of onset, attempt to increase retinal blood flow even though chances of recovering vision are poor. Emergency treatment aims to reduce IOP by ocular massage, surgical removal of aqueous from the anterior chamber, or the use of intraocular hypotensive treatment. There is no universally accepted emergency treatment and one analysis failed to show a difference between the aforementioned interventions and observation.[40] Long-term management involves primary prevention of CVS risk factors to minimize further events.

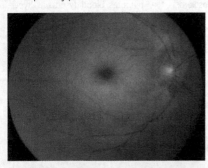

Fig 4.29 Central retinal artery occlusion. With arterial occlusion note retinal pallor and the cherry-red macula.

We thank Dr R K Reddy, Dr Badrinath, and Dr Ravishankar (Sankara Nethralya, Chennai, India) for their help with this page, and for permission to reproduce this image.

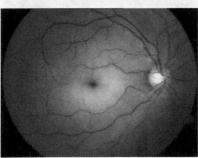

Fig 4.30 Another example of central retinal artery occlusion. Note the retinal pallor and cherry-red macula.

We thank Dr R K Reddy, Dr Badrinath, and Dr Ravishankar (Sankara Nethralya, Chennai, India) for their help with this page, and for permission to reproduce this image.

4 Ophthalmology

Further reading

Guevara M, Kollipara CS (2018). Recent advances in giant cell arteritis. *Curr Rheumatol Rep* 20:25.
Unwin B (2006). Polymyalgia rheumatica and giant cell arteritis. *Am Fam Physician* 74:1547–54.

Retinal vein occlusion (RVO)

The 2nd most common retinal vascular disease after diabetic retinopathy.[41] Vein occlusion causes an increase in retinal capillary pressure resulting in retinal haemorrhage and loss of vision secondary to retinal ischaemia (which causes neovascularization) ± macular oedema. Classification is by anatomical location of occlusion:

Central retinal vein occlusion (CRVO)

(fig 4.31 & 4.32) Occurs at the level of the optic nerve, presenting with sudden-onset painless blurring of vision in one eye.

Branch retinal vein occlusion (BRVO)

Occurs when occlusion is at an arteriovenous crossing and may be asymptomatic if the macula is not affected, although most experience visual field defect corresponding to the area of occlusion.

CRVO

Further divided into *ischaemic* (poor vision, RAPD, cotton wool spots, swollen optic nerve, macular oedema, and risk of neovascularization) and *non-ischaemic* (more common with a better visual prognosis, however 30% convert to the ischaemic).

Causes/associations: Arteriosclerosis, ↑BP,[42] diabetes, blood dyscrasias, hyperlipidaemia, hyperhomocysteinaemia, glaucoma (all types), and systemic inflammatory diseases.[43] Incidence increases with age.[41] Associated with ↑ risk of stroke and increased mortality.[43] *Investigations:* FBC, glucose, BP, ESR. Look for systemic causes.[43] Fundus fluorescein angiography to investigate for retinal ischaemia.

Management: ▶▶Refer to on-call ophthalmologist. Retinal photocoagulation if retinal ischaemia has caused neovascularization (new vessel formation),[43] fig 4.33. The aim is to prevent loss of vision secondary to rubeotic glaucoma (blind painful eye), tractional retinal detachment, and vitreous haemorrhage. Anti-VEGF therapy such as ranibizumab, aflibercept, or dexamethasone implant can be used to treat macular oedema.[43] Macular laser can be considered in macular oedema secondary to BRVO.

Prognosis: Recovery of vision is most likely in BRVO and in the absence of ischaemia.

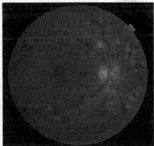

Fig 4.31 Central retinal vein occlusion: note hyperaemia and haemorrhages.

Courtesy of Miss Tsaloumas and University Hospitals Birmingham NHSFT, with thanks to Mark Lane for image collection.

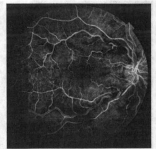

Fig 4.32 Fluorescein fundus angiogram of CRVO, note black areas of hypoperfusion.

Courtesy of Miss Tsaloumas and University Hospitals Birmingham NHSFT, with thanks to Mark Lane for image collection.

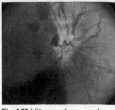

Vitreous haemorrhage (VH)

May arise from retinal neovascularization (2° to diabetic retinopathy, BRVO, or CRVO), retinal tears, retinal detachment, or trauma. *Presentation:* A small amount of bleeding will result in vitreous floaters (fig 4.33), seen by the patient as small black dots (with normal visual acuity). A large haemorrhage can completely obscure the vision and lead to absence of red reflex. *Examine:* Visual acuity, pupil reactions, fundi, then refer. *Management:* Depends on underlying cause. If the haemorrhage prevents visualization of the retina then urgent vitrectomy may be required

Fig 4.33 Vitreous haemorrhage (bottom left) from new vessels (top right).

to remove the vitreous haemorrhage and obtain a view of the retina since visual loss can rapidly progress in the presence of a retinal tear.[44]

Wet age-related macular degeneration (AMD)

Is a common cause of rapidly progressive visual loss in the elderly (see 'Macular degeneration', pp. 352–3).

Optic neuritis

Subacute loss of vision: Unilateral loss of vision occurs over hours or days with pain which is typically worse on eye movement. Reds appear less bright (red desaturation; + reduced colour vision). The pupil shows an RAPD (p. 366). Vision usually recovers over 2–6wks, but is rarely complete. The 15yr probability of MS increases from 25% if normal MRI at baseline to 72% if >1 white matter lesion[45] (*OHCM* p. 496). R̥: High-dose **methylprednisolone** for 72h (1000mg/24h IV), then **prednisolone** (1mg/kg/d PO) for 11 days may be of benefit, however this is still controversial.[46,47]

> #### Optic neuropathies
>
> May be acute (such as AION described here) or insidious (such as nutritional). Damage to the optic nerve typically produces:
> • Monocular vision loss with a central scotoma.
> • Afferent pupillary defects (unilateral lesions).
> • Dyschromatopsia (colour blindness, see p. 325).
> • Papillitis on fundoscopy which eventually progresses to optic atrophy (pale disc, indicates long-term damage).
>
> There are many causes of optic neuropathies beyond this section.[5]

Other causes of sudden monocular loss of vision

• Retinal detachment (pp. 356–7)
• Acute glaucoma (painful, pp. 331)
• Migraine.

Stroke patients may complain of monocular blindness but visual field testing will usually reveal a homonymous hemianopia. Sudden bilateral visual loss is unusual (may be CMV infection in HIV patients).

Further reading

Balcer LJ (2006). Optic neuritis. *NEJM* 354:1273–80.

Denniston A and Murray PI (2018). *Oxford Handbook of Ophthalmology 4th edition.* Oxford: Oxford University Press; pp666–7, 670–80.

Phillpotts BA (2013). *Vitreous Haemorrhage.* Medscape. http://emedicine.medscape.com/article/1230216

Rucker JC et al. (2004). Ischaemic optic neuropathies. *Current Opin Neurol* 17:27–35.

Sivaprasad S *et al.* (2015). RCO guidelines on retinal vein occlusions: executive summary. *Eye* 29:1633–8.

Wong TY *et al.* (2010). Retinal vein occlusion. *NEJM* 363:2135–44.

5 Other causes of optic neuropathy: infective (eg meningitis), inflammatory (eg systemic autoimmune diseases), genetic, compressive (eg neoplasm, abscess), trauma, toxic (eg alcohol excess, radiation), nutritional.

For most people, sight is the most precious of the senses, and for many who are losing vision the thought of going blind is a dominant but unspoken fear—make sure you give the opportunity to talk about this.

Causes of gradual loss of vision
- Cataract (p. 350)
- Glaucoma
- Macular degeneration ('dry' form) (p. 352)
- Diabetic retinopathy (p. 370)
- Uveitis (intermediate, posterior, or panuveitis)
- Optic atrophy (p. 358)
- Retinal dystrophies (eg retinitis pigmentosa)

Primary open-angle glaucoma

Glaucoma is responsible for ~10% of blind registrations in the UK. It affects ~2% of the population >40yr-old and almost 10% of the population >75yr-old.[48] Glaucoma is a progressive optic neuropathy with characteristic changes in the optic nerve head and corresponding loss of visual field. It represents a final common pathway for a number of conditions of which (for most) raised IOP is the most important risk factor. (See fig 4.11 on p. 331 for circulation of aqueous humour.) It is asymptomatic until visual fields are badly impaired; hence the need for screening. If ↑IOP is found, life-long follow-up is needed. Visual field loss may be dangerous eg difficulty spotting while crossing busy roads.[49] *Risk factors:* Include ↑IOP, black ethnicity, family history, ↑ age, and low diastolic perfusion pressure.[50]

Diagnosis Requires: • IOP measurement using tonometry • Central corneal thickness measurement (tonometry overestimates IOP if ↑ corneal thickness) • Peripheral anterior chamber configuration and depth assessments using gonioscopy • Visual field measurement • Optic nerve assessment using a slit lamp with fundus examination.

Routine eye tests The NHS recommends routine eye tests every 2yrs,[51] and offers free eye tests to patients >40yrs old with a family history of glaucoma.[51] Regular eye tests are extremely important as glaucoma is asymptomatic until the advanced stages when loss of vision is irreversible. Screening examination involves tonometry, visual fields, and optic disc examination.

Follow-up Once diagnosed, lifelong monitoring is required to ensure visual damage is detected and limited. Once lost, sight cannot be restored. NICE guidance takes into account evidence of progression and whether IOP has been controlled. Intervals between visits may vary from 1 to 18 months depending on these factors.

Drug treatment Glaucoma is a heterogeneous disease process which may or may not progress to symptomatic vision loss. One study suggested that 12 patients with ↑IOP would need to be treated to prevent 1 case of glaucoma.[52] Compliance with eye drops is difficult when patients are asymptomatic. Aim to reduce IOP by 30% of baseline. Surgery is used if drugs fail.

- *Prostaglandin analogues:* (Latanoprost; travoprost.) ↑ uveoscleral outflow. Dose: once daily (evenings). SE: red eye, iris colour change, periocular skin pigmentation, eyelash growth.
- *β-blockers:* (Timolol 0.25–0.5% or betaxolol 0.25–0.5%.) Use twice daily (once daily for Timoptol LA®) to ↓ production of aqueous. They are β-blockers (∴ caution in asthma or heart failure; systemic absorption occurs with no 1st-pass liver metabolism). SE: dry eyes, corneal anaesthesia, ↓ exercise tolerance, sometimes nightmares.
- *α-adrenergic agonists:* (Brimonidine, apraclonidine.) ↓ production of aqueous and ↑ uveoscleral outflow. SE: lethargy, dry mouth.
- *Carbonic anhydrase inhibitors:* (Dorzolamide & brinzolamide drops, acetazolamide PO.) ↓ production of aqueous. SE of acetazolamide: lassitude, dyspepsia, ↓K+, paraesthesiae. Avoid if pregnant.

- *Miotics:* (Pilocarpine 0.5–4% drops.) ↓ resistance to aqueous outflow. Causes miosis, ↓ acuity, and brow ache from ciliary muscle spasm. Use 4×/day.
- *Fixed-dose combination drops:* Can give the best 24h efficacy. NB: dorzolamide + timolol may reduce pressure more than brimonidine + timolol.[53]

Laser therapy (trabeculoplasty) ↑ aqueous outflow = ↓IOP. Long-term efficacy is comparable to medical treatment and may be more cost-effective.[54]

Surgery Trabeculectomy is a filtration surgery that establishes a pressure valve at the limbus so aqueous can flow into a conjunctival bleb. Problems include early failure, hypotony, bleb leakage, infection. Newer miniature (1mm × 0.33mm) implants such as the iStent®, can be inserted through a single incision into the trabecular meshwork to create a communication between the aqueous and Schlemm's canal, thus reducing IOP.

Optic disc cupping Characterized by loss of disc substance which makes the cup look larger. Normal cup:disc ratio is commonly 0.4–0.7 but this depends on the size of the disc: ►a large cup in a small disc is probably pathological. As damage progresses, the disc pales (atrophies), and the cup widens and deepens, so vessels emerging from the disc appear to have breaks as they disappear into the cup and are then seen at the base again (fig 4.34). Notching of the cup and haemorrhage at the disc may occur. As cupping develops, the disc vessels are displaced nasally. Nasal and superior fields are lost first (temporal last) and central vision tends to be maintained. Asymmetric cupping suggests glaucoma. Notching at the neuroretinal rim is usually inferior, and best seen where the vessels enter the disc. Glaucomatous optic nerve damage affects the anterior visual pathway up to the optic chiasm. See p. 358 for other optic disc abnormalities.

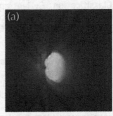

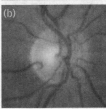

Fig 4.34 The right disc (a) is grossly cupped and atrophic, the left disc (b) has been unaffected by the open angle glaucoma.

Courtesy of University Hospitals Birmingham NHSFT, with thanks to Mark Lane for image collection.

Pathogenesis Susceptibility of a patient's retina and optic nerve to IOP-related damage is very variable. IOP ≥21mmHg may or may not correlate with cupping, nerve damage, and field loss. Since the central field is intact, good acuity is maintained, so presentation is often delayed until irreversible optic nerve damage has occurred. Control of IOP does stop visual field loss but does not reverse it.[55] The visual defects tend to be bilateral, although are not always symmetrical. Some get glaucoma with normal IOP (normal tension glaucoma).[56]

Educating people about their glaucoma

It is common for people to be seen regularly for years in the glaucoma clinic and yet understand almost nothing about their condition. In one study, 48% believed symptoms would warn them of disease progression. 30% of new patients believed that blindness was likely.[57] So, try to explain what happens in glaucoma, and give printed details (check the patient can read them!).

Further reading

Denniston A and Murray PI (2018). *Oxford Handbook of Ophthalmology 4th edition.* Oxford: Oxford University Press; pp382–441.

NICE (2017). *Glaucoma: Diagnosis and Management* (NG81). London: NICE.

Quigley HA (2009). Glaucoma. *Lancet* 377:1367–77.

Vas C *et al.* (2007). Medical interventions for primary open angle glaucoma and ocular hypertension. *Cochrane Database Syst Rev* 4: CD003167.

Cataract describes the loss of transparency of the lens and is the leading cause of blindness worldwide. Cataract surgery is spectacular to observe, especially if the opportunity arises to do so down the viewing arm of the microscope where everything is 3D and magnified.

Risk factors Most cataracts are age related, but may occur early in systemic disease (eg diabetes), ocular disease (eg uveitis), and after specific exposures such as smoking, alcohol excess, UV light, trauma, radiotherapy, or HIV.[58] In children, many are genetic. ▶When a cataract is found, measure fasting plasma glucose; in a younger patient consider additional risk factors such as steroid use; and consider specific syndromes such as myotonic dystrophy.[59]

Classification By lens appearance. With immature cataracts the red reflex still occurs; in dense cataracts there is no red reflex, or visible fundus. *Nuclear cataracts* change the lens refractive index (='second sight' as the patient becomes more myopic and regains reading vision). They are common in old age. *Cortical cataracts* are spoke-like wedge-shaped opacities which have milder effects on vision. *Posterior subcapsular cataracts* typically progress faster and cause the classic glare from bright sunlight and lights while driving at night, which can be troublesome even when visual acuity is only mildly affected. Subcapsular opacities (eg from steroid use) are just deep to the lens capsule—in the visual axis. Dot opacities are common in normal lenses but are also seen in fast-developing cataracts in diabetes or myotonic dystrophy.

Presentation Clouded/blurred vision. Unilateral cataracts are often unnoticed, but loss of stereopsis affects distance judgement. Bilateral cataracts cause gradual painless loss of vision (frequent spectacle changes as refraction changes) ± dazzle (esp. in sunlight) ± monocular diplopia. Patients describe difficulties driving at night and haloes around street lights. In children they may present as squint, or a white pupil, or as nystagmus (infants)/amblyopia.

Management Often up-to-date refraction helps a bit, but if symptoms are troubling, lifestyle is restricted, or if unable to read a number plate at 20m (and they need to drive) offer surgery. Explain risks: 2% get serious complications; even if surgery may vastly improve vision, eyes may not be entirely normal afterwards (dazzle/glare often remains). Spectacles are often needed post operatively too, especially for reading. Some have coexisting macular degeneration, or other ophthalmic pathology which limits outcome.

Surgery is usually performed as a day case using local anaesthesia (either injection or drops). Younger people, high myopes, and the squeamish may prefer general anaesthesia. An incision of 2–3mm is made, and the lens is removed by phacoemulsification (ultrasound breaks it up: it is then aspirated into a cannula). The lens capsule is carefully left in place. The incision is fractionally enlarged and a folded artificial lens (eg of Perspex®, acrylic, or silicon) is implanted and unrolled into the empty capsule. The patient can usually return home immediately afterwards. With phacoemulsification, full activities can be resumed the next day. With complicated surgery or extracapsular extraction, a larger incision is needed and there may be more limitations. Patients use antibiotic & anti-inflammatory drops for 3–6 weeks postoperatively. Then they need to change spectacles to get the full benefit of surgery. Multifocal intraocular lenses exist and in appropriately selected patients they can be helpful. *Postoperative complications:* Posterior capsule opacification is common occurring in ~20%, over months to years. It seems 'like my cataract returning' or 'I'm looking through frosted glass'. It is easily treated by capsulotomy with a YAG laser as an outpatient. Astigmatism can be corrected during surgery by using a toric lens, or an incision in the cornea to reduce the steepness in one meridian. Endophthalmitis is a potential serious complication, which can lead to loss of vision, or the eye.

Prevention/photoprotection Use sunglasses (↓UV-B).[60] Reduce oxidative stress (with antioxidants eg vitamin c).[61] Stop smoking![62]

Pre-and postoperative care Prior to surgery, *ocular biometry* must be done. This is a measurement of the curvature of the cornea and the length of the eye which enables prediction of the suitable intraocular lens implant (fig 4.35). In most cases it aims to leave the patient emmetropic (in focus for distance), or just slightly myopic, but this may vary considerably depending on patient preference and pre-existing refraction. It is not an exact science as the clinical measurements vary and many people do continue to wear spectacles postoperatively for some degree of residual refractive error.[63]

▶If patients develop a painful red eye or loss of vision postoperatively, think *endophthalmitis* and refer back to the ophthalmologist immediately for same-day management with vitreous biopsy and intravitreal antibiotics.

Some *eye irritation* needing additional or altered drops postoperatively is common. Many experience awareness of the eye or dry/gritty sensations. Lubricants such as carbomer gel, eg Viscotears,® may help. Some may have *anterior uveitis* requiring new medication. Rarely, there may be vitreous haemorrhage, retinal detachment, or glaucoma (± permanent visual loss), risk of endophthalmitis (<1/1000).[64] If vision deteriorates with time they should initially see if they need a new prescription change; and thereafter see an ophthalmologist to consider YAG laser capsulotomy and to exclude other problems.

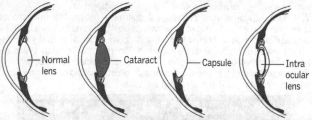

Fig 4.35 Position of the intraocular lens after cataract surgery.

Cataracts at birth: ▶act quickly!

If there is a congenital cataract the patient needs to be referred *urgently* to ophthalmology for surgical consideration. Intervention needs to be done within the latent period of visual development (1st 6 weeks of life) to prevent significant deprivation amblyopia. Do a TORCH screen too (pp. 78–9).[65]

Claude Monet

'Halo' refers to a circle of light, white or coloured, seen around *any* luminous body (not just saints). Also call to mind Monet, his cataracts (a cause of haloes) and his paintings and their 'investments in light' (another meaning of halo). In the poem, Monet refuses surgery

> *D*octor, you say there are no haloes around the streetlights in Paris and what I see is an aberration caused by old age, an affliction. I tell you it has taken me all my life to arrive at the vision of gas lamps as angels.
>
> Lisel Mueller: *Monet Refuses the Operation.*
> MF McLellan (1996). *Lancet* 348:1640.

for his cataracts: how differently doctors and artists see the world! So before we advise surgery it's wise to get to know our patients, and to keep an eye on posterity. Visual changes are also thought to have influenced other painters including Vincent Van Gogh and Rembrandt van Rijn.[86]

Further reading
Asbell PA *et al.* (2005). Age-related cataract. *Lancet* 365:599–609.
Denniston A and Murray PI (2018). *Oxford Handbook of Ophthalmology 4th edition*. Oxford: Oxford University Press; pp336–79.
Keay L *et al.* (2011). Routine preoperative medical testing for cataract surgery. *Cochrane Database Syst Rev* 3:CD007293.
NICE (2017). *Cataracts in Adults: Management* (NG77). London: NICE.

Macula (fig 4.38) An area 5.5mm across, just lateral to the optic disc. In the middle of the macula is a 1.5mm pit, the fovea (fovea centralis). In the middle of the fovea is the foveola where the cones are narrow, long, and densely packed (up to 300,000/mm²). This cone gradient correlates with acuity. Any disturbance in this region can impact vision greatly. Test visual acuity and use an Amsler grid (fig 4.37) to assess visual distortion.

Age-related macular degeneration (AMD) The leading cause of blindness in the developed world in those >50yrs. *Risk factors:* Increasing age, family history, smoking, ↑BP, ↑BMI, diet low in omega 3 & 6, carotenoids, and minerals, lack of exercise. Diagnosis and monitoring have been revolutionized by optical coherence tomography (OCT) which provides retinal resolution down to a few microns.

Dry AMD Accounts for 90% of cases, with a gradual deterioration in central vision, usually over decades. Associated with the presence of drusen (fig 4.42) and pigmentation at the macula. With time this can progress to atrophy of the macula (geographic atropy, see fig 4.36) and visual acuity of counting fingers or worse. *Presentation:* Gradual-onset loss of central vision (fig 4.37) leading to difficulty reading, making out faces, ↓ night vision, visual fluctuations (good vision one day, worse the next). Symptoms gradually worsen over years. *Treatment/prevention:* See BOX 'Managing AMD'.

Wet AMD (Neovascular) pathological choroidal neovascular membranes (CNVM) develop under the retina. The CNVM can leak fluid and blood and cause a central disciform scar. *Presentation:* Rapid deterioration of central vision associated with distortion (metamorphopsia). Ophthalmoscopy shows fluid exudation, localized detachment of the pigment, and sometimes haemorrhage. *Treatment:* Prompt treatment is essential as substantial visual loss may occur while the patient waits (see BOX 'Managing AMD').

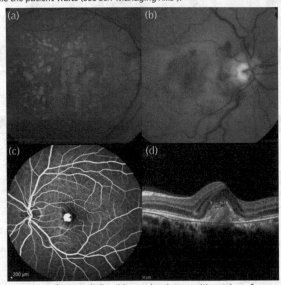

Fig 4.36 Images of AMD including (a) macular drusen with patches of geographic atrophy, (b) fundus photograph of wet AMD, (c) fluorescein angiogram showing fluid leak from wet AMD, (d) OCT image of wet AMD.

(a) and (b) courtesy of Mr Keane and Moorfields Eye Hospital NHS Foundation Trust; (c) and (d) courtesy of Dr Hina Khan and the Amanat Eye Hospital, Pakistan, with thanks to Mark Lane for image collection.

Managing AMD

Wet AMD Urgent fluorescein angiogram is performed to determine the type of new vessels, alongside OCT, to examine for extent of intraretinal and subretinal fluid.

Treatment VEGF is a secreted protein that leads to angiogenesis, blood vessel leakage, and inflammation. Anti-VEGF therapy ↓ formation of new blood vessels, ↓ vascular leaks, and hence ↑ visual acuity. Ranibizumab and aflibercept have NICE approval and form the mainstay of treatment superseding previous therapies such as photodynamic therapy and laser photocoagulation.[67] Intravitreal injections are given on a monthly basis in the first instance, although long-acting versions are being trialled. Bevacizumab is not licensed for use in wet AMD, however it is significantly cheaper and has sparked an interesting debate regarding the use of 'off-label' medication.[68]

Screening In patients with early signs of AMD, ask patients to report any new signs of neovascularization: a good self-test is 'Do window and door frames appear straight?' Refer if distortions or sudden blank spots.

All patients with AMD Most must rely on visual aids (eg magnifiers) to read, along with sufficient lighting. Up-to-date refraction is essential. Prompt referral to the low vision service and registration as visually impaired can facilitate appropriate support.

Diet/supplements AREDS (Age-Related Eye Disease Study) showed dietary supplementation with zinc, β-carotene, and vitamins C & E slowed AMD progression. AREDS 2 demonstrated that oral supplementation with macular xanthophylls (lutein & zeaxanthin) in place of β-carotene (risk of lung cancer in smokers) decreased risk of progression but omega-3 made no difference. Patients should also be advised to stop smoking and have a diet rich in green vegetables.[69,70]

4 Ophthalmology

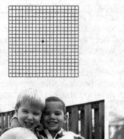
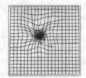
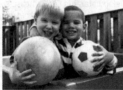
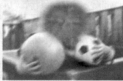

Fig 4.37 Use of Amsler grids: as wet ARMD (pp. 352–3) progresses, the patient experiences distortion of straight lines (metamorphopsia); this is detected using an Amsler grid. Central vision is distorted when the fovea is involved. These images demonstrate the visual deterioration the patient experiences.

'Eye disease simulation, age-related macular degeneration' by National Eye Institute, National Institutes of Health: http://www.nei.nih.gov/photo/keyword.asp?narrow=Eye+Disease+Simulation&match=all (TIFF image). Licensed under Public Domain via Commons.

Further reading

For a very detailed overview of AMD see: http://www.rcophth.ac.uk/wp-content/uploads/2014/12/2013-SCI-318-RCOphth-AMD-Guidelines-Sept-2013-FINAL-2.pdf

For a patient friendly version see: https://www.rcophth.ac.uk/wp-content/uploads/2015/02/RCOphth-RNIB-Understanding-Age-Related-Macular-Degeneration-AMD-2013.pdf

4 Ophthalmology

Macular hole (fig 4.38)

A small break in the macular region of the retinal tissue. It involves the fovea therefore affecting the visual acuity causing blurred and distorted central vision. *Prevalence:* 3.3/1000 in persons >55yrs old. There is a 10–15% lifetime risk of developing a macular hole in the other eye—the patient must undergo surveillance. *Pathogenesis:* Usually idiopathic; with ageing, the vitreous starts to lose some of the 80% water content, which causes it to shrink causing traction on the retinal tissue. Other risk factors include high myopia, injury to the eye, and retinal detachment. *Presentation:* Distorted vision with visual loss. The effect on visual acuity is dependent on the site of macular damage. On examination, look for a tiny punched-out area in the centre of the macula; there may be yellow-white deposits

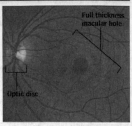

Fig 4.38 The macula lies lateral to the optic nerve and contains the structures enabling high visual acuity.

Reproduced from Sundaram V. *et al.*, *Oxford Specialty Training: Training in Ophthalmology* (2009) with permission from OUP.

at the base. Slit-lamp exam with a convex lens shows a round excavation with well-defined borders interrupting the slit-lamp beam. The hole is typically surrounded by a grey halo of detached retina (fig 4.37 p. 353). *Tests:* Amsler grids (fig 4.37 p. 353) reveal visual distortion; optical coherence tomography (OCT) diagnoses and stages macular holes. *Treatment:* ▶Refer urgently to a specialist vitreoretinal surgeon. In stage 1 (impending hole seen as a yellow spot on the fovea), 'watch and wait' (no treatment if there is spontaneous resolution or no progression). ~50% of holes progress to stage 2—when treatment is needed. *Surgery:* A vitrectomy is done to remove the vitreous and the internal limiting membrane over the hole is peeled. A gas bubble is introduced to nudge (tamponade) the macula back into position. Postoperatively the patient will need to spend time 'posturing' (eg 50mins in every hour being face down for 1–2 weeks). Success is also possible if the hole is long-standing (>6 months). However, in some patients, more than one operation is needed to close the hole, and adverse effects may occur. *Early complications:* iatrogenic retinal tears and detachments, postoperative IOP spikes, and rarely endophthalmitis. *Later:* most patients develop cataracts (76% of cases requiring extraction within 2yrs). *Non-surgical measures:* If a patient declines/is not suitable for surgery consider whether they need low-vision support eg visual aids.[71]

Retinitis pigmentosa

The commonest inherited retinal disorder affecting 1:3000–7000. Rod photoreceptors are lost initially, with cone photoreceptors being lost later. Eventually there is atrophy of all retinal cells with the retinal nerve fibre layer preserved until last (this is of use in retinal implant technology). Since rod photoreceptors are lost first, the initial symptoms are of night blindness, followed by tunnel vision. Visual acuity is preserved until later stages. *Fundus examination* reveals mid-peripheral 'bone spicule' pigmentation of the retina, a waxy pallor to the optic disc, and attenuation of the retinal arterioles. There are a multitude of mutations responsible for RP which can be inherited in either AD, AR, or X-linked forms. 50% of cases occur in patients with no family history. Retinitis pigmentosa most commonly occurs in isolation, however it can form part of a syndrome. Usher syndrome (AR, retinitis pigmentosa, and deafness) accounts for ~50% of patients who are both blind and deaf. Bardet–Biedl syndrome (p. 842) should also be considered.[72] Throughout life, 25% of retinitis pigmentosa patients retain ability to read, with reduced visual fields. Only a few have acuity ≤6/60 at age 20yrs; but by 50, many are reduced to this level.[72] *Novel non-standard therapies* include neural prosthetics (artificial vision by stimulating retinal ganglion cells electrically) (p. 382).

Posterior uveitis (Including choroiditis, chorioretinitis, and retinitis.) The choroid is the most posterior part of the uveal tract. Inflammation of the choroid and/or the overlying retina usually presents subacutely with any of central visual loss, blind spots (may be blurry rather than absolute), 'floaters', and/or visual distortion. It may be due to 1 *inflammation*, either purely ocular, or systemic (eg sarcoidosis) or 2 *infection* (herpes virus family, toxoplasma, tuberculosis). Posterior uveitis usually requires systemic therapy and/or injection therapy, in line with the underlying cause.

Seen, unseen, and seer—and the indifferent pixel

'The greatest thing a human soul ever does in this world is to see something, and tell what it saw in a plain way. Hundreds of people can talk for one who can think, but thousands can think for one who can see.' John Ruskin *Modern Painters;* vol. III

Interpreting but not over-interpreting our visual sensations entails the almost impossible task of seeing the indifferent pixels as well their patterns. When a classicist, revising for her exams, says 'I'm preparing for my Unseen' she means 'I'm preparing for a surprise. I'm going to have to translate, without warning, some unknown ancient passage (our primordial unconscious) into modern parlance (current sensations).' To do well, she (and we) have to expect the unexpected, or else the snake will bite us. More deeply, all visual experience is ambiguous, yet we believe and act on it all the time. Seers, philosophers, and, above all, poets know that the issue here is the role our imagination plays in seeing. *'I have seen sometimes what men imagine they see.'* (J'ai vu quelquefois ce que l'homme a cru voir!) *The Drunken Boat* Arthur Rimbaud

How is this important clinically? Just as we are born expecting to hear each other's voices, so we are born expecting to see each other's faces. If in later life we lose our vision, then the brain, with exaggerated zeal, compensates by creating fictive visual percepts, almost always involving faces—a surprisingly common non-psychotic hallucination named after Charles Bonnet, who first described it in his 89-year-old grandfather in 1769.

Charles Bonnet's grandfather might say with insight: *'I have imagined sometimes what other men know they see'*—le the mirror-image of Arthur Rimbaud's formulation. The point is that neither Rimbaud nor Bonnet can pinch themselves to see if their hallucinatory state is real. By their systematic derangement of their senses they teach us something universal about our place in our external and internal worlds, namely that we can never fully disentangle what we see from what we expect to see. It is as if our propensity for illusions validates and authenticates our experience of being us.

So don't get too annoyed with your patients when they give ambiguous answers to your questions about floaters, flashes, and more complex fictive visual percepts. Just smile to yourself and to Rimbaud in his embodiment as a drunken, waterlogged boat (*Le bateau ivre*) and remember that *the boat is in the drink and the drink is in the boat.*

Further reading

Denniston A and Murray PI (2018). *Oxford Handbook of Ophthalmology 4th edition*. Oxford: Oxford University Press; pp476–518, 550–2, 574–91.

Ferrari S *et al.* (2011). Retinitis pigmentosa, genes and disease mechanisms. *Curr Genomics* 12:238–49.

Hartong DT *et al.* (2006). Retinitis pigmentosa. *Lancet* 368:1795–809.

Macular Society: https://www.macularsociety.org/macular-hole

New-onset 'flashes and floaters' should be assumed to be due to a retinal tear + detachment until proven otherwise—although it will be more commonly due to posterior vitreous detachment (PVD).

Flashes

Due to retinal pathology or migraine. 1 Retinal stimulation eg by traction during the normal age-related process of a posterior vitreous detachment (p. 357) in which the vitreous jelly separates from the retina; it is often accompanied by ≥1 floaters. More seriously, 5% go on to develop retinal tears, which in turn may lead to retinal detachment. Retinal damage is usually peripheral and hard to see—refer *immediately* for specialist help. 2 Migraine—classically has the appearance of 'fortification spectra' of spreading zig-zag lines and is not accompanied by floaters. Ask about headache, nausea, or previous migraine.

Floaters

Very common visual symptom, usually arising simply due to physiological (age-related) degeneration of the vitreous resulting in imperfections in the gel (occurs younger in myopes, after trauma or ocular surgery) and/or the normal age-related process of a PVD in which the vitreous jelly separates from the retina.
Common pathological causes: 1 Blood—ie vitreous haemorrhage (diabetic retinopathy; vein occlusions; trauma; retinal tear/traction on a retinal vessel). 2 Inflammation (intermediate, posterior, or panuveitis) or infection (bacterial or fungal endophthalmitis). 3 Intraocular malignancy.

Management: Floaters present as small dark spots in the visual field, particularly noticeable against a bright background (fig 4.39). Often, they are just annoying, but harmless, and may settle with time. Examine the vitreous and retina, and treat the cause before reassuring. *Sudden showers* of floaters in one eye (± flashing lights) may be due to blood. ▶*Refer immediately* (specialist assessment within 24h) due to possibility of retinal tear + detachment (see next section).

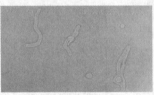

Fig 4.39 A simulated image of the appearance of floaters while looking at blue sky. You may notice floaters yourself eg when staring at a white wall.

Retinal detachment

(RD, fig 4.40) The separation of the neurosensory retina from the underlying retinal pigment epithelium (RPE). *Types:*

1 *Rhegmatogenous retinal detachment:* a tear in the retina allows fluid to pass from the vitreous space into the subretinal space between the sensory retina and the retinal pigment epithelium. These tears occur due to abnormal vitreoretinal adhesions often in areas of pre-existing retinal weakness, which

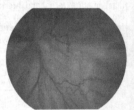

Fig 4.40 RD; note retinal folds.
© Bristol Eye Hospital.

fail to withstand the normal ageing process of vitreous shrinkage and separation from the retina (known as 'posterior vitreous detachment'). Myopic eyes are more prone to detachment due to ↑ axonal length. The higher the myopia, the greater the risk. Cataract surgery for myopia carries ↑ risk of detachment.

2 *Exudative retinal detachment:* the retina detaches without a tear, eg hypertension, vasculitis, macular degenerative conditions, tumours.

3 *Tractional retinal detachments:* pulling on the retina, eg proliferative diabetic retinopathy.

Presentation: The 4 'F's : Floaters, Flashes (in ~50%), Field loss, and Fall in acuity—painless and may be as a curtain falling over the vision (the curtain falls down as the lower half of the retina detaches upwards). Field defects indicate position and extent of the detachment (in superior detachments field loss is inferior). *Ophthalmoscopy:* grey opalescent retina, ballooning forward. Extensive detachment of the retina will pull off the macula. If it does detach, central vision is lost and doesn't always recover completely—even if the retina is successfully fixed. Superior detachments progress faster due to gravitational effects.

Prognosis: Depends on:
• Site and extent of detachment.
• Time to definitive treatment.
• Nature of underlying pathology.

Differential diagnosis: 'Flashes and floaters'—posterior vitreous detachment (p. 357); vitreous haemorrhage (p. 347). 'Flashes' in a spreading pattern is *more typical* of migraine.

Management: This is an emergency. ▸▸Refer for immediate assessment and urgent surgery: vitrectomy and gas tamponade (or silicone oil); scleral silicone implants. Cryotherapy or laser coagulation is used to secure the retina. Postoperatively, re-detachment occurs in 5–10%.

Posterior vitreous detachment (PVD)

Degenerative changes in the vitreous lead to its eventual separation from the retina. This is part of normal ageing. Patients describe monochromatic photopsia in the peripheral temporal field. This is more obvious in dim light and with eye movements. There is an increase in floaters but vision remains unchanged and there are no field defects. Refer for fundus check as retinal tears can happen as a consequence of a PVD.

Further reading

Denniston A and Murray PI (2018). *Oxford Handbook of Ophthalmology 4th edition*. Oxford: Oxford University Press; pp522–41.

Hollands H *et al.* (2009). Acute onset floaters and flashes: is this patient at risk for retinal detachment? *JAMA* 302:2243–9.

Kahawita S *et al.* (2014). Flashes and floaters—a practical approach to assessment and management. *Aust Fam Physician* 43:201–3.

4 Ophthalmology

Optic disc (fig 4.43 p. 360) Represents the head of the optic nerve which can be seen clinically; the rest of the optic nerve extends towards the optic chiasm. *Examination* of the optic disc aims to describe the Contour (borders should be well defined, the disc may appear oval in astigmatic eyes, and appear abnormally large in myopic eyes), Colour (should be pink-yellow with a pale centre, the disc colour is more pallid in optic atrophy), and Cup (see p. 360).[73] The disc has a physiological cup which lies centrally and should occupy ~⅓ of the disc diameter. Cup widening and deepening occurs in glaucoma. Blood vessels radiate away from the disc. The normal arterial/venous width ratio is 2:3. Venous engorgement appears in retinal vein thrombosis; abnormal retinal pallor with artery occlusion; and haemorrhages + exudates in hypertension and DM (pp. 370–1).

Causes of disc swelling
• Papilloedema
• Malignant hypertension (*OHCM* p140)
• Cavernous sinus thrombosis
• Optic neuritis
• Cranial space-occupying lesion
• Optic neuropathy
• Central vein occlusion
• Opaque myelinated nerve fibres (fig 4.47 p. 361)
• Disorders of the nerve sheath (fig 4.45 p. 361)

Papilloedema (fig 4.44 p. 360) Swelling of the optic disc caused by ICP; bilateral, but not necessarily symmetrical. ►Papilloedema should be your main differential for optic disc swelling until proven otherwise. *Presentation* is usually due to symptoms of raised ICP: nausea/vomiting. Headaches worse in the mornings, centred in the frontal region, aggravated by bending down or coughing. Double vision 2° to CN VI palsy. Enquire about transient visual obscurations (vision goes black very briefly and then returns) and pulsatile tinnitus. Check colour vision and visual fields. *Investigations:* An intracranial space-occupying lesion must be ruled out; MRI with contrast is gold standard, but CT head is often quicker to obtain. Measure the BP; any hypertensive changes or haemorrhages? Any signs of CRVO (p. 346)? In young obese women, think of idiopathic intracranial hypertension (*OHCM* p. 498). If neuroimaging is normal (= no risk of coning) then consider lumbar puncture to establish opening pressures and facilitate CSF analysis.[74] NB: Foster–Kennedy syndrome occurs where there is unilateral visual loss from a compressive optic neuropathy in 1 eye (pale disc) with papilloedema of the other disc (eg from meningioma of the optic canal pressing on 1 optic nerve and extending sufficiently to cause raised ICP resulting in contralateral papilloedema (fig 4.45 p. 361) in the eye with optic atrophy; in practice, the usual cause is consequential ischaemic optic neuropathy). *Nystagmus* suggests a lesion in the posterior fossa; *Sixth nerve palsy* may be a false localizing sign. *Causes* of disc swelling—see MINIBOX 'Causes of disc swelling'.

Pseudopapilloedema (see fig 4.46) One or both discs appear elevated/have unclear margins but there is no optic nerve axon swelling. Caused by a small or tilted disc or optic disc drusen. Usually the appearance does not change over time.[75] Treat as papilloedema until otherwise proven; fluorescence angiography (FA), US, and OCT can help to determine the cause.

Diabetic papillopathy Rare but can affect both type 1 and 2 DM irrespective of glycaemic control. Presents with progressive mild visual impairment and optic disc swelling ± features of diabetic retinopathy. 30% of patients develop non-arteritic ischaemic optic neuropathy.[76]

Optic atrophy (fig 4.41) Discs are pale (degree doesn't correlate with visual loss). Causes are diverse including ↑IOP (glaucoma), or retinal damage (choroiditis, retinitis pigmentosa, cerebromacular degeneration), ischaemia (retinal artery occlusion, GCA), Leber optic atrophy (p. 852), multiple sclerosis (MS), syphilis, external pressure on the nerve (intraorbital or intracranial tumours, Paget disease affecting the skull, pituitary adenoma).

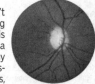

Fig 4.41 Optic atrophy.

Optic disc drusen

Optic disc drusen[75] (fig 4.42) (See also fig 4.48.) Consist of acellular deposits in the optic nerve head that become calcified over time making the optic disc edge irregular and lumpy. They are typically buried in early life and become more prominent in later childhood. Drusen can be associated with abnormal branching of the retinal vessels (trifurcation) and absence of the optic cup. Misdiagnosis of optic disc drusen may lead to unnecessary work up for papilloedema (see p. 358). Ultrasound, fluorescein angiography, fundus autofluorescence, and OCT examination may help to determine the cause. They can be associated with a visual field defect which can lead to added diagnostic confusion.

(a)

(b)

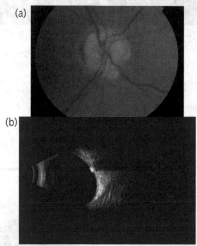

Fig 4.42 Optic drusen. (a) Fundus appearance; (b) ultrasound appearance.

a) Courtesy of Prof Shah and University Hospitals Birmingham NHSFT; b) Courtesy of Peter Good and Sandwell and West Birmingham Hospitals NHS Trust, with thanks to Mark Lane for image collection.

Normal optic disc

(fig 4.43) The neuroretinal rim should be well defined and pink; if it looks pale, consider optic atrophy. If the border looks fuzzy, the disc may be swollen.

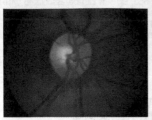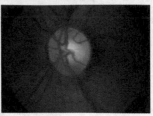

Fig 4.43 The normal optic disc has a pink neuroretinalrim outside with a central pale depression called the optic cup (see p. 349 for cupping).

Image reproduced with permission from Medscape Drugs & Diseases (http://emedicine.medscape.com/), Optic Atrophy, 2019, available at: https://emedicine.medscape.com/article/1217760-overview.

Papilloedema

Optic disc swelling due to raised ICP. The discs are swollen forwards and also outwards into the surrounding retina. Disc margins are hidden and in places retinal vessels are concealed, because oedema has impaired the translucency of the disc tissues. In fig 4.44a the retinal veins are congested and there are a few haemorrhages at 9 o'clock.

►Urgently rule out an intracranial space-occupying lesion (eg brain tumour). Papilloedema is almost always bilateral. Rare causes of unilateral papilloedema include meningioma of one optic nerve (fig 4.45).

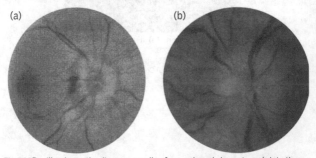

Fig 4.44 Papilloedema: the discs are swollen forwards and also outwards into the surrounding retina. Disc margins are hidden and in places retinal vessels are concealed, because oedema has impaired the translucency of the disc tissues. In (a) the retinal veins are congested and there are a few haemorrhages at 9 o'clock.

We thank Mr J F Cullen FRCS for permission to use the image.

4 Ophthalmology

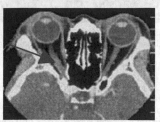

Fig 4.45 Meningioma of right optic nerve sheath.

We thank Mr J F Cullen FRCS for permission to use the image.

Pseudopapilloedema

(figs 4.46 & 4.47) Occurs when there is an elevated appearance to the optic nerve head without oedema of the nerve fibre. A variety of abnormalities can create this appearance including optic disc drusen (fig 4.48).

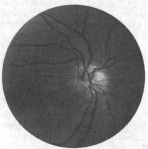

Fig 4.46 Pseudopapilloedema.
Reproduced from *Brain's Diseases of the Nervous System*, with permission from OUP.

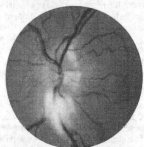

Fig 4.47 Myelinated nerve fibres mimicking papilloedema.
We thank Mr J F Cullen FRCS for permission to use the image.

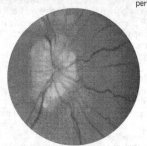

Fig 4.48 Optic drusen, which can be mistaken for papilloedema.
We thank Mr J F Cullen FRCS for permission to use the image.

Further reading

Denniston A and Murray PI (2018). *Oxford Handbook of Ophthalmology 4th edition*. Oxford: Oxford University Press; pp728–63.

Ong HS *et al.* (2014). Acute visual loss in papilloedema: the diagnostic pitfalls. *Int Ophthalmol* 34:607–12. [2 interesting case reports.]

Optic-disc.org: www.optic-disc.org

Pane A *et al.* (2017). *The Neuro-Ophthalmology Survival Guide* (2nd ed). Edinburgh: Elsevier.

When assessing for visual field defects, it is important to ask focused questions to correctly classify the defect: ▶*Because of* CNS *plasticity, people often think that the area of defect (scotoma) is smaller than it is.*

1 Is the defect unilateral or bilateral?
2 Does the defect have sharp or blurred boundaries?
3 Does the defect lie in the vertical or horizontal meridian?
4 What is the current acuity?
5 Onset? Lesions of sudden onset are often due to a vascular cause.

Anatomy of the visual pathway Superior parts of the visual field fall inferiorly on the retina; temporal fields on the nasal retina, and vice versa. Fibres from the nasal retina of both eyes cross in the optic chiasm to join uncrossed temporal retinal fibres. As fibres cross they maintain position (superior fibres stay superior). From the optic chiasm fibres pass in the optic tract to the lateral geniculate body, then as the optic radiation to the visual cortex.

Tests *Finger confrontation:* The patient closes one eye, fixes on your eye, and notes the presence of a finger in all fields mapped, against your vision. It is used for testing peripheral fields. *Hat-pin confrontation:* The patient fixes on your eye (sit ~1m away). Red (central vision) or white (peripheral vision) hat-pins are used to define any vertical meridian, the size of the blind spot, and the boundaries of any scotomas. More reliable mapping of visual fields is done by perimetry, usually using automated presentation of lights at different locations of varying brightness. *Amsler grids:* Detect distortion in central vision, eg from macular disease. The chart is 10 × 10cm square with 5mm squares drawn on it and a dot in the centre. With the chart held at 30cm the patient is instructed to look at the dot and report any distorted squares or wavy lines (metamorphopsia) (fig 4.37, p.353).

Optic nerve (fig 4.49 number 1.) Lesions of the optic nerve may cause a range of scotomas varying from enlargement of the normal 'physiological blind spot' to complete blindness. This will be associated with increasing severity of RAPD, to the point where there may be no direct response (but the consensual will remain intact). Acuity and colour vision tends to be affected.

Optic chiasm (fig 4.49 number 3.) Central lesions in the chiasm will produce a bitemporal hemianopia (eg from pituitary enlargement). This is due to the fact that the fibres coming from the nasal halves of both retinas are involved.

Optic tracts (fig 4.49 number 5.) A lesion on the optic tract causes a contralateral homonymous hemianopia eg a right-sided optic tract lesion causes a left temporal hemianopia and a right nasal hemianopia.

Optic radiation Optic radiation lesions produce a contralateral homonymous hemianopia. Lesions over the lateral portions of the lateral geniculate body which receives impulses from the inferior retinal quadrants cause a superior quadrantic hemianopia (fig 4.49 number 4). Lesions in the nerve fibres passing more directly posterior to the cortex cause an inferior quadrantic hemianopia.

Visual cortex Lesions at the primary visual cortex produce contralateral homonymous hemianopia. A contralateral upper homonymous quadrantanopia may be caused by temporal lobe tumours. A contralateral inferior homonymous quadrantanopia may be caused by a parietal lobe lesion.[77] In the visual cortex the macular is represented at the tips of the occipital lobes, a lesion affecting the tip of the lobe produces a central homonymous scotoma (fig 4.49 number 6). The anterior visual cortex deals with peripheral vision and is supplied by the posterior cerebral artery. If the cause is posterior cerebral artery ischaemia then the macula (and so visual acuity) may be spared as it has an overlap of flow via the middle cerebral artery.[77]

Causes of visual field defects *Ocular:* Glaucoma, macular diseases (eg AMD), optic nerve diseases (eg ischaemic, nutritional, hereditary), retinitis pigmentosa. *CNS:* Ischaemia (TIA, migraine, stroke), glioma, meningioma, abscess, AV malformation, *drugs*, eg ciclosporin.[78]

NB: cortical visual defects may be fundamentally capricious—in that when an object is presented to the affected field of view, the patient announces that they cannot see it—yet 'guesses' correctly that it is there (non-cortical visual pathways): there are some things we know we can see; other things we see without knowing (blindsight); and others that we know without seeing (eg that a table has 4 legs when we can only see 3 at any one time).

Scotomata

Arcuate scotoma: moderate glaucoma

Unilateral defect found with:
Arterial occlusion
Branch retinal vein thrombosis
Inferior retinal detachment

Central scotoma: Macular degeneration or macular oedema

The visual pathways

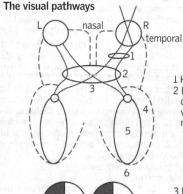

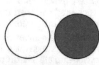

1 R optic nerve lesion
2 Lesion of chiasm—complicated defects depending upon which of the fibres are most affected

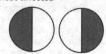

3 Bitemporal hemianopia due to eg pituitary pathology

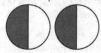

4 Left superior quadrantanopia due to R temporal lobe lesion

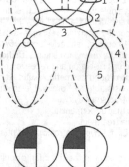

5 Homonymous hemianopia from lesions affecting all R optic radiation or visual cortex

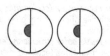

6 L homonymous scotoma due to lesion at tip of R occipital lobe

Fig 4.49 The retina, the optic nerve, the optic chiasma, the optic tracts, the lateral geniculate bodies, the optic radiations, and the visual cortical areas make up the visual pathway. They are all part of the central nervous system. Lesions of many pathological causes in these areas can cause visual impairment.

To maintain single vision, fine coordination of movement of both eyes is necessary (fig 4.50). Abnormality of the coordinated movement is called squint. *Other names for squint: strabismus; eso/exotropia.* Strabismus can have a significant impact on quality of life including finding a partner, job prospects, and interaction with peers.[79] There are 2 broad categories of squint: non-paralytic and paralytic; either can be convergent or divergent and/or vertical.

Non-paralytic squints These usually start in childhood. Squints may be constant or not. All squints need ophthalmological assessment as vision may be damaged, visual development may stop, and the child may become amblyopic if not treated.

Convergent squint (esotropia): One or both eyes turn inward. This is the commonest type in children. Commonly due to hypermetropia (p. 376) or no cause found (idiopathic). It may lead to amblyopia in which the brain suppresses the deviated image, and the visual pathway does not develop normally.

Divergent squint (exotropia): One eye is turned out. Usually in older children, often intermittent.

Diagnosis *Screening tests:*
1 *Corneal reflection:* reflection from a bright light falls centrally and symmetrically on each cornea if no squint, asymmetrically if squint present.
2 *Cover test:* movement of the uncovered eye to take up fixation as the other eye is covered demonstrates manifest squint; latent squint is revealed by movement of the covered eye as the cover is removed (see fig 4.51).

Management Remember 3 'O's: Optical; Orthoptic; Operation. Treatment starts as soon as the squint is noticed. *Optical:* Assess the refractive state after cyclopentolate 1% drops; the cycloplegia allows objective determination of the refractive state; the mydriasis allows a good view into the eye to exclude abnormality eg cataract, macular scarring, retinoblastoma, optic atrophy. Spectacles are then provided to correct refractive errors. *Orthoptic:* Patching the good eye encourages use of the one which squints. Orthoptic review charts progress. *Operations:* (Such as resection and recession of rectus muscles.) These help alignment and give good cosmetic results. NB: use of botulinum toxin in some patients is reasonable and preferable to surgery.[80] Best results are achieved in childhood strabismus by:
• Early detection; if >7yrs old, amblyopia may be permanent.
• Conscientious and disciplined amblyopia treatment.
• Optimal glasses (especially correcting the full hypermetropic prescription in patients with esotropia).[81]

Paralytic squint Diplopia is most on looking in the direction of pull of the paralysed muscle (see table 4.4). When the separation between the two images is greatest the image from the paralysed eye is furthest from the midline and faintest.
• *3rd nerve palsy (oculomotor nerve):* Ptosis, proptosis (as recti tone ↓), fixed pupil dilatation, with the eye looking down and out. *Causes*: p. 366. This is an emergency.
• *4th nerve palsy (trochlear nerve):* There is diplopia and the patient may hold their head tilted (ocular torticollis). Eye movements may look relatively normal but there is a slight upward deviation of the affected eye, and difficulty looking down and in (superior oblique paralysed). *Causes*: trauma 30%, diabetes 30%, tumour, idiopathic.
• *6th nerve palsy (abducens nerve):* There is diplopia in the horizontal plane. The eye is medially deviated with reduction in lateral movement from midline, as the lateral rectus is paralysed. *Causes*: tumour causing ↑ICP (compresses the nerve on the edge of the petrous temporal bone), trauma to base of skull, vascular, or multiple sclerosis. Diabetes is a risk factor.

Table 4.4 Direction of action of the extraocular muscles

Muscle	Primary action	Secondary action
Medial rectus	Adduction (towards nose)	None
Lateral rectus	Abduction (away from nose)	None
Superior rectus	Moves gaze up	Intorsion*
Inferior rectus	Moves gaze down	Extorsion**
Superior oblique	Intorsion*	Moves gaze down
Inferior oblique	Extorsion**	Moves gaze up

* Intorsion = rotates the top of the eye towards the nose.
** Extorsion = rotates the bottom of the eye towards the nose.

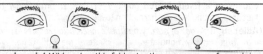

```
              Right eye              Left eye
         SR          IO         IO          SR
           ╲        ╱             ╲        ╱
         LR  ╳  MR              MR  ╳  LR
           ╱        ╲             ╱        ╲
         IR          SO         SO          IR
```

Fig 4.50 The 6 cardinal positions of gaze (from observer's perspective).

Reproduced from Denniston A. and Murray P.I. *Oxford Handbook of Ophthalmology* (2018), with permission from OUP.

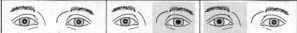

Pseudosquint Wide epicanthic folds give the appearance of a squint in the eye looking towards the nose. That the eyes are correctly aligned is confirmed by the corneal reflection.

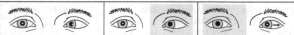

Normal Corneal reflection shows correct alignment. Neither eye moves as they are alternately covered.

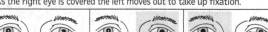

Left convergent squint Corneal reflection shows misalignment. As the right eye is covered the left moves out to take up fixation.

Left divergent squint Corneal reflection shows misalignment. As right eye is covered the left moves in to take up fixation.

Fig 4.51 The *cover test* relies on the ability to fixate. If there is *eccentric fixation* (ie foveal vision is so poor that it is not used for fixation), the deviating eye will not move to take up fixation. Corneal reflection shows that misalignment is present.

Further reading

Denniston A and Murray PI (2018). *Oxford Handbook of Ophthalmology 4th edition*. Oxford: Oxford University Press; pp820–53.

Montgomery TM (2015). *The Extraocular Muscles.* http://www.tedmontgomery.com/the_eye/eom.html

Nield LS *et al.* (2011). *Strabismus: A Close-Up Look.* http://www.pediatricsconsultant360.com/content/strabismus-close-look

Pupil reflexes Light detection by the retina is passed to the brain via the optic nerve (afferent pathway) and pupil constriction is mediated by the oculomotor (3rd) cranial nerve (efferent pathway). The sympathetic nervous system is responsible for pupil dilatation via the ciliary nerves.

Afferent defects (Absent direct response.) The pupil won't respond to light, but constricts to a beam in the other eye (consensual response). Constriction to accommodation still occurs. *Examine with the 'swinging flashlight' test:* (fig 4.52) On beaming light to the normal eye, both pupils constrict (direct & consensual response); if, on swinging the light to the affected eye, the pupil *dilates* it is a *relative afferent pupillary defect* (RAPD). *Causes:* Damage to the optic nerve prevents transmission of light signal to the brain eg optic neuritis, optic atrophy, retinal disease. The pupils are the same size (consensual response unaffected). Compression of the optic nerve can cause a reduction in colour vision (see fig 4.4 p. 325 for examples of Ishihara colour plates).

Efferent defects The 3rd nerve also mediates eye movement and eyelid retraction. With complete palsy there is complete ptosis, a fixed dilated pupil, and the eye looks down (superior oblique still acts) and out (lateral rectus acting). *Causes:* Cavernous sinus lesions, superior orbital fissure syndrome, diabetes, posterior communicating artery aneurysm. The pupil is often spared in vascular causes (diabetes; hypertension). Pupillary fibres are peripheral and are the first affected by compressive lesions eg tumour; aneurysm.

Other causes of a fixed dilated pupil Mydriatics, trauma (blow to iris), acute glaucoma, coning ie uncal herniation (OHCM p830).

Tonic (Adie) pupil *A lack of parasympathetic innervation results in poor constriction to light.* Initially monolateral, then bilateral, pupil dilatation with delayed responses to near vision effort, with delayed redilation. *Typical patient:* A young woman, with sudden blurring of near vision, and a dilated pupil, with slow responses to accommodation, and, especially, to light (looks unreactive). *Slit-lamp exam:* Iris shows spontaneous wormy movements (*iris streaming*). Can be caused by damage to local structures, but most are idiopathic. *Holmes–Adie syndrome:* Tonic pupil, absent knee/ankle jerks, and impaired sweating.[82] The pupil's size may fluctuate, and get smaller than the other (if both pupils are involved they may be confused with Argyll Robertson pupils. See later for other tonic pupils.[6]

Horner syndrome Occurs on disrupting sympathetic fibres, so the pupil is miotic (smaller) with no dilation in the dark and there is partial ptosis. Unilateral facial anhidrosis (sweating ↓) may indicate a lesion proximal to the carotid plexus—if distal, the sudomotor (*sudor* = sweat) fibres will have separated, so sweating is intact. Congenital Horner's includes iris heterochromia (fig 4.8 & 4.9 p.329).

Causes of Horner's
• Posterior inferior cerebellar artery or basilar artery occlusion
• Multiple sclerosis
• Cavernous sinus thrombosis
• Pancoast's tumour
• Hypothalamic lesions
• Cervical adenopathy
• Mediastinal masses
• Pontine syringomyelia
• Klumpke's palsy (p.556)
• Aortic aneurysm

Argyll Robertson pupil Occurs in neurosyphilis and diabetes; there is bilateral miosis, poor pupillary dilation, pupil irregularity, and light-near dissociation (LND, −ve to light +ve to accommodation). Pupil accommodates but does not react to light: 'prostitute's pupil'.

Causes of light-near dissociation Argyll Robertson pupil; Holmes–Adie and Parinaud syndromes;[7] meningitis; alcoholism; tectal lesions, eg pinealoma; mesencephalic or thalamic lesions.[8]

Anisocoria: an emergency?

Anisocoria—unequal pupils—should always be taken seriously. It may herald life-threatening pathology such as an acute CN III palsy secondary to a posterior communicating aneurysm. It may, however, be benign[8]. Physiological anisocoria is present in 20% of people. Additionally anisocoria may arise from previous eye disease/surgery. Identification of the 'normal' side is the first step; is it the small (impaired dilation) or large pupil (impaired constriction) which is abnormal? Sympathetic lesions tend to cause a small pupil, often associated with Horner syndrome. Parasympathetic causes include CN III palsy, drugs, and trauma.

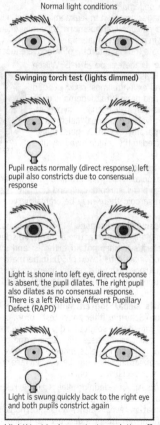

Normal light conditions

Swinging torch test (lights dimmed)

Pupil reacts normally (direct response), left pupil also constricts due to consensual response

Light is shone into left eye, direct response is absent, the pupil dilates. The right pupil also dilates as no consensual response. There is a left Relative Afferent Pupillary Defect (RAPD)

Light is swung quickly back to the right eye and both pupils constrict again

Fig 4.52 'Swinging flashlight' test to demonstrate a relative afferent pupillary defect.

6 Migraine; syphilis; diabetes; chickenpox; arteritis; sarcoid; myasthenia; hamartoma; anti-Hu autoantibodies to neural nuclei; Sjögren's; Meige syndrome; botulism; dermatomyositis; amyloidosis; paraneoplasia.

7 Light near dissociation + nystagmus, upward gaze palsy, and eyelid retraction (Collier's sign).

8 The path from the optic tract to the Edinger–Westphal nucleus is disrupted but deeper cortical connections remain intact, so accommodation is spared.

Systemic disease often manifests itself in the eye and, in some cases, eye examination will first suggest the diagnosis. (See *OHCM* p560.)

Vascular retinopathy This may be *arteriopathic* (*arteriovenous nipping*: arteries nip veins where they cross—they share the same connective tissue sheath) or *hypertensive* (arteriolar vasoconstriction and leakage) producing *hard exudates, macular oedema, haemorrhages*, and, rarely, *papilloedema*. Thick, shiny arterial walls appear like wiring (called 'silver' or 'copper'). Narrowing of arterioles leads to infarction of the superficial retina seen as cotton wool spots and flame haemorrhages. Leaks from these appear as hard exudates ± macular oedema/papilloedema (rare).

Retinal haemorrhages are seen in leukaemia; retinal new vessel formation and comma-shaped conjunctival haemorrhages may occur in sickle cell disease; optic atrophy in pernicious anaemia.

Note also Roth spots (retinal infarcts) of infective endocarditis (*OHCM* p150).

Metabolic disease Diabetes: pp. 370–1. Wilson disease (Kayser–Fleischer ring, fig 4.53). Hyperthyroidism, and exophthalmos: *OHCM* p219. In myxoedema, eyelid and periorbital oedema is quite common. Lens opacities may occur in hypoparathyroidism. Conjunctival and corneal calcification may occur in hyperparathyroidism. In gout, monosodium urate deposited in the conjunctiva may give sore eyes.

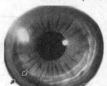

Fig 4.53 Kayser–Fleischer ring.
Courtesy of Jon Miles.

Granulomatous disorders (TB, sarcoid, leprosy, brucellosis, toxoplasmosis.) All produce inflammation in the eye (uveitis). TB, congenital syphilis, sarcoid, CMV, and toxoplasmosis may all produce choroidoretinitis. In sarcoid there may be cranial nerve palsies and lacrimal gland swelling.

Collagen and vasculitic diseases These also cause inflammation. Conjunctivitis is found in SLE and reactive arthritis; episcleritis In polyarteritis nodosa and SLE; scleritis in rheumatoid arthritis; and uveitis in ankylosing spondylitis and reactive arthritis (*OHCM* p550). In dermatomyositis there is orbital oedema & heliotrope rash with retinal haemorrhages. Behçet syndrome causes uveitis & retinopathies. Temporal arteritis leads to ischaemic damage to the optic nerve.

Keratoconjunctivitis sicca/Sjögren syndrome (*OHCM* p710) There is reduced tear formation (Schirmer filter paper test), producing a gritty feeling in the eyes. Decreased salivation also gives a dry mouth (xerostomia). ►It occurs in association with collagen diseases. Pilocarpine and cevimeline help sicca features and topical ciclosporin helps moderate or severe dry eye. Silicone punctal plugs help maintain tears on the eye surface for longer. All these named treatments are specialist use only.

HIV/AIDS *CMV retinitis:* An AIDS-defining illness and is responsible for 40% of cases of loss of vision in HIV⁺ patients. It most commonly occurs when CD4 <50/mm³. Fundus examination reveals either a haemorrhagic retinitis ('pizza pie' appearance), a granular retinitis or a perivascular retinitis. Treatment is with HAART (↑CD4 count) and antivirals such as IV ganciclovir or its prodrug (oral valganciclovir). *HIV retinopathy:* Cotton wool spots, telangiectasia, intraretinal haemorrhages, and venous or arterial occlusions. This is a microvasculopathy rather than a *retinitis*. Candida endophthalmitis is hard to treat. Kaposi's sarcoma (fig 6.43 p. 457) may affect the lids or conjunctiva.[83]

Other causes of retinopathy (*Haemorrhages, microaneurysms, hard exudates.*)[84] Radiation; diabetes; carotid artery disease; central or branch retinal vein occlusion; retinal telangiectasia/Coats disease; Leber's miliary aneurysms; and drugs (p.372).

Pregnancy presents significant physiological changes to the mother which enable her body to cope with the increased demands from the fetus. These changes are usually transient and benign, but can become damaging in the presence of pre-existing pathology.

Physiological changes in the eye

Eyelids don the 'mask of pregnancy'; increased pigmentation, due to hormonal changes, around the eye called chloasma. This is reversible and fades postpartum. Eyes become drier in 80% of women as *tear production* is affected. Women previously unable to tolerate contact lenses may now be able to as *corneal sensitivity* decreases towards the end of pregnancy, but advise them to wait 6 weeks postpartum to get new glasses as corneal refraction may also have changed. On the same note, *lens refraction* may also change subtly. Women with autoimmune eye disease may experience temporary relief as the *immune system* is depressed to facilitate embryo implantation. *Visual field* changes may not always be physiological and warrant further investigation

Pre-existing ocular disease

Glaucoma: Patients may show improvement due to the reduction in IOP—do involve an ophthalmologist in their care as evidence on safety of glaucoma medication in pregnancy is lacking. It is common to avoid β-blockers, prostaglandin agonists, and carbonic anhydrase inhibitors in the first trimester due to potential harms (including teratogenicity); brimonidine may be the safest pharmacological option. Laser treatment or surgical intervention (p. 349) can be offered to minimize reliance on medication.[85]

Diabetic retinopathy: (DR) (See also p. 370.) Pregnancy is a notorious risk factor in worsening the progression of DR, especially for type 1 DM. Other influences include degree of retinopathy at time of conception, glycaemic control, and coexisting hypertension. The pathogenesis is unclear, but likely related to the altered retinal haemodynamics and circulating growth factors/hormones. Proliferative changes develop in ~20% of women; those with pre-existing non-proliferative retinopathy are especially at risk.[86] Laser photocoagulation prior to conception protects against DR progression; counsel patients to pursue this prior to pregnancy if possible. If DR first develops during pregnancy it tends to be less severe; 50% undergo complete regression and 30% partial regression of DR after delivery.[86] NICE guidelines state that all women seeking preconception care should be offered annual retinal assessment. During pregnancy, further assessment should be at the booking clinic, 16–20 weeks (if DR was present at booking clinic), and at 28 weeks. DR is not a contraindication to rapid optimization of glycaemic control.[87]

Ocular involvement in pregnancy-related complications

Pre-eclampsia and eclampsia: (pp. 50-1) Ocular sequelae occur in up to ⅓ of pre-eclampsia and ½ of women with eclampsia. Visual blurring is most common, but scotoma, photopsia, and diplopia are also reported.[88] The majority of women experience complete resolution after delivery, cortical blindness is a rare complication.

Occlusive vascular disorders: Pregnancy is associated with changes to platelets, clotting factors, and haemodynamics generating a hypercoagulable state. Subsequently women are at higher risk of retinal vein/artery occlusion (p. 348), DIC (*OHCM* p352), TTP (*OHCM* p315), amniotic fluid embolism (p. 100), and cerebral venous thrombosis (*OHCM* p480).

Further reading

Denniston A. and Murray (2018). *Oxford Handbook of Ophthalmology 4th edition*. Oxford: Oxford University Press; pp. 794–802.

Schultz KL *et al.* (2005). Ocular disease in pregnancy. *Curr Opin Ophthalmol* 16:308–14.

Somani S (2015). *Pregnancy Special Considerations*. Medscape. https://emedicine.medscape.com/article/1229740-overview

1 in 11 adults have diabetes of whom ½ are undiagnosed, and ⅔ are of working age.[89] Diabetic eye disease is silent until the late stages and as a result it is one of the commonest causes of blindness in the working population.

Diabetic retinopathy *Pathogenesis:* Capillary microangiopathy causes vascular occlusions which lead to ischaemia ± new vessel formation. Ischaemia causes cotton wool spots (ischaemia of nerve fibres), new vessels can form on the retina or disc, which can bleed and cause reduced vision secondary to vitreous haemorrhage. Retraction of fibrous tissue running with new vessels leads to a risk of tractional retinal detachment, which can cause permanent loss of vision. As pericytes are lost, capillaries bulge forming microaneurysms. Fluid leaks from the vessels leading to retinal oedema and hard exudates (deposits of lipoprotein and lipid-filled macrophages). Rupture of microaneurysms causes flame-shaped haemorrhages at the retinal nerve fibre layer (haemorrhage runs parallel to nerve fibres) or blot haemorrhages when rupture occurs deep in the retina. *Classification:* There are essentially 2 levels of diabetic retinopathy, non-proliferative and proliferative, although some grading schemes use the term 'pre-proliferative' to describe more advanced non-proliferative retinopathy. *Non-proliferative diabetic retinopathy (NPDR):* Rated as mild, moderate, or severe depending on the degree of ischaemia. Signs comprise microaneurysms (seen as 'dots'), haemorrhages (flame shaped or 'blots'), hard exudates (yellow patches), engorged tortuous veins, cotton wool spots, large blot haemorrhages (the latter 3 are signs of significant ischaemia). NPDR can progress to sight-threatening proliferative retinopathy. *Proliferative diabetic retinopathy (PDR):* Sufficient ischaemia for fine new vessels to appear on the optic disc and retina. *Diabetic maculopathy:* Leakage from the vessels close to the macula cause oedema and exudates that can significantly threaten vision (clinically significant macular oedema). It can exist with otherwise mild diabetic retinopathy. ►Refer those with maculopathy, severe NPDR, or proliferative retinopathy urgently for assessment and treatment to protect vision. ►*Presymptomatic screening:* Enables timely treatment. Diabetic patients should have their eyes screened at time of diagnosis and at least annually thereafter.[90] Screening is by dilated fundus photography. Referrals are then made accordingly (see BOX 'Results of retinal screening'). Lesions are mostly at the posterior pole and can be easily seen by ophthalmoscopy.

Management ►Pregnancy, dyslipidaemia, ↑BP, renal disease, smoking, and anaemia may accelerate retinopathy. Good control of diabetes prevents new vessels forming and reduces future macro- and microvascular complications. Argon laser photocoagulation is used to treat both maculopathy (focal or grid) and proliferative retinopathy (panretinal photocoagulation). Intravitreal dexamethasone implants & anti-VEGF drugs (p. 353) are used with laser to treat macular oedema. See figs 4.54 & 4.55 and BOX 'Results of retinal screening'.

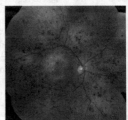

Fig 4.54 Severe non-proliferative diabetic retinopathy.

Reproduced from Sundaram V. et al., *Oxford Specialty Training: Training in Ophthalmology* (2009) with permission from OUP.

Other complications: *The lens:* Accelerated formation of age-related cataract. Younger patients can develop 'snowflake' cataract, or 'osmotic' cataract due to rapid changes in fluid and electrolyte balance (reversible). *The iris:* New blood vessels growing on the iris (rubeosis) can block drainage of aqueous leading to *rubeotic glaucoma*, which can lead to a painful blind eye. *The CNS:* Cranial nerve palsies can occur (typically III and VI). In diabetic CN III the pupil may be spared as fibres to the pupil run peripherally in the nerve, receiving blood supply from the pial vessels. Argyll Robertson and Horner's may also occur (p. 366).

Results of retinal screening: *National Screening Committee* UK *guidelines for when to refer to the Hospital Eye Service*

1 *Maculopathy*—NSC grade 'M1': • Exudate or retinal thickening within one optic disc diameter of the centre of the fovea • Circinate or other group of exudates within the macula • Any microaneurysm or haemorrhage within 1 disc-diameter of the centre of the fovea, if best visual acuity is <6/12.

2 *Pre-proliferative retinopathy*—NSC grade 'R2' (venous beading; venous loops); multiple deep, round, or blot haemorrhages.

3 *Proliferative diabetic retinopathy*—NSC grade 'R3'; presence of new vessels of the disc or elsewhere (urgent treatment within 2 weeks).

Management of diabetic retinopathy Proliferative diabetic retinopathy should be treated within 2 weeks with panretinal (scatter) laser photocoagulation (PRP). This involves treating the peripheral retina which is not receiving adequate blood flow in order to remove the stimulus driving the neovascular process. As this treatment involves many laser applications (eg >1000) it may be divided into ≥2 sessions, although pattern lasers which apply blocks of spot treatment may speed this. NB: panretinal photocoagulation does not improve vision. It is intended to help prevent blindness. It may cause some loss of peripheral field (if severe may preclude driving), colour, and night vision. Some patients get generalized blurring of vision which is usually transient but may persist.

Source: data from National Screening Committee
UK guidelines for when to refer to the Hospital Eye Service

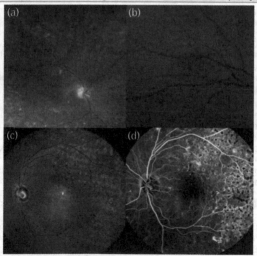

Fig 4.55 (a) Proliferative diabetic retinopathy and previous panretinal photocoagulation. Note blot haemorrhages and new vessels on the inferior temporal arcade. (b) New vessels on the temporal arcades. (c) Multicolour image showing PRP scars in a patient with treated proliferative diabetic retinopathy. (d) Corresponding FFA showing PRP scars in a patient with treated proliferative diabetic retinopathy.

Images (a) and (b) courtesy of Mr Keane and Moorfields Eye Hospital NHS Foundation Trust.;
Images (c) and (d) courtesy of Dr Hina Khan and the Amanat Eye Hospital, Pakistan,
with thanks to Mark Lane for image collection.

4 Ophthalmology

Further reading

Denniston A and Murray PI (2018). *Oxford Handbook of Ophthalmology*. Oxford: OUP; pp794–802.

Free ebook on diabetic retinopathy: www.drcobook.com

Mohamed Q *et al.* (2007). Management of diabetic retinopathy: a systematic review. *JAMA* 298:902–16.

Ockrim Z *et al.* (2010). Managing diabetic retinopathy. *BMJ* 341:c5400.

The eye does not retain drops for as long as ointments and hourly applications may be needed. Eye ointments are well suited for use at night. Allow 5min between doses of drops to prevent overspill. Always consider the manual dexterity of your patients—the elderly may struggle to accurately apply topical medication (eye dropper dispenser tools/applicators are available—speak to a pharmacist).

Common topical eye drops used in ophthalmology

- *Antibiotics:* Chloramphenicol, fusidic acid, neomycin, ofloxacin.
- *Mydriatics:* (=Cycloplegics.) They dilate the pupil. They also cause cycloplegia (paralysis of ciliary muscles), hence blurred near/intermediate vision. ►Warn the patient not to drive. Use 0.5% or 1% tropicamide to dilate the eye 15mins before you wish to examine the fundus; the effect lasts 3–4 hours. These drugs may also be used to prevent synechiae formation in anterior uveitis. The risk of precipitating an attack of angle closure glaucoma is low; the risk of missing pathology because you haven't looked is high.
- *Miotics:* eg pilocarpine. These constrict the pupil and increase drainage of aqueous. They are used in the treatment of acute glaucoma (p. 331).
- *Local anaesthetics:* Proxymetacaine hydrochloride 0.5% is commonly used to allow examination of the eye. An eye pad to occlude the unaffected side may help reduce painful eye movements. Oral analgesia also helps.
- *Steroids and NSAID drops:* Used with care in ophthalmic inflammation and under ophthalmologist guidance for treatment in allergy, episcleritis, scleritis, or iritis. ►Care is needed when using steroid drops as they may increase IOP (beware glaucoma) or induce catastrophic progression of infected corneal ulcers (see p. 373). Ophthalmoscopy may miss corneal ulcers, and slit-lamp inspection is essential if steroid drops are being considered. Some drops have less effect on IOP. Fluorometholone causes less IOP increase than dexamethasone & prednisolone acetate. NSAID drops, eg ketorolac, may obviate the need for some steroid drops and do not affect the IOP.

Systemic drugs that cause ophthalmological issues

- *Dry eyes:* β-blockers, anticholinergics, any eye drop (can affect the tear film).
- *Corneal deposits:* Amiodarone, chloroquine, chlorpromazine.
- *Lens opacities:* Steroids (including high-dose inhaled).
- *Glaucoma:* Steroid drops, mydriatics, & anticholinergics (tricyclics and some Parkinson's drugs).
- *Floppy iris syndrome:* Loss of iris muscle tone leading to poor dilation, fluttering and bellowing of the iris, and a tendency to prolapse during surgery associated with α1-adrenoceptor antagonists such as tamsulosin.
- *Papilloedema:* Raised ICP from eg vitamin A derivatives, tetracyclines, steroids, oral contraceptive pill.
- *Retinopathy:* The following drugs are culprits if used chronically. *Chloroquine* (CQ)/*hydroxychloroquine* (HCQ) can cause (untreatable) retinopathy if high doses are used. Risk of toxicity is increased by excessive daily dose by weight, and increases with continued use. At recommended doses the risk of toxicity up to 5yrs is under 1% and up to 10yrs is under 2%, but it rises to 20% at 20yrs. *Screening schedule:* baseline exam on starting with OCT, autofluorescence, and central visual fields—may contraindicate therapy. Start annual screening at 5yrs (or sooner if there are unusual risk factors). Automated visual fields and spectral domain OCT are recommended for screening.[92]
- *Optic neuropathy: Vigabatrin; ethambutol:* warn patients to report any visual SE (loss of acuity, colour blindness). ~10% report new visual problems, and in 10% of these the cause is optic neuropathy (which may be irreversible).[91] *Isoniazid:* ↓ red-green perception; pyridoxine co-administration prevents this.

Eye drops as a cause of systemic symptoms

Drugs applied to the eye may be absorbed systemically producing SE—eg bronchospasm or bradycardia in susceptible individuals using anti-glaucoma β-blocking drops, eg timolol, carteolol, betaxolol. ►Symptoms may be subtle and insidious—eg gradually decreasing exercise tolerance, or falls from arrhythmias. Serious problems are more likely if there is comorbidity (eg respiratory infection).

Other anti-glaucoma drops (pp. 348–9) cause headaches, and a bitter taste in the mouth; urolithiasis is reported with dorzolamide.

Pilocarpine may cause parasympathetic sweating. Accommodation spasm may lead to brow-ache (worse if <40yrs old, or just starting treatment). Other SE: flu-like syndrome, sweating, urinary frequency; more rarely: urinary urgency, D&V (or constipation ± flatulence), dyspepsia, flushes, ↑BP, palpitations, rhinitis, dizziness, lacrimation, conjunctivitis, visual disturbances, ocular pain, rash, pruritus.

Even highly selective α2-receptor agonists used in glaucoma, eg brimonidine, can cause effects such as dry mouth (in 33% of patients), headache, hypertension, fatigue, and drowsiness.

Steroid eye drops

Be careful when initiating steroid eye drops they can be used for allergic eye disease but are associated with increased ocular pressure (risky in glaucoma patients) and cataract formation. Steroids can potentially prolong the course of viral conjunctivitis by increasing the latency of adenovirus.

►There are disastrous consequences if a corneal ulcer is missed and steroid drops are used as they can accelerate the ulcer causing corneal melt and blindness.

Contact lenses: hygiene and wear tips

See also p. 378.

►Pay attention to contact lens containers, as well as lenses.

Can I reuse my daily disposable contact lenses?

No! Overnight storage in blister-pack saline results in contaminated lenses and infections (esp. staphs and esp. in men). We must educate patients in correct use of contact lenses. Patients should also be advised not to swim or shower wearing contact lenses.

►Do not assume that because a person uses disposable lenses there can be no nasty acanthamoebae infections. These free-living protozoa (found in soil and water, including bathroom tap water) may cause devastating keratitis even with disposable lenses.

• Follow the manufacturer's instructions in how you regularly clean the lens case; tap water should be avoided because of risk of acanthameoba.
• Wash your hands before handling the contact lens container.
• Replace the container at least every 3 months.
• Protozoa may survive new '1-step' solutions of 3% hydrogen peroxide. Amoebae are difficult to treat.
• Follow instructions about getting used to extended wear. Most corneal ulcers from contact lenses are in people who are not used to extended wear and sleep overnight with their contact lenses in, or napped with them on a plane (or elsewhere) for as little as 2–3h.
• Losing the lens within the eye. Hard lenses may be lost in any fornix, soft lenses are usually in upper outer fornix.
• Corneal abrasion is common while adjusting to wear. Pain ± lacrimation occurs some hours after removing the lens.

Xerophthalmia This is dry eyes associated with deficient vitamin A. If left untreated can progress to keratomalacia where the cornea softens, thins, and eventually ulcerates. Blindness can occur. Peak incidence: 2–5yrs; 40 million children worldwide. *Signs:* Night blindness (nyctalopia), tunnel vision, poor acuity, and dry conjunctivae (xerosis). The cornea is unwettable and loses transparency. Small foamy plaques occur, raised from interpalpebral conjunctiva. Vitamin A may reverse changes. *Tests:* Visual fields; dark-adapted electroretinography, plasma vitamin A ↓. R: Just hand out the vitamins? It's not so simple. Every Bitôt spot is a stain on the soul of politics, and as each represents a failure of education and aid, we are all implicated. Examine the cultural web that led to the deficiency, and try to take *whatever* steps are needed to correct it. Improve diet & address associated causes: alcoholism, nutrition, poverty.

Trachoma Caused by *Chlamydia trachomatis* (serotypes A, B, or C). Spread mainly by flies, where it is hot, dry, and dusty and the people are poor, living near cattle. Trachoma is the most common infectious cause of blindness (onchocerciasis is the 2nd, see p. 374-5), 160 million people live in endemic areas.[93] It causes scarring on the inner eye lids (fig 4.56) which directly damages the cornea (fig 4.56), and later causes the eyelid to roll inwards (entropion) so the lashes directly rub on the cornea causing it to scar and ulcerate. *Management:* The WHO has developed the SAFE strategy (Surgery (for trichiasis), Antibiotics, Facial cleanliness, Environmental improvement). WHO recommends either 1 dose of PO **azithromycin** (20mg/kg stat) or **tetracycline** 1% eye ointment both eyes BD for 6 weeks to clear infection.[93] Mass anti-trachoma treatment is initiated in communities where prevalence of follicular trachoma is >10%. There is no point in just treating individuals as reinfection between family members is high. Azithromycin is especially useful as clinics can observe the ingestion of a stat dose, ensuring compliance with eye drops is not as easy. Facial cleanliness and improved sanitation ↓ transmission. *Lid surgery:* Can ↓ progression of corneal scarring and entropion. The WHO trains local health workers to perform bilamellar tarsal rotation operations.

Onchocerciasis (river blindness) (*OHCM* p439.) This is caused by the nematode parasite *Onchocerca volvulus*, transmitted between humans (definitive host) by black flies of the *Simulium species* (vector). Of the 20–50 million people affected, 99% live in Africa. It may cause blindness in up to 40%. Unless the eye is affected, problems are mostly in the skin. Having entered the subcutaneous tissue, larvae mature into adult worms up to 80cm long and mate to produce microfilaria within subcutaneous nodules. Microfilariae then spread to nearby tissues before being ingested by blackfly. Invasion of the conjunctiva, cornea, ciliary body, and iris (rarely retina or optic nerve) can occur. Sometimes they may be seen swimming in the aqueous or dying in the anterior chamber. Microfilariae initially excite inflammation; fibrosis then occurs around them; if in the cornea, corneal opacities (nummular keratitis) occur. Chronic iritis causes synechiae ± cataracts and a fixed pupil. R: See BOX 'Neglected tropical diseases (NTDs)' for the Mectizan Donation Program. **Ivermectin** is the chief microfilaricide but has no effect on adult worms. Give ~150mcg/kg to 200mcg/kg PO stat annually.[94] Give a 3-day course of steroids prior to ivermectin in severe eye involvement. Macrofilariae are adults living in lymphatics.[94] Reports have started to question the rise of resistance to ivermectin.[95,96] A recent clinical trial has shown that a single dose of moxidectin results in a lower microfilarial skin load than a single dose of ivermectin, which may be a promising step towards elimination.[97]

Neglected tropical diseases (NTDs)

In 2005 the WHO identified a list of NTDs which principally impacted the poorest populations and caused significant morbidity and mortality; in sub-Saharan Africa the disease burden may be comparable to TB and malaria in addition to making HIV infection more dangerous.[98] The economic and health impact of ignoring these diseases is huge. These are often debilitating, chronic disease processes with associated stigma (eg leprosy). They are of particular importance in ophthalmology, since 4 key NTDs affect the eyes; trachoma, onchocerciasis, cysticercosis, and Chagas disease. Improving education and school attendance is impossible if students and workers are going blind. Research funding and treatment has been overshadowed by the international focus on the big three named above. It simply wasn't financially viable for pharmacy companies to invest in long trials for medication unlikely to generate financial gain. In recent years, awareness has risen and schemes set in place to encourage treatment for the NTDs where mass drug administration is possible (trachoma, onchocerciasis, lymphatic filariasis (OHCM p421), soil-transmitted helminths, and schistosomiasis), although drug resistance may be becoming a problem. Many of the drugs can be given together, as stat doses, which makes distribution more efficient. Combine praziquantel, ivermectin, and albendazole to treat schistosomiasis, onchocerciasis, and soil-transmitted helminths respectively. Delivery of drugs to a rural community is challenging, not only is infrastructure and funding lacking, but locals may be mistrusting of 'free drugs' and there are significant compliance issues. The leading example of mass drug administration is for onchocerciasis; in 1987 Merck started a remarkable donation programme of ivermectin with a view to eradicate this disease (Mectizan Donation Program[99]) and which has recently extended to include ivermectin as part of the regimen for eliminating lymphatic filariasis.

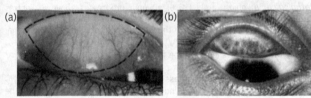

Fig 4.56 Trachoma: (a) dots outline the area to be examined; (b) follicular trachomatous inflammation causes intense inflammation and trachomatous scars (white bands or sheets in the tarsal conjunctiva).

Reproduced from the *Oxford Textbook of Medicine*, with permission from OUP.

Further reading

Utzinger J et al. (2012). Neglected tropical diseases: diagnosis, clinical management, treatment and control. *Swiss Med Wkly* 142:w13727.

World Health Organization: www.who.int

A normal eye will focus light from a distant object onto the retina. If that object is moved closer to the eye the ciliary muscles will relax, the lens will become more convex (curved), the refractive power of the eye will be increased, and the image will be focused on the retina. The loss of this ability with age results in the need for reading glasses (presbyopia). Refractive errors arise when the image is focused in front of (myopia) or behind (hypermetropia) the retina (see fig 4.57).

Myopia (short sightedness) The eyeball is too long, or the refractive surface of the eye is too powerful, so the image of the object falls in front of the retina (unless it is very close). This can be corrected with a concave lens which displaces the image backwards. *Causes:* Genetic.[100] Very close work in the early decades (not just at school) may lead to changes in the synthesis of mRNA and the concentration of matrix metalloproteinase, resulting in myopia. Acetylcholine, dopamine, and glucagon are triggers for eye growth.[101]

In normal growth, changes in eyeball and lens curvature compensate for the eye getting longer as it grows, but in myopic children, such compensations may not be occurring, so myopia worsens with age. Most do not become myopic until the age of ~6yrs (a few are born myopic). Myopia will then usually continue to worsen until the late teens, when changes stop above 6 dioptres in most people. It is important, therefore, for children with myopia to have their eyes regularly checked, as spectacle changes are to be expected, perhaps every 6 months. In later life, increasing myopia may indicate developing cataracts. Myopes are at higher risk of posterior vitreous detachment and retinal detachment (pp. 356-7).

NB: when aboriginal people are exposed to Western education, rates of myopia rise from ~0 to Western levels (eg 50%) and there appears to be a dose-response curve relating hours spent indoors to degree of myopia.[102]

Pathological myopia: Rarely (≤3%), myopia progresses above 6 dioptres (sometimes up to >20 dioptres). This has serious consequences later in life because secondary degeneration of the vitreous and retina can lead to retinal detachment, choroidoretinal atrophy, and macular bleeding.

Management: Concave lenses in the form of spectacles or contact lenses; or refractive surgery (p. 379).

Hypermetropia (long sightedness) The eyeball is too short, or the refractive surface is too weak resulting in the image being focused behind the retina when the eye is at rest. In mild cases when the ciliary muscles contract the lens gets more convex and the refractive power is sufficiently increased to bring the object into focus on the retina. Since accommodation is linked to convergence, this excessive accommodation can be a cause of convergent squint in children.

Management: Convex lenses in the form of spectacles or contact lenses; or refractive surgery (p381).

Astigmatism A common eye condition that occurs when the cornea does not have the same degree of curvature across its surface. This means when light rays strike the cornea, they do not focus together in one point resulting in a blurred image. Correcting lenses compensate accordingly. It can occur alone or be associated with myopia or hypermetropia. Specific causes include trauma, surgery, or keratoconus.

Presbyopia The ciliary muscle reduces tension in the lens, allowing it to get more convex, for close focusing. Young lenses can go from far to near in 0.4sec (going out of focus at ~7cm). With age, the lens stiffens and can't change shape so convex lenses are needed for reading. These changes start in the lens at ~40yrs and are complete by 60.

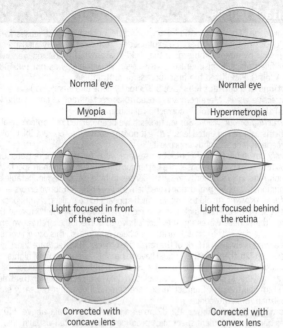

Normal eye

Normal eye

Myopia

Hypermetropia

Light focused in front of the retina

Light focused behind the retina

Corrected with concave lens

Corrected with convex lens

Fig 4.57 Myopia and hypermetropia. Concave lenses can be referred to as 'minus' lenses, convex lenses are referred to as 'plus' lenses.

Further reading

Denniston A and Murray PI (2018). *Oxford Handbook of Ophthalmology 4th edition*. Oxford: Oxford University Press; pp926–9.

Powell C (2005). Screening for correctable visual acuity deficits in school-age children and adolescents. *Cochrane Database Syst Rev* 1:CD005023.

Wojciechowski R (2011). Nature and nurture: the complex genetics of myopia and refractive error. *Clin Genet* 79:301–20.

Leonardo da Vinci first outlined the principle behind contact lenses in his 1508 'Codex of the eye' where he explained a method of directly altering corneal power by either submerging the head in a bowl of water, or wearing a water-filled glass hemisphere over the eye.[103] However it was not until 1888 that Adolf G. Fick fitted the first successful contact lens.

Functions of a contact lens (See p. 373 for hygiene and wear tips.)

- *Corrective vision:* More commonly used to correct refractive error (spherical lens), they also have a role in correction of astigmatism.
- *Correcting colour vision:* Some studies have been carried out on colour-blind patients using a red tinted lens. While it doesn't completely correct their colour perception, it does slightly improve it.[104]
- *Purely cosmetic:* 80% of contact lenses are worn for cosmetic reasons. Only 20% are worn because lenses are better for the eye condition than spectacles. Among this 20% a minority wear the lenses to hide disfiguring inoperable eye conditions, a greater proportion have them for very high refractive errors.
- *Orthokeratology:* An old technique which appears to be making a comeback. It uses gas-permeable contact lenses at night which reshape the cornea so that when the patient wakes up, they don't have to correct their refractive error during the day as the corneal surface has been remoulded. This occurs because the cornea is involved in 60% of the refractive process. Its effects are short lived, averaging 72h, therefore they would have to be worn every couple of nights.
- *Therapeutic:* Contact lenses may be used as 'bandage contact lenses' or increasingly being considered as vehicles to deliver directed ocular treatment eg stem cell therapy. Contact lenses are commonly used in the early stage treatment of keratoconus.

Indications Myopia above −12 dioptres and hypermetropia above +10 dioptres because equivalent spectacles produce quite distorted visual fields.

Types of lens Hard lenses are 8.5–9mm in diameter and are made of polymethylmethacrylate (PMMA). Gas-permeable hard lenses are larger and allow gas to permeate through to the underlying cornea. They can only cope with a limited degree of astigmatism and do not wet as well as standard hard lenses, so may mist up in the day. Soft disposable lenses can be worn during the day for up to 4 weeks. Disposable contact lenses are now more common for convenience and lower risk of ocular infections.

Complications CLARE: Contact Lens-Induced Red Eye reaction typically presents as an acute inflammatory response of the anterior segment of the eye defined by severe conjunctival and circumlimbal hyperaemia. It is very common to see both diffuse and focal subepithelial infiltrates.[105] *Keratoconjunctivitis* or *giant papillary* change in the upper tarsal conjunctiva, possibly due to sensitization to the cleansing materials used, or to the mucus which forms on the lens (fig 4.17). *Sensitivities:* Cleaning solutions made by different manufacturers should not be mixed. The storage solution should be washed off before the lens is inserted. Soft contact lenses, being permeable, tend to absorb chemicals, so weaker cleaning agents are used. Sensitivity to cleaning agents usually presents as redness, stinging, ↑ lens movement, ↑ mucus production, and thickened lids. It may be necessary to stop wearing lenses for several months. *Infection:* It is always imperative that when taking an eye history, you ascertain if the patient wears contact lenses as it hugely increases the risk of corneal infections and the susceptibility to specific organisms. Acanthamoeba infection is 10× more likely in contact lens wearers and is most likely if contact lenses are over used, not cleaned properly, worn while sleeping or swimming (peak incidence of infection is in the summer months). Clinical presentation is variable, leading to the diagnosis often being missed until infection is well established which can result in loss of vision, or the eye.

Further reading

Denniston A and Murray PI (2018). *Oxford Handbook of Ophthalmology 4th edition*. Oxford: Oxford University Press; pp936–45.

Juárez MM *et al.* (2018). Acanthamoeba in the eye, can the parasite hide even more? Latest developments on the disease. *Cont Lens Anterior Eye* 41:245–51.

4 Ophthalmology

Refractive procedures

Refractive procedures are increasingly undertaken as an alternative to wearing spectacles; mostly for cosmetic reasons. Occasionally they are undertaken for anisometropia (imbalance of prescriptions); for astigmatism after surgery; or for intolerance of spectacles or contact lenses. LASIK (see later) is now the most common procedure. Modern refractive surgery is associated with good outcomes and with a low rate of complications, but there are possible complications and it is certainly not suitable for everyone. It should be noted that most ophthalmologists wear spectacles! The following provides an outline of some of the commonest techniques.

Corneal techniques

LASIK (Laser-Assisted In Situ Keratomileusis):
- *Indication*: myopia (+6DS to –12DS of myopia with up to 5D cyl of astigmatism).
- *Procedure*: this is a 'flap-based' technique in which a partial thickness superficial corneal flap is created with a microkeratome or femtosecond layer, the stroma is selectively ablated with an excimer laser and then the flap replaced.
- *Outcome*: it is relatively painless, settles quickly, and is fairly predictable in its outcome. Corneal sensitivity recovers after ~6 months.[106] Serious complications are rare but trauma to or infection of the flap may result in permanent corneal scarring. The improved acuity tends to wane over time[107] and does not overcome the problem of presbyopia (ie they may still need reading glasses). Intraocular pressure often falls (eg by 4mmHg).

PRK (Photorefractive Keratectomy):
- *Indication*: +6DS to –12DS of myopia with up to 5D cyl of astigmatism.
- *Procedure*: this is a 'surface ablation' technique in which the epithelium is removed, the stroma selectively ablated with excimer laser, before insertion of a bandage contact lens.
- *Outcome*: it is less predictable than LASIK. Corneal haze with reduced vision, glare, and haloes are occasional problems. In most low myopes it gives good outcome but it is very painful for a few days.

LASEK (Laser-Assisted Sub-Epithelial Keratectomy):
- *Indication*: +6DS to –12DS with up to 5D cyl of astigmatism.
- *Procedure*: this is a 'surface ablation' technique in which the epithelium is removed as a sheet using alcohol, the stroma selectively ablated with excimer laser, before insertion of a bandage contact lens.

SMILE (SMall Incision Lenticule Extraction):
- *Indication*: –1DS to –10DS with up to 5D cyl of astigmatism.
- *Procedure*: an intrastromal lenticule is created with a femtosecond laser, as is a small exit channel. Surgical instruments are used to remove the lenticule of corneal stroma through the exit channel. There is no flap.

Lens techniques

Phakic IOL insertion:
- *Indication*: typically for high myopia (≥10DS); sometimes used where corneal techniques are contraindicated.
- *Procedure*: the insertion of a prosthetic intraocular lens, while leaving the original lens in place.

Refractive lens exchange:
- *Indication*: typically for higher refractive error, especially in older patients or where corneal techniques are contraindicated.
- *Procedure*: identical to modern cataract surgery but with the removal of the normal lens. Accommodation is lost, so reading needs correction.

Further reading

Denniston A and Murray PI (2018). *Oxford Handbook of Ophthalmology 4th edition*. Oxford: Oxford University Press; pp946–75.

NICE (2006). Photorefractive (laser) surgery for the correction of refractive errors (IPG164). London: NICE.

4 Ophthalmology

4 Ophthalmology

Registration Approximately 360,000 people are registered partially sighted or blind in the UK. It is estimated that a total of 2 million people are living with visual impairment. Blindness may be voluntarily registered in England, making one eligible for certain concessions. Visual acuity levels take into account both level of acuity and degree of field loss. *Criteria for sight impaired ('partially sighted') registration:* Acuity is <6/60 (or >6/60 with visual field restrictions). *Criteria for severely sight impaired (blind) registration:* Acuity <3/60 with a full visual field, or >3/60 but with substantial visual field loss (as in advanced glaucoma).[108]

Why register? In England, responsibility for blind registration lies with the local authority. Application is made by a consultant ophthalmologist and is voluntary, not statutory. The register is confidential. Registration as blind entitles one to extra tax allowances, 50% reduction in TV licence fees, some travel concessions, and access to audio books. It does not automatically entitle patients to welfare benefits, but it does make it easier for them to claim. Special certification from an ophthalmologist is necessary for the partially sighted to receive talking books. At one time it was statutory that the registered blind should receive a visit from a social worker but this is no longer the case, although the social services employ social workers who specialize in care of the blind. The Royal National Institute of Blind People[109] will advise on aids, such as guide dogs.

Living with blindness and partial sight This can be socially isolating and challenging. Getting back to work and finding suitable employment and education requires a lot of motivation and support. The elderly are at high risk of falls. People value vision very highly. One review has suggested that people with 6/9–6/12 vision would be willing to pay 19% of their lifetime to get back normal visual acuity. Patients with 6/60 visual acuity will give up 48% of their lifetime, and blind people would release 60%. DVLA: see p. 807.[110]

If patients have severe bilateral sight loss, ask specifically about whether they are getting visual hallucinations (often of faces). These occur without psychiatric signs and are often related to failing vision in the elderly: Charles Bonnet syndrome (see BOX 'Seen, unseen, and seer—and the indifferent pixel', p. 355).[111]

Use of services by older patients with failing vision

There is good evidence in the UK of underuse of services by older people. Population-based cross-sectional studies in primary care show that prevalence of bilateral visual impairment (acuity <6/12) is ~30%. Most of these are not in touch with ophthalmic services. ►Three-quarters of these have remediable problems. In one study, 20% had acuity in one or both eyes of <6/60. Typical causes were found to be cataract (30%), macular degeneration (8%), and undiagnosed chronic glaucoma.[112] Despite the good availability of NHS-funded eye examinations for many people (including all those >60 years), many of these patients in the UK do not engage in these free services. Efforts need to focus on raising public understanding regarding the purpose of eye examinations in terms of other causes of preventable sight loss (such as diabetes or glaucoma).[113]

Further reading
Read about Helen Keller—a remarkable story about deafness and blindness. https://www.britannica.com/biography/Helen-Keller

Common causes of blindness in the world

'An eye for an eye only ends up making the whole world blind.' Mahatma' Gandhi

The pattern of blindness around the world differs considerably. 90% of the world's blind live in developing countries—and 80% would not be blind if trained eye personnel, medicines, ophthalmic equipment, and patient referral systems were optimized.[114] Global estimates of visual impairment in 2010 report that 285 million people are visually impaired (visual acuity <6/18, ≥3/60) of whom 39 million are blind (visual acuity <3/60). The global distribution of blindness is as follows; China (20.9%), India (20.5%), Africa (15%), Eastern Mediterranean (12.5%), South East Asia (10.1%), Americas (8%), Europe (7%), Western Pacific (6%).[115]

Global causes of visual impairment including blindness

(As a percentage of total global visual impairment.)[115]

1 Uncorrected refractive errors (42%)
2 Cataract (33%)
3 Glaucoma (2%)
4 Age-related macular degeneration (1%)
5 Diabetic retinopathy (1%)
6 Corneal opacities (1%)
7 Trachoma (1%)
8 Childhood causes (1%)
9 Undetermined (18%)

Global causes of blindness

(As a percentage of total global blindness.)[115]

1 Cataract (51%)
2 Glaucoma (8%)
3 Age-related macular degeneration (5%)
4 Corneal opacity (4%)
5 Refractive error (3%)
6 Trachoma (3%)
7 Diabetic retinopathy (1%)
8 Undetermined (21%)

Causes of avoidable blindness in the least developed countries	Causes of blindness in developed countries
1 Cataract	1 Cataract
2 Glaucoma	2 Age-related macular degeneration
3 Corneal opacities	3 Glaucoma
4 Trachoma	4 Diabetic retinopathy
5 Childhood blindness	
6 Onchocerciasis	

The most common cause of irreversible blindness and partial sight in developed countries is age-related macular degeneration. In patients of working age, diabetic retinopathy is the leading cause in the West.

Over the past 20yrs there have been significant efforts by the WHO to decrease visual impairment worldwide; especially in reducing the disease burden of onchocerciasis and trachoma-related blindness.

Causes of blindness in the UK have changed considerably over the last 70yrs. Whereas in the 1920s ophthalmia neonatorum (p. 41) was responsible for 30% of blindness in English blind schools, this is now a rare but treatable disease. Retinopathy of prematurity was common in the 1950s,[116] monitoring of intra-arterial oxygen in premature babies tries to prevent this.[117]

The prevalence of sight loss and blindness in the UK is estimated to have increased by 7.5% since 2008. This, in addition to an ageing population means that the estimated number of people with sight loss within the UK is expected to increase to 4.1 million by 2050.[118]

3D bioprinting Corneal transplantation restores vision in patients with severe corneal scarring. Worldwide, the demand for donor corneas outweighs the supply. Research is currently under way to print a 3D bio-cornea which could be tailor-made to fit each patient's eye. This would revolutionize the world of corneal transplant surgery improving availability of tissue and refractive outcomes.[119]

The bionic eye The bionic eye has historically been considered as science fiction; however, over the past years significant advances have been made towards making the restoration of vision a clinical reality. These devices target various components of the visual pathway (see p. 362); specifically the cortex, subcortex, optic nerve, and retina. Retinal devices are especially beneficial for degenerative retinal diseases such as retinitis pigmentosa (p. 354), for which there is no current cure. The Argus II® is a retinal implant that has been approved by the FDA and EMA (fig 4.58). It is approved for adults with profound retinitis pigmentosa who have previously had some useful vision but currently minimal or no vision in both eyes. The device consists of a small video camera mounted on a pair of glasses worn by the patient. A small computer processes the images and sends the information back to the glasses via a cable. The information is then transmitted wirelessly from the glasses to a pre-inserted retinal implant which stimulates the retina's remaining cells to create perceptions of light. Watch the videos of the experimental outcomes at www.2-sight. com. Learning to interpret the patterns of light with the retinal implant takes time and currently technology enables patients to simply gain an appreciation of light flashes to detect motion. The visual outcomes so far are basic, but represent significant progress.[120,121] More recently the Orion® Cortical Visual Prosthesis System, a cortical implant which uses the same device to stimulate the visual cortex directly, has qualified for the FDA's voluntary breakthrough programme.[122] With the potential to bypass the optic nerve this device may provide help to end-stage glaucoma patients.

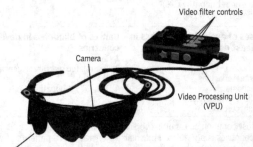

Fig 4.58 The Argus II™ system.

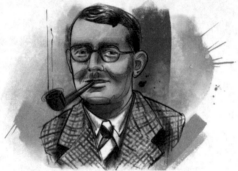

Fig 5.1 Ronald Macbeth was appointed as the first ENT surgeon to the Radcliffe Infirmary, Oxford in 1932. The initial years were hard—in just one night in 1935, during a serious outbreak of group A β-haemolytic streptococci, Macbeth undertook five acute cortical mastoid operations in the primitive conditions of a school sanatorium. By 1937 he had formed a fully equipped department and in 1941 was the first ENT surgeon to infuse penicillin into infected mastoid cavities, seeing remarkable recoveries in the treatment group. He helped inspire the Macintosh laryngoscope blade (working with anaesthetist Sir Robert Macintosh) and was the first British surgeon to inject sclerosant into oesophageal varices caused by portal hypertension. He described the definitive surgical method for frontal sinus obliteration (of which his name is still associated) and together with Esme Hadfield showed a conclusive link between hardwood dust and the development of adenocarcinoma of the sinuses in furniture workers. Macbeth had an amazing career which covered a vast array of subspecialty interests. Allow his interest in teaching and learning, his passion for international collaboration, and his energy and enthusiasm to inspire you to ask questions, to share your knowledge with others and to introduce new ideas.[1]

Artwork by Gillian Turner.

With many thanks to our junior reader Hassan Maimouni for their contribution to this chapter.

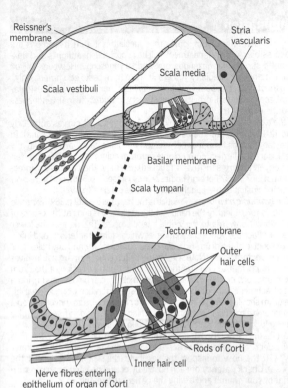

Reissner's membrane

Stria vascularis

Scala vestibuli

Scala media

Scala tympani

Basilar membrane

Tectorial membrane

Outer hair cells

Rods of Corti

Inner hair cell

Nerve fibres entering epithelium of organ of Corti

Fig 5.2 A cross-section of the cochlea. The basilar membrane is stiffer at the broad, outer end, so different frequencies peak at different positions along it. Hearing and balance rely on the ability of hair cells to sense tiny mechanical stimuli. Outer hair cells are actively motile structures that feed energy into the vibration of the inner ear and enhance sensitivity to sound and movement. The sounds they produce are called otoacoustic emissions (OAEs). Detecting OAE is a good test of a healthy inner ear and is used in neonatal screening tests. OAES and other hair cell functions are impaired by various types of hereditary deafness, syndromic hearing loss, and inner ear disease (eg Ménière disease).

From the index... ENT emergencies

Examination in ENT differs from some other specialties in that its regions are rather inaccessible. An ENT department will have portable headlights and flexible fibre-optic scopes for nasendoscopy and laryngoscopy. However, if you are working in another specialty you are likely to have basic equipment only.

The ear *Inspect:* Pinna (p.388); any deformity? Look for *scars*—postauricular or endaural scars suggest previous ear surgery. *Palpate:* Tragal tenderness points to otitis externa (p.392).

Examine the external auditory canal (EAC): Anatomically it curves anteriorly and inferiorly. In adults, pull the pinna up and back to straighten the canal. In infants, the canal bends forwards only, so pull the pinna backwards. Swab any discharge. Insert the largest comfortable aural speculum (don't probe too far, the inner bony ⅔ is very sensitive if touched). Examine the canal. Any infection/inflammation? Wax? Foreign bodies? Or exostoses? (p.388). NB: there may be complete occlusion of the canal in severe otitis externa (p.392).

Examine the tympanic membrane: Practice is the key (figs 5.6–5.12 p.389). Examine the quadrants in turn. Identify the handle of the malleus, this ends at the centre of the drum. Follow it upwards to the visible lateral process. This defines the lower limit of the pars flaccida. Notice the light reflex which radiates anteriorly and inferiorly from the centre of the drum. Note the colour, translucency, and any bulging or retraction. Any **perforations**? (Note size; position; site: central or marginal, involves the annulus?) Important to visualize the pars flaccida or attic region of the drum to look for retractions or cholesteatoma. Drum mobility can be assessed using a pneumatic attachment. Lack of movement suggests perforation or middle ear effusion (the drum should move with changes in EAC pressure). Drum movement on a Valsalva manoeuvre means a functional Eustachian tube. Consider: free field voice testing; tuning forks (see BOX 'Free field voice testing & tuning forks').

The nose (Testing smell is often omitted, but often fascinating.[1]) Sit face to face. Inspect the external nose: skin, size, shape, scars? Deviations? Deformity? Lift the nose to inspect the vestibule (the skin-lined cavity of the anterior nose). Check patency of each nostril by occluding each nostril in turn with the flat of your thumb and asking the patient to breathe in.

Inspect the nose internally: Assess mucosa and septum (Is it straight? Any bleeding points, crusting, or perforations?). Assess the size of the inferior turbinates (are they hypertrophied? Do they have a blue tinge?). Any nasal polyps visible (see p.407)? The inferior & middle turbinates, and the space beneath them (the inferior & middle meatus), along with the Eustachian tube and postnasal space can be examined with a *Thudicum's speculum*.

Examination of the posterior nose: Using a nasendoscope ± LA/decongestant spray. Check middle meatus (site of drainage of frontal, ethmoid, and maxillary sinuses) for obstruction, pus, polyps. The postnasal space (nasopharynx) containing the Eustachian tube orifice may contain adenoids or nasopharyngeal cancer in a lateral space behind Eustachian cushion (fossa of Rosenmüller). A postnasal mirror can be used to examine the nasopharynx via the oral cavity. Examine the palate—it is the floor of the nose.

The throat (fig 5.3) • Position yourself as for nasal examination; remove any dentures • Inspect lips and perioral region. Ask the patient to open their mouth without protruding the tongue. Use a tongue depressor and a headlight to assist in performing a thorough examination of the oral cavity. Inspect the buccal mucosa, the parotid duct opening (opposite the upper 2nd molar), gums, teeth, floor of the mouth, and the retromolar trigone (mucosa behind the 3rd molar over the ramus of the mandible—also known as 'coffin corner' as lesions are easily missed) • Depress the tongue; say 'ah then aye' (checks palate movement and exposes more mucosa). Check gag reflex bilaterally. Is uvula elongated? • Examine the tonsils (deep crypts with debris can be normal) • Put on a glove for bimanual examination of any oral lesion • Palpate the floor of the mouth (any submandibular gland stones or masses?).

Cardinal ear symptoms	Cardinal nose symptoms	Cardinal throat symptoms
• Ear pain/discharge: pp. 390–395	• Nasal congestion: p. 406	▶▶ Stridor: pp. 416–17
• Hearing loss: pp. 400–1	• Epistaxis: pp. 412–13	• Hoarseness: p. 418
• Tinnitus/vertigo: pp. 402–405		• Dysphagia: p. 420
		• Neck lumps: p. 426

Prevalence of ENT symptoms

In a UK study of >15k people, ~20% report current hearing troubles eg difficulty with speech in background noise; 20% report tinnitus lasting >5 minutes. ~15% report hayfever in the last year and 31% had severe sore throat/tonsillitis. ~21% report ever having had dizziness (things spinning around them) and 13% reported dizziness in which they seemed to move.[2]

Free field voice testing & tuning forks

Free field testing Examiner stands behind seated patient + speaks into test ear while rubbing tragus to mask sounds in non-test ear. Tests ear until 50% words identified. Whisper at 60cm then 15cm. Conversational voice at 60cm then 15cm. Loud voice at 60cm. Hearing loss normal <30dB (hears whisper at 60cm), moderate 30–70dB (whisper at 15cm –conversation at 15cm) and severe >70dB.

Phone apps Can mimic free field testing.

Tuning fork tests These tests are popular in exams! Use a 512Hz tuning fork. (Lower frequencies stimulate vibration sensation.) Activate by tapping elbow or knee. Rinne and Weber tests are performed together as a 'package' to help identify the type of hearing loss. Tragal rub for masking to avoid false-negative Rinne's test.

Weber test Place the activated tuning fork on the vertex or forehead. Patient localizes sound to left, right, or midline. Sound localizes to the affected ear with conductive hearing loss, and to the contralateral ear in sensorineural hearing loss (SNHL), and to the midline if both ears are normal (or there is bilateral SNHL).

Modified Rinne test Place activated tuning fork behind the ear against the mastoid process (tests bone conduction), then move to 2cm from the external auditory meatus (tests air conduction). Tips of tines of fork parallel to EAC. Ask 'Which is louder?' Positive test: air conduction is better than bone (=normal or SNHL). Negative test: bone conduction is better than air conduction (=conductive deafness). False-negative test: bone conduction is being detected in opposite ear with sound travelling across skull. Blocked by masking opposite ear with a tragal rub.

▶If tuning fork tests suggest SNHL in sudden hearing loss refer the same day (p. 400).

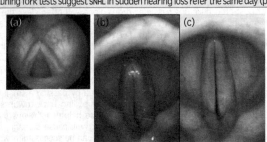

Fig 5.3 Vocal cords abducted for inspiration (a) and adducted for low- (b), and high-pitch phonation (c). NB: elongation to raise pitch is done by the cricothyroid muscle.

Courtesy of James Thomas.

1 *Sweat, darkness, dirt, and lust.* Smells are as hard to name as emotions: when we are told by a novelist or a chef, we say 'Yes: that's it!' Smells and emotions go hand in hand with memory. When we re-smell the smells of youth we are transported back to that moment. In his novel *À la recherche du temps perdu*, Proust describes a character vividly recalling long-forgotten childhood memories after smelling a tea-soaked madeleine biscuit.

The external ear (fig 5.5). The pinna is fibroelastic cartilage, covered by skin. The ear drum (figs 5.4 & 5.6) is set obliquely, the external auditory canal is ~3cm. The canal's outer ⅓ is cartilage, having hairs and ceruminous (wax) glands in the skin; its inner ⅔ is bony and lined with sensitive skin.

Congenital anomalies The pinna develops from 6 hillocks derived from the 1st and 2nd branchial arches that appear at 4–6wks, with the intervening 1st branchial groove forming the external auditory canal. Any malfusion may give rise to accessory tags/auricles or a preauricular pit, sinus, or fistula. An infected sinus may be mistaken for an infected sebaceous cyst, but there is often a deep branching subcutaneous tract. It can be removed to avoid further infection.
►Auricular anomalies are frequently associated with middle ear anomalies.

Chondrodermatitis nodularis helicis This Latin term describes an exquisitely tender, cartilaginous, inflamed nodule dwelling on the upper helix or antihelix (fig 5.5). It is commoner in men working outdoors and (legendarily) wimple-wearing nuns. *Cause:* Unknown. ?Poor blood flow (avascular chondritis) from prolonged pressure; or vasoconstriction from cold. The affected side is usually the one on which the patient lies. *R:* Relieve pressure. If not helpful, excise skin and underlying cartilage (eg 'wide excision' or 'deep shave').[3]

Pinna haematoma Blunt trauma may cause bleeding in the subperichondrial plane elevating the perichondrium to form a haematoma. *R:* Arrange incision of the haematoma with primary closure (+ packing, to prevent accumulation). Aspiration is rarely adequate due to the thickness of the clot. Poor treatment leads to ischaemic necrosis, then fibrosis (cauliflower ear, p. 546). Secondary infection may cause major loss of cartilage; cover with antibiotics (eg ciprofloxacin).

Auditory exostosis (surfer's ear) These are smooth, multiple, bilateral swellings of the bony canals that represent local bone hypertrophy from cold exposure. *Symptoms:* None, so long as the lumen is sufficient for sound conduction (they are often picked up incidentally). If they hinder migration of wax or debris, occlude the canal to cause conductive deafness, or there is recurrent infection, surgical removal is indicated. Osteomas (p. 505) are usually solitary.

Wax (cerumen) Cerumen is the natural protective wax produced and secreted in the outer ⅓ of the canal. The amount of wax produced varies greatly from person to person. Excess wax may become impacted causing dulled hearing and a feeling of fullness in the ear ± tinnitus. Due to epithelial migration, the ear is self-cleaning; cotton buds are unnecessary. *R:* Optimal treatment for wax removal is suction under direct vision using a microscope. Irrigation (syringing) usually works too eg after softening with olive oil or bicarbonate drops. Warn of post-procedure dizziness. Ear drops alone will often clear the wax. Instil the drops while lying with the affected ear uppermost. Pour in a few drops 2–3 times each day for 3–7 days. ►Avoid irrigation if the drum is perforated; if grommets (or within 1½yrs); cleft palate; or after mastoid surgery. *Complications:* Pain; otitis externa; vertigo (0.2%); perforated drum (≤0.2%).

Ear foreign bodies (FBs) FBs are most common in children. There are many possible methods of removal. Soft FBs (eg cotton wool) may be grasped with crocodile forceps. Solid FBs are best removed by passing a small blunt wax hook beyond the object then rotating and pulling back towards you. Microsuction attachments for FB removal can be helpful ►*Always use instrumentation under direct vision.* Blind probing will cause damage. Avoid pushing objects deeper into the canal. *Irrigation* can be successful if you are sure there is no trauma to the ear canal or drum. Flapping insects can be killed with olive oil. The first attempt at FB removal will usually be the best tolerated. Difficult patients (eg children; the anxious) are best referred to ENT directly, without inexpert attempts at removal. This will increase the chance of successful removal with few complications.[4]

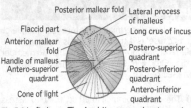

Posterior mallear fold Lateral process
                        of malleus
Flaccid part   Long crus of incus
Anterior mallear
fold   Postero-superior
Handle of malleus   quadrant
Antero-superior   Postero-inferior
quadrant   quadrant
Cone of light   Antero-inferior
                        quadrant

Fig 5.4 Left drum. The 4 arbitrary quadrants are indicated by solid lines and by the handle of the malleus. The light reflex points to the feet.

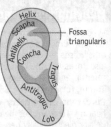

Helix
Scapha
Antihelix   Concha   Fossa
                          triangularis
            Tragus
Antitragus
      Lob

Fig 5.5 The pinna.

Fig 5.6 Normal right
drum. If only patients
could see how beautiful
and delicate the drum
is, amateur instrumen-
tation of the ear would
be far less common!
Courtesy of Nicholas
Steventon FRCS.

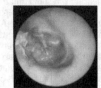

Fig 5.7 The right drum has *retracted*, as has the handle of
the malleus (appears short).
The lateral process will also
become more prominent than
normal. The long process of
the incus has eroded.
Courtesy of Nicholas
Steventon FRCS.

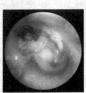

Fig 5.8 (Right drum.)
This crust in the
attic represents a
large underlying
cholesteatoma.
Courtesy of Nicholas
Steventon FRCS.

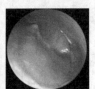

Fig 5.9 The (right) drum
is opaque. There is
prominence of blood
vessels suggesting a
middle ear effusion. This
is one of several appear-
ances of glue ear.
Courtesy of Nicholas
Steventon FRCS.

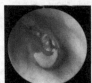

Fig 5.10 (Right drum.)
White patches are usually *tympanosclerosis* (calcium deposits)
eg after infection or trauma.
They are often of no significance; if severe, can cause
mild conductive hearing loss.
Courtesy of Nicholas
Steventon FRCS.

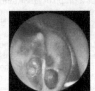

Fig 5.11 (Right drum.)
Posterior retraction revealing
head of stapes and erosion
of long process of the incus.
Posterior retractions/per-
forations may signify serious
underlying disease, but this
one is dry, and its posterior
margin is defined. Traumatic
perforations (eg barotrauma)
are often posterior and linear,
like a tear rather than a hole.
Courtesy of Nicholas
Steventon FRCS.

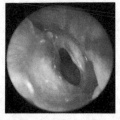

Fig 5.12 *Anterior perforation* of the right tympanic
membrane. These images may look surprisingly
clear: this is because they were taken through a
Hopkins rod, rather than an otoscope.
Courtesy of Nicholas Steventon FRCS.

When assessing suspected hearing loss, determine its nature (conductive or sensorineural), its severity, and its cause: is it treatable, and is it part of some other disease process—eg unilateral SNHL in acoustic neuroma? Remember also to assess the degree of disability. ►If sudden sensorineural deafness, refer urgently (same day) to ENT (see p. 400).

Tuning fork test See p. 387.

Pure tone audiometry (PTA) The most common method used to assess hearing. It quantifies hearing loss and determines its nature. Headphones deliver electronically generated tones at different sound pressure levels over frequencies of 250–8000Hz in a sound-proofed room. Air-conducted sound is initially played above the hearing threshold and then decreased in 10dB increments until it is no longer heard. The sound intensity is then increased in 5dB increments until a 50% response rate is obtained. A bone conduction threshold is also obtained by using a transducer over the mastoid process. NB: masking (=narrowband noise to the untested ear) prevents cross-stimulation of the non-test ear. The results are recorded on a chart, with frequency (in Hz) on the x-axis and decibels hearing level (dBHL = deviation from normal) on the y-axis—see figs 5.14-5.20. See also BOX "The bounds of 'normal' hearing", p. 401.

Tympanometry (acoustic impedance audiometry) An objective way of measuring pressure in the middle ear and establishing the cause of conductive deafness. *Principles:* Admittance of sound to the middle ear is greatest when the air pressure in the EAC is the same as the middle ear space. So the peak of the tympanometry curve, which measures admittance, reflects middle ear pressure. *Procedure:* A probe with an airtight seal is introduced into the meatus; it measures the amount of a 226Hz sound signal which is reflected back off the tympanic membrane as the pressure of air in the EAC is varied. It generates a graph of admittance (fig 5.13). *Results:* A normal ear (middle ear space filled with air; ossicles intact) will show a normal peak with normal compliance (TYPE A, PURPLE).If there is disruption of the ossicular chain, or if part of the drum is flaccid, a large amount of energy will be absorbed into the drum which is free to move a lot—and it will move most when canal pressure = middle ear pressure (high compliance; TYPE AD, RED). Fluid in the middle ear is incompressible. The admittance will not vary and the tympanogram is flat (low compliance, TYPE B, GREEN). TYPE C (BLUE): shift in peak of the curve to the left found with negative middle ear pressure eg as in developing or resolving otitis media and Eustachian tube dysfunction. Ear canal volume is indirectly calculated by the tympanometer: if normal ≈ otitis media; if low ≈ wax occlusion; if high ≈ grommets or perforation.[5]

Speech audiometry (In conjunction with PTA) assesses speech discrimination (how well speech is understood and heard)—measured as a percentage.

Otoacoustic emissions (OAEs) Used to assess function of the cochlea by recording sound vibration produced by the outer hair cells in the cochlea. It is most commonly used in neonatal screening (see p. 398).

Auditory brainstem responses (ABRs) Record electrical activity along the auditory pathway in response to a sound stimulus (see p. 398).

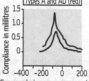
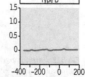
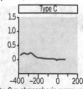

Ear canal air pressure—as set by the tympanometer in decapascals (daPa; 0 = atmospheric pressure)

Fig 5.13 Acoustic impedance audiometry (tympanometry).

Courtesy of Jane Jones, Oxford Radcliffe Hospitals NHS Trust.

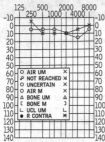

Fig 5.14 Normal hearing. © C Potter.

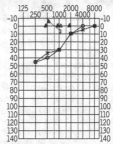

Fig 5.15 Bilateral middle ear congestion (air–bone gap due to conductive loss).
© C Potter.

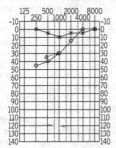

Fig 5.16 Right-sided Ménière's (p. 404). Hearing loss is low frequency.
© C Potter.

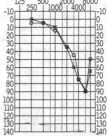

Fig 5.17 Noise-induced hearing loss (p. 403). Audiometric notch at 4kHz. © C Potter.

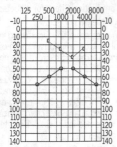

Fig 5.18 Right-sided otosclerosis, with Carhart's notch at 2kHz on masked bone conduction. © C Potter.

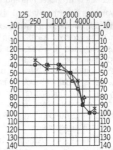

Fig 5.19 Typical presbycusis—bilateral, symmetrical, high-frequency SNHL. © C Potter.

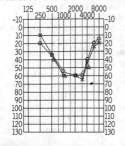

Fig 5.20 Cookie-bite loss: as if someone took a bite out of the top of the audiogram (isolated mid-range hearing loss). It is likely to be hereditary. Test siblings. Referral to a geneticist may be indicated. © C Potter.

Abbreviations:
Right ear (red)
Left ear (blue)
m = masked
um = unmasked
►See also p. 401 'normal hearing'.

5 ENT

The cause is often non-otological (in 50%); look for sources of referred pain (BOX 'Referred otalgia') eg throat and teeth: *does grinding/tapping hurt?*— see pp. 430-1.

Otitis externa (OE) Discharge, itch, pain, and tragal tenderness due to acute inflammation of the skin of the meatus, usually caused by excess canal moisture. Other causes: trauma eg fingernails (from itchy conditions eg eczema/ psoriasis); high humidity; absence of wax (from self-cleaning); a narrow ear canal; and hearing aids. *Pseudomonas* is the chief organism, though *Staphylococcus aureus* is another common offender. ΔΔ: Contact eczema.

• *Mild OE:* Scaly skin with some erythema. Normal diameter of external auditory canal (EAC). ℞: for all OE, cleaning the EAC is key (see BOX 'Cleaning the external auditory canal'. Ears should be kept water free during treatment. In mild OE, use hydrocortisone cream to the pinna and EarCalm® Spray (2% acetic acid, lowers pH and may favour non-pyogenic bacteria).

• *Moderate OE:* (fig 5.21) Painful ear, narrowed EAC with malodorous creamy discharge. ℞: swab for microscopy. Clean the canal. Prescribe topical antibiotic/ ± steroid drops (eg Otosporin®; Sofradex®; Gentisone HC®) Although topical aminoglycosides are theoretically ototoxic, their use in the presence of grommets or perforation of the tympanic membrane is not contraindicated providing that infection is present and that the course does not exceed 10 days. Topical ciprofloxacin drops are not licensed for treating OE but there is less potential for ototoxicity in those with grommets or perforation. Use drops for ≤7 days, as troublesome fungal infections can arise if used for longer (treat with clotrimazole 1% solution). If there is pinna cellulitis start antibiotics and refer.

• *Severe OE:* (fig 5.22) The EAC is occluded. A thin ear wick can be inserted with eg aluminium acetate (may require ENT referral). After a few days, the meatus will open up enough for either microsuction or careful cleansing.

Furunculosis Painful staphylococcal abscess arising in a hair follicle within the canal. Lance with sucker fine end. Treat with oral antibiotics. Check for diabetes.

▶Beware persistent unilateral otitis externa. ?NOE (below) or SCC.

Necrotizing (malignant) otitis externa (NOE) An aggressive, life-threatening infection of the external ear that can lead to temporal bone destruction and base-of-skull osteomyelitis. 90% have diabetes. *Presentation:* Otorrhoea. Severe otalgia not in keeping with appearance of EAC. Granulations in floor of EAC at junction of bony and cartilaginous canal. ?CN VIIth palsy and CN VI and IX-XII as disease progresses. The cause is usually *Pseudomonas aeruginosa. Management:* Swab for MC&S. Biopsy EAC to exclude SCC. CT scan to evaluate severity of disease. ?Nuclear medicine scan to reveal extent. *Treatment:* Aural toilet. Topical and oral ciprofloxacin antibiotics length depending on response (Cipro resistance increasing). Diabetes control. Surgical debridement unusual. Hyperbaric oxygen therapy.

Barotrauma If the Eustachian tube is occluded, middle ear air pressure cannot be equalized during descent in an aircraft or diving, so causing damage. *Symptoms:* Severe pain as the drum becomes indrawn initially then a secondary effusion may occur as a transudate or haemotympanum. *Prevention:* Not flying with an URTI; decongestants into the nose (eg xylometazoline); repeated yawns/swallows/jaw movements. ℞: Supportive if simple; effusions usually clear spontaneously, and most perforations heal.

Temporomandibular joint (TMJ) dysfunction *Symptoms:* Earache, facial pain, and joint clicking/popping related to teeth-grinding or joint derangement, and, importantly, stress, making this a biopsychosocial disorder which may become a chronic pain syndrome. *Signs:* Joint tenderness exacerbated by lateral movement of the open jaw, or trigger points in the pterygoids. ℞: Most patients improve without treatment. Reassure and explain. Simple analgesia. *Specialist treatment:* Dental occlusion therapy (eg oral splinting); physiotherapy; cognitive behavioural therapy (p.754); surgery (rarely needed).[7]

Cleaning the external auditory canal

Cleaning the ear canal facilitates application and effectiveness of topical treatment. Options include:
- *Gentle syringing or irrigation* to remove debris (provided the TM is intact). Not suitable if otitis externa—water often exacerbates condition.
- *Dry mopping* under direct vision using the reverse end of a Jobson Horne probe. A wisp of cotton wool is wound around the reverse end of a Jobson Horne probe or orange stick to resemble a paint brush. The cotton wool is used to clean the auditory meatus with a gentle rotary action; don't touch the drum. Replace the cotton wool at intervals and continue until the wool is returned clean. Attend to the anterior-inferior recess, which often harbours debris. NB: patients who have mastoid cavities (a surgical widened canal done to treat infection) should be followed up by ENT for irrigation and drying.
- *Microsuction* is very effective but not readily available in primary care, so may need referral to ENT. ▶Patients who have mastoid cavities are treated by microsuction, not irrigation.

Referred otalgia: when the cause is not in the ear

Referred (secondary) pain can arise from disease processes in the territories of the sensory nerves supplying the ear:
- *CN V* —the auriculotemporal nerve (a branch of the trigeminal nerve which supplies lateral upper half of pinna) may refer pain from dental disease and TMJ dysfunction (p.392).
- *CN VII* —a sensory branch of the facial nerve (supplies lateral surface of ear drum) refers pain in geniculate herpes (Ramsay Hunt syndrome, p.856).
- *CN IX* —primary glossopharyngeal neuralgia is a rare cause of pain often induced by talking or swallowing.
- *CN IX & X* —the tympanic branch of the glossopharyngeal nerve and the auricular branch of the vagus (supplies medial surface of drum) refer pain from the posterior ⅓ of the tongue, pyriform fossa, or larynx eg from cancer, or from the throat to the ear eg in tonsillitis or quinsy. Otalgia is common post tonsillectomy (esp. in adults), so it is worth warning all patients.
- *Spinal nerves c2 and c3* —the great auricular nerve (C2, C3, supplying lower ½ of pinna) refers pain from soft tissue injury in the neck and from cervical spondylosis/arthritis.

5 ENT

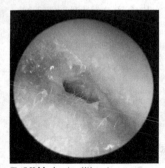

Fig 5.21 Moderate otitis externa.
Courtesy of Michael Hawke, MD, University of Toronto, hawkelibrary.com.

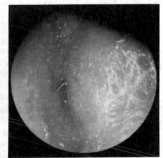

Fig 5.22 Severe otitis externa: the EAC is completely occluded.
Courtesy of Michael Hawke, MD, University of Toronto, hawkelibrary.com.

The character of the discharge provides clues:

- *External ear*—inflammation ie otitis externa (OE) produces a scanty discharge, as there are no mucinous glands—see p.392. Blood can result from trauma to the canal. Liquid wax can sometimes 'leak' out.

Causes of discharge to consider
• Otitis externa/media.
• Cholesteatoma (rare but important). NB: crust in the attic/postero-superior quadrant often hides pathology.

- *Middle ear*—mucous discharges are almost always due to middle ear disease. Serosanguinous discharge suggests a granulation tissue on the tympanic membrane. Offensive discharge suggests *Pseudomonas*.

- *CSF otorrhoea*—CSF leaks may follow trauma: suspect if you see a halo sign on filter paper or pillowcase. Sample tests positive for β_2 (tau) transferrin.

Acute otitis media (OM) Entails middle ear inflammation; it presents with rapid onset of pain, fever ± irritability, anorexia, or vomiting often after a viral upper respiratory infection. Common organisms: *Pneumococcus, Haemophilus, Moraxella*. In acute OM, bulging of the tympanic membrane causes pain (fig 5.23), which eases if the drum perforates (there is associated purulent discharge). R: Analgesia. Acute OM resolves in 60% within 24h without antibiotics. Consider immediate antibiotics if systemically unwell; immunocompromised; or no improvement in symptoms >3 days. Patients with otorrhoea or <2yrs old with bilateral OM are more likely to benefit from antibiotics (NB: seek advice for any infant <3 months with a temp of ≥38°c). Give amoxicillin (erythromycin if penicillin allergic) for 5–7 days. If less likely to benefit from antibiotics, consider a 'delayed' prescription (to start if more unwell or after 3 days if ongoing symptoms).

Continuing discharge may indicate complications eg mastoiditis which is rare. Mucopus may continue to drain when there is no mastoiditis, especially if grommets are in place. Clean the EAC to remove infected material from the meatus. ▶*If discharge continues, get expert help.*

Otitis media with effusion (glue ear) This occurs when an effusion is present after regression of the symptoms of acute OM, see pp.396–7.

Chronic otitis media (COM) A variety of terms are used to categorize chronic infectious or inflammatory conditions of the middle ear. COM is defined as an ear with a tympanic membrane perforation in the setting of recurrent or chronic infections.¹ Associated symptoms include hearing loss, otorrhoea, fullness, and otalgia.

- *Benign (or inactive) COM* is characterized by a dry tympanic membrane perforation without active infection.
- *Chronic serous otitis media* is characterized by continuous serous drainage.
- *Chronic suppurative otitis media (CSOM)* is diagnosed when there is persistent purulent drainage through a perforated tympanic membrane.

R: Topical/systemic antibiotics (based on swab results); aural cleaning; water precautions; careful follow-up. Surgery may be required (myringoplasty; cortical mastoidectomy—see BOX 'Surgery for CSOM'). *Complications:* Prolonged low middle ear pressure allows for the development of a retraction pocket of the *pars flaccida* (fig 5.7), as this enlarges, squamous epithelium builds up and can no longer escape from the neck of the sac, resulting in a cholesteatoma.

Eustachian tube dysfunction The Eustachian tube can cause problems by being closed (blocked) or constantly open (patulous). Interestingly the symptoms can have considerable overlap. See table 5.1. The tympanic membrane of a patient with a patulous tube can be withdrawn and have apparent retraction pockets. These are 'the sniffers'. Constant sniffing stops the sensation of the patulous tube and leads to retracted drum. *Blocked tube* R: Grommet insertion. Balloon dilation of Eustachian tube. Eustachian cushion surgery to open orifice. *Patulous tube* R: Topical intranasal irritants eg oestrogen or potassium iodide nose drops to cause oedema of Eustachian tube orifice. Surgical augmentation of Eustachian tube opening to close tube with cartilage or filler.

Cholesteatoma (fig 5.24) Serious rare complications (meningitis; cerebral abscess; hearing loss; mastoiditis; facial nerve dysfunction). *Incidence:* 1:10,000. Peak age: 5–15yrs. It is a misnomer as it is neither cholesterol nor a tumour (it *is* locally destructive around and beyond the *pars flaccida*—from the release of lytic enzymes). Δ: Discharge ± deafness; headache, pain, facial paralysis, and vertigo indicate impending CNS complications. ℞: Mastoid surgery (see BOX 'Surgery for CSOM') is needed to make a safe dry ear by removing the disease (preserving hearing is secondary).

Mastoiditis Middle ear inflammation leads to destruction of air cells in the mastoid bone ± abscess formation. Beware intracranial extension. Giving antibiotics for otitis media can prevent mastoiditis (NNT >4000). *Signs:* Fever; tenderness, swelling and redness behind the pinna (mastoid) + protruding auricle. *Imaging:* CT. ℞: Admit for IV antibiotics, myringotomy ± definitive mastoidectomy.

Surgery for chronic suppurative otitis media (CSOM)

In patients with CSOM, surgery may be considered if aural cleaning and antibiotic treatment fail, and there is persistent perforation/discharge, conductive hearing loss, chronic mastoiditis, or cholesteatoma formation.[s]

Myringoplasty (= Repair of the tympanic membrane alone.) A perforation in the tympanic membrane is patched using a graft (often using temporalis fascia or tragal perichondrium), and applied (usually) underneath the tympanic membrane. It acts as a scaffold for the tympanic membrane to grow across and has a ~90% success rate.

Mastoidectomy For patients with mastoiditis or advanced cholesteatoma, mastoid surgery and *tympanoplasty* (= surgical repair of the tympanic membrane and ossicles) is used to eradicate the source of chronic infection, excise the cholesteatoma, and reconstruct the hearing mechanism. 'Canal wall up' mastoidectomy removes mastoid air cells while retaining the posterior canal wall. It leaves normal ear anatomy intact and prevents problems associated with a mastoid cavity (eg ongoing requirement for microscopic cleaning).

Table 5.1 Symptoms associated with Eustachian tube dysfunction

Symptoms	Patulous	Blocked
Autophony*	x	
Muffled hearing	x	x
Ear blockage	x	x
Tinnitus	x	x
Vertigo	x	x

* Autophony is hearing one's breathing, heartbeat, voice loudly.

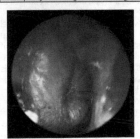

Fig 5.23 Acute otitis media. There is erythema and bulging of the pars flaccida and dilated circumferential vessels.
Courtesy of Nicholas Steventon FRCS.

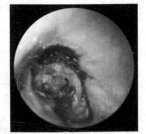

Fig 5.24 Attic cholesteatoma. Featureless erythematous tympanic membrane inferiorly with a large retraction pocket full of keratin superiorly in the attic
Courtesy of Nicholas Steventon FRCS.

Further reading

NICE (2018). *Clinical Knowledge Summaries: Otitis Media*. http://cks.nice.org.uk/otitis-media-acute

This is detected by otoscopy (fluid level or bubbles behind the drum) or indirectly, by tympanometry (p. 390). 50% of 3yr-olds have ≥1 ear effusion/yr. *In adults, exclude a postnasal space tumour as the cause of middle ear fluid.*

Otitis media with effusion (OME)/glue ear ►*Hearing impairment noticed by parents is the mode of presentation in 80%.* The fundamental problem lies with dysfunction of the Eustachian tubes. The exact cause is unclear, but there are associations with upper respiratory tract infections, oversized adenoids, narrow nasopharyngeal dimensions, and presence of bacterial biofilms on the adenoids. OME is more common in boys; Down syndrome; cleft palate; winter season; atopy; children of smokers; and primary ciliary dyskinesia.[2] OME is the chief cause of hearing loss in young children, and can result in significant learning and behavioural problems. OME may cause no pain, so its presence may not be suspected.

History: Focus on poor listening, poor speech, language delay, inattention, poor behaviour, hearing fluctuation, ear infections/URTIs, balance problems, and poor progress at school.

Examination: There is a variable appearance of the tympanic membrane on otoscopy (fig 5.25) eg retracted or bulging drum. It can look dull, grey, or yellow. There may be bubbles or a fluid level, or superficial radial vessels and ↓ drum mobility when tested with a pneumatic attachment. Otoscopic diagnosis is very inaccurate.

Tests: Refer for formal assessment of hearing, which should be appropriate for the child's developmental stage. *Audiograms:* look for conductive defects. *Tympanometry:* look for flat type B tympanogram (fig 5.13 p. 390). This helps distinguish OME from other causes eg otosclerosis. Also consider coexisting causes of hearing loss (pp. 398–9).

Treatment:[10] OME is usually mild, transient, and resolves spontaneously: 50% of children with bilateral hearing loss of 20dB are likely to resolve in 3 months.
- *Active observation for 3 months:* if bilateral OME is confirmed, there should be a 3-month period of active observation. Give advice on strategies to minimize impact of hearing loss (eg reducing background noise (turn off the TV); sit at the child's level, and give short, simple instructions). Reassess with repeat hearing tests at 3 months.
- *Autoinflation* of the Eustachian tube may help during this period (eg using an Otovent® device—which involves inflating a special balloon via the nose).
- *Topical and systemic methods:* NICE doesn't recommend antibiotics, changes to diet, antihistamines, decongestants, steroids, or acupuncture, etc.
- *Surgery:* if persistent bilateral OME + hearing level in better ear of 25–30dBHL (=decibel hearing level) or worse is confirmed over 3 months, consider insertion of ventilation tubes (AKA tympanostomy tube or grommets; fig 5.26). Surgery is also an option if hearing loss is less severe but there is a significant impact on development or education. The main complications of grommets are infections and tympanosclerosis (fig 5.10 p. 389). Treat infections with aural cleaning and topical antibiotic/steroid ear drops; grommet removal may be needed. Adjuvant adenoidectomy at the time of grommet insertion should not be performed routinely.
- *Adults* with longstanding OME can be treated with tympanostomy tubes.
- *Hearing aids* should be reserved for persistent bilateral OME and hearing loss if surgery is not accepted. *Post-op:* It is OK to swim with grommets, but avoid forcing water into the middle ear by diving. Pain on swimming or swimming-related discharge will necessitate ear plugs/swim hats. Grommets extrude after ~3–12 months; recheck the hearing at this point; ~25% need re-insertion. Rarely, a small perforation may persist after the grommet has come out, which may require surgery.

2 PCD/Kartagener syndrome (p. 850) often causes otitis media and OME throughout childhood (due to loss of ciliary function in the Eustachian tube and middle ear), despite fairly continuous antibiotics. After 18yrs of age, the ear improves somewhat. Grommet placement does not improve middle ear function.

Grommets and hearing gain

Use of grommets to ventilate the middle ear is common but how much do they improve hearing? A Cochrane review[11] found the effect of grommets on hearing in children with OME, as measured by standard tests, was small (~12dB) and diminished after 6 months (4dB)—by which time natural resolution had led to improved hearing in non-surgically treated children. The raw numbers may look unimpressive, but due to the logarithmic decibel scale, even a 3dB increase in sound equates to a doubling of intensity and hearing sensitivity. For reference, a 16 to 25dB hearing loss may be mimicked by plugging the ears with the index fingers. In the classroom setting, this level of hearing loss presents an appreciable educational difficulty (see also BOX "The bounds of 'normal' hearing", p. 401).[12]

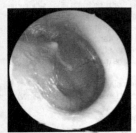

Fig 5.25 Glue ear with dull retracted drum.
Courtesy of Nicholas Steventon FRCS.

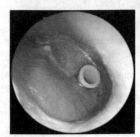

Fig 5.26 A grommet.
Courtesy of Nicholas Steventon FRCS.

Further reading

NICE (2008). *Surgical Management of Children with Otitis Media with Effusion* (CG60). London: NICE. https://www.nice.org.uk/guidance/cg60

1 in every 500 newborns has bilateral permanent sensorineural hearing loss ≥40dB. Half of all prelingual deafness is genetic, 25% non-genetic, and 25% idiopathic.[13] ▶*If you or a parent are worried, refer to audiology.*

Genetic hearing loss (50%)
Conductive hearing loss—CHL: Congenital anomalies of pinna, external ear canal, drum, or ossicles; Treacher Collins (p. 859); Pierre Robin (p. 854); Goldenhar syndrome (oculoauriculovertebral (OAV) syndrome)—causes CHL and SNHL.

Sensorineural hearing loss—SNHL:
* *Autosomal dominant:* Waardenburg syndrome (SNHL, heterochromia iridis + wide nasal bridge); Klippel–Feil syndrome (p.850); Alport syndrome (p.842); branchio-oto-renal (BOR) syndrome (outer, middle, & inner ear + kidney malformations).
* *Autosomal recessive:* Pendred syndrome (SNHL with goitre); Usher syndrome (SNHL+ retinitis pigmentosa); Jervell and Lange-Nielsen syndrome (SNHL + ↑QTc).
* *Non-syndromic SNHL:* accounts for 70% of genetic hearing loss. Many genes are implicated are different patterns of inheritance (most are autosomal recessive). The degree of hearing loss and age of onset varies with type.
* *x-linked:* Alport syndrome (p.842); Turner syndrome (p.859).

Non-genetic hearing loss (25%)
* *Intrauterine TORCH infection:* eg CMV; rubella; toxoplasmosis; HSV; syphilis.
* *Perinatal causes:* Prematurity; hypoxia; IVH; kernicterus; infection (see below).
* *Infections:* eg meningitis, encephalitis, measles, mumps.
* *Other causes:* Ototoxic drugs; acoustic or cranial trauma.

Universal newborn hearing screening (UNHS) Screening within weeks of birth is the best way to ensure deafness is diagnosed and managed. Tests:
* *Otoacoustic emissions (OAEs):* A microphone placed in the external meatus detects tiny cochlear sounds produced by movement of the outer hair cells, which occur spontaneously or in response to an auditory stimulus. OAE evaluates function of the peripheral auditory system, the area most often involved in SNHL (ie the sensory part of the cochlea and not the neural pathway, which is tested using ABR). OAE is abnormal or equivocal in 3–8%. Most of these 'failures' (84%) have external ear canal obstruction (collapsed ear canal or debris). For these patients arrange a repeat test or measure ABR.
* *Auditory brainstem response (ABR):* The ears are covered with earphones that emit a series of soft clicks. Electrodes on the infant's forehead and neck measure brain wave activity in response to the clicks. ABR tests the auditory neural pathway from CN VIII to the lower brainstem.

Prevalence of deafness found at UNHS: 0.9–3.24:1000 for permanent bilateral hearing loss of >35dB; 5.95:1000 when unilateral and moderate hearing loss.[14]

Subjective hearing tests in older children
* *Distraction testing:* (6–18 months; not very accurate.) An assistant in front of the child attracts their attention while a tester attempts to distract them by making noises behind and beside the child eg with a rattle, or voice.
* *Visual reinforced audiometry:* (6 months–2½yrs.) The child turns their head to a sound stimulus and a toy lights-up to reward the listening behaviour.
* *Speech discrimination:* (At 24–60 months.) The child touches selected objects cued by acoustically similar phrases eg *key/tree*.

Management Give support, advice, and information to the patient and family. Maximize the hearing a deaf child may have by use of hearing aids or cochlear implant (see BOX 'Cochlear implants'). Provide support to develop spoken or signed communication.

Further reading
NHS newborn hearing screening programme (NHSP): www.gov.uk/topic/population-screening-programmes/newborn-hearing

Smith RJH *et al.* (2014). Deafness and hereditary hearing loss overview. *GeneReviews®*. ncbi.nlm.nih.gov/books/NBK1434/

Cochlear implants

NICE recommends cochlear implants for children and adults with profound sensorineural deafness who do not benefit from a conventional hearing aid. Normal cochlear structure is essential, as is preoperative multidisciplinary assessment.

Cochlear implants comprise a multichannel electrode inserted surgically into the cochlea that directly stimulates the auditory nerve when electrical signals are applied. The electrode is attached to an external auditory processor through the skin via a magnetic coupler. The signal is not normal sound and intensive therapy is needed to understand the new sounds. Implants allow better lip-reading, provision and recognition of environmental sounds, and relief of isolation. Quality is now sufficient for previously deaf people to have excellent hearing and eg use the phone.

BAHA: the bone-anchored hearing aid

Sound is transmitted to the cochlea via bone conduction (fig 5.27).

Indications Intolerance of conventional hearing aids (eg persistent draining ear; mastoid cavity; topical sensitivity); congenital malformations (eg microtia; atresia); single-sided deafness. BAHAs are becoming more widely used and have a special benefit in some children with complex disorders because the children do not physically feel the presence of the hearing aid. On quality of life measures BAHAs do very well. **Complications** Include skin regrowth around the titanium screw and non-osseointegration. **Contraindications** Average bone threshold worse than 65dB; non-compliance; poor hygiene; lack of bone volume.

5 ENT

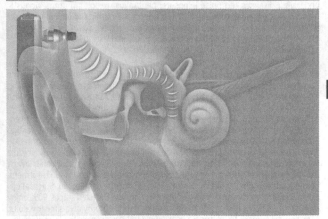

Fig 5.27 A bone-anchored hearing aid allows sound to be transmitted to the cochlea via bone conduction. A titanium screw implanted into bone allows attachment of the hearing aid.   © Cochlear Limited 2012.

> I t is not the actual sound itself that matters, but the reverberations that it makes as it travels through our mind. These are often to be found far away, strangely transformed; but it is only by gathering up and putting together these echoes and fragments that we arrive at the true nature of our experience.   Virginia Woolf, 1926.

Deepening the emotional content of music, for example, by associating melody with concrete events in our lives, depends on dealings in ancient subneocortical limbic regions such as the hippocampus, amygdala, and anterior cingulate cortex, which form the hub of all our emotions, passions, and delights.

Many cope well with mild hearing loss if given comprehensive rehabilitation.

Classification Classify the type and possible cause of hearing loss:

- *Conductive hearing loss (CHL):* There is impaired sound transmission via the external canal and middle ear ossicles to the foot of the stapes through a variety of causes: external canal obstruction (wax, pus, debris, foreign body, developmental anomalies); drum perforation (trauma, barotrauma, infection); problems with the ossicular chain (otosclerosis, infection, trauma); and inadequate Eustachian tube ventilation of the middle ear (eg with effusion secondary to nasopharyngeal carcinoma). All result in conductive deafness.

- *Sensorineural hearing loss (SNHL):* Results from defects central to the oval window in the cochlea (sensory), cochlear nerve (neural) or, rarely, more central pathways. Ototoxic drugs (eg streptomycin, vancomycin, gentamicin, chloroquine and hydroxychloroquine, vinca alkaloids), post-infective (meningitis, measles, mumps, flu, herpes, syphilis), cochlear vascular disease, Ménière's (p. 404), trauma, and presbycusis are all sensorineural. *Rare causes:* Acoustic neuroma (p. 403), vitamin B12 deficiency, multiple sclerosis, brain metastases.

▶ If unilateral SNHL, exclude an acoustic neuroma (MRI).

Sudden hearing loss • *If sensorineural: Definition:* loss of ≥30dB in 3 contiguous pure tone frequencies over 3 days. Hearing loss may be sudden and abrupt, or rapidly progressive. Incidence: 5–20 per 100,000/yr. It is usually unilateral and the prognosis for some recovery is good (partial or complete spontaneous recovery occurs in 30–65%). *Management:* ▶▶immediate specialist referral for investigation and management (see BOX 'Managing sudden sensorineural deafness'). Sudden SNHL has many possible aetiologies. Detailed evaluation reveals underlying diseases (eg noise exposure; gentamicin toxicity; mumps; acoustic neuroma; MS; vasculopathy; TB) in 10%. Diagnose idiopathic sudden SNHL (ISSNHL) if no cause is found. Negative prognostic factors include: age <15yrs or >65yrs, ↑ESR, vertigo, hearing loss in the opposite ear, severe hearing loss.

• *Conductive:* A cause is 'always' found: infection, occlusion, trauma, fracture.

Otosclerosis New spongy bone is formed around the stapes footplate. Calcification leads to its fixation and a progressive conductive hearing loss. The disease process may also enter the cochlea directly causing a high-frequency SNHL. *Prevalence:* 0.5–2% clinically, 10% subclinically. *Cause:* Autosomal dominant with incomplete penetrance; 50% have a family history. 85% are bilateral; ♀:♂ ≈ 2:1

Symptoms: Usually appear in early adult life and can be accelerated by pregnancy. There is conductive deafness, ~75% have tinnitus; mild, transient vertigo is common too. 10% have Schwartze's sign—a flamingo pink blush seen through the posterior superior segment of the drum showing active disease in the middle ear space around the ossicles; audiometry with masked bone conduction shows a dip at 2kHz (Carhart's notch—see fig 5.18, p.391). *Treatment options:* No treatment, hearing aid (including BAHA), or surgery after a trial of a hearing aid. Surgical options include stapedectomy or stapedotomy, to replace the fixed stapes. 90% enjoy an improvement in hearing. Microdrill and laser stapedotomy give similar results. Many prefer surgery to wearing a hearing aid but careful selection is required as one complication of surgery is complete SNHL (1–4%). Surgery is only performed on the worse hearing ear; contralateral SNHL is a contraindication. Cochlear implant is another option (if patient has poor speech discrimination scores).

Presbycusis Age-related, bilateral, high-frequency SNHL. The exact mechanism is unclear but loss of high-frequency sounds starts before 30yrs and the rate of loss is progressive thereafter. Deafness (loss of hair cells: see fig 5.2, p.385) is gradual and we do not usually notice it until hearing of speech is affected with loss of high-frequency sounds (consonants at ~3–4kHz are needed for speech discrimination). Hearing is most affected in the presence of background noise (try where possible to decrease this). Hearing aids are the usual treatment. See pure tone audiogram on p.391 (fig 5.19).

▶▶Managing sudden sensorineural deafness

- ▶▶ Take a full history, including drug history.
- ▶▶ Examine the EAC and TM to exclude wax/effusion. Perform tuning fork tests (p. 387; Weber goes to the other ear; Rinne AC >BC in affected ear).
- ▶▶ Get expert ENT help.
- ▶▶ Look for causes: FBC; ESR/CRP; U&E; LFT; TSH; autoimmune profile; clotting studies; fasting glucose; cholesterol.
- ▶▶ Arrange audiology: audiometry ± auditory brainstem responses.
- ▶▶ Treatment depends on the cause (if found). There are varied treatment regimens for ISSNHL—no single treatment has been shown to be effective.
- ▶▶ High-dose steroids are commonly used (presumed inflammatory cause). One starting regimen is **prednisolone** 60mg/24h PO for 7 days then 7 day taper days. Intratympanic dexamethasone has a salvage role in treatment failure.
- ▶▶ There may be a response to hyperbaric O_2 therapy, if given promptly.
- ▶▶ Routine prescribing of antivirals, thrombolytics, vasodilators, vasoactive substances, or antioxidants to patients with ISSNHL is not recommended.[18]

5 ENT

The bounds of 'normal' hearing

Both frequency (Hz) and sound pressure (decibels, dB) are important for the detection of sound by the human ear, though the relationship between the two is also important. A person with normal hearing will hear sound frequencies between 20 and 20,000Hz. Sound frequencies between 250 and 8000Hz are the most important for speech interpretation. Vowel sounds have low frequencies (250–1000Hz) and are easier to hear. Consonants, at higher frequencies (1500–

Is your hearing reduced?
• Do people 'mumble'?
• Do you keep saying 'What?'
• Do you misunderstand names?
• Is your TV volume 'too loud'?
• Are noisy rooms a problem?

6000Hz) convey most of the meaning of what we say, which is why those with higher frequency loss (eg presbycusis) have such difficulty (see also fig 5.28).

The normal range of hearing is 0–140dB. Hearing is measured in decibels of hearing level (dBHL)—decibels relative to the quietest sounds heard with normal hearing. Normal hearing level = –10 to 25dBHL ('0' is average, hence minus scores are better than average). Hearing loss is categorized into mild (26–40dBHL); moderate (41–70dBHL); severe (71–90dBHL); and profound, which is defined as >90dBHL. Remember that decibels are a logarithmic scale, and that the range from 0 to 120dBs actually represents a million times relative increase in sound pressure. At high intensity (≥130dB), sound can also be a *painful* stimulus, showing an interesting (and variable) threshold relationship between useful information from special senses and painful stimuli (also present in the eye).

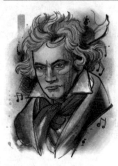

Fig 5.28 Composer **Ludwig van Beethoven's** hearing loss is well documented and his gradual deafness may have influenced his compositions. Researchers argue that as his hearing worsened, he favoured lower- and middle-frequency notes, which he could hear better. Once totally deaf, he began to compose using high-frequency notes again.[18] It seems a cruel twist of nature that one of the greatest composers should retreat into an ever quieter world, yet even more remarkable that in spite of this, his work flourished. ▶Try to encourage those struggling to overcome adversities of physical disease to engage in positive activities to help break through the barriers hindering them (whether perceived or real).

Artwork by Gillian Turner.

Further reading

Mathur NN (2019). *Sudden Hearing Loss*. Medscape. http://emedicine.medscape.com/article/856313

Tinnitus (Latin *tinnire*, meaning to ring) is a perception of sound, typically in the absence of auditory stimulation. Tinnitus is often a symptom of an underlying abnormality. **Prevalence** 15% (0.5% severe). ⅔ of patients have associated sensorineural hearing loss (SNHL). ⅓ have no identifiable cause.

Tinnitus character This may help identify aetiology. It may be unilateral or bilateral, pulsatile or non-pulsatile. Ringing, hissing, or buzzing suggests an inner ear or central cause. Popping or clicking suggests problems in the external or middle ear, or the palate. Pulsatile tinnitus is often objective (see later) but can also simply reflect an increased awareness of blood flow in the ear.

Classification Tinnitus may be objective or subjective.[17]
- *Objective tinnitus* (which is audible to the examiner) is rare and occurs due to:
  - *Vascular disorders:* pulsatile vibratory sounds from eg AV malformations; carotid pathology; glomus tumours (fig 5.29) • *High-output cardiac states:* Paget's; hyperthyroidism; anaemia, causing pulsatile tinnitus • *Myoclonus* of palatal or stapedius/tensor tympani muscles, resulting in an audible click • *Patulous Eustachian tube:* prolonged opening, causing abnormal sound transmission to the ear.
- *Subjective tinnitus* is audible only to the patient. *Associations:* • most commonly associated with disorders causing SNHL eg presbycusis; noise-induced hearing loss; Ménière's (unilateral) • *Conductive deafness* is less commonly associated eg from impacted wax; otosclerosis • *Ototoxic drugs:* cause bilateral tinnitus with associated hearing loss. Cisplatin and aminoglycosides can cause permanent hearing loss. Aspirin, NSAIDs, quinine, macrolides, and loop diuretics are associated with tinnitus and reversible hearing loss ± *Otitis media* ± effusion • *Other associations:* hyper/hypothyroidism; diabetes; MS; ►acoustic neuroma (unilateral); trauma to the head or neck. Anxiety and depression is frequently associated with and may exacerbate tinnitus.

Pathophysiology Poorly understood. Possible mechanisms include spontaneous otoacoustic emissions; altered or increased spontaneous activity in the auditory nerve or central structures; plastic reorganization of central pathways; inappropriate feedback via descending pathways, and auditory–limbic interactions (see BOX 'The Jastreboff model of tinnitus'). Usually we are able to habituate tinnitus. If not, it becomes problematic.[18]

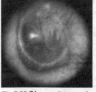

Fig 5.29 Glomus tympanicum tumour: note red anterior mass and a small fluid meniscus around it.

Courtesy of Rory Herdman FRCS.

Tests Audiometry; tympanogram. ►Investigate unilateral tinnitus (MRI) to exclude acoustic neuroma (p. 403; 10% present this way).

℞ Treat any underlying cause. Take time to explain tinnitus—it is common and usually improves with time (via habituation). Ask their beliefs about tinnitus and address any underlying concerns. Manage depression, anxiety, or insomnia. Positive attitudes help. Treat the whole person, not just a malfunctioning ear. Treatment is aimed at reducing the impact of symptoms:
- *Hearing aids:* If hearing loss >35dB, a hearing aid that improves perception of background noise makes tinnitus less apparent.
- *Psychological support:* Psychoeducational counselling together with *sound therapy* (the use of background sound to reduce the impact of tinnitus by partially masking it eg from a radio or fan) are the mainstay of rehabilitation.
- *Cognitive behavioural therapy:* (p. 754) To identify and modify unhelpful thoughts and behaviours.

5 ENT

An indolent, histologically benign tumour. It is a misnomer as it usually arises from the Schwann cells of the superior vestibular nerve (*vestibular schwannoma*). Originating in the internal auditory canal, it causes local pressure on the auditory, vestibular, and facial nerves in the narrow space of the canal. Continued growth leads to medial extension into the cerebellopontine angle where it acts as a space-occupying lesion. 95% sporadic. 5% related to neurofibromatosis type 2 (NF2). **Symptoms** Unilateral hearing loss 70%, unilateral non-pulsatile tinnitus 50%, balance problems 20%. Larger tumours can lead to paraesthesia of the face including loss of corneal reflex, headaches, cerebellar dysfunction, facial nerve palsy, ↑ICP signs, and other cranial nerve palsies. **Tests** ►Pure tone audiogram and speech audiogram. MRI scan. ΔΔ Meningioma 10%, epidermoid tumours 5%, lower nerve schwannomas 2%, and arachnoid cysts 1% **Management** Watchful waiting with interval MRI scans in small slow growing tumours. Surgical removal for large or rapidly growing tumours using translabyrinthine, middle fossa, or retrosigmoid approaches. Stereotactic radiosurgery is increasingly popular.

Noise-induced hearing loss (NIHL)

Exposure to loud noise will cause damage to the inner ear resulting in hearing loss. This can be a one-time exposure to an intense sound (= acoustic trauma eg from an explosion) or, more commonly in occupational NIHL, continuous exposure to loud sounds that causes hearing loss over time. There is a relationship between volume of sound and its duration: 8 hours' exposure to a sound level ≥85dB usually causes damage. Acoustic trauma is caused by sounds >180dB. Rupture of the drum and ossicular fracture may occur.

Symptoms There is bilateral symmetrical sensorineural hearing loss ± tinnitus. There may be noise-induced temporary threshold shift, which occurs when hearing improves away from the source of exposure.

Audiometry Typically shows a 'notch' at 4kHz with recovery at 8kHz (see fig 5.17, p. 391).

Management Reduce risk of occupational exposure: abide by health and safety law; provide ear defenders; and screen occupations at risk. In established hearing loss use hearing aids.

The Jastreboff model of tinnitus

The Jastreboff neurophysiological model

This model proposes that the limbic and autonomic nervous systems are the primary systems for the development of tinnitus annoyance, with the auditory system playing a secondary role in tinnitus manifestation.

Tinnitus retraining therapy

Therapy is based on this model and is aimed at habituating tinnitus-evoked reactions and perception. The 2 main components are educational counselling (to reclassify and neutralize tinnitus), and sound therapy (via constant low level broad band sound). Successful treatment results in patients who are not bothered by their tinnitus, even though they are aware of it.

Further reading

McKenna L et al. (2014) A scientific cognitive-behavioral model of tinnitus: novel conceptualizations of tinnitus distress. Front Neurol 2014;5:196. Pubmed ID: 25339938. https://www.ncbi.nlm.nih.gov/pubmed/25339938

NICE (2017). *Clinical Knowledge Summaries: Tinnitus*. http://cks.nice.org.uk/tinnitus

Vertigo is a symptom—the sensation that you, or the world around you, is moving or spinning.

Vestibular (peripheral) vertigo is often severe, and may be accompanied by loss of balance, nausea, vomiting, ↓ hearing, tinnitus, nystagmus (usually horizontal), and diaphoresis. Hearing loss and tinnitus are less common in *central vertigo* (usually less severe), nystagmus may be horizontal or vertical.

Is the symptom vestibular? 'I'm dizzy' is ambiguous. Elicit the illusion! Ask 'Did you or the world seem to spin (like getting off a playground roundabout?)' or 'Which *way* are things going?' Those with vertigo often know without hesitation; if not, this is a cue to pursue other causes (lightheadedness ± a 'sense of collapse' can be vascular, ocular, musculoskeletal, metabolic, or claustrophobic). ►Ask about duration of vertigo: seconds to minutes ≈ BPPV; 30min to 30h ≈ Ménière's or migraine; 30h to a week ≈ acute vestibular failure.

Causes (often multifactorial)
Peripheral:
• Ménière disease
• Benign paroxysmal positional vertigo (BPPV)
• Vestibular failure
• Labyrinthitis
• Superior semicircular canal dehiscence
Central:
• Acoustic neuroma
• Multiple sclerosis
• Head injury
• Migraine-associated dizziness
• Vertebrobasilar insufficiency
Other:
• Multifactorial disequilibrium (causing falls in elderly)

Examination/tests Full otoneurological examination. *Assess:* nystagmus, gait, Romberg's test (+ve if balance is worse when eyes are shut, implying defective joint position), and Unterberger's test. *Do provocation tests (head thrust test; Dix–Hallpike test,* see BOX 'Vestibular testing'). Request audiometry and MRI. If diagnostic doubt, consider caloric testing and electronystagmography.

Benign paroxysmal positional vertigo (BPPV) Commonest cause of vertigo. Attacks of sudden vertigo lasting <30sec are provoked by head-turning or turning over in bed. Other otological symptoms are rare. *Pathogenesis:* Displacement of otoconia (= otoliths) stimulate the semicircular canals. *Causes:* Idiopathic; head injury. *Diagnosis:* Establish important negatives. No other otoneurological symptoms. *Dix–Hallpike test* is +ve. Rotatory nystagmus which is fatiguable (BOX 'Vestibular testing'). ℞: Usually self-limiting; if persistent, try: • Epley manoeuvre (fig 5.30) is 70–80% effective • Home repositioning manoeuvres/vestibular habituation exercises (BOX 'Treatment of BPPV') • *Drugs:* vestibular suppressant medication does not stop the vertigo • *Last resort:* surgery eg semicircular canal plugging (rare).

Vestibular migraine 2nd commonest cause of vertigo. Vertigo attacks last from minutes to hours. Often associated with blurred vision, flashing lights (fortification spectra), sensitivity to light and sound. 50% have headaches associated with attacks. May have mild hearing loss on PTA. Treatment with vestibular suppressants. Triptans for prolonged symptoms and headaches. Consider migraine prophylaxis regimes.

Ménière disease 2 or more episodes of vertigo lasting between 20min and 12h. Low-frequency SNHL of 30dB at 2 contiguous frequencies. Fluctuating aural symptoms within 24h of attack eg fluctuating hearing, tinnitus, and aural fullness. Absence of other causes. *Cause:* Abnormality of endolymph production leading to endolymphatic hydrops in inner ear. Δ: History, audiogram, and normal MRI. ℞: *Acute:* prochlorperazine (eg Buccastem® 3mg/8h buccal; short term as vestibular sedative) *Prophylaxis:* Betahistine 16mg/8h PO. *Interventional approaches for disabling frequent symptoms (balances success of vertigo control against potential hearing loss and morbidity of procedure):* instillation of gentamicin via a grommet (achieves chemical labyrinthectomy via round window absorption from middle ear space) 80% success, 1–10% hearing loss; endolymphatic sac decompression or shunt 70% success but 10% hearing loss. Surgical labyrinthectomy is 95% effective in controlling vertigo but causes total ipsilateral deafness; posterior cranial fossa approach for vestibular nerve section (90% effective; 5% risk of hearing loss; 0.5% mortality).

5 ENT

Acute vestibular failure (*AKA vestibular neuronitis/labyrinthitis*) (NB: the cochlea and semicircular canals = the labyrinth.) Sudden attacks of unilateral vertigo and vomiting in a previously well person, often following a recent URTI. It lasts 1–2 days, improving over a week. Full recovery may take several months. Often suffer from episodes of decompensation before full recovery. *Signs:* Nystagmus away from the affected side. *Investigations:* Audiogram; MRI scan. ℞: Vestibular suppressants eg **Buccastem®** 3mg/8h buccal or **cyclizine** 50mg/8h PO. **Prochlorperazine** 10mg IM 8hrly PRN for acute symptom control. Use only for vertiginous symptoms not disequilibrium. Can slow rehabilitation.

Vestibular testing

Unterburger's test The patient stands with arms outstretched and eyes closed and marches (high knee lift if possible) on the spot for 1min. Positive test = rotation >30° or movement >2m.

Head thrust test Patient sits opposite the examiner and is asked to fixate on the examiner's nose. The examiner rapidly turns the patient's head to one side. This is repeated on the opposite side. A positive test is where saccadic movement occurs to correct fixation.

Dix–Hallpike test For details of how to perform see ☞www.thebsa.org.uk. The test can produce a positive response for any peripheral vestibular disorder. It is important to make sure that the positive features of the test show rotatory nystagmus with a latency of onset of 5–10sec and lasts for between 5 and 60sec. The nystagmus is fatiguable with repeat testing.

Treatment of BPPV

- *Epley manoeuvre,* see fig 5.30.
- A *modified Epley manoeuvre* can be taught to patients to perform at home. It is helpful in those who have frequent recurrence of vertigo or who do not respond quickly to therapist-led manoeuvres.
- *Semont manoeuvre* and *Roll manoeuvre* are clinician-led repositioning exercises.
- *Brandt–Daroff* exercises were developed as a series of home exercises to reduce symptoms of BPPV. They are thought to work through habituation from repeated exposure. Take longer to achieve results.
- Cochrane review suggests repositioning manoeuvres are more effective than exercise-based vestibular rehabilitation eg *Cawthorne Cooksey exercises*, although a combination of the two is effective for longer-term recovery.[13]

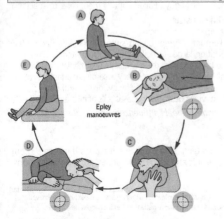

Epley manoeuvres

Fig 5.30 The *Epley manoeuvre*. The therapist moves the patient's head through 4 sequential positions, resting for ~30sec between each movement. The aim is to reposition otoconia away from the sensitive posterior canals. This works in ~80% (a 2nd go may help). Some evidence supports postural restrictions post procedure (upright head posture for 48h, avoid lying on affected side for 7 days).

These are air-filled cavities in the bones around the nose, in continuity with the nasal cavity (fig 5.33). They are lined by ciliated mucosa, which sweep debris and mucus towards and through the ostiomeatal complex into the middle meatus (fig 5.34). Obstruction impairs drainage and is due to anatomical problems (eg septal deviation/polyps), or mucosal problems (viruses cause mucosal oedema and ↓ cilia action). Recognizing and correcting drainage problems is important.

Rhinosinusitis

In adults this is defined as inflammation in the nose and paranasal sinuses with ≥2 symptoms, one of which must be nasal blockage/obstruction/congestion, or nasal discharge, ± facial pain or pressure, reduction or loss of smell, and either endoscopic (polyps, pus, mucosal obstruction in middle meatus) and/or CT signs of sinus or middle meatus obstruction.

Rhinosinusitis may be acute (ARS) or chronic (CRS if >12 weeks). Severity of symptoms is classified using a 10cm visual analogue scale (VAS; a 10cm line is drawn with the labels 'not troublesome' and 'worst thinkable troublesome' at either end. The patient then marks a point on the line to signify how the disease is affecting them. Measuring the position of the mark from the 'not troublesome end' classifies the disease as mild (0–3cm), moderate (>3–7cm) or severe (>7cm). Severe group also includes at least 3 of discoloured discharge, severe local pain, fever, ↑ESR/CRP, and double sickening (ie a deterioration after an initial milder phase of illness).

Differential diagnosis of sinusitis

(Non-sinus pain): migraine, TMJ dysfunction (p. 392); dental pain; neuropathic pain; temporal arteritis; herpes zoster. Pain in the absence of symptoms described previously is unlikely to be sinusitis.

Acute rhinosinusitis

Mild (common cold): Many episodes are self-limiting. Symptomatic relief with simple analgesics, nasal saline irrigation, and decongestants. If symptoms persist >10 days, trial of intranasal corticosteroids (eg mometasone; fluticasone; advise on correct technique, see fig 5.31 p. 408). If still persists after further 7–14 days consider specialist referral.

Moderate (post viral): Symptomatic relief and intranasal steroid spray. If no improvement in 14 days refer to specialist.

Severe (incl. bacterial): Topical steroids and antibiotics. Reassess at 48 hours. If improved continue treatment for 14 days. Failed improvement refer to specialist.

Causes of acute bacterial sinusitis

►Most follow viral infection. Other causes:

1 Direct spread (dental root infection or diving/swimming in infected water).
2 Odd anatomy: septal deviation, large ethmoidal bulla, polyps, lateralized uncinate process (part of ethmoid bone forming the maxillary sinus medial wall).
3 ITU causes: mechanical ventilation; recumbency; use of nasogastric tubes.
4 Systemic causes: Kartagener's; immunodeficiency; or general debility.
5 Biofilms:[3] type of infection which destroys mucosal cells of cilia and goblet cells.

Common organisms: S. pneumoniae, H. influenzae; and *S. aureus, Moraxella catarrhalis,* fungi.[4]

Specialist management

Nasal endoscopy, culture, imaging. Admit for IV antibiotics if severe or complications. Consider oral steroids and surgery if severe and/or complications.

---

3 Free-floating organisms become anchored to a living or inert surface (eg sinus mucosa; urinary catheter) and form a biofilm. This progressive organization facilitates further attachment and hinders removal.
4 Fungi can be isolated from the sinuses of almost every patient, so its causality is questionable.

Chronic rhinosinusitis without nasal polyps

Mild: VAS 0–3. No serious mucosal disease at endoscopy. ℞: intranasal cortico-steroids *and* nasal saline irrigation.

Moderate/severe: VAS >3. Mucosal disease at endoscopy. Topical steroids, saline irrigation, culture, and long term antibiotics (if not ↑IgE) eg macrolide for 12 weeks. CT scan and possible surgery if severe or not resolving.

Chronic rhinosinusitis with nasal polyps

Polyps are pale, mobile, and insensitive to gentle palpation (fig 5.32). They can fluctuate in size. Turbinates are pink, mobile, and sensate.

Children: ►Nasal polyps are rare if <10yrs old; rule out neoplasms, cystic fibrosis, and meningocele/encephalocele (esp. if unilateral and <2yrs old).

Mild: VAS 0–3. No serious mucosal disease at endoscopy. ℞: intranasal cortico-steroids. Review at 3 months. If improvement, continue topical steroids and review every 6 months.

Moderate: VAS >3–7. Mucosal disease at endoscopy. Trial of steroid spray. Consider ↑ dose of steroid spray. Steroid drops may be more efficacious. Consider **doxycycline** 200mg loading dose (day 1) followed by 100mg OD for 20 days.

Severe: VAS >7–10. Mucosal disease at endoscopy. Trial of topical steroids. Short course of oral steroids eg **prednisolone 60mg OD for 1 week**. Review at 1 month. If symptomatic improvement, continue topical therapy. If no improvement, CT scan then possible surgery.

Complications of sinusitis

► *Orbital cellulitis/abscess:* This is an emergency, p. 342.

► *Intracranial involvement:* Meningitis, encephalitis, cerebral abscess, cavernous sinus thrombosis. *Mucoceles:* (Esp. frontal sinus.) May become infected pyoceles (pus-filled cavity). *Osteomyelitis:* Classically staph. eg frontal bone. *Pott's puffy tumour:* A subperiosteal abscess arising from frontal osteomyelitis.

Other causes of chronic rhinorrhoea/rhinitis

Foreign body (see later), CSF (eg after head injury), bacteria (eg TB), HIV, CF, age ('old man's drip'[5]), pregnancy, decongestant overuse, antibody deficiency (p. 244), non-allergic rhinitis with eosinophilia (NARES), ASA triad (*A*spirin *S*ensitivity and late-onset *A*sthma with nasal polyps).

Other causes of nasal congestion

Child: Large adenoids; choanal atresia (congenital blockage of one or both nasal passages by bone or tissue); postnasal space tumour (eg angiofibroma); foreign body (►refer same day if *unilateral* obstruction ± foul/bloody discharge).

Adult: Deflected nasal septum; granuloma (TB, syphilis, granulomatosis with polyangiitis, leprosy); topical vasoconstrictors; tricyclics. ►*Refer urgently if:* • Numbness • Tooth loss • Bleeding • Unilateral obstructing mass. *Ask:* do symptoms vary? Is it both sides? Any effects on eating, speech, smell, or sleep (snoring)? Assess nasal deflection. Is either nostril completely blocked (occlude each nostril)? Examine the postnasal space (nasal endoscope or mirror).

Further reading

British Society for Allergy & Clinical Immunology (BSACI). *Guideline for the diagnosis and management of allergic and non allergic rhinitis* (2017). https://onlinelibrary.wiley.com/doi/full/10.1111/cea.12953

Fokkens WJ *et al.* (2020). EPOS 2020: European position paper on rhinosinusitis and nasal polyps 2020. A summary for otorhinolaryngologists. *Rhinology* 50:1–12.

---

5 Old man's drip often occurs on eating, and ipratropium nasal spray (Rinatec®) may help.

Allergic rhinosinusitis May be seasonal (hay fever, prevalence ≈20%, common in childhood) or perennial (more common in adults). *Cause:* IgE-mediated inflammation from allergen exposure to nasal mucosa causing inflammatory mediator release from mast cells eg from house dust mite (perennial), pollens or animal dander. *Symptoms:* Sneezing; pruritus; nasal discharge (bilateral & variable); bilateral itchy red eyes. Check for asthma. *Signs:* Turbinates (fig 5.34) may be swollen and mucosa pale or mauve; nasal polyps (fig 5.32). ℞: • *Allergen/irritant avoidance* • *Nasal saline irrigation* (p. 411) • *Antihistamines* (non-sedating eg **loratadine** 10mg OD).[20] If moderate/persistent symptoms: • *Intranasal corticosteroid sprays* (see fig 5.31)—use non-systemically bioavailable corticosteroids (eg mometasone; fluticasone).

A short course of **prednisolone** can help rapid resolution of severe symptoms eg during exams (eg adults 10–20mg/24h; children 10mg/24h for 5–10 days). *Immunotherapy:* Can induce long-term tolerance to allergens eg once-daily sublingual immunotherapy (SLIT) for grass pollen-induced rhinosinusitis. The future for some patients may lie in same-season ultra-short course allergy vaccine (eg 4 injections of Pollinex Quattro®).[21]

Functional endoscopic sinus surgery (FESS) May be performed when maximum medical therapy has failed or as part of treatment for the complications of acute or chronic rhinosinusitis.

The aim of surgery is to improve the drainage of the sinuses (table 5.2). A systematic approach is followed using the preoperative CT findings as a guide to the type and extent of surgery required. Surgical opening of the maxillary, ethmoid, frontal, and sphenoid sinuses is possible. The septum can be straightened (septoplasty) and the inferior turbinates reduced at the same time to improve nasal airflow. Surgery is performed under a GA using endoscopes and microinstruments. A microdebrider is often used to help with surgery. Advanced surgery on the skull base can be augmented using an image guidance system.

Postoperatively: 'Don't blow your nose until you are better'. Watch for bleeding. Abide by epistaxis advice (pp. 412-13). Rest for 1 week. Saline irrigation as required.

Complications: Complications of endoscopic surgery are rare. Bleeding is the commonest problem which may require packing. Infection can occur but routine use of antibiotics in the absence of purulent sinus secretions is not obligatory. Orbital complications can include breach of the medial orbital wall leading to periorbital bruising, an orbital haematoma requiring immediate drainage, or damage to the medial rectus muscle. The optic nerve can be bruised or transected as it travels in the lateral wall of the sphenoid sinus. The development of a CSF leak is uncommon due to breach of the skull base.

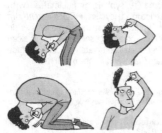

Fig 5.31 The left 2 images show how we should use nose drops; both the methods on the right are *equally* useless.

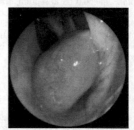

Fig 5.32 A polyp arising from left middle meatus. NB: the lower part of septum deviates to this side.
Courtesy of Nicholas Steventon FRCS.

5 ENT

Cancer of the paranasal sinuses
Suspect when chronic sinusitis presents for the first time in later life. *Early signs:* Blood-stained nasal discharge and nasal obstruction; cheek swelling. *Ix:* MRI/CT ± endoscopy (with biopsy). *Differential histology:* Squamous cell (50%), lymphoma (10%), adenocarcinoma, adenoid cystic carcinoma, olfactory neuroblastoma, or chondrosarcoma, benign tumours. *R̩:* Radiotherapy ± radical surgery.

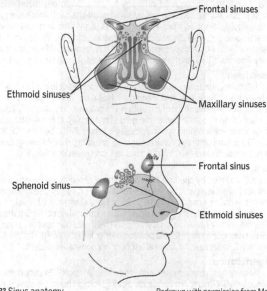

Frontal sinuses

Ethmoid sinuses

Maxillary sinuses

Frontal sinus

Sphenoid sinus

Ethmoid sinuses

5 ENT

Fig 5.33 Sinus anatomy.   Redrawn with permission from Medtronic.

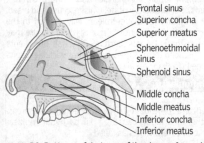

Frontal sinus
Superior concha
Superior meatus
Sphenoethmoidal sinus
Sphenoid sinus
Middle concha
Middle meatus
Inferior concha
Inferior meatus

Fig 5.34 The nasal turbinates (conchae) and meati. Table 5.2 shows the patterns of drainage of the sinuses & nasolacrimal duct.

Table 5.2 Patterns of drainage of the sinuses & nasolacrimal duct

Sinus (drains to →)	Meatus
Maxillary	Middle
Anterior ethmoidal	Middle
Middle ethmoidal	Middle
Posterior ethmoidal	Superior
Sphenoid	Sphenoethmoidal recess
Frontal	Middle
Nasolacrimal duct	Inferior

Nasal injury and foreign bodies

Nasal fractures

►Always exclude significant head or c-spine injury. The most common cause is direct trauma from a punch, clash of heads, or a fall, often with brief but short-lived epistaxis. *Diagnosis:* New nasal deformity, often with associated facial swelling & black eyes. Examine the patient from behind & above, looking along the nose. x-rays are not required, but may help exclude other facial fracture. Look for a septal haematoma (a boggy swelling of the septum causing near-total nasal obstruction). ►If present it requires urgent incision and drainage. R: Treat epistaxis (pp. 412-13); advise on analgesia/using ice; close any skin injury. Reassess 5–7d post-injury (once swelling has resolved). If MUA is required, it can be performed 10–14d after the injury (before the nasal bones set).[22]

CSF rhinorrhoea

Ethmoid fractures disrupting dura and arachnoid can result in CSF leaks. ►If not associated with trauma, ask: is it a tumour? Nasal CSF discharge tests +ve for glucose (dipstick unreliable; confirm with a lab glucose). CSF uniquely contains β_2 (tau) transferrin (needs >0.5mL; the gold standard). R: If traumatic, conservative management has high spontaneous resolution: 7–10d bedrest (head elevated 15–30°) ± lumbar drain. Avoid coughing, sneezing, nose-blowing. Surgery is often not needed. Cover with antibiotics and pneumococcal vaccine.

Foreign bodies

Most are self-inserted by children. Organic material presents early with purulent unilateral discharge; inorganic bodies may remain inert for ages. Use an auroscope to examine the child's nose. R: Ask the child to blow their nose (if able) or ask a parent to try a 'parental kiss' by blowing the mouth while occluding the other nostril (success rate >70%). If a child is cooperative it may be possible to grasp the object with crocodile forceps (avoid pushing deeper into the nose). Batteries need urgent removal. Refer to ENT if failed attempt or uncooperative patient.

Septal perforation

Septal surgery is the most common cause (BOX 'Septoplasty and septorhinoplasty'). *Others: Trauma* (nose picking; foreign body; laceration; septal haematoma); *inhalants* (nasal steroid/decongestant sprays; cocaine abuse); *infection* (TB; syphilis; HIV); *inflammation/malignancies* (SCC; Churg–Strauss; granulomatosis with polyangiitis). Perforations irritate, whistle, crust, and bleed. R: Symptomatic. Saline nasal irrigation (p. 411); petroleum jelly applied to the edge of the perforation. Progressive enlargement is a risk. Surgical closure may be via placement of a septal prosthesis ('silastic button'). Only half of patients find this tolerable and continue use long term. Surgical repair has variable results (even in experienced hands). See fig 5.35 for nasal septal anatomy.

Septoplasty and septorhinoplasty

Septoplasty

Corrects a deviated nasal septum. It is most often performed where there is nasal obstruction with no other identifiable cause (eg polyps, hypertrophied turbinate) and where conservative treatment has failed.

Septorhinoplasty

Aims to straighten and/or refashion the shape of the nose—for cosmesis and to help breathing by improving the airway.

Postoperative care: Avoid nose blowing for 1 week. Saline nasal irrigation (p. 411) with saline sniffs ×4/day for 2 weeks (prevents crusting). *Complications:* Bleeding; CSF leakage; altered sensation of lips, gums, and incisors. If a septal haematoma develops, incise and drain + give antibiotics to prevent a septal abscess (formal drainage may be needed, and may not prevent septal perforation). Adhesions between the septum and the lateral nasal wall may develop and may require division.

Nasopharyngeal cancer (NPC)

Rare in the UK. **NPC** differs significantly from other cancers of the head and neck (HNSCC, pp. 422–3). *Signs/symptoms:* Neck lump (cervical lymphadenopathy in 90%); nasal symptoms (bleeding/obstruction/discharge). Hearing loss (usually unilateral due to conductive deafness from Eustachian tube blockage); cranial nerve palsies (not I, VII, VIII) due to base of skull extension. *Δ:* Endoscopy/biopsy. NB: submucosal spread may mean the area *looks* normal. Stage by MRI. *R̵:* Radiotherapy is mainstay ± chemotherapy ± surgery (radical neck dissection). *Prognosis:* 5yr survival >80% for stage I; <30% for advanced tumours.

Nasal saline irrigation (AKA nasal douching; 'saline sniffs')

Nasal irrigation

A simple procedure that requires patients to 'sniff' a saline solution into the nostril. It helps keep the nose clean and removes any debris. It also prevents crusts from forming after surgery or epistaxis and is used in the management of rhinitis (p. 406), clearing away irritant allergens.

To make the saline solution: Place 1 flat teaspoon of salt and 1 flat teaspoon of bicarbonate of soda into a bowl and add ~1 pint of cooled boiled water. Stir until the salts have dissolved.

To use the solution: Pour some cooled solution into a *neti pot* or squeezy bottle with a nozzle (more effective than sniffing from the 'cup' of your hand). Close one nostril using your hand and pour or squeeze the solution up into your nose and let it run out. Repeat this action ~4 times up each nostril.[29]

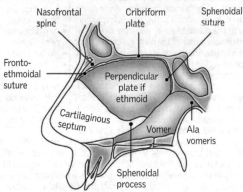

Fig 5.35 Nasal septal anatomy.
Reproduced from Warner *et al*, *Oxford Specialist HandBook of Otolaryngology and Head and Neck Surgery* (2009) with permission from OUP.

Respect all nosebleeds. While they are common, they can be life-threatening. Epistaxis is *anterior* or *posterior.* Anterior bleeds that can be easily seen with rhinoscopy are simpler to treat and are usually less severe. Proceed as follows: G-up (gown, goggles, gloves), then:

▶▶ Assess blood loss and resuscitate as needed eg if BP↓ or dizzy on sitting. ABC; IVI, SaO2, etc. Monitor vital signs.

▶▶ History: which side? Trauma? How much loss? On warfarin/aspirin? Note past medical history.

▶▶ Ask the patient to apply pressure by pinching the *lower* part of nose for 10min. Repeat if still bleeding. Breathe through the mouth; sit forward and spit blood into a bowl.

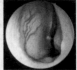
Fig 5.36 Vessels in Little's area (left side of septum). These are the main cause of epistaxis in children.
Courtesy of Nicholas Steventon FRCS.

▶▶ Place an ice pack on the dorsum of the nose (ice may also be sucked). If this doesn't work ...

▶▶ Prepare to cauterize the nose with silver nitrate.

▶▶ Use headlight and Thudicum's speculum.

▶▶ Look inside; remove clots (gentle suction).

▶▶ Apply a cotton ball soaked in 1:200,000 adrenaline for 2 minutes (causes vasoconstriction); or use local anaesthetic spray (eg lidocaine).

▶▶ Find bleeding points (often on the anterior septum). They look like small volcanoes. Apply cautery for 2sec at a time, work around the base of the volcano moving in a circle before proceeding to the top (this treats any feeding vessel). Several silver nitrate sticks will be required.

▶▶ Remember: 'silver nitrate cauterizes everything it touches'. Avoid using if actively bleeding as this will wash the chemical away and may cause unwanted discolouration of the nostril and philtrum.

▶▶ Be careful cauterizing large areas on both sides of the septum, as this risks perforation.

▶▶ If you cannot see the bleeding point, refer to ENT.

▶▶ If bleeding continues, try an *anterior nasal pack* (eg Rapid Rhino®; Merocel®). This should be 10cm long to pack entire nasal cavity. Lubricate/soak the pack as instructed; advance it into the nose horizontally and parallel to the hard palate (**not** up) keeping close to nasal septum and medial to the inferior turbinate. Inflate if required, and tape securely to the face. If all is well, remove after 24h. If bleeding continues pack the other nostril. Pressure can be applied to the nose with packs *in situ*. If bleeding continues, consider a *postnasal pack*—a variety are available, however a Foley urinary catheter (16–18G) is effective. Pass via the nostril into the nasopharynx. Inflate the balloon with >10mL water and pull anteriorly to occlude the posterior choana. Clamp (with padding over the skin) at the nasal vestibule, to prevent it falling backwards into the airway. The anterior nose will now have to be packed with ribbon gauze.

Causes/associations
• Local trauma (eg nosepicking)
• Facial trauma
• Dry/cold weather
• Dyscrasia/ haemophilia*et al*
• Septal perforation

After the bleed ...
• Don't pick or blow!
• If you sneeze, send it through your open mouth
• Avoid bending, lifting, or straining.
• No hot food or drink[6]
• If it restarts, apply ice to the bridge of the nose, and hold the soft lower part *continuously* for 20min; get help if this fails.

Anterior epistaxis

Almost invariably septal; Little's area (Kiesselbach's plexus) is used to describe the area where anterior ethmoidal, sphenopalatine, and facial arteries anastomose to form an anterior anastomotic arcade (figs 5.36 & 5.37).

6 Clearly no one will follow this advice, so suggest each mouthful is washed down with ice cold water to help keep the mouth cold and prevent vasodilatation.

5 ENT

Continued epistaxis despite adequate packing
More invasive procedures may be required:
1 *Examination under anaesthesia:* If a discrete bleeding point is found it can be treated directly eg with diathermy, otherwise repacking may be needed. Correction of septal deviation may improve access.
2 *Arterial ligation:* Endoscopic ligation of eg the sphenopalatine artery is the cornerstone of serious epistaxis management in specialist units.
3 *Embolization:* Of eg the internal maxillary or facial artery can be lifesaving—but this can cause a stroke if there is communication between the internal and external carotid circulation.

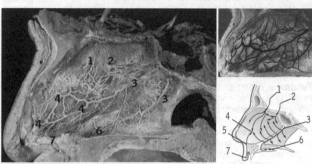

Fig 5.37 Blood supply to the nasal septum. 1 Anterior ethmoidal artery 2 Posterior ethmoidal artery 3 Sphenopalatine artery (≥2 branches, as on the dissection) 4 Little's area (anterior ethmoidal, sphenopalatine, and facial arteries anastomose to form this anterior anastomotic arcade) 5 Septal branch 6 Greater palatine artery 7 Superior labial artery and branches (from facial artery).

Courtesy of Prof Tor Chiu who performed the dissection.

An acute sore throat can be due to *acute pharyngitis* (inflammation of the oropharynx), or *tonsillitis* (fig 5.38).[23] It is commonly caused by a viral or bacterial infection and is generally self-limiting. Symptoms resolve in 40% within 3 days and within 1 week in 85%.

Causes • *Viral:* 'The common cold' eg rhinovirus, coronavirus, and parainfluenza virus account for ~25% of all sore throats; influenza type A and B (4%); adenovirus (4%); herpes simplex virus (2%); Epstein–Barr virus (glandular fever; 1%) • *Bacterial:* Group A β-haemolytic *Streptococcus* (GABHS) may cause pharyngitis, tonsillitis, or scarlet fever (see later). It cannot be diagnosed on clinical features alone but the *Centor criteria* (see 'Treatment') can be used to assist the decision on whether antibiotics should be prescribed. GABHS accounts for ~15–30% of sore throats in children and ~10% in adults • *Rarer infectious causes: Haemophilus influenzae* type B (▶epiglottitis, p. 416) *Tests:* Throat swabs should not be taken routinely. Antistreptococcal antibody tests have no role in diagnosis, but can help confirm a history of GABHS in patients with suspected poststreptococcal glomerulonephritis or rheumatic fever.

Treatment Reassure. *Symptomatic relief:* Regular ibuprofen ± paracetamol to relieve pain and fever. Consider mouthwashes or spray (benzydamine eg Difflam®). *Antibiotics:* Do not routinely prescribe antibiotics (see BOX). Most cases are viral. Antibiotics won't provide symptomatic relief and should not be given to prevent complications. If *Centor criteria* are 3 or 4 (below), consider phenoxymethylpenicillin for 10 days (lower relapse). Or clarithromycin or erythromycin for 5 days if penicillin allergic. Avoid amoxicillin, which causes a pathognomonic rash in almost all whose pharyngitis is from EBV. If immunosuppressed (eg leukaemia, aplastic anaemia, asplenia, or HIV/AIDS), seek urgent specialist advice. If on DMARDs or carbimazole, check FBC urgently. *Centor criteria:* • Presence of tonsillar exudate • Presence of tender anterior cervical lymphadenopathy • History of fever • Absence of cough. The presence of 3 or 4 of these criteria suggests infection due to *Streptococcus* (positive predictive value ~50%) and patients may benefit from antibiotics. If all 4 are absent, the negative predictive value is 80%. FeverPAIN is an alternative scoring system.

Complications of tonsillitis Associations: • *Otitis media:* p.394 • *Sinusitis:* p.406.

• *Peritonsillar abscess (quinsy):* Presents with sore throat, dysphagia, peritonsillar bulge, uvular deviation, trismus, and muffled voice. Antibiotics and aspiration (preferred to surgical drainage) are needed.

• *Parapharyngeal abscess:* A serious but rare complication, presenting with diffuse swelling in the neck, dysphagia, head turned towards side of abscess due to irritation of sternomastoid muscle. R: CT/US to identify site; IV antibiotics and/or incise and drain under GA if symptoms do not resolve.

• *Lemierre syndrome:* Acute septicaemia and jugular vein thrombosis secondary to infection with *Fusobacterium* species + septic emboli (to lungs, bone, muscle, kidney, liver). Rare.

Differential diagnosis of unilateral tonsillar enlargement

• Apparent enlargement may be due to tonsillar shift because of peritonsillar abscess/parapharyngeal mass.

• If true asymmetry, perform excision biopsy to exclude malignancy (squamous cancer in 70%).

Scarlet fever (Notifiable disease.) Caused by exotoxins released from *Strep. pyogenes* (a GABHS). If a rash develops on the chest, axillae, or behind the ears, 12–48h after initial sore throat and fever, you are probably observing scarlet fever. *Signs:* Red 'pin-prick' blanching rash; facial flushing with circumoral pallor; a 'strawberry tongue'. R: Phenoxymethylpenicillin (clarithromycin if allergic) for 10 days. *Complications:* Sydenham chorea (p. 858) or even a postinfectious demyelinating disorder eg acute disseminated encephalomyelitis. Scarlet fever used to be a major cause of infant mortality, but is now generally self-limiting in developed countries.

☙ A holistic approach to the person with a sore throat

Don't focus on the throat, the swab, or the microbiology: home in on people's health beliefs and work to harmonize these beliefs with your own.

We often think patients expect antibiotics, and will be disappointed if they are not given. Often this is not the case. Do they attend with *every* sore throat? If not, why now? Symptoms may be worse than usual and ibuprofen may help. But what may *really* help is dialogue. Rich dialogue reduces symptoms rather than merely making them more acceptable.

But improving symptoms is not the only aim: dialogue may promote patients' trust in their own body and may be a stepping stone to active health rather than passive disease.

Don't do tonsillectomy unless you are sure that …

- Recurrent sore throat is in fact due to tonsillitis.
- The episodes of sore throat are disabling and prevent normal functioning.
- ≥7 well-documented, clinically significant, adequately treated sore throats in the preceding year; ≥5 episodes in each of the last 2 years or ≥3 in the last 3 years.

NB: there is now a risk that too few tonsillectomies are being done as more adults and children are being hospitalized for throat infections.

Other indications: children with OSA; suspicion of malignancy.

▶▶ Complications of tonsillectomy

- Primary haemorrhage (<24h) often requires a return to theatre.
- Secondary haemorrhage (>24h, but typically after 5–10 days) due to infection of the tonsillar fossae. As with primary haemorrhage, this is an ENT emergency and a common ED presentation. Use the ABC approach; gain IV/IO access; cross-match and give fluid boluses; summon an experienced anaesthetist and ENT surgeon. Major haemorrhage protocols vary. Surgery may be required. If bleeding stops, admit for hydrogen peroxide gargles, IV antibiotics, and observation.

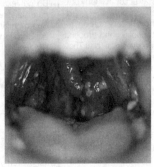

Fig 5.38 Tonsillitis.
Courtesy of Nicholas Steventon FRCS.

5 ENT

Further reading

NICE (2018). *Clinical Knowledge Summaries: Sore Throat – Acute.* http://cks.nice.org.uk/sore-throat-acute

SIGN (2010). *Management of Sore Throat and Indications for Tonsillectomy* (Guideline No. 117). Edinburgh: SIGN. www.sign.ac.uk/guidelines/fulltext/117/

Stridor This is a high-pitched noise heard in inspiration from partial obstruction at the larynx or large airways. **Stertor** is an inspiratory snoring noise, coming from obstruction of the pharynx.

▶*Children's airways are narrower than adults, so obstruction happens faster and more dramatically.* Poiseuille's law: resistance varies inversely with the 4th power of the radius, so 1mm of oedema in a neonate's 4mm diameter airway increases resistance 16-fold.

▶**Look for** Swallowing difficulty/drooling; pallor/cyanosis; use of accessory muscles of respiration; downward plunging of the trachea with respiration (tracheal tug): all are grave signs and mean impending obstruction. Birth marks or strawberry naevi.

Causes • *Congenital:* Laryngomalacia, web/stenosis, vascular rings.
• *Inflammation:* Laryngitis, epiglottitis, croup, anaphylaxis.
• *Tumours:* Haemangiomas (usually disappear without treatment). Laryngeal papillomata HPV related but malignant transformation rare.
• *Trauma:* Thermal/chemical—or from intubation.

Laryngotracheobronchitis/ croup This is the leading cause of stridor (predominantly inspiratory) with a barking cough ± respiratory distress due to upper airway obstruction. It is often worse at night. 95% are

Severity grading of croup
Mild: Occasional cough; no stridor at rest
Moderate: Frequent cough; stridor at rest
Severe: As moderate + respiratory distress

viral eg parainfluenza. ℞: Give all children with mild, moderate, or severe croup a single dose of **dexamethasone** 0.15mg/kg (**prednisolone** 1–2mg/kg is an alternative). Advise parents it is usually self-limiting and resolves within 48h. Warn to seek help if severe signs. Humidified air (steam inhalations) are not recommended. Admit if moderate (and not settling), or severe croup. See also p. 208.

▶▶ **Acute epiglottitis** This is rapidly progressive inflammation of the epiglottis and adjacent tissues (fig 5.39). It's an emergency as respiratory arrest can occur abruptly due to airway obstruction. Children (2–4 years old) present with a short history of fever, irritability, sore throat, pooling and drooling of saliva, and a muffled voice or cry. They prefer to lean forward and breathe tentatively. Cough is absent. It is now rare in children in the UK (*Haemophilus influenzae* type b vaccination has reduced prevalence). The typical patient now presenting is an adult, with severe sore throat and painful swallowing. See also p. 208.

Managing epiglottitis
▶▶Keep the patient upright.
▶▶Do not examine the throat or cause distress.
▶▶Summon an anaesthetist and ENT surgeon.
▶▶Diagnosis is made by laryngoscopy in the operating theatre and the patient intubated and treated with dexamethasone and antibiotics.
▶▶A surgical airway may be required if oral intubation is not possible.
The tracheostomy set is open and ready with appropriate tracheostomy tube prepared with appropriate connectors.

Laryngomalacia This is the main congenital anomaly of the larynx and is often noticeable within hours of birth (or up to a few months old). There is excessive collapse and indrawing of the supraglottic airways during inspiration leading to stridor, and breathing and feeding difficulties. Stridor may be most noticeable in certain positions, during sleep, or if excited/upset. In 85%, no treatment is needed and symptoms usually improve by 2yrs of age. May be associated with acid reflux. Feeding may be prolonged and sleep disturbed. Failure to thrive and or cyanotic episodes necessitate further investigation. Microlaryngoscopy and bronchoscopy for diagnosis under GA. Surgery can help in severe cases (aryepiglottoplasty).

Vocal cord palsy (laryngeal paralysis) Accounts for 15–20% of all those with congenital laryngeal anomalies. *Cause:* Often unknown, but might be from vagal stretching at birth. *Unilateral:* May manifest during the first few weeks of life with a hoarse, breathy cry that is aggravated by agitation, feeding difficulties ± aspiration. *R:* supportive; most recover by 2–3 years. *Bilateral:* Inspiratory stridor at rest that worsens upon agitation ± significant respiratory distress. *R:* urgent airway intervention may be needed (intubation, tracheotomy) ± surgery.

▶▶Acute airway obstruction: management in adults

▶▶Give O_2 or Heliox® (a mixture of helium and O_2 that is less dense than air and *may* reduce work of breathing/respiratory distress).

▶▶**Nebulized adrenaline** (1mL of 1:1000 with 1mL saline).

▶▶Note O_2 saturation, respiratory rate, pulse, and blood pressure.

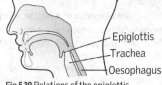
Fig 5.39 Relations of the epiglottis.

▶▶Call the on-call ENT registrar and anaesthetist for help.

▶▶Take a brief history from relatives, keeping in view the common causes of stridor.

Endotracheal intubation should be the 1st line of intervention where possible. Move on quickly if it proves difficult.

Emergency needle cricothyroidotomy and cricothyroidotomy kits eg MiniTrach II® are temporary measures pending formal tracheostomy. A wide-bore cannula is inserted through the cricothyroid membrane. This will sustain life for 30–45min as jet insufflation oxygenates rather than ventilates and CO_2 builds up.

Surgical cricothyroidotomy is quicker and easier to perform than emergency tracheostomy but is not usually performed in children <12 years.

Why is this child drooling?

Drooling is often normal if <3yrs old (eg associated with teething). So don't assume that drooling + stridor must mean epiglottitis if drooling predated the stridor. Is drooling due to reduced cerebral control of oral function, hypersalivation, or an obstruction to swallowing?
• ▶▶Angio-oedema/anaphylaxis. ▶▶Rabies (*OHCM* p437). ▶▶Epiglottitis
• Neurodisability eg cerebral palsy, bulbar palsy (↓ oro-motor control).
• Muscle problems (oesophageal dysmotility; cricopharyngeal achalasia).
• Ingestion of a foreign body or chemical toxin.
• Head and neck trauma.
• Enlarged tonsils or adenoids.
• Congenital lesions/nasal masses (eg an encephalocele or glioma).

Hoarseness entails difficulty producing sound, with change in voice pitch or quality ('breathy', 'scratchy', 'husky'). The majority of voice problems are due to viral upper respiratory tract infection and settle with little treatment. ▶Investigate hoarseness (esp. in smokers) lasting >6wks, as it is the chief (and often the only) presentation of laryngeal carcinoma (pp. 422–3). **Ask about:** gastro-oesophageal reflux (GORD), dysphagia, smoking, stress, singing, & shouting. Voice overuse is a common cause.

Tests Laryngoscopy to assess cord mobility, inspect the mucosa, and exclude local causes. Video flexible or rigid endoscopy with stroboscopy can aid in diagnosis.

Differential diagnosis of a hoarse voice

Laryngeal cancer: Progressive and persistent gruff voice (see pp. 422–3).

Vocal cord palsy: A weak 'breathy' voice. Often due to cancer (see BOX 'Laryngeal nerve palsy').

Laryngitis: (fig 5.40) This is often viral and self-limiting, but there may be secondary infection with streps or staphs. It can also be secondary to GORD (see later) or autoimmune disease eg rheumatoid arthritis. *Symptoms:* pain (hypopharyngeal, dysphagia; pain on phonation); hoarseness; fever. ℞: supportive.

Reflux laryngitis (laryngopharyngeal reflux, LPR): There are chronic laryngeal signs and symptoms associated with GORD. ~15% of all visits to ENT clinics are because of LPR. ℞: PPI; diet/lifestyle modification; elevate the head of the bed; weight loss ± surgical fundoplication.

Reinke's oedema: Chronic cord irritation from smoking ± chronic voice abuse may cause a gelatinous fusiform enlargement of the cords, resulting in a deep gruff voice. Women often say they sound like a man. Seen almost exclusively in hypothyroid, elderly, female smokers. ℞: if conservative treatment fails (stop smoking, SALT), laser therapy may help.

Vocal cord nodules: Caused by vocal abuse (eg poor singing technique, shouting, or voice abuse) and result in a variable husky voice. Fibrous nodules (often bilateral) form at the junction of the anterior ⅓ and posterior ⅔ of the cords. This is the middle of the membranous vocal folds (the posterior portion of the vocal fold is cartilage), and it may receive most contact injury during speech. ℞: speech therapy (if used early), or surgical excision. *Other causes:* Before saying 'no cause can be found', consider generalized infiltrating entities of the larynx, such as hyperkeratosis (as a result of smoking, alcohol abuse, pollution), leukoplakia, granulomata, papillomata (arising from HPV infection), polyps, and cysts. Dysphonia can be caused by high-dose inhaled corticosteroids (rinsing mouth with water after inhaling + using spacer devices may improve symptoms).

Disorders of speech articulation causing a hoarse voice

• *Spasmodic dysphonia* is a focal laryngeal dystonia of unknown cause (a similar focal dystonia is blepharospasm = involuntary blinking of the eye). Involuntary spasms of the vocal cords produce strained strangled breaks in connected speech. Symptoms vary from day to day and can be worse with anxiety. ℞: Botox® injections into laryngeal muscles; no treatment is proven.

• *Muscle tension dysphonia* is a functional disorder due to abnormal laryngeal muscle tension. Patients complain of a husky, hoarse voice that tires easily. It is associated with voice misuse and psychological stress. Globus-type symptoms are common (a feeling of a lump in the throat; frequent clearing of the throat). ℞: reassurance and explanation ± speech therapy.

• *Children with functional speech disorders* have difficulty with specific speech sounds (eg /r/ /s/ /z/ /l/ and/or 'th'). Try to distinguish articulation disorders from phonological disorders and speech dyspraxia.

Laryngeal nerve palsy

The recurrent laryngeal nerve supplies the intrinsic muscles of the larynx (apart from the cricothyroid muscle which is supplied by the external branch of the superior laryngeal nerve) and is responsible for both abduction and adduction of the vocal fold. It originates from the vagus nerve and has a complex course making it susceptible to damage. Symptoms of vocal cord paralysis are:

• A weak 'breathy' voice with a weak cough.
• Repeated coughing/aspiration.
• Exertional dyspnoea (a narrow glottis reduces air flow). NB: while at rest the contralateral cord can compensate by increased abduction.

Causes 30% are due to cancers (larynx; thyroid; oesophagus; hypopharynx; bronchus). 25% are iatrogenic ie after parathyroidectomy, oesophageal, or pharyngeal pouch surgery. *Other causes:* CNS disease (polio; syringomyelia); TB; aortic aneurysm; 15% are idiopathic (postviral neuropathy).

Investigations If there is no history of recent surgery request a CXR. If this is normal, proceed to: CT (skull base to hilum) ± US thyroid ± OGD.

Treating non-malignant causes Unilateral palsies can be compensated for by movement of the contralateral cord, but may need formal medialization via injections, or thyroplasty. *Reinnervation techniques* are also possible eg ansa cervicalis-to-recurrent laryngeal nerve (eg after damage during thyroidectomy).

Vocal hygiene ... Don't whisper! Don't shout!

• Drink plenty (eg 2L of fluid each day prevents dehydration of the cords).
• Get plenty of sleep: tiredness kills the voice.
• Take adequate deep breaths while speaking.
• Steam inhalations help keep the vocal cords hydrated.
• Avoid shouting or whispering. If your voice feels tired or strained, rest it!
• Avoid excessive throat clearing (it bashes the vocal cords together).
• Avoid irritants (spicy foods, tobacco, smoke, dust, alcohol).
• Avoid eating late at night, as indigestion may affect the voice.
• Avoid throat lozenges; these numb the throat, and menthol is drying.

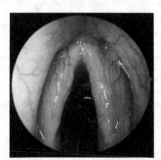

Fig 5.40 Laryngitis secondary to fungal overgrowth.
Courtesy of Nicholas Steventon FRCS.

5 ENT

Dysphagia is difficulty in swallowing: unless it is associated with a transitory sore throat, it is a serious symptom: ►*endoscopy is essential*. *Painful swallowing* is termed 'odynophagia'.

The patient As examination is typically normal (unless anaemic), the history is key. Dyspepsia? Weight loss? Lumps? Progressive dysphagia?

1 Can fluid be drunk as fast as usual, except if food is stuck?
   YES: suspect a stricture (benign/malignant).
   NO: think of motility disorders (achalasia, neurological causes).

2 Is it difficult to make the swallowing movement?
   YES: suspect bulbar palsy, especially if cough on swallowing.

3 Is the dysphagia constant and painful?
   YES (either feature): suspect a malignant stricture.

4 Does the neck bulge or gurgle on drinking?
   YES: suspect a pharyngeal pouch (food may be regurgitated).

Malignant causes
• Oesophageal cancer
• Pharyngeal cancer
• Gastric cancer
• Extrinsic pressure eg from lung cancer or node enlargement

Neurological causes
• Bulbar palsy (*OHCM* p507)
• Lateral medullary syn.
• Myasthenia gravis
• Syringomyelia (*OHCM* p516)

Other causes
• Benign strictures
• Pharyngeal pouch
• Achalasia (*OHCM* p250)
• Systemic sclerosis
• Oesophagitis
• Iron-deficient anaemia

Tests FBC; ESR; CXR; barium swallow; endoscopy with biopsy; oesophageal motility studies (requires swallowing a catheter containing a pressure transducer).

Nutrition Dysphagia can cause malnutrition. Nutritional support may be needed pre- and post-treatment eg via a percutaneous endoscopic gastrostomy (PEG). Get expert dietician help; see *OHCM* p586.

Oesophageal carcinoma This is associated with achalasia, alcohol, smoking, Barrett's oesophagus (*OHCM* p695), tylosis (a hereditary condition causing hyperkeratosis of the palms), Patterson–Brown–Kelly (Plummer–Vinson) syndrome. *Symptoms:* Dysphagia, weight loss, hoarseness, cough. *R̶:* Surgery ± chemo/radiotherapy. Post-resection 5yr survival is poor (*OHCM* p618).

Benign oesophageal stricture *Causes:* Oesophageal reflux; swallowing corrosives; foreign body; trauma. *Treatment:* Dilatation (endoscopic or with bougies eg under GA). **Barrett's oesophagus** *OHCM* p695. **Achalasia** *OHCM* p250.

Pharyngeal pouch The pharyngeal mucosa herniates through an area of weakness known as 'Killian's dehiscence', possibly due to incoordination of swallowing and increased pressure above the closed upper oesophageal sphincter. Often reflux associated. *Signs:* Dysphagia with gurgling, and regurgitation of undigested food; a nocturnal cough from spillage into larynx; aspiration/pneumonia; a lump in the neck. Often seen in elderly men. *Imaging:* Barium swallow (fig 5.41). Endoscopy must also be performed to exclude malignancy within the pouch (rare). *Treatment:* (if symptomatic), endoscopic stapling of the wall that divides the pouch from the oesophagus.

Globus pharyngeus (AKA globus hystericus) This is a sensation of a lump in the throat that is most noticed when swallowing saliva (rather than swallowing food or liquid). Patients may also complain of mucus in the throat which they are unable to clear. There is no primary swallowing difficulty and symptoms tend to come and go (worse when stressed or tired). *Cause:* Unclear. Possibly due to excess muscle tension in the pharynx, or ↑ acid exposure at the laryngopharyngeal junction. *Treatment:* Reassure. It is worsened by anxiety, and stress can form a vicious circle, but don't dismiss these patients as '*globus hystericus*'. Endoscopy may be required to exclude malignancy (eg if unilateral symptoms, otalgia, neck lump, or progressive swallowing difficulty).

5 ENT

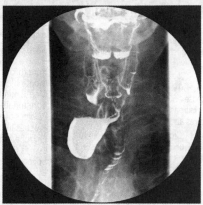

Fig 5.41 A pharyngeal pouch (called Zenker's diverticulum in the USA) 'I've got this cough... seems to get worse watching the news on TV'. When we hear this sort of absurdity, ask 'What are you doing *before* the news comes on?' 'Eating my dinner...' At this point ask about dysphagia, choking, chronic cough, regurgitation of undigested food, halitosis, weight loss, and aspiration. Listen to the neck after eating: any gurgles? Any lateral fullness/swelling? Oesophageal mucosa is herniating backwards between cricopharyngeus and inferior pharyngeal constrictors. *Typical patient*—a man over 60. *Incidence*—2/100,000/yr. *Treatment*—surgery eg day-case endoscopic stapling; note that flexible endoscopy can cause perforation when a pouch is unsuspected; hence the need for barium imaging.

Reproduced from E.E. McGrath, J. McCabe & A. Ududu. *Zenker's diverticulum. QJM: An International Journal of Medicine* (2008) 101 (9): 747–748, by permission of OUP.

90% of head and neck cancers are squamous cell carcinomas (HNSCC).[a] HNSCC develops from the linings of the upper aerodigestive tract, comprising the:

- Oral cavity.
- Oropharynx.
- Hypopharynx, larynx, and trachea (see fig 5.43).

>80% arise in those >50yrs old, but incidence among young people is increasing. Disease typically invades adjacent structures and spreads via lymphatics.

Symptoms of HNSCC
• Neck pain/lump
• Hoarse voice >6wks
• Sore throat >6wks
• Mouth bleeding
• Mouth numbness
• Sore tongue
• Painless ulcers
• Patches in the mouth
• Earache/effusion
• Lumps (lip, mouth, gum)
• Speech change
• Dysphagia

Associations • Cigarette smoking =10× ↑ risk • HPV 70% of oropharyngeal cancers • ↑ alcohol consumption • Vitamin A & C deficiency • Nitrosamines in salted fish • GORD • Deprivation.

Diagnosis Patients with suspicious symptoms (MINIBOX 'Symptoms of HNSCC') should be referred urgently for ENT review. Investigations include fibreoptic endoscopy of the upper aerodigestive tract; fine-needle aspiration or biopsy of any masses and CT or MRI of the primary tumour site to stage the neck for nodal metastatic disease. Treatment and surgery is discussed and planned by a multidisciplinary team. *Staging:* Uses the 'TNM' system:

- *Tumour* (extent of primary tumour): T1 = <2cm; T4 = extension to bone, muscle, skin, antrum, neck.
- *Node* (involvement of regional lymph nodes): N0 = no involvement; N3 = any lymph node >6cm. For the purposes of surgical neck dissection, the lymph nodes of the neck are divided into 6 areas (levels) (see fig 5.42).
- *Metastases* (presence of metastases): M0 = no mets; M1 = distant mets.

Oral cavity and tongue Uncommon in the UK. Associated with smoking and chewing betel nut (paan). *Signs/symptoms:* Persistent, painful ulcers; white or red patches on the tongue, gums, or mucosa; otalgia; odynophagia; lymphadenopathy. *R̩:* Surgery/radiotherapy. >80% 5yr survival in early disease.

Oropharyngeal carcinoma Often advanced at presentation. ♂:♀≈5:1. Increasing incidence and younger age of presentation due to HPV. 70% HPV +ve. *Typical older patient:* Smoker with sore throat, sensation of a lump, referred otalgia. *Risk factors:* Smoking and alcohol. 20% are node +ve at presentation. *Imaging:* MRI. *R̩:* Surgery and radiotherapy. Chemoradiotherapy may be 1st line if the tumour is T1 (<2cm) or T2 (>2cm but <4cm). *Prognosis:* 5yr survival ~50% for stage I. Tonsillar cancer has a better prognosis. *High-risk* HPV (esp. type 16) has been linked to cancer of the tongue, tonsil and pharynx. HPV16 is most commonly transmitted during oral sex and cancer risk relates (partly) to number of partners. Cancers associated with HPV occur in younger people, and carry a better prognosis (only in the oropharynx) than those associated with smoking. Vaccination may ↓ risk.

Hypopharyngeal tumours Rare. They can present as a lump in throat, dysphagia, odynophagia, pain referred to the ear, and a hoarse voice. The anatomic limits of the hypopharynx are the hyoid bone to the lower edge of the cricoid cartilage. *Premalignant conditions:* Leukoplakia (hyperkeratosis ± underlying epithelial hyperplasia); Patterson–Kelly–Brown syndrome (Plummer–Vinson)—pharyngeal web associated with iron deficiency: 2% risk postcricoid cancer. *R̩:* Radiotherapy and surgery. *Prognosis:* Poor (60% mortality at 1yr).

Laryngeal cancer (fig 5.44) *Incidence:* 2300/yr (UK). *Typical older patient:* Male smoker with progressive hoarseness, then stridor, difficulty or pain on swallowing ± haemoptysis ± ear pain (if pharynx involved). *Typical younger patient:* HPV +ve. *Sites:* Supraglottic, glottic, or subglottic. Glottic tumours have the best prognosis as they cause hoarseness earlier (spread to nodes is late). *Diagnosis:* Laryngoscopy + biopsy; HPV status; MRI staging. *R̩:* Radical *radiotherapy* for small tumours. Larger tumours are treated with partial/total *laryngectomy* ± block dissection of neck glands. See BOX 'Voice restoration after laryngectomy'. 5yr survival rate is 66%. *Neck dissection techniques:* Include *radical neck dissection:* all neck lymph nodes removed (level I–V) + spinal accessory nerve, internal jugular vein, and sternocleidomastoid muscle; *modified radical neck dissection:* as radical but with preservation of 1 or more non-lymphatic structures; *selective neck dissection:* 1 or more of the lymphatic groups is preserved, based on the patterns of metastases which are predictable for each site of disease; *extended neck dissection:* additional lymph node groups or non-lymphatic structures are removed.[25]

Voice restoration after laryngectomy

Patients may fear not only losing 'their' voice, but that they will be unable to communicate after laryngectomy. While surgery for small tumours may conserve a patient's voice, if the larynx is removed and the trachea brought to the skin as an end-stoma in the neck, a patient will require voice restoration.

Oesophageal speech The patient gulps down an air bolus then belches it up. The pharyngeal mucosa vibrates producing a noise which can be modified by the tongue and mouth to produce useable speech. Can be difficult to learn.

Transoesophageal puncture (TEP) A one-way valve (voice prosthesis) is inserted between the trachea and the pharynx/oesophagus, which vibrates the pharyngeal-oesophageal (PE) segment. The valve is activated when the patient occludes their stoma and breathes out. Exhaled air is modified and shaped with the lips and teeth into speech.

Artificial larynx (Servox®) If the above-listed forms of speech are not achieved, an artificial vibrating larynx can be held firmly against the patient's neck, which causes the tissues (and as a result the air within the pharynx) to vibrate, producing a distinct electronic voice sound.

5 ENT

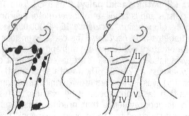

Fig 5.42 Lymph node levels in the neck. *The lymph nodes of the neck are described in 6 levels: level 1 (submandibular and submental), levels 2, 3, and 4 (high, mid, and low jugular chain), level 5 (posterior triangle), and level 6 (central neck).*
Reproduced from Corbridge et al., Oxford Handbook of ENT and Head and Neck Surgery (2010), with permission from OUP.

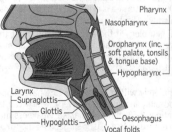

Pharynx
Nasopharynx
Oropharynx (inc. soft palate, tonsils & tongue base)
Hypopharynx

Larynx
Supraglottis
Glottis
Hypoglottis

Oesophagus
Vocal folds

Fig 5.43 Anatomy of the head and neck.

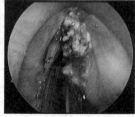

Fig 5.44 Laryngeal cancer along right vocal cord.
Courtesy of Nicholas Steventon FRCS.

Arising from motor and sensory nuclei in the pons and exiting the brainstem at the pontomedullary junction, the facial nerve passes through the posterior fossa and runs through the middle ear before emerging from the stylomastoid foramen to pass into the parotid. Lesions may be at any part of its course.

Intracranial branches 1 The greater superficial petrosal nerve (lacrimation) 2 Branch to stapedius (lesions above this cause hyperacusis) 3 The chorda tympani (supply taste to anterior ⅔ of the tongue).

Extracranial branches (All are motor fibres that branch after emerging from the stylomastoid foramen.) • Posterior auricular nerve • Branch to posterior belly of digastric muscle and stylohyoid muscle. There are 5 major branches within the parotid: • Temporal • Zygomatic • Buccal • Marginal mandibular • Cervical.

Causes of facial palsy
Intracranial: Brainstem tumours; strokes; polio; multiple sclerosis; cerebellopontine angle lesions (acoustic neuroma, meningitis).
Intratemporal: Otitis media; Ramsay Hunt syndrome; cholesteatoma.
Infratemporal: Parotid tumours; trauma leading to a complete palsy is an indication for urgent CT—if the nerve canal is disrupted, surgical exploration is advised.
Others: Lyme disease; sarcoid; diabetes; Bell's palsy.

Signs Lower motor neuron lesions can paralyse all of one side of the face; but in upper motor neuron lesions (eg CVA), the forehead muscles and closing the eyes may still work (they are bilaterally represented).

Tests ESR; glucose; Lyme disease serology. Examine the parotid for lumps and the ears to exclude cholesteatoma and Ramsay Hunt syndrome (p. 856). Any head trauma? *MRI:* Space-occupying lesions; CVA; MS; temporal bone fracture.

Bell's palsy (AKA idiopathic facial palsy) (figs 5.45 & 5.46) This is the cause of 70% of facial palsies and is a unilateral lower motor neuron facial palsy. It is partly a diagnosis of exclusion. *Incidence:* 15–40/100,000/yr. Risk ↑ in pregnancy (×3) and diabetes (×5). *Features:* The cause is unclear but is thought to be due to inflammatory oedema from entrapment of the facial nerve in the narrow bony facial canal. Onset is abrupt (eg overnight or after a nap), with complete weakness at 24–72h. The mouth sags and there is dribbling and watering (or dry) eyes + impaired brow-wrinkling, blowing, whistling, lid closure, cheek-pouting, taste, and speech ± hyperacusis from stapedius palsy. *Treatment:* There is good evidence that **prednisolone** results in improved rate of recovery and shorter time to recovery for people presenting within 72h of symptom onset. There is no consensus on the optimum dosing regimen. Options include 25mg/12h for 10 days, or 60mg/24h for 5 days reduced by 10mg each day thereafter. There is no role for antiviral treatment either alone or in combination with prednisolone—it has shown no effect on either rate of recovery or time to recovery. *Protect the eye* by keeping it well lubricated (drops during the day; ointment at night). If the cornea is exposed on trying to close the eye seek urgent ophthalmology advice.[26,27,28]

Referral: Refer urgently to ENT or neurology if there is any doubt about the diagnosis; if recurrent Bell's palsy (~7%); in bilateral facial palsy (common causes: Lyme disease, Guillain–Barré syndrome, leukaemia, sarcoidosis, EBV, trauma, myasthenia gravis); and if paralysis shows no sign of improvement after 1 month.

Prognosis: ~80% will recover completely within 3 months. ~15% have axonal degeneration with delayed and possibly incomplete recovery, which can be complicated by aberrant reconnections. ~5% have permanent weakness that is cosmetically and clinically apparent (refer to a plastic surgeon >6 months).

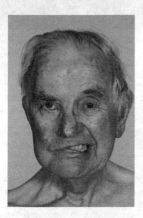

Fig 5.45 Right-sided Bell's palsy: the patient is trying to smile, but his right lower lid is drooping, the nasolabial fold is slack, and the lips do not move.

© OUP data bank.

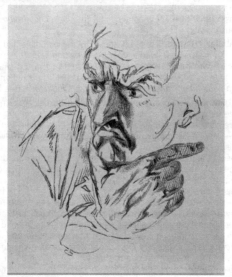

Fig 5.46 'Peevish melancholy' by Scottish surgeon, anatomist, and neurologist, Sir Charles Bell (1774–1842) from his work 'Essays on the Anatomy of Expression in Painting' (1806). 'In discontent the brow is clouded, the nose peculiarly arched, and the angle of the mouth drawn down very remarkably.'

Bell is best known for describing the facial palsy that bears his name, but also first described the trajectory of the facial nerve. He combined neuroanatomy with practice and studied in detail the emotions of facial expression. A talented artist, he undertook numerous anatomical drawings, including many of injuries seen while operating on the wounded at the battle of Waterloo in 1815.

Further reading

Gagyor I et al. (2015). Antiviral treatment for Bell's palsy (idiopathic facial paralysis). *Cochrane Database Syst Rev* 11:CD001869.

Madhok VB et al. (2016). Corticosteroids for Bell's palsy (idiopathic facial paralysis). *Cochrane Database Syst Rev* 7:CD001942.

▶Refer urgently any possibly malignant neck lump to ENT.

Diagnosis First, ask *'How long has the lump been present?'* If <3 weeks, re-active lymphadenopathy from a self-limiting infection is likely, and extensive investigation is unwise. Next ask: *'Which tissue layer is the lump in?'* Is it intra-dermal (eg from sebaceous cyst with a central punctum, or a lipoma)?

If the lump is not intradermal, and not of recent onset, you are about to start a diagnostic hunt over complex terrain. But remember—you are vastly outnum-bered by a pack of diseases and possible pathology.

Tests US shows lump architecture and vascularity and allows guidance of FNAC. CT defines masses in relation to their anatomical neighbours. Do virology and Mantoux test. CXR may show malignancy, or in sarcoid reveal bilateral hilar lymphadenopathy. Fine-needle aspiration cytology has a pivotal role in investigating suspicious lymph nodes (fig 5.51) in the neck (FNAC, figs 5.53 & 5.54).

Midline lumps • In patients <20yrs old, the likely diagnosis is a *dermoid cyst* • If it moves *up* on protruding the tongue and is below the hyoid, it is likely to be a *thyroglossal cyst* (a fluid-filled sac resulting from incomplete closure of the thyroid's migration path; treated by surgery) • If >20yrs old, it could be a thyroid mass (fig 5.48) • If it is bony hard it may be a *chondroma* (a benign cartilaginous tumour).

Submandibular triangle (Bordered above by the mandible and below by digastric.) • If <20yrs, self-limiting *reactive lymphadenopathy* is likely • If >20yrs, exclude *malignant lymphadenopathy* (eg firm and non-tender; any B symptoms: fever, night sweats, weight loss?) • ▶Is TB likely? • If it's not a node, think of *submandibular salivary stone, tumour,* or *sialadenitis* (see fig 5.52).

Anterior triangle (Between the midline, anterior border of sternomastoid, and the line between the 2 angles of the mandible.) • *Lymphadenopathy* is common: remember to examine the areas which they drain (is the spleen enlarged?—this ± B symptoms may indicate lymphoma) • *Branchial cysts* (fig 5.47) emerge under the anterior border of sternomastoid where the upper ⅓ meets the middle ⅓. The popular theory is that they are due to non-disappearance of the cervical sinus (where the 2nd branchial arch grows down over 3rd and 4th) but this is not universally accepted. Lined by squamous epi-thelium, their fluid contains cholesterol crystals. Treat by excision • If the lump is in the superoposterior area of the anterior triangle, is it a *parotid tumour* (more likely if >40yrs)? • *Laryngoceles* are an uncommon cause of lumps in the anterior triangle: they are painless, more common in males, and are made worse by blowing. If the lump is pulsatile it may be a: • *Carotid artery an-eurysm* • *Tortuous carotid artery* or • *Carotid body tumour* (chemodectoma). These are very rare, move from side to side, but not up and down, and splay out the carotid bifurcation. They are firm and pulsatile, and do not usually cause bruits. They may be bilateral, familial, and malignant (5%). Suspect in any mass just anterior to the upper third of sternomastoid. Diagnose by US/MRA. Treatment: extirpation by a vascular surgeon. Fig 5.49 & fig 5.50 show superficial and deep infections.

Posterior triangle (Behind sternomastoid, in front of trapezius, and above the clavicle.) • *Cervical ribs* p. 468 may intrude into this area. These are enlarged costal elements from C7 vertebra. The majority are asymp-tomatic but can cause neurological symptoms from pressure on the bra-chial plexus or Raynaud syndrome by compressing the subclavian artery • *Pharyngeal pouches* can protrude into the posterior triangle on swallowing (usually left sided) • *Cystic hygromas* are macrocystic lymphatic malfor-mations that transilluminate brightly. Treat by surgery or hypertonic saline sclerosant • If there are many small lumps, think of *lymphadenopathy*—TB or viruses eg HIV or EBV or, if >20yrs, consider lymphoma (any B symptoms?) or metastases.

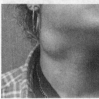

Fig 5.47 Branchial cyst.
© Bechara Ghorayeb.

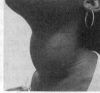

Fig 5.48 Goitre.
© Bechara Ghorayeb.

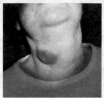

Fig 5.49 Infected cyst.
© Bechara Ghorayeb.

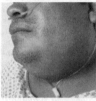

Fig 5.50 Deep cervical abscess.
© Bechara Ghorayeb.

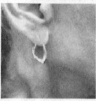

Fig 5.51 Lymph node metastases.
© Bechara Ghorayeb.

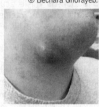

Fig 5.52 Submandibular abscess.
© Bechara Ghorayeb.

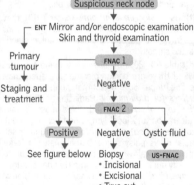

Fig 5.53 Fine-needle aspiration cytology (FNAC) in the investigation of a neck node.

Balm *et al.* 'Diagnosis and treatment of a neck node swelling', *International Journal of Surgical Oncology*, 2010.

Fig 5.54 Procedure for suspicious node if FNAC is positive. EGA: examination under GA; LCUC: large cell undifferentiated cancer; MDT: multidisciplinary team; SCC: squamous cell cancer.

Balm *et al.* 'Diagnosis and treatment of a neck node swelling', *International Journal of Surgical Oncology*, 2010.

The 3 major pairs of salivary glands are: *parotid* (on the side of the face in front of the ear), *submandibular* (just under and deep to the mandible body), and *sublingual* (in the floor of the mouth). Many additional minor salivary glands are distributed throughout the mouth and throat.

Examination Look for external swellings, palpate for stones, test facial nerve function. Note size, mobility, and extent of any mass, as well as fixity to surroundings. Any tenderness? Assess surrounding skin as regional metastases from skin or mucosal malignancies may present as salivary gland masses.

Sialadenitis This is acute infection of the submandibular or parotid glands. It usually occurs in elderly or debilitated patients, who may be dehydrated and have poor oral hygiene. *Symptoms:* Painful diffuse swelling of the gland + fever. Pressure applied over the gland may lead to pus leaking out of the duct. *R:* Antibiotics + good oral hygiene. Sialagogues are helpful (eg lemon drops, which stimulate salivation). Surgical drainage may be required. Chronic inflammation or recurrent attacks may occur due to strictures (from previous infection) or salivary gland stones. Pain and swelling on eating are common.

Salivary stones (sialolithiasis) Usually affect the submandibular gland where secretions are richer in calcium and thicker. *Signs and symptoms:* Pain and tense swelling of the gland during/after meals. A stone may be palpable in the floor of the mouth. *Imaging:* Plain x-ray or sialogram if diagnostic doubt. *R:* Small stones may pass spontaneously (sialagogues may help). Larger stones may need surgical removal. Endoscopic removal is possible.

Other inflammatory conditions • *Sjögren syndrome* (OHCM p710) may cause diffuse enlargement of the parotid • *Viral infections* eg mumps and HIV may cause inflammation of the parotid or submandibular glands • *Granulomatous disease* eg TB and sarcoidosis.

Salivary gland tumours See table 5.3. '80% of all salivary gland tumours occur in the parotid gland; 80% of these are benign pleomorphic adenomas; 80% of these are in the superficial lobe.' 50% of submandibular gland tumours are malignant. *Risk factors for malignancy:* Radiation to the neck; smoking. *Symptoms suggestive of malignancy:* Hard, fixed mass ± pain. There may be overlying skin ulceration and local lymph node enlargement. Tumours do not vary in size (eg when eating), as seen in inflammation or salivary stones. An associated facial nerve palsy suggests malignancy. ►Refer all patients with unexplained persistent salivary gland swelling, or any unexplained neck lump (or any previously undiagnosed neck lump that has changed over a period of 3–6 weeks). *Investigations:* US/MRI, FNAC/CT-guided biopsy. *R:* Surgery, radiotherapy. *Pleomorphic adenoma:* A slow-growing benign tumour occurring in middle-age that may turn malignant if present for many years. Usually diagnosed by FNAC. *Treatment:* surgical removal. *Warthin's tumour (adenolymphoma):* Usually occur in elderly men, most commonly in the parotid gland. May be bilateral. *Treatment:* partial parotidectomy. *Mucoepidermoid carcinoma:* Aggressive high-grade tumours require excision + radiotherapy. Low-grade tumours usually only need surgery. *Adenoid cystic tumours:* Painful slow-growing tumours that tend to spread along the nerves ('perineural infiltration') + distant metastases and late recurrence. *Treatment:* surgical excision + postoperative radiotherapy.

Table 5.3 Salivary gland tumours

Benign tumours	Low-grade malignant	High-grade malignant
Pleomorphic adenoma	Mucoepidermoid (grade I or II)	Mucoepidermoid (grade III)
Adenolymphoma	Acinic cell tumours	Adenocarcinoma
(Warthin's tumour)		Squamous cell cancer
Rarer: oncocytomas		Adenoid cystic

The dry mouth (xerostomia)

Signs • Dry, atrophic, fissured oral mucosa; also:
• Discomfort, causing difficulty eating, speaking, and wearing dentures.
• No saliva pooling in floor of mouth.
• Difficulty in expressing saliva from major ducts.

Complications Dental caries; candida infection.

Management • ↑ oral fluids; take frequent sips.
• Good dental hygiene; no acidic drinks or foods that demineralize teeth.
• Try saliva substitutes/dry mouth products (eg Biotène® products).

Typical causes

• Hypnotics & tricyclics
• Antipsychotics
• β-blockers; diuretics
• Mouth breathing
• Dehydration
• ENT radiotherapy
• Sjögren syndrome
• SLE and scleroderma
• Sarcoidosis
• HIV/AIDS
• Parotid stones

5 ENT

Łucja Frey and her misconnection syndrome

'Doctor … when I eat, or even just *think* of food, a sweaty rash crops up on my cheek.' (fig 5.55)

Duphenix first described gustatory sweating in 1757, but its cause was mysterious until 1923, when a soldier presented to Łucja Frey, a pioneering Polish neurologist.[7] Her soldier had a bullet in his parotid, and with it, gustatory sweating. Frey's brilliant dissections showed how the auriculotemporal branch of the trigeminal nerve sends parasympathetic fibres to the parotid and sympathetic fibres to facial sweat glands. During resprouting after injury, fibres switch course to cause gustatory sweating.

You don't have to be shot to get Frey syndrome. Other causes: birth trauma; parotid surgery (in 23%, so preoperative counselling is vital but only understood fully by neuroanatomists). Management is difficult, but not always needed. Botulinum toxin has been tried.

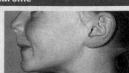
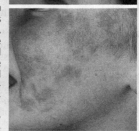

Fig 5.55 Frey syndrome before and after eating.

Reproduced with permission from Hussain N *et al.* Frey's syndrome: a masquerader of food allergy. *Postgraduate Medical Journal* 2010;86:62. doi: http://dx.doi.org/10.1136/pgmj.2009.090225. Copyright © 2010, British Medical Journal.

---

7 Łucja Frey was the first female neurologist we know of, and the most tragic. She was murdered by the Nazis in the Lwów ghetto in 1942.

▶Any oral ulcer which has not healed in 3 weeks should receive specialist assessment for biopsy to exclude malignancy (*оncm* p246).

Causes of facial pain Tooth pathology, sinusitis, temporomandibular joint (TMJ) dysfunction, salivary gland pathology, migraine, trigeminal neuralgia, atypical facial pain (no clear cause), trauma, cluster headache (*оncm* p457), angina, frontal bone osteomyelitis (post sinusitis), ENT tumours.

When helping a patient with a dental infection pay attention to the following features, before consulting a dentist, or a maxillofacial surgeon:

1 *Is it the teeth?* History: *Is the pain …*

- Worse with sugar and heat? ⎫ ► Tooth is alive
- Worse or better with cold? ⎬ (pulpitis)
- Intermittent? ⎭

Is the pain …
- Worse with percussion? ⎫ ► Tooth dead
- Constant/uninterrupted? ⎬ (osteitis/abscess)

Is the pain …
- Exacerbated by movement ⎫ ► Abscess
  between finger and thumb? ⎭

x-ray (usually helpful): orthopantogram (OPT) is useful for imaging molars and pre-molars. If incisors are suspected, request periapical x-rays of the tooth in question. Interpretation of x-ray: fig 5.56.

2 *Trismus:* (Opening mouth is difficult because of spasm or pain.) This is a sign of severe infection. Ask the patient to open mouth wide and measure how many fingers' breadth between the incisor teeth. Trismus always requires maxillofacial advice. Other causes: tetanus; neoplasia.

3 *Facial swellings due to dental infection:* Usually subside with oral antibiotics. ▶If swelling is related to the lower jaw, assess for airways obstruction; if spreading to the eye, assess the 2nd cranial nerve. If in any doubt, refer to a maxillofacial surgeon.

4 *Vital signs:* Check temperature, pulse, and blood pressure. Patients who are systemically unwell require maxillofacial advice/admission.

5 *Systemic disease complicating dental infection:* Any immunocompromise (eg HIV, leukaemia, diabetes, patients on steroids); patients at risk of endocarditis; coagulopathy (eg haemophilia or warfarin) ▶Seek specialist advice.

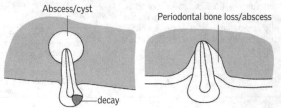

Fig 5.56 Distinguishing between (left) abscess of the tooth and (right) periodontal disease.

Dental caries Declining in the West due primarily to fluoride, this condition is increasing exponentially in developing countries. Causes: bacteria (esp. *Strep. mutans*), substrate (sugars), and susceptible tooth surface. In otherwise healthy individuals it is an entirely preventable disease.

Radiation caries (eg post head & neck radiotherapy eg with jaw osteoradionecrosis.) *Treatment and complications:* Pain ± infection. Toothache pain responds best to NSAIDS eg **ibuprofen** 200–400mg/8h PO after food, and dental infection to penicillin and metronidazole, but drug treatment is never definitive, and a dental referral is required.

Periodontal disease Virtually all dentate adults have gingivitis, caused by bacterial and polysaccharide complexes at the tooth–gingival interface (= plaque). Toothbrushing is the only answer. Pathogens: herpes; streps etc. *Vincent's angina:* (Necrotizing ulcerative gingivitis.) A smoking- or HIV-associated, painful, foul-smelling gingivitis, caused by anaerobes (*Fusobacteria*) ± spirochetes (*Borellia vincenti*). ℞: **amoxicillin** 500mg/8h PO + **metronidazole** 400mg/8h PO + dental referral. *Causes of gingival swelling:* Fibrous hyperplasia (congenital; or from phenytoin, ciclosporin, nifedipine); pregnancy, HIV, scurvy, leukaemic deposits. *Periodontitis (pyorrhoea):*

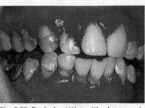

Fig 5.57 Periodontitis with damage to supporting tissue including bone.

Reproduced with permission from Coventry J, *et al.* Periodontal disease *BMJ* 2000; 321:36. doi: https://doi.org/10.1136/bmj.321.7252.36. Copyright © 2000, British Medical Journal Publishing Group.

(fig 5.57) A progression of localized inflammation from the gums into the ligament supporting a tooth. *Associations:* anaerobes; calcified bacterial deposits (calculi, tartar); poor oral hygiene. It needs a dentist.

HIV and periodontal disease: HIV causes candida, ulcers, linear gingival erythema, necrotizing ulcerative gingivitis, and necrotizing ulcerative periodontitis. *Causes of juvenile periodontitis:* Poor nutrition; immunosuppression; ↓WCC; neutrophil dysfunction (leucocyte adhesion deficiency, Chediak–Higashi or Papillon–Lefèvre syndrome with palmar keratosis), granulomatous disease.

Malocclusion Inappropriate positioning of the teeth in the jaws or between the jaws themselves is common. Those with prominent upper teeth are particularly prone to trauma, and those at risk (eg in epilepsy or involved in contact sports) should see an orthodontist. Those with severe facial or jaw disharmony who may be unable to chew or have psychological difficulty with their appearance may be amenable to surgical correction.

Wisdom teeth These declare themselves in early adult life. Like the appendix, they are something of a vestigial organ. Impaction can cause pain (fig 5.58). If asymptomatic and not exposed to contamination by the mouth, they don't usually need removal. Complications are pain and infection and they may be involved in fractures of the mandible. Postoperative recovery is often complicated by pain and swelling; pain responds well to NSAIDs and poorly to opiates. Infection complicates up to 30% not receiving antibiotics.

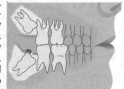

Fig 5.58 Impacting wisdom teeth.

Amoxicillin and metronidazole (as previously described) are standbys.

Teething An acute sore mouth during tooth eruption is often caused by viral infections. The onset of eruption of first deciduous teeth correlates with the fall-off in transferred maternal antibody.

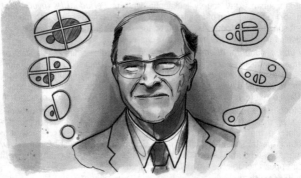

Fig 6.1 At the age of 23, while still a medical student, Frederic Mohs started to develop a surgical technique that would change the practice of dermatological surgery forever. In 1933, while working as a research assistant, he found that tissue could be 'fixed' for microscopic examination using zinc chloride. This allowed him to map and remove not just the visible parts of a skin cancer but also any microscopic spread. Mohs performed the technique on human patients for the first time in 1936. Although it took several days to fully excise skin cancers using this technique in those early days, the methods have been modified over the years and the procedure is now carried out as a day treatment. The Mohs Micrographic Surgery technique allows patients to have their skin cancers excised with a 99% cure rate while maximizing the preservation of normal tissues and therefore offering the best cosmetic results. This is particularly important in the treatment of skin tumours in challenging sites, such as those in close proximity to the eyes or nose. Mohs' story illustrates that astute observations and innovative thinking from medical students and trainee doctors can lead to major shifts in practice and improvements in patient care. We can all take inspiration from him![1,2]

Artwork by Gillian Turner.

With many thanks to our junior reader Bernard Ho for their contribution to this chapter. We also thank and acknowledge Dr Susan Burge for her kind permission to use images from the Oxford Handbook of Medical Dermatology.

☘ Holistic approaches to dermatology

Because our skin is our most superficial organ, dermatology is never given due weight; but the skin is also our heaviest organ, and although its wounds may only seem skin deep, their effects can cast long shadows: people judge our health and beauty by the condition of our skin.

Our skin displays a more varied range of signs and reaction patterns than any other organ, but dermatologists do not confine themselves to the skin. Skin disorders such as psoriasis and eczema may be worsened by emotional stress (psychophysiological disorders) and skin symptoms are features of many systemic diseases (p. 438). Primary psychiatric disorders may manifest as skin complaints, such as dermatitis artefacta and delusions of parasitosis (see BOX 'Delusions of parasitosis', p. 460).

Common skin conditions such as eczema (p. 446) and psoriasis (p. 444) are not only the domain of dermatologists but are likely to be encountered by us all, regardless of our speciality. A practical knowledge and clinical confidence in diagnosing skin disease is a most valuable asset—and we *all* need to know how the dermatological aspects of our patients' lives interact with complex biological, social, and psychological events.

Dermatology terminology—it's all Greek[G] (and Latin[L]) to me!

Alba[L]=white (as in albino).

Alopecia[G]='fox-mange' (which causes patches of hair loss).

Atopy/Atopic[G]=out of place/unusual (a predisposition to allergic responses).

Atrophy[G]='without food' (thinning and loss of skin substance).

Cutis[L]=skin (sub[L]=under eg subcutaneous).

Derma[G]=skin (intra[L]=within).

Eczema[G], from *ekzein*, to break out, boil over.

Erythema[G]=redness. Blanches with pressure.

Filiform[L]=thread (long, irregular projections, seen in warts).

Impetere[L]=to attack (as in impetigo).

Indurare[L]=to harden (as in induration).

Lichen[L]=tree moss (thick, bark-like skin caused by scratching, fig 6.2).

Livedo[L]=furious, red/blue.

Reticulum[L]=net.

Lupus[L]=wolf. The cutaneous manifestations of SLE appear similar to a wolf-bite.

Macula[L]=stain/spot.

Papilla[L]=nipple or teat (papule; papilloma).

Pilus/pili[L]=hair.

Pityriasis[G]=grain husk, flaky scales.

Psoriasis[G]=psora=itch; NB: psoriasis often does not itch.

Purpura[L]=purple (imperial) colour. Does not blanch with pressure.

Rosea[L]=pink.

Seborrhoeic=making

Sebum[L]=(suet, grease).

Telangiectasia[G] ... *telos*=end; *angeion*= vessel; *ekstasis*=extension (fig 6.3).

Topicos[G]=surface (hence creams are *topical*).

Vesica[L]=purse, bladder (fluid-filled blister).

Vitellus[L]=spotted calf (as in vitiligo).

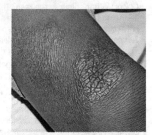

Fig 6.2 Lichenification.

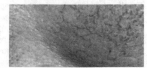

Fig 6.3 Telangiectasia.
Reproduced from *Longmore et al. Oxford Handbook of Clinical Medicine* (2014) with permission from OUP.

History See table 6.1.

Table 6.1 Important points to elicit in a dermatological history

	Rashes	Lesions
Presenting complaint	Duration, site, spread, evolution, distribution, symptoms (itch, pain, bleeding), aggravating/relieving factors (sunlight/heat), preceding trauma	
Past medical history	Atopy (eczema/hay fever/asthma), history of skin disease	History of skin cancer/premalignant lesions. Skin type—burns easily?
Family history	Atopy, history of skin disease	Skin cancers
Drug history	Regular medication, any new medications and timeline	Immunosuppressive drugs (↑ risk of skin cancer), anticoagulants
Social history	Pets, foreign travel, smoking, alcohol use, sexual history (if relevant), occupation, QOL impact	History of sun exposure, use of sunbeds, occupation, ever lived abroad?

Examination Examine all the skin, scalp/hair, nails, and mucous membranes. Try to be as accurate as possible in describing lesions (see fig 6.4 on p. 435 for terminology). Is the problem epidermal or dermal?

• *Shape:* What shape are the lesions? Monomorphic (one form or shape) or polymorphic? Ring-like (annular) eg in fungal infections—active edge with healing centre, p. 448? Linear, eg from excoriations? Discoid (coin-like)?

• *Pattern:* Are lesions grouped, scattered, or generalized? Are there crops of lesions (eg varicella)? Target-like (in erythema multiforme)? Does it demonstrate a Köbner phenomenon (a predilection for areas of skin injury)?

• *Border:* Is the border distinct and well demarcated or indistinct?

• *Surface:* Is the surface scaly (suggesting epidermal pathology, eg in psoriasis) or smooth (dermal)? Are there excoriations or erosions from scratching? Lichenified skin looks thickened (from chronic rubbing). Any scarring?

• *Elevation:* Are the lesions raised or flat? If raised, is it due to a solid mass or fluid? Are blisters tense (subepidermal), or do they rupture easily (intraepidermal)?

• *Colour:* What colour is the rash? If red, does it blanch on pressure (suggesting erythema from increased blood in small vessels)? Non-blanching indicates purpura (from leakage of blood in the dermis)?

• *Temperature:* Does the affected skin feel hotter or cooler than normal?

• *Evolution:* Ask to look at lesions at different stages.

Distribution • Symmetrical (suggesting an endogenous/systemic cause), or asymmetrical (suggesting an external cause eg insect bites, infection, trauma, or contact dermatitis)? • Is there a predilection for certain areas? eg flexural in atopic eczema (fig 6.28 on p. 447), or extensor in psoriasis (p. 444) • Areas in contact with jewellery or cosmetics (allergic contact dermatitis) • Areas exposed to sun, eg backs of hands, face, neck (photosensitivity; solar keratosis).

Ointments, creams, lotions: the spectrum of emollients

Emollients Ointments, lotions, creams, or sprays that soothe and hydrate the skin. Use in all dry, eczematous, and scaling disorders. The best emollient is the one the patient likes most. Apply frequently and liberally (in the direction of hair growth) + use as soap substitutes or bath additives. If a large area of skin is involved, a large volume of emollient is needed, eg 500g/week. Most come as pump dispensers, which avoids bacterial contamination.

Ointments Greasy preparations that have no added water, more occlusive than creams. They consist of soft, hard, or liquid paraffin, and are suitable for chronic, dry lesions. Low risk of contact allergy as no preservatives.

Creams Emulsions of oil and water, well absorbed into the skin. They are generally more acceptable to patients than ointments because they are less greasy and easier to apply. Require preservatives to extend shelf life.

Lotions Less commonly used and have a cooling effect eg calamine lotion.

6 Dermatology

Describing a lesion

Flat, non-palpable changes in skin colour

Macule
Flat, non-palpable change in skin colour <0.5cm diameter.
'Freckles' are pigmented macules

Patch
Flat, non-palpable change in skin colour >0.5cm diameter

Elevation due to fluid in a cavity

Vesicle
Fluid within the upper layers of the skin <0.5cm diameter

Bulla
Large, fluid-filled lesion below the epidermis >10cm diameter

Blister
Fluid within the upper layers of the skin >0.5cm diameter

Pustule
Visible collection of pus in the subcutis

Elevation due to solid masses

Papule
A raised area <0.5cm diameter

Plaque
A raised area >2cm diameter

Nodule
A mass or lump >0.5cm diameter

Wheal
Dermal oedema

Callus
Hyperplastic epidermis, often found on the soles, palms, or other areas of excessive friction/use

Loss of skin

Erosion
Partial epidermal loss
Heals without scarring

Ulcer
Full thickness skin loss

Fissure
A linear crack

Atrophy
Thinning of the epidermis
Loss of tissue (epidermis/dermis +/or subcutis)

Surface changes

Scale
A small thin piece of horny epithelium resembling that of a fish

Crust (scab)
Dried exudate of blood/plasma or tissue fluid

Excoriation
A scratch mark

Lichenification
Thickening of the epidermis with exaggerated skin markings (bark-like) usually due to repeated scratching

Vascular changes

Telangiectasia
Easily visible superficial blood vessels

Spider naevus
A single telangiectatic arteriole in the skin

Purpura
A rash caused by blood in the skin—often multiple petechiae

Petechia
Micro-haemorrahge 1–2mm diameter

Ecchymosis
A 'bruise'. Technically a form of purpura

Erythema
A reddening of the skin due to local vasodilatation

Fig 6.4 To communicate with a dermatologist, it is customary to translate your findings into the descriptive terms shown in the figure.

6 Dermatology

Hypopigmented (reduced pigment) and depigmented (absent pigment) lesions

- *Pityriasis versicolor:* Superficial slightly scaly infection with the yeast *Malassezia furfur.* Appears hypopigmented on darker skin. ℞: p. 448.
- *Pityriasis alba:* Post-eczema hypopigmentation, often on children's faces.
- *Vitiligo:* (fig 6.5) Smooth white depigmented patches or macules. *Associations:* autoimmunity—particularly thyroid disease. ℞: sun protection, cosmetic camouflage. Management is difficult: potent topical steroids/calcineurin inhibitors may induce some repigmentation if recent onset; UVB phototherapy/PUVA (p. 445).

Hyperpigmented lesions

- *Lentigos:* Persistent brown macules, often larger than freckles, see p. 437.
- *Café-au-lait spots:* Faint brown macules; if >5, consider neurofibromatosis.
- *Melasma (AKA chloasma):* Smooth brown patches especially on the face, may be associated with pregnancy or oral contraceptive use.
- *Melanocytic naevi:* Pigmented moles (p. 443).
- *Seborrhoeic warts/keratoses:* Benign, greasy-brown, warty lesions usually on the back, chest, and face; very common in the elderly, fig 6.6.
- *Systemic diseases:* Addison's (palmar creases, oral mucosa, scars); haemochromatosis; porphyria cutanea tarda (+ skin fragility and blisters).

Ring-shaped lesions

- *Basal cell carcinoma:* (p. 440) Typically a pearly papule ± central ulcer.
- *Tinea:* (p. 448) Ringworm lesions are round, scaly, & itchy with central clearing.
- *Granuloma annulare:* (fig 6.7) Chronic, non-infectious, inflammatory, ~1cm ring-shaped, smooth plaques, often with raised edges. Cause unknown.
- *Erythema multiforme:* (p. 438) Target-like lesions, often on extensor surfaces. Most common causes: infections (HSV, mycoplasma); drugs.

Round, oval, or coin-shaped (discoid) lesions

- *Bowen's disease (AKA squamous cell carcinoma in situ):* (p. 440; fig 6.16, p. 441) Slow-growing, red, scaly plaque.
- *Discoid eczema:* Itchy, crusted/scaly eczema, worsened by heat.
- *Psoriasis:* Well-defined scaly red/pink plaques (p. 444). Distribution on extensor surfaces, scalp, and natal cleft distinguishes it from discoid eczema. Can affect nails.
- *Pityriasis rosea:* (p. 452) Herald patch; oval, red lesions with scaly edge.
- *Erythema migrans:* (p. 438) Pathognomonic of Lyme disease (fig 6.8).
- *Impetigo:* Well-defined red patches, with honey-coloured crust (fig 6.9). Common superficial bacterial skin infection.

Linear lesions

- *Köbner phenomenon:* Lesions (eg psoriasis) related to skin injury (fig 6.10).
- *Dermatitis artefacta:* (p. 460) Bizarre-shaped lesions induced by the patient.
- *Herpes zoster:* (p. 448) Shingles: vesicles/pustules in a dermatomal distribution.
- *Scabies burrows:* (p. 458). • *Cutaneous larva migrans:* OHCM p433.

Itch (pruritus) ►*Itch can be very distressing.* Skin will usually be scratched or rubbed and a number of secondary skin signs are seen: excoriations (scratch marks); lichenification (skin thickening, fig 6.2 on p. 433); papules or nodules (local skin thickening). *Causes:* Dry (and older) skin tends to itch. Determine if there is a primary skin disease or if itch is due to systemic disease (see also BOX 'Pruritus in the elderly', p. 455).

- *Itchy lesions: scabies* (burrows in finger-webs, wrists, groin, buttock; p. 458); *urticaria* (transient wheals, dermographism); *atopic eczema* (flexural eruption, lichenification; fig 6.2 on p. 433); dermatitis herpetiformis (very itchy blisters on elbows, shoulders); lichen planus (flat violaceous papules often on wrists).
- In ~22%, itch is caused by a systemic disease:[3] *iron deficiency* (koilonychia, pallor); *lymphoma* (nodes, hepatosplenomegaly); *hypo/hyperthyroidism; liver disease* (jaundice, spider naevi); *chronic renal failure* (dry sallow skin); *malignancy* (clubbing, masses); *drugs* (statins, ACE inhibitors, opiates, antidepressants). *Workup:* FBC, ESR, ferritin/iron studies, LFT, U&E, glucose, TSH, CXR.

Treatment: Treat any primary disease; emollients (eg Diprobase®) to soothe dry skin; sedating antihistamines at night may be helpful. Some patients find creams containing menthol helpful in relieving itch.

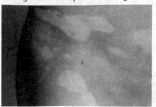

Fig 6.5 Vitiligo.
Reproduced from Burge S, *Oxford Handbook of Medical Dermatology* (2016), with permission from OUP.

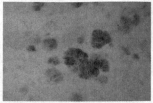

Fig 6.6 Seborrhoeic warts.
© DermNet New Zealand, reproduced with permission.

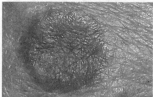

Fig 6.7 Granuloma annulare.
Courtesy of Dr Jonathan Bowling.

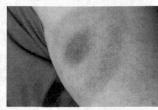

Fig 6.8 Erythema migrans (p. 438).
CDC/James Gathany.

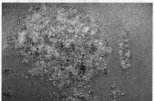

Fig 6.9 Impetigo (honey-coloured crusts).
Courtesy of Dr Samuel Da Silva.

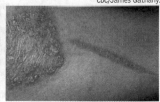

Fig 6.10 Köbner—psoriasis in a scratch.
Reproduced from Burge S, *Oxford Handbook of Medical Dermatology* (2016), with permission from OUP.

Lentigos Brown macules/patches that persist in winter (unlike freckles). *Solar lentigos* are found on sun-damaged skin in older patients. *Lentigo maligna* (fig 6.11) is a subtype of *melanoma in situ* and in ~5% may progress (over months or years) to *lentigo maligna melanoma* (a type of invasive melanoma; p. 442). Typical patient: Caucasian >40yrs with sun-damaged skin due to occupational exposure. The lesion is irregular, and variably pigmented (darker areas may be invasive). Not all show ABCDE signs of malignancy (p. 442). Use dermatoscope[1] ± full-thickness biopsy in equivocal lesions. Excision is best.

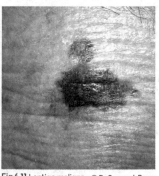

Fig 6.11 Lentigo maligna. © Dr Susannah Baron.

1 The dermatoscope is a handheld microscope using epiluminescence for evaluating pigmented skin lesions. It allows vision through the stratum corneum.

Diabetes *Flexural candidiasis; necrobiosis lipoidica* (waxy, shiny yellowish area on shins); *acanthosis nigricans* (pigmented, rough thickening of axillary, neck or groin skin); generalized *granuloma annulare* (fig 6.7); *folliculitis*.

Coeliac disease *Dermatitis herpetiformis* (very itchy/'burning' blisters on elbows, scalp, shoulders, ankles). *Treatment:* long-term gluten-free diet. It responds quickly to dapsone (specialist use).

Inflammatory bowel disease • *Erythema nodosum* (tender ill-defined subcutaneous nodules, eg on shins; other causes: sarcoidosis, drugs, pregnancy, TB, strep) • *Pyoderma gangrenosum:* rapidly growing, very painful recurring nodulo-pustular ulcers, with tender red/blue overhanging necrotic edges. Often preceded by a tender pustule. Site: leg; abdomen; face. Other causes: rheumatoid arthritis; myeloproliferative disorders (50% have no underlying disease).

Systemic lupus erythematosus (SLE) *OHCM* p554. *Facial butterfly rash; photosensitivity* (face, dorsum of hands, v of neck); *diffuse alopecia*. Patients may have cutaneous lupus erythematosus (see BOX 'Connective tissue diseases and the skin').

Erythema multiforme (EM) (fig 6.12) A type of hypersensitivity reaction triggered most often by herpes simplex. *Minor form:* Erythematous well-defined round lesions appear on extensor surfaces of peripheries, palms, and soles and evolve at different stages (multiform) into pathognomonic target lesions. There is minimal mucosal involvement. *Major form:* (Regarded as distinct from Stevens–Johnson syndrome/ toxic epidermal necrolysis, p. 451.) There is associated systemic upset, fever, and severe mucosal involvement. *Causes:* Herpes simplex (70%); mycoplasma; cytomegalovirus; drugs. *R:* No treatment is required in the majority of cases. Potent topical steroid may relieve any rash discomfort (but does

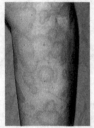

Fig 6.12 Erythema multiforme.

not speed resolution). If needed, treat the cause eg aciclovir for HSV; antibiotics for mycoplasma; oral steroids if severe (controversial); supportive care. EM resolves spontaneously without scarring within 4 weeks. In recurrent disease, consider aciclovir prophylaxis.

Erythema migrans (fig 6.8 p. 437) This is the best way to diagnose Lyme disease, as serology is difficult. ▶ <50% give history of a tick bite. The lesion is seen in 80% of cases and develops 7–10 days after the tick bite. A papule becomes a spreading red ring, lasting weeks to months. *R:* Get advice from someone experienced in managing Lyme disease. Antibiotics of choice are doxycycline, amoxicillin (unlicensed), or cefuroxime for 2–4 weeks.

Cutaneous vasculitis *Signs:* Variable; palpable purpura, eg on legs; nodules; painful ulcers; *livedo reticularis* (next paragraph p. 438). *Causes:* Idiopathic (often); systemic vasculitis, eg polyarteritis nodosa (PAN), Henoch–Schönlein purpura (vasculitic rash on legs/buttocks); granulomatosis with polyangiitis.

Livedo reticularis (fig 6.13) Non-blanching vague pink-blue mottling caused by capillary dilatation and stasis in skin venules, like diamond-shaped holes in a net, most often on the legs. *Causes:* A continuous network is physiological & disappears when the skin is warmed. Persistent and discontinuous is seen in connective tissue disease, vasculitis, cholesterol emboli, & hyperviscosity states. *R:* Treat the cause.

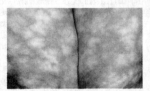

Fig 6.13 Livedo reticularis.
Reproduced from Wilkinson *et al., Oxford Handbook of Clinical Medicine* (2017) with permission from OUP.

6 Dermatology

Connective tissue diseases and the skin

Lupus erythematosus (LE) An uncommon group of skin disorders:

1 *Chilblain LE:* Cold-induced plaques on fingers and toes.
2 *Chronic cutaneous (discoid) LE:* Inflamed scaly plaques + scarring ± atrophy often localized to the head & neck. Most do not have significant systemic disease.
3 *Subacute cutaneous LE:* Widespread, non-scarring round or psoriasis-like plaques in a photosensitive distribution. 50% fulfil criteria for SLE.
4 *Acute SLE:* Seen in active SLE. Specific malar butterfly rash or widespread indurated erythema on upper trunk.
5 *Non-specific cutaneous LE phenomenon:* Vasculitis, alopecia, oral ulcers, palmar erythema, periungual erythema, Raynaud's phenomenon.

Systemic sclerosis Features scleroderma (skin fibrosis) and vascular disease:

- *Limited cutaneous systemic sclerosis:* (formerly CREST syndrome) **C**alcinosis (subcutaneous tissues), **R**aynaud's, oesophageal and gut dysmotility, **S**clerodactyly (swollen tight digits), and **T**elangiectasia. Skin involvement is 'limited' to the face, hands, and feet.
- *Diffuse cutaneous systemic sclerosis:* 'Diffuse' skin involvement (affecting the whole body if severe) and early organ fibrosis.

Sarcoidosis A multisystem granulomatous disorder. Skin is affected in 25% and lesions include • Hypopigmented patches • Yellow-brown firm (periorbital) papules • Scarring alopecia • Sarcoid in scars • Firm subcutaneous nodules (*Darier–Roussy sarcoid*) • *Lupus pernio* (fig 6.14) is diagnostic of sarcoidosis: chronic sarcoid plaques on nose, ears, lips, and cheeks ± permanent scarring.

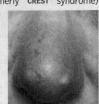

Fig 6.14 Lupus pernio of the nose.

Reproduced from Warrell et al., *Oxford Textbook of Medicine* (2010), with permission from OUP.

Paraneoplastic skin phenomena

If a tumour makes transforming growth factor (similar to epidermal growth factor and binds the same receptors), it is proposed that distant keratinocytes can flourish and a range of proliferative paraneoplastic signs erupt. Most are uncommon and are seen also in non-malignant conditions.[4]

Leser–Trélat sign: Sudden eruption of multiple *seborrheic keratoses* seen rarely in association with GI adenocarcinomas & genitourinary cancers.

Acanthosis nigricans: Darkened velvety skin, most commonly due to diabetes/obesity but can be associated with gastric cancer and lymphoma.

Dermatomyositis: Heliotrope (red/purple) eyelids (see fig 12.26 in *OHCM* p563); Gottron's papules (flat violet knuckle papules). 10–30% have an associated malignancy eg breast & ovary (♀), lung & prostate (♂), and colorectal.

Paraneoplastic pemphigus: (Rare) severe mucosal and cutaneous erosions associated with lymphoreticular malignancy.

Acquired ichthyosis: Dry scaly skin seen in lymphoproliferative disorders.

Hypertrichosis lanuginosa: An increase in downy lanugo hair, most often associated with GI adenocarcinomas and lung cancer.

Tripe palms: Ridged velvety lesions on the palms, often in association with acanthosis nigricans & associated with GI adenocarcinoma and lung cancer.

Actinic (solar) keratoses (AK) (fig 6.15) Premalignant crumbly, yellow-white scaly crusts on sun-exposed skin from dysplastic intra-epidermal proliferation of atypical keratinocytes. *UK prevalence:* 23% of those ≥60yrs old (NICE figures). *Natural history:* May regress/recur. Progression to SCC risk is <1% per year. This risk increases over time and with larger numbers of lesions. ΔΔ: Bowen's, psoriasis, BCC, seborrhoeic keratosis. If in doubt, biopsy. *Treatment:* See BOX 'Options in actinic keratoses (AK)'. *Prevention:* Education; hats; sunscreens. Advise all patients to monitor their skin as AK is a marker for risk of developing skin cancer.

Bowen disease (SCC *in situ*, fig 6.16) A well-defined, slowly-enlarging red scaly plaque with a flat edge (asymptomatic). *Histology:* Full-thickness dysplasia/carcinoma *in situ*. 3–5% progress to SCC (but the risk of metastases from the SCC is high). *Cause:* UV exposure; radiation; immunosuppression; arsenic; HPV infection is associated with the development of anogenital disease. ℞: Options include cryotherapy; topical fluorouracil or imiquimod (unlicensed); photodynamic therapy; curettage + cautery; excision.[5]

Basal cell carcinoma (BCC, rodent ulcer) The commonest skin cancer. *Nodular:* Typically, a pearly nodule with rolled telangiectatic edge on the face or a sun exposed site ± central ulcer (fig 6.17). Metastases are very rare. It slowly causes local destruction if left untreated. *Superficial:* Lesions appear as red scaly plaques with raised smooth edge, often on the trunk or shoulders. *Cause:* UV exposure; immunosuppression. ℞: Depends on type, site, and whether primary or recurrent. Excision is often the treatment of choice. Other options: cryotherapy, curettage, radiotherapy, photodynamic therapy. Topical **imiquimod** or **fluorouracil** are reasonable options for superficial lesions at low-risk sites.[6]

Squamous cell cancer (fig 6.18; the commonest skin cancer after BCC.) A persistently ulcerated or crusted, firm, irregular lesion often on sun-exposed sites. It is locally invasive and may metastasize (↑ risk if lip, ear, or non-sun exposed site; >2cm diameter; poor histological differentiation or host immunosuppression). Also related to chronic inflammation, eg leg ulcers, and HPV (eg genital area or periungual). ℞: Local complete excision in primary SCC.

Other malignancies & skin

Metastatic cancer Skin metastases (from direct tumour invasion or lymphatic/haematogenous spread) are uncommon but well recognized. The most commonly associated cancers causing cutaneous metastases are: • Breast (fig 6.20; skin of chest & scalp) • Stomach and colon (skin of abdominal wall—esp. periumbilical) • Lung (skin of chest & scalp) • Genitourinary system (uterus, ovary, kidney, bladder: skin of scalp, lower abdomen & external genitalia). Non-Hodgkin's lymphoma and leukaemia can also metastasize to the skin. Metastases are usually firm, intradermal, or subcutaneous nodules of varying colour.

Mycosis fungoides The commonest cutaneous T-cell lymphoma, which progresses from well-defined itchy, red, scaly patches and plaques to red-brown infiltrated plaques and ulcerating tumours. Δ: Biopsy. ℞: *Early stage:* potent topical steroids, PUVA. *Late stage:* radiotherapy. Sézary syndrome is a leukaemic form of cutaneous T-cell lymphoma characterized by erythroderma, lymphadenopathy, and malignant circulating CD4 positive T-cells (Sézary cells).

Paget disease of the nipple (fig 6.19) An itchy, red, scaly, or crusted nipple, from direct extension of intraductal adenocarcinoma. Δ: Biopsy. ΔΔ: Eczema (but eczema is bilateral, non-deforming, and waxes and wanes), so … ►*always consider a biopsy in 'nipple eczema'* + check for a breast lump. *Surgery:* Mastectomy or lesser surgery ± radiotherapy.

Options in actinic keratoses (AK)

- *No treatment* or *emollient* is a reasonable option for mild AK.
- *Diclofenac gel* (3%) is moderately effective (mechanism unknown); used twice daily for 60–90 days it is well tolerated and cheap.
- *Fluorouracil* (*5FU*) 5% cream once or twice daily for up to 6 weeks is effective in clearing the majority of non-hypertrophic lesions for up to 12 months. It works by causing erythema→vesiculation→erosion→ulcers→necrosis→healing epithelialization and leaves healthy skin unharmed.
- *Imiquimod* 5% 3× a week for 4wks to lesions; assess after a 4wk treatment-free gap; repeat once if persisting; allow cream to stay on for 8h, then wash. It augments cell mediated immunity by inducing interferon-α and causes a similar inflammatory reaction to fluorouracil + occasionally 'flu-like' symptoms.
- *Cryotherapy:* effective for up to 75% of lesions.
- *Photodynamic therapy:* effective in up to 91% but availability is limited. Useful if located at sites of poor healing eg lower leg.
- *Surgical excision and curettage + cautery:* excise AKs if atypical, unresponsive to treatment, or invasive SCC is suspected.

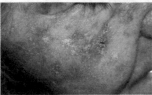

Fig 6.15 Actinic (solar) keratosis.
Courtesy of Dr Samuel da Silva:
www.atlasdermatologico.com.br

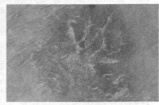

Fig 6.16 Bowen disease.
Courtesy of Dr Jonathan Bowling.

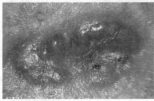

Fig 6.17 Basal cell carcinoma.
Courtesy of Dr Samuel da Silva:
www.atlasdermatologico.com.br

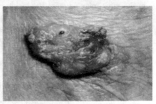

Fig 6.18 Squamous cell carcinoma.

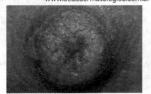

Fig 6.19 Paget disease of nipple.
Courtesy of Dr Samuel da Silva:
www.atlasdermatologico.com.br

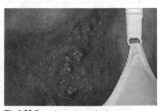

Fig 6.20 Breast cancer metastases.
Courtesy of Dr Samuel da Silva:
www.atlasdermatologico.com.br

Further reading

de Berker D et al. (2017). British Association of Dermatologists' guidelines for the care of patients with actinic keratosis. *Br J Dermatol* 176:20–43.

Morton CA et al. (2014). British Association of Dermatologists' guidelines for the management of squamous cell carcinoma in situ (Bowen's disease) 2014. *Br J Dermatol* 170:245–60.

Telfer NR et al. (2008). Guidelines for the management of basal cell carcinoma. *Br J Dermatol* 159:35–48.

6 Dermatology

Malignant melanoma (figs 6.21 & 6.22) The 5th commonest cancer in the UK. *UK incidence:* Incidence of melanoma has quadrupled since the 1970s. Incidence is expected to reach 32 per 100,000 people by 2035 (Cancer Research UK figures). Nearly ⅓ occur in those aged <50yrs and melanoma accounts for 75% of deaths associated with skin cancer. Most arise *de novo*, not in pre-existing melanocytic naevi.

Risk UV exposure ↑; sunburn, fair complexion, many (>50) melanocytic or dysplastic naevi, +ve family history, previous melanoma, old age (the highest incidence is in those >80yrs old). *Early diagnosis* ►Everyone should know what early melanomas look like, and know how to get help.

Signs Use the ABCDEF criteria to identify suspicious pigmented lesions:
• **A**symmetry in the outline of the lesion.
• **B**order irregularity or blurring.
• **C**olour variation with shades of black, brown, blue, or pink.
• **D**iameter >6mm (cannot be covered by the end of a pencil).
• **E**volution (all changing moles—in size, elevation, and/or colour, are suspect).
• **F**unny looking mole—'the ugly duckling sign'—a mole that stands out or is different from others is better than ABCDE criteria for identifying nodular melanoma, which can be symmetrical, have regular borders, and be uniform in colour. Nodular melanomas are **E**levated, **F**irm, and **G**rowing.

►► Refer urgently (under the 2-week rule in the UK) any pigmented lesion you are concerned about. Prognosis is determined primarily by Breslow thickness and mortality is significantly improved if the tumour is removed when it is thin.

ΔΔ: Benign melanocytic lesions (see BOX 'Common benign melanocytic naevi'); non-melanocytic pigmented lesions, eg *seborrhoeic keratoses*, common if >50yrs.

Types of melanoma:
• *Superficial spreading melanoma* (70%): presents as a slowly enlarging pigmented lesion with colour variation and an irregular border. Initially growth is in the radial plane, where the lesion remains thin, but this may be followed by vertical invasion. Common on the trunks of men or legs of women.
• *Nodular melanoma* (15%): the most aggressive type of melanoma. There is no radial growth phase and lesions grow rapidly, invade deeply, and metastasize early. It is often darkly pigmented but may be amelanotic in 5%.
• *Acral lentiginous melanoma* (10%): occur on the palms, soles, and subungual areas. It is the most common type of melanoma in black and Asian skin. Refer urgently any new pigmented line in a nail, or growing under a nail (especially if it extends from the nailbed to the nailfold=*Hutchinson's nail sign*).
• *Lentigo maligna melanoma* (5%): arises within a lentigo maligna (p.437).

Treatment: Surgery is the only curative treatment.[1] For *any* unusual, growing, or changing pigmented lesion, excision biopsy of the whole lesion must be considered (with a 2mm *margin of normal skin* around the lesion + a cuff of subcutaneous fat). This allows for histological diagnosis and measurement of tumour depth (Breslow thickness). If malignant melanoma is confirmed, a wider excision margin is taken (up to 3cm) to ensure complete removal (° sentinel lymph node biopsy).

Prognosis: Depends on excision completeness and Breslow thickness. If <0.75mm thick, 5yr survival is >95%; if >4mm it is 45%. Metastatic disease has a 5yr survival of <10%. *Metastatic melanoma:* Adjuvant therapy eg interferon alfa (IFN-α) is used to minimize the risk of relapse in patients with resected node-positive (stage III) disease. There is no curative treatment for stage IV disease. Treatment (aimed at palliating symptoms and maximizing quality of life) includes chemotherapy, biological therapy (IFN-α; IL-2) and novel therapies targeting specific molecular abnormalities eg vemurafenib/dabrafenib for those with BRAF mutations. Immunotherapy with ipilimumab (anti-CTLA-4), nivolumab, or pembrolizumab (both anti-PD1) can result in prolonged survival in some patients who respond. Melanoma is not responsive to radiotherapy.

Prevention: ► Don't just diagnose today's melanoma: prevent tomorrow's.

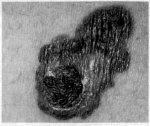

Fig 6.21 Superficial spreading melanoma.
© Dr Susannah Baron.

Fig 6.22 Nodular melanoma.
© Dr Susannah Baron.

Common benign melanocytic naevi (naevus = mole)

Congenital melanocytic naevi (Usually >1cm.) Present at birth or in the early neonatal period. If >20cm there is increased risk for malignant change.[9]

Acquired melanocytic naevi Present in childhood or in young adults and have a characteristic evolution (fig 6.23). They start as flat, evenly pigmented naevi, in which 'nests' of melanocytes collect along the basal layer of the epidermis (=junctional naevi). As melanocytes migrate from the epidermis to the dermis, moles evolve into raised evenly pigmented dome-shaped naevi (=compound naevi). Finally, the epidermal component is lost and moles change into pale brown papules (=intradermal naevi), before disappearing in old age.[9]

Halo naevi Common in adolescence. A 'white' halo develops around a benign melanocytic naevus. It is not sinister and results from loss of melanocytes by lymphocyte action. Halo naevi in adults (age 40–50yrs) may indicate melanoma elsewhere—check skin, eyes, and mucosal surfaces.[9]

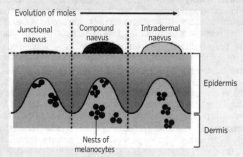

Fig 6.23 The life of a mole: evolution of melanocytic naevi.
Reproduced from Burge S, *Oxford Handbook of Medical Dermatology* (2016), with permission from OUP.

Further reading

Marsden JR *et al.* (2010). Revised UK guidelines for the management of cutaneous melanoma 2010. *Br J Dermatol* 163:238–56.

6 Dermatology

Psoriasis A chronic inflammatory skin condition characterized by scaly ery-thematous plaques, which typically follows a relapsing/remitting course. *Pathogenesis:* The epidermis in psoriatic plaques is hyperproliferative. There is proliferation and dilatation of blood vessels in the dermis + infiltration of in-flammatory cells (T-cells ± neutrophils). Plaque psoriasis is the commonest form (~90%). *Prevalence:* 1–3% (varying among ethnic groups eg 0.3% in China). 75% are affected before 46yrs old (uncommon in children). ♂:♀≈1:1. Susceptibility is inherited—if both parents have psoriasis, risk to offspring is ~50%. *Triggers:* Stress, infections (esp. streps), skin trauma (Köbner phenomenon), drugs (lithium, NSAIDs, β-blockers, antimalarials), alcohol, obesity, smoking, and climate.

⚙Psychological and social effects of psoriasis are common and can be profound. 20% are depressed. Consider the impact on body image, mood, relationships, work/school, and any problems caused by treatment. DLQI (Dermatology Life Quality Index) scoring can be helpful.

Types of psoriasis • *Chronic plaque psoriasis:* (fig 6.24) Symmetrical, well-defined red plaques with silvery scale on extensor aspects of the elbows, knees, scalp, and sacrum • *Flexural psoriasis:* Plaques in moist flexural areas (axillae, groins, submammary areas, and umbilicus) are less scaly and often misdiagnosed as fungal infection (symmetry suggests psoriasis) • *Guttate psoriasis:* (fig 6.25) Large num-bers of small plaques <1cm over the trunk and limbs are seen in the young (espe-cially after acute streptococcal infection), usually lasting 3–4 months • *Pustular psoriasis:* (Palmoplantar psoriasis.) Yellow-brown pustules within plaques affecting the palms & soles; ♀:♂≈9:1 •*Generalized (erythrodermic) psoriasis:* (and generalized pustular psoriasis) May cause severe systemic upset (fever, ↑wcc, dehydration)—both are a medical emergency requiring urgent hospital referral. NB: Also triggered by rapid withdrawal of steroids •*Nail changes:* (In 50%.) Pitting, onycholysis (sep-aration from nail-bed, fig 6.26), thickening, and subungual hyperkeratosis (fig 6.27).

Psoriatic arthropathy 7% develop a seronegative arthropathy. Screen an-nually using PEST questionnaire. 5 types: 1 Asymmetrical mono/oligoarthritis 2 Symmetrical polyarthritis (RA-like) 3 Psoriatic spondylitis 4 Distal predom-inant 5 Arthritis mutilans (destructive). Joint disease can precede skin disease.

ΔΔ Eczema; tinea (solitary or few lesions; asymmetrical; expanding); mycosis fungoides (asymmetric, less scaling, do biopsy); seborrhoeic dermatitis.

Management *Education* is vital; control, not cure, is realistic. Assess severity and proportion of skin affected (Psoriasis Area Severity Index is a useful tool). Consider phototherapy or systemic therapy if >10% body area affected. *Emollients* reduce scale and help relieve irritation. For all topical treatment select a base the patient prefers (ointment, cream, lotion, gel, or foam).

Topical treatment[10] • *Plaque psoriasis:* Use a topical corticosteroid (eg Betnovate®) each morning *plus* a topical vitamin D preparation (which affects cell division; eg Dovonex®) at night. NB: Dovobet® is a combined once-daily ointment or gel. Enstilar® is a combined foam formulation and some patients prefer this. Review at 4wks (advise patient to stop steroid before if skin is clear). If response is good, continue until the skin is clear or nearly clear. Potent corticosteroids should not be used for more than 8wks + there should be a treatment break of 4wks be-fore being restarted (during which vitamin D analogues can be continued). 1% coal tar lotion (eg Exorex®) is easier if widespread thin-plaque disease (not limited to use on affected skin). Monitor FBC, U&E, LFT, glucose, and fasting lipid profile. • *Scalp psoriasis:* Potent topical steroid lotion (OD for max 8wks) or vitamin D analogue scalp preparation. Coal tar shampoos may help. Diprosalic® (combined steroid and salicylic acid) softens and lifts scale, allowing the steroid to exert its effect under-neath • *Flexural psoriasis:* Use a mild–moderate potent topical steroid for up to 2wks (± antifungal/antibiotic combination). Break for 4wks between courses • *Localized pustular psoriasis & nail psoriasis:* Best managed by a dermatologist • *Psoriatic arthropathy:* NSAIDs, DMARDs (eg methotrexate), and anti-TNF agents.

Phototherapy, systemic, & biological treatment

Phototherapy *Narrowband uvb phototherapy:* Most suitable for guttate or plaque psoriasis that cannot be controlled with topical treatments or when disease is widespread (± topical adjunctive or systemic treatment). PUVA: Psoralen + UVA is suitable for extensive large plaque psoriasis (oral psoralen) or localized pustular psoriasis (topical psoralen). There is increased risk of skin cancer (esp. squamous cell carcinoma).

Non-biologic oral drugs Severe psoriasis often needs oral drugs (refer to dermatology). *Methotrexate:* 10–20mg/week PO; also useful in psoriatic arthropathy. Monitor FBC & LFT. *Ciclosporin:* 2.5–5mg/kg/day PO; good, but SE can be severe (BP↑; ↓U&E). *Acitretin:* Oral retinoid; useful for moderate/severe disease; SE: teratogenic; dry skin and mucosae; ↑ lipids; ↑LFT (reversible). Monitor FBC, U&E, LFT, glucose, and fasting lipid profile. In the UK, use is limited to specialists. Starting at 25–30mg/24h PO. Exclude pregnancy, avoid donating blood for >1yr and pregnancy until >3yrs after the last dose.

Biological drugs[11] Inhibit T-cell activation and function, or neutralize cytokines. They have revolutionized treatment of severe psoriasis that hasn't improved with systemic treatments or light therapy (or where these are contraindicated/have caused SE). First-line agents are ustekinumab, adalimumab, and secukinumab. Adalimumab should be considered first-line particularly if psoriatic arthritis is coexistent. All are specialist use only.

6 Dermatology

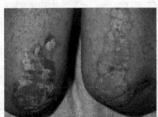

Fig 6.24 Plaque psoriasis on extensor surfaces.
Reproduced from Burge S, *Oxford Handbook of Medical Dermatology* (2016), with permission from OUP.

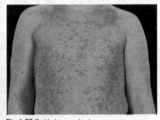

Fig 6.25 Guttate psoriasis.
Reproduced from Lewis-Jones, *Paediatric Dermatology* (2010), with permission from OUP.

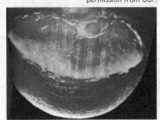

Fig 6.26 Onycholysis. Nail pitting may also be present.
© Dr Susannah Baron.

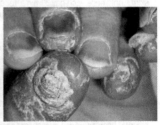

Fig 6.27 Psoriasis affecting the nails.
© Dr Susannah Baron.

Further reading

NICE (2012, updated 2017). *Psoriasis: The Assessment and Management of Psoriasis* (CG153). London: NICE.

Smith CH *et al.* (2017). British Association of Dermatologists' guidelines for biologic therapy for psoriasis 2017. *Br J Dermatol* 177:628–36.

Acute eczema causes a rash with inflamed red skin that is poorly demarcated and less scaly than psoriasis. The barrier function of the epidermis is abnormal and skin is easily irritated. Eczema is itchy and there is often associated excoriation. The pathophysiology is poorly understood and there are a number of patterns: eczema may be *endogenous* eg *atopic, seborrhoeic, varicose* (from venous stasis), or *discoid*; or *exogenous* eg *allergic contact* (type IV hypersensitivity), or *irritant contact*. Different types may coexist. Ask about impact on quality of life, school/work, and sleep.

Atopic eczema (fig 6.28)[12,13] *Causes:* Multifactorial: • *Genetic:* a family history of atopy is common (70%) • *Infection:* staphs colonize lesions, suggested by weeping, crusting, or pustules • *Allergens:* Avoidance of allergens eg house dust mite or animal dander is difficult and of limited benefit. Food allergy is rarely the cause of eczema. Consider if there is a clear trigger with immediate symptoms (eg confirm a dairy allergy with specific IgE test; if +ve, get a dietician's help); or, in poorly controlled eczema associated with GI symptoms or failure to thrive. *Diagnosis:* A child must have itchy skin (or parents report scratching) + ≥3 of:[14] 1 Onset before 2yrs 2 Past flexural involvement 3 History of generally dry skin 4 Personal history of other atopy (or history of atopy in 1st-degree relative if <4yrs) 5 Visible flexural dermatitis (or on cheeks/forehead and outer side of limbs if <4yrs). There may be lichenification (fig 6.2, p. 433, from chronic rubbing) or post-inflammatory hypo- or hyperpigmentation. Atopic eczema typically spares the nappy area. *Severity:* Mild, moderate, or severe, based on signs and symptoms, and quantity/strength of treatment required. 50% of children grow out of atopic eczema by puberty.

Management:
• *Explain:* management involves control, not cure. Discuss the cause (multifactorial, causing a breakdown of the skin barrier). Eczema fluctuates and can be frustrating to treat. Say to report any severe weeping rash eg around the mouth: this may be ▶▶*eczema herpeticum* a primary herpes infection which may be fatal (get urgent help). Discourage elimination diets.
• *Emollients & soap substitutes:* dry skin itches and is susceptible to irritants. Use emollients liberally (at least ×3–4/day), even when eczema is less active. They treat dryness and act as a barrier. The best emollient is the one the patient likes the most. Prescribe in large quantities (>500g/wk). Use emollient soap substitutes and bath oils. Intensive use ↓ need for topical steroids.
• *Topical corticosteroids:* use for exacerbations and only on active eczematous skin. Apply once each day 30min after emollient. Steroid phobia and underuse are common. Explain treatment is safe if used as prescribed. Potent corticosteroids may be needed—step up or down using the weakest steroid which is fully effective. Many dermatologists have moved towards a 'Get Control. Keep Control' regimen for use of topical steroids. This involves once-daily use of topical steroid for a period of 2wks, followed by twice-weekly use as maintenance therapy to previously affected skin. Haelan® tape (fludroxycortide) is good at healing fissured digits. Treat secondary bacterial infection (fig 6.29) with oral antibiotics. Topical pimecrolimus or tacrolimus can be used if eczema is not controlled with topical steroids or as steroid-sparing agents. Systemic treatments such as azathioprine, ciclosporin, or methotrexate may be indicated in severe disease. Dupilumab (biologic therapy) has recently been approved by NICE for the treatment of moderate to severe eczema, in those who have failed at least one conventional systemic therapy.[15]
• *Itch:* sedating antihistamines eg hydroxyzine used intermittently at night can reduce the itch/scratch cycle. Keep fingernails short and advise pressing the skin rather than scratching or rubbing.

Adult seborrhoeic dermatitis This common red, scaly rash affects scalp (dandruff), eyebrows, nasolabial folds, cheeks, and flexures. *Cause:* eg overgrowth of skin yeasts (*Malassezia*). It can be severe if HIV+ve. ℞: Mild topical steroid/antifungal preparations, eg Daktacort® or ketoconazole 2% cream or shampoo. Treat intermittently, as needed.

6 Dermatology

Irritant and allergic contact dermatitis

Irritant dermatitis We are all susceptible to irritants. Hands are often affected; redness ± weeping precedes dry fissuring. *Common irritants:* Detergents, soaps, oils, solvents, alkalis; water (if repeated). It often affects bar staff and cleaners. ℞: Avoid all irritants; hand care (soap substitutes; regular emollients; careful drying; cotton or cotton-lined rubber gloves for dry and wet work respectively); as-needed use of topical steroids for acute flare-ups.

Allergic contact dermatitis (fig 6.30) (Type IV reaction.) *Common allergens:* Nickel (jewellery, watches, coins, keys); chromates (cements, leather); lanolin (creams, cosmetics); rubber (foam in furniture); plants (primulas); topical neomycin, framycetin, antihistamines, or anaesthetics (haemorrhoid creams). The pattern of contact gives clues to the allergen. There is often a sharp cut-off where contact ends. Secondary spread elsewhere can occur (auto-sensitization). ℞: Consider patch testing and avoidance of implicated allergens; use a topical steroid appropriate for severity (↓ strength and stop as it settles).

Potency & side effects of topical corticosteroids

Mild Hydrocortisone 0.5%, 1%; *with antimicrobials* eg Canesten HC®, Daktacort®.
Moderate eg Betnovate–RD®, Eumovate®; *with antimicrobials* eg Trimovate®.
Potent eg Betnovate®, Elocon®; *with antimicrobials* eg Fucibet®, Betnovate-N®.
Very potent eg Dermovate®, Etrivex®.
Side effects Mild/moderate are associated with few. SE depend on potency (caution in potent/very potent) and duration of use. *Local:* Skin thinning, irreversible striae, telangiectasia, worsening of untreated infection, contact dermatitis. *Systemic:* Adrenal suppression (rare).

The amount of topical steroid required can be estimated using the fingertip unit (FTU=the amount of cream squeezed from a standard 5mm nozzle along the palmar surface of the distal phalanx of an adult finger). 1FTU will cover an area equivalent to the palmar surface of 2 adult hands (including fingers).

6 Dermatology

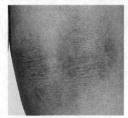

Fig 6.28 Atopic eczema.
© Dr Susannah Baron.

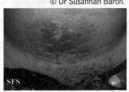

Fig 6.30 Contact dermatitis.
Courtesy of Dr Samuel da Silva:
www.atlasdermatologico.com.br

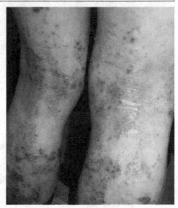

Fig 6.29 Atopic eczema with secondary bacterial infection causing crusting and weeping.
Reproduced from Burge S, *Oxford Handbook of Medical Dermatology* (2016), with permission from OUP.

Further reading

British Association of Dermatologists & Primary Care Dermatology Society (2015). *Management of Atopic Eczema.* http://www.pcds.org.uk/clinical-guidance/atopic-eczema

NICE (2007). *Atopic Eczema in Under 12s: Diagnosis and Management* (CG57). London: NICE.

6 Dermatology

Dermatophyte infections *(Ringworm; 'tinea'):* Fungal infections that invade and grow in dead keratin. Spread is most often transmitted indirectly from man to man. Species that infect only humans (=anthropophilic, eg *Trichophyton rubrum*, fig 6.31) are the most common. Fungi that infect animals (=zoophilic, eg *Microsporum canis*) cause a more inflamed rash in humans. Geophilic (soil) species rarely infect humans (eg *Microsporum gypseum*). A ringworm infection is a round, scaly, itchy lesion whose edge is more inflamed than its centre. It is called *tinea* followed, in Latin, by the part affected, eg tinea pedis (foot); cruris (groins); capitis (scalp); unguium (nail); corporis (body, fig 6.32). *Δ:* Send skin scrapings (from the active edge of a lesion), scalp brushings, or nail clippings/ scrapings of subungual debris for microscopy (rapid result) and culture (4–6wks). *R̃: Skin:* topical antifungal eg terbinafine or imidazole creams (eg clotrimazole) twice daily for 2wks. *Scalp:* treat empirically with oral griseofulvin or terbinafine + ketoconazole shampoo until culture results are known (*M. canis* responds to griseofulvin; *T. tonsurans* responds better to terbinafine). *Nails:* nail infection is difficult to treat. Confirm diagnosis (microscopy/culture) before starting treatment. Amorolfine paint may be effective if mild (use for 6 months for fingernails; 9–12 months for toenails). Terbinafine PO for 6wks–3 months (fingernail); or 3–6 months (toenails) if deemed essential. Explain about SE and interactions.

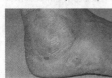

Fig 6.31 Tinea pedis. *Trichophyton rubrum.* Courtesy of Dr Jonathan Bowling.

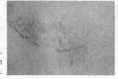

Fig 6.32 Tinea corporis. Courtesy of Dr Susannah Baron.

Yeast *Candida albicans:* A commensal in the mouth and GI tract, it commonly infects skin, mainly affecting the mouth, vagina, glans of penis, skin folds/ toe web, & nail areas. They are often pink and moist ± satellite lesions. Oral candida wipes off with a spatula (unlike lichen planus, p. 452) *R̃: Skin:* imidazole creams. Mouth: **nystatin** (eg oral suspension, 1mL/6h for 1 week) or miconazole oral gel. Vagina: imidazole cream ± pessary (eg Canesten Combi®). *Pityriasis versicolor:* *Malassezia* species (eg *M. furfur*) cause multiple hypopigmented scaly macules on the upper trunk and back. The commensals produce azelaic acid which inhibits melanogenesis and prevents affected skin from tanning. *R̃:* Imidazole cream BD for localized disease; 2% ketoconazole shampoo daily for 5 days (wash off after 5min). Relapses are frequent. Oral antifungals can be used in resistant/extensive disease.

Bacteria *Impetigo:* Contagious superficial infection caused by *Staph aureus* (± *Strep pyogenes*). *Peak:* 2–5yrs. Lesions (often well defined) usually start around the nose & face with honey-coloured crusts on erythematous base (± superficial flaccid blisters; fig 6.9, p. 437). *R̃:* Try topical fusidic acid for localized infection. Give oral antibiotics (eg **flucloxacillin** QDS for 7 days) if severe. Hygiene advice.

Erysipelas: Sharply defined superficial infection caused by *Strep pyogenes*. Often affects the face (unilateral) with fever and ↑WCC. *R̃:* See following 'Cellulitis' section. *Cellulitis:* Acute infection of skin and soft tissues (eg legs). *Cause:* β-haemolytic streps & staphs. It is deeper and less well defined than erysipelas. *Signs:* pain, swelling, erythema, warmth, systemic upset, and lymphadenopathy. *R̃:* ► Elevate the affected part. **Benzylpenicillin** 600mg/6h IV (or **phenoxymethylpenicillin** 500mg/4–6h PO) + **flucloxacillin** 500mg/6h PO. If penicillin-allergic, try **erythromycin** 500mg/12h PO (check local protocols).

Skin TB: Lupus vulgaris (a red-brown scarring plaque); scrofuloderma (suppurating nodules from direct extension of TB in lymph nodes); TB *verrucosa cutis* (indolent warty plaques); TB *gumma* (extension of TB from underlying foci); *tuberculids* (generalized exanthems eg erythema induratum/lichen scrofulosorum).

Common viral infections

Warts (fig 6.33) Caused by human papillomavirus (HPV) in keratinocytes. *Common warts and plantar warts (verrucae):* Papules or nodules with a hyperkeratotic or filiform surface, most commonly seen at sites of trauma (fingers, elbows, knees, and pressure points on soles) in children. Warts may coalesce into confluent lesions (mosaic warts). Warts are contagious but risk of transmission is low. They rarely cause symptoms and will disappear spontaneously (within months–2yrs) without treatment and without scarring. *R:* Consider if painful, unsightly, or persisting. Any treatment should not cause more problems than the wart itself. • Topical salicylic acid (keratolytic), eg Salatac® gel daily for 12wks • Cryotherapy (not in younger children as it is painful) once every 3–4wks for up to 4 cycles • Duct tape occlusion—leave in place for 6d at a time for up to 8wks.[16] There is also some evidence for oral zinc supplementation.[32]

Plane warts: Flat skin-coloured or brown lesions; tend to Köbnerize (p. 437) in scratch marks; they often resist treatment.

Genital warts (condylomata acuminata): Sexually transmitted. *R:* NB: there is significant treatment failure and relapse rate • No treatment (⅓ resolve within 6months) • Self-applied podophyllin or imiquimod cream (not if pregnant or in children) • Cryotherapy. Screen for other STIs. If a child, suspect abuse.[17]

Molluscum contagiosum *(Pox virus)* These pink papules have an umbilicated (depressed) central punctum. Common in children. They resolve spontaneously (may take months). Treatment is often not recommended. Gentle cryo or squeezing/piercing may be tried.

Herpes simplex Recurrent genital or perioral infection, often preceded by symptoms of burning/itching. *Signs:* Grouped painful vesicles on erythematous base which heal without scarring (fig 6.34). *Treatment: Oral:* often none required. The benefits of topical aciclovir are small. *Genital:* oral **aciclovir** (200mg 5×/day PO for 1wk, within 5 days of lesion onset). Hygiene measures + abstain from sex until lesions have cleared. Consider prophylaxis if >6 attacks/yr. Get expert advice if immunosuppressed or pregnant.

Herpes zoster Varicella-zoster virus becomes dormant in dorsal root ganglia after *chickenpox* infection has subsided. Recurrent infection affects one or more dermatomes (=*shingles*) (fig 8.36, p. 552, esp. if immunosuppressed). Pain and malaise may precede the rash. *Signs:* Polymorphic red papules, vesicles, pustules (fig 6.35). *R:* If mild, none. If >50yrs, ophthalmic involvement, severe, or immunosuppressed, use an antiviral (eg **aciclovir** 800mg 5×/day PO for 1wk) starting within 72h of rash onset, to reduce pain and severity. Seek specialist advice if pregnant, immunocompromised or ophthalmic involvement. Varicella-zoster vaccine (eg Zostavax®) helps protect against herpes zoster and is given to those aged 70–79 (UK). Immune globulin can be used postexposure. *Complications:* Post-herpetic neuralgia; meningitis; encephalitis.

6 Dermatology

Fig 6.33 Common wart.

OUP.

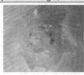

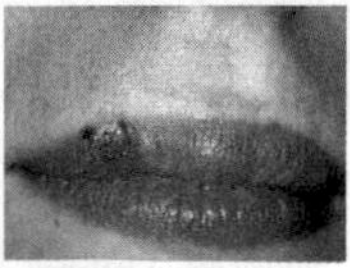

Fig 6.34 Herpes simplex.

Reproduced from Robinson et al., *Oral Pathology* (2018), with permission from OUP.

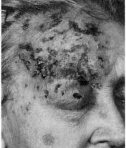

Fig 6.35 Ophthalmic zoster (shingles).

The 5 pillars of acne 1 Basal keratinocyte proliferation in pilosebaceous follicles (androgen- and corticotropin-releasing hormone driven) 2 ↑ sebum production 3 *Propionibacterium acnes* colonization 4 Inflammation 5 Comedones (white- & black-heads) blocking secretions, hence papules, nodules, cysts, and scars (face, neck, upper torso). It is almost universal in teenagers: it causes much angst (nature picks the fairest skin at its weakest moment for her fiercest pustules). Most with acne don't have ↑ androgens but their sebaceous glands are more sensitive to androgens.

℞ Be holistic; subtle doctors use acne consultations to promote mental health by giving patients a vocabulary to describe their misery, and so to control it. Dispel myths: it is NOT due to dirt, lack of washing, etc. & not infectious/contagious. Diet has little or no effect on acne. Ask about mood, effect on body image/self-esteem, & fears of social rejection. Suicidal ideation is a red flag.

Mild acne Mainly facial comedones. *℞:* Topical benzoyl peroxide eg 2.5%, 5%, or 10% (start with a low strength), or topical retinoid (avoid in pregnancy) eg isotretinoin, or topical antibiotic alone (eg Dalacin T®). If poorly tolerated, try azelaic acid (15% gel). Treatment takes up to 8 weeks to be effective. If response is poor, consider a topical antibiotic combined with benzoyl peroxide or topical retinoid (eg Duac®, Isotrexin®).

Moderate acne Inflammatory lesions (papules and pustules) dominate, affecting face ± torso. *℞:* • Topical antibiotic combined with benzoyl peroxide or topical retinoid (reduces bacterial resistance; for max. 12wks) • Oral antibiotic—tetracycline, oxytetracycline, doxycycline, or lymecycline are 1st line (erythromycin if pregnant or <12yrs old). Use for ≥4–6 months *with* topical benzoyl peroxide (start at 2.5% to avoid irritation). Do not use topical antibiotics at the same time • A topical retinoid with benzoyl peroxide (Epiduo® gel) is an alternative that can be used • In females, consider a standard COCP if contraception required; or if treatment has failed, a COCP with antiandrogen activity (if no CIs) eg co-cyprindiol (eg Dianette®).[18,19]

Severe acne There are nodules, cysts, scars, and inflammatory papules and pustules. Refer to a specialist. *℞:* Isotretinoin may be the best option (↓ sebum production & pituitary hormones; specialist prescribing in UK). Marked benefit occurs in virtually all patients (permanent ~65%). SE: teratogenic (contraception must be used during + for 1 month before and after); skin & mucosal dryness; depression.

Rosacea

Rosacea A chronic relapsing/remitting disorder of blood vessels and pilosebaceous units in central facial areas typically in fair-skinned people. *Prevalence:* 10%. *Pre-rosacea features:* Flushing triggered by stress/blushing, alcohol, & spices. *Signs:* A central facial rash (usually symmetrical) with erythema, telangiectasia, papules & pustules (without comedones), inflammatory nodules ± facial lymphoedema, blepharitis/conjunctivitis (ocular rosacea). In men, rhinophyma (swelling + soft tissue overgrowth of the nose) may occur. *Cause:* Unknown. *Demodex* mites are sometimes observed in papules but their role is unclear.

℞: Use soap substitutes; avoid sun overexposure & use sun-block.

• *Mild disease:* topical metronidazole gel (0.75%) or cream (1%) ×2/day for 3–4 months or topical 15% azelaic acid gel (may cause transient stinging). Topical ivermectin (eg Soolantra®) can be used for papulopustular rosacea.[20] It is both anti-inflammatory and controls *Demodex* mites.

• *Moderate or severe disease:* an oral tetracycline (or erythromycin if contraindicated) taken for 4 months helps control extensive papules or pustules but has little effect on redness. Low-dose **doxycycline** (40mg ×1/day) is also licensed and effective. Oral isotretinoin (see earlier) and lasers are rarely needed.

• *Ocular rosacea:* eyelid hygiene, ocular lubricants ± ciclosporin 0.5% (specialist use).[20]

Further reading

American Academy of Dermatology (2016). Guidelines of care for the management of acne vulgaris. *J Am Acad Dermatol* 74:945–73.

NICE (2018). *Clinical Knowledge Summary: Acne Vulgaris.* http://cks.nice.org.uk/acne-vulgaris

Cutaneous drug reactions are common, so know the main culprits & how to treat.

- *Morbilliform:* (=Measles-like) or *exanthematous* (fig 6.36). The commonest drug reaction, presenting with generalized erythematous macules and papules eg on the trunk ± mild fever, within 1–3wks of drug exposure. No mucosal involvement. *Drugs:* amoxicillin (especially if the patient has glandular fever), cephalosporins, antiepileptics, sulfonamides, allopurinol, captopril, thiazides. *ΔΔ:* Measles, scarlet fever, viral exanthema.

- *Urticaria:* *Signs:* see p. 453. *Drugs:* penicillins and cephalosporins, opiates, NSAIDS, ACEI, thiazides, phenytoin. *R:* antihistamine ± IV hydrocortisone/IM adrenaline if anaphylaxis.

►► *Erythroderma (exfoliative dermatitis):* *Signs:* widespread erythema and dermatitis affecting ≥90% body surface. *Causative drugs:* sulfonamides, allopurinol, carbamazepine, gold. Discuss management with a dermatologist.

►► *Stevens–Johnson syndrome (SJS):* vague upper respiratory tract symptoms occur 2–3 weeks after starting a drug and ~2 days before a rash that affects <10% body surface. *Signs:* painful erythematous macules evolving to form target lesions. Severe mucosal ulceration of ≥2 surfaces eg conjunctivae, oral cavity, labia, urethra. *Drugs:* sulfonamides, antiepileptics, penicillins, NSAIDS. *R:* See following TEN section.

►► *Toxic epidermal necrolysis (TEN):* flu-like symptoms may precede skin involvement which affects >30% body surface. *Signs:* widespread painful dusky erythema, then necrosis of large sheets of epidermis (fig 6.37). Mucosae severely affected. Mortality: ~30%. *Drug causes:* sulfonamides, antiepileptics, penicillins and cephalosporins, allopurinol, NSAIDS. *R:* Essentially supportive. Manage in ICU, HDU, or burns unit. Systemic treatments such as IVIG, ciclosporin, and systemic steroids have been tried but there is a lack of conclusive evidence demonstrating clear benefit. Early withdrawal of the culprit drug and high-quality multidisciplinary care are the priorities. Relieve pain; protect skin (do not debride).

- *Lichenoid:* similar to lichen planus. Itchy flat-topped purple–red papules. *Drugs:* β-blockers, thiazides, gold, antimalarials. *R:* potent topical steroids.

- *Fixed drug eruption:* lesions recur in the same area each time a particular drug is taken. *Drugs:* paracetamol, tetracyclines, sulfonamides, aspirin.

Management principles A clear history of the onset and duration of the rash is essential. Record *all* drugs taken with timelines (date started, date rash appeared, etc.). Stop the likely offender. Drug withdrawal is not diagnostic—urticarial reactions settle in a few days; morbilliform in 7–10 days; most others last >8 weeks. Document the signs and symptoms including mucosal/systemic involvement. Assess the likelihood of this being a serious reaction and consider if it is likely to evolve A peripheral eosinophilia may be suggestive of a drug reaction. Close attention should be paid to derangements in U&E and LFT. Give regular emollients for dryness or itch. Potent topical steroids reduce itch in widespread morbilliform, eczematous, or lichenoid reactions. More severe eruptions are best managed by specialists. Rechallenge with the suspected drug is generally inadvisable.

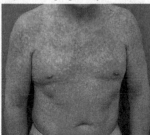

Fig 6.36 Morbilliform rash.
© DermNet NZ, reproduced with permission.

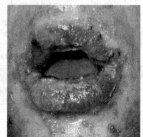

Fig 6.37 TEN/Stevens–Johnson syndrome.
© Dr Susannah Baron.

Lichen planus Lesions (eg on flexor aspects of wrists, forearms, ankles, and legs) are purple, pruritic, poly-angular, planar (flat-topped) papules, seen at any age + white lacy markings (known as Wickham's striae). Lesions elsewhere: scalp (scarring alopecia), nails (longitudinal ridges), tongue, mouth (lacy white areas on inner cheeks), and genitals. Lesions often arise at sites of trauma. Usually persists for 6–18 months. ℞: Topical steroids (± topical antifungals) are 1st line (esp. in oral disease, eg fluticasone spray).

Strawberry naevi (infantile haemangiomas) Occur in neonates as a rapidly enlarging red spot. Most resolve by the age of 5–7yrs. No treatment is required unless a vital function is impaired, eg obscuring vision, impairing suck, or airway compromise.

Pyogenic granuloma (fig 6.38) A vascular lesion thought to arise as a result of minor trauma, typically occurring on fingers. It appears as a fleshy moist red lesion which grows rapidly and often bleeds easily. ΔΔ: ► Amelanotic malignant melanoma. ℞: Curettage and cautery.

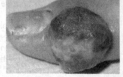

Fig 6.38 Pyogenic granuloma.
Courtesy of Dr Jonathan Bowling.

Pityriasis rosea A common, self-limiting rash which often may have a viral cause. The rash is preceded by a *herald patch* (oval red scaly patch, similar to, but larger than later lesions). It affects the neck, trunk (distributed in a 'Christmas tree' pattern), and proximal limbs. There is no treatment. It will resolve in 2–12wks.

Alopecia Hair loss is *non-scarring* or *scarring*. Non-scarring causes may be reversible, but scarring alopecia implies irreversible loss.

• *Non-scarring alopecia: Alopecia areata:* smooth, well-defined round patches of hair loss on scalp; hairs like exclamation marks (short & tapering) are a typical feature; spontaneous regrowth occurs within 3 months in 80%. Total scalp hair loss = *alopecia totalis*; total body hair loss = *alopecia universalis*. ℞: difficult. Consider topical or intralesional steroids. Psychological support. *Telogen effluvium* is shedding of telogen phase hairs after a period of stress, eg childbirth, surgery, severe illness. Other causes: nutritional (↓Fe or Zn); *androgenetic* (♀ & ♂ pattern). ℞: minoxidil.

• *Scarring alopecia:* Inflammatory disease damages follicular stem cells (eg lichen planus; discoid lupus); or follicles are damaged by trauma or tumour (BCC, SCC).

Blistering disorders *Causes:* Infection (eg herpes); insect bites; friction/trauma; eczema; drugs (ACEI; furosemide); immunobullous (dermatitis herpetiformis, pemphigoid, pemphigus). *Bullous pemphigoid:* The chief autoimmune blistering disorder in the elderly—due to IgG autoantibodies to basement membrane. *Signs:* tense blisters (1–3cm in size) on inflamed or normal skin. *Skin biopsy:* +ve immunofluorescence (linear IgG and C3 along the basement membrane). ℞: Very potent topical steroids eg clobetasol (applied to lesions); prednisolone 0.3–1mg/kg/day PO (+bone & gastric protection; ↓ dose gradually after 4 weeks if no new blisters).[21,22] Blisters heal without scarring but the disease runs a relapsing/remitting course over 5–10yrs. The BLISTER trial showed that tetracycline antibiotics can lead to effective control of pemphigoid in 74% of patients at 6 weeks, with a reduced risk of serious/life-threatening side effects at 52 weeks, when compared with oral steroids, and are therefore used as first line treatment in some centres.[22] *Pemphigus:* Affects younger people (<40yrs). It is due to IgG autoantibodies against desmosomal components (desmoglein 1 & 3), which leads to acantholysis (keratinocytes separate from each other). *Signs:* flaccid superficial blisters which rupture easily to leave widespread erosions. The oral mucosa is often affected early. *Skin biopsy:* +ve immunofluorescence (intercellular IgG giving a crazy-paving effect). ℞: **Prednisolone** (40–60mg/day PO, with gradual tapering). Steroid-sparing agents: mycophenolate mofetil and azathioprine. Rituximab and IV immunoglobulin in resistant cases.[23]

Photosensitivity denotes conditions triggered by light. Rashes affect sun-exposed areas eg face, 'v' of neck, dorsum of hands and arms. They may be *primary* (rare, eg cutaneous porphyrias, xeroderma pigmentosum) or *acquired*.

Drug-induced photosensitivity Often due to phototoxicity (causing an exaggerated sunburn response ± blisters), or photoallergy (delayed hypersensitivity reaction). Drugs may also cause pseudoporphyria or lichenoid reactions. Frequent offenders: thiazides; tetracyclines/sulfonamides; tricyclics; phenothiazines; NSAIDs; amiodarone.

Photoaggravated skin disease Cutaneous features of a disease are more severe on sun exposure eg rosacea, autoimmune blistering diseases, SLE.

Phytophotodermatitis Reactions from contact with light-sensitizing chemicals in plants (eg psoralens) cause linear erythema and blistering.

Polymorphic light eruption A common idiopathic disorder typically affecting young women in spring. After light exposure, itchy red papules, vesicles, and plaques develop on exposed sites, fading after 1–6 days. It often improves over the summer due to a phenomenon called 'hardening'. ℞: Sun-avoidance; sun-protection (high factor UVA + UVB sunscreen). Acute attack: potent topical steroids ± **prednisolone** 15–20mg/day for 3 days (eg to control if on holiday). Desensitization using UVB phototherapy or PUVA therapy (in severe cases).

Porphyria cutanea tarda (The commonest porphyria.) Reduced enzyme activity of uroporphyrinogen decarboxylase results in overproduction of photoactive porphyrins. Presentation is subacute and the relationship to sun exposure is easily missed. *Causes:* Triggers eg HIV; hepatitis C; alcohol; OCP/HRT, ↑ iron levels initiate disease in those genetically susceptible. *Signs:* Vesicles/bullae in sun-exposed sites, hypertrichosis, hyperpigmentation, skin fragility, and scarring (milia). *Tests:* faecal & urinary porphyrins; skin biopsy. ℞: Remove precipitants; sun avoidance/protection; regular venesection; low-dose chloroquine.

Urticaria

Ordinary urticaria *Acute:* Smooth, erythematous, itchy hives and wheals are precipitated by eg infections and parasites (helminths); chemicals (insect bites, latex, drugs, or food); or systemic disease. Skin prick or blood RAST tests may help. *Chronic:* (=Urticaria lasting >6wks.) Idiopathic in most, and lasts months–years (continuous or episodic). ~30% have histamine-releasing autoantibodies. Non-sedating antihistamines can be up-titrated to 4 times the recommended dose if required.[33,34]

Physical urticaria Induced reproducibly by an external trigger, eg *dermographism* (a wheal develops on rubbing/stroking the skin); *cold contact* (occurs on exposure to cold air/water); *delayed pressure* (sustained pressure causes wheals after a delay of 30min–6h); *solar urticaria* (occurs on UV exposure). ℞: Antihistamines (response to the different antihistamines varies from patient to patient so several may have to be tried before the one that provides benefit is found!).

Urticarial vasculitis Cutaneous lesions resemble urticaria (tender wheals), and small-vessel cutaneous vasculitis (palpable purpura). If complement levels are low, it may be associated with SLE. ℞: Antihistamine, NSAIDS, but some patients may need immunosuppressive therapy.

Further reading

Harman KE *et al.* (2017). British Association of Dermatologists' guidelines for the management of pemphigus vulgaris. *Br J Dermatol* 177:1170–201.

Venning VA *et al.* (2012). British Association of Dermatologists' guidelines for the management of bullous pemphigoid 2012. *Br J Dermatol* 167:1200–14.

6 Dermatology

Venous ulcers

Venous leg ulcers (fig 6.40) *Risk factors:* Varicose veins, DVT, venous insufficiency, poor calf muscle function, arteriovenous fistulae, obesity, leg fracture. Venous hypertension from damaged valves of the deep venous system causes superficial varicosities and skin changes (lipodermatosclerosis, fig 6.41). Minimal trauma, typically over the medial malleolus, causes ulcers. *Management:* Graded compression bandaging promotes healing.[24] Pressure reduces from the ankle (40mmHg) to the calf (15–20mmHg). This reduces superficial venous pressure. Do Dopplers first to exclude arterial disease (ensure the ankle–brachial pressure index is >0.8). Ulcers heal more quickly with occlusive dressings which absorb exudate and improve comfort. Infection should be treated with systemic antibiotics until definitive sensitivities are available (swab only if

Typical causes of ulcers
• Neuropathy
• Vascular: venous 75%; arterial 10%; mixed 15%
• Trauma

Rarer causes
• Pyoderma gangrenosum (eg with Crohn's; UC)
• Sickle cell disease
• Vasculitis (eg SLE)
• Cryoglobulinaemia
• Malignancy
• Infection eg leishmaniasis
• Drugs eg nicorandil

signs of infection). Avoid topical antibiotics as they ↑ the risk of resistance and contact dermatitis. Ensure adequate analgesia. Involve tissue viability nurses. **Pentoxifylline** 400mg TDS PO for up to 6 months can be considered to promote healing (unlicensed and not commonly used). Ulcers which don't heal on adequate treatment for 3 months must be investigated further (eg biopsy for malignancy). Once an ulcer is healed, patients should follow advice aimed at preventing recurrence: wearing compression stockings, skin care, leg elevation, calf exercises, and good nutrition.

Pressure ulcers

Pressure ulcers Result from uninterrupted pressure on the skin, leads to ulcers and extensive, painful, subcutaneous destruction, eg on the sacrum, heel, or greater trochanter.[25,26] Shearing forces (from sliding down the bed); friction (when a patient is dragged across a bedsheet); and moisture (eg from incontinence) are implicating factors. See table 6.2 for staging. *Risk factors:* Extremes of age, reduced mobility and sensation, vascular disease, and chronic or terminal illness make this more likely, particularly if nursing is poor. A full-thickness sacral sore causes much misery and extends hospital stay by *months.* ► This should make prevention a central preoccupation.

Table 6.2 Staging of pressure ulcers

Stage		
I	Non-blanching erythema over intact skin
II	Partial thickness skin loss, eg shallow crater
III	Full thickness skin loss, extending into fat
IV	Destruction of muscle, bone, or tendons

Prevalence: ~3–14% of inpatients have pressure sores; most are over 70yrs. The prevalence in nursing homes is similar. 1/5 of pressure ulcers develop at home. Those with spinal injury are significantly at risk: 20–30% have a pressure ulcer within 1–5yrs of injury. *Complication:* Osteomyelitis.

Treatment: • Pressure-relieving mattresses and cushions • Frequent repositioning (turning charts help) • Optimize nutrition (get specialist help) • Treat systemic infection with antibiotics • Use modern dressings (eg hydrogels, hydrocolloids, films) to create an optimum environment to aid wound healing • Debride dead or necrotic tissue • Topical negative pressure treatment.

Prevention: Most pressure ulcers are avoidable. Initial and ongoing assessment of risk is vital, along with regular inspection of the skin + minimizing excess moisture. Proper positioning and regular turning (eg every 2h, alternating between supine, and right or left lateral position). Use pillows to separate the knees and ankles, and lifting devices to move patients.

6 Dermatology

Pruritus in the elderly

Pruritus A common complaint in the elderly:
- *Skin causes:* Eczema (including asteatotic eczema, see BOX 'Asteatotic eczema (eczema craquelé)'); scabies (appearance can be similar in the elderly); pemphigoid/pre-pemphigoid eruptions; generalized xerosis.
- *Medical causes:* Anaemia; polycythaemia; lymphoma; solid neoplasms; hepatic and renal failure; hypo- and hyperthyroidism; diabetes (candidiasis). Excluded by blood tests.

Asteatotic eczema (eczema craquelé)

Commoner in the elderly, this particularly affects the lower legs with a dry eczema that polygonally fissures into a crazy-paving pattern (fig 6.39). Emollients and soap substitutes help + moderately potent steroid (eg eumovate) for affected itchy inflamed areas. Rare (paraneoplastic) association is lymphoma (suspect if the eczema is difficult to treat).

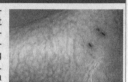

Fig 6.39 Eczema craquelé.
© Dr Susannah Baron.

6 Dermatology

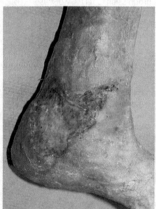

Fig 6.40 Venous leg ulcer (with eczema). Is there healthy granulation tissue on the ulcer floor? Remove all that over-ripe camembert pus to find out. Pain is frequent in these patients (who are often obese, so compounding immobility).

© Dr Susannah Baron.

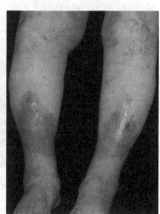

Fig 6.41 Varicose eczema with hyperpigmentation and lipodermatosclerosis (inflammation of layer of fat under the dermis and an ill-defined band resembling an inverted champagne bottle causing leg tapering down towards the ankle).

© Dr Jonathan Bowling.

Further reading

Grey GJ (2006). Pressure ulcers. *BMJ* 332:472.

NICE (2014). *Pressure Ulcers: Prevention and Management* (CG179). London: NICE.

SIGN (2010). *Guideline 120: Management of Chronic Venous Leg Ulcers*. Edinburgh: SIGN.

Skin disease is a burdensome stigma for HIV patients.[27] Skin problems are markers of HIV progression, so understanding them is vital. Highly active anti-retroviral therapy has helped HIV-related skin disease become less common, but it may trigger inflammatory reactions (immune reconstitution inflammatory syndrome; IRIS)—see later.

Acute seroconversion Occurs 1–3 weeks after exposure; 70% experience symptoms. Features include an acute mononucleosis-type illness, usually accompanied by a non-specific maculopapular eruption affecting the upper trunk, associated with lymphadenopathy, malaise, headache, and fever. There may be oral or genital ulcers or candidiasis.

Infections There is increased risk from common pathogens and commensal organisms that don't normally cause disease. Signs may be florid and atypical.
- *Herpes virus:* See BOX 'Herpes viruses and HIV'.
- *Epstein–Barr virus:* Implicated in causing oral hairy leucoplakia (fig 6.42).
- *Warts:* Widespread on oral mucosa, face, perianal region, + genital tract.
- *Molluscum contagiosum:* Widespread and atypical eg unusual sites; face, genitals. R: (difficult): cryotherapy, topical retinoids, cautery, or curettage.
- *Candidiasis:* May be severe, disseminated, and treatment resistant, involving the oropharynx, vagina, and skin. R: topical nystatin; systemic imidazoles.
- *Tinea:* Generalized dermatophytosis/tinea capitis is common.
- *Syphilis:* Multiple ulcers (primary); rapid progression to tertiary disease.
- *Cryptococcosis:* Looks like facial molluscum contagiosum. R: fluconazole.
- *Demodicosis:* Inflamed pruritic papular eruptions on face and upper trunk caused by *Demodex* (mite) folliculitis.
- *Scabies:* Severe variants, eg crusted are more common in advanced HIV disease. Paradoxically, patients may not complain of severe itch. A widespread scaly, crusted eruption occurs (highly infectious p. 458). R: permethrin lotion.

Inflammatory disorders
- *Seborrhoeic dermatitis:* Widespread inflammatory red scaly patches on hairy areas and nasolabial folds & flexures. R: Daktacort®/ketoconazole cream.
- *Acquired ichthyosis:* (Scaly skin) and keratoderma (thickened palm/soles).
- *Psoriasis:* HIV may lead to psoriasis, or cause pre-existing disease to worsen. Treating HIV will often improve response to standard therapy (p. 444).
- *Eosinophilic folliculitis:* The cause of this intensely itchy, papulopustular eruption of sterile pustules is unknown. Δ: Biopsy. R: 0.1% tacrolimus, topical steroids, UVB therapy, PUVA therapy.
- *Drug reactions:* Common in HIV especially co-trimoxazole's maculopapular eruptions or erythema multiforme; toxic epidermal necrolysis, p. 451.
- *Pruritic papular eruption (PPE):* Common; small symmetrical red or skin-coloured itchy papules. Cause unknown. 80% have advanced immunosuppression.

HIV & nail changes Onychomycosis (eg *Trichophyton rubrum*; multiple fungi are often cultured in a single patient); nail pigmentation; Beau's lines.

HIV & hair Diffuse alopecia or alopecia areata is associated with HIV.

HIV & skin neoplasia Kaposi's sarcoma (see BOX 'Herpes viruses and HIV'), BCC, SCC, melanoma, skin lymphomas, Merkel cell cancer (a rare, aggressive neuro-endocrine skin malignancy).

IRIS *(immune reconstitution inflammatory syndrome):* With antiretrovirals, immunity begins to recover, but then responds to previously acquired opportunistic infection with a powerful inflammatory response, paradoxically worsening symptoms, often involving the skin. You may confuse this with serious HIV progression.

Lipodystrophy Subcutaneous fat is lost from the face and limbs (+ deposited on the trunk), as an effect of treatment with protease inhibitors.

Herpes viruses and HIV

Herpes simplex This can be increasingly troublesome as HIV progresses. Painful chronic ulcers and erosions develop, eg around mouth and genitals. ℞: High-dose aciclovir (oral or IV).

Varicella zoster This may occur with atypical signs (eg ≥1 dermatome; folliculitis; verrucous lesions). Ulceration and post-herpetic neuralgia may be more frequent and severe. In advanced disease, disseminated infection occurs. ℞: High-dose aciclovir (IV if systemic disease).

Kaposi's sarcoma (KS) An abnormally vascularized spindle cell tumour derived from capillary endothelial cells. Cause: HHV-8 (human herpes virus). It presents as purple papules or plaques on the skin and mucosa of any organ (fig 6.43). It metastasizes to nodes. 4 types: classic KS (typically on legs); endemic (African) KS; KS in immunosuppression (eg organ transplant recipients); and AIDS-related KS, often multiorgan (skin is not always involved). Incidence is falling thanks to HAART. ℞: *(if HIV +ve)* optimize HAART; radiotherapy can palliate symptomatic disease (esp. if unable to tolerate chemotherapy). Local treatment: intralesional chemotherapy, cryo, laser, photodynamic treatment, and excision. Systemic interferon alfa or chemotherapy (eg pegylated-liposomal anthracyclines & paclitaxel).

6 Dermatology

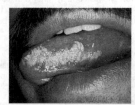

Fig 6.42 Oral hairy leucoplakia (adherent white plaques) is thought to be caused by Epstein–Barr virus. 'Corrugated' would be a better term than 'hairy' as there are no hairs. Associations: HIV (esp. if CD4 <200/mm³); immunosuppressants; lamotrigine.

© Prof D. Rosenstein.

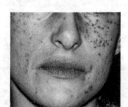

Fig 6.43 Kaposi's sarcoma.
© Dr Susannah Baron.

Further reading

Schwartz RA *et al.* (2013). *Cutaneous Manifestations of HIV.* Medscape. http://emedicine. medscape.com/article/1133746-overview

6 Dermatology

Scabies (*Sarcoptes scabei*; fig 6.44) A highly contagious, common disorder particularly affecting children and young adults. *Spread:* Direct person to person, eg by holding hands, sharing a bed. The ♀ mite digs a burrow (patho-gnomonic sign—a short, wavy, grey or red line on the skin surface) and lays eggs which hatch as larvae. The itch and subsequent red rash is probably due to allergic sensitivity to the mite or its products. *Signs:* It presents as very itchy papules, vesicles, pustules, and nodules affecting finger-webs (esp. first), wrist flexures, axillae, abdomen (esp. around umbilicus and waistband area), buttocks, and groins (itchy red penile or scrotal papules are virtually diagnostic). In young infants, palms and soles are characteristically involved. The eruption is usually excoriated and becomes eczematized. Mites can sometimes be extracted from burrows and visualized microscopically; eggs can be seen in skin scrapings. Crusted or Norwegian scabies is the same mite, but seen in the elderly or immuno-compromised who harbour ~2 million mites, and are highly contagious. *Management:* Treat all members of the household and all close contacts at the same time, even if asymptomatic. A good explanation (verbal + written) will aid concordance and promote the chances of successful cure. Permethrin 5% dermal cream is probably the most effective topical agent. It is also the drug of choice for pregnant women. Malathion is a good second choice (but not if pregnant or <6 months old). Oral ivermectin is recommended for severe scabies (200mcg/kg stat, repeated after 7–14 days). The rash and symptoms of itch will take a few weeks to settle, occasionally longer. A suitable anti-pruritic such as crotamiton cream (eg Eurax®) (which also has anti-scabetic activity) can be useful during this period. *Example of advice to give for treating scabies:*
• Take a warm bath and soap the skin all over.
• Scrub the fingers and nails with a firm brush. Dry your body.
• Apply permethrin (or malathion 0.5% liquid) to *all* body parts from the neck down, including soles (+ scalp, face, and ears if <2yrs old, elderly, or immunosuppressed). Avoid the eyes! Save a small amount of cream and use this to reapply to any body part (eg hands) that is washed before the 24h is up.
• Wash off after 24h.
• Wash all sheets, towels, and clothing in a hot wash.
• Repeat treatment after 7 days.
• Treatment may worsen itch for 2 weeks—so use calamine lotion or crotamiton cream (eg Eurax®).

Headlice (*Pediculus capitis*; fig 6.45) Common in children. Spread is only by head-to-head contact. Lice are 3mm long and have legs adapted to cling to hair shafts. Eggs (nits) are bound firmly to the scalp hairs & when empty appear white. *Signs:* Usually asymptomatic (presentation is upon seeing lice). Itch ± papular rash on the nape. *R:* All require 2 applications, 7 days apart. • Malathion 0.5%: apply to the hair from the roots to the tips. Leave lotion on overnight, then shampoo & rinse off • Dimeticone 4%: leave lotion on overnight, then shampoo & rinse off. Resistance is a problem • Isopropyl myristate and cyclomethicone: Leave on hair for 10min, then systematically comb using a fine-toothed comb to remove lice before washing with shampoo. (Not suitable if <2yrs old or in those with skin conditions.) *Combing* (see box 'Detection combing'). Only treat head-to-head contacts (over the past 5wks) if they have live lice (say to have a careful look).

Crab lice (*Phthiriasis pubis*) Often sexually transmitted and affect pubic hairs. Eyebrows, eyelashes, and axillae may also be involved. *Management:* Topical malathion 0.5% or permethrin to all affected areas. Wash off after 12h and repeat after 7 days. Screen for other sexually transmitted diseases.

Flea bites (*Pulicidae*) Spread plague, typhus, and cat-scratch disease. The animal (eg cat or dog) which spreads the flea may not itch or scratch itself. Flea bites cause a papular urticaria in a sensitized individual. *Treatment:* De-flea pets; de-flea household carpets and soft furnishings.

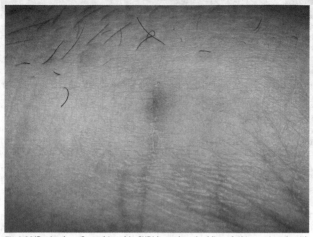

Fig 6.44 'Doctor, have I caught scabies?' 'Did you share bedding, clothing, or towels with anyone 4–6 weeks ago? Have you cuddled a pet? Or been to an institution? Is the itching worse at night?' Look for rows of irregular or s-shaped red furrows in web spaces, axillae, ventral skin on wrist or knee (also palms & soles in children). Here is a scabies burrow with a mite just visible (with the eye of faith) beyond the red area.

© Dr Jonathan Bowling.

Detection combing and combing treatment for head lice

Seeing lice[28] is hard; a special fine comb (prescribable or bought at a chemist) can be used for detecting and treating lice. Here's what to do:
- Wash hair with ordinary shampoo, rinse, and apply lots of conditioner. Comb the hair with a normal comb to untangle it; then use the fine-toothed comb. Slot its teeth into the hair roots so they touch the scalp; draw it through to the hair tips.
- Ensure all hair is combed; check comb for lice after each stroke (use a magnifying glass). If lice are seen, clean comb by wiping it on a tissue, or rinse it before the next stroke. NB: nits (empty eggshells) don't mean live lice, as they can stick to hair even if lice have gone.
- After all hair is combed, rinse out conditioner.
- Treatment is only needed if ≥1 live lice are seen.
- *Wet combing treatment* involves the above steps with repeat combing at least 4 times every 4 days; only stop when no more lice have been seen for 12 days.
- For topical treatments—see p. 458.
- All affected people in the household need to be treated at the same time.

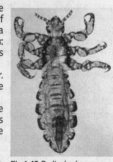

Fig 6.45 *Pediculus humanus.*
© Prof S. Upton, Kansas Univ.

Further reading
Knott L (2013). *Head Lice*. Patient. http://patient.info/doctor/head-lice-pro

⊛ To construct a coherent identity, we must distinguish what belongs to the external, perceived world from what belongs to our inner world. The skin marks this boundary and can become the battlefield where different identities fight for dominance. A range of self-destructive skin phenomena exist, in which the primary problem is psychological:

Neurotic excoriations[29] Conscious compulsive picking, scratching, or gouging of the skin. It may be initiated by minor skin problems such as an insect bite or folliculitis, but it also occurs with previously normal skin. There is no known problem with the skin, so this is a physical manifestation of an emotional problem. Picking causes distress and there are often repeated attempts to stop. Lesions are usually similar in size and shape, and are grouped on easily accessible and exposed sites. Management is challenging.

Acne 'excoriée de la jeune fille' A form of neurotic excoriation, typically affecting young girls with mild acne who obsessively pick at the skin causing scarred, infected lesions. The picking may continue long after the original acne has healed.

Trichotillomania Persistent and excessive hair-pulling resulting in noticeable hair loss, most frequently on the scalp, eyebrows, and eyelashes. It is common in children, who often deny hair-pulling. It is frequently precipitated or exacerbated by stress.

Dermatitis artefacta The deliberate and conscious production of self-inflicted skin lesions to satisfy an unconscious psychological or emotional need.[30] Patients deny responsibility for the lesions and are resistant to the idea that they are important unconscious non-verbal messages (eg dealing with emotional deprivation), and as such are reluctant to accept psychiatric help.

Associations: Any chronic medical or skin condition, eg acne, alopecia, leg ulcer (which they may encourage); also psychosocial problems, eg emotionally unstable personality, see table 12.7, p. 745; stress; unemployment; depression; anorexia nervosa (in 33%); chronic pain syndrome; sexual conflicts. There is overlap with Münchausen's and other pathomimicry, factious, or somatizing syndromes.

Epidemiology: ♀:♂ ≈ 6:1. In conscript armies, sex ratios may reverse (there is usually obvious secondary gain).

Signs: Variable (simply showing images can be very misleading). The morphology depends on how the lesions are induced but the outline is often different from the smooth outline of endogenous skin disease (eg irregular, jagged, linear geometric shapes). Look for unusual/inexplicable features. *Histology:* Non-specific, but may help establish a definite diagnosis.

ΔΔ: Always consider an alternative diagnosis eg pyoderma gangrenosum, contact dermatitis, photodermatitis, infection, or fixed drug eruption.

Treatment: Provide symptomatic care of skin lesions. Supportive care will only gain traction once issues surrounding emotional deprivation, isolation, insecurity, and other psychological states are addressed. Try to avoid confrontation—don't just prescribe antidepressants or antipsychotics and move on. Spend time with your patient and develop a therapeutic alliance. Include the family. Find a specialist (GP, dermatologist, or psychiatrist) who enjoys a holistic challenge of epic ectodermal proportions and who can roll skin and brain into a single unified management plan.

Delusions of parasitosis

In this rare disorder,[31] patients have a fixed firm belief that they are infested with an insect or parasite which is causing pruritus. You will be shown excoriations and nodules, all caused by picking and scratching, that are produced by the 'insects'. Patients will often present pieces of skin, scale, or other debris (often contained in a matchbox) with the belief it is a carefully collected specimen of the parasite—and as proof of their affliction.

Primary skin lesions are not present and there is no true infestation or primary cause of pruritus. There is no obvious cognitive impairment. It typically occurs in white, middle-aged or older women.

Treatment is challenging. The patient believes there is a real and physical cause for a psychological problem. Try to encourage them to see a psychiatrist (this will be difficult). Olanzapine and risperidone are antipsychotics of choice. Do not use the delusion to encourage the patient to take medication 'in order to help kill the parasites'.

Morgellons disease is related to delusional parasitosis and affected individuals describe filaments or fibres growing from the skin that cause painful lesions (± biting or crawling sensations). Patients mistakenly believe they are infested with a parasite and present collected 'fibres' for examination and may pick at lesions with tweezers.

Skin type

The Fitzpatrick skin type is a numerical classification dependent on the amount of melanin pigment in the skin (determined by constitutional skin colour) and the response of this skin type on exposure to ultraviolet radiation (tanning). See table 6.3.

Table 6.3 Fitzpatrick classification of skin type

Skin type	Do you burn or tan?	Those affected
I	Always burns, never tans	White/pale skin (freckles, blond/red hair)
II	Burns easily, tans poorly	Pale skin (blond hair, blue eyes)
III	May burn, tans lightly	Darker white skin (dark hair, brown eyes)
IV	Burns minimally, tans easily	Olive skin eg Mediterranean
V	Rarely burns, always tans	Asian, Middle Eastern, Latin American
VI	Never burns, tans darkly	Black African

Further reading

Koo JYM (2013). *Dermatitis Artefacta*. Medscape. http://emedicine.medscape.com/article/1121933

Scheinfeld NS (2014). *Delusions of Parasitosis*. Medscape. http://emedicine.medscape.com/article/1121818

Scheinfeld NS (2015). *Excoriation Disorder*. Medscape. http://emedicine.medscape.com/article/112204

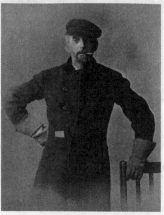

Fig 7.1 Huw Owen Thomas. With the exception of penicillin, the most lifesaving medical intervention thus far developed was invented by a Welshman accepted as the 'Father of Orthopaedics'. Huw Owen Thomas' Thomas splint was originally intended for the management of tuberculosis of the knee, but in 1916 it was used on the front in WWI by his nephew, Robert Jones, for the management of femoral fractures on the battlefield. This simple device, often applied under fire, changed the mortality of open femoral fractures from over 80% to less than 20%. Thomas died in 1891, so did not see the results of his device, but his influence over orthopaedic surgery remains today, with the Thomas test still used to detect fixed flexion deformities of the hip. He was beloved in Liverpool, where he lived and practised, and was known to treat patients for free every Sunday, well before the advent of the NHS.

Further reading and other relevant pages

www.orthoworld.com
www.anatomy.tv
Metabolic bone disease: OHCM pp682–685;

www.wheelessonline.com
www.e-anatomy.org
Rheumatology: OHCM p538–63
Trauma/PHEM management: Chapters 8 and 9

With many thanks to our junior reader Sophie Howarth for their contribution to this chapter.

A small collection of orthopaedic-related mnemonics

For the reflexes: (p. 550)
1,2 Buckle my shoe: *S1/S2* ankle.
3,4 Kick the door: *L3/L4* knee.
5,6 Pick up sticks: *C5/C6* biceps & brachioradialis.
7,8 Shut the gate: *C7/C8* triceps.

Serratus anterior: Is supplied by the long thoracic nerve.
C5, 6, & 7 Raise your arms up to heaven (Nerve root for Long Thoracic Nerve).

Musculocutaneous nerve: Supplies the 'BBC' (p. 550):
Biceps, **B**rachialis, & **C**oracobrachialis.

Superficial forearm flexors: **P**layers **F**ollow **P**imps **F**or **F**un:
Pronator teres, **F**lexor Carpi Radialis, **P**almaris longus, **F**lexor carpi ulnaris, **F**lexor digitorum superficialis.

Radial nerve: Supplies the 'BREAST':
Brachio**R**adialis, **E**xtensors, **A**nconeus, **S**upinator, **T**riceps.

Median nerve in the hand: Supplies 'LOAF' (p. 555 & p. 477):
Lateral 2 lumbricals, **O**pponens pollicis, **A**bductor pollicis brevis, **F**lexor pollicis brevis.

The hand interossei: 'PAD/DAB': **P**almar **AD**duct, **D**orsal **AB**duct.

Hand deformities: 'DR CUMA' (p. 550):
Drop wrist **R**adial nerve, **C**law hand **U**lnar nerve, **M**edian nerve **A**pe hand.

Femoral sheath: Lateral to medial 'NAVeL': **N**erve, **A**rtery, **V**ein, (empty space), **L**ymph nodes.

Femoral triangle: **S**o **I** **M**ay **A**lways **L**ove **S**urgery:
Superior (**I**nguinal), **M**edial (**A**dductor longus), **L**ateral (**S**artorius).

External hip rotators: **P**retty **G**irls **O**ften **G**row **O**ld **Q**uickly:
Piriformis, **G**emellus **S**uperior, **O**bturator internus, **G**emellus inferior, **O**bturator externus, **Q**uadratus femoris.

Foot Evertors: **E**: p**E**rineus longus/br**e**vis/t**e**rtius.

Foot Invertors: **I**: T**I**bialis posterior/anterior.

Structures behind medial malleolus: **T**om, **D**ick and **A** **V**ery **N**ervous **H**arry:
Tibialis posterior, Flexor **D**igitorum longus, **A**rtery (posterior tibial), **V**ein (posterior tibial), **N**erve (posterior tibial), Flexor **H**allucis longus (fig 7.61, p. 517).

Salter–Harris fractures: I–V—SALTR *(in relation to epiphysis)* (p. 469):
Separation, **A**bove, **L**ower, **T**hrough, **R**ammed (Compression).

Age of ossification in paediatric elbow: CRITOL:
Capitellum: 1 year.
Radial head: 3 years.
Internal (medial) epicondyle: 5 years.
Trochlea: 7 years.
Olecranon: 9 years.
Lateral epicondyle: 11 years.

x-ray features of OA: LOSS (p. 499):
Loss of joint space, **O**steophytes, **S**ubchondral sclerosis, and **S**ubchondral cysts.

Typical presenting features of musculoskeletal disease

- Trauma
- Sequelae from previous trauma
- Pain (traumatic or atraumatic)[1]
- Deformity
- Swelling
- Weakness
- Loss of function
- Stiffness
- Neurological.

A patient's report of pain, stiffness, swelling, and weakness/loss of function are key components of any orthopaedic story. Careful dissection of details within these sections is required.

Questions to ask Any recent or past trauma to site? Hand dominance? Assessment of the patient's baseline function and expectations is also essential, is she expecting to regain the ability to perform fine needlework? Occupation and hand dominance plays a major role, is he a professional piano player reliant on fine finger movements or a builder dependent on physical strength?[2] General health OK? If aches and pains all over, is it fibromyalgia or polymyalgia?

Medical conditions affecting orthopaedic function (See *OHCM* chapter 12.)

Mnemonic: RPT—MSK—DHS.[3]

- **R**heumatic fever (or childhood arthritis).
- **P**soriasis (think of psoriatic arthritis).
- **T**B (affects joints as well).
- **M**usculoskeletal disorders (such as SLE, hypermobility, bone malignancy, osteoarthritis).
- **D**iabetes.
- **H**ypo/**H**yperthyroidism and other metabolic bone disease.
- **S**exually transmitted diseases may cause reactive arthritis (Reiter syndrome).

Also consider:

- Medications (eg steroids aggravating osteoporosis and subsequent bisphosphonate treatment).
- Smoking (reduced healing time).
- Neuromuscular disease.

'Look, Feel, Move' and special tests

Going through clinical examination with an expert is the best way to learn, but this experience can be reinforced by taking principles and background reading with you into the arena. Most orthopaedic examinations can be developed by following the '**LOOK, FEEL, MOVE**' structure.

- **LOOK** for swelling, deformity and resting joint position, skin changes (scars/erythema/bruising) and soft tissues (muscle wasting/contractures).
- **FEEL** for anatomical landmarks, warmth, swelling, and tenderness.
- **MOVE** joint actively first before you assess passive range of movement and power (see table 7.1 MRC scale). With respect to movement limitation: *active loss* = neuromuscular deficit; *passive loss* = bony/soft tissue is blocking movement.

Special tests Finally assess joint function and include any special tests (eg knee meniscal tests, hip fixed flexion deformities). Establish neurovascular status by capillary refill time (CRT) and sensation/power of local nerves.

Key points • Always examine *the joint above* and *below* the joint being examined ie for the hip, examine the knee and lumbar spine. This will uncover any referring pathology • Always compare with the same joint on the other side • Assess the neurovascular status (especially in trauma) • Exposure should be appropriate but remember to respect patient dignity.

---

1 Use SOCRATES to help take a history of pain. Site, Onset (Sudden, gradual), Character (Ache? Stabbing? Burning?), Radiation, Associated symptoms, Time (When did it start?), Exacerbating/Relieving factors, Severity (use a scale out of 10).

2 Be aware of patient expectations. *Patient*: Will I be able to play the piano after these bandages come off? *Doctor*: Yes, you can expect full recovery. *Patient*: Great! I've never been able to play the piano …

3 See p.540 for why the acronym DHS will stick in your mind!

Table 7.1 Quantifying strength: the UK MRC scale

Grade 0	No muscle contraction	Grade 3	Active movement against gravity but not against resistance
Grade 1	Flicker of contraction	Grade 4	Active movement against resistance but not achieving full power.
Grade 2	Active movement with gravity eliminated	Grade 5	Normal power

Grades 4–, 4, and 4+ describe movement against slight, moderate, and strong resistance. To test proximal muscle power: ask patient to sit from lying and to rise from squatting. ►Observe gait (easy to forget, even if the complaint is of walking difficulty!). See p. 488 and OHCM p467 for gait disorders.

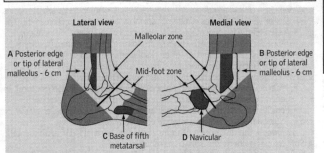

Fig 7.2 Use the Ottawa ankle rules to guide the need for an x-ray. Ankle x-rays are required only if there is pain in the malleolar zone and tenderness at either point *A*, point *B*, or inability to weight bear both immediately and in the ED. Foot x-rays are required if there is pain in the midfoot zone and tenderness at either point *C*, point *D*, or inability to weight bear both immediately and in the ED.   Reproduced with permission from Bachmann LM, et al. Accuracy of Ottawa ankle rules to exclude fractures of the ankle and mid-foot: systematic review *BMJ* 2003; 326:417. Copyright © 2003, British Medical Journal Publishing Group.

When you examine, it's useful to have a picture in your mind's eye of the pathology you are looking for and which investigations could help. Here are the *Ottawa ankle rules* (fig 7.2); a decision aid for excluding fractures of the ankle and midfoot. They have a sensitivity of almost 100%, which allow you to confidently rule out fractures in ankle sprains without the need for an x-ray. As a consequence though, the specificity is somewhat lower. In this case, specificity is an indicator of the number of unnecessary x-rays which could be avoided if following these rules.

Three wise men

Reaching the correct diagnosis can be difficult and this paper[1] gives a very thought-provoking overview in the diagnostic challenges faced in clinical medicine. Diagnostic errors are the leading cause of litigation in the USA. Is this new lesion a metastasis from the existing lung cancer or is it a new primary? The answer dictates your treatment. The authors draw inspiration from 3 wise men. *Occam's razor* states that a simple unifying diagnosis is likely the cause of all the symptoms. In contrast, *Hickam's dictum* quotes that 'patients can have as many diseases as they damn well please'. *Crabtree's bludgeon* puts the latter 2 into perspective and reminds us of the risk of ignoring key facts as we insist on finding evidence to support our ideal diagnosis instead. How many times have you diagnosed a rarity and then enthusiastically searched the case notes to find further evidence to back your claim, while ignoring features supportive of another theory? As patients live longer and chronic diseases are more prevalent, Hickam's dictum may be more appropriate and Occam's razor better applied to the younger, healthier population. Reflect on those approaches as you embark on your own diagnostic journey.

►►If you suspect a cervical spine injury, immobilize the neck with 3-point immobilization: collar, blocks, and tape.

Imaging Supervise all movements closely during transport to radiology. If there is a clear spinal cord injury, and the patient is stable, CT is the 1st line of imaging. Image the whole spine as there may be more than one injury. MRI shows fractures, subluxations, disc disruption and protrusion, and cord contusion—and helps establish prognosis. ►NB: it is hard to arrange in emergency settings, and takes a lot longer than CT (eg 20min vs 20sec). Consider CT myelography if MRI is contraindicated.

When examining the image, follow 4 simple steps (ABCS):

1 *Alignment*—check alignment of the following: • Anterior vertebral bodies • Posterior vertebral bodies • Posterior spinal canal • Spinous processes (fig 7.4).
  • A step >3mm is abnormal (<25%=unifacet; >50%=bifacet dislocation).
  • Atlas–dens interval (ADI)—normal if <3mm (adults) or <5mm (children).
  • 40% of <7yr-olds have anterior displacement C2 on C3 (in this pseudo-subluxation the posterior spinal line is maintained).
2 *Bone contour*—trace around each vertebra individually.
  • Anterior/posterior height difference of >3mm (implies *wedge fracture*). In general, <25% difference is stable and >25% difference is unstable.
  • Pedicles (*hangman's #*, fig 7.7) & spinous processes (*clayshoveller's #*).
  • Avulsion fractures of the vertebral body (*teardrop #*).
3 *Cartilages*—the disc space margins should be parallel (>11° is abnormal).
4 *Soft tissues*—check the soft tissue shadows:
  • Retropharyngeal—C1–C3 <7mm; C4–C7 <22mm/1 vertebral body (fig 7.5).
  • Spinous process separation (interspinous ligament rupture). CT can help diagnose fractures here.

►All 7 cervical vertebrae must be seen, along with the C7–T1 junction: do not accept an incomplete image—a 'swimmers' view of C7–T1 or CT may be needed.
►A cross-table lateral in the best hands will still miss at least 15% of injuries.

Other views and investigations
• Open mouth 'peg' view (OMV, fig 7.6) for suspected odontoid peg fractures and C1 fractures (*total* lateral mass overhang of C1 on C2 should be <8mm).
• CT is used to image areas not adequately assessed on plain films.
• MRI is vital for assessing ligamentous disruption, disc prolapse, and the neural elements (spinal cord and nerve roots), all of which can only be inferred from CT and plain x-ray. Whole spine assessment is best.

Spinal cord injury with out radiological abnormality (SCIWORA) This is becoming less common as pathology may be visible on MRI (fig 7.3). It is a condition in which there is a neurological deficit in the absence of a lesion on plain x-rays. It typically occurs in paediatric cervical spine injuries and is treated in the same manner as a spinal fracture with appropriate immobilization and referral. Clinical evidence of the injury in children may be delayed in up to 50%, so always consider spinal cord injury if the mechanism is appropriate.[2]

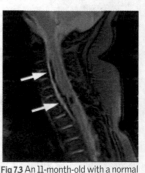

Fig 7.3 An 11-month-old with a normal CT neck on admission, developed paraplegia 6 hours after his stroller was hit by a car. An urgent MRI was performed; T1-weighted image showing anterior subdural haemorrhage from C2 to C7 (arrows).

Reproduced with permission from *Western Journal of Emergency Medicine*, copyright remains with the original authors.

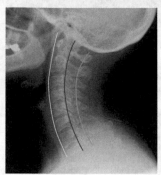

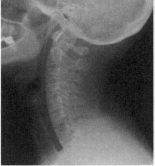

Fig 7.4 The lines to check for discontinuity on a lateral c-spine x-ray:
Yellow = anterior spinal line.
Red = posterior spinal line.
Green = spinolaminar line.
Blue = tips of spinous processes.
Note that we can see all the way to C7–T1.
Courtesy of The Norfolk and Norwich University Hospitals (NNUH) Radiology Dept.

Fig 7.5 More important areas.
Yellow = ADI should be <3mm in adults.
Red = before C1–C3 should be <7mm.
Blue = before C4–C7 should be <22m.
ADI is the distance between the anterior aspect of the odontoid peg and the posterior of the anterior arch of C1.
Courtesy of The Norfolk and Norwich University Hospitals (NNUH) Radiology Dept.

▶ *Do a detailed neurological examination in all fractures of the c-spine and seek advice from the on-call neurosurgical or spinal team.*

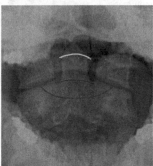

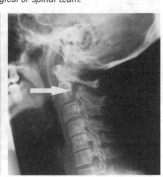

Fig 7.6 Odontoid peg fractures are best seen on the OMV. There are 3 types:
Type I (yellow) = through the tip (stable).
Type II (red) = through the base (unstable).
Type III (blue) = into the body of C2 (?stability).
Remember to check for the overhang of C1 on C2 (<8mm in total).
Courtesy of The Norfolk and Norwich University Hospitals (NNUH) Radiology Dept.

Fig 7.7 Lateral x-ray of the c-spine showing a fracture through the pedicles of the C2 vertebra—the hangman's fracture, which is traumatic spondylolisthesis of C2.
Courtesy of Professor Peter Scally.

The paediatric cervical spine

Below the age of ~9yrs, the cervical spine needs to be assessed as an entirely different entity, as it creates very different patterns of normality and abnormality. The most important point to make here is it is best to ask a specialist's opinion—ie ask a paediatric radiologist. Nonetheless, remember:
▶▶ Injury is commonest in the upper spine.
▶▶ SCIWORA (see p468).
▶▶ Growth plates (physes) and synchondroses can be mistaken for fractures.
▶▶ C2–3 and C3–4 can demonstrate pseudosubluxation.
▶▶ C7–T1 does not need to be visualized unless ≥8yrs old or clinical suspicion requires.

7 Orthopaedics

Cervical spondylosis (See *OHCM* p508.) Degenerative changes of the cervical spine (eg featuring degeneration of the annulus fibrosus and bony spurs) tend to narrow the spinal canal and intervertebral foramina. Very common: ~90% of men >60yrs and women >50yrs. Usually asymptomatic, but can cause neck and arm pain with paraesthesiae. 5–10% of symptomatic patients develop *cervical myelopathy* (progressive cord compression with spastic weakness). Acute myelopathy requires urgent neurosurgical referral. See *OHCM* p508.

Cervical spondylolisthesis Displacement of one vertebra upon the one below. *Causes:* 1 Congenital failure of fusion of the odontoid process with the axis, or fracture of the odontoid process (skull, atlas, & odontoid process slip forward on axis) 2 Inflammation softens the transverse ligament (fig 7.9) of the atlas (eg rheumatoid, or complicating throat infections), so the atlas slips forward on the axis 3 Instability after injuries. The most important consequence of spondylolisthesis is the possibility of spinal cord compression. Treatments used include traction, immobilization in plaster jackets, and spinal fusion.

Prolapsed cervical disc (See p. 482 on back pain.) Central protrusions (typically C5/6 & C6/7) may give symptoms of spinal cord compression (p. 562). Posterolateral protrusions may cause a stiff neck, pain radiating to the arm, muscle weakness, and depressed reflexes. *Tests:* MRI if possible (fig 7.10). *Treatment:* Analgesia (NSAIDs 1st line), postural alteration, and pillow reduction[4]. As pain subsides, physiotherapy may help to restore mobility. Surgery is rarely indicated, in the light of CT/MRI findings.

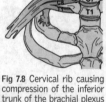

Cervical rib Congenital development of the costal process of the C7 vertebra is often asymptomatic but may cause thoracic outlet compression (figs 7.8 & 7.11). Similar symptoms with no radiological abnormality is called a scalenus or 1st rib syndrome. Thoracic outlet[4] compression involves the lowest trunk of the brachial plexus (fig 8.37, p. 557) ± the subclavian artery. Pain or numbness may be felt in hand or forearm (often on the ulnar side); there may be hand weakness and muscle wasting (thenar or hypothenar). *Diagnosis:* Weak radial pulse ± forearm cyanosis. Specific manoeuvres (eg Adson's test) are not reliable. x-rays may not reveal cervical ribs, as symptoms may be caused by fibrous bands. Arteriography may show subclavian compression. *Treatment:* Physiotherapy to strengthen the shoulder elevators may improve symptoms, but rib removal or band division may be needed.

Fig 7.8 Cervical rib causing compression of the inferior trunk of the brachial plexus (p. 557). The distal part of the rib can also cause stenosis in the subclavian artery, with post-stenotic dilatation (visible on arteriography).

Spasmodic torticollis (cervical dystonia) The commonest adult focal dystonia. Episodes of a sudden stiff painful neck with torticollis are due to trapezius and sternocleidomastoid spasm. Social withdrawal can be a problem. *Causes:* Idiopathic; genetic; trauma. *Treatment:* Is notoriously challenging. 20% experience spontaneous recovery within 5 years of symptoms but generally it is a life-long disorder. Heat, manipulation, relaxants, and analgesia offer limited benefit. Try anticholinergics, benzodiazepines, and baclofen. Botulinum toxin is a safe and effective option.[3] Surgical intervention is becoming more successful and includes selective ramisectomy for cervical musculature, deep brain stimulation from electrodes,[5] and selective peripheral denervation of the cervical musculature which participates in the abnormal neck postures.[6]

Infantile torticollis A congenital packaging deformity caused by contracture of sternocleidomastoid. *Typical age:* 0–36 months. *Treatment:* Self-limiting in 97%. If persistent, physio helps by lengthening the muscle; surgical division is more drastic.[7]

4 The thoracic outlet is the space between the 1st rib and clavicle.

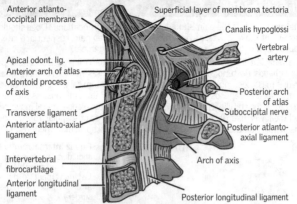

Anterior atlanto-occipital membrane

Superficial layer of membrana tectoria

Canalis hypoglossi

Vertebral artery

Apical odont. lig.
Anterior arch of atlas
Odontoid process of axis

Posterior arch of atlas
Suboccipital nerve

Transverse ligament
Anterior atlanto-axial ligament

Posterior atlanto-axial ligament

Intervertebral fibrocartilage
Anterior longitudinal ligament

Arch of axis

Posterior longitudinal ligament

Fig 7.9 Cut-away sagittal view of the atlas and the axis cervical vertebrae, showing the ligaments around the odontoid peg.

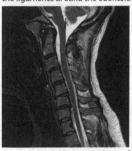

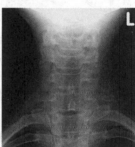

Fig 7.10 T2-weighted sagittal MRI of the cervical spine showing intervertebral disc protrusion at the C5/6 level.
Courtesy of The Norfolk and Norwich University Hospitals (NNUH) Radiology Dept.

Fig 7.11 AP x-ray of the cervical spine showing bilateral rudimentary cervical ribs in the form of prominent transverse processes (the condition is a spectrum). They are usually a unilateral x-ray finding, though the contralateral side may still have a ligamentous band present. The presence of a cervical rib increases the likelihood of the brachial plexus being *prefixed*—ie arising from C4–C8 rather than C5–T1. Courtesy of The Norfolk and Norwich University Hospitals (NNUH) Radiology Dept.

Whiplash injury

This is cervical strain caused by sudden neck extension with rebound flexion. It is common, often in rear-end crashes. Hyperextension causes damage to the anterior musculoligamentous structures. Subsequent protective muscle spasm causes pain and stiffness, which may be severe. *Treatment* Reassure physical injury is rare. Emphasize positive attitudes to prognosis and recovery are important. Encourage prompt return to usual activity and occupation. Suggest active mobilization. Aim to prevent chronicity and 'disuse syndrome' through advocating self-management with analgesia. Collars, rest, and negative attitudes can contribute to delayed recovery and chronicity. If symptoms last for >1yr, they are likely to be permanent.[8] Always give a patient information leaflet.

Further reading

Jinnah HA *et al.* (2013). The focal dystonias. *Mov Disord* 28:926–43.
National Spasmodic Torticollis Association: www.torticollis.org
ST Dystonia: www.spasmodictorticollis.org/index.cfm

History Where is the pain: shoulder or neck? Past dislocations? Does shoulder movement make it worse? If all movements worsen pain, suspect arthritis or capsulitis; if only some movements, suspect impingement.

Examination Strip to waist. *LOOK:* Wasting of rotator cuff muscles, deltoid, pectorals, hands. Posterior glenohumeral dislocation causes internal rotation, anteromedial mass seen on anterior dislocation. *FEEL:* Anatomically, the glenohumeral joint is lax and depends far more on surrounding rotator-cuff muscles than bony structures for stability (figs 7.13 & 7.14). *MOVE:* To assess glenohumeral movement, feel the lower half of the scapula to estimate degrees of scapular rotation over the thorax. Half the range of normal abduction is by scapula movement (fig 7.12).

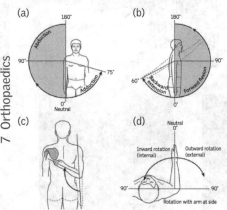

Fig 7.12 Internal rotation of shoulder: 'imagine you are doing up a bra'. This is the last movement to recover after shoulder soft tissue surgery.

Reproduced from Bowden et al., *Oxford Handbook of Orthopaedics and Trauma* (2010), with permission from OUP.

The muscles used for movement at the shoulder joint
* *Flexion:* (Forward movement.) Pectoralis major, deltoid (ant. ⅓), coracobrachialis.
* *Extension:* Deltoid (posterior ⅓); latissimus dorsi, pectoralis major, and teres major begin the extension if the shoulder starts out flexed.
* *Abduction:* Supraspinatus for first 20°, then deltoid.
* *Adduction:* Pectoralis major, latissimus dorsi, teres major, subscapularis.
* *Medial rotation:* Pectoralis major, deltoid (middle ⅓), latissimus dorsi, teres major, subscapularis.
* *Lateral rotation:* Teres minor, infraspinatus.

Scapula movement on the chest wall NB: serratus anterior prevents 'winging' of the scapula as pressure is placed on the outstretched hand.
* *Elevation:* (Shrug shoulders.) Levator scapulae, trapezius.
* *Depression:* Serratus anterior, pectoralis minor.
* *Forward action:* (=protraction, eg punch.) Serratus anterior, pectoralis major.
* *Retraction:* (Brace shoulders.) Trapezius, rhomboid.

The importance of shoulders
We shrug our shoulders to show we don't know, or don't care. We give the cold shoulder to someone we dislike yet we offer our shoulder for a friend to cry on and we help shoulder their burden. We stand shoulder-to-shoulder, united, in a common cause. We pull onto the hard shoulder of the motorway when our car breaks down. Take any shoulder pathology seriously as loss of upper limb function can have a large impact on many aspects of life.

Further reading
www.shoulderdoc.co.uk

7 Orthopaedics

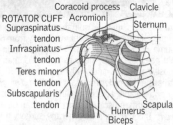

Fig 7.13 Shoulder anatomy (without deltoid: anterior view). Rotator cuff muscles: Supraspinatus (abduction), Subscapularis (internal rotation), Infraspinatus (external rotation), Teres Minor (external rotation + extension). Mnemonic: sits (supraspinatus, infraspinatus, teres Minor, subscapularis). Biceps' long head traverses the cuff attaching to top of the glenoid cavity.

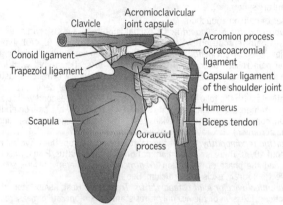

Fig 7.14 Shoulder and acromioclavicular (ac) joint ligaments: anterior view.

Some specific specialist shoulder examination tests

There are >100 shoulder tests, many of which are not performed as they were first described. Here is a useful quotient for the budding orthopod.

Tests for impingement A painful arc between 60° and 120° abduction; exacerbated by thumb pointing down (empty can) and better with thumb pointing up (full can). *Hawkins test:* Shoulder and elbow both flexed to 90°, pain on passive internal rotation as the rotator cuff rubs on the undersurface of the acromion.

Tests for rotator cuff tears *Jobe test (supraspinatus):* Patient internally rotates arm while in 45° abduction and 30° forward flexion with an extended elbow (like emptying a can). Attempt to resist downward pressure results in pain. *Belly-press test (subscapularis):* patient presses on their abdomen (+ve if elbow drops posteriorly as there is pain on internal rotation of shoulder). *Infraspinatus and teres minor:* Flex elbow to 90° and externally rotate against resistance. *Drop arm sign:* Patient lowers arm slowly from 160° abduction. If patient can't control the arm, and it drops quickly to the side = rotator cuff tear.

Test for ac joint disease *Scarf test:* Forced adduction of arm across the neck.

Biceps tendonitis *Speed's test:* Patient starts with arm flexed forward 60°, elbow extended and forearm in supination, and attempts to flex shoulder forward against resistance. Pain on palpation of long head of biceps tendon during this manoeuvre.

Rotator cuff tears Tears in supraspinatus tendon (fig 7.15) or adjacent subscapularis and infraspinatus may present insidiously from degeneration in the elderly or after trauma in younger patients. Patients complain of shoulder *weakness* and pain. Night pain may affect sleep as patient is unable to keep the arm in a comfortable position. Typical age: >40yrs, patients <50 years need urgent investigation and treatment in order to regain function⁹. *Imaging:* US and MRI are useful; US is quicker and cheaper to perform and gives information about tear or no tear, but MRI can quantify muscle wasting which can be a useful prognostic indicator.¹⁰ *Treatment:* Incomplete: physiotherapy, surgery if symptoms persist. Complete: prompt referral for assessment for open or arthroscopic repair.

Impingement syndrome (On abducting 45°–160°.) Only a proportion will have a painful arc (others have increasing pain up to full abduction), which is why the term *impingement syndrome* (as the tendon catches under the acromion during abduction between eg 70° and 140°) is preferred (rather than painful arc syndrome).

Causes of pain on abduction:

1 *Supraspinatus tendinopathy:* Or partial rupture of supraspinatus tendon gives pain reproduced by testing supraspinatus strength (p. 470). Typical age: 35–60. *Treatment:* active shoulder movement with physiotherapy and pain relief; subacromial bursa injection of corticosteroid with local anaesthetic may help.¹¹ Refer patients with refractory symptoms lasting 6 months for consideration of arthroscopic subacromial decompression.¹² Patients with the following features are most likely to respond well to surgery: temporary benefit following steroid injection, mid-arc pain on abduction, consistently positive Hawkins test.¹³ The 'sourcil sign' (sclerosis under the acromion) on x-ray does not aid diagnosis.¹⁴

2 *Calcific tendinopathy:* One of the acute calcific arthropathies. Typical age about 40yrs. There is acute inflammation of supraspinatus. Pain is maximal during the phase of resorption. *Treatment:* physiotherapy, NSAIDs; steroid injection; rarely, excision of calcium. See fig 7.16.

3 *Acromioclavicular joint osteoarthritis: Treatment:* Rest; NSAIDs; steroid injections. Excision of the ACJ only if resistant to non-operative measures.

Long head of biceps tendinopathy Pain is in the anterior shoulder and characteristically ↑ on forced contraction of biceps. *Treatment:* Pain relief; corticosteroid injection to the tendon may help, but risks tendon rupture.

Rupture of long head of biceps Discomfort occurs after 'something has gone' when lifting or pulling. A 'ball' appears in the muscle on elbow flexion, like a 'Popeye' muscle. *Treatment:* repair is rarely indicated as function remains.⁵

Frozen shoulder (adhesive capsulitis) Normally has no obvious triggers. Pain may be severe and worse at night (eg unable to lie on one side). The natural history is divided into: 1 The painful phase (6 weeks–9 months). Active and passive movement range is reduced. Abduction ↓ (<90°) ± external rotation ↓ (<30°) 2 Frozen phase where pain usually settles but the shoulder remains stiff (6–12 months) 3 Thawing phase as the shoulder slowly regains range of movement (1–3 years). It may be associated with diabetes, thyroid disease, and cervical spondylosis (more global restriction of movement). *Treatment:* Early physiotherapy and NSAIDs if tolerated. Corticosteroid joint injections may reduce pain in early phases.¹⁵ Oral steroids provide short-term improvement but benefits are not maintained beyond 6 weeks and therefore not used in clinical practice.¹⁶ Surgical release with arthroscopic arthrolysis ± manipulation under anaesthesia is currently the most effective treatment. Resolution may take years.

5 Conversely, if it is the biceps *insertion* that is avulsed, surgical repair will be required.

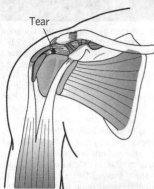

Tear

Fig 7.15 Rotator cuff tear in the supraspinatus tendon. See fig 7.13, p. 471 for muscle names. Distinguishing between tendinopathy and partial tears can be difficult as both cause a painful arc syndrome as the tendon catches in the subacromial space during abduction. Partial tears cause a painful arc (below); complete tears limit shoulder abduction to the 45–60° given by scapular rotation. NB: tendon rupture can also be asymptomatic.[18] If the arm is passively abducted beyond 90° deltoid's contribution to abduction comes into play, which is then possible from this point. Full-range passive movement is present.

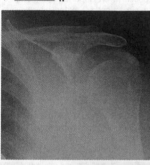

Fig 7.16 AP x-ray of the left shoulder showing calcific tendinopathy in the left supraspinatus. The glenohumeral joint also appears subluxed, though this is most likely 'deltoid inhibition' caused by pain. Supraspinatus involvement is common since the tendon is susceptible to minor trauma due to poor vascularity at the insertion point.

Courtesy of The Norfolk and Norwich University Hospitals (NNUH) Radiology Dept.

Shoulder osteoarthritis

►Remember that the neck may refer pain via C5 to the deltoid region and via C6, C7, and C8 to the superior border of the scapula, so consider MRI in patients with neck and shoulder pain. If aches & pains all over; think about polymyalgia rheumatica or fibromyalgia. If shoulder tip pain is present, examine for diaphragmatic irritation. Shoulder OA (fig 7.17) is not so common as hip or knee OA. Good success rates (especially for pain relief) are being achieved by joint replacement. Timing of surgery is important, so that the rotator cuff and glenoid are not too worn for good stability.[17] See Fig 7.48 p. 499 for features of OA on x-ray.

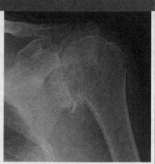

Fig 7.17 AP x-ray of the left shoulder showing osteoarthritis: loss of joint space, subchondral sclerosis, osteophytes, glenoid erosion, and humeral head deformity are all present.

Courtesy of The Norfolk and Norwich University Hospitals (NNUH) Radiology Dept.

Further reading

Favejee MM et al. (2011). Frozen shoulder: The effectiveness of conservative and surgical interventions – systematic review. Br J Sports Med 45:49–56.

Lateral epicondylitis (tennis elbow) Inflammation where the common extensor tendon arises from the lateral epicondyle of the humerus (fig 7.19). *Presentation:* Often a clear history of repetitive strain. Pain is felt at the front of the lateral condyle, and is exacerbated when the tendon is most stretched (wrist and finger flexion with hand pronated). With the patient's elbow fully extended, ask them to extend their wrist against resistance: is pain elicited? *Treatment:* Most cases will naturally resolve through restriction of activities which overload the tendons. Cases typically last 6–24 months and 90% recover within 1 year. Physiotherapy in motivated patients is the most effective non-surgical treatment, using eccentric loading exercises, acupuncture, and deep friction manual therapy. Epicondylitis braces have no proven efficacy but are helpful in some patients. Corticosteroid joint injections are no longer recommended; although giving excellent short-term results (6wks) they are disruptive in the long term (>3 months). One study showed that success rates at 1yr for physiotherapy and 'wait and see' policies were superior to injections.[19] Novel therapies such as platelet-rich plasma injections are expensive, invasive, and not currently recommended by NICE.[20] Only severe cases unresponsive to conservative management should be considered for surgical tendon release.

Medial epicondylitis (golfer's elbow) Inflammation of the forearm flexor muscles at their origin on the medial epicondyle. Most common cause of medial elbow pain, but ⅕ as common as tennis elbow. Pain is exacerbated by pronation and forearm flexion. Occasionally associated with ulnar neuropathy as the ulnar nerve runs behind the epicondyle. Treatment and prognosis is similar to tennis elbow.

Olecranon bursitis (student's elbow) This is a traumatic bursitis following pressure on the elbows eg while engrossed in a long book. There is pain and swelling behind the olecranon. If there is overlying skin cellulitis then consider antibiotics. A rare complication of olecranon bursitis is abscess formation; septic bursitis should be formally drained by the orthopaedic team and will need IV antibiotics. Send aspirate fluid for Gram stain and microscopy for crystals. Other causes include gouty bursitis (look for tophi).

Osteoarthritis of the elbow (fig 7.18) Osteochondritis dissecans[6] and fractures involving the joint are risk factors. *Tests:* Flexion, extension, and forearm rotation may be impaired. Loose bodies may cause restriction of movement eg loss of full extension. *Treatment:* Surgery is indicated for pain or stiffness not responding to conservative measures or if there are signs of locking. While total elbow replacement in rheumatoid arthritis is very effective, it is less so in the treatment of OA.

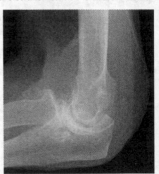

Fig 7.18 Lateral x-ray of the elbow showing degenerative changes of osteoarthritis. There is loss of joint space, osteophyte formation, bony deformity, and subchondral sclerosis. Movement is painful and severely restricted.

Courtesy of The Norfolk and Norwich University Hospitals (NNUH) Radiology Dept.

6 *Osteochondritis dissecans:* subchondral bone becomes avascular, and may progress to fragments of bone and overlying cartilage (osteochondral fragments) breaking away from the bone to form loose bodies. *Cause:* unknown. *Typical site:* lateral side of the medial femoral condyle of 13–21-year-olds. *Symptoms:* pain after exercise with intermittent knee swelling. *Treatment:* stable lesions are treated conservatively, as spontaneous healing can occur. Unstable fragments may be pinned.

7 Orthopaedics

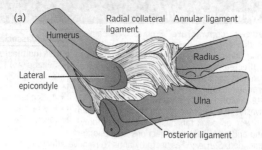

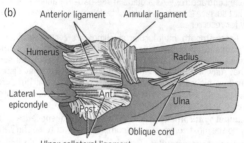

Fig 7.19 The ligaments around the elbow joint—posterolateral view of the right elbow (a) and anteromedial view of the left elbow (b). Stability of this joint is mainly from bony factors, though ligaments do play an important part—eg the annular ligament wraps around the head of the radius (which can pop out in a 'pulled elbow' and also allows smooth pronation/supination). Remember that the joint is made up from 3 articulations: radiohumeral, proximal radioulnar, and humeroulnar. The elbow joint is formed by an articulation of the distal humerus with the proximal radius and ulna. Flexion/extension occurs at the ulnohumeral joint and is possible through a range of 0°–150°. With the elbow flexed, supination/pronation of 90° should be possible—this occurs at the radiohumeral and proximal radioulnar articulations. Pain at the elbow may radiate from the shoulder.

Ulnar neuritis (cubital tunnel syndrome) Osteoarthritic or rheumatoid narrowing of the ulnar groove and constriction of the ulnar nerve as it passes behind the medial epicondyle, or friction of the ulnar nerve due to cubitus valgus (a possible sequel to childhood supracondylar fractures) can cause fibrosis of the ulnar nerve and ulnar neuropathy. *Presentation:* Sensory symptoms usually occur first, eg ↓ sensation over little finger and medial half of ring finger. Patients may experience clumsiness of the hand and weakness of the 4 small muscles of the hand innervated by the ulnar nerve (see p. 550). *Tests:* Nerve conduction studies may confirm the site of the lesion. *Treatment:* Surgical decompression. See p. 554 for nerve compression syndromes.

Pulled elbow (subluxation of radial head) Typical patient: 1–4yr-old who has been lifted by the arm in play, causing the radial head to slip out of the annular ligament. The arm is held slightly flexed and twisted inwards. Reduction can be achieved through the examiner cradling the elbow, with thumb/forefingers over the radial head and either hyperpronating or supinating (limited evidence to support that pronation may be less painful) and flexing the elbow and function is quickly restored. Imaging is not needed. Caution parents to avoid future pulling of the arm, as this condition recurs in up to 25%.

Further reading

Orchard J et al. (2011). The management of tennis elbow. *BMJ* 342:d2687.

Dupuytren's contracture Progressive, painless fibrotic thickening of the palmar fascia with skin puckering and tethering. Ring and little fingers are chiefly affected. It is often bilateral and symmetrical. As thickening occurs there may be MCP joint flexion. If interphalangeal joints are affected the hand may be quite disabled. Early disease may benefit from less invasive treatments eg injectable *Clostridium histolyticum* or percutaneous needle fasciotomy.[21] Splinting and corticosteroid injections are no longer recommended. *Surgery:* Fasciectomy aims to remove affected palmar fascia and release contractures.[18] As a guide, if the patient cannot place their palm flat on a flat surface (Hueston's tabletop test), refer for surgery. There is a high tendency for recurrence.

Causes/associations
Often multifactorial:
• Genetic (AD)
• Smoking
• Diabetes
• Antiepileptics
• Peyronie disease (OHCM p708)

Ganglia These smooth, multilocular swellings are cysts containing jelly-like fluid in communication with joint capsules or tendon sheaths. Treatment is not needed unless they cause pain or pressure (eg on median or ulnar nerve at the wrist). They may disappear spontaneously. Local pressure may disperse them (traditionally a blow from a Bible!). Aspiration may work, but surgical dissection gives less recurrence.[22] Problems include painful scars, neurovascular damage (esp. in palmar wrist ganglia), and recurrence (up to 50%).

Carpal tunnel syndrome (See p. 555.) The most frequent cause of hand pain at night and the most common nerve compression syndrome (fig 7.20).

De Quervain's tenosynovitis Refers to thickening and tightening of the first extensor compartment (there are 6 in total) which contains the abductor pollicis longus and extensor pollicis brevis tendons as they cross the distal radial styloid (fig 7.20). Pain is worst when these tendons are stretched (eg lifting a teapot), and is more proximal than that from osteoarthritis of the 1st carpometacarpal joint. *Finkelstein's sign:* Pain elicited by gripping the thumb into the palm of the same hand with passive ulnar deviation. *Cause:* Unknown but symptoms can be exacerbated by overuse of the tendons (eg wringing clothes). *Treatment:* First try rest (thumb spica splint), ice, and NSAIDs. Corticosteroid injection (p.514) at tendon site during the 1st 6 months of symptoms is effective in 90% of patients. If conservative measures fail, decompression of the tendons is provided by splitting the tendon sheaths. >80% do well postoperatively.[23]

Volkmann's ischaemic contracture Is fortunately now rare. It follows poorly managed compartment syndrome or interruption of the brachial artery near the elbow (eg after supracondylar fracture of humerus, p. 533). Muscle necrosis (esp. flexor pollicis longus and flexor digitorum profundus) results in contraction and fibrosis causing a flexion deformity at wrist and elbow. *Treatment:* See p. 528 for compartment syndrome. *Treating contractures:* Prevention is key! To restore lost function, surgery to release compressed nerves ± tendons.

"You have strong, clever hands ..." She looked up at me questioningly. *"What do you do for a living?"* *"I play the lute"* /Patrick Rothfuss *The Wise Man's Fear* There are no minor injuries of the fingers or hand, especially for those who rely on dexterity for a living. This musician would not only be stripped of his ability to earn, but also of his coping mechanism. What is your coping mechanism to survive the turmoil medicine throws at you? In the UK, alcohol and tobacco use are common coping strategies and in Pakistan, students reported music and sports. Stress among undergraduates is prevalent; ensure that you find and protect a *positive* coping mechanism.

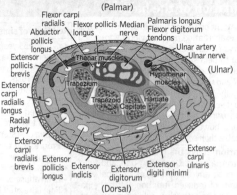

(Palmar)

Flexor carpi radialis
Abductor pollicis longus
Flexor pollicis longus
Median nerve
Palmaris longus/ Flexor digitorum tendons
Extensor pollicis brevis
Thenar muscles
Ulnar artery
Ulnar nerve
(Ulnar)
Hypothenar muscles
Trapezium
Extensor carpi radialis longus
Trapezoid
Capitate
Hamate
Radial artery
Extensor carpi radialis brevis
Extensor pollicis longus
Extensor indicis
Extensor digitorum
Extensor digiti minimi
Extensor carpi ulnaris
(Dorsal)

Fig 7.20 Cross-sectional view of the wrist showing the contents of the carpal tunnel and the extensor tendons of the hand. When trying to describe local anatomy of the hand, it is easier to use the terms *ulnar* and *radial (thumb side)*, rather than medial and lateral, which can cause confusion. *Dorsal* refers to the posterior surface, while *palmar* (*also known as volar*) refers to anterior surface.[7] See p. 555 for carpal tunnel syndrome.

Flexor tendons pulley mechanisms

In order to stop the long flexor tendons of the hand bowing when the fingers are flexed, the fingers have a number of pulleys (well-placed thickenings in the flexor sheath) attached to the bones and palmar plates beneath. Named morphologically as either 'A' for annular, or 'c' for cruciate, there are 5 A-pulleys and 3 c-pulleys. The most important are A2 (which is at the proximal end of the proximal phalanx) and A4 (at the middle of the middle phalanx), both of which need to be preserved during any surgery to prevent bowing of the flexor tendons. Sometimes mountaineers, and others hanging on by their fingertips, partially damage the A2 pulley (typically). Apply ice and buddy-taping/splinting. Then do only light exercises (rubber doughnut squeezes; mild stretches) until 2wks after pain and swelling subside. Visible bowing of the tendon may indicate that surgery is needed. See fig 7.21.

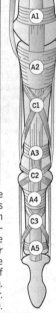

Trigger finger (tendon nodules) Caused by a swelling of the flexor tendon or tightening of the sheath. Ring and middle fingers most commonly affected, but trigger thumb is more common in children. Swelling of the tendon sheath, along with nodule formation on the tendon, proximal to the A1 pulley (fig 7.21) prevents the tendon gliding smoothly and instead 'catches' causing the finger to lock in flexion. As extension occurs, the nodule moves with the flexor tendon, but then becomes jammed on the proximal side of the pulley, and has to be flicked straight, so producing triggering. Much more common in diabetes where recurrence is also higher. ℞: Steroid injection is usually successful. See p. 515 (fig 7.59). Surgery is curative if recurrent.[24]

Fig 7.21 Pulley system.

Further reading

Black EM *et al.* (2011). Dupuytren disease: an evolving understanding of an age-old disease. *J Am Acad Orthop Surg* 19:746–57.

Pettitt DA *et al.* (2012). Clinical review: Volkmann's ischaemic contracture. *Eur J Trauma Emerg Surg* 38:129–37.

7 The International Federation for Societies for Surgery of the Hand recommends the term 'palmar'.

7 Orthopaedics

History Attention should be paid to the nature of the pain, exacerbating and relieving factors, and the history of onset. Review the sinister causes of back pain to help structure your history taking. ▶You must document the presence of red flags (pp. 486-7 and MINIBOX 'Red flags of sinister pain'). These signify cord or cauda equina compression and should set alarm bells ringing: refer at once (needs an MRI in <4h). Remember that motor deficits and bowel or bladder disturbances are more reliable than sensory signs.

Red flags of sinister pain
• ≤20 or ≥55 years old
• Violent trauma
• Minor trauma in osteoporosis
• Alternating or bilateral sciatica
• Weak legs
• Weight loss/fever
• Taking oral steroids
• Progressive, continuous, non-mechanical pain
• Systemically unwell
• Drug abuse or HIV +ve
• Pain unrelated to mechanical events
• Local bony tenderness
• CNS deficit at more than one root level
• Thoracic spine pain
• Worse pain while supine
• Previous neoplasia

Examination Starts the moment your patient walks into the room. Observing gait and function can elicit any discrepancies in a patient's descriptions of reduced function. With the patient standing and wearing only underwear, inspect the back for abnormality or surgical spinal scars. Palpate bony landmarks (fig 7.22) for local tenderness and deformity. Localized sacroiliac joint tenderness suggests spondyloarthropathy (sacroiliitis is suggested when there is pain on hip adduction as the hip and knee are flexed). Spinal movements assessed are *forward flexion* (stretch forward to touch toes with knees straight)—look to see how much movement is due to back flexion and how much by flexion at the hips—with back flexion the back has a gently rounded contour. On bending fully forwards, the distance between vertebral spines should increase. *Schober's test* determines any limitations to forward flexion. Locate where L5 lies, then place one finger 5cm vertically below and another finger 10cm above. Lumbar flexion is considered limited if the distance increase is <5cm as the patient leans forward to touch their toes. Look for a rib hump—a sign of scoliosis (p. 480); *extension* (arch spine backwards); *lateral flexion* (lean sideways so hand moves down corresponding thigh); and *rotation* (keep pelvis fixed but move shoulders round to each side in turn—mostly from the thoracic spine). Movement at the costovertebral joints is assessed by the difference in chest expansion between maximal inspiration and expiration (normal=5cm). Iliac crests are grasped by the examiner and compressed to move sacroiliac joints and see if this reproduces the pain. Compare leg length; quantify discrepancy and muscle wasting (measure thigh and calf circumference). If there are leg symptoms ensure *neurological assessment* of L4 (knee reflex), L5 (weakness of ankle and great toe dorsiflexion, sensory loss in medial foot and 1st/2nd toe web space), and S1 (ankle reflex, weakness of plantar flexion) roots.

Testing for nerve root irritation (ie sciatica) Most commonly at the L4–S1 levels. You can try to incorporate these tests into the rest of your examination as they may prove pain free if the patient is not genuine. *Straight leg raising:* Aims to stretch the sciatic nerve and reproduce root pain (a characteristic stabbing pain distributed in the relevant dermatome, and made worse by coughing or sneezing). Keeping the knee extended, lift the patient's leg off the couch and note the angle to which the leg can be raised before eliciting pain. If 30–70°, Lasègue's sign is said to be positive. The crossed straight leg raise involves lifting the unaffected leg. If this reproduces pain in the affected side it is said to be positive. It is less sensitive but more specific for an underlying herniated disc. All these tests may still give false positives and negatives, hence the importance of a good history combined with the examination. Other causes of sciatica include spinal stenosis, cauda equina syndrome, and pregnancy.

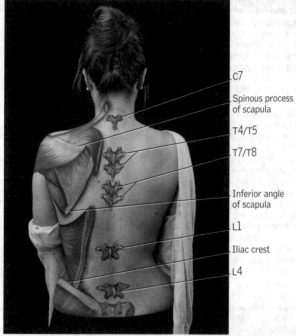

Fig 7.22 Surface anatomy of the back.

Reproduced courtesy of Art and Anatomy Edinburgh. Copyright © Art and Anatomy Edinburgh. Contributors Kimmie Dunlop, Nichola Robertson, Megan Anderson, Philip Stewart, and Alex Haddon.

Other causes of back pain

The commonest musculoskeletal complaint is back pain, yet do not apply your orthopaedic blinkers until other causes of back pain have been ruled out:

- Retroperitoneal (duodenal ulcer, AAA; pain is often lumbo-dorsal and spine movements pain-free and full).
- Local infection or systemic TB causing osteomyelitis.
- Renal colic or pyelonephritis.
- Neoplasia (eg myeloma, pancreatic cancer).
- Bone metastases—the commonest tumours to metastasize to bone are: breast, bronchus, kidney, thyroid, and prostate so it may be relevant to examine these. <1% of patients presenting to primary care have spinal malignancy as a cause for back pain. Historically, if the following features were absent then spinal malignancy was considered unlikely: >50yrs old, PMH of cancer, pain >1 month, raised ESR, and low Hb. However, a Cochrane review in 2013 questioned the diagnostic accuracy of these screening questions. Only a PMH of cancer increased the likelihood of spinal malignancy.

Other parts of the body to examine ►Remember to examine gait and hip joints (pp. 488–9) as hip flexion can reproduce nerve root pain. Other relevant areas are the iliac fossae (important in days when tuberculous psoas abscesses were common), abdomen, pelvis, rectum, and major arteries.

Further reading

Sandella BJ (2014). *Examination of Low Back Pain Technique.* Medscape. http://emedicine. medscape.com/article/2092651-technique

Kyphosis Excessive curvature of spine in the sagittal plane (>40°), typically the thoracocervical spine, sometimes with a lordosis of the lumbar spine. Less common than scoliosis, but potentially more dangerous are dislocations of the spinal column into cord which can cause cord compression and paraplegia, which sometimes develops rapidly eg during adolescence.

Causes of kyphosis
• Congenital
• Osteoporosis
• Spina bifida
• Calvé's vertebra
• Cancer; wedge fractures
• Tuberculosis; polio
• Paget disease
• Ankylosing spondylitis

Scheuermann disease One of the osteochondroses (pp. 508-9).[8] The commonest cause of kyphosis in 13–16yr-olds. It typically presents when parents notice poor posture and kyphosis. Aetiology remains unknown. The normal ossification of ring epiphyses of several thoracic vertebrae is affected. Deforming forces are greatest at their anterior border, so vertebrae are narrower here, causing kyphosis. During the active phase, vertebrae may be tender. Patients appear round shouldered and 'hunched'—they tend to present for deformity rather than pain. *x-rays:* Irregular vertebral endplates, Schmorl's nodes (herniations of the intervertebral disc through the vertebral endplate), and ↓ disc space ± anterior wedging causing thoracic kyphosis of >40°. 3 adjacent vertebral bodies of at least 5° of wedging is pathognomonic. *Treatment:* Involves posture control and exercise (eg swimming). Physiotherapy ± spinal braces can help, though curvature may recur after discontinuation of bracing. Surgery may be tried for severe kyphosis (>75°) with curve progression, refractory pain, or neurological deficit.

Scoliosis This is lateral spinal curvature with vertebral rotation. There is lateral curvature (Cobb angle) of the thoracic or lumbar spine of >10° accompanied by a degree of rotation of the spinal column. The chief cause is idiopathic with no serious underlying pathology. The UK screening programme was discontinued in 2012 since clinically significant cases would have been detected anyway. *Classification:*
• Idiopathic (may be infantile, juvenile, adolescent, or adult onset).
• Neuromuscular (neuropathic eg neurofibromatosis) or myopathic).
• Other (eg tumour, osteoporosis, infection etc.).

Adolescent idiopathic scoliosis The most common spinal deformity, most frequently affecting girls. Complications in later life revolve around pain, cosmesis, and impaired lung function. Curvature increases while the affected person continues to grow, so usually the earlier the onset the worse the deformity. Risk of progression is also higher with greater Cobb angles at presentation (>25°), double curves progress more than single curves, and a scoliosis in girls is more likely to progress than one in boys. *Treatment:* All should be referred to specialist clinics for observation and measurements of Cobb angle. ~1/6 patients require treatment and only ¼ of those treated need surgery. When curvatures are progressing, attempts to halt it may be made using braces but benefit is limited by psychosocial issues and adherence to wearing a brace for the optimal ≥20h/day. Bracing will not correct the deformity but has a role in slowing/preventing curve progression. Surgery in <8yr-olds attempts to optimize lung development, as alveoli stop multiplying after age 8,[25] however surgery in older patients is only indicated if existing deformity is causing problems or progression is likely. Surgery involves deformity correction with spinal fusion and stabilization (fig 7.24). Intraoperative spinal cord monitoring reduces the most feared post-op complication—paralysis (it now occurs in 0.2%). ►When scoliosis in youth gives pain (especially at night), exclude osteoid osteoma (p. 505), osteoblastoma, spondylolisthesis (p. 482), and spinal tumours.

---

8 Scheuermann also described a separate condition involving lumbar disc spaces (now called juvenile disc disorder to avoid confusion between disease processes).

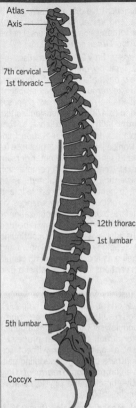

Atlas
Axis

7th cervical
1st thoracic

12th thoracic
1st lumbar

5th lumbar

Coccyx

Fig 7.23 The spine.

During development, the vertebral column initially has a *primary curvature* (anteriorly concave, as for the thoracic and sacral curvatures in red), then goes on to develop *secondary curvatures* in the cervical and lumbar regions (in **blue**, fig 7.23). The normal vertebral body count is 7 cervical, 12 thoracic, 5 lumbar, 5 sacral, and then some coccygeal (3–5). There is some variation, eg L5 can be fused to the sacrum (sacralization) or S1 can be distinct from the sacrum (lumbarization), though total numbers remain constant (even across some mammalian species, especially in the cervical region—eg the giraffe also has 7 cervical vertebrae).

Remember that there are 8 cervical spinal nerve roots, with the C1 root arising from above the C1 vertebra, the C8 root from above the T1 vertebra, and from T1 onwards the root exiting below the corresponding vertebra. This occurs because during development the incipient spinal nerves develop through the embryonic sclerotomes, with the upper part of the C1 sclerotome joining with the last occipital sclerotome to form the base of the occipital bone, and the lower part of the C1 sclerotome forming the C1 vertebra with the upper C2 sclerotome—and so on. Failure of formation and segmentation during development can lead to *congenital scoliosis* (rare). Defective induction of vertebral body formation on one side of the body (=hemivertebra) may cause a severe *scoliosis*, and incorrect or absent induction of vertebral arch closure by the neural tube causes the degrees of *spina bifida* (p. 285).

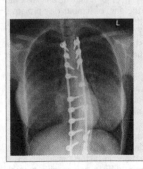

Fig 7.24 Kyphoscoliosis.
This chest x-ray of a 21-year-old female demonstrates spinal stabilization surgery with pedicle screws and longitudinal rods performed aged 11. Thoracic problems tend to give more severe deformity than lumbar. Rib deformity causes a characteristic hump on the convex side of the curve which manifests on asking the patient to bend forwards, see www.sauk.org.uk (Scoliosis Association UK) for examples.

© Nina Hjelde.

Further reading

Tribus C (2010). *Scheuermann Kyphosis*. Medscape. http://emedicine.medscape.com/article/1266349-overview

Backache is often from low back strain or degenerative disease. *Local pain* is typically deep and aching (from soft tissue and vertebral body irritation). *Radicular pain* is stabbing, and is caused by compression of the dorsal nerve roots, and projects in a dermatomal distribution. *Other causes* include:

Intervertebral disc disorders 1 *Disc prolapse:* (fig 7.25) Lumbar discs are those most likely to rupture (esp. L4/5 & L5/S1). Typically, one is seized by severe pain on coughing, sneezing, or twisting a few days after back strain (onset may be insidious). Pain may be confined to the lower lumbar area (lumbago), or may radiate to buttock or leg (sciatica) if the herniated nucleus pulposus compresses a nerve root. *Signs:* forward flexion (p. 478) and extension limited, ± lateral flexion—unilaterally and inconstantly. With L5/S1 prolapse, S1 root compression causes calf pain, weak foot plantar flexion, ↓ sensation (pin-prick) over sole of foot and back of calf, and ↓ ankle jerk. With L4/5 prolapse (L5 root compression), hallux extension is weak and sensation ↓ on outer dorsum of foot. If lower lumbar discs prolapse centrally, cauda equina compression (p. 487) may occur. *Tests:* MRI (or CT) if intervention is contemplated—▶▶an emergency if cauda equina compression is suspected—or if rest fails and symptoms are severe, with CNS signs such as reflex or sensory changes, or muscle wasting. *Treating disc prolapse:* brief rest and early mobilization + pain relief is all that is needed in 90% (± physiotherapy). Discectomy is needed in cauda equina syndrome, progressive muscular weakness, or continuing pain 2 *Degenerative disc disease:* The exact aetiology remains unknown and is likely multifactorial and not only due to ageing as it occurs in young people too. It may lead to herniation. Surgical interventions include prosthetic disc replacement 3 *Discitis:* (see p. 486).

Spondylolisthesis There is displacement (usually forward) of one lumbar vertebra upon the one below (usually L5 on S1, sometimes palpable). *Causes:* Spondylosis (age-related degeneration resulting from joint deformity, associated with osteophyte formation), spondylolysis (results from a defect in the pars interarticularis), congenital malformation of articular processes, osteoarthritis of posterior facet joints. Onset of pain with or without sciatica is often in adolescence ± hamstring tightness causing a waddling gait. *Diagnosis:* By x-rays and MRI to assess nerve compression. *Treatment:* Only temporary relief is achieved with conservative bracing and physio, curative treatment involves spinal fusion (essential for slips >50%).

Lumbar spinal stenosis (LSS) and lateral recess stenosis (figs 7.26 & 7.27) Generalized narrowing of the lumbar spinal canal or its lateral recesses causing nerve ischaemia. Typically caused by facet joint OA (the only synovial joints in the back) and osteophytes. Unlike the pain of lumbar disc prolapse, this can cause: • Pain worse on walking with aching and heaviness in one or both legs causing the person to stop walking (= 'spinal claudication') • Pain on extension • Negative straight leg raising test • Few CNS signs. Watch out for the patient who prefers to lean over shopping trollies, walk uphill rather than down, and cycle as these activities help flex the back and release tension on compressed nerves. *Tests:* MRI is preferred, but when insufficient or contra-indicated, myelography (injection of contrast into subarachnoid space) is available. *Treatment:* Decompressive laminectomy gives good results if NSAIDs, epidural steroid injections, and corsets (to prevent exaggerating the lumbar lordosis of standing) fail to help.

Inflammatory back pain: spondyloarthropathies (p550 OHCM) (figs 7.28 & 7.29) Inflammatory diseases which affect axial and peripheral joints. The most common is ankylosing spondylitis. Key questions in history: insidious onset over months, early morning stiffness >45min, diffuse non-specific buttock pain, pain improves with activity and worsens on rest, other joint, bowel, or eye involvement.

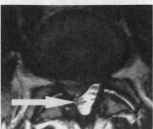

Fig 7.25 Axial MRI image at the L5/S1 level showing a right-sided paracentral disc prolapse. Observe the displaced nerve roots within the CSF-filled dural sac (arrow). Remember that CSF is white on T2-weighted MRI.

Courtesy of Mr Mark Brinsden, FRCS.

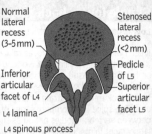

Normal lateral recess (3–5 mm)

Stenosed lateral recess (<2 mm)

Inferior articular facet of L4

Pedicle of L5

Superior articular facet L5

L4 lamina

L4 spinous process

Fig 7.26 L5 cross-section showing lateral recess stenosis. This is usually caused by degenerative disease of the facet joint, but rarely can be from congenitally shortened pedicles.

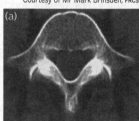
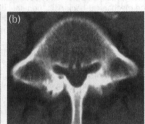

Fig 7.27 (a, b) Cross-section CT images at L5, one with spinal stenosis (b). Observe the difference in spinal canal shape and dimensions caused by osteoarthritis of the facet joints posterolaterally. Factors contributing to spinal stenosis: disc prolapse, spondylolisthesis, hypertrophy of the ligamentum flavum. Identify the spinal canal contents at this level, including the thecal sac and the 2 L5 nerve root sheaths that occupy the lateral recesses. Courtesy of Mr Mark Brinsden FRCS.

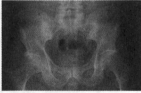

Fig 7.28 x-ray findings in a patient with established ankylosing spondylitis. Bilateral sacroiliitis with subchondral erosions and sclerosis. x-ray examination is used as a diagnostic criterion for ankylosing spondylitis. MRI is useful in cases with normal x-rays but high clinical suspicion.

Reproduced from Inman R et al., Oxford Textbook of Axial Spondyloarthritis (2016), with permission from OUP.

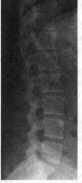

Fig 7.29 Lateral view of the lumbar spine demonstrating early changes of ankylosing spondylitis. There is squaring of the vertebral bodies with associated sclerosis of the corners (Romanus lesions).

Reproduced from Watts RA et al., Oxford Textbook of Rheumatology (2013), with permission from OUP.

Further reading

Hughes SP et al. (2012). The pathogenesis of degeneration of the intervertebral disc and emerging therapies in the management of back pain. *J Bone Joint Surg Br* 94:1298–304.

Issack PS et al. (2012). Degenerative lumbar spinal stenosis: evaluation and management. *J Am Acad Orthop Surg* 20:527–35.

Lower back pain Extremely common; ~80% of people in the UK suffer at some stage in their lives. 50 per 1000 industrial workers have time off work because of it each year, with each employee taking an average of 19 days off work. In the UK it accounts for 4.9 million lost working days/yr.[26] A GP expects 20 people per 1000 on her list to consult with it each year (only ~10% are referred to hospital of whom <10% need surgery). ~90% of backache can be attributed to non-specific lower back muscular strain or degenerative disease. Typically affects 30–50yr olds. The spine is a complex series of articulations (p. 481), with spongy discs between vertebral bodies acting as shock absorbers, and a multitude of articulating facet joints. Problems in one part affect function of the whole. Spasm of vertebral muscles can cause significant pain. Upright posture provokes big forces on the spine eg when lifting, and discs may rupture (if young), vertebrae fracture (elderly), or soft tissues tear (low back strain). NB: with low back strain the exact mechanism may be elusive. It is not uncommon for patients to develop sciatica (p. 482) or other nerve root signs. *A variety of terms* can be used to describe mechanical back pain; non-specific, uncomplicated, or simple back pain. Be cautious of telling your patient you have diagnosed 'simple' back ache since, for them, the pain is everything but 'simple'! Carefully explain that these terms simply declare a lack of sinister features (pp. 478–9). *Key questions to ask:* The goal is to rule out serious pathology (pp. 478–9). Were there any triggers to pain starting? Any previous back problems? Adequate analgesia taken? What are their expectations for recovery and current coping mechanisms? (See 'Yellow flags' in BOX 'Why do some people get Intractable back pain?')

Imaging Plain x-rays correlate poorly with symptoms; only consider in the acute setting if suspecting malignancy or fractures (ie trauma, osteoporosis)[27] as a 2-view lumbar spinal x-ray irradiates gonads and can be the equivalent radiation dose of 1 CXR every day for a year. Reserve CT/MRI and bloods for when symptoms are chronic (>4 weeks) or in sinister causes.[9]

Why do some people get intractable back pain?

The worldwide prevalence of chronic back pain is 23%.[28] Much energy is expended on frequently fruitless searches for pathology. Imaging may be non-specific. The patient's attitude towards rehabilitation is pivotal and the following list demonstrates potential psychosocial issues which can prolong recovery and spiral into chronic back pain.[29]

Yellow flags
- Belief that pain and subsequent activity are harmful.
- Pain behaviour (such as extended rest, avoidance of normal activities).
- Over-reliance on passive treatments (such as ice packs, analgesia, etc.).
- Depression, anxiety, personality disorders.
- Unsupportive home environment or overprotective family.
- Inappropriate expectations and failing to actively engage with treatment.

Other risk factors for chronicity Poor work conditions, low income/social class, and number of children (for women and men). Be cautious of blaming sedentary lifestyles, sitting at work, or occupational carrying as studies do not find in favour of this popular association.[30-32] Associations with smoking and coexisting cardiorespiratory disease may be due to vascular problems, and pain may be maintained by involvement of the sympathetic chain, which mediates hyperaesthesia, hyperpathia (excess pain from minor noxious stimuli), allodynia (pain from minor skin stimulation)—but surgical sympathectomy often only provides temporary relief. This implies central neuromodulation of stimuli producing a complex regional pain syndrome (p. 529). Dorsal horn receptor fields may expand and have their thresholds changed by peripheral injury, so pain is more intense, and appreciated over a wider area than simple anatomy would predict.

---

9 Only offer MRI for non-specific lower back pain if assessing patient for potential spinal fusion.

Management of lower back pain See also table 7.2. Most simple back pain is self-limiting: of those attending GPs, 70% are better after 3 weeks, 90% by 6 weeks, irrespective of treatment. Lower back pain is especially challenging to manage as it disrupts patients physically, socially, and psychologically. Focus on:

- Pain relief.
- Identifying yellow flags which impede recovery (see BOX 'Why do some people get intractable back pain?').
- Exercises to improve function.
- Lifestyle changes to prevent recurrence.

'Get on with your life within the limits of the pain' gives better results than physiotherapy with lateral bending exercises. Encourage patients to return to work. Avoid bed-rest after the 1st 48h (a board under the mattress helps). *Analgesia* breaks the pain–muscle spasm cycle (NSAID eg **ibuprofen** 400mg/8h PO or **naproxen** 500mg/12h PO ± **paracetamol** ≤4g/24h PO). Opioids may be needed early. *Warmth* helps, as does swimming in a warm pool. If acute spasm persists, try a *muscle relaxant* such as **diazepam** 2–4mg/8h PO for 3 days and warn about side effects (eg drowsiness). *Cognitive therapy in groups* (p. 764) helps tackle unhelpful beliefs about backache and fears about restarting activity. The role of *antidepressants* is disputed but may help refractory pain, but not level of functioning.[33] *Physiotherapy* in the acute phase can ↓ pain and spasm. Many consult osteopaths or physiotherapists or chiropractors for manipulation, but studies show that it is unlikely to provide relief beyond that attained from other standard therapies. Referral for epidural anaesthesia. Note that orthopaedic referral for spinal fusion is no better than intensive rehabilitation.

A large RCT compared early surgery (<12 weeks) versus conservative treatment for sciatica caused by lumbar disc herniation. Although early surgery generated faster pain relief (especially if sitting aggravated pain), at the end of 1 year both groups had similar rates of dissatisfaction.[34]

Table 7.2 Referral criteria to specialist services (orthopaedics or spinal surgeons). The current guidelines advocate earlier referral than previously practised.

'Red flags' present =	Immediate referral
Progressive/severe neurological deficit =	To be seen by specialist within 1 week
Disabling pain >2 weeks =	Early referral to physio, consider corticosteroid injections
Disabling pain >6 weeks (despite physio & analgesia) =	To be seen by specialist within 2 weeks

Laid flat by a wealth of evidence

Entering the search term 'back pain' in PubMed for the previous edition of this book delivered 49,498 entries, with 558 meta-analyses. At the time of writing, the same search now yields 64,305 entries and 647 meta-analyses! How much of this is relevant to your practice? Where do you start in your quest for answers? What do you look for, and how can you filter? Does this wealth of evidence exist because back pain is such a common condition, because there are so many different treatment options, or because we are not yet able to offer definitive therapy to our patients?

As we stand up to the challenge laid down by evolution (and search engines alike), those without back pain can count themselves lucky, while those struck horizontal by our primitive postural problems try not to think of the irony that we are lying in the plane in which our vertebral column originally worked!

Further reading

Knott L (2013). *Lower Back Pain and Sciatica*. Patient. http://patient.info/doctor/low-back-pain-and-sciatica

NICE (2017). *Clinical Knowledge Summaries. Scenario: Management of Sciatica*. https://cks.nice.uk/sciatica-lumbar-radiculopathy#!scenario

Sahrakar K (2015). *Lumbar Disc Disease*. Medscape. http://emedicine.medscape.com/article/249113-overview

Age is important (see table 7.3): only 3% of those aged between 20 and 55 have 'spinal pathology' (eg tumour, infection, inflammatory disease) compared with 11% of those <20yrs, and 19% >55yrs. ▶Pain brought on by activity and relieved by rest is rarely sinister. If cancer or infection is suspected, refer promptly.

Spinal tumours These may be of spinal cord, meninges, nerves, or bone. They may be primary, secondary, lymphoma, or myeloma. They may compress the cord, causing pain, lower motor neuron signs at the level of the lesion, upper motor neuron signs and sensory loss below—or bowel and bladder dysfunction. Peripheral nerve function may be impaired resulting in pain along the course of the nerve, weakness, hyporeflexia & ↓ sensation (p.552). With cauda equina involvement there is saddle anaesthesia ± urinary retention (see box 'The *cauda equina* (=horse's tail)'). When the deposit is in the spinal canal and there is no bone involvement, there may be no pain, just long tract signs. When bones of the back are involved there is progressive, constant pain and local destruction of bone. Metastases tend to affect cancellous bone, but focal lesions cannot be seen on x-rays until 50% of bone mass is lost. There may be muscle spasm and local tenderness to percussion. Bone collapse may result in deformity, or cause cord or nerve compression. *Tests:* ▶Do FBC, ESR, LFT, bone profile in presence of red flags or whenever pain lasts >4 weeks, whatever the age. Do a myeloma screen if >50 years. Plain x-rays; CT; MRI; isotope bone scans; bone biopsy. In those with past cancer and current back pain, it is best to do a bone scan first (fig 7.30), with plain x-rays of any hot spots suggesting metastases.

Pyogenic spine infections This is a notoriously difficult diagnosis as all signs of infection may be absent (eg no fever, tenderness, or wcc↑, but the ESR is often ↑). It may be secondary to other septic foci. Pain occurs, and movement is restricted by spasm. It is usually an infection of the disc space (discitis). *Risk factors:* Diabetes mellitus, immunosuppression, urinary surgery, or catheterization. Half of infections are staphylococcal. *Streptococcus, Proteus, E. coli, Salmonella typhi,* and TB also occur. *Tests:* ESR↑; wcc↑; x-rays show bone rarefaction or erosion, joint space narrowing ± subligamentous new bone formation. Technetium bone scans and MRI (fig 7.31) are better. *Treatment:* As for osteomyelitis (pp. 502-3), resting the back with bed rest or brace if tolerated. Surgery may be needed if unresponsive to medical therapy.

Pott disease (spinal TB) A frequent form of extrapulmonary TB (represents 1–3% of all TB and incidence is rising), especially if co-infected with HIV. Tends to affect young adults who present with systemic symptoms, gradual onset localized back pain, and stiffness of all back movements. Most commonly affects T10–L1. Spinal deformity is common, especially kyphosis when thoracic vertebrae are affected. Abscesses (esp. of psoas muscle) and cord compression may occur (Pott's paraplegia). *Differential diagnoses:* See table 7.3. Malignancy; other infections; gout; rheumatoid. *Tests:* ESR↑. x-rays tend to be normal until >50% bone mass, later images show narrow disc spaces, local osteoporosis, and bone destruction leading to wedging of vertebrae. MRI is more specific than CT in the diagnosis of spinal TB and is the ideal way to delineate cord compression. Bone scans can help differentiate from malignancy. One meta-analysis showed PET to be superior to all other forms of imaging, with a sensitivity of 96% and a specificity of 91%.[35] Considering the imaging resources available in each country though, naturally the majority of research into spinal TB is based on x-rays. Cultures of synovial tissue or bone from needle biopsy are often needed. Always do CXR to check for coexisting pulmonary TB. *Treatment:* See pp. 502-3, 'Osteomyelitis'. There is insufficient evidence for the routine use of surgery alongside medical treatment.[36]

Table 7.3 Typical causes of back pain according to age

15–30yrs	Prolapsed disc, trauma, fractures, ankylosing spondylitis (*OHCM* p550), spondylolisthesis, pregnancy
>30yrs	Prolapsed disc, malignancy (lung, breast, prostate, thyroid, kidney)
>50yrs	Degenerative, osteoporosis, Paget disease (*OHCM* p685), malignancy, myeloma (*OHCM* p368), lumbar artery atheroma (which may itself cause disc degeneration)

The *cauda equina* (=horse's tail)

The cord tapers to its end, the *conus medullaris*, at approximately (can be variable) L1 in adults. Lumbar and sacral nerve roots arising from the *conus medullaris* form the *cauda equina*. These spinal nerve roots separate in pairs, exiting laterally through the nerve root foramina, providing motor and sensory innervation of the legs and pelvic organs. Compression is most frequently from large prolapses or herniation of lumbar discs, but may be from extrinsic tumours, primary cord tumours, spondylosis, spinal stenosis. Compression to the cauda equina clinically produces a lower motor neuron lesion. Keep an eye out for the following danger signs: ▶▶Poor anal tone (do PR) ▶▶Severe back pain ▶▶Saddle-area (perineal) sensation ↓ ▶▶Incontinence/retention of faeces or urine ▶▶Paralysis ± sensory loss. Diagnosis can be tricky. See p. 562 for the functional anatomy. Although most patients present with sudden-onset back pain and neurological signs progressive over hours/days, the syndrome can be painless and develop over weeks. Although this syndrome is rare (affects 2% of herniated lumbar discs) it must always be considered because delay in diagnosis can lead to permanent neurological damage to sexual, bladder, and bowel function. Subsequently, for medicolegal purposes, it is critical that clinical documentation *must always* make comment on these signs whenever a patient presents with back pain. If suspected, refer to neurosurgery/spinal teams immediately who will expect an MRI within 4 hours. See *OHCM* p466 for metastatic spinal cord compression.

7 Orthopaedics

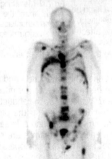

R   L

Fig 7.30 Bone scan showing multiple metastases from prostatic cancer, including infiltration of the pelvis, ribs, left femur, and spinal column. Bone scans in spinal TB are not as useful since infection typically causes a hotspot but avascular bony fragments from TB can be cold spots.
Courtesy of The Norfolk and Norwich University Hospitals (NNUH) Radiology Dept.

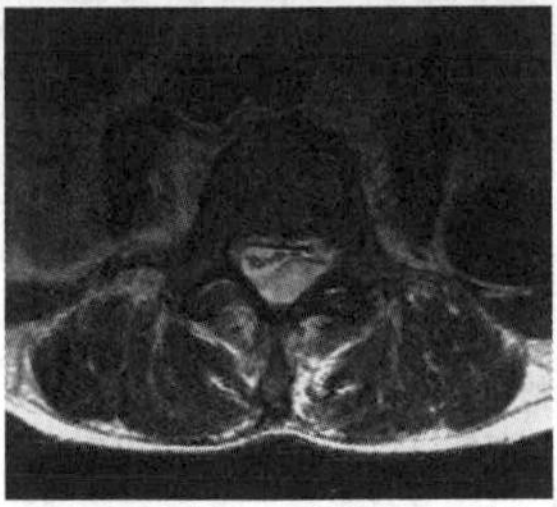

Fig 7.31 Axial T2-weighted MRI of the lumbar spine showing an epidural abscess in the posterior portion of the spinal canal causing mild stenosis.
Courtesy of The Norfolk and Norwich University Hospitals (NNUH) Radiology Dept.

Further reading

Gardner A *et al.* (2011). Cauda equina syndrome: a review of the current clinical and medico-legal position. *Eur Spine J* 20:690–7.

Garg RK *et al.* (2011). Spinal tuberculosis: a review. *J Spinal Cord Med* 34:440–54.

Jutte PC *et al.* (2006). Routine surgery in addition to chemotherapy for treating spinal tuberculosis. *Cochrane Database Syst Rev* 5:CD004532.

Problems with the hip joint usually remain clinically silent until patients present with secondary dysfunction, often of lower limb and back, arising from long-term compensatory movements. (For hip prostheses, see p. 510.) It can be difficult to differentiate between hip and back pathology. Pain in the knee may be referred from the hip (and vice versa). The movements examined at the hip are described in fig 7.33. Internal rotation is often the first movement to be restricted by hip disease. **Questions** Are activities of daily living affected?—Walking distance, ability to climb stairs (only one at a time possible?), difficulty getting out of low chairs. **Examination** Follow the routine for joint examination (pp. 464-5). **Also examine** spine, knee, sacroiliac joints/pelvis.

Measurements Apparent leg length disparity (with the lower limbs parallel and in line with the trunk) is called either 'apparent shortening' (eg due to pelvic tilt or fixed adduction deformity—which gives the apparent shortening on that side) or 'apparent lengthening' (eg due to fixed hip abduction). In these cases, there is no true disparity, as detected by measuring between the anterior superior iliac spine and medial malleolus on each side with the pelvis held square (fig 7.32) and the lower limbs held equally adducted or abducted or by comparing leg length by positioning the lower limbs perpendicular to a line joining the anterior superior iliac spines.

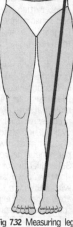

Fig 7.32 Measuring leg length: from the anterior superior iliac spine to the medial malleolus.

Fixed deformity Joint or muscle contractures prevent limbs from being put in the neutral position. With fixed adduction deformity, the angle between the limb and the transverse axis of the pelvis (line between both anterior superior iliac spines) is <90° but with fixed abduction deformity it is >90°. Fixed flexion deformity is detected by the *Thomas test* — with the patient supine on an examination couch, flex the good hip up towards the chest until the lumbar lordosis is obliterated (check by finding it impossible to pass a hand between the patient and the couch in the small of the back). If there is a fixed flexion deformity the thigh on the affected side will lift off the couch as the lumbar lordosis is obliterated. NB: to assess the full range of extension, have the patient prone or lateral on the table and then extend the hip.

The Trendelenburg test A test of the function of hip abduction and the ability to support the pelvis when standing on one leg. In this state, it is normal for the pelvis to rise on the side of the lifted leg. Weakness of the abductors on the weight-bearing leg cause a 'positive' Trendelenburg test; the pelvis falls on the side of the lifted leg. A common mnemonic is 'sound side sags'. *Causes:* 1 Abductor muscle paralysis (gluteus medius and minimus are supplied by the superior gluteal nerve) ie nerve root lesions, pain, postoperative nerve damage, weakened muscles due to OA 2 Upward displacement of the greater trochanter (severe coxa vara, fig 7.34, or dislocated hip) 3 Absence of a stable fulcrum (eg un-united fractures of the neck of femur).

Gait If a hip is unstable or painful, a stick is used on the opposite side (the reverse is true for knees) so as to off-load the hip abductors on the affected side. *Antalgic gait:* Shortening of the stance phase[10] on the painful leg occurs, with quick and short steps. *Short-leg gait:* Discrepancy in length is compensated for by adduction of the long leg at the hip and abduction of the short leg creating pelvic drop, or an *equinus* deformity. *Trendelenburg gait:* A waddling gait caused by weak hip abductors, in which the trunk tilts over the weakened side (can be bilateral) in the stance phase. See *OHCM* p467.

10 The *stance phase* of gait starts when the forward foot makes contact with the ground. Then there is loading, mid-, and terminal stance (+ pre-swing)—before the shorter *swing phase* starts.

7 Orthopaedics

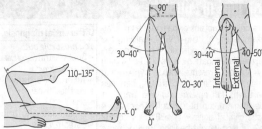

Fig 7.33 Ball and socket (eg the hip) joints have 3 axes of movement: flexion–extension (left); ab- & adduction (middle); and external & internal rotation. External rotation of the ball in the socket is achieved by movement of the shin across the midline, as in the diagram (40–50°).

Fig 7.34 Coxa vara and coxa valga. Coxa vara is more common; the angle between the neck and the shaft of femur is less than the normal 125°; causes true shortening of limb and Trendelenburg 'dip' on walking with resultant limp. Causes: congenital; SUFE, malunion # of neck of femur or trochanteric #; softening of bones (rickets, osteomalacia, Paget disease).

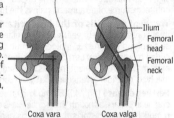

Coxa vara   Coxa valga

7 Orthopaedics

Osteoarthritis of the hip

In addition to the secondary risk factors for OA mentioned on p. 498, hip OA can follow AVN (see p. 541) and paediatric hip disease (see pp. 490–1). Note that BMI does not increase risk of hip OA as it does in knee OA. See also *OHCM* p544.

History Pain is poorly localized around groin, thigh, or buttocks. Pain can be referred to the knee. Worse on weight-bearing with stiffness when attempting activities which flex the hip (eg tying shoe laces).

On examination Antalgic gait with a positive Trendelenburg sign. Expect reduced ROM (especially on internal rotation). Figs 7.35 & 7.36 show examples of hip arthroplasty. Most patients won't know what type of prosthesis they have, you must become familiar with the x-ray appearances. Re-surfacing of the hip is rarely performed now but there remains a cohort of patients with them *in situ*.

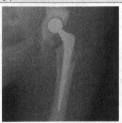

Fig 7.35 AP x-ray of a cemented total hip arthroplasty.
Courtesy of The Norfolk and Norwich University Hospitals (NNUH) Radiology Dept.

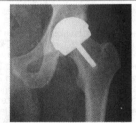

Fig 7.36 AP x-ray of the left hip after Birmingham hip resurfacing.
Courtesy of The Norfolk and Norwich University Hospitals (NNUH) Radiology Dept.

Further reading

Byrd JW (2007). Evaluation of the hip: history and physical examination. *N Am J Sports Phys Ther* 2:231–40.
Sabharwal S *et al.* (2008). Methods for assessing leg length discrepancy. *Clin Orthop Relat Res* 466:2910–22.

►When a child complains of pain in the knee, always examine the hip (fig 7.38). Localizing the source of pain can be difficult. Any limp warrants further investigation (see BOX 'The limping child'). A 4yr-old presents with a pyrexia and a limp due to hip pain; differentiating between septic arthritis (an emergency) and transient synovitis (benign) can be difficult. There are 4 prognostic clinical signs: • T° >38.5° • WCC >12 • CRP >20 • Non-weight-bearing. If 3 or more are present, then there is >93% chance of septic arthritis.[37] If so, do urgent blood culture ± US-guided aspiration. The hip is a deep joint so local

Differential diagnosis

You must rule out:
• Septic arthritis (OHCM p544)
Then consider:
• Tubercular arthritis[2-5YRS]
• Perthes disease[4-7YRS]
• SUFE[10-16YRS]
• Inflammatory arthritis
• Osteomyelitis
And by exclusion:
• Transient synovitis

signs (eg warmth, erythema) will appear late in the disease process. The most common source of atraumatic pain is the hip, here are some important causes:

Transient synovitis of the hip (irritable hip) The chief cause of hip pain in children aged 4–10 years but is a diagnosis of exclusion. Acute onset and self-limiting with rest ± analgesia. Aetiology considered to be viral illness preceded by recent viral URTI or autoimmune. On examination there is pain in the extremities of movement, bloods and radiology are normal. If other joints are involved, consider juvenile idiopathic arthritis (see 'Still disease', p. 858).

Perthes disease (fig 7.40) For no known reason, avascular necrosis of the femoral head occurs, although this ischaemia is self-healing, it is the subsequent bone remodelling that distorts the epiphysis and generates abnormal ossification. It affects those aged 3–11yrs (typically 4–7yrs). It is bilateral in 10–15%. ♂:♀ ≈ 4:1. It presents with pain in hip or knee and causes a limp. On examination, all movements at the hip are limited, especially internal rotation and abduction. Early x-rays ± MRI show joint space widening. Later there is a decrease in size of the femoral head with patchy density. Later still, there may be collapse and deformity of the femoral head with new bone formation. Long-term prognosis is governed by the risk of OA in the deformed hip. Severe deformity of the femoral head risks early arthritis and likely need for joint replacement. The younger the patient (<6yrs) the better the prognosis (due to increased ability to remodel). For those with less severe disease (<½ the femoral head affected on lateral x-rays, and joint space depth well preserved) treatment is non-weight-bearing with crutches and NSAIDs until pain-free, followed by x-ray surveillance. If prognosis poorer (>½ femoral head affected, narrowing of total joint space) surgery may be indicated.

Slipped upper femoral epiphysis (SUFE) Affects those aged 10–16yrs, although not unheard of in patients as young as 6yrs. 20% are bilateral. ♂:♀ ≈ 3:1. The exact cause is unknown, though it is likely to be a combination of hormonal & biomechanical factors.[11] About 50% are obese. There is displacement through the growth plate (fig 7.39) with the femoral neck slipping upwards and forwards in relation to the epiphysis. It usually presents after minor injury (or atraumatic) with limping and pain in the groin, anterior thigh, or knee. 90% are able to weight bear (stable) and 10% are not (unstable). Flexion, abduction, and medial rotation are limited (eg lying with foot externally rotated). Δ: Anteroposterior (fig 7.37) + frog-leg lateral x-rays of both hips. Delayed diagnosis can lead to progression of slip with increased risk of early OA and stable lesions becoming unstable. Treatment is surgical with early internal fixation to stabilize any slippage and encourage physeal closure. Prophylactic fixation remains controversial and assessed on individual basis. If untreated, consequences may be avascular necrosis of the femoral head (p. 541) or malunion predisposing to arthritis. ►Symptoms may be mild so have a high index of suspicion if in correct age group. If occurring in those <10 or >16yrs then consider an endocrinopathy, eg hypothyroidism or growth hormone imbalance.

11 It may be that unrecognized SUFE can cause later osteoarthritis of the hip.

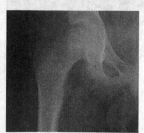

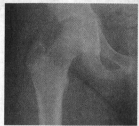

Fig 7.37 AP x-ray of the right hip showing a SUFE. The changes are subtle, but note that a line (the line of Klein) drawn along the upper edge of the femoral neck in fig 7.38 would intersect the femoral head, but would not in fig 7.37. More reliable, though even harder to appreciate, is the widening of the physis—most prominent at the lateral edge.

Courtesy of The Norfolk and Norwich University Hospitals (NNUH) Radiology Dept.

Fig 7.38 Normal AP x-ray of the right hip. Practise your saccadic eye movements between the two to appreciate the slip downwards and medially.

Courtesy of The Norfolk and Norwich University Hospitals (NNUH) Radiology Dept.

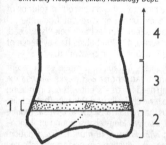

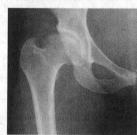

Fig 7.40 Right hip x-ray showing modelling deformity of the femoral head, consistent with prior Perthes disease.

Courtesy of The Norfolk and Norwich University Hospitals (NNUH) Radiology Dept.

Fig 7.39 Bones such as the femur grow from a cartilaginous growth plate called a *physis* (1); the end of a bone beyond the growth plate is called the *epiphysis* (2); the shaft of a long bone is called the *diaphysis* (4); the ossified portion of bone in a transitional zone between the epiphysis and diaphysis is called the *metaphysis* (3) and it should always have a smooth cortex. The diaphysis continues (arrow) to the metaphysis at the other end of the bone. The stem, *-physis*, comes from the Greek for 'growth'. An *apophysis* is a bony outgrowth independent of a centre of ossification. Epiphyseal injuries: p527. Courtesy of Tom Turmezei

The limping child

Pain in the hip is the main cause for a limp in children, a presentation which must be taken seriously. You must assume it is septic arthritis until proven otherwise (see MINIBOX 'Differential diagnosis'). Examination can prove difficult since children will often inadvertently exaggerate their limp and are poor historians. Challenging a little one to race you down the hall or see who can jump the highest is an excellent motivator to make children forget their ailment and engage in activity with you. This trick was learned from an ED consultant who got the child I had been desperately trying to mobilize, leap out of the room. She simply suggested that the noise outside meant that the new toys had arrived. Other non-hip causes of limp in children: malignancy (leukaemia), infection (discitis), metabolic (rickets), and inflammatory (reactive arthritis, juvenile idiopathic arthritis).

Further reading

BMJ Best Practice (2015). *Assessment of Gait Disorders in Children*. http://bestpractice.bmj.com/best-practice/monograph/709.html

Shah H (2014). Perthes disease. *Orthop Clin North Am* 45:87–97.

Walter KD (2015). http://emedicine.medscape.com/article/91596-overview

DDH refers to a spectrum of pathology from stable acetabular dysplasia to established hip dislocation. It has replaced the term congenital dislocation of the hip (CDH) to reflect the progressive course of this condition. Affects 1–3% of newborns. ♀:♂ ≈ 6:1; left/right hip incidence ≈ 4:1; bilateral in ⅓.

At-risk babies
• Breech birth
• Caesar for breech
• Other malformations
• Sibling with DDH
• Birth weight ↑
• Oligohydramnios
• Primip/older mother
• Postmaturity

Diagnosis Early diagnosis is important since, if appropriately aligned in the first few months of life, a dysplastic hip may spontaneously resolve.[12] Delays in diagnosis (termed >7 weeks late) require more complex treatment and have less successful outcomes. A Norwegian study showed that DDH was responsible for 29% of hip replacements in patients aged <60yrs.[38] All babies should have their hips examined in the 1st days of life and at 6 weeks (fig 7.41). If high risk (see MINIBOX 'At-risk babies'), the infant should have an US at 2–4 weeks, with treatment instigated by 6 weeks if not spontaneously resolved. ►Be alert to DDH throughout child surveillance (p. 256) as a hip may be normal at birth, and become abnormal later.

Ultrasound The imaging of choice, up to 4.5 months, as it is non-invasive and dynamic. Pelvic x-rays are better for older infants. Routine US screening for DDH remains controversial on account of the high rate of spontaneous resolution of dysplasia and due to insufficient evidence (based on a recent Cochrane review);[39] however, targeting high-risk babies (BOX 'HIp tests for DDH') is advised. Bear in mind though that in a large UK series, 40:1000 babies had evidence of instability on routine US screening; only 3:1000 required treatment.

Treatment If neonatal examination suggests instability, arrange US. A recent Cochrane review confirmed that delaying treatment by 2–8 weeks allows time for spontaneous resolution, thus reducing need for treatment without increasing risk of later complications in infants who have clinically unstable hips (but not dislocated) or have mild dysplasia on US. Hips that remain unstable at 6 weeks require prompt treatment. Typically treatment involves long-term splinting in flexion–abduction in a Pavlik® harness (see fig 7.42). *From 6–18 months:* Examination-under-anaesthetic, arthrography, and closed reduction are performed followed by a period of immobilization in a *spica* hip bandage (*spica* refers to the pattern of bandaging, from the Latin for an 'ear of corn'), as the harness is <50% successful beyond 6 months of age. Open reduction is sometimes required if closed techniques fail. *After 18 months:* (Delayed presentation.) Open reduction is required with corrective femoral/pelvic osteotomies to maintain joint stability.

Club foot (talipes equinovarus)

A common congenital deformity with unknown aetiology. Mostly an isolated idiopathic finding, but 20% are associated with genetic syndromes or other congenital conditions. ♂:♀ >1:1; bilateral in 50%. The foot deformity consists of: 1 Inversion 2 Adduction of forefoot relative to hindfoot (which is in varus) 3 Equinus (plantarflexion) deformity. The foot cannot be passively everted and dorsiflexed through the normal range. The preferred treatment, starting as early as possible, is the *Ponseti method*, in which the foot is manipulated and placed in a long leg plaster cast (which aims to correct the forefoot adduction and hindfoot varus deformity) on repeated occasions. It is important that deformity correction is *gradual*. If this does not work, soft tissue release between ages 6–12 months (with further surgery on bones if required in later childhood).[40]

---

12 The importance behind picking up DDH is that for a hip to develop normally the femoral head must articulate with the acetabulum. Failure to identify the problem early means that there is no development of the acetabulofemoral joint, posing real problems for any prospect of surgical correction.

7 Orthopaedics

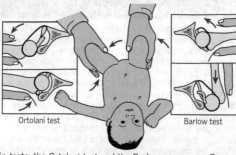

Ortolani test   Barlow test

Fig 7.41 Hip tests: the Ortolani test and the Barlow manoeuvre. Beware repeated Ortolani and Barlow manoeuvres which may induce instability.

Hip tests for DDH

Clinical detection of DDH is user dependent, but improves with training and guidance.⁴ The manoeuvres in fig 7.41 detect unstable hips, but will both be negative in an irreducible dislocated hip, so use other tests as well.

Ortolani manoeuvre Relocates a subluxed or partially dislocated hip. With the child's hips flexed and abducted, place your fingers on the greater trochanter and try to lift up the femoral head and relocate it into the acetabulum. The test is positive when there is a palpable 'clunk' as the hip relocates. The test will be negative if there is an *irreducible* dislocation.

Barlow manoeuvre Aims to sublux or dislocate an unstable hip. Start with hip flexed and adducted slightly. Gently apply axial load to the femur and try to dislocate the femoral head with the thumb. The test is positive when the femoral head is felt to dislocate; may be accompanied by a 'clunk'.

Galeazzi test Looks for apparent shortening of femur caused by dislocation of femoral head. The child lies supine on an examination table with the hips flexed, the feet flat on the table, and the ankles touching the buttocks. The test is positive when the knees are at different heights. This test will be negative if both hips are dislocated as there will be no apparent discrepancy.

Other signs A widened perineum and buttock flattening on the affected side. Unequal leg length and asymmetrical groin creases may also suggest DDH (although not present in bilateral cases). If >3 months old, limited abduction (<60°) of hip while in flexion may be the most sensitive test for DDH. Signs in older children: delay in walking and waddling gait (affected leg is shorter). Bilateral involvement will increase the lumbar lordosis.

Pavlik® harness

A Pavlik® harness is adjusted during growth to help maintain hip reduction and stability (fig 7.42). Excess abduction (in splint) may cause *avascular necrosis* of the head of femur—the worst possible outcome of treatment. Monitor patient carefully to ensure that harness fits well and hips are adequately reduced; us is helpful here. Continue to wear harness until hip remains stable both clinically and on us. Contraindicated if >4.5 months old or hips are irreducible.

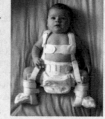

Fig 7.42 The Pavlik® harness. © Anna Williams 2012.

Further reading
Eastwood DM *et al.* (2010). Clinical examination for developmental dysplasia of the hip in neonates: how to stay out of trouble. *BMJ* 340:c1965.

Sewell MD *et al.* (2009). Developmental dysplasia of the hip. *BMJ* 339:b4454.

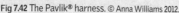

The knee is the largest human joint in terms of volume and surface area of cartilage and is most susceptible to injury, age-related wear, inflammatory arthritis, and septic arthritis. It consists of a hinge joint between the femur and tibia. The patella is the largest sesamoid bone and is embedded in the quadriceps tendon. It articulates with the trochlear groove of the femur and increases the mechanical advantage of the quadriceps. **History** Traumatic? (Think ligament/meniscal damage.) Atraumatic? (Think overuse problem or degenerative changes.) Did patient hear/feel a pop? (Often occurs with anterior cruciate ligament (ACL) tears.) How long did swelling take to develop? (Immediate: # eg tibial plateau/ACL tear; overnight: meniscal tear.) Does the knee lock? Is squatting difficult? (Both potentially present when meniscal tears flip in/out of joint.) Does the knee give way? (Non-specific for muscle weakness, meniscal tears, or ligament instability.)

Examination Fully expose the leg. *LOOK FOR:* Alignment, quadriceps wasting, and for swelling. Even 5–10mL of fluid will 'fill in' the medial and lateral peripatellar dimples giving the knee a general fullness. *FEEL:* Confirm by placing the palm of one hand above the patella over the suprapatellar pouch, and thumb and forefinger of the other hand below the patella. Fluid can be moved between the two by squeezing one hand, then the other. If >15mL fluid is present it may be possible to feel a *patellar tap* (milk fluid towards centre of knee then ballott patella against the anterior surface of the femur). Palpate the medial and lateral joint lines (for osteoarthritis/meniscal/plateau injuries), the patella, the popliteal fossa, and femoral condyles. *MOVE:* Flexion should be enough for the heel to touch the buttock (depending on habitus). Check to see no evidence of crepitus or 'locking'. Ensure extensor mechanism is intact by examining active knee extension/straight leg raise.

Examine the *medial* and *lateral collateral ligaments* (fig 7.43) with the knee in full extension and flexed 20–30° (to relax the posterior capsule and the cruciate ligaments); one hand lifts the ankle, the other stabilizes the knee. Stress the knee by abducting the ankle while pushing the knee medially with the hand behind the knee (tests the *medial* ligament with a *valgus* stress force). Reverse the pressures to give adducting force to test *lateral* ligament (ie *varus* stress). If these ligaments are torn the knee joint opens more widely when the relevant ligament is tested (compare knees against each other, as general laxity may be present). Tenderness over lateral joint line could be iliotibial band tendinitis.

Test the *cruciate ligaments* (figs 7.44 & 7.45) with the knee 90° flexed (anterior/posterior drawer tests); immobilize the patient's leg by sitting on their foot, and then with the knee in flexion, grip the upper tibia and try to draw it towards you, away from the femur. At 20° flexion, Lachmann's test involves flexing the patient's knee over your own, stabilizing the femur with one hand, and using the other to draw the tibia towards you. The ACL prevents *anterior* glide of the tibia on the femur; the posterior cruciate ligament (PCL) prevents *posterior* glide. Excessive glide in one direction suggests damage to the relevant ligament. The 'pivot shift test'[13]—a more sensitive test to determine if symptoms really are due to cruciate damage (can be asymptomatic).

McMurray's rotation test is an unreliable way of detecting pedunculated *meniscal tears.*[14] With the knee flexed, the tibia is externally rotated, then the knee is extended. This is repeated with varying degrees of knee flexion, and then again with the tibia medially rotated on the femur. The test is designed to jam the free end of a torn meniscus in the joint—a click being felt and heard and it is positive if pain is experienced by the patient as the jammed tag is released as the knee straightens. NB: normal knees often produce patellar clicks. Apley's grinding test is more reliable and easier to perform; with the patient lying prone, flex the knee to 90° and rotate the tibia with axial pressure while distracting the femur.[42]

13 This is so called because it was found to be positive in patients (eg American Football players) who reported to their surgeon that 'When I pivot (on my leg) something shifts'.
14 Meniscal tears are especially difficult to clinically diagnose because the menisci are avascular and only the outer ⅓ is innervated; there can be little pain or swelling after injury.

Arthroscopy Enables internal structures of the knee to be seen and a definite diagnosis may be made. It also enables a wide range of operations to be done as day-case surgery. This is routinely preceded by MRI.

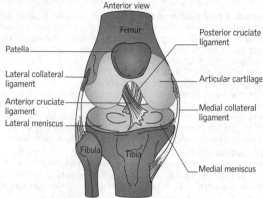

Fig 7.43 The anatomy of the right knee—as seen from in front. The medial collateral ligament is much broader than the lateral ligament, and its deep fibres are firmly attached to the medial meniscus. The lateral ligament and the lateral meniscus are interposed by the popliteal tendon (see fig 7.44), and hence are not connected. 4 ligaments stabilize the knee: anterior and posterior cruciate ligaments, medial and lateral collateral ligaments. The secondary stabilizers include the menisci, iliotibial band, and biceps femoris.

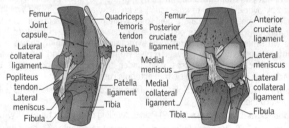

Fig 7.44 The synovium of the right knee joint: lateral (left) and posterior views. Note that the synovium extends up behind the patella (remember for joint aspiration, p.512), and that both cruciate ligaments are extrasynovial (but are intracapsular). NB: the joint capsule is distended in these images by infusion of fluid.

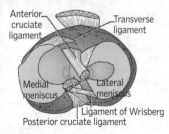

Fig 7.45 Tibial plateau and ligaments. The ACL prevents anterior translation and rotation of the tibia on the femur. The PCL prevents posterior subluxation of the tibia on the femur.

The medial meniscus is securely attached to the joint capsule, and consequently more frequently torn compared to the lateral meniscus which is more mobile.

Further reading

Rossi R et al. (2011). Clinical examination of the knee: know your tools for diagnosis of knee injuries. *Sports Med Arthrosc Rehabil Ther Technol* 3:25.

The common symptoms are anterior knee pain and swelling. Anterior knee pain can be due to many causes:

Patellofemoral pain syndrome (PFPS) Common in young athletes and may be associated with overuse as well as lower limb malalignment, muscle imbalance, and patellar tracking abnormalities. Patellar aching is felt after prolonged sitting or on climbing/descending stairs. There may have been a recent increase in sporting activity or trauma, ask about a history of patella subluxation/dislocation. Effusion is rare. Diffuse retropatellar tenderness and pain on patellofemoral compression occur: +ve Clarke's test = pain on patellofemoral compression with tensed quadriceps muscles. There may be either decreased or increased patellar mobility. *Diagnosis* is clinical. *Treat* by relative rest—if due to increased training employ a structured rehabilitation. Quadriceps and hip strengthening exercises are the mainstay of treatment. NSAIDs may only reduce pain for a few months. Surgery is rarely indicated.[43]

Bipartite patella (fig 7.46) Congenital fragmentation of the patella, found in ~1%. Usually an incidental x-ray finding (often falsely interpreted as a fracture pattern), but may give pain if the superolateral fragment is mobile with tenderness over the junction. Excision of fragment may relieve refractory pain.

Patellar tendinopathy (jumper's knee) Usually initiated by micro- or macro patellar tendon tears, eg associated with repetitive sporting loads. It can occur anywhere in the patellar tendon, and settles with rest ± NSAIDs. Steroid injections are contraindicated due to the risk of patellar tendon rupture).[44] Eccentric contraction exercises (tension while lengthening the muscle) and bracing may also help.[45]

Hoffa's fat pad syndrome Very painful impingement of the infrapatellar (Hoffa's) fat pad thought to be caused by maltracking of the patella. Typically caused by over-extension of knee (such as an awkward fall or lifting weights with locked knees). Extending a bent knee while putting pressure on the patellar tendon margins elicits pain and a defensive behaviour.[46] Think of it in those with meniscus or ligament-type symptoms when imaging shows they are intact. MRI may show a hypertrophic Hoffa pad impinging between articular surfaces (which causes pain under the patella). There may be hydrarthrosis or haemarthrosis (from arteriole rupture).

Chrondromalacia patellae Softening of the articular cartilage of the patella. Usually grouped with PFPS.

Osgood–Schlatter disease (p. 509) Pain ± swelling over tibial tuberosity.

Bursitis (fig 7.47) The *prepatellar bursa* is the most commonly affected causing anterior knee pain following trauma or overuse (kneeling for prolonged periods of time) earning it the name 'housemaid's knee'. May also occur with infection, crystal arthropathies, and rheumatoid arthritis. Typically presents with swelling and tenderness anterior to patella, and pain on kneeling. Prepatellar bursae may be aspirated, ± corticosteroid injected to decrease recurrence. If very persistent it may need excision. Pain may be relieved by topical NSAIDs. Aspiration distinguishes friction bursitis from infected bursitis, which needs drainage and antibiotics. ▶ Always consider septic arthritis of joint (OHCM p544).

The *infrapatellar bursa* leads to 'clergyman's knee' as they kneel more upright. The *semimembranous bursa* lies in the popliteal fossa (a popliteal cyst which differs from the 'Baker's cyst' which is a herniation from the joint synovium) and causes popliteal discomfort.

You will notice the strong association of overuse injuries with occupation—housemaid's knee has also been referred to as nun's knee, miner's knee, etc. So remember to ask about occupation or repetitive sport movements such as tennis or golf in elbow injuries.

Further reading

LLopis E *et al.* (2007). Anterior knee pain. *Eur J Radiol* 62:27–43.

'All these hags'

Once, after a stay in hospital with a fracture, a patient who was not quite as deaf as she was supposed to be, told one of us (JML) how she had overheard a newly arrived orthopaedic surgeon say to the ward nurse 'What are we going to do with all these hags?'. As he progressed down the ward, turning first to the left and then to the beds on the right, his mood became morose, then black—as if he was getting angry that all these 'hags' were clogging up his beds, preventing his scientific endeavours. But what was really happening, my patient suspected, was that, as he turned to left and right, he was really nodding goodbye to his humanity, and, dimly aware of this, he was angry to see it go. On this view, these rows of hags were like buoys in the night, marking his passage out of our world. We all make this trip. Is there any way back? The process of becoming a doctor takes us away from the very people we first wanted to serve. Must medicine take the brightest and the best and turn us into quasi-monsters?

The answer to these questions came unexpectedly in the months that followed: sheer pressure of work drove this patient's observations out of my mind. It was winter, and there was 'flu. In the unnatural twilight of a snowy day I drifted from bed to bed in a stupor of exhaustion with a deepening sense of a collapse that could not be put off ... It was all I could do to climb into bed: but when I awoke, I found I had somehow climbed into a patient's bed, who had kindly moved over to make space for me, and was now looking at me with concern in her eyes. Herein lay the answer: the hag must make room for the doctor, and the doctor must make room for the hag: *we are all in the same bed*.

7 Orthopaedics

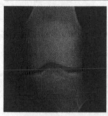

Fig 7.46 Bipartite patella at the usual position of the superolateral edge. This x-ray has been 'windowed' to make the lesion more obvious (the bean-sized fragment is between 1 and 2 o'clock). This has been one of the major advantages of digitized image viewing.
Courtesy of The Norfolk and Norwich University Hospitals (NNUH) Radiology Dept.

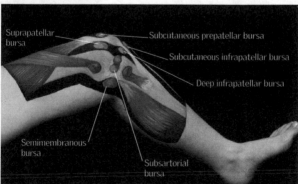

Suprapatellar bursa
Subcutaneous prepatellar bursa
Subcutaneous infrapatellar bursa
Deep infrapatellar bursa
Semimembranous bursa
Subsartorial bursa

Fig 7.47 Bursa around the knee joint. Bursae are small fibrous sacs of fluid with a synovial lining, typically found around joints and between tendons and ligaments where they pass over bones. They function to reduce friction. Bursitis is inflammation of a bursa with consequent increases in synovial fluid production & swelling. There are ~16 bursae surrounding the knee, see p. 496 for those most commonly affected.

Reproduced courtesy of Art and Anatomy Edinburgh. Copyright © 2015 Art and Anatomy Edinburgh.
Contributors Kimmie Dunlop, Nichola Robertson, Megan Anderson, Philip Stewart, and Alex Haddon.

Osteoarthritis (OA) (Also see *OHCM* p544) Knee OA is the most common joint disease in Europe. Women (especially if >55yrs old) are at greater risk.[47] Knee swelling may occur with any arthritic process.

Secondary OA causes
• Post-traumatic
• Postoperative
• Post-infective
• Malposition
• Mechanical instability
• Osteochondritis dissecans (p. 508)

Primary osteoarthritis can be defined as degeneration of the articular cartilage and surfaces of a joint with no predisposing factors—in this sense, the disease is idiopathic, though current research is suggesting many of these cases have subtle underlying congenital/developmental defects. In *secondary* OA there is an underlying precipitant to the degenerative process (see MINIBOX 'Secondary OA causes'). OA is associated with ↑BMI, genetic factors, age, and occupation. Weight loss in women reduces risk of getting OA symptoms.[48][n=796] Patients complain of pain on initiating movement. Stiffness follows inactivity, but often resolves in <30min. In the knee, OA particularly affects the posterior patella and the medial compartment, so tending to varus deformity (osteotomy is an attractive alternative to total knee replacement (TKR) for early OA in young, active patients since a prosthesis may only last ~15 years). Osteotomies can delay TKR for up to 10 years. On examination, an arthritic knee will have a limited range of motion with crepitus during both active and passive movements. There may be joint deformity and bony overgrowth from osteophytes. x-ray findings are shown in fig 7.48. *Treatment:* NSAIDs (topical ibuprofen may be as good as oral in older patients, and has fewer SE), quadriceps strengthening exercises, weight loss, local steroid injections (gives some benefit in the short term, but long-term benefit is unclear).

Knee replacement Consists of resection of articular surfaces of the knee, then resurfacing with metal and polyethylene components. Replacement may be total or partial (unicompartmental). Pain correlates poorly with radiological signs. Success rate: 95%. Consider referral for joint surgery in those patients with significant disabling pain (even at rest or disturbing sleep) which has a detrimental impact on QOL despite adequate conservative approaches. Postoperative knee swelling is relatively common; due to the close proximity of the joint to the external environment any suspicion of infection must be dealt with seriously. ►►Prosthetic joints must only be aspirated in an orthopaedic theatre; never in ED or clinic. *Joint survival:* 90% last 15yrs (better than hips). Revision rates are similar. Quality of life can be transformed, even if >80yrs old. TKR is highly cost-effective with respect to QALYs gained.[49]

Meniscal cysts *Typical patient:* A young man, with past trauma, then insidious development of cyst. *Pain:* Over the joint line. Lateral cysts are 5–10× more common than medial. Swelling may disappear with full flexion. The meniscus is often torn radially (an otherwise unusual direction) so there may be knee clicking and giving way. Δ MRI. *Treatment:* Arthroscopic decompression.

Ligament tears, meniscus lesions, patellar dislocation See p. 543.

Baker's cyst The most common swelling of the popliteal fossa. Primary cysts in young people tend to be asymptomatic. Secondary cysts are a misnomer, since they result from fluid building up within the semimembranosus bursa associated with chronic knee effusions from OA. Patients present with posterior knee swelling and aching. ►►Always consider DVT, especially if cyst has ruptured causing calf swelling. US helps determine nature of cystic lesions and presence of vascular flow. Treatment is mostly conservative with analgesia, spontaneous resolution can occur in young people. To date, there is no gold standard approach and treatment is aimed at the underlying articular disorders.

The acutely swollen hot joint

►You must suspect septic arthritis (p544 *OHCM*) in any acutely painful and swollen joint as this is the most serious diagnosis. See table 7.4 for differential diagnosis

Osteoarthritis, many of the rheumatological conditions, and malignancy can also present with chronic swelling. Note that acute polyarthritis is associated with multiple systemic rheumatological and infective disease processes.

►►Always ask if other joints are affected and if patient is systemically unwell.

Examination Feel the joint margins for bogginess (suggestive of chronic inflammatory arthritis) and palpate for effusions. Look for erythema and feel for warmth.

Investigations *Aspiration of synovial fluid from the affected joint:* The key investigation. Analysis (see table 7.7, p. 513) helps to diagnose haemarthrosis, infectious and crystal arthropathies. Be mindful that one cannot rule out sepsis simply because crystals are present or initial Gram staining is negative—use your clinical judgement and treat if you suspect infection. ►Aspiration of a replaced joint must be done under sterile conditions in theatre. See p. 512. *Bloods:* Do CRP, FBC, U+Es, LFTs, bone profile (for calcium and phosphate) and blood cultures. Also request a serum urate but note it may be normal in acute attacks of gout. Consider rheumatoid factor, anti-CCP, and antibody titres if rheumatological cause is suspected. Ask the rheumatology team for help if no obvious cause.

X-rays: Usually normal in septic arthritis but may show signs of chronic gout (well-defined 'punched out' erosions in juxta-articular bone, see fig 12.6 on p541 in *OHCM*).

Table 7.4 Differential diagnosis of an acutely swollen joint

Inflammatory disease	Disorders in bone/cartilage
Septic arthritis	Trauma
Crystal arthropathy (gout and pseudo-gout (CPPD)) (*OHCM* p548)	Haemarthrosis (associated with high bleeding tendency)
Rheumatoid arthritis	Fracture
Reactive arthritis	
Psoriatic arthropathy	

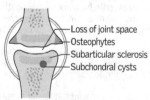

— Loss of joint space
— Osteophytes
— Subarticular sclerosis
— Subchondral cysts

Fig 7.48 Radiological features of osteoarthritis.
Courtesy of Dr DC Howlett

Further reading

Eid AS *et al.* (2012). As we managing knee effusion well? *BJMP* 5:a504. www.bjmp.org/files/2012-5-1/bjmp-2012-5-1-a504.pdf

7 Orthopaedics

Examination 25° of dorsiflexion and 30° of plantarflexion are the norm at the tibiotalar joint. Inversion and eversion are from the subtalar and midtarsal joints. Toes should have between 60° and 90° dorsiflexion. Note callosities. Examine the arches (fig 7.62 p. 517). Watch as the toes are lifted off the ground, and on standing on tiptoe. Examine gait and shoes (normal wear pattern: medially under ball of foot, posterolaterally at heel).

Hallux valgus (bunion) The big toe deviates laterally at the metatarsophalangeal joint (fig 7.49). Typically present bilaterally. Pressure of the deformed metatarsophalangeal joint against the shoe leads to bunion formation; some have gross relatively painless deformity which only causes problems with shoe-fittings, others can report high levels of pain with minimal deformity. Risk factors include female gender, age, type of footwear, a positive family history, conditions causing joint hypermobility, and neuromuscular disease. Secondary OA in the joint is common. Educate the patient on appropriate footwear (wide, low-heeled shoes). Bunion pads and plastic wedges between great and second toes may relieve pain, but this is a progressive condition and correction of deformity requires surgery. Painful bunions which inhibit lifestyle should be considered (surgery should not be for cosmetic reasons). Many different operations are used

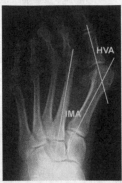

Fig **7.49** Weight-bearing AP image showing a hallux valgus deformity and the hallux valgus angle (HVA) and intermetatarsal angle (IMA).

Courtesy of Professor Peter Scally.

with no accepted gold standard and each patient is considered individually. Surgery achieves toe alignment and alleviates pain in ~90%.[50] Complications include chronic pain, recurrence, and joint stiffness.

Lesser toe deformities May accompany a hallux valgus as they have similar biomechanical risk factors. All present with painful calluses when walking and difficulties finding shoes that are comfortable. Typically affects >60-year-olds. Initially the deformity will be flexible, over time the joint stiffens and becomes fixed. ►Always investigate for diabetic neuropathy. Examine the lower limb neurovascular status and musculature. Management is similar to hallux valgus with orthotics and surgery reserved to correct painful, debilitating deformities.

1 *Hammer toes:* Extended at the MTP joint, hyperflexed at the PIP joint, and extended at the DIP joint. The toes look curled. Associated with contracture of flexor digitorum longus tendon. 2nd toes are most commonly affected.

2 *Claw toes:* Extended at the MTP joint but flexed at PIP and DIP joints giving a clawed appearance where the toe digs into the sole of the foot. The operative treatment for both hammer and claw toes is metatarsal shortening (flexible deformity) or PIP joint arthrodesis (fixed deformity).

3 *Mallet toes:* Flexion deformity of the DIP joint in isolation treated with flexor tenotomy (flexible deformity) or DIP joint arthrodesis (fixed deformity).

Our feet have carried us through the history of mankind. Although many of our problems today arise from the strained biomechanics of walking on 2 feet, the foot remains a remarkable structure. Historically, pain in the foot has not captured much interest among the medical profession and research has moved slowly. Often dismissed as trivial, we now increasingly have started to recognize the importance of physical inactivity and how very limiting chronic foot pain can be.[51] So just like we tend to forget to nurture our souls, don't leave these soles out of your assessment.[15, 52,53]

Ingrowing toenails (onychocryptosis) Typically the big toe in young adults. Incorrect nail cutting ± pressure of shoes predispose to the lateral nail digging into its fleshy bed, which reacts by becoming heaped up infection—'proudflesh'. *Conservative treatment* involves tucking cotton-wool soaked in surgical spirit under the proudflesh and awaiting nail growth (then cut it straight with edges protruding beyond flesh margins). However, a 2012 Cochrane review has shown that *surgical interventions* (whole-nail avulsion or wedge resection of affected side) are more effective in preventing recurrence, especially when combined with the application of phenol.[54]

Adult forefoot pain (metatarsalgia) Increased pressure on the metatarsal head causes pain in the ball of the foot. Associated with ↑BMI, high heels, toe deformities, high-impact sports, and inflammatory arthritis. Orthotic supports for shoes may help. Advise rest and gentle strengthening exercises. Surgery other than for rheumatoid arthritis is unpredictable.

Morton's neuroma: A common cause of metatarsalgia in women. Pain is from pressure from an interdigital neuroma[16,55] between the metatarsals (eg from tight-fitting shoes). Pain usually radiates to the lateral side of one toe, and the medial side of its neighbour (eg toes 3 & 4). Compressing the affected web space is quite specific. MRI helps diagnosis, as does US if by an experienced operator. Neuroma excision may be needed.[56]

March (stress) fractures Occur in the shaft of 2nd or 3rd metatarsals. May follow excessive walking: the history should raise suspicion and prompt a scouring search of the metatarsi. x-rays may be normal, or have subtle periosteal changes. Radionuclide bone scans are more discriminating. Treatment is rest and analgesia, crutches for a few weeks may be useful. If pain is severe, try a plaster cast or walking boot while awaiting healing.

Pain in the heel Can be a diagnostic challenge, consider use of x-rays (to see calcaneal spurs), MRI (to highlight degenerative tendon changes), or bone scans (diffuse uptake in inflammatory arthritis or stress fractures). *Causes:*

- Diseases of the calcaneum
- Rupture of calcaneal tendon (p. 516)
- Postcalcaneal bursitis (back of heel)
- Post-traumatic (eg calcaneal #)
- Arthritis of the subtalar joint
- Systemic diseases
- Seronegative spondylarthopathy
- Infection.

Plantar fasciitis The plantar fascia supports the arch of the foot. The most common cause of plantar heel pain. Repetitive trauma causes microtears and inflammation in the origin of the plantar fascia on the heel. Obesity, inactivity, and excessive walking are risk factors. Treatment should be instigated promptly (immobility is a risk factor for chronicity). No clear superiority between stretching of the Achilles tendon, orthotics, and shockwave therapy. Corticosteroid injections have a role in recalcitrant pain, and surgical release can be effective in people who have not responded to conservative measures.[57] Prognosis is usually good with minimal treatment, the trick is to encourage athletes to be patient and discourage immobility in inactive patients.

15 Corns: focal friction-dependent hyperkeratotic intradermal nodules develop at bony pressure points. A bursa-like structure may form around these islands. Likelihood ↑ if neuropathy eg diabetes. Unlike calluses (thickened areas of skin) they have a core of keratin, occur only on the foot, and cause pain. Optimize footwear, chiropody, or excise the corn.

16 It is not a true neuroma, but rather inflammatory and degenerative changes to the interdigital nerve resulting in entrapment neuropathy.

7 Orthopaedics

This is an infection of bone. Incidence is reducing as living standards rise. It can be categorized as acute haematogenous, secondary to contiguous local infection (with or without the presence of vascular disease), or direct inoculation from trauma or surgery. All forms can progress to chronic osteomyelitis. Infection may spread from boils, abscesses, pneumonia, or genitourinary instrumentation, though often no primary site is found.

Common organisms
• *Staphylococcus aureus*
• *Pseudomonas*
• *E. coli*
• Streptococci

Other organisms
• *Salmonella* (esp. with sickle cell disease)[58]
• Mycobacteria
• Fungi

▶Always look for osteomyelitis in diabetic feet and deep pressure sores.

Clinical features See box 'Clinical features of osteomyelitis'. **Tests** ESR/CRP↑, WCC↑. Blood culture (only +ve in 50%) and most useful in haematogenous spread of infection. Bone biopsy and culture is gold standard for pathogen identification and if diagnosis remains uncertain—but rarely required for acute osteomyelitis. Swabs from discharging sinuses, or needle aspiration of material near bone, may give misleading results.[59] x-ray changes are not apparent for 10–14 days but then show haziness ± loss of density of affected bone, then subperiosteal reaction, and later, sequestrum and involucrum (see box 'Clinical features of osteomyelitis' & figs 7.50-7.52). NB: infected cancellous bone shows less change. MRI is sensitive and specific (88% and 93%)—and avoids ionizing radiation. Nuclear medicine white cell scans are becoming popular and have comparable sensitivity and specificity to MRI (80–90%).[60]

Treatment Before antibiotics, the treatment was amputation, now surgery aims to drain abscesses and remove sequestra (culture all sequestra). The key is 6 weeks of antibiotics following local empirical guidelines until the organism and its sensitivities are known. Be guided by sensitivities and a microbiologist, as organism profiles may differ between areas, and according to patient risk factors. In children, prevalence of *Haemophilus*

Complications
• Septic arthritis
• Fractures
• Deformity
• Chronic osteomyelitis

influenzae osteomyelitis is reducing due to the HIB vaccination.

Chronic osteomyelitis Poor treatment results in pain, fever, sequestra (infected dead bone), and sinus suppuration (presence of a sinus tract is pathognomic) with long remissions. Always suspect chronic development in vascular insufficiency with non-healing tissue ulceration overlying bony prominences. Diabetic ulcers have a high risk of osteomyelitis, even before bone becomes exposed. If bone can be felt on probing the ulcer, then this is sufficient to diagnose chronic osteomyelitis.[61] x-rays show thick irregular bone. Treatment involves radical excision of sequestra, skeletal stabilization, 'dead-space' management (often needs plastic surgical input), and antibiotics (modified according to sensitivities) for ≥12 weeks. *Complications:* Amyloid, squamous carcinoma development in sinus track.

Bone TB (eg vertebral body = Pott disease, see pp. 486–7.[17]) Represents 1–3% of all TB; incidence is rising, but remains rare in UK. Spread is haematogenous or via nearby nodes. *Treatment:* Drain abscesses, immobilize affected large joints. Standard 6-month courses (OHCM p394) of eg **isoniazid** (300mg/day), **rifampicin** (600mg/day), and **pyrazinamide** (1.5g/day) may not be long enough and treatment is likely needed for 1 year. Bed rest and bracing is no longer recommended, and gentle exercise is encouraged. A Cochrane review has found no evidence to support routine surgical intervention; it is only necessary in advanced cases with marked deformity, abscess formation, or paraplegia.[38] Prognosis in patients with no neurological defecit tends to be good.

7 Orthopaedics

Clinical features of osteomyelitis

Patterns of infection Cancellous bone is typically affected in adults—commonly in vertebrae and feet (diabetics). In children, vascular bone is most affected (eg in long-bone metaphyses—esp. distal femur, upper tibia). Infection leads to cortex erosion, with holes (*cloacae*). Exudation of pus lifts up the periosteum interrupting blood supply to underlying bone and necrotic fragments of bone may form (*sequestrum*). The presence of sequestra is typical of chronic infection. New bone formation created by the elevated periosteum forms an *involucrum*. Pus may discharge into joint spaces or via sinuses to the skin.

Risk factors
• Diabetes
• Vascular disease
• Impaired immunity
• Sickle cell disease
• Surgical prostheses
• Open fractures

The patient Pain of gradual onset and unwillingness to move over the course of a few days. Local findings include tenderness, warmth, erythema, and slight effusion in neighbouring joints. Look for signs of systemic infection. All signs are less marked in adults.

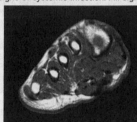

Fig 7.51 Axial T1-weighted MRI of the foot through the metatarsals, showing reduced signal within the first metatarsal (from replacement of the marrow fat with pus) consistent with osteomyelitis.

Courtesy of The Norfolk and Norwich University Hospitals (NNUH) Radiology Dept.

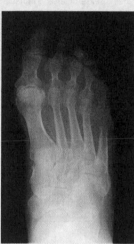

Fig 7.50 Osteomyelitis causing destruction of the 5th metatarsal head and the base of the 5th proximal phalanx. Note also the vascular calcification in this patient, who had diabetes.

Courtesy of The Norfolk and Norwich University Hospitals (NNUH) Radiology Dept.

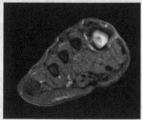

Fig 7.52 Axial T1-weighted MRI of the same patient as fig 7.51, this time with FAT SAT (fat saturation) and IV gadolinium contrast. The effect of this technique is to suppress the marrow fat and enhance the infection.

Courtesy of The Norfolk and Norwich University Hospitals (NNUH) Radiology Dept.

7 Orthopaedics

Further reading

Howell WR *et al.* (2011). Osteomyelitis: an update for hospitalists. *Hosp Pract (1995)* 39:153–60.

Termaat MF *et al.* (2005). The accuracy of diagnostic imaging for the assessment of chronic osteomyelitis: a systematic review and meta-analysis. *J Bone Joint Surg Am* 87:2464–71.

17 Mr Percivall Pott has an interesting story, he's not only famous for Pott disease of the spine. https://edu.rsc.org/feature/percivall-pott-chimney-sweeps-and-cancer/2020205.article

Bone is a common site for secondaries (prostate, thyroid, lung, kidney, breast)[18] while primary bone neoplasia is rare: incidence of 9 per million population/year. Delays in diagnosis are common. Metastases are blood-borne and usually arise in the lungs or other bones. Investigation is with MRI (to define the lesion), bone scan (to look for other lesions), and CT (to find the primary). Treatment of these rare and highly aggressive primary tumours is best carried out in multidisciplinary specialist treatment centres.

Bone sarcoma presentation
• Non-mechanical bone or joint pain
• Bone pain at night
• Bony swellings
• Pathological fractures

Multiple myeloma (OHCM p368) The most common primary malignant bone tumour and accounts for 45% of all malignant bone tumours. Bony manifestations include multiple punched-out osteolytic lesions.

Osteosarcoma The 2nd most common primary malignant bone tumour.[19] Primary osteosarcoma typically affects adolescents and arises in the metaphyses of long bone, especially around the knee. Secondary osteosarcoma may arise in bone affected by Paget disease or after irradiation. Classically presents between ages 10–20 with a peak in adolescent growth spurt. *Imaging:* Bone destruction and new bone formation (sunray spiculation), often with marked periosteal elevation (Codman's triangle). 50% of lesions are around the knee joint. Patients often present with pain before a mass develops. Staging MRI of the area will assess intramedullary spread. Do an HRCT chest to screen for pulmonary metastases, especially if ALP is raised. *Treatment:* Historically, the affected extremity was usually amputated but >80% of patients developed recurrent disease (typically pulmonary metastases) which highlights that most patients probably have micrometastatic disease at diagnosis. Neoadjuvant (prior to surgery) chemotherapy is advised. A 5-year survival rate of ~60–70% is achievable.[62]

Ewing sarcoma This malignant round-cell tumour of long bones (typically diaphysis) and limb girdles, usually presents in adolescents. See MINIBOX 'Radiological features'. MRI is helpful. Typically patients have a T11:22 chromosomal translocation. *Treatment:* Chemotherapy, surgery, and radiotherapy are required. The key adverse prognostic factor is metastases at diagnosis (5-year recurrence-free survival is 22%—vs 55% if no metastases).[63,975]

Radiological features
• Bone destruction
• New bone formation in concentric layers: 'onion layer' sign
• Soft tissue swelling
• Periosteal elevation

Chondrosarcoma May arise *de novo* or from malignant transformation of chondromas. It is usually associated with pain, or a lump, and presents in the axial skeleton of the middle-aged. 'Popcorn calcification' is typical on x-ray. MRI/CT will better define tumour extent. *Treatment:* No response to chemotherapy or radiotherapy, so treatment is by excision. Inadequate surgery is accompanied by local recurrence, often of a higher grade of malignancy. The cure rate depends on the type and grade of chondrosarcoma at diagnosis.

Limb-sparing surgical reconstruction (After excising a bone tumour) may involve replacing affected bone with a metal and polyethylene endoprosthesis—as an alternative to amputation. Excellent and durable reconstruction is possible using massive endoprostheses or bone allografts. Amputation is reserved for exceptional cases. 85% of patients now have limb salvage following chemotherapy for primary bone tumours.

18 Mnemonic for tumours which commonly metastasize to bone: Particular Tumours Love Killing Bone.
19 There are many different subtypes, including intramedullary, periosteal, parosteal, & telangiectatic.

Osteochondroma The commonest benign bone tumour, usually occurring about the knee, proximal femur, or proximal humerus.[20] Presents as a painful mass associated with trauma. Seen on x-ray as a bony spur arising from the cortex and usually pointing away from the joint. *Treatment:* Remove if causing symptoms, eg pressure on adjacent structures. Any osteochondroma continuing to grow after skeletal maturity must be removed because of risk of malignancy (arises rarely in solitary osteochondromas but in up to 10% of patients with *multiple hereditary exostoses*—an autosomal dominant inherited condition causing short stature as well as forearm, knee, and ankle deformity, see p. 506).

Osteoid osteoma Painful benign bone lesion that occurs most commonly in long bones of males 10–25yrs old (and also often in the spine). It appears as local cortical sclerosis on x-rays with a central radiolucent nidus. Within the nidus there may be a small nucleus of calcification. The nidus produces prostaglandins leading to pain unrelated to activity, and relieved by ibuprofen (and other prostaglandin inhibitors). *Treatment:* CT-guided biopsy and radiofrequency ablation.[64] Plain x-rays may miss these tumours. CT is the best imaging modality.[65]

Chondroma These benign cartilaginous tumours may arise from bone surfaces or within the medulla (=enchondromata). They may cause local swelling or #. *Treatment:* Rarely needed, exclude malignancy (chondosarcoma).

Fibrous dysplasia of bone Developmental abnormality where bone is not properly formed. May lead to pain and increased risk of fracture. Surgical stabilization is sometimes needed. In the polyostotic form bisphosphonates may help relieve symptoms.

Sarcoma versus carcinoma

A sarcoma is any malignant neoplasm arising from mesenchymal cells (which give rise to connective and non-epithelial tissue). There are 3 broad categories: 1 Soft tissue cancers 2 Primary bone cancers 3 Gastrointestinal stromal tumours (GIST). Carcinomas affect epithelial cells and frequently cause breast, bowel, and lung cancers.

Soft tissue sarcomas (STS)

STS are uncommon (~1500/yr in UK) but can arise in any mesenchymal tissue, originating from fat, muscle, etc. presenting as a painless enlarging mass. Risk factors include neurofibromatosis type 1 (*OHCM*, p514) and previous radiotherapy. **Diagnosis** Any lump that has any feature from the following MINIBOX is to be considered malignant until proved otherwise. **Imaging** MRI followed by needle biopsy. Pathological diagnoses include rhabdomyosarcoma (most common in

Consider STS malignant if
• Bigger than 5cm
• Increasing in size
• Deep to the deep fascia
• Painful

children), liposarcoma, leiomyosarcoma, fibrosarcoma, etc. Gene expression profiling is helping to improve diagnosis and indicate tumours which may respond to chemotherapy. **Treatment** Excision with wide margins followed by radiotherapy for most. Adjuvant chemotherapy with doxorubicin may be appropriate, trabectedin has a role.[66] **Prognosis** Related to histological grade, size and depth of the tumour. High-grade, large, deep tumours have <50% 5yr survival. STS in children often respond well to chemotherapy; survival is better.

Further reading

Skinner HB *et al.* (2015). *Current Diagnosis & Treatment in Orthopaedics* (5th ed). New York: McGraw-Hill Medical.

20 Cartilage tumour classification: is the lesion benign or malignant? Is the lesion a pure or impure cartilaginous tumour? Is the epicentre of the lesion intraosseous, juxtacortical, or in the soft tissues? The most common bone tumours are enchondroma, osteochondroma, chondroblastoma, and chondromyxoid fibroma. Chondrosarcoma is malignant.

7 Orthopaedics

Osteogenesis imperfecta (OI) 'brittle bone disease' Inherited disorder of type I collagen that results in joint laxity and fragile, low-density bones which recurrently fracture. It affects 1 in 20,000. OI has historically been classified into 4 forms (table 7.5, although type IV has recently been expanded into IV–VII). Since patients initially present with inconsistent histories of injury frequency and severity, this condition can be mistaken for child abuse (pp. 196-7). *x-rays:* Many fractures, osteoporotic bones with thin cortex, and bowing deformity of long bones. *Histology:* Immature unorganized bone with abnormal cortex. *Treatment:* Prevent injury. Physio, rehab, and occupational therapy are key. Osteotomies may correct deformity. Intramedullary rods are sometimes used in long bones. Bisphosphonates may increase cortical thickness.[67] As OI is a genetic disease, gene therapy is being explored in hopes to alter the course of the collagen mutations. This is especially challenging due to genetic heterogeneity and that most OI mutations are dominant negative (the mutant allele product interferes with normal allele function).[68]

Table 7.5 Categories of osteogenesis imperfecta

I	The mildest and most common form. It is autosomal dominant (AD). Associated with blue sclerae (due to increased corneal translucency) and 50% have hearing loss. Fractures typically occur before puberty. Normal life expectancy
II	Lethal perinatal form with many fractures, blue sclera, & dwarfism. Recessive
III	Severe form—occurs in about 20%. Recessive. Fractures at birth + progressive spinal and limb deformity, with resultant short stature; blue or white sclera; dentinogenesis imperfecta common (enamel separates from defective dentine, leaving teeth transparent or discoloured); life expectancy is decreased
IV	Moderate form. AD. Fragile bones, white sclerae after infancy

7 Orthopaedics

Achondroplasia (fig 7.53) Most common form of disproportionate short stature. It occurs due to reduced growth of cartilaginous bone. It is AD, but ~80% are from spontaneous mutation.[69] Gross motor skills develop later—only 50% sit unsupported at 9 months, and only 50% walk alone at 18 months. *x-rays:* Short proximal long bones & wide epiphyses. *Treatment:* Involves monitoring for potential complications. Growth hormone has been tried.[70]

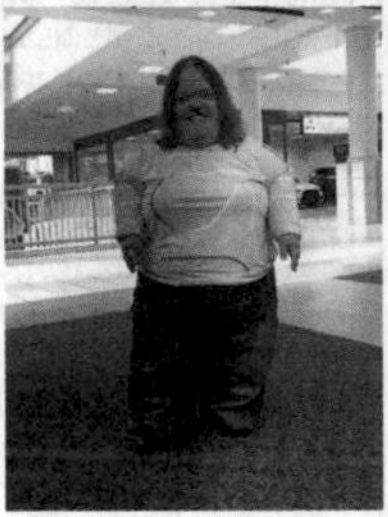

Multiple hereditary exostoses AD disorder in which certain proteins accumulate leading to cartilage-capped tumours (exostoses/osteochondromata) developing from affected cartilage at the end of long bones. These point away from the nearby joint. If severe, bones are badly modelled, causing short stature as well as forearm, knee, and ankle deformity. Beware of malignant transformation to chondrosarcomas or osteosarcomas (see p. 504). *Treatment:* Remove symptom-producing exostoses.

Osteopetrosis Failure of osteoclastic bone resorption results in very hard, dense 'marble' bones that are brittle. Anaemia and thrombocytopenia may result from decreased marrow space. Deafness and optic atrophy can result from compression of cranial nerves. Lack of remodelling preserves variations of ossific density causing the characteristic 'bone within a bone' appearance.

Fig **7.53** Adults with achondroplasia are short with ↑ lumbar lordosis, bow legs, and short proximal arms & legs. Lifespan & mental & sexual development are normal. Complications include tibial bowing, joint hypermobility, hydrocephalus, foramen magnum compression (5–10%), recurrent otitis media, hearing loss, sleep apnoea (75%), & ↑BMI.

© Nina Hjelde.

See Neurofibromatosis (*OHCM* p514), Marfan's (*OHCM* p706), Ehlers–Danlos p. 846 & Morquio's (p. 854).

Developmental bone biology

Because bone is ossified, we tend to think of it as the architectural rock around which our living tissues are constructed. But bone maintenance and development is a highly dynamic and regulated process sensitive to a wide variety of hormones, inflammatory mediators, growth factors, and genetic influences which become aberrant whenever there are deletions, insertions, and missense mutations. The concept of a *master gene* is useful to indicate how genes relate and interact. Master genes encode proteins that can control other genes by directly binding to their DNA; eg the transcription factor OSF2 (osteoblast specific transcription factor 2) gene is thought to serve as a master gene regulating expression of other genes, allowing mesenchymal stem cells to differentiate into osteoblasts. NB: master genes make a mockery of genes vs environment questions. One gene is an environment for another, and the effects of each may be catastrophic in some environments or negligible in others.

Remain in light ... the different types of bone

- *Lamellar*—the overall normal type of adult bone (subdivided into cancellous and compact), characterized by repeating architectural patterns (fig 7.54).
- *Cancellous (spongy bone)*—trabeculations form a network of parallel lamellae, the spaces being filled with connective tissue or bone. This type of bone does not make callus when healing (a type of lamellar bone).
- *Compact*—non-cancellous bone that is formed from Haversian canals and concentric lamellae (a type of lamellar bone).
- *Cortical*—superficial layer of compact bone.
- *Endochondral*—develops in cartilage that has been destroyed by calcification and subsequent resorption.
- *Heterotopic*—forms outside the normal skeleton either from a pathological process (eg in the heart) or as a reaction to local trauma/surgery.
- *Membranous*—formed from intramembranous ossification (eg clavicle).
- *Sesamoid*—bone formed in a tendon where it passes over a joint (eg the pisiform bone in flexor carpi ulnaris, and the patella).
- *Cartilaginous*—formed from growth plates (p. 491).

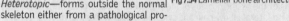
Fig 7.54 Lamellar bone architecture.

Cement — Lamellae
Haversian canal
Lacuna

Remain in light ... the different types of joint

- *Cartilaginous, primary*—hyaline cartilage between the bone ends. Only types are the costochondral and sternochondral (1st rib) joints.
- *Cartilaginous, secondary*—as for primary, but with a layer of fibrocartilage between the layers of hyaline cartilage. Only types (that all lie in the midline) are the manubriosternal, intervertebral, pubic symphysis, xiphisternal, and sacrococcygeal joints.
- *Fibrous*—fibrous tissue between bones; eg radio-ulnar interosseous membrane.
- *Synovial*—joint cavity containing synovial fluid, with hyaline cartilage on the bone surface; eg acetabulofemoral, glenohumeral.
- *Synovial, atypical*—joint cavity containing synovial fluid, with fibrocartilage on the bone surface ± a fibrocartilage disc; eg acromioclavicular and sternoclavicular joints (with discs). NB: fibrocartilage is found on the articulating surface of any bone that undergoes intramembranous ossification.

Further reading

Glorieux FH (2008). Osteogenesis imperfecta. *Best Pract Res Clin Rheumatol* 22:85–100.

Renaud A *et al.* (2013). Radiographic features of osteogenesis imperfecta. *Insights Imaging* 4:417–29.

Wright MJ *et al.* (2011). Clinical management of achondroplasia. *Arch Dis Child* 97:129–34.

The osteochondroses (table 7.6) are a group of conditions characterized by the abnormal endochondral ossification of epiphyseal growth during childhood. Osteochondrosis (also called osteochondritis) occurs in the wrist, elbow, hip, knee, ankle, fingers, toes, and spine. The underlying cause of most osteochondroses is unknown, although inheritance, overuse/trauma, rapid growth, and anatomic configuration may be predisposing factors. All osteochondroses undergo an interruption of blood supply to the epiphysis, followed by bone and cartilage necrosis, revascularization, and regrowth of bone.

Kienböck disease Avascular necrosis of the lunate bone. Affects young adults 20–40 years; typically gymnasts. Thought to be due to repetitive trauma combined with abnormal wrist biomechanics (ie negative ulnar variance) Pain is felt over the lunate (esp. during active wrist movement). Grip is impaired due to pain. *x-rays:* (fig 7.55) Sclerotic lunate with a little depth reduction early; more marked flattening later, leading later to osteoarthritis. *Treatment:* Early disease is managed symptomatically with splinting and analgesia; if sufficiently symptomatic then surgery attempts to ease compression of the lunate by ulnar lengthening or radial shortening and fusion of the capitate. Late, symptomatic presentation: proximal row carpectomy, intercarpal arthrodesis, total wrist arthrodesis. Vascularized bone graft is showing good early results, but no long-term data as yet. Wrist arthrodesis is the last resort.

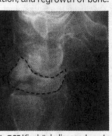

Fig 7.55 Kienböck disease. Lunate sclerosis with central lucency.

Reproduced from Bulstrode et al., *Oxford Textbook of Trauma and Orthopaedics* (2011), with permission from OUP.

Panner disease/osteochondritis dissecans (OCD) of the elbow Represent a continuum of disease of the capitellum. Panner disease is the avascular necrosis of the ossific nucleus of the capitellum. Mostly presents in boys <10yrs, causing lateral elbow pain and swelling. Conservative management is usually all that is required. OCD of the elbow affects the surface below the cartilage of the anterior capitellum. A loose body is formed from a convex joint surface when a segment of subchondral bone and cartilage becomes avascular and separates from underlying bone. Adolescents experience early aching and effusions after use and sudden painful locking of joints once pieces have separated to make loose bodies. *x-rays:* Look for lucent areas in a piece *about* to separate, the defect from which the piece *has* separated, and loose bodies *after* separation. *Treatment:* Stable lesions are managed conservatively with activity modification. Unstable lesions may need fixation ± removal of loose bodies. Closed wedge resection may lead to revascularization.

Köhler disease Rare, affects the navicular bone.[21] Children affected are 3–5yr-olds. Pain is felt in the mid-tarsal region and they limp. *x-rays:* Dense, deformed bone. *Treatment:* Symptomatic: resting the foot or wearing a walking plaster. *Prognosis:* Excellent, with few long-term problems.

Freiberg disease Infarction and fracture of the lesser metatarsal heads (commonly the 2nd). Presents as forefoot pain that worsens with pressure. Usually starts around the time of puberty. There may be microfractures at the junction of the metaphysis and the growth plate—precise aetiology is unknown, but associated with a long 2nd metatarsal. *x-rays:* Epiphysis of a metatarsal head becomes granular, fragmented, and flattened. *Treatment:* Good shoes ± metatarsal pad. Limit activity for 4–6 weeks. If severe, consider removal of affected bone with bone grafting or arthroplasty and use of a walking plaster.

21 The navicular is the bone at the top of the foot and is separated from the metatarsals by the 3 cuneiform bones with which it articulates. Moving proximally, it articulates with the talus. Navicula is Latin for a small ship. The term carpal navicular was formerly used for the scaphoid bone in the wrist.

Osgood–Schlatter disease Tibial tuberosity apophysitis affecting children 10–15yrs old. ♂:♀ ≈ 3:1. The 'accepted theory' suggests that repeated traction causes inflammation and chronic avulsion of the secondary ossification centre of the tibial tuberosity, leading to inflammation, hence its association with physical overuse. The pain below the knee is worse on strenuous activity and quadriceps contraction (lift straight leg against resistance). The tuberosity looks enlarged and is tender. Osgood–Schlatter disease is self-limiting in >90% of cases. *x-rays:* Tibial tuberosity enlargement (±fragmentation) (fig 7.57). Note the appearance of a normal immature tibial tuberosity, fig 7.56. MRI shows the tendonitis. NB: diagnosis is clinical, not simply radiological. *Treatment:* Standard treatment is limitation of activity, ice, oral anti-inflammatories, knee padding, and physiotherapy. Plaster cast immobilization is only used for severe pain which does not settle with simple measures. Tibial tubercle excision once skeletally mature may be recommended if these measures fail.[71]

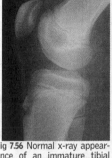

Fig 7.56 Normal x-ray appearance of an immature tibial tuberosity.

Courtesy of The Norfolk and Norwich University Hospitals (NNUH) Radiology Dept.

Sinding–Larsen disease (jumper's knee) Similar pathophysiology and treatment to Osgood–Schlatter disease but the onset tends to be 1–2yrs earlier. Traction tendinopathy with calcification in the proximal attachment of the tendon, which may be partially avulsed.

Sever disease This common calcaneal apophysitis is probably from strained attachment of the Achilles tendon. It is usually self-limiting. Typical age: 8–13yrs. There is pain behind the heel (bilateral in 60%) ± limping, and tenderness over the lower posterior calcaneal tuberosity. *x-rays:* Often normal. *Treatment:* Activity moderation, Achilles stretching, heel pads, and NSAIDs. If needed, a below-knee walking plaster may give pain relief. Most are well after 5 weeks.[72]

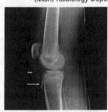

Fig 7.57 Osgood–Schlatter disease. Patellar tendon oedema (small arrow) and thin osseous density anterior to the apophysis of the tibial tuberosity (large arrow).

Reproduced with permission. Maher PJ, Ilgen JS Osgood-Schlatter disease *Case Reports* 2013;2013:bcr2012007614. doi: http://dx.doi.org/10.1136/bcr-2012-007614. Copyright © 2013, British Medical Journal.

Table 7.6 Eponyms of osteochondroses

Eponym	Site affected
Blount disease	Proximal tibial epiphysis
Freiberg disease (p. 508)	Head of 2nd or 3rd metatarsal
Friedrich disease	Clavicle
Köhler disease (p. 508)	Navicular bone
Osgood–Schlatter disease (p. 509)	Tuberosity of the tibia
Panner disease (p. 508)	Capitellum of humerus
Perthes disease (p. 490)	Hip
Scheuermann disease (p. 480)	Vertebral ring epiphyses
Sever disease (p. 509)	Calcaneal apophysis
Sinding–Larsen disease (p. 509)	Secondary patellar centre

Further reading

Cooper G (2014). *Osteochondritis Dissecans.* Medscape. http://emedicine.medscape.com/article/1253074

Maher PJ et al. (2013). Osgood-Schlatter disease. *BMJ Case Reports.* http://casereports.bmj.com/content/2013/bcr-2012-007614.full

The first recorded attempts at joint replacement were over 100 years ago. However, joint replacements as we would recognize them today have been performed since the 1960s. In 2017, 232,746 joint replacements were performed in England, Wales, and Northern Ireland. The number of procedures has risen annually and is predicted to continue rising. 93% of hips and 96% of knees were done for OA with a median age of 63 (hips) and 70 (knees).[73]

Early complications
• VTE[4%]
• Dislocation[3%]
• Deep infection[2%]
• Fracture[1%]
• Nerve palsy[1%]
• Limb-length discrepancy[1%]
• Death[0.4–0.7%] [75]

Preoperative assessment (6wks prior to operation.) Preoperative assessment of co-morbidities and ability to cope with rehabilitation must be thorough; it is likely to be complicated in this patient population. Give written information.[74]

Hip replacement Carried out to relieve pain and disability caused by arthropathies of the hip. Other conditions which may result in replacement are: rheumatoid arthritis; avascular necrosis of head of femur; congenitally dislocated hip; fractured neck of femur. 60% are women but incidence in men is increasing. *Total hip replacement (THR)* is where both the articular surfaces of femur and acetabulum are replaced. *Hip resurfacing* where only the joint surface is replaced is now rarely performed. *Hemiarthroplasty* where only the articular surface of femoral head is replaced is only indicated in patients with intracapsular #NOF p. 542. Many prostheses are available; most consist of a metal femoral component with an intramedullary stem which may be held in place by bone cement, or through a specially textured metal which encourages bone growth onto the stem. The acetabular 'cup' is either plastic, or metal with a plastic or ceramic liner—fig 7.35 on p. 489. 57% of UK hip replacements are cemented.[73] Younger patients typically receive uncemented prostheses. *Outcomes* can be determined by persistence of pain or proportion of patients who require revision. Early success of operation occurs in 90%. Later problems of loosening or infection are heralded by return of pain. If plain x-rays are inconclusive in the case of loosening, strontium or technetium scans may reveal increased bone activity. Suspected sepsis should be investigated by WCC, ESR, and aspiration in theatre. Revision arthroplasty is more successful for loosening than for infection.[76,77] *Joint survival:* 95% of primary hip replacements should still be *in situ* at 10 years[78]. Although there are occasions where it is indicated, be cautious in recommending replacement to those <60 years old as they will have a high chance of revision in their lifetime. Revision operations are more demanding both for surgeon and patient than the primary operation. Earlier replacement is used for rheumatoid arthritis as joints tend to be grossly affected at a younger age—and excessive delay may result in technically difficult surgery upon very rarefied osteoporotic bone.

Other joints Total joint arthroplasty is now used with success in many joints, including shoulder, elbow, wrist, finger, and ankle. The National Joint Registry records data on every joint arthroplasty implanted in the UK. It is critical in evaluating which areas of the body and which prostheses are successful. Joint spacers are used in finger joints for rheumatoid.

Knee replacement See p. 498.

Thromboembolic events See p. 528.

22 CRP returns to normal after 3 weeks and ESR returns to <20mm/h after 6 weeks.

Dislocation (mostly THR) Occurs in 0–5% of primary THR but risk is higher with revision surgery due to existing weakening of surrounding tissues. Causes for recurrent dislocations are multifactorial and include neuromuscular disease, inappropriate choice, or incorrect placement of implants. Typically relocation takes place under GA and rarely needs open surgery, but recurrent dislocations may require surgical revision. Preventable by comprehensive patient education and rehabilitation programmes.

Prosthetic loosening Most common contributor to failure of TKR in the long term. It can present with chronic pain or increased risk of fracture. Metal-on-metal hip replacement where all components are metal have a high incidence of loosening and pain. In addition they can cause aseptic lymphocyte dominated vasculitis-associated lesion (ALVAL), pseudotumours, and soft tissue reactions.

Periprosthetic fractures Occur most commonly around hip arthroplasties (1% after primary but 4% after revision[79]) and incidence is likely to rise as the age of the population increases. Typically present after trauma which can be minor (especially if prosthesis has started to loosen). Factors predisposing to periprosthetic fractures are osteoporosis and loosening of the implant (both septic and aseptic). Recently bisphosphonates have also been implicated.[80]

Infection Disastrous complication of joint replacement. Occurs in 1–2% of cases. It can be early (<3 months) or late. May present acutely with fever and suppuration or in a more indolent fashion with pain and loss of function due to loosening of components. Perioperative wound complications, obesity, increased age, diabetes mellitus, steroid use, and rheumatoid arthritis increase risk. Coagulase-negative staphylococci are the common infective organisms. *Investigations:* Although essential in diagnosis of chronic infection, CRP[22] is not helpful in early stages due to recent traumatic surgery, but joint aspiration with high WCC and clinical findings of acute joint swelling, erythema, and warmth with a fever is indicative.[81] Take blood cultures. Plain x-rays may show periprosthetic loosening. CT/MRI may be of limited use due to artefact. Gallium/labelled leucocyte imaging may be useful in hard to diagnose cases. *Treatment:* Early on, debridement + antibiotics may be enough. Later, with loosening of components, radical debridement must include removal of all prosthetic material, as well as any involved bone and soft tissue. Antibiotics may be needed for months. The joint is usually washed out and a 2-stage revision is performed which involves removing the prosthesis and cement mantle to debride the debris from the inside of the bone followed by implantation of an antibiotic-loaded cement spacer. This is functionally debilitating for the patient. If the infection is cleared, then reimplantation after >2 months can occur.

Antibiotic prophylaxis against prosthesis infection

- *Dentistry:* Infection with oral bacteria is rare; prophylaxis is not needed.[82]
- *Colonoscopy + polypectomy:* This may be more risky than dentistry; some recommend prophylaxis, if <6 months since replacement.
- *Antibiotic-impregnated cement?* The best prophylaxis might be achieved with a combination of gentamicin-impregnated cement, systemic antibiotics intraoperatively, and surgery performed in ultra-clean environments (laminar air flow theatres/surgeons in 'space suits').

Further reading

Buckley R (2014). *General Principles of Fracture Care Treatment & Management*. Medscape. http://emedicine.medscape.com/article/1270717

NICE (2011). *The Management of Hip Fractures in Adults (CG124)*. London: NICE.

Norris R et al. (2012). Occurrence of secondary fracture around intramedullary nails used for trochanteric hip fractures: a systematic review of 13,568 patients. *Injury* 43:706–11.

7 Orthopaedics

Joint aspirations *Diagnostic role:* Any blood, crystals, or pus? (See table 7.7 on p. 513 for diagnostic analysis.) *Therapeutic role:* For tense effusions, septic effusions, and haemarthroses. Approaches for specific joints are given here and on pp. 514-15. ▶Remember that aspiration of a joint with a prosthesis should only be done under the strictest sterile conditions (ie in the operating theatre) to minimize risk of introducing infection. *Equipment:* Check you have swabs, needles, and sterile bottles. For aspiration of viscid fluid (eg haemarthrosis) use a 19G needle. Use a 19G (white) needle for knees and hips, a 21G (green) needle for ankles, elbows, and shoulders. Locate joint margins carefully before cleaning; once the skin is clean, use scrupulous aseptic no-touch technique but even then, the skin is clean but not sterile. Samples for microbiology should be sent in sterile containers (also for cytology) and blood culture bottle. Radiological guidance may be needed for certain joints (eg hip, spine).

Steroid injections Injections to inflamed joints, bursae, or tendon sheaths aim to ↓ inflammation and relieve pain, perhaps by ↓ prostaglandin synthesis, stabilizing mast cells, or ↓ tissue calcification, or increasing vascularization and permeability of synovium. *Preparations:* Include methylprednisolone and triamcinolone (intermediate acting). They may be mixed with 1% lidocaine. When triamcinolone is used for injecting near short tendons, 10mg strength is preferred to 40mg as tendon rupture has been reported after the latter. Despite our best intentions, 'joint' injections often fail to meet their target (50% in one study in which contrast material was also injected); those off-target are less likely to relieve symptoms.[83]

Conditions responding to steroid injection Localized subacromial bursitis; large and small joint arthritis eg hip, knee, acromioclavicular, and sternoclavicular joints; arthritis of elbow, radioulnar, acromioclavicular, and sternoclavicular joints; ganglia; trigger fingers; de Quervain disease; suprapatellar, infrapatellar, and Achilles tendinopathy; plantar fasciitis; traumatic arthritis of metatarsophalangeal joints; and sesamoid 1st metatarsal joint, rheumatoid arthritis.

Be cautious In immunosuppressed patients, diabetics, blood clotting disorders, active infection, and nearby tumours. ▶ Never inject through cellulitis or into a prosthetic joint.

Side effects: Typically include pain at the injection site and skin atrophy/fading of skin pigment. Other side effects include: haemarthrosis, facial flushing, urticaria, post-injection flare syndrome (synovitis with fever), paresis, and septic arthritis (≤1 in 14,000 injections). ▶*It is essential that steroids are not used in septic conditions* and, if any doubt at all exists, results of synovial fluid culture should be awaited. Remember the possibility of tuberculous synovitis—especially in recent foreign travel. Repeated injections increases the risks of side effects: beware ligamentous laxity, joint instability, calcification, or tendon rupture.

Further reading

Courtney P *et al.* (2009). Joint aspiration and injection and synovial fluid analysis. *Best Pract Res Clin Rheumatol* 27:137–69.

Peterson C *et al.* (2011). Adverse events from diagnostic and therapeutic joint injections: a literature review. *Skeletal Radiol* 40:5–12.

Synovial fluid in health and disease

See table 7.7.

Blood, crystals, or pus? Aspiration of synovial fluid is used to diagnose haemarthroses, or infectious or crystal (gout and calcium pyrophosphate deposition CPPD—old name = pseudogout) arthropathies.

Table 7.7 Analysis of synovial fluid

	Appearance	Viscosity	WBC/m³	Neutrophils
Normal	Clear, colourless	High	<200	<25%
Non-inflammatory eg OA	Clear, straw	High	<5000	<25%
Haemorrhagic eg tumour, haemophilia, trauma	Bloody, xanthochromic	Variable	<10,000	<50%
Acute inflammatory*	Turbid, yellow	Decreased		
• Acute gout			~14,000	~80%
• Rheumatic fever			~18,000	~50%
• Rheumatoid arthritis			~16,000	~65%
Septic	Turbid, yellow	Decreased		
• TB			~24,000	~70%
• Gonorrhoeal			~14,000	~60%
• Septic (non-gonococcal)**			~16,000	~95%

* Includes eg Reiter syndrome, pseudogout, SLE, etc.
** Includes staphs, streps, Lyme disease, and Pseudomonas (eg post-op).

Managing carpal tunnel syndrome (CTS)

See p. 555 for clinical features.

Tests Nerve conduction studies can be helpful in complex or mixed symptoms as well as monitoring responses to surgery. Ultrasonography and MRI can help identify lesions.[84]

Management Treat any treatable association (see MINIBOX 'CTS associations'). Rest, weight reduction, and wrist splints are 1st line for both alleviation of symptoms and also reducing risk of recurrence. 20% of cases will spontaneously resolve. *Splinting* in a neutral position alone was sufficient to relieve symp-

CTS associations
• Hypothyroidism
• Pregnancy; the pill
• Gout & pseudogout
• Diabetes; obesity
• Cardiac failure
• Acromegaly
• Rheumatoid arthritis
• Premenstrual state
• Amyloidosis

toms and avoid surgery in 37% of patients.[85=176] *Corticosteroid injections* are widely used for short-term (10 weeks) pain relief in mild to moderate disease but when compared to placebo at 1 year there was no difference and 75% of patients still needed surgery within 1 year.[86] There are no adequate guidelines for repeated injections after the first successful injection wears off. Seek expert help before injecting patients with clinically severe or complex disease, diabetes, or the elderly as outcome may be worse.

Injection technique: Introduce the needle angled at ~45° just proximal to the distal wrist crease, to the ulnar side of palmaris longus. ▶Do not use local anaesthetic. If the patient reports an 'electric shock' then you are probably touching the nerve. Redirect the needle towards the ulnar side and then inject 25mg **hydrocortisone acetate**. The intention is to deliver steroid around the flexor tendons and not into the carpal tunnel itself. A splint worn for the next few days may mitigate symptoms which can occur at the time of injection. *Carpal tunnel decompression:* Release of the flexor retinaculum has a well-documented success rate for more permanent results.[87] Endoscopic release is as effective as the standard open approach in terms of symptom relief and functional status, although the endoscopic approach may be associated with better grip strength and a faster return to work.[88] Complications are rare, but persistence of symptoms, reduced grip, and pillar pain (deep aching pain at the base of the thenar eminence and across wrist) can persist up to 2 years and must be explained to the patient.

Shoulder injection As shoulder pain from soft tissue causes are common (lifetime incidence ~10%), and pain can be chronic (≤23% resolve within 4wks), this is one of the most commonly injected joints. There is no difference between 40mg and 80mg of steroid; however, use large volumes eg 5–10mL as small volumes are at risk of being injected into structures rather than around them.

Subacromial injection: (Impingement syndrome, calcific tendinitis, see p. 472.) While standing behind, seat the patient with arm resting on lap. Palpate 2cm medial and inferior to the end of the spine of the scapula (easily palpable). Aim tip of needle towards the anterolateral tip of the acromion. *Intra-articular injection:* (Arthritis, frozen shoulder.) While standing behind, seat the patient with arm resting on lap. Palpate 2cm medial and inferior to the end of the spine of the scapula (easily palpable). Aim needle directly towards the coracoid process felt anteriorly. If the needle hits bone, then external rotation of the arm will help the needle drop into the joint. ►*Do not go medial to the coracoid process (neurovascular structures, p. 557 figs 8.38 & 8.39).*

Lateral approach: (Subacromial bursitis, impingement syndrome.) Inject 25–50mg **hydrocortisone acetate** with lidocaine just below the lateral tip of the acromion, pointing downwards and advancing medially. If the needle is withdrawn from touching the head of humerus with slight pressure on the plunger, a drop in pressure is felt as the bursa is entered.

Knee joint The patient lies with knee supported, slightly flexed and muscles relaxed. Palpate the joint space behind patella either medially or laterally—the lateral approach may be less reliable.[88] Insert a needle between the patella and femur, aiming slightly posteriomedially. Slight resistance is felt on traversing the synovial membrane; it should be possible to aspirate fluid, and injection fluid should flow easily. Ultrasound guidance may result in less procedural pain, greater synovial fluid yield, and improved clinical outcomes.[90] *Usual doses:* 25–50mg **hydrocortisone acetate**, 40mg **methylprednisolone**, 20mg **triamcinolone**. Repeat injections should be longer than 3 months apart. If injection is used for prepatellar bursitis, give 25mg **hydrocortisone acetate** into the most tender spot.

The ankle Plantar flex foot slightly, palpate joint margin between tibialis anterior (the most medial) and extensor hallucis longus (lateral to tibialis anterior) tendons just above the top of medial malleolus. Inject 25mg **hydrocortisone acetate** into the joint. See fig 7.58a.

Biceps tendinopathy No longer injected as the risk of biceps tendon rupture is high, us-guided injection lessens the risk.[91]

Wrist injection Locate Lister's tubercle (bony prominence on the dorsal aspect of the radius) and inject 25mg **hydrocortisone acetate** into the 'soft spot' just above to this, 1–1.5cm deep.

De Quervain's tenosynovitis Extensor pollicis brevis and abductor pollicis longus tendons—on traversing the extensor retinaculum on the dorsal wrist—may cause a tender swelling (p. 476). With needle almost parallel to skin pointing proximally, inject 25mg **hydrocortisone acetate** slowly just distal or proximal to the radial styloid, at the site of maximum tenderness. If needle in tendon, injection is difficult so withdraw until easy flow occurs. See fig 7.58b.

Trigger finger (fig 7.59) Insert needle at MCP skin crease parallel to flexor tendon, pointing to palm. Palpate tendon thickening in palm; proceed as for de Quervain's. See p. 477 for more information on trigger fingers. ►When injecting a trigger finger, ask the patient to flex and extend the finger to ensure that the tip of the needle is not in the tendon.

1st carpometacarpal joint of thumb Avoiding radial artery, inject 25mg **hydrocortisone acetate** at base of 1st metacarpal at 1cm depth in anatomical snuffbox (aim at base of little finger). ►In all areas, learn from an expert.

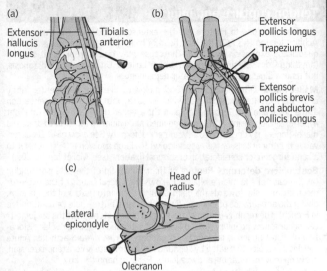

Fig 7.58 (a) Dorsal aspect of the right ankle indicating anatomical landmarks—shown here is the anterior ankle approach. (b) Dorsal aspect of the right wrist indicating anatomical landmarks—shown here from left to right are the injection sites for the wrist joint, de Quervain's tenosynovitis, & the 1st carpometacarpal joint. (c) The right elbow, flexed—shown from left to right the posterior and lateral approaches.⁹⁷

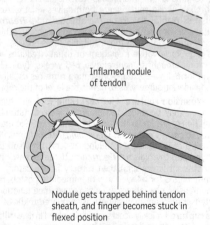

Fig 7.59 Trigger finger.

Further reading

Vitale MA (2014). Doc, will this injection make my trigger finger go away? *Bone Joint Surg Am* 96:e191.

The main tendons to rupture are the extensor tendons of the fingers, the Achilles tendon (fig 7.61), the long head of biceps, the supraspinatus, and the quadriceps expansion (fig 7.60). The cause may be sharp or blunt trauma (anything from sporting injuries to rubber bullets). Ultrasound aids diagnosis, but its usefulness is largely operator dependent.

Mallet finger Often caused by a sudden blow to an extended finger (eg hit by cricketball on outstretched finger) which leads to rupture of the extensor tendon at the distal phalanx. *Treatment:* Splint the affected digit for 6 weeks (in slight hyper-extension) using a Stack or moulded aluminium splint. If untreated, the mallet finger may develop into a swan-neck deformity. See *OHCM* p540. If conservative treatment fails, or it is associated with a large avulsion # (>30%), refer to a hand surgeon for consideration of surgical fixation[93] (see 'Mallet toes', p. 500.)

Boutonnière deformity Rupture of the central slip of the extensor tendon (at the base of the middle phalanx) allows the lateral bands of the extensor mechanism to slip towards the palm, turning them into flexors of the PIP joint, giving the appearance of poking a finger through a button hole (= boutonnière in French). The result is flexion at the PIP and hyperextension of the DIP joint. It can occur following injury (forced flexion of extended PIP joint or volar dislocation of distal finger at PIP joint) or secondary to rheumatoid arthritis. Acute injuries are typically treated by splinting PIP in complete & constant extension, allowing movement at DIP and MCP joints. Refer to hand therapy.

Achilles (calcaneal) tendon rupture Typified by sudden pain at the back of the ankle during running or jumping as the tendon ruptures. Pain may be perceived as a 'kick' rather than actual pain. It is possible to walk (with a limp), and some plantar flexion of the foot remains, but it is impossible to raise the heel from the floor when standing on the affected leg. A gap may be palpated in the tendon course (particularly within 24h of injury). *The squeeze test* (Simmonds' or Thompsons' test) is sensitive: ask the patient to kneel on a chair, while you squeeze both calves—if the Achilles is ruptured, there is less plantar flexion on the affected side. *Treatment:* Tendon repair (percutaneous or open) is often preferred by young, athletic patients. Conservative treatment may be most suitable for smokers, diabetics, and those >50yrs old. Conservative management usually requires initial casting in equinus position brought to neutral over 6–8 weeks. Typically there is no weight-bearing for 6–8 weeks. Late-presenting ruptures usually need reconstructing. If considering surgery, US to define the level of the rupture.[94]

Quadriceps expansion rupture (fig 7.62) Quite rare and typically affects >40yr-olds. Injury may be direct (eg blow) or indirect (stumbling causing sudden contraction of the apparatus). Jumper's knee (p. 496) may predispose. *Look for systemic causes of tendon weakening:* Steroid abuse (especially in spontaneous rupture in athletes); pseudogout (CPPD); Wilson disease; renal failure with hyperparathyroidism.[95] *Treatment:* If the extensor mechanism is disrupted (no straight leg raising) then surgery is mandatory. After repair, the knee is immobilized for >4 weeks with immediate postoperative weight-bearing; then intensive physiotherapy helps regain knee function. Many have persistent extensor mechanism weakness as compared to the other leg.

Distal biceps rupture Typically occurs in men involved in heavy lifting. Presents with a history of something 'tearing' or 'popping' and pain in the antecubital fossa with bruising over the medial forearm. Needs urgent surgical repair.

Further reading

Taylor DW *et al.* (2011). A systematic review of the use of platelet-rich plasma in sports medicine as a new treatment for tendon and ligament injuries. *Clin J Sport Med* 21:344–52.

Wilkins R *et al.* (2012). Operative versus nonoperative management of acute Achilles tendon ruptures. A quantitative systematic review of randomized controlled trials. *Am J Sports Med* 40:2154–60.

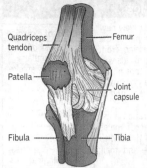

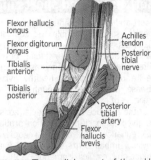

Fig 7.60 The quadriceps (extensor) expansion encloses the patella and inserts into the tibial tuberosity as the patellar tendon. Rupture can occur at the site of quadriceps insertion to the patella, through the patella by fracture, or by avulsion of the patellar tendon from the tibial tuberosity.

Fig 7.61 The medial aspect of the ankle, showing the extensor and flexor tendons of the foot. The Achilles tendon tends to rupture ~5cm proximal to its insertion into the calcaneus. Also note the ordering of the flexor tendons posterior to the medial malleolus, from anterior to posterior—this can be remembered with the mnemonic on p. 463: **T**om, **D**ick and **A V**ery **N**ervous **H**arry.

The foot arches

Pes planus (flat feet) The medial longitudinal arch (fig 7.62) collapses—leading to the whole sole nearly coming in contact with the ground. Flat feet are normal when a child is learning to walk. The medial arch develops over the next few years. In adults flat feet are associated with dysfunction of the posterior tibialis tendon (PTT) (a dynamic stabilizer of the medial arch). In most, it is asymptomatic and may not need intervention if the arch restores itself on standing on tiptoe (eg a 'mobile' flat foot). Pain may develop medially over the PTT and there may be

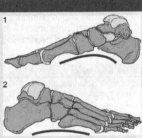

Fig 7.62 The medial (1) and lateral (2) longitudinal arches of the foot.

progressive forefoot abduction and hindfoot valgus deformity with loss of ability to heel rise, as the condition progresses. Weight loss, supportive shoes (with insoles), orthosis may help in mild cases.[96] Pain and limitations in sport tend to be post-op complications so don't advise surgery lightly.

Pes cavus Accentuated longitudinal foot arches which do not flatten with weight-bearing. May be idiopathic, or associated with an underlying neurological condition (see MINIBOX 'Pes cavus associations'). Claw toes may occur, as weight is taken on metatarsal heads when walking (hence causing pain). *Other symptoms:* Difficulty with shoes; foot fatigue; mobility ↓; ankle instability/sprains; callosities. *If foot used to be normal, refer to a neurologist.* If orthoses and custom footwear fail, surgical procedures include soft tissue releases, tendon transfers, arthrodesis.[97]

Pes cavus associations
• Spina bifida
• Cerebral palsy
• Polio
• Muscular dystrophy
• Charcot–Marie–Tooth dis.
• Syringomyelia
• Friedreich's ataxia
• Spinal tumour

Sport and exercise medicine (SEM) is a relatively new medical specialty. While the central theme is the diagnosis and management of injury arising from participation in sport, including but not exclusively elite athletes, it has an increasingly important public health role: promoting healthy living and chronic disease management through exercise (see MINIBOX 'Benefits of exercise').[98]

Benefits of exercise
Reduced risk of:
• Cardiovascular disease and stroke
• Diabetes
• Obesity
• Osteoporosis
• Dementia
• Certain cancers
Improved:
• Immune response
• Psychological well-being
• Sleeping patterns

In the practice of SEM, special consideration must be given to specific population groups—eg females (± pregnancy), children, older people, and those with physical impairments/spinal cord injury—and their unique physiological demands.[23]

Pre-participation Preparation and safety is paramount in minimizing risk of injury and improving performance outcomes both recreationally and at an elite level; avoiding adverse outcomes should always be regarded as preferential to their management (see table 7.8). You should carefully consider the impact of known medical conditions but also those that are potentially undiagnosed eg the need for cardiac screening in elite athletes.

The medical practitioner should encourage the patient to control factors that can be controlled and prepare for those that cannot. Initial measures to be taken include: appropriate training and technique prior to participation; comprehensive warming up and cooling down to protect the participant from soft tissue and joint injuries; the correct use of strapping for the provision of additional joint support and proprioceptive feedback; and extra care if over-reaching to avoid overtraining syndrome.

Table 7.8 Potential factors influencing risk of injury and performance

External factors	Internal factors
Environment (climate, altitude, playing surface)	Pre-existing health conditions
Sports type	Previous injury
Opponent	Current fitness level and correct technique
Equipment	Hydration and nutrition
Technology	Warm up and cool down

Injury assessment SEM spans primary to tertiary care and encompasses a large multidisciplinary team: medics, surgeons, radiologists, physiotherapists, nutritionists, psychologists, epidemiologists, orthotics, and sports scientists, among others. Each sport and activity possesses a particular injury profile, whereby certain injuries are more likely due to the nature of the specific sport eg shoulder injuries are more frequent in contact sports such as rugby than they are in football, due to the physicality required in the tackle. As in other areas of medicine, a thorough history and understanding of the injury mechanism is paramount, and is complemented by appropriate clinical examination. Investigations are more readily available at the elite level, with near-patient US a desirable skill of the sports medicine doctor.[99]

When working 'pitch-side' for a sports team be aware of the variety of complaints and injuries that may emerge; you can find yourself as general practitioner, emergency doctor, and musculoskeletal specialist. In one afternoon the sports medic may have to deal with earache, a traumatic eye injury, head injury with loss of consciousness, and knee pain, highlighting the importance of versatility and a broad knowledge base.

23 We thank Dr Gemma Phillips for help with this topic.

7 Orthopaedics

Concussion and sport-specific protocols

Concussion is a minor traumatic brain injury. It has a variable presentation that includes (to name a few) nausea, dizziness, headache, unsteadiness, and visual disturbance. It is not always associated with loss of consciousness and when subtle can be very tricky to spot. Emerging evidence has suggested not only immediate concerns of subsequent increased injury risk and second impact syndrome, but a long-term potential for chronic neurological impairment. Many sports have implemented specific guidance for the assessment and management for head injuries/concussion, including a graduated return to play—protecting players and empowering medical teams. Please refer to the 2017 Zurich consensus statement on concussion in sport for more information.[100]

Injury management Overuse injuries are widely seen in all levels of SEM, where repetitive mechanical stress outweighs the body's mechanism for recovery. An example would be *iliotibial band (ITB) syndrome*. The ITB passes over the lateral tibial tuberosity during knee flexion, friction here causes local inflammation producing lateral knee pain on movement and direct palpation. As with all soft tissue injuries, a protocol of 'RICE' (rest, ice, compression, and elevation) is recommended in the first instance (NB: icing should be limited to maximum of 20-minute sessions, with a barrier between the cold surface and skin, to limit local cold injuries). Judicial use of NSAIDs in those without contraindications in the short term can be helpful for analgesia and treatment, followed by a suitable rehabilitation programme: stretching exercises of the ITB, gluteal strengthening, and a graduated return to the ITB-stressing activity. In severe cases, specialist review and steroid injection is an option but the risk of tendon rupture must be balanced.[101] For elite athletes, the threshold for specialist intervention and active management (including surgery) is lower for all injuries. In professional sport always be aware of antidoping regulations, it is highly recommended to become an accredited UK Antidoping (UKAD) Advisor (www.ukad.org.uk).

Ethics in sports medicine

A fundamental aspect of medicine is to first do no harm, a principle that can be difficult to define, let alone follow, when the objective of the patient is personal and professional success in a career that is anything but health promoting. Ethics is a pertinent feature of SEM with the typical doctor–patient relationship mixed with potentially competing interests. You should consider the individual's understanding of, and capacity to make, each decision in a given situation bearing in mind the combined personal and external (coach/team/media/fans/timing) pressures. Remember, careers are often short lived, athletes are competing for their livelihoods—a drive which must not be underestimated or ignored. Consider their perspective: 'If I come off the pitch injured today does it compromise my first-team position? I have a family that needs to be supported, will this impact my future contract and income? How will I be perceived by my team mates and coaches?' You may find yourself deciding during the half time break of a cup final, whether you should permit the star-player carrying an injury to remain on the field despite the potential for longer-term adverse implications. As an SEM practitioner in a professional sporting environment it is inevitable that a fine line will exist between maintaining doctor–patient trust, prioritizing patient welfare, and protecting your own professional integrity, all the while trying to balance good working relations with coaches and management. At times, you may find yourself advocating for the athlete's longer-term interests—often these decisions are the most difficult.

Further reading

British Association of Sport and Exercise Medicine: www.basem.co.uk

Holm S *et al.* (2009). Ethics in sports medicine. *BMJ* 339:b3898.

McCrory P *et al.* (2017). Consensus statement on concussion in sport: the 5th International Conference on Concussion in Sport. *Br J Sports Med* 2017;51:838–47.

Managing trauma patients involves having a systematic approach. These patients commonly have both internal and external injuries which are potentially life-threatening. When assessing major trauma patients, a focused history and C A (+ c-spine) B C D E examination is mandatory (as per Advanced Trauma Life Support (ATLS®) principles, see p. 587). Appropriate imaging must be arranged urgently but this must not delay the treatment of life-threatening issues.

This chapter aims to guide you through orthopaedic trauma, look to the 'Emergency medicine' chapter to address major trauma (see p. 586).

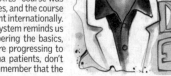

Fig 8.1 Dr James K Styner. After crashing his light aircraft (in which his wife was instantly killed and 3 of his 4 children left unconscious), Dr James K Styner flagged down a passing car to be taken to the local hospital, which on arrival was closed. The doctors that did assemble had little training in managing serious trauma. Following this personal tragedy, Styner knew the system had to change and collaborated with colleagues to develop the Advanced Trauma Life Support (ATLS®) process which has revolutionized the management of trauma patients. In 1978, the first ATLS® course was taught by Styner and his colleagues, and the course is now in its 10th edition, and taught internationally. The simple ABCDE (now CAcBCDE) system reminds us all of the importance of remembering the basics, and managing one problem before progressing to the next. When managing trauma patients, don't panic, stick to your system, and remember that the patient is twice as frightened as you.

Artwork by Gillian Turner.

Further reading
Image bank: www.trauma.org
www.radiologymasterclass.co.uk

With many thanks to our junior reader Aung Oo for their contribution to this chapter.

Describing a fracture over the phone can be intimidating. Know your anatomy and the following basic descriptive terms before you start.

Description *Site:* Bone(s) involved; which part of the bone is broken (proximal, middle, or distal—useful to split the bone into thirds for this). *Is a joint involved ('intraarticular')? Is the growth plate involved ('epiphyseal'—in children)?* (See table 8.2 for Salter–Harris classification.) *Obliquity:* Transverse; short oblique; spiral; multi-fragmentary. *Displacement:* Can be described in terms of rotation, angulation, shortening, and translation. Compare placement (in degrees or %) of distal fragment with respect to proximal fragment so when giving a displacement description, this refers to the *distal* fragment. For angulated fractures, the terms 'apex dorsal' and 'apex palmar' can be used in the hand. *Fracture pattern:* Can be simple (spiral, oblique, or transverse), buckle, greenstick, wedge, comminuted (splintered fragments), or segmental (multiple breaks in the bone creating at least 3 fragments). Avulsion of a fragment occurs when a tendon or ligament pulls a fragment of bone away. *Impaction:* Can occur if the 2 sides of the fracture are 'rammed' together and may cause shortening, try and estimate the extent. *Dislocation* may occur along with a fracture. Does the joint look normal? *Soft tissues:* Typically assessed on examination. Neurovascular status? Always consider compartment syndrome (see BOX 'Compartment syndrome', p. 528). *Open:* (Formerly known as compound). The Gustilo classification is most commonly used for open fractures (table 8.1 p. 524).

▸▸Take a full history. Was a fall due to sudden dizziness that may need an ECG and a medical review? Is the fracture you are focusing on part of a larger trauma case (see p. 586 for ATLS® principles)? Look for more occult signs of injury.

8 Trauma

A game of trauma?

We encourage you to think about the mechanism of injury when assessing a fracture (see p. 628, 'Read the wreckage'). Is it a little grandmother who FOOSH (fell on outstretched hand) (see p. 534 for Colles-type fractures)? Or is it a young chap falling off a horse (see pp. 558-9 for spinal cord injuries)? Each era has been associated with different accidents (fig 8.2). Consider the Hangman's fracture (forced hyperextension of the neck causing fracture of both c2 pedicles; fig 7.7 p. 467). This was historically named after judicial hangings, yet postmortem studies showed that only a few hangings actually demonstrated this injury pattern.[1] The majority of eponyms arise from recent times, but the medieval era was a vicious and bloody one—yet there are no residual eponyms. This time was called the Dark Ages, not because there were so many (k)nights, but because there is a paucity of historical records kept as compared to the wealth of knowledge which is now documented. It is likely they did have eponymous fracture patterns among each community. Next time you watch any battles onscreen, pay attention to the mechanisms of injury. Archaeological studies have demonstrated that fracture immobilization and reduction likely took place[2] and that farming injuries were very common.

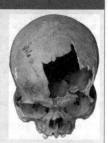

Fig 8.2 This adult skull was found amid medieval remains in Norway. Just like modern medicine, the clues to aetiology lie in noting the surroundings. Was farming equipment used in defence against a Viking raid, or was this a more formal battle scene?

Reproduced with permission from Brødholt, E. T. and Holck, P. (2012), Skeletal trauma in the burials from the royal church of St. Mary in medieval Oslo. *Int. J. Osteoarchaeol.*, 22: 201–218. doi:10.1002/oa.1198. Copyright © 2010 John Wiley & Sons, Ltd.

The aim is to provide information that will alter management, without exposing patients to unnecessary radiation—think especially of the radiation exposure to thyroid in c-spine x-rays, gonads in pelvic views, and to the eyes in skull and facial x-rays (lens cataracts are the risk). It is impossible to protect the ovaries. For example, each lumbar spine x-ray=2.2mSv=40 cxRs. The Sievert (Sv) is the si unit of radiation absorbed by biological tissues—see *OHCM* p719. This dose may be expected to cause 16 malignancies/yr in the UK at current rates of exposure. Guidelines which help clinicians make sensible radiology requests yield substantial savings in costs and in patients' waiting times, without compromising patient care.
▶Remember to treat and assess the patient, not just the radiological findings.

When an x-ray is indicated, consider the 'Rule of 2s':
• 2 views (often AP and lateral views, but some need joint-specific views such as the AP mortise view[1] for ankles and the odontoid peg for c-spine).
• 2 joints (above and below the fracture site of an extremity).
• 2 times (pre- and post any intervention to the dislocation or fracture).

Twisting injury of foot/ankle Follow the Ottawa rules & fig 7.2 on p.465 but all rules have exceptions, and, on occasion, we've all seen patients walk on a fractured ankle.

Injury to the cervical spine The consequences of a missed c-spine injury are disastrous, and so imaging is always performed for major trauma. Remember that you should be able to see the top of T1 vertebra on a c-spine x-ray.

In patients who have been subjected to less violent trauma, when should imaging be requested? Based on the *Nexus criteria*[3] for imaging of blunt injury, the following factors (mnemonic NSAID) are important, though may have the drawback of a low sensitivity if applied as the sole criteria for imaging:
• Neurological exam reveals a focal deficit.
• Spine exam reveals tenderness (posterior midline).
• Alteration in consciousness.
• Intoxication.
• Distracting injury—ie long bone #, clavicle #, chest trauma, etc.

The Canadian c-spine[4] rules are more specific but more complicated. High-risk factors (dangerous mechanism, age >65, focal neurology) mandate an x-ray. Absence of these allows consideration of low-risk factors (simple rear-end RTC, sitting up in ED, ambulatory at any time, delayed onset of pain, absence of midline c-spine tenderness)—the presence of any 1 low-risk factor allows clinical examination of the neck: if the patient can rotate their neck 45° left and right they do not need an x-ray. Don't rely on mobile equipment; if possible, take to the radiology department, supervising all movements closely. If there is a clear spinal cord injury, and the patient is stable, CT is the 1st line of imaging (see p.523). Image the whole spine as there may be >1 injury. MRI shows fractures, subluxations, disc disruption and protrusion, and cord contusion—and helps establish prognosis. ▶NB: MRI is hard to arrange in emergency settings, and takes a lot longer than CT (eg 20min vs 20sec). Consider CT myelography if MRI is contraindicated.

See pp.590–1 for head injury associated with neck injury.

Nose injury Imaging in ED is not indicated in simple nasal injury.

Rib injury A CXR is only indicated if you suspect a pneumothorax; rib views are not needed in uncomplicated blunt injury as presence of a rib fracture will not alter your management.

Lumbar spine pain Avoid x-rays in 1st 6 weeks if there are no factors suggesting serious disease eg trauma, focal neurology, fever, malignancy. See pp.486–7.

Foreign bodies Always x-ray if the presence of glass is possible (glass is usually radiopaque). Ultrasound can also be used in foreign body detection and to guide removal, especially for those that are not radio opaque (eg splinters).

1 AP mortise view (foot is held in 15° internal rotation) to assess presence of talar shift.

Quick, accurate, and available: good reasons to think of CT as 1st-line imaging for trauma patients. But there are caveats, as any radiologist who has seen images arriving at their workstation monitor, only to have to comment that the patient's heart has stopped, will tell you. The appropriateness of scanning in an acute trauma must be decided on the balance of risk and benefit to the patient. It is not that radiologists don't want sick patients in their department; radiology departments just aren't the best place to be if you are very sick. ►*Ensure that the patient is haemodynamically stable before moving them to the relatively resource-poor radiology department.* Some centres have tried to overcome this problem by bringing CT to the ED. A CT is no substitute for a stethoscope. Remember that *radiation can do harm:* it cannot be used limitlessly (OHCM p719). *Imaging is just a snapshot:* a 'normal' scan mustn't allow for complacency in patient observation. ►*Always be on the lookout for clinical deterioration requiring prompt intervention. Imaging takes time:* transfers and interpretation take the longest: CT itself may only take 20sec. This is time that the patient is at risk and also time delaying definitive management.

CT in major trauma Performed according to a specific protocol in most departments, and should include the head, c-spine, thorax, abdomen, and pelvis. It is indicated when the mechanism of injury suggests a high possibility of serious injury, or there is obvious severe injury on clinical assessment.

CT of the cervical spine Quick and effective. Meta-analysis suggests that CT be used as the 1st-line investigation in those with a depressed mental status, though not as a matter of course for less severe injury, in which plain x-ray should still be used.[5] It is also indicated if an injury is seen on the plain film series and if there is inadequate visualization (C7/T1 can be difficult to image in full with plain x-ray.) Remember that MRI may still be needed to assess the vital soft tissue structures.

CT guidelines for head injury See p. 591.

CT of the chest Evidence of traumatic injury on CXR that warrants further imaging: • Haemothorax • Pneumothorax • Widened mediastinum (all difficult to spot on a supine film) • Pneumomediastinum • Posterior rib fractures • Fractures of ribs 1 or 2 • Pulmonary contusion.

CT of the abdomen and pelvis Usually done together. Indications may include: • Free fluid noted on FAST scan (p. 587) • Suspicion of retroperitoneal haemorrhage • Renal trauma (macroscopic haematuria, microscopic haematuria + shock).

►*Remember to think of patterns of injury:* eg rib fractures with bilateral pulmonary contusions have a high coincidence of intra-abdominal injury.

CT of the appendicular skeleton Part of preoperative planning for complex injury patterns.

MRI Especially useful for bony lesions such as tumours, osteomyelitis, or osteonecrosis and soft tissue pathology such as meniscal or shoulder rotator cuff tears.

Further reading

Royal College of Radiologists. *Standards of Practice and Guidance for Trauma Radiology in Severely Injured Patients* (2nd ed). www.rcr.ac.uk/standards

Stiell JG *et al.* (2001). The Canadian c-spine rule for radiography in alert and stable trauma patients. *JAMA* 286:1841–8.

Vinson DR (2001). Nexus cervical spine criteria. *Ann Emerg Med* 37:237–8.

A fracture is a soft tissue injury with an associated break in the bone. Remember that although terminology around fractures may be familiar to the patient, thanks to the plethora of hospital-based drama and reality TV available, the meanings of these terms will differ from one person to the next. While some patients will be comforted to know that 'it's only a fracture' others will think the same word means major surgery is required, and be terrified. Explore what they think you mean when you tell them about their injury. In many cases, it doesn't matter whether patients know that a fracture and a broken bone are the same thing, what matters to them is what this means for their function, their job, and their home life. Although jargon is to be approached with caution in this situation, always use appropriate terminology when *describing x-rays to colleagues* (p. 521).

Fracture healing (fig 8.3) In adults, x-ray changes showing callus formation around the fracture site can be seen 8–12 weeks post injury. A rule of thumb for fracture healing is given by the 'rule of 3s'. A *closed, paediatric, metaphyseal, upper limb* fracture is the simplest and will heal in 3 weeks. Any 'complicating factor' *doubles* the healing time ie adult; diaphyseal; lower limb; open injury. For example, an *adult (6), diaphyseal (12) forearm* fracture may take 12 weeks to heal. Likewise an *open (6), adult (12), diaphyseal (24), tibia (48)* may be expected to take 48 weeks (almost a year!) to heal. Metaphysis and epiphysis are defined on p. 491 (fig 7.39). See also fig 8.4.

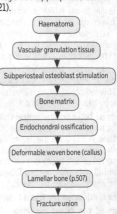

Fig 8.3 Bone healing.

Fracture healing depends on the position and stability of the bone segments, but is also influenced by the patient's general health (MINIBOX 'Risk factors for poor healing') and difficulties with wound such as local infection and neurovascular compromise.

Use the *Gustilo classification* (table 8.1)[6] to describe the severity of open fractures. (see also p. 527) Note that grade 3 implies significant neurovascular compromise. It is the most commonly used, but other classification systems may offer enhanced evaluation (eg Tscherne and Hanover fracture scales).

Pathological fractures See p. 567.

Risk factors for poor healing
• Older age
• Co-morbidities (esp. diabetes)
• Recent trauma
• Smoker (see p. 525)
• Osteoporosis
• Corticosteroids
• NSAIDs
• Local complications to fracture

Table 8.1 Gustilo classification of open fractures

Type I	*Low-energy* wounds <1cm long eg caused by bone piercing skin
Type II	*Low-energy* wounds >1cm, causing moderate soft tissue damage
Type III	All *high-energy* injuries irrespective of wound size:
	• IIIA fractures have *adequate* local soft tissue coverage
	• IIIB fractures have *inadequate* local soft tissue coverage
	• IIIC implies arterial injury needing repair

Source: data from Gustilo RB *et al.* Prevention of infection in the treatment of one thousand and twenty-five open fractures of long bones: retrospective and prospective analyses. *Journal of Bone & Joint Surgery*, 1976, Volume 58(4), pp.453–8 and Gustilo RB et al. Problems in the management of type III (severe) open fractures: a new classification of type III open fractures. *Journal of Trauma and Acute Care Surgery*, 1984, Volume 24(8), pp.742–6.

8 Trauma

Smoking and tissue healing—the consequences of a cigarette break

Trauma patients need to knit back together well, and they face a number of complications without adding tobacco into the physiological equation. Smokers have increased risk of perioperative complications (VTE, respiratory tract infection, & cardiac ischaemia) and reduced fracture healing.

What damage are smokers doing? Nicotine increases the time it takes for a fracture to unite *and* reduces quality of bone healing. Tobacco smoking also reduces tissue oxygenation and wound healing. This is particularly pertinent for operations on the lower extremities—eg Achilles tendon repair (p. 516) or calcaneal fracture ORIF—because of the precarious local blood supply combined with a propensity for compartment syndrome, ▶p. 528.

Is it justifiable to withhold surgery from smokers? Perhaps 'yes', if a given problem has a non-operative alternative with similar outcome yet potentially disastrous complications exacerbated by smoking: eg a calcaneal ORIF spiralling out of control into an amputation. Also perhaps 'yes', if resources must be distributed across a population in whom smokers are shown to fare much worse with a given operative management. The ethical counterpoise would be from a discriminatory angle, both in terms of costs and the concept of self-inflicted harm—eg in comparison to dangerous sporting activity.[2]

How to approach the issue Careful informed consent will be vital, though whether scare tactics are allowed is another matter altogether. Abstaining for 6–8 weeks prior to elective surgery will reduce many of the side effects of smoking, but this is not a luxury afforded to trauma patients, and for some the stresses of what has happened may be too much to place on top of stopping smoking.[3] Do smokers mobilize more keenly in the post-op period in response to their craving to get off the ward for a cigarette? There appear to be no studies to answer this yet! For giving *advice on stopping smoking*, see p. 825.

Salter and Harris classification of epiphyseal injury

See fig 8.4 and table 8.2. Injuries to and around the growth plate can be difficult to distinguish from normal appearances, especially when they are viewed obliquely. Most physes are in a plane that makes it relatively easy to diagnose the injury (eg distal radius, and to a lesser extent proximal femur), whereas some cross the plane of the x-ray at multiple angles (eg proximal humerus). With these trickier physes, it is wise to liaise with someone with experience. Also consider comparison with the contralateral side.

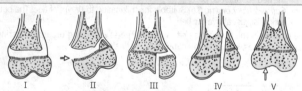

Fig 8.4 Salter and Harris classification of epiphyseal injury.

Table 8.2 Salter and Harris classification

I	Seen in babies or pathological conditions (eg scurvy)
II	The commonest injury, with the fracture line *above* the growth plate
III	There is a displaced fragment, with the fracture line *below* the growth plate
IV	Fracture across the growth plate, may interfere with bone growth
V	Compression of the epiphysis causes deformity and stunting

2 With pressure to provide a cost-effective and fair service in the NHS, there are strong arguments from both parties. The debate certainly does not allow for smoke without fire ...
3 Though even stopping just 1 day before surgery has been shown to improve outcome.

8 Trauma

The following principles of fracture management aim to restore the limb to its maximal biomechanical function:

1 Anatomical reduction (realignment) of fracture fragments.
2 Stabilization of fragments to enable normal activity (eg surgical fixation or splinting in a cast).
3 Maintaining neurovascular (NV) supply.
4 Encouraging early rehabilitation.

Conservative management Uses splints (see p. 526), casts, slings, and traction to realign and stabilize displaced fractures. This may also allow neurovascular structures trapped or damaged by the fracture to function. ▶▶Occasionally reduction will be required immediately to preserve NV status ie in ED before an x-ray is even taken (eg for fracture-dislocation of the ankle or knee). Manipulation under anaesthesia (for analgesia and muscle relaxation) and x-ray screening. NB: if under GA, obtain consent for ± ORIF in case closed reduction is unsuccessful.
▶▶Remember to emphasize the importance of elevation of the casted limb, as swelling within a cast can be dangerous and very painful!

Methods of traction Rarely used as definitive management in adults, but it is still used in the initial post-injury phase, and for children. Traction or fixation helps hold the reduced fracture in place for healing, and pain relief.

- *Skin traction:* Uses adhesive strapping to attach the load to the limb. The load cannot be very great, as it may tear the skin.
- *Skeletal traction:* Using a pin through bone, bigger forces can be employed such as fixed and balance traction:
  - *Fixed traction:* The Thomas' splint (fig 8.5, see also p. 640). Weight can be added over a pulley (at the foot end) to relieve pressure on ischial tuberosity.

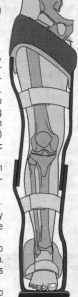

Fig 8.5 Thomas' splint.

  - *Balanced traction:* (fig 8.6) The weight of the limb balanced against the load. This can enable the patient to easily lift the leg off the bed eg for a bed pan.
  - *Gallows traction* (fig 8.6) Suitable for children up to $1\frac{1}{2}$yrs of age. The buttocks rise just above the bed.

The nurses on the specialist units will be experts at setting up and adjusting traction devices, so ask if you can watch and help.

Complications of casts
• Avoid these by providing education on good cast care and rehabilitation courses
• Muscle atrophy
• Stiff joints
• Pressure ulcers
• NV disturbance
• Osteoporosis

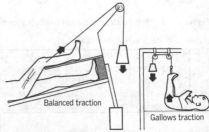

Balanced traction

Gallows traction

Fig 8.6 Traction: balanced traction, and gallows traction.

8 Trauma

►►Open fractures (Excerpts from British Orthopaedic Association & British Association of Plastic, Reconstructive and Aesthetic Surgeons standards for trauma[2-5].)

- Patients with open fractures of long bones, hindfoot, or midfoot should be taken directly or transferred to a specialist centre that can provide orthoplastic care.
- Intravenous prophylactic antibiotics should be administered as soon as possible, ideally within 1h of injury.
- The examination of the injured limb should include assessment and documentation of the vascular and neurological status. This should be repeated systematically, particularly after reduction manoeuvres or the application of splints.
- The limb should be realigned and splinted.
- In patients where an initial 'trauma CT' is indicated, the initial sequence should include a head to toes CT scan. This should be used with clinical correlation to direct further specific limb sequences during that initial CT examination.
- Prior to formal debridement the wound should be handled only to remove gross contamination and to allow photography, then dressed with a saline-soaked gauze and covered with an occlusive film.
- Debridement should be performed immediately for highly contaminated wounds (agricultural, aquatic, sewage) or where there is an associated vascular compromise (compartment syndrome or arterial disruption causing ischaemia). Within 12h of injury for solitary high-energy open fractures, or within 24h for low-energy open fractures.

Open reduction internal fixation (ORIF)

If possible, fractures involving joint articulations should be treated by ORIF which allows rigid fixation of the joint surfaces such that immediate rehabilitation can occur—see MINIBOX 'Indications for ORIF'. The aim is to achieve stable internal fixation in order to facilitate healing and also reduce serious complications (p. 528). *Plates* provide strength & stabilize

Indications for ORIF
• Failed conservative R $_x$
• 2 #s in 1 limb
• Bilateral identical #s
• Intra-articular #s
• Open #
• Displaced unstable #

#. Specifically designed types exist to counteract the various forces experienced in different joints & long bone shafts (eg compression plates for long bones). *Screws* are often combined with other devices. Many different types and sizes exist. *Closed reduction internal fixation:* Sometimes, fractures require fixation to improve the position for healing, but do not need to be held rigidly using a plate. *Intramedullary nails:* Placed in the medullary cavity (centre) of long bones, typically in femoral and tibial shaft fixation. They span the length of the bone, & are inserted away from the fracture site. *Kirschner wires (κ-wires):* Often used for closed reduction & percutaneous fixation of fractures, rarely ORIF. κ-wires are less rigid than plates & screws but can easily be removed after use.

External fixation Useful when there are burns, loss of skin and/or bone, or in case of open fractures since it avoids disruption to the fracture site and associated soft tissue. It can be definitive or temporary. Pins/wires are placed away from the zone of injury in various configurations giving varying degrees of stability. Pins are inserted into the bones directly; either just through the far bone cortex or directly through the opposite side of the limb. Pins are connected using a series of clamps and rods. Stability of fixation can be increased in a number of ways—use additional or larger diameter pins, move rods closer to the bone, insert pins in different planes, etc.

Damage control orthopaedics (DCO) Used in haemodynamically unstable polytrauma patients who receive temporary external fixation (eg pelvis) to facilitate haemorrhage control and resuscitation in order to optimize the patient for more permanent surgery later. Immediate invasive surgery provokes further inflammatory damage already induced by trauma so DCO aims to perform the minimal amount of orthopaedic surgery to achieve haemodynamic stability (p. 595).

Further reading

Taljanovi MS *et al.* (2003). Fracture fixation. *Radiographics* 23:1569–90.

See MINIBOX 'Complications'. **Fat embolism** Typically after pelvic or femur #. The mechanical theory—fat emboli are released from disrupted bone marrow. The biochemical theory—release of free fatty acids directly damage the pneumocytes. Usually arises on day 2–3. *Signs:* Altered mental state (few have fits), pyrexia (even low grade), SOB, hypoxia, tachycardia, petechial rash. ▶▶Consider ITU. Treatment is mainly supportive for respiratory failure. Mortality is 5–15%. Early immobilization has reduced incidence in femoral shaft #. ▶▶Major differential is PE.

Neurovascular injury Increasingly likely as deformity worsens, vascular injury is common in knee dislocations and supracondylar humeral #.

Infection The most common complication following # surgery is infection <1% in elective surgery to 20% in open fractures. Cellulitis, osteomyelitis, and sepsis can occur. See p. 511 on prosthetic infections.

Delayed union When the # has not healed within the expected time (see p. 524). *Causes:*
- # in a bone which has finished growing.
- Poor blood supply (eg tibia) or avascular fragment (eg scaphoid).
- Comminuted/infected fracture.
- Systemic disease (eg malignancy or infection).
- Smoking.
- Distraction of bone ends by muscle; ORIF prevents this.

Non-union This is said to have occurred when fracture healing is not complete by 9 months, with no evidence of progression towards healing, clinically or radiologically, for 3 months. Broadly, a non-union occurs from inadequate or abnormal biology or mechanics. Management is aimed at optimizing biology (infection, blood supply, bone graft) or the mechanics (skeletal stabilization). Avascular necrosis is also a cause, seen typically in femoral neck (p. 542) and scaphoid fractures (p. 537).

Complications
Immediate:
• Internal bleeding
• External bleeding
• Organ injury
• Nerve or skin injury
• Vessel injury (limb ischaemia: OHCM p657)
Later—local:
• Skin necrosis/gangrene
• Pressure sores
• Infection
• Non- or delayed union
Later—general:
• Venous/fat embolism
• Pulmonary embolism
• Pneumonia
• Arthritis

Malunion Occurs when the fragments have not healed in anatomical positions, risking loss of function, secondary OA, and contractures.

Thromboembolic events DVT occurs in ~⅔ of major orthopaedic events, but fatal PE in only 0.1–0.2%. Patients undergoing repair of hip # have the highest risk of fatal PE. LMWH halves DVT rate and lowers risk of fatal PE by ~75%.[7] Compression stockings are less effective. Initiate **enoxaparin** 40mg 12–24h post-op and a further 7–10 days (minimum) to reduce risk of VTE while minimizing risk of bleeding. Warfarin can also be used (INR 2–3) but has 33% higher risk of DVT and bleeding compared to LMWH. **Fondaparinux** 2.5mg/day may be better than enoxaparin.[8]n=1049

Late complications: Include • CRPS (p. 529).
- *Failure of fixation:* eg plates or nails break, or dislodge.
- *Psychological problems in mobilizing:* eg 'compensation neurosis'.

Compartment syndrome

▶▶Life- and limb-threatening. Occurs when swelling of tissues in an anatomical compartment (can occur anywhere, most commonly in the leg) occludes the vascular supply leading to hypoxia and eventually necrosis. On examination there is swelling, redness, and *pain on passive muscle stretching*. Pain is often disproportionate to injury. Subsequent rhabdomyolysis can cause renal failure. Correct hypovolaemia vigorously. Watch out for ↓ urine output & ↑ plasma K+. Intracompartmental pressures can be measured >30mmHg indicates compartment syndrome, this should not delay surgical review as the diagnosis is clinical and prompt fasciotomy is life/limb-saving.[9]

8 Trauma

A controversial, poorly understood diagnosis, and a condition that is notoriously difficult to treat.

CRPS *type I* is a deranged sensitivity to stimuli following limb trauma *without* nerve injury (CRPS I ≈ algodystrophy ≈ reflex sympathetic dystrophy, RSD). *CRPS type II* has an identifiable nerve lesion. Both local and central nervous systems play a part. Patients diagnosed with CRPS show substantial reorganization of somatotopic CNS maps—leading to mislocalization of tactile stimuli.[10].

CRPS I is a 'complex disorder of pain, sensory abnormalities, abnormal blood flow, sweating, and trophic changes in superficial or deep tissues'. The central event may be loss of vascular tone or supersensitivity to sympathetic neurotransmitters. Pathogenesis is obscure, the idea of exaggerated regional inflammatory responses is supported by the fact that IgG labelled with indium (^{111}In) is concentrated in the affected extremity.[11]

Causes Injury esp. distal and esp. upper limb—eg fractures, carpal tunnel release, operations for Dupuytren's, tendon release procedures, mastectomy, transradial cardiac catheterization, knee surgery, crush injury, ankle arthrodesis, amputation, hip arthroplasty, rotator cuff injury, zoster, myocardial infarction, stroke, cancer, spontaneous/idiopathic.

Presentation Typically patients have initial trauma—commonly in a hand or foot—which may be trivial or severe. This is followed weeks or months later by pain, allodynia/hyperalgesia, vasomotor instability, and abnormal sweating. Pain is often burning in nature and may extend to the whole limb. The limb may be cold and cyanosed, or hot and sweating (locally). T° sensitivity may be heightened. The skin of the affected part may be oedematous, or, later, shiny and atrophic. Hyperreflexia, dystonic movements, and contractures may occur. Symptoms are often worse after exercise, and may include weakness, hyperalgesia, clumsiness, inability to initiate movements, spasms, dystonias, and allodynia (a stimulus not usually painful now hurts). There are no systemic signs (no fever, tachycardia, or lymphadenopathy).

Imaging *x-rays:* Patchy osteopenia greater than expected from disuse; joint space *not* narrowed (*no* thinned cartilage)—see fig 8.7. *Bone scintigraphy:* Characteristic uniform uptake, with increased limb perfusion on the dynamic phase.

Treatment ▶Refer to pain clinic/multidisciplinary team (physio + OT).

- Encourage optimism and pleasurable things. Ultimately, with appropriate care, CRPS is self-limiting.
- Avoid bad habits of trying to protect the affected limb by keeping it immobile (leads to stiffness). Educate on using the limb in activities of daily living.
- Effective painkillers eg **amitriptyline** 25mg ON PO ± NSAIDs.
- Remember that CRPS can mask other pathology. Just because the patient is already in pain, doesn't mean they don't have a new injury!

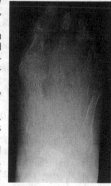

Fig 8.7 CRPS type I, with diffuse osteopenia and destruction of the 2nd and 3rd metatarsals.

Courtesy of The Norfolk and Norwich University Hospitals (NNUH) Radiology Dept.

Further reading

Singh JA *et al.* (2011). Cardiac and thromboembolic complications and mortality in patients undergoing total hip and total knee arthroplasty. *Ann Rheum Dis* 70:2082–8.

Talbot M *et al.* (2006). Fat embolism syndrome: history, definition, epidemiology. *Injury* 37(Suppl 4):S3–7.

8 Trauma

Fracture of the clavicle Historically thought to be caused by a fall onto an outstretched hand (FOOSH), most seem to occur after a direct blow to the clavicle and is common in cyclists. Fractures are most common in the middle ⅓ where proximal fragment is pulled superiorly by sternocleidomastoid. Management is typically a polysling with follow up x-rays at 6 weeks to ensure union. ORIF of displaced # significantly reduces the risk of non-union; deformity may lead to functional problems in adulthood (figs 8.8–8.10).

►Examine the skin overlying the fracture site carefully, 'tented' skin is at risk of necrosis.

►Remember the possibility of neurovascular injury (brachial plexus; sub-clavian vessels) + pneumothorax as complications.

Scapula and acromion fractures Rarely need fixation. These represent high-energy transfer injuries, so assess carefully to exclude other injuries.

Acromioclavicular (AC) joint dislocation Typically caused by a direct blow to top of the shoulder in young contact-sport athletes. The patient has a tender prominence over the AC joint. Assess neurovascular status. *Imaging:* On x-ray check for congruity of the underside of the acromion with the distal clavicle. Radiography may be normal. R: Depends on displacement of the AC joint on x-rays. Minimal displacement can be rested in a sling, more severe disruption may require open reduction and ligament reconstruction.[12]

Anterior shoulder dislocation Most common (95%) (fig 8.11). Typically young males present following contact sports which have forced the arm into abduction, extension, and external rotation. Elderly patients can simply have a history of falling on an outstretched hand. *Signs:* Loss of shoulder contour (flattening of deltoid), an anterior bulge from the head of the humerus, which may also be palpated in the axilla. ►Check pulses and nerves (including the axillary nerve supplying sensation over lower deltoid area) pre- and post-reduction. Before reduction, do x-ray (*is there a fracture?*). Relieve pain (eg intra-articular local anaesthetic, parenteral opioid, Entonox®) throughout the procedure. *Treatment: Simple reduction:* apply longitudinal traction to the arm in abduction, and replace the head of the humerus by gentle pressure. *Risk:* humeral #. Remember to obtain an x-ray post reduction. Support the arm in internal rotation with a broad arm sling and refer to fracture clinic for follow-up. Surgery may be needed eg if young/athletic, or recurrent dislocation.

Posterior dislocation of the shoulder Rare and presents with a limitation of external rotation. May be associated with epileptic seizures or electrical shocks. It may be hard to diagnose from an anteroposterior x-ray ('light-bulb' appearance of humeral head, Fig 9.19 p. 615); lateral x-ray views are essential.

Fracture of the proximal humerus Most are stable osteoporotic fractures in the elderly following a fall on an outstretched arm. Minimally displaced fractures may be managed conservatively in a collar and cuff with the wrist above the level of the elbow. Multifragmented fractures, open fractures, pathological fractures, fracture-dislocations, or those with neurovascular injury (brachial plexus/axillary artery) will need operative management. Prognosis and complications (eg avascular necrosis) worsen with ↑ number of fragments.

Fracture of the humeral shaft Typically after a fall onto the arm. Most do not need surgery; splinting with a humeral brace and gravity traction by means of 'collar and cuff' sling usually gives satisfactory reduction. Immobilize for 8–12 weeks. Surgical options include humeral nailing or plating. ►Radial nerve injury may cause wrist-drop, but damage can also be a complication of surgery, so *document function preoperatively*.

Fractures of the distal humerus See p. 532.

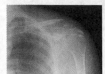

Fig 8.8 Comminuted distal clavicular fracture—an injury requiring ORIF.

Courtesy of The Norfolk and Norwich University Hospitals (NNUH) Radiology Dept.

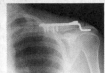

Fig 8.9 Hook plate repair of Fig 8.8-type injury. Remember nearby vessels!

Courtesy of The Norfolk and Norwich University Hospitals (NNUH) Radiology Dept.

Fig 8.10 Healed mid-clavicular # (different patient)—note deformity. Often, surgical repair is not needed for clavicle #, as healing and long-term function are good.

Courtesy of The Norfolk and Norwich University Hospitals (NNUH) Radiology Dept.

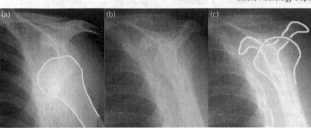

Fig 8.11 Due to the ligamentous laxity (see pp. 472–3) the shoulder joint comprises 45% of all dislocated joints. Anterior dislocation of the shoulder (a)[4] and a post-reduction image (b)—copied and highlighted (c). The dislocation can be painful, so positioning is difficult for the radiographer. These are attempted lateral views of the scapula. After reduction, the head of the humerus lies in the centre of the 'Y' with the coracoid process anterior and the acromion posterior.

Courtesy of Prof Peter Scally.

Recurrent shoulder dislocation

Is there an underlying connective tissue disorder? 2 types: **Atraumatic** (5%.) Often a teenager with no history of trauma, but having general joint laxity. Remember **AMBRI**: **A**traumatic (ie 'born loose'); **M**ultidirectional; **B**ilateral; treat by: **R**ehabilitation; **I**nferior capsular shift surgery only if rehab fails. Beware of habitual dislocations; a patient who deliberately causes dislocations as their 'party trick' (less likely to respond to operative intervention). **Traumatic** Dislocation is anterior (sometimes inferior, rarely posterior) and secondary to trauma (may be mild); abduction + lateral rotation of the arm (eg donning a coat) may cause dislocation. Remember **TUBS**: **T**raumatic (ie 'torn loose'); **U**nilateral; **B**ankart lesion; **S**urgical treatment. Recurrent dislocations cause further instability through the creation of damaged joint capsule components: *Bankart lesions* arise from avulsion of the glenoid labrum from the glenoid *Hill–Sachs lesions;* an impaction # of the humeral head following anterior dislocations (seen on x-rays with arm medially rotated). Those <25 years have a higher risk of recurrent events compared to >40-year-olds, but this latter group requires imaging of rotator cuff as high risk of traumatic rupture rather than labral injury. **Treatment** Depends on the cause and typically requires arthroscopic investigation. Both open and arthroscopic repair is possible, the latter however is gaining popularity, further supported by a recent study suggesting that the majority of patients have successful outcomes and relatively low risk of recurrence with arthroscopic fixation too.[13] Care of elderly patients focuses more on physio exercises to strengthen rotator cuff muscles.

4 The humeral head can sometimes lie low in the glenoid fossa with surgical neck fractures, from 'deltoid inhibition'—relaxation of the muscle from pain, causing subluxation; it is *not* a fracture-dislocation.

► Look for neurovascular compromise! The antecubital fossa contains (from lateral to medial) the radial nerve, biceps brachii tendon, brachial artery and median nerve (typically anterior interosseous branch). The ulnar nerve passes posteriorly at the medial epicondyle.

The elbow *Imaging:* Presence of an elbow fracture is suggested by an 'anterior sail sign' or 'posterior fat pad sign' fig 9.18 (p. 615).[5] *Management:* If no # obvious, but an effusion is present, treat initially with a collar and cuff. Re-x-ray after 10 days (# more easily seen): if clear, start mobilization. For fractures, internal fixation may be needed. Physiotherapy & early mobilization are vital in preventing stiffness.

Fractures of the distal humerus • *Supracondylar fractures:* See p. 533.
• *Fracture of the medial epicondyle:* These may require surgery if a fragment is in the joint or if there are ulnar nerve compression symptoms.
• *Fracture of the lateral epicondyle:* Surgical fixation may be required. Complications include cubitus valgus and ulnar nerve palsy.
• *τ-shaped intercondylar humerus fracture:* This is a supracondylar fracture with a break between the condyles. Difficult to surgically fix; requires rigid plate fixation to allow early mobilization.

Fractures of the radial head 33% of elbow fractures. Caused by a fall onto outstretched hand. The elbow is swollen and tender over the radial head; flexion/extension may be possible but pronation & supination hurt. Radiography often shows an effusion, but minor fractures are often missed. Undisplaced fractures can be treated in a collar and cuff for a short period, followed by mobilization. If displaced or fragment prevents supination/pronation then internal fixation or excision of the radial head may be needed. *Complications:* 35% are associated with another bony/ligamentous injury, 3–14% are associated with the 'terrible triad' of radial head fracture, elbow dislocation, and coronoid process #.

Elbow dislocations Commonly posterior (90%) and result from a fall on a not yet fully outstretched hand, with forearm supinated; this causes posterior ulnar displacement on the humerus, and a swollen elbow, fixed in flexion.
► Associated fractures, brachial artery and nerve injury must be considered. *Closed reduction (±GA):* Stand behind the patient; flex the elbow to relax biceps brachii. With your fingers around the epicondyles, push forwards on the olecranon with your thumbs, and down on the forearm. Hearing a clunk heralds success. This may be aided by traction at the wrist. A post-reduction image is needed to exclude fractures. Immobilize for 10 days. *Complications:* Stiffness, instability, radio-ulnar joint disruption, failure to identify neurovascular compromise leading to severe morbidity with limb ischaemia, compartment syndrome, and neurological changes.[14]

Olecranon fractures (fig 8.12) Can be a simple avulsion injury when triceps (which inserts onto olecranon) contracts during a fall on the outstretched arm, or comminuted, usually following a direct blow. Treat displaced fractures with ORIF eg tension band wiring if simple, and plate if comminuted.

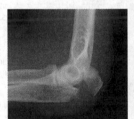

Fig 8.12 Displaced olecranon fracture needing fixation.
Courtesy of The Norfolk and Norwich University Hospitals (NNUH) Radiology Dept.

5 The *anterior fat pad* can be seen on lateral elbow x-ray as a radiolucent triangle in front of the distal humerus. It can be present in a normal elbow, and is only abnormal when raised off the bone by an effusion. A visible *posterior fat pad* is always abnormal. Absence of either of these signs makes a fracture very unlikely. Other things to check on the lateral x-ray: *anterior humeral line* (which should cross the anterior third of the capitellum) and *alignment of the radial shaft* with the capitellum (which it should bisect) fig 9.18 (p. 615).

The Salter–Harris classification of physeal injuries (see p. 525) helps predict the risk of growth disturbance. Paediatric elbow x-rays can be difficult to interpret because of the ossification centres (see mnemonic p. 463). Physeal #s tend to heal quickly (~4 weeks) but monitor carefully to ensure normal growth has not been disrupted. Paediatric bone is softer and leads to unique # patterns not seen in adults eg: *greenstick #* (cortex fails in tension and develops a partial transverse crack), *torus #* (buckle of one cortex as it fails in compression), *plastic deformation* (the bone bends with no evidence of #). Typically these are treated with closed reduction (if needed) and cast immobilization.

Pulled elbow (subluxation of radial head) See p. 475.

Supracondylar fracture The most common # of childhood (rare in adults). Presents with pain, swelling, and inability to move elbow. Most (95%) are due to hyperextension. The Gartland classification (fig 8.13) uses lateral x-rays to describe the severity of displacement from extension injuries. Gartland type IIIA is *posteromedial* and threatens the radial nerve. IIIB is *posterolateral* and threatens the median nerve, esp. the anterior interosseous branch, which innervates deep flexors to the index finger and flexor pollicis longus (pincer grip); entirely a motor nerve, so injury is easily missed. *Management:* ▶ Check neurovascular status. Keeping the elbow in extension after injury prevents exacerbating brachial artery damage from the time of injury. Type I fractures can be managed with and above elbow back slab and sling. Type II fractures may require reduction under sedation/GA. Type III fractures generally require GA and fixation with κ-wires.[15] *Complications:* A cubitus varus deformity of the elbow can result from malunion.

Examining neurovascular status in children

Median nerve (via anterior interosseous nerve): Supplies flexor pollicis longus, and radial half of flexor digitorum profundus—'*Can you make an OK sign?*'

Radial nerve (via posterior interosseous nerve): Supplies extensor pollicis longus (among others)—'*Can you put your thumbs up?*'

Ulnar nerve: Supplies the interossei (among others)—'*Can you cross your fingers?*'

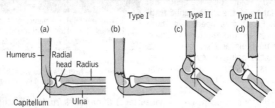

Fig 8.13 (a) In a normal elbow, a line drawn along the anterior surface of the humerus. (b) Gartland type I: the anterior humeral line passes through the middle of the capitellum. Non-displaced. Difficult to see on x-ray so look for the fat pad signs. See footnote 5 on p. 532. (c) Gartland type II: the anterior humeral line passes anterior to the middle of the capitellum. The distal fragment is angulated with an intact posterior cortex. (d) Gartland type III: unstable posterior displacement.

Republished, with permission, from resources at The Royal Children's Hospital, Melbourne, Australia http://www.rch.org.au/clinicalguide/guideline_index/fractures/Supracondylar_fracture_of_the_humerus_Emergency_Department/

Further reading

Chen HW *et al.* (2014). Complications of treating terrible triad injury of the elbow: a systematic review. *PLoS One* 9:e97476.

Jie KE *et al.* (2014). Extension test and ossal point tenderness cannot accurately exclude significant injury in acute elbow trauma. *Ann Emerg Med* 64:74–8.

Distal radial and ulnar fractures Very common, especially in osteoporotic postmenopausal women who fall on an outstretched hand. ► Compartment syndrome can occur in forearm injuries, as can damage to the ulnar, radial, and median nerves (especially the anterior osseous branch). *Treatment:* Guided by evidence of neurovascular compromise and patient criteria. Traditionally, the majority of wrist fractures were 'pulled' (closed reduction) in the ED using either a haematoma block or Bier's block (IV regional anaesthetic using an inflatable cuff around the upper arm). The general consensus in the literature is that Bier's blocks are more effective overall then haematoma blocks and are preferable.[16] Current practice, however, varies and there is an increasing number of wrist # undergoing surgical fixation; there remains dispute over whether ORIF or K-wires (not strictly ORIF) is best.[17] Closed reduction in the ED is being reserved more and more for those patients with neurovascular compromise or where manipulation in the department is likely to be the definitive treatment (eg frail patients with low functional demands). See p. 535 for procedure. If closed manipulation is performed, x-rays must be obtained.

Use your eponyms wisely (Also see *OHCM* p695.) It is so tempting to fire off 'Colles' fracture' or other names that spring to mind whenever faced with an x-ray suggestive of distal radial injury... Have a quick think before scrambling for eponyms; modern practice has shifted towards simply describing the anatomical fracture pattern that you see (see p. 521) as eponyms are frequently incorrectly applied. Here are a few in the forearm: *Colles' fracture:* An extra-articular # of the distal radius with dorsal displacement of the distal radius. Note that Colles originally based his descriptions solely on clinical examination (since Röntgen only discovered x-rays in 1895) and described this injury as a wrist dislocation with 'dinner-fork' deformity (the fingers are the prongs). Avulsion of the ulnar styloid process may also occur. *Smith's fracture:* (Reverse Colles'.) Volar displacement and angulation of the distal radial fragment. Fixation is needed in these fractures as the fracture is inherently unstable and fragment tends to migrate palmarly, even if casted. *Barton's fracture:* Intra-articular fracture involving the dorsal aspect of the distal radius (fig 8.14 is a re-

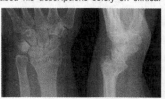

Fig 8.14 AP and lateral views of the left wrist. Does it matter what eponym denotes which type of wrist fracture this is? Colles', Smith's, or Barton's? Try describing it anatomically instead.

Courtesy of The Norfolk and Norwich University Hospitals (NNUH) Radiology Dept.

verse Barton's, involving the palmar surface). *Chauffeur's fracture:* Fracture of the radial styloid (historically seen in drivers who drove old cars which needed cranking to engage the engine). *Monteggia/Galeazzi fractures:* See p. 854 & p. 848. *Night-stick fractures:* Isolated ulnar shaft #s, typically associated with a direct blow to a forearm held up in self defence against a truncheon (a 'night stick'). Look for other injuries as this fracture pattern requires a large force.

Wrist dislocation Although wrist injuries are very common, dislocations are in the minority. They most commonly involve the carpal bones, especially at the scapholunate or lunotriquetral junctions. May be anterior or posterior. Typically high-energy injuries in young athletes. x-rays help rule out fracture. Manipulation and usually open reduction, and plaster immobilization eg for 6 weeks. Median nerve compression may occur.[18] See p. 537 for scaphoid fractures.

Further reading

Hoynack BC (2015). *Wrist Fracture in Emergency Medicine*. Medscape. http://emedicine.medscape.com/article/828746

8 Trauma

Reduction of a fracture of the distal radius (Colles' type)

- Ensure that there is adequate regional anaesthesia. Traction should be applied to the hand via the 1st and 5th metacarpals with an assistant providing counter-traction at the elbow. The fracture can often be felt to disimpact with a 'clunk' (figs 8.16 & 8.17).
- *Exaggerate* dorsal angulation while maintaining distal traction to stop the inelastic dorsal periosteum from preventing reduction by longitudinal traction.
- Correct dorsal and radial angulation, again maintaining distal traction. Aim for anatomical alignment.
- Apply plaster backslab, moulded to maintain reduction with some wrist flexion and a small amount of ulnar deviation. Backslabs are safer than full casts; as you do not need to split the cast to accommodate swelling.

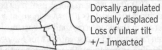

Dorsally angulated
Dorsally displaced
Loss of ulnar tilt
+/– Impacted

Fig 8.15 View before reduction (radius shown alone in lateral view only).

- Maintain traction while the POP is applied. This is most easily done by pulling on the thumb and 1st finger against counter-traction. This applies to both palmar and ulnar deviation.
- Support in a sling, once an x-ray has shown a good position (fig 8.18).
- Check x-ray in 5 days, when swelling has reduced; the plaster is then completed.

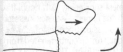

Fig 8.16 Apply traction and exaggerate dorsal angulation.

- ▶ Inability to get a good position may indicate soft tissue interpositioning.
- ▶ Practice is needed to maintain traction and reduction while a plaster is applied. Ask your local plaster room for help!

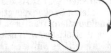

Fig 8.17 Then correct dorsal and radial angulation.

8 Trauma

A-P views

Normal
15–20°

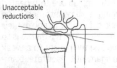

0–2 mm

The articular surface of the radius is level with, or proud of, the ulna and is tilted towards the ulna.

Unacceptable reductions

Note loss of radial length and reduction in ulnar tilt of the radius.

Lateral views

Normal 0–10°

Acceptable

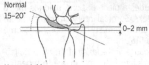

Dorsal

Palmar

The distal radial articular surface is vertical.

Unacceptable

The distal radial surface is dorsally angulated. If allowed to heal in this position it will cause a marked restriction in function.

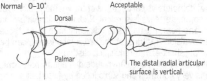

Fig 8.18 Acceptable positions post-reduction of wrist fractures (dorsal tilt <10°; radial shortening <2mm; radial inclination >15°; articular step <2mm; and distal radioulnar joint congruence).

5th metacarpal fractures Typically caused by a punch injury ('boxer's fracture'). Up to 40° of volar angulation can be accepted in the shaft, and more at the head. Distal fractures can be managed by strapping the small finger to the ring finger ('neighbour strapping') with more proximal fractures managed in a plaster splint (see 'Metacarpal fractures').

Metacarpal fractures The base of the 2nd and 3rd metacarpals (MCs) form the functional centre of the hand around which the movement of the hand is centred (fig 8.20). Thus, while malalignment may be tolerated in the 5th MC, far less is permitted in the 2nd MC (<10°). Management may vary depending on whether the fracture is in the head/neck/shaft or base of the MC, however, stable closed fractures can be managed in a splint/cast for ~2 weeks, with the wrist in partial extension (20–30°), MCP joints in 70–90° flexion with fingers in extension. Unstable fractures may require K-wires/ORIF. Longer periods of splinting in plaster can cause a stiff hand eg from joint adhesions/contracture, flexor tendon fibrosis, and collateral ligament shortening. Rotational fractures disclose themselves by producing a rotation of the fingers—see BOX 'Assessing rotational deformity'; they require operative fixation, as do fractures of ≥2 MCs. ▶Beware wounds overlying metacarpophalangeal joints (often contaminated from the punched victim's teeth, and may communicate with the joint). These always need washout and exploration in theatre.

Fractures of the proximal phalanx Spiral or oblique fractures occurring at this site are likely to be associated with a rotation deformity—and this must be corrected (see BOX 'Assessing rotational deformity'). The only way to do this accurately is by open reduction and fixation.

Middle phalanx fractures Manipulate these if needed; splint in flexion over a splint or plaster, with neighbour strapping. The aim is to control rotation, which interferes with later finger flexion.

Distal phalanx fractures May be caused by crush injuries and are often open. If closed, symptoms may be relieved by trephining the nail (see p. 539).

Mallet finger The tip of the finger droops because of avulsion of the extensor tendon's attachment to the terminal phalanx or rupture of the terminal part of the tendon. If the avulsed tendon includes a piece of bone, union is made easier—using an extension splint for 6 weeks. Surgical intervention may be indicated if the fracture fragment is >30% of the joint surface. Poorer outcome is associated with delay in splinting (see p. 516).

Gamekeeper's thumb This is so called because of the laxity of the ulnar collateral ligament of the metacarpophalangeal joint of the thumb due to repeated forced thumb abduction that occurs when wringing a pheasant's neck. The same injury is described acutely in skiers who fall and catch their thumb in their pole, or ski matting ('skier's thumb'). Diagnosis can be difficult as the thumb is so painful to examine, but to miss this injury may condemn the patient to a weak pincer grip—inject 1–2mL 1% **lidocaine** around the ligament to facilitate examination, and try to radially deviate the thumb at the MCPJ in extension and 30° of flexion. Increased deviation compared to the uninjured side indicates complete injury. Differentiation of complete vs partial tears of the ligament is crucial because the treatment for complete tears is surgical. Radiographic evaluation will detect a bony avulsion fragment. Partial tears (clinically stable), or those associated with undisplaced avulsion fractures of the proximal phalanx, can be adequately treated using simple short-arm thumb spica casting.

Fingertip amputation Distal to the DIP joint, can include damage to nail, bone, and soft tissues. This injury is very common and surrounded by false belief that the severed tip should be placed directly in ice—discourage this first-aid practice. Transport of tip should be made in a clear bag near ice for preservation; however, it is rarely appropriate to reattach a damaged fingertip. Look for associated fracture or foreign bodies. Minor soft tissue loss is treated conservatively with dressings as it will likely heal by secondary intention after 3–5 weeks.[6] More significant injury requires skin grafting, or shortening of the finger ('terminalization').

Assessing rotational deformity

Refer any fractures with obvious rotational deformity (a clinical, not a radiological decision, fig 8.19), as this can be disabling. Assessing for rotational deformity in finger and metacarpal fractures is essential. Ask the patient to flex their fingers: they should all point to the scaphoid. Alternatively, look at and assess the nails end on in this position. Refer to a specialist if rotation is detected, as manipulation may be required; function and perhaps livelihood are at stake.

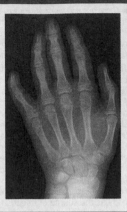

Fig 8.19 Salter–Harris II fracture of base of 5th proximal phalanx. The finger can be appreciated to be angulated, but the degree of rotation must still be assessed clinically. See p. 525, 'Salter–Harris fractures'.

Image courtesy of The Norfolk and Norwich University Hospitals (NNUH) Radiology Dept.

Scaphoid fractures

Common and easily missed on x-ray; results from falls on the hand. *Signs:* Tender in anatomical snuff box and over scaphoid tubercle, pain on axial compression of the thumb. *Imaging:* Request a dedicated 'scaphoid' series. If –ve, and fracture is suspected, MRI has been shown to be sensitive and cost-effective.[20] If MRI is unavailable, cast and re-x-ray in 2 weeks. Non-displaced fractures involving the waist of the scaphoid may be immobilized in a neutral forearm cast for several weeks until union. Percutaneous cannulated screw fixation allows the patient to return to work earlier but does not affect the long-term outcome. *Complications:* Avascular necrosis: the proximal pole relies on interosseous supply from the distal part.

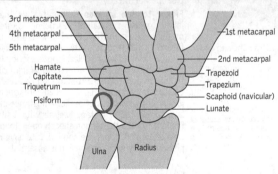

Fig 8.20 Naming the carpal bones doesn't have to be tedious, there are several mnemonics. Some less appropriate than others and we encourage you to seek them out! One more sensible option to describe the carpal bones in the proximal row, then distal row is: She Left The Party To Take Cathy Home (Scaphoid, Lunate, Triquetrum, Pisiform, Trapezium, Trapezoid, Capitate, Hamate).

Further reading

Mallee WH *et al.* (2014). Clinical diagnostic evaluation for scaphoid fractures: a systematic review and meta-analysis. *J Hand Surg Am* 39:1683–91.

6 This link shows an excellent demonstration of fingertip healing post injury.[19]

▶*There are no minor injuries to the hand.* Any breach of the integument may be the start of a chain of events that leads to loss of our most useful appendage. *Hands are very frequently injured simply because they are how we tend to explore our surroundings. The complexity of anatomy and biomechanics in our hand truly deserves its own chapter but here are a few things to consider.*

Infections *Staph aureus* is the most common bacteria associated with hand infection (80%). Others include streps and Gram –ves. *Paronychia:* Infection causing painful cellulitis around the fingernail (see fig 8.21). In the early stages, antibiotics may cure this, but once a collection forms, drainage of the abscess is required. Chronic fungal infections typically develop in workers whose hands are repeatedly exposed to wet conditions. They describe a history of

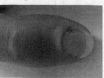

Fig 8.21 Acute paronychia.
© DermNet New Zealand, reproduced with permission.

frequent bacterial infections with abscess formation and nail deformities. *Felon:* An abscess in the pulp of the distal finger. x-ray to look for a foreign body as the source of infection. Incise into area of maximal fluctuance; blunt dissection is needed to break up septa, and a drain left in place and treat with IV antibiotics.[21] *Infective flexor tenosynovitis:* Bacterial infection of flexor tendon sheath—which can spread via the carpal tunnel to the forearm; this potential for rapid spread makes it a surgical emergency. Look for 'Kanavel's 4 signs': 1 Fusiform swelling of the finger(s) 2 Tenderness over flexor sheath 3 Pain on passive extension of fingers so the patient preferentially chooses to 4 hold the finger in slight flexion. Treat urgently with IV antibiotics and either repeated visits to theatre or postoperative in-dwelling catheter irrigation (fig 8.22). Even previously healthy patients can expect residual digital stiffness despite optimal therapy.

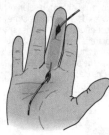

Fig 8.22 Drainage and closed irrigation for flexor sheath infection. The antibiotic solution drips in through the distal catheter and drains out the proximal one.

Reproduced with permission of Way LW ed. 'Current Surgical Diagnosis and Treatment', 10th ed. Appleton & Lange 1994 © McGraw Hill.

Flexor tendon injuries Failure to flex the DIP joint against resistance ≈ flexor digitorum profundus division (fig 8.23). If this is intact but flexion of the PIP joint is affected, there is division of superficialis. Flexor pollicis longus section leads to inability to flex the interphalangeal joint of the thumb. In general, flexor tendon injuries are best treated by primary repair (most are open injuries). If there is loss of tendon substance or delayed presentation, a staged repair with a silastic implant to keep the tendon sheath open, followed by a tendon graft, may be needed. Intensive hand physiotherapy with supervision is essential.

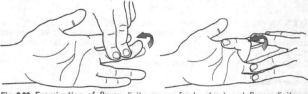

Fig 8.23 Examination of flexor digitorum profundus (FDP) and flexor digitorum superficialis (FDS).

Reproduced from Warwick et al., *Hand Surgery* (2018), with permission from OUP.

8 Trauma

In the absence of fingernails, the ability to manipulate small objects is significantly reduced, the distal phalanx is rendered defenceless, and the cosmetic appearance is flawed. Yet injuries to the nail are still frequently ignored when multiple injuries affect the hand.[22] The anatomy of the nail is far more complex than people initially consider. The nail bed is adherent to the periosteum of the distal phalanx below and the nail plate above. This rich vascular layer enables nail plate growth; allowing the average nail to completely regrow within 3 months. Note that various systemic diseases can also affect the nail (eg psoriasis, liver disease, thyroid disease).

Injury to the nailbed Often associated with subungual haematomas and damage to the distal phalanx ►Always do an x-ray as 50% of nail bed injuries are associated with fractures of the distal phalanx. Crush injuries (such as door closures or hammers) are the most common cause.

Subungual haematoma: Seen under the nail when the highly vascular nailbed is disrupted after trauma to the fingertip. The nail is often still intact. Small, pain-free haematomas tend to settle spontaneously and patients do not attend the doctor. It can become painful if the build-up of blood increases the pressure under the nail. Trephination of the haematoma (fig 8.24) should be considered to release this pressure, approaches include electric cautery, 18-gauge needle, and a heated paper clip. This can be performed without anaesthesia in the ED. The key question to ask before attempting this: is there evidence of complex laceration to the nail bed? Lacerations may require suturing and exploration of the nail bed. Studies have suggested that when the haematoma covers >50% of the nail then further examination may be warranted.[23] Failure to address nailbed injuries appropriately can result in nail bed deformities and abnormal growth, and infections of both soft tissue and bone (osteomyelitis). ► Trephination performed in the presence of a fracture converts it into an open fracture. Do an x-ray if in doubt!

Nail bed repair: Required when repairing avulsed nails, bed lacerations, and after injuries which have crushed the fingertip. Use a digital nerve block[7] and sterilize the area well. Elevate (avulse) the nail using fine scissors or a Mitchell elevator (usually available from theatres). Use fine absorbable sutures and keep debridement to a minimum to reduce scarring. Replace the nail to serve as a splint and secure it with sutures. Refer to hand surgeons in complex injuries.

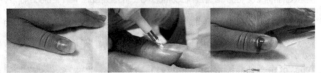

Fig 8.24 Trephination of a subungual haematoma. Clean the site well to minimize risk of infection. Once the trephination device reaches the collection of blood you will see it ooze out, multiple trephination holes may be required. Watch this video for the technique.[8][24]

Image reprinted with permission from Medscape Drugs & Diseases (http://emedicine. medscape.com/), 2015, available at: http://emedicine.medscape.com/article/827104-overview

Further reading

BMJ Best Practice (2015). *Paronychia.* http://bestpractice.bmj.com/best-practice/monograph/350.html

British Society for Surgery of the Hand: www.bssh.ac.uk

Haneke E (2006). Surgical anatomy of the nail apparatus. *Dermatol Clin* 24:291–6.

7 A ring block (digital block) which anaesthetizes the distal phalanx is required for treating most painful fingertip injuries. Inject 1% lidocaine on both medial and lateral midpoints of the middle phalanx. Do not mix the lidocaine with adrenaline which can cause end-artery spasm and fingertip ischaemia.

8 https://emedicine.medscape.com/article/82926-overview

Fractures of the femoral shaft and distal femur (supracondylar femur) usually involve significant trauma in young adults while relatively minor trauma in the elderly can cause neck of femur (NOF) fractures.

Intracapsular fractures Occur just below the femoral head and may be subcapital (most common) or transcervical (fig 8.25). These often cause *external rotation & shortening of the affected leg*.[9] The injuring force can be trivial and the patient is usually unable to walk. In elderly patients with a fall and hip pain, an MRI scan should be requested if the x-ray is normal, but suspicion is high for a #NOF.[4] Intracapsular # have a higher incidence of AVN and non-union due to the femoral head blood supply (p. 541). If displacement is minimal, internal fixation *in situ* gives the best outcome (rate of displacement, risk of AVN, and non-union are all reduced). In displaced # the head is excised and a prosthesis inserted. NB traumatic hip # tend to receive a hemiarthroplasty, predominantly due to patient comorbidity. The acetabulum is not replaced unlike elective THR.

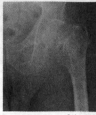

Fig 8.25 AP x-ray of the left hip showing a subcapital fracture of the femoral neck. This may be easily appreciated on this view, but a lateral is vital for less obvious injuries.

Courtesy of The Norfolk and Norwich University Hospitals (NNUH) Radiology Dept.

Garden classification for intracapsular femoral neck fractures (table 8.3) Is based purely on the AP x-ray and correlates with prognosis, IV being the worst risk of AVN. The key is to differentiate between undisplaced (I & II) versus displaced (III & IV).

Table 8.3 Garden classification for intracapsular femoral neck fractures

I	Incomplete undisplaced fracture with the inferior cortex intact
II	Complete undisplaced fracture through the neck
III	Complete neck fracture with partial displacement
IV	Fully displaced fracture

Reproduced with permission and copyright © of the British Editorial Society of Bone and Joint Surgery, Garden RS. Low-angle fixation in fractures of the femoral neck. *J Bone Joint Surg [Br]* 1961;43-B:647–663 (the Garden classification).

Extracapsular fractures (Between insertion of the hip joint capsule & 5cm below the lesser trochanter, fig 8.26.) These are subclassified as basicervical, pertrochanteric or subtrochanteric. Compared to intracapsular #s, the blood supply to the femoral head is not disrupted so AVN/# non-union is rarer. Fixation uses either intramedullary nails or sliding hip screws (for which the trade name Dynamic Hip Screw (DHS) is often used). A DHS will stabilize the # but allow compression at the site due to sliding of the screw in the femoral head, on weight-bearing.

Types of proximal femoral fractures (fig 8.26)

Intra-int and extra-ext-capsular fractures:[25] 1 Subcapitalint; 2 Transcervicalitn; 3 Basicervicalext; 4 Intertrochanteric/pertrochanteric-ext; 5 Reverse oblique/transtrochanteric-ext; 6 Subtrochanteric.-ext

Fracture type (eg displaced/undisplaced) and site determines management:
- Undisplaced intracapsular (1 or 2) → cannulated hip screw,
- Displaced intracapsular (1 or 2) → (hemi)arthroplasty or THR if normally ambulant & medically fit,
- Basicervical (3)/intertrochanteric (4) → DHS fixation,
- Transtrochanteric (5)/subtrochanteric (6) → intramedullary hip screw (but note that a DHS can be used in selected cases).

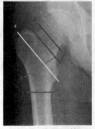

Fig 8.26 Fracture patterns in the proximal femur.

Courtesy of The Norfolk and Norwich University Hospitals (NNUH) Radiology Dept.

Blood supply to the femoral head

The primary blood supply to the femoral head are the retinacular arteries from the medial and lateral femoral circumflex arteries (arising from profunda femoris artery) (fig 8.27). This blood supply can be compromised by intracapsular fractures and SUFE (pp. 490–1) and place the femoral head at risk of *avascular necrosis* (*AVN*). There is a small contribution from the foveal artery which runs in the ligament attached to head of femur, but this is either inadequate or not present in adults. Risk of AVN is <10% if undisplaced, but can be >80% if displaced.[26] NICE recommends that surgery should be performed on the day or day after admission.[25] *Imaging:* MRI is best. *Local causes:* Trauma;

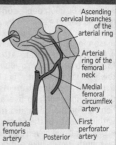

Fig 8.27 Blood supply to the femoral head.

secondary to rheumatoid, severe OA, psoriatic arthropathy, or neuropathic joints. *Systemic:* Atraumatic AVN can initially be painless and incidentally discovered on x-rays, make sure you educate this patient group to report symptoms promptly. Thalassaemia, sickle-cell (+ any cause of microthrombi eg platelets ↑ in leukaemia), NSAIDs/steroids (eg post-transplant). *Treatment:* Immobilization; analgesia; for hips, arthroplasty. >50% will require operative intervention within 3 years. AVN will eventually cause necrosis with bone collapse and secondary OA.[27]

More femoral and hip injuries

Femoral shaft fracture ►Requires considerable force—look for injuries elsewhere. 500–1500mL of blood may be lost in a simple #; check distal pulses (possible femoral artery injury). Sciatic nerve injury may also occur. The proximal bone fragment is flexed by iliopsoas, abducted by gluteus medius, and laterally rotated by gluteus maximus. The lower fragment is pulled up by the hamstrings and adducted (with external rotation) by the adductors. *Treatment:* Stabilize patient in ED and traction with a Thomas' splint (fig 8.5 p. 526) to relieve pain and minimize blood loss. Definitive treatment is typically with a locked intramedullary nail introduced over a guide wire. This allows early mobilization.

Distal femoral & proximal tibial fractures Divided into intra- or extra-articular (supracondylar). Intra-articular # needs internal fixation with anatomically contoured locking plate. Tibial plateau # are intra-articular and difficult to treat; non-operative treatment may be appropriate in the elderly, however internal fixation is normally required to restore the articular surface and minimize later OA. Hinged cast braces locked in extension can reduce the risk of chronic flexure contracture following tibial plateau fractures.[28]

Posterior hip dislocation (eg to front-seat passengers if the knee strikes the dashboard.) Feel for the femoral head in the buttock. The leg is *flexed, internally rotated, adducted,* and *shortened.* Frequently associated with # of femoral head, neck, or shaft. ►The sciatic nerve may be lacerated or stretched/compressed; early MRI diagnosis may prevent later equinus foot deformity. *Treatment:* CT scan, as long as this does not delay theatre. Reduction under GA within 4 hours to reduce risk of AVN. Traction for 3 weeks promotes joint capsule healing.[29]

Further reading

Baker PN (2014). Evolution of the hip fracture population: time to consider the future? *BMJ Open* 4:e004405.

BMJ Best Practice (2014). *Hip Fractures.* http://bestpractice.bmj.com/best-practice/monograph/387/resources.html

9 This is opposed to the internal rotation found in hip dislocation. These positionings are explained by the changes in the fulcrum for the force applied by iliopsoas to the proximal femur in either condition.
►NB: *pathological fractures* are discussed in BOX 'Pathological fractures', p.567.

►Around 80,000 people suffer a hip fracture annually in the UK. This number is set to rise to >100,000 by 2020 in line with the predicted 88% rise in people >65 years old over the next 25 years. Hip fractures are the most common reason for admission to the orthopaedic ward.[30]

Amid your desperate attempts at identifying and describing the type of fracture that you think you might see, take a peek past the computer screen towards your patient. This is most likely a life-changing injury. ~¼ of patients are admitted from institutional care and ~20% of those previously independent enough to live at home will eventually need to move into care homes. The mortality and morbidity is vast with hip fractures. ~8% will die within 1 month of this fracture; 30% will die within 1 year. Be kind, and gently explain that we haven't offered a cup of tea because she needs to remain nil by mouth (NBM). Take a moment to explain the severity of this injury to the family also; in those patients who had significant morbidity and frailty prior to this injury it might be worth discussing issues surrounding resuscitation.

Management

Assess obs. Treat shock with crystalloid, but beware of incipient heart failure.

- Relieve pain (eg **morphine** 0.1mg/kg IV + femoral nerve block or a fascia iliaca compartment block + an antiemetic).
- Imaging: a good quality lateral is essential (see fig 8.25, p. 540). 2–10% of fractures can be missed on x-ray, consider CT/MRI.[31]
- Prepare for theatre: FBC, clotting, U&E, CXR, ECG, crossmatch 2u, consent.
- Sort out medical problems pre-op: ►get help from an ortho-geriatrician.

Preventing hip fractures

Preventing hip fractures is the best approach to reducing mortality, elective hip replacements have a 0.5% 30-day mortality risk while those following traumatic hip fractures have ~8% risk.[32]

- Prevent falls: eg good lighting, less sedation, & falls prevention programmes.
- Teach exercise and balance training: eg with tai chi classes for the elderly. This lessens fear of falling, and can halve rates of multiple falls.
- Treat and/or prevent osteoporosis: eg exercise, bisphosphonates.
- Ensure good vitamin D intake (plasma levels ≥30nmol/L; esp. in northern climes). A lack of vitamin D and calcium is associated with hip fractures whether or not patients are osteoporotic.
- Follow-up meta-analyses have cast doubt over whether hip protectors decrease risk of hip fracture in the elderly. Acceptability by users remains a problem, because of discomfort and practicality.[33]

The following may prevent complications after hip injury

- Early mobilization and post-procedure anticoagulation (p. 528).
- Coordinated multidisciplinary inpatient rehabilitation.
- Good nutrition—but meta-analyses do not provide much support for specific multi-nutritional commercial food supplements.

Further reading

Butler M et al. (2011). Evidence summary: systematic review of surgical treatments for geriatric hip fractures. J Bone Joint Surg Am 93:1104–15.

Hu F et al. (2012). Preoperative predictors for mortality following hip fracture surgery: a systematic review and metaanalysis. Injury 43:676–85.

Ongley D (2014). Fractured NOF Patient: Killing Me Softly with My Song ... http://www.aqua.ac.nz/upload/resource/NOF%20patient%20killing%20me%20softly.pdf

The patella *Dislocation:* Is typically lateral—often as the result of twisting the lower leg, combined with contraction of the quadriceps. The knee is flexed with a lateral deformity. Reduction is achieved with firm medial pressure while extending the knee. Post reduction: do x-rays to check for patellar # and check the extensor mechanism of the knee. Ensure a period of immobilization in cast/posterior splint or brace. Rehabilitation will require quadriceps strengthening exercises. *Recurrent patellar subluxation:* May be related to developmental abnormalities around the knee. A tight lateral retinaculum causes the patella to sublux laterally, giving medial pain. The knee may give way. It is commoner in girls and with valgus knees. It may be familial, or associated with joint laxity, a high-riding patella (*patella alta*), or a hypotrophic lateral femoral condyle. *Signs:* Increased lateral patellar movement, accompanied by pain and the reflex contraction of quadriceps (ie a +ve patellar apprehension test). It may warrant surgery to strengthen the medial expansion.[34] *Patellar fracture* usually results from a fall onto a flexed knee or due to dashboard injury in motor vehicle collision. Non-displaced fractures with an intact extensor mechanism may be managed conservatively. Displaced fractures are likely to require operative fixation.

The knee *Injury to a collateral ligament:* Common in sport. *Mechanism:* the medial ligament is most commonly injured by a blow to the lateral aspect of the knee while the foot is fixed (putting valgus stress on the knee); vice versa for the lateral ligament. *Signs:* effusion ± tenderness over affected ligaments. Rest is needed, then firm support. NB: surgery is rarely needed for isolated medial collateral ligament injury. Lateral injury is less common but tends to be more extensive and involve cruciates and common peroneal nerve injury; surgery is required if there is instability. *Anterior cruciate ligament (ACL) tear:* Typically follows a twisting injury to the knee with the foot fixed to the ground. There is immediate swelling and inability to continue playing. *Signs:* effusion; haemarthrosis; +ve 'draw' sign (p. 494). Examination under GA may be needed. *Treatment:* this is problematic. 3 weeks' rest and physio may help. In the young, or ↑ knee instability, consider ligament reconstruction (autograft).[35] Chronic ACL deficiency results in the knee giving way with laxity on examination and risk of OA. *Posterior cruciate ligament (PCL) tear:* The PCL is twice as strong as ACL and less frequently damaged. Menisci are rarely involved. Occurs in car crashes as the knee strikes the dashboard. Often missed in the acute injury. Do a posterior draw test (p. 494). Most are treated conservatively, PCL reconstruction is more difficult and less predictable than ACL reconstruction.[36] *Meniscal tears:* Most common reasons for knee arthroscopy. See p. 495 for anatomy. Medial meniscus tears (eg 'bucket-handle') follow twists to a flexed knee (eg in football). Adduction + internal rotation causes lateral meniscus tears. Extension is limited (knee locking) as the displaced segment lodges between femoral and tibial condyles. The patient must stop what they are doing, and can only walk on tiptoe, if at all. The joint line is tender, and McMurray's test is +ve (p. 494). If the 'handle' of the 'bucket' becomes free at one end (= 'parrot beak' tear), the knee suddenly gives way, rather than locking. MRI gives tear location, morphology, length, depth, and stability, and helps predict tears requiring repair. Look for avulsions on x-ray. Management is conservative when possible, small asymptomatic tears tend to heal spontaneously, though arthroscopy is usually needed for locked knees, cysts, or persisting symptoms after injury. Surgery aims to preserve the meniscus. Peripheral tears in young, stable knees can be considered for meniscal repair, but repairs do not do well with a combined ACL tear and the knee remains unstable; the meniscus must then be reconstructed.[37] *Typical injury triad:* ACL + medial collateral ligament + medial meniscus following valgus stress with rotation of the knee.[10][38]

10 Also known as O'Donoghue's unhappy triad.

8 Trauma

The ankle is composed of 2 joints: the subtalar joint (consists of calcaneus and talus to facilitate eversion/inversion) and the 'true' ankle joint (consists of tibia, fibula, and talus to facilitate dorsi- and plantar flexion).

Ankle ligament strain Usually (85% of sprains) an inversion injury which injures the *anterior talofibular part* of the lateral ligament (ATFL). 5% are eversion sprains (damaging medial deltoid ligament) and 10% are syndesmotic injuries.[39] *Signs:* Stiffness, tenderness over the lateral ligament, pain on inversion. ►Follow the Ottawa ankle rules to decide if an x-ray is needed to rule out # (see fig 7.2 on p. 465). *Treatment:* Consists of 'POLICE' (Protection from further injury, Optimal Loading, Ice, Compression, Elevation) for simple sprains, ensure good analgesia to enable patient to gently exercise ankle as early as pain allows. In contrast, severe sprains (ligament is completely ruptured with inability to weight bear) require below knee immobilization for at least 10 days. Rehabilitation is advised to reduce recurrent injury. Advise patient to return if there is evidence of neurovascular compromise or pain hinders any weight on injured limb by 24 hours and not full weight-bearing by 4 days.

Ankle fractures In general, stable fractures only involve one side of the ankle (Weber A/B fractures—see fig 8.28). Stable or minimally displaced fractures may be treated non-operatively in a cast. Unstable or displaced fractures require surgery. See fig 8.29 for identifying individual bones on x-ray. *Maisonneuve fracture:* fig 9.20 p. 617 *Proximal* fibular fracture + syndesmosis rupture, and medial malleolus fracture or deltoid ligament rupture. If 2 bones dislocate where no true joint exists, the term *diastasis* ('standing apart') is used. ►Always examine the proximal fibula with 'ankle sprains'. ℞ is surgical as fractures are unstable and require fixation to restore the ankle mortise and placement of 1–2 suprasyndesmotic screws.

Foot fractures: *Lisfranc fracture-dislocation:* ►A commonly missed fracture in multitrauma patients. It may cause compartment syndrome of the medial foot (± later arthritis and persistent pain) and instability, so must be treated promptly. *Imaging:* on x-ray look for widening of the gap between the base of the 1st & 2nd metatarsals. Because of the overlapping bones, subluxations can be hard to see. MRI helps. ℞: achieve *precise* anatomical reduction with screw fixation across the 2nd tarsometatarsal joint (Lisfranc joint).[40] *Fractured neck of talus:* Can occur after forced dorsiflexion, and is a serious injury because interruption of vessels may lead to avascular necrosis of the body of the talus. ℞: displaced fractures require ORIF. *Calcaneus (os calcis) fractures:* Often bilateral, after serious falls. The outcome is frequently poor and many patients are left disabled and unable to return to their previous work. ►Always look for associated spinal fracture. *Signs:* swelling; bruising; inability to weight bear. ℞: ►Does the fracture enter the subtalar joint? For years there has been debate and insufficient evidence to distinguish between conservative and operative approaches; a recent RCT[n=151] reported that operative treatment compared to non-operative care (POLICE, splints, and early mobilization) showed no advantage after 2 years in patients with typical displaced intra-articular fractures of the calcaneus. The risk of complications was also higher post surgery.[41] *2nd metatarsal fracture:* ►Look for Lisfranc dislocations. Usually heal well with non-operative cast and weight-bearing as pain allows. *5th metatarsal fracture:* Two main types: proximal avulsion # typically associated with ankle inversion (treat conservatively) and Jones # (transverse fracture near base) which may require surgical intervention due to risk of non-union. See p. 501 for march fractures.

►►Consider venous thromboprophylaxis in all immobilized lower limbs.

The Danis–Weber classification defines ankle fractures by the level of fibula fracture relative to the tibiofibular syndesmosis. Involvement of the medial/lateral/posterior[11] malleoli are described as malleolar, bimalleolar, or trimalleolar. The Lauge–Hansen classification is more complicated (involves mechanism of injury, position of foot at time of injury in addition to x-ray findings).

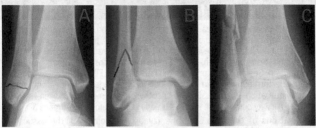

Fig 8.28 A simplification of the *AO Weber classification* of malleolar fractures.
A Below.   **B** At the level of   **C** Above.

Images courtesy of Professor Peter Scally.

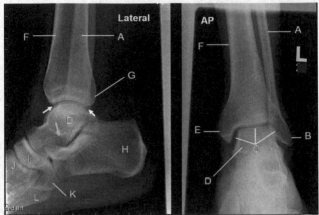

Fig 8.29 Identifying individual bones on x-ray (AP and lateral views of the left ankle). Labelled are the fibula (A), lateral malleolus (B), mortise joint of ankle (C), talus (D), medial malleolus (E), tibia (F), posterior malleolus of talus (G), calcaneus (H), navicular (I), superimposed cuneiforms (J), cuboid (K), base of 5th metatarsal (L).

Reproduced with permission of Nicholas Joseph, CEO CE Essentials.

Further reading

Bleakley CM *et al.* (2012). PRICE needs updating, should we call the POLICE? *Br J Sports Med* 46:220–1.
Kaminski TW *et al.* (2013). National Athletic Trainers' Association position statement: conservative management and prevention of ankle sprains in athletes. *J Athl Train* 48:528–45.

11 The posterior malleoli refers to the posterior part of the distal tibia.

Assault is the commonest cause of facial trauma; young men are most affected.[42] Facial laceration and mandible fracture are the most frequent injuries. Always consider associated neck, eye, or head injury. Remove blood, loose/false teeth, and vomit from the mouth. Lie in the semi-prone position to prevent airway obstruction. See pp. 466-7 for assessing neck injuries. Fibreoptic nasoendoscopy can be performed by the ENT team to look for pharyngeal/laryngeal trauma; try gentle intubation—if impossible, do cricothyrotomy (OHCM p772), then tracheostomy. ▸Airway compromise requires urgent expert help (anaesthetics & ENT).

Lacerations of the face Clean meticulously. Alignment of the tissues and antisepsis must be exact to produce a good cosmetic result.
• *Simple lacerations:* Consider glue or skin closure strip (eg Steri-Strips™) (p.621).
• *Complex lacerations:* Ask for a plastic/ENT/maxillofacial surgeon.
• *Animal bites:* See p. 618.
• *Ruptured ear drum:* NSAIDs for analgesia, and advise to keep ear dry (pp. 394–5).
• *Eye injury (pp. 548–9), nose fractures (p. 410), and nose bleeds (pp. 412–13).*

Mandible injury *Signs:* Local tenderness and swelling; jaw malocclusion; a mobile fragment; bone may protrude into the mouth in open fractures; if comminuted, the tongue may make airway management extremely difficult, so get expert help. *Diagnosis:* Orthopantogram (OPG) x-rays. Enlist dental help. *Treating TMJ dislocations:* Place (gloved) thumbs over the back teeth and press downwards, while at the same time levering the chin upwards with your fingers (both hands). Consider midazolam sedation: see p. 581. Blows to the chin may cause fracture at the impact site, or indirect fractures near the temporomandibular joint. *Fractures:* Usually require ORIF with miniplates in theatre; conservative treatment involves wiring teeth together for 6 weeks. Complicated fractures may benefit from lag osteosynthesis. *Complications:* Infection; nonunion. *Avulsed teeth:* May be replaced (p. 622). If inhaled, do expiratory CXR. *Bleeding socket:* Ask patient to bite on adrenaline-soaked pads, or suture.

A badge of honour? A common facial injury in wrestlers and rugby players is a direct blow to the pinna, the resultant shearing force causes separation of the auricular perichondrium from the underlying cartilage. The adherent network of perichondrial blood vessels tear and cause a haematoma to develop (see also p. 388). This vascular disruption leads to compromised cartilage viability giving rise to a 'cauliflower' ear deformity; players can be surprisingly proud of these (fig 8.30). If the patient presents within 7 days attempt to drain the haematoma, beyond this, formation of scar tissue complicates drainage. There is no preferred method of drainage, options include needle aspiration and incision & drainage. Review after 24 hours to check for re-accumulation and re-drain if needed. Apply a pressure bandage after drainage by stuffing saline-soaked gauze in the external auricular crevices and wrap bandages around the head. Specialist bandages also exist. Give broadspectrum antibiotics to cover soft tissue infection.[44]

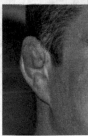

Fig 8.30 Cauliflower ear. See this excerpt from a UK newspaper which shows an interesting display of cauliflower ears.[43]

Nils Jorgenson/ Shutterstock.

Further reading

Bell RB *et al.* (2004). Management of cerebrospinal fluid leak associated with craniomaxillofacial trauma. *J Oral Maxillofac Surg* 62:676–84.

Laski R *et al.* (2004). Facial trauma: a recurrent disease? The potential role of disease prevention. *J Oral Maxillofac Surg* 62:685–8.

Reuben AD *et al.* (2005). A comparative study of evaluation of radiographs, CT and 3D reformatted CT in facial trauma: what is the role of 3D? *Br Jr Rad* 78:198–201.

Bony injuries to the face

The face forms a shock absorber which protects the brain from injury. The most common #s to the facial bones lie along 2 hoops, from ear to ear. One is formed by the zygomatic arch, body, infraorbital rim, and nose. The other is formed by the mandible (fig 8.31). Major blunt trauma can cause a # to the entire middle ⅓ of the face, which has been classified by *Le Fort*, but since the advent of seat belts these are less common.

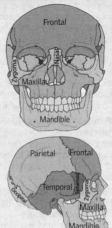

Zygoma fractures *The arch:* Before swelling arrives, there is a depression in front of the ear, and lateral jaw excursions or jaw opening may be limited and painful. A suitable x-ray is the submentovertex view (SMV). *The complex:* The zygoma's body has 4 extensions: 1 frontozygomatic 2 Arch 3 Maxillary buttress (in mouth) 4 Infra-orbital rim. Fractures may be palpated at these points, or disproportionately severe pain elicited on palpation. Occipitomental views are most suitable. *Orbital floor injuries:* Blunt trauma around the eye can cause # to the orbital floor. Imaging: CT is best, but OM views may show trap door sign in the maxillary sinus (fig 8.32).

Fig 8.31 Skull: (a) AP, (b) lateral.

Clinical exam for periorbital trauma:
• Is there CSF rhinorrhoea (yes in ≤25%)? See p. 410.[45]
• Check zygomatic arch by assessing range of mandibular lateral excursions and opening. Also palpate over the arch (just under the skin) and compare with the unaffected side.
• Patient sitting, doctor standing above and behind, place index fingers on the cheeks and look down from above for asymmetry.

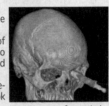

Fig 8.32 3D CT of a nasty injury to the eye. ▶▶On no account remove the knife.
Courtesy of Prof Peter Scally.

• Check the orbit floor for: diplopia on upward gaze (≈trapped orbital contents); enophthalmos; numbness in the distribution of the infraorbital nerve (suggests fracture).
• Small risk of retrobulbar haemorrhage: catastrophic if missed: severe pain at back of eye; proptosis; loss of visual acuity. ▶Prompt eye exam is essential.

NB: if the eye is very swollen, application of a rubber glove filled with ice is invaluable, especially if you ask a specialist to travel to check patient; they can no more open a swollen eye than you. *Treatment:* Unless vision ↓, or there is significant risk of infection, admission on presentation is not mandatory: seeing at the next fracture clinic is adequate. If in doubt, consult the relevant specialist. Explain about not blowing the nose in fractures in continuity with the maxillary sinus (risks periorbital emphysema and infection).

▶*Medicolegal issues:* Facial injuries commonly result from assault. Your notes may be used in criminal injuries claims or as evidence in court. Often the individual is drunk and abusive, it is late, and you are busy, but you must make accurate notes with diagrams. Other people will definitely take time to study and criticize what you have written. Don't forget photographs if assault is particularly serious or children are involved. Document that the patient has given, or refused, permission for statements to be made to the police or legal professionals (the medical notes are confidential).

▶Prevention is the key eg wearing goggles, or plastic glasses when near small, moving objects or using tools (avoids splinters, fish-hooks, and squash-ball injuries). *Always record acuity* (both eyes; if the uninjured one has poor vision the implications of this injury are even greater). Take a detailed history of the event.

If unable to open the injured eye, instil a few drops of local anaesthetic (**tetracaine** 1%): after a few minutes, comfortable opening may be possible. Examine lids, conjunctiva, cornea, sclera, anterior chamber, pupil, iris, lens, vitreous, fundus, and eye movement. An irregular pupil may mean globe rupture. Afferent pupil defects (p. 366) do not herald well for sight recovery. Note pain, discharge, or squint. CT may be very useful (foreign bodies may be ferromagnetic, so avoid MRI).

Penetrating trauma Refer immediately: delays risk of ocular extrusion or infection. Uveal injury risks sympathetic ophthalmia in the other eye. ▶A history of flying objects (eg work with hammers and chisels) prompts careful examination + x-ray to exclude intraocular foreign bodies (± skull x-ray or CT to exclude intracranial involvement). ▶*Don't* try to remove a large foreign body (knife; dart). Support the object with padding. Transport supine.

Foreign bodies (FBs) (fig 8.33) *Have a low threshold for getting help*; FBs often hide, so examine *all* the eye and evert the lid. FBs cause chemosis, subconjunctival bleeds, irregular pupils, iris prolapse, hyphaema, vitreous haemorrhage, and retinal tears. If you suspect a metal FB discuss with radiology; traditional x-ray of orbits is largely now replaced with 1st-line CT depending on level of suspicion; orbital US is useful but is usually provided by ophthalmology rather than radiology (pick-up rate is 90% vs 40% for x-rays but skill is needed as there is a risk of worsening a ruptured globe with pressure on the eye). Low-risk, superficial FBs may be removable with a triangle of clean card (**chloramphenicol** 0.5% drops after, to prevent infection), but if in any doubt refer to somebody with experience of using a 'slit-lamp' who can assess the depth of penetration, and remove it under direct magnified vision.

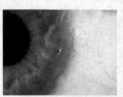

Fig 8.33 Corneal FB (centre).
© Bristol Eye Hospital.

Corneal abrasions (fig 8.34; often from small fast-moving objects eg children's fingernails; twigs.) They may cause intense pain. Apply a drop of local anaesthetic, eg 1% **tetracaine** before examination. Abrasions will show fluorescein staining. Remember to evert the lid to ensure the offending FB isn't lodged beneath. Look carefully for any retained corneal FB, and for any fluid leak from the eye (Seidel's test, see p. 326).

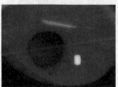

Fig 8.34 Corneal abrasion just above the pupil.
© Bristol Eye Hospital.

The anterior chamber should be well formed. Send the patient home with oral analgesics and **chloramphenicol** ointment 1% QDS. If still having a FB sensation after removing the pad, stain again with fluorescein. If the cornea stains, repeat the procedure after 24h. If it still stains after 48h, refer. NB: a Cochrane review of small corneal abrasions does not favour using pads.[48] See also p. 334.

Burns Treat chemical burns immediately: irrigate, irrigate, irrigate until a neutral pH is reached; instil anaesthetic drops (**tetracaine** 1%) until the patient is comfortable. Often the lids close tight from severe pain, but watch out for particulate chemicals which may be trapped in the lid fornices. Late serious sequelae: eg corneal scarring, opacification, and lid damage. Alkali burns penetrate more deeply than acid, and so may be more destructive to intraocular structures. Seek expert advice.

8 Trauma

Photokeratitis, 'arc eye' Welders and sunbed users who don't use uv protection may damage the cornea (FB sensation, watering, blepharospasm). Intense pain (has been compared to child birth!) starts 6–12h after uv exposure. *R:* Generous oral analgesics, analgesic eye drops for home use are not advised due to ocular toxicity if overused. Give antibiotic ointment and it will recover in 24h.[47]

Major trauma Very rare, but think of *fat embolus* in major trauma patients with visual problems.

Contusions and intraocular haemorrhage

Our eyes are protected by bony orbital ridges; significant force is needed to fracture these so look for associated peripheral and head injuries. Severe contusions from large objects may damage the eye, but smaller objects such as squash balls and airgun pellets cause local contusion eg resulting in lid bruises, subconjunctival haemorrhage, retinal contusion (may be associated with breaks or tears and lead to retinal detachment), or even globe perforation.

Intraocular bleeds ►*Get expert help:* acuity may be affected. Blood is often found in the anterior chamber (hyphaema, fig 4.5, p. 326): small amounts clear spontaneously but if filling the anterior chamber, evacuation may be needed. It is often recognizable by pen-torch examination. Even small hyphaemas must be carefully evaluated (so refer): it may signify serious injury. *Late complications:* Glaucoma; corneal staining; rebleeding. Vitreous haemorrhage may cause a fall in visual acuity, and loss of red reflex on fundoscopy if severe, as may retinal detachment. Sometimes the iris is paralysed and dilated due to injury (called traumatic mydriasis). This usually recovers in a few days but sometimes it is permanent. Consider relative afferent pupillary defect and optic nerve damage as an alternative cause of a dilated pupil (p. 366). Lens dislocation, tearing of the iris root, splitting of the choroid, detachment of the retina, and damage to the optic nerve may be other sequelae; they are more common if contusion is caused by smaller objects rather than large.

Blows to the orbit Blunt injury (eg from a football) can cause sudden ↑ in pressure within the orbit, and may cause blowout fractures with the orbital contents herniating into the maxillary sinus. Tethering of the inferior rectus and inferior oblique muscles causes diplopia. Test the sensation over the lower lid skin. Loss of sensation indicates infra-orbital nerve injury, suggesting a blowout fracture. CT may show the depressed fracture of the posterior orbital floor. Fracture reduction and muscle release is necessary.[48]

Acknowledgement

We thank Professor Alastair Denniston and Priscilla Matthewson for their help with this page.

8 Trauma

Further reading

Magarakis M *et al.* (2012). Ocular injury, visual impairment, and blindness associated with facial fractures: a systematic literature review. *Plast Reconstr Surg* 129:227–33.

Roth FS *et al.* (2010). Pearls of orbital trauma management. *Semin Plast Surg* 24:398–410.

Wipperman JL *et al.* (2013). Evaluation and management of corneal abrasions. *Am Fam Physician* 87:114–20.

Table 8.4 Testing peripheral upper limb nerve motor function

Nerve root	Muscle	Test by asking the patient to:
C3,4	Trapezius	Shrug shoulder (via accessory nerve)
C4,5	Rhomboids	Brace shoulder back
C5,6,7	Serratus anterior	Push arm forward against resistance
C5,6	Pectoralis major (clavicular head)	Adduct arm from above horizontal, and push it forward
C6,7,8	Pectoralis major (sternocostal head)	Adduct arm below horizontal
C5,6	Supraspinatus	Abduct arm the first 15°
C5,6	Infraspinatus	Externally rotate arm, elbow at side
C6,7,8	Latissimus dorsi	Adduct arm from horizontal position
C5,6	Biceps	Flex supinated forearm
C5,6	Deltoid	Abduct arm between 15° and 90°
Radial nerve (C5–8)		
C6,7,8	Triceps	Extend elbow against resistance
C5,6	Brachioradialis	Flex elbow with forearm half way between pronation and supination
C5,6	Extensor carpi radialis longus	Extend wrist radially with fingers extended
C6,7	Supinator	Arm by side, resist hand pronation
C7,8	Extensor digitorum	Keep fingers extended at MCP joint
C7,8	Extensor carpi ulnaris	Extend wrist to ulnar side
C7,8	Abductor pollicis longus	Abduct thumb at 90° to palm
C7,8	Extensor pollicis brevis	Extend thumb at MCP joint
C7,8	Extensor pollicis longus	Resist thumb flexion at IP joint
Median nerve (C6–T1)		
C6,7	Pronator teres	Keep arm pronated against resistance
C6,7	Flexor carpi radialis	Flex wrist towards radial side
C7,**8**,T1	Flexor digitorum superficialis	Resist extension at PIP joint (while you fix his proximal phalanx)
C8,T1	Flexor digitorum profundus I & II	Flex the DIP of the index finger, with the PIP held in extension
C8,T1	Flexor pollicis longus	Resist thumb extension at interphalangeal joint (fix proximal phalanx)
C8,T1	Abductor pollicis brevis	Abduct thumb (nail at 90° to palm)
C8,T1	Opponens pollicis	Thumb touches base of 5th fingertip (nail parallel to palm)
C8,T1	1st and 2nd lumbricals	Extend PIP joint against resistance with MCP joint held in flexion
Ulnar nerve (C7–T1)		
C7,**8**,T1	Flexor carpi ulnaris	Flex wrist towards ulnar side
C7,C8	Flexor digitorum profundus III & IV	Flex the DIP of the little finger, with the PIP held in extension
C8,**T1**	Dorsal interossei	Abduct fingers (use index finger)
C8,**T1**	Palmar interossei	Adduct fingers (use index finger)
C8,T1	Adductor pollicis	Adduct thumb (nail at 90° to palm)
C8,T1	Abductor digiti minimi	Abduct little finger
C8,T1	Flexor digiti minimi	Flex the little finger at MCP joint
The musculocutaneous nerve (C5–6)		
C5,6	This may be injured at the brachial plexus, causing weakness of biceps, coracobrachialis, and brachialis. Forearm flexion is weak, ± some loss of sensation	

Sources MRC Handbook; www.rad.washington.edu/atlas; www.medmedia.com/05/324.htm

See p. 552 for dermatomes and peripheral nerve distributions.

NB: root numbers in **bold** indicate that root is more important than its neighbour. ►Sources vary in ascribing particular nerve roots to muscles—and there is some biological variation in individuals. The tables are a reasonable compromise, and are based on the MRC guidelines.

8 Trauma

Table 8.5 Testing peripheral lower limb nerve motor function

Nerve root	Muscle	Test by asking the patient to:
L**4,5**, S1	Gluteus medius & minimus	Internal rotation at hip, hip abduction
L5, S1,2	Gluteus maximus	Extension at hip (lie prone)
L**2,3**,4	Adductors (obturator nerve)	Adduct leg against resistance
Femoral nerve (L2–4, posterior division)		
L1,2,3	Iliopsoas	Flex hip with knee flexed and lower leg supported: patient lies on back
L2,3	Sartorius	Flex knee with hip external rotated
L2,3,4	Quadriceps femoris	Extend knee against resistance
Obturator nerve (L2–4, anterior division)		
L2,3,4	Hip adductors	Adduct the leg
Inferior gluteal nerve		
L5,S1,S2	Gluteus maximus	Hip extension
Superior gluteal nerve		
L4,5,S1	Gluteus medius & minimus	Abduction and internal rotation of hip
Sciatic nerve (including the common peroneal nerve^{cP} & tibial nerve^{T})		
L**4,5**^{cP}	Tibialis anterior	Dorsiflex ankle
L**5**,S1^{cP}	Extensor digitorum longus	Dorsiflex toes against resistance
L**5**,S1^{cP}	Extensor hallucis longus	Dorsiflex hallux against resistance
L5,S1^{cP}	Peroneus longus & brevis	Evert foot against resistance
L5,S1^{cP}	Extensor digitorum brevis	Dorsiflex 2nd–4th toes (muscle of foot)
L5,S1,2^{T}	Hamstrings	Flex knee against resistance
L4,5^{T}	Tibialis posterior	Invert plantarflexed foot
S1,2^{T}	Gastrocnemius	Plantarflex ankle joint
L5,S1,2^{T}	Flexor digitorum longus	Flex terminal joints of toes
S1,2^{T}	Small muscles of foot	Make sole of foot into a cup

Table 8.6 Quick screening test for muscle power

Shoulder	Abduction	c5	Hip	Flexion	L1,2
	Adduction	c5,7		Extension	L5,S1
Elbow	Flexion	c5,6	Knee	Flexion	S1
	Extension	c7		Extension	L3,4
Wrist	Flexion	c7,8	Ankle	Dorsiflexion	L4
	Extension	c7		Plantarflexion	S1,2
Fingers	Flexion	c7,8			
	Extension	c7			
	Abduction	T1 (ulnar)			

See table 7.1 on p. 465 for MRC grading of muscle power, see also fig 8.35, the motor homunculus.

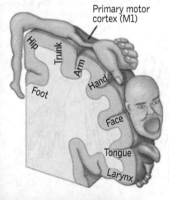

Fig 8.35 The motor homunculus—a pictorial representation of the anatomical divisions of the primary motor cortex. © BrainHQ from Posit Science.

Primary motor cortex (M1)

Hip · Trunk · Arm · Hand · Foot · Face · Tongue · Larynx

8 Trauma

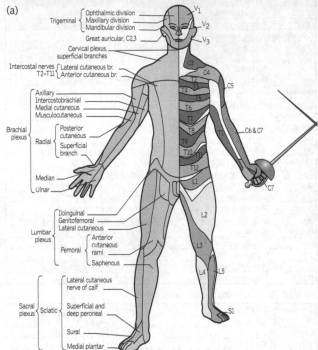

(a)

Fig 8.36 (a) These images reflect the 2011 evidence-based dermatomes, which have revealed much more individual variation than originally thought, so much so that some areas have been left blank (white) because no single best option can be given. (b) Feet and hands (c) Posterior view. (d) Perineal dermatomes.. See p.550 for testing peripheral motor nerves.

Reproduced with permission from M.W.L. Lee, R.W. McPhee, M.D. Stringer, An evidence-based approach to human dermatomes, *Clinical Anatomy*, Volume 21, Issue 5, pp.363–373, Copyright © 2008 John Wiley & Sons.

(b)

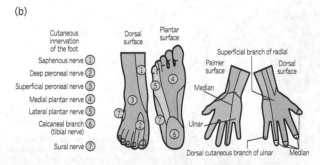

553

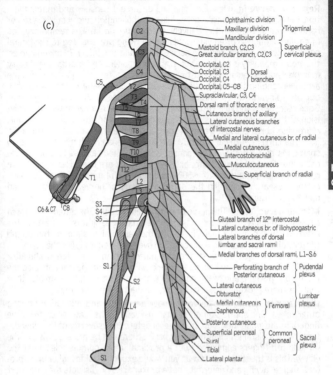

(c)

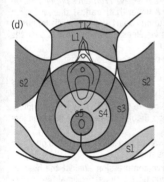

(d)

Aim to keep a few key dermatomes up your sleeve

C3–4	Clavicles
C6–7	Lateral arm/forearm
T1	Medial side of arm
C6	Thumb
C7	Middle finger
C8	Little finger
T4	Nipples
T10	Umbilicus
L2–L3	Anterior & inner leg
L5	Medial side of big toe
L5, S1–2	Posterior & outer leg
S1	Lateral margin of foot and little toe
S2–4	Perineum

The above is a rough approximation

8 Trauma

Repair of nerve injuries Examine and document sensory and motor function. Repair of any peripheral nerve injury is challenging and requires a senior hand or plastic surgeon to be involved. *Neurapraxia* implies temporary loss of nerve conduction often via ischaemia following pressure (eg to the lateral popliteal nerve as it crosses the neck of the fibula, see later). In mixed nerves, the motor modality is the more vulnerable component eg Saturday night palsy (compression of radial nerve at the spiral groove after falling asleep with the arm overhanging the chair). *Axonotmesis* entails damage to the nerve fibre but the epineural tube is intact, providing guidance to the regrowing nerve. Good recovery is the rule. Growth rate is 1–3mm/day. *Neurotmesis* means division of the whole nerve. As there is no guidance from the endoneural tube, regrowing fibrils cause a traumatic neuroma if they are unable to bridge the gap. The current surgical standard is epineural repair with nylon sutures. To span gaps that primary repair cannot bridge without excess tension, nerve-cable interfascicular autografts or nerve transfers are used. Results of nerve repair are fair (at best), with ~50% regaining useful function. There is much current research regarding the pathophysiology of nerve regeneration and how to optimize repair.[49]

Median nerve (C5–T1) The nerve of *grasp*. Injury above the antecubital fossa causes: • Inability to flex index finger interphalangeal joints on clasping the hands (Ochner's test) • Inability to flex the terminal phalanx of the thumb (flexor pollicis longus) • Loss of sensation over the thenar half of the palm.

If the lesion is at the wrist, the only muscle reliably affected is abductor pollicis brevis. Test it by holding the hand palm up. Can the patient raise the thumb out of the plane of the hand? The area of sensory loss is smaller than that for more proximal lesions. See BOX, 'Median nerve anatomy'.

Ulnar nerve (C8–T1) The nerve of finger abduction and adduction (among other roles). One subtle sign of an ulnar nerve lesion is inability to cross the fingers in the 'good luck' sign. Injury level determines severity of the claw deformity. In a distal lesion of the ulnar nerve, there will be more clawing of the 4th and 5th fingers compared with a proximal, more complete lesion at the elbow. This is the *ulnar paradox* as you would expect a lesion higher up to produce more clawing and deformity, but a proximal lesion disrupts the ulnar part of flexor digitorum profundus leading to unopposed extension and therefore less clawing; the closer the paw the worse the claw. *Froment's paper sign:* On holding a piece of paper between thumb & finger (both hands), there is flexion of the thumb's distal phalanx on trying to pull apart (flexor pollicis longus, is recruited to overcome adductor pollicis weakness). Sensory loss is over the little finger & a variable area of the ring finger.

Radial nerve (C5–T1) The nerve of extension of the elbow, wrist, and fingers. It opens the fist. Injury will produce wrist-drop. Test for this with the elbow flexed and the forearm pronated. Sensory loss is variable, but always includes the dorsal aspect of the root of the thumb.

Lateral popliteal (common peroneal) nerve (L4–S2) The commonest lower limb nerve injury. Lesions lead to foot drop, inability to evert the foot, and loss of sensation over the dorsum of the foot.

Tibial nerve (S1–3) Loss causes calcaneovalgus and inability to stand on tiptoe or invert the foot. Sensory loss is over the sole.

Common peroneal compression Nerve compression against the head of fibula (eg plaster casts, thin patients lying unconscious, proximal fibula fracture, squatting, obstructed labour) causes inability to dorsiflex the foot. Sensation may be ↓ over the dorsum of the foot. *Treatment:* Most recover spontaneously but surgical decompression may be needed (eg if >3 months without improvement). Physiotherapy and splint until foot-drop recovers.

Carpal tunnel syndrome (CTS) ►The commonest cause of hand pain at night. It is due to compression of the median nerve as it passes under the flexor retinaculum.[12] ♀:♂ >1:1. *Signs:* These are in the median nerve distribution:
• Tingling or pain is felt in the thumb, index, and middle fingers.
• When the pain is at its worse, the patient characteristically flicks or shakes the wrist to bring about relief. Pain is especially common at night and after repetitive actions. Affected persons may experience clumsiness.
• Wasted thenar eminence & ↓ sensation over the lateral 3½ digits (*not* 5th).
• Lateral palmar sensation is spared as its supply (the palmar cutaneous branch of the median nerve) does not pass through the tunnel.
• *Phalen's test:* holding the wrist hyperflexed for 1min reproduces the symptoms. (This is more reliable than *Tinel's test*—tapping over the tunnel to produce paraesthesiae. Note: Phalen's flexing, Tinel's tapping.)
Investigations and management: See p. 513 and fig 7.20.

Median nerve anatomy

The median nerve arises from C5, C6, C7, C8, & T1 as a condensation of lateral & medial cords of brachial plexus (fig 8.37, p. 557). It crosses medial to the brachial artery in antecubital fossa. It has no branches above the elbow. ~5cm distal to elbow it gives off its anterior interosseous branch (motor to flexor pollicis longus (FPL), flexor digitorum profundus (FDP), index finger & pronator quadratus). The palmar cutaneous branch (sensory to thenar skin) arises ~5cm proximal to wrist and overlies the flexor retinaculum. The recurrent motor branch to the thenar muscles arises at the distal end of carpal tunnel. The median nerve is motor to PT (pronator teres), FCR (flexor carpi radialis), PL (palmaris longus), FDS (flexor digitorum superficialis), LOAF (see p. 463). Sensation: radial 3½ digits. See fig 7.20, for a cross-sectional diagram of the carpal tunnel.

Anterior interosseous nerve compression This median nerve branch may be compressed under the fibrous origin of flexor digitorum profundus, causing weakness of pinch and pain along the forearm's radial border. The patient will be unable to flex the DIP joint of the index finger and PIP joint of the thumb to make a rounded 'o' shape *Treatment:* Initial conservative management with surgical decompression if required.

Posterior interosseous nerve (PIN) compression This branch of the radial nerve is compressed on passing through the proximal supinator muscle eg after forearm fracture or excessive exercise. Patients experience weakness of thumb and finger extension. Electromyographic studies are typically positive.

Radial tunnel syndrome Involves compression of the same nerve, but presents with lateral forearm pain rather than weakness. Electrodiagnostic studies tend to be negative. *Examination:* May show weakness of long finger extensors, and short and long thumb extensors, but no sensory loss. *Treatment:* Rest, splints, NSAIDs are 1st line. Steroid injections may help. In resistant cases surgical decompression of areas of potential compression of the PIN.

Ulnar nerve compression at the wrist Uncommon. See *OHCM* p502.

Meralgia paraesthetica (lateral femoral cutaneous nerve) A symptom complex of numbness, paraesthesiae, and pain (eg burning/shooting) in the anterolateral thigh. Most cases are idiopathic. ΔΔ: Lumbar disc hernia. R̝: (often self-limiting but may recur). Lose weight if needed, rest, NSAID ± carbamazepine ± cortisone and local anaesthetic injection at the anterior superior iliac spine gives unpredictable results.[50]

Further reading

Heaton S *et al.* (2012). Entrapment syndromes. In Simpson DM *et al.* (eds) *Neuropathic Pain: Mechanisms, Diagnosis and Treatment*, pp281–305. New York: OUP.

Sawardeker P *et al.* (2015). Nerve compression: ulnar nerve of the elbow. In Trail IA *et al.* (eds) *Disorders of the Hand*, pp243–65. New York: Springer.

12 Ulnar nerve compression at elbow, p. 475; brachial plexus injury, p. 556; peripheral nerve injury, p. 550 & p. 554.

8 Trauma

The brachial plexus extends from the intervertebral foramina to the axilla via Roots, Trunks, Divisions, Cords, and Branches ('Remember To Drink Cold Beer') spanning a distance of ~15cm. Useful landmarks on its route from cord to arm worth remembering are:
- The roots leave the vertebral column between the scalenus medius and anterior muscles (see fig 8.38).
- The creation of divisions from trunks takes place under the clavicle, *medial* to the coracoid process.
- The plexus has an intimate relationship with the subclavian and then axillary arteries, with the median nerve forming from the medial and lateral cords anterior to the latter. Look for the characteristic 'M' formation: see fig 8.39.

Traumatic causes *Direct:* eg shoulder girdle fracture, penetrating or iatrogenic. *Indirect:* eg avulsion/traction injuries, due to excessive lateral flexion of the neck—as may occur in motorcycle injuries, or to the newborn during delivery.

Atraumatic causes Tumours (eg Pancoast, from lung), radiation, neuropathy.

Root injuries There are 4 types: high, middle, low, or complete. The position of the arm at time of injury determines the nerves involved.
- *High lesions—Erb's palsy:* (c5, c6) Damage affects the suprascapular, musculocutaneous and axillary nerves. This leads to paralysis of supraspinatus (abduction), infraspinatus (external rotation), biceps (supination), brachialis (flexion of elbow), deltoid (abduction), and teres minor (external rotation). As a result the arm is held internally rotated, pronated, extended and adducted in the *'waiter's tip'* position. Sensation is impaired over deltoid, lateral forearm, and hand. Difficult deliveries (or any trauma in a downwards direction) can produce this sign in neonates.
- *Low lesions—Klumpke's paralysis:* (c8, t1) Occurs when the arm is pulled superiorly (forced abduction)—eg trying to break a fall from height by grabbing onto something. Damage to the c8, t1 roots leads to a combination of median and ulnar nerve injury which may produce 'claw hand' (extension at MCP joints, with flexion at DIP/PIP joints) due to loss of lumbrical function. The arm is held in adduction. Horner' syndrome (p. 366) may also occur.

Injury to the cords
- *Injury to the lateral cord of the plexus:* Absent power in the biceps and brachioradialis (flexes the forearm at the elbow).
- *Posterior cord injury:* Teres major & deltoid inaction; radial nerve palsy.
- *Medial cord injury:* Affects the ulnar and median nerves. Sensation is absent over the medial arm and hand. See fig 8.37.

Recovery Difficult to determine as each lesion and patient must be assessed individually. Intensive rehabilitation with physiotherapy and occupational therapy is needed to encourage spontaneous healing if nerves are not completely disrupted. Minimize contracture development by using braces. With incomplete trunk lesions recovery may take >5 months. Prognosis is poor in lesions proximal to the dorsal root ganglion (DRG). Surgical intervention is complex. Early liaison with a regional centre is advised as early exploration improves the outcome of nerve repair. Surgical options include nerve grafting of viable roots, nerve transfer (from intercostal or phrenic nerves), free functioning muscle transfers, and tendon transfers.[51]

Further reading
British Orthopaedic Association (2012). BOAST 5: *Peripheral Nerve Injury.* https://www.boa.org.uk/wp-content/uploads/2014/12/BOAST-5.pdf

8 Trauma

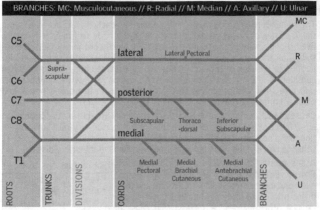

BRANCHES: MC: Musculocutaneous // R: Radial // M: Median // A: Axillary // U: Ulnar

Fig 8.37 The brachial plexus, the *bête noire* of medical students. This diagram should be just memorizable the night before an exam.   Image courtesy of Luke Famery.

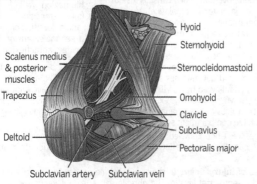

Fig 8.38 The proximal brachial plexus. The purpose of this Figure and Fig 8.39, is to show *where* the brachial plexus is, and not *what* the brachial plexus is.

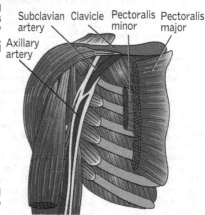

Fig 8.39 The distal brachial plexus: note the relationship with the axillary artery.

The spinal cord is a precious bundle of nerves which travels down through the 33 bones of the spinal column to enable the body to function normally. Even though <5% of spinal injuries result in spinal cord injury (sci), the resulting motor, sensory, and autonomic dysfunction are too devastating to ignore. It is the lack of motor function that one immediately thinks of when considering life in a wheelchair. However, most patients with significant sci prioritize their wishes for restoration of functions in this order: bowel and bladder control; sexual function; hand function; breathing.

Causes Most commonly due to trauma; especially RTCs but as the population ages, falls are becoming more frequent. For this reason, pay particular attention to the need for examining and imaging the neck in head injuries (pp. 590-1). Other causes include tumours, prolapsed discs (p. 587), and inflammatory disease.

Assessment Follow the ATLS® principles (p. 587). Plan movements carefully and use the log-roll technique and c-spine immobilization. Prevent and treat hypotension (aim for SBP >90mmHg). Look for, and exclude other injuries before assigning cause of hypotension to neurogenic shock. Restore intravascular volume (don't overload) then consider use of vasopressors (see later for fluid balance). Monitor and treat symptomatic bradycardia. Monitor and regulate temperature. ▶Perform and document serial neurological examinations to assess for deterioration; test for root lesions (see MINIBOX 'For

For root lesions, test
• C5: shoulder abduction
• C6: elbow flexion
• C7: elbow extension
• C8: finger flexion (grip)
• T1: finger abduction
• L2: hip flexion
• L3: knee extension
• L4: ankle dorsiflexion
• L5: great toe extension
• S1: ankle plantarflexion

root lesions, test'); test the reflexes: (biceps C5; brachioradialis C6; triceps C7). Motor nerve roots and dermatomes are given on pp. 550–553. The main sites of injury are C6 & C7, followed by C2. ~10% of c-spine fractures will have another spinal fracture elsewhere, so always examine the whole spine. ▶▶NB: Remember that a spinal cord injury causing anaesthesia may be masking serious injury below the lesion (eg compartment syndrome, acute abdomen).

Imaging See p. 466. Good knowledge of anatomical and developmental variation is also required when assessing x-rays—eg pseudosubluxation of C2 on C3 mimicking injury.

Consequences of injury Injury to the cervical spine causes tetraplegia, but injury above the segmental level of the phrenic nerve (C3, 4, 5 keeps the diaphragm alive) results in paralysis of the diaphragm. Intubate and ventilate patients with high tetraplegia early on. Thoracic spine damage causes paraplegia and lumbar spine lesions give rise to symptoms of cauda equina compromise. Lesions above T6 can be associated with autonomic dysreflexia (see p. 564). Incomplete spinal cord injuries display specific patterns (see p. 560). *Respiratory insufficiency:* Arises both from neurological dysfunction and associated trauma to chest wall or head. Check vital capacity repeatedly. If <500–600mL, intubation and ventilation will be needed. Monitor arterial blood gases. Intubation may produce vagal bradycardia, so consider **atropine** 0.3–0.6mg IV before intubation and suction. If abdominal distension is causing respiratory compromise, pass an NGT as there is high risk of aspiration. *Fluid balance:* There is likely to be hypotension below the lesion (sympathetic interruption and resultant *neurogenic shock*—↓BP and pulse rate). This is not due to hypovolaemia, and it is dangerous to give large volumes of fluid. Use IV not oral fluids for 48h and while ileus persists. *The skin:* Turn every 2h between supine and right/left lateral positions. The Stoke Mandeville bed does this electronically. Use pillows to separate the legs and maintain a lumbar lordosis. *The bladder:* Pass a urinary catheter before the bladder volume exceeds 500mL (overstretching of detrusor can delay the return of automatic bladder function).

Treatment Starts on-scene with controlled movement of the patient and optimizing conditions in head injury in order to minimize secondary insults.

▶Arrange early transfer to a spinal injuries unit. *Steroids:* ☞ May marginally improve motor strength if given within 8 hours.[52] Seek specialist advice. *Early surgical decompression and stabilization:* ☞ Should be attempted when feasible but there may be no difference in neurologic or functional improvement with early vs late surgery.[53] *Traction:* Skeletal traction will be needed for cervical injuries. Spring-loaded Gardner–Wells skull tongs are preferable to Crutchfield calipers, which need incisions. *Anticoagulation:* Acute cord injury patients are at very high risk of developing VTE, with asymptomatic DVT demonstrable in 60–100% of patients. LMWH (eg **enoxaparin** 40mg/24h SC) is currently recommended over unfractionated heparin regimens for prevention of VTE.[54] Start warfarin later and continue for at least 3 months or until completion of inpatient rehabilitation.[55]

Immobilization of the cervical spine

Which patients should be immobilized? In trauma with a significant mechanism of injury (eg high-speed RTC), head injury with neck pain, or patients found collapsed with suspected trauma then a c-spine injury should be assumed until otherwise proven. Patients who are GCS 15, sober with no neurology, no distracting injuries, and no neck pain or midline tenderness do not need collars. **When can I remove the collar?** If your patient is pain free, GCS 15, cooperative, with no neurological signs then remove the collar for examination: note the posture of the neck and any bone tenderness (midline and over the spinous processes). If safe to remove collar, check the range of movements: flexion & extension (mainly atlanto-occipital joint); rotation (mainly atlanto-axial joint); lateral flexion (whole of cervical spine). Rotation is the movement most commonly affected. **When are x-rays indicated?** (see p. 466 for imaging) Follow the Canadian c-spine rules. Use the NICE 2014 head injury guidance to see if imaging of the neck is needed in head injury (p. 591). If x-rays are normal but patient still complains of midline tenderness, then consider CT imaging. **Is full immobilization truly possible?** ☞There is no evidence that applying cervical collars reduces c-spine injury, in fact some evidence suggests collars actually cause more harm.[56] The incidence of significant cervical spine injuries in high-risk trauma patients is 0.7%, but application of a collar can inhibit airway management (think of vomiting and the risk of aspiration) and also place the jugular veins under pressure and subsequently increase the ICP (esp. problematic in head injuries see p. 591). Have someone apply a collar to you—it's very uncomfortable and doesn't stabilize the neck as much as you would want. A cadaver study demonstrated that application of collars in cadavers with inflicted cervical injuries increased the fracture separation by 7mm![57] **A revolution in trauma care?** ☞ A pre-hospital care unit in Norway have removed the collar from routine practice and only utilize it temporarily during extrication). Many other countries are adopting this proposal that optimal immobilization avoids collars and just uses spinal board, head blocks with straps, and ideally a spinal vacuum mattress. Transporting patients in the lateral trauma position has also been proposed.[58] **So what should I do now?** For now, you must follow the local protocol of practice and work within the accepted practice of your employer. New hypotheses are always popping up and guidelines are only ever established once safe, evidence-based practice is identified. Hopefully we have challenged you to reflect on current practice in any specialty and not just take what has 'always been done' as gospel.

Further reading

Sansam KAJ (2006). Controversies in the management of traumatic spinal cord injury. *Clin Med* 6:202–4.

Sundstrøm T et al. (2014). Prehospital use of cervical collars in trauma patients: a critical review. *J Neurotrauma* 31:531–40.

The spinal cord originates from the brainstem at the base of the skull and terminates at L1 where the cauda equina starts (fig 8.40) (see p. 487). Most SCI do not completely sever the cord, instead the ability of the cord to function is compromised to varying degrees (figs 8.41–8.43). The American Spinal Injury Association (ASIA) scale (table 8.7) can be used to describe the completeness of the injury. Someone without an initial SCI does not receive an ASIA grade. Determining the neurological level of injury (NLI) refers to the most caudal segment of the cord with intact sensation and >3 muscle function strength.

Table 8.7 The ASIA International Standards of Spinal Cord Injury

A	Complete; no sensory or motor function is preserved in the sacral segments S4–S5
B	Sensory incomplete. Sensory but not motor function is preserved below the neurological level and includes sacral segments S4–5 (light touch/pin prick at S4–5 or deep anal pressure) AND no motor function preserved >3 levels below the motor level on either side
C	Motor incomplete. Motor function is preserved at the most caudal sacral segments for voluntary anal contraction (VAC) and less than half of key muscle functions below the single NLI have a muscle grade ≥3
D	Motor incomplete but at least half (half or more) of key muscle functions below the single NLI having a muscle grade >3
E	Normal motor and sensory function

© 2019 American Spinal Injury Association. Reprinted with permission.

Sacral sparing is confirmed by flexion of the great toe and a PR to assess perianal sensation and anal tone. Preservation of sacral function (S4–5) is a prognostic indicator confirming the integrity of the cord and can be the only neurological finding to help differentiate between incomplete and complete SCI.

Does this patient have a spinal cord injury?

At the accident In any unexplained trauma, suspect cord injury if:

- Responds to pain only above clavicle.
- Dermatomal pattern of sensory loss.
- Breathing—diaphragmatic without use of accessory respiratory muscles.
- Muscles—hypotonic, including reduced anal tone (do a PR).
- Reflexes—hyporeflexic.

- Absence of movement in both legs.
- Slow pulse and ↓BP, but in the presence of normovolaemia.
- Priapism[13] or urinary retention.
- Unexplained ileus.
- Clonus in an unconscious trauma patient without decerebrate rigidity.

Use this 2-page work sheet from the 'International Standards for Neurological Classification of Spinal Cord Injury' to formally assess spinal cord injuries: http://www.asia-spinalinjury.org/elearning/isncsci_worksheet_2015_web.pdf

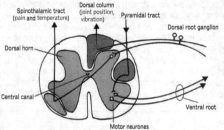

Fig 8.40 Cross-section of the spinal cord. The only neurons to decussate at (or near) their spinal cord level are those in the spinothalamic tract. Pyramidal tract fibres decussate in the medulla and the dorsal column fibres decussate after the gracile and cuneate nuclei of the medulla.

Adapted from Donaghy, M. *Oxford Core Texts: Neurology* (2008) with permission from OUP.

8 Trauma

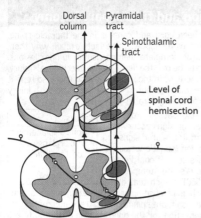

Fig 8.41 *Brown–Séquard* syndrome (*онсм*, p696). In this rare injury pattern, there is hemisection of the spinal cord (more often seen after penetrating rather than blunt trauma), causing ipsilateral loss of dorsal column sensation and motor function below the lesion and contralateral loss of spinothalamic sensation from a few levels below the lesion.

NB: spinothalmic tract fibres ascend for a few levels on the same side as cord entry before they decussate.

Adapted from Donaghy, M. *Oxford Core Texts: Neurology* with permission from OUP.

8 Trauma

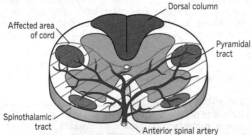

Fig 8.42 Anterior cord syndrome. There is infarction of the spinal cord in the distribution of the anterior spinal artery, causing complete loss of motor function and pain and temperature sensation below the lesion. Vibration and joint position sense are retained. This injury pattern has the worst prognosis of the incomplete injuries.

Adapted from Donaghy, M. *Oxford Core Texts: Neurology* with permission from OUP.

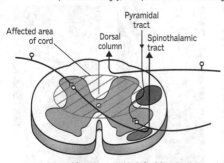

Fig 8.43 Central cord syndrome. Usually seen after a hyperextension injury in someone with pre-existing spinal canal stenosis (most often in the cervical region). There is greater loss of motor power in the upper extremities compared to the lower extremities combined with varying patterns of sensory loss and sphincter dysfunction.

Adapted from Donaghy, M. *Oxford Core Texts: Neurology* with permission from OUP.

---

13 *Priapism* is when pathologic stimuli (eg cervical cord lesions) cause prolonged erection (>4h), or when normal stimuli occurring under pathologic circumstances eg stasis from sickle-cell disease or leukaemia with leucostasis (wcc↑↑) cause prolonged erections. As it can cause permanent damage, get help. Bilateral shunting between the corpus cavernosum and corpus spongiosum may be needed.

Priapism is named after Priapus, the son of Aphrodite (the goddess of love). He, though, is ugly in most depictions—with a penis so large that he is generally relegated to the position of a scarecrow in the fields. From this position he is happy to be the god of gardens, bees, goats, sheep—and fertility.

The area of 'tightest fit' between cord and canal is in the thoracic spine; this region also has the poorest blood supply. These facts explain why thoracic lesions are more likely to be complete than cervical or lumbar lesions. Ischaemic injury often spreads below the level of the mechanical injury. Neurological symptoms often increase in the hours following injury, so repeat examinations are essential. For the segment of the cord involved with injury at a specific vertebra, see the following & table 8.8.

Cord compression See MINIBOX 'Causes'. Root pain (pp. 486-7) and lower motor neuron signs occur at the level of the lesion with upper motor neuron signs and sensory changes below the lesion (spastic weakness, brisk reflexes, upgoing plantars, loss of coordination, joint position sense, vibration sense, temperature, and pain). Cord anatomy (p. 560) is such that dorsal column sensibilities (light touch, joint position sense, vibration sense) are affected on the same side as the insult, but spinothalamic tract interruption affects pain and temperature sensation for the opposite side of the body 2–3 dermatome levels lower than the affected sensory level. As the cord ends at L1, compression at this vertebral level affects information in the cord relating to lower dermatomes. To determine the cord level affected behind a given vertebra, add the number in blue to that of the vertebra concerned, thus:

Causes
• Bone displacement
• Disc prolapse
• Local tumour
• Abscess
• Haematoma

- C2–7: **+1**.
- T1–6: **+2**.
- T7–9: **+3**.
- T10 has L1 and L2 levels behind it.
- T11 has L3 and 4.
- L1 has sacral and coccygeal segments.

It can be difficult to determine the level: MRI will help clarify this (fig 8.44).

Lower lumbar problems can cause cauda equina compression (►►BOX 'The cauda equina (=horse's tail)', p. 487) characterized by muscular pain, dermatomal sensory changes (if the lowest sacral dermatomes are affected the genitals are anaesthetic), and retention of urine ± faeces. ►*These signs indicate urgent neurosurgical referral with imaging eg to confirm or exclude a tumour or extradural abscess.*

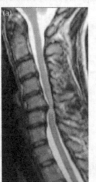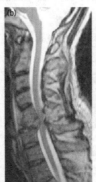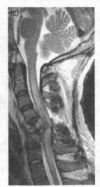

Fig 8.44 Cord compression. Because of different technical settings, MRI images can be called T1 or T2 weighted. These images can be recognized as T2 weighted because the CSF is white (see *OHCM* p734). Compression of the cord has occurred as a result of: (a) disc protrusion, (b) metastatic deposit, and (c) trauma.

Courtesy of Prof Peter Scally.

8 Trauma

Restoring lost function: is it possible?

Inducing repair of the spinal cord must take into account the complex pathophysiology involved during spinal cord damage. Primary injury is the direct mechanical damage to the neural elements, the resultant oedema and vascular disruption triggers secondary damage. Secondary injury is the delayed and prolonged response to neurotoxins and subsequent apoptosis; this secondary injury can be minimized with prompt emergency care. The 4 key principles of spinal cord repair are:

• Neuroprotection (to protect the surviving cells from further damage).
• Regeneration (targeting the correct neuronal connections).
• Replacement (of damaged nerve cells).
• Retraining CNS circuits to restore body functions.[59]

Novel therapies aim to optimize the environment both to minimize further damage and encourage repair. Often these options seem a long way off, but note that only 10% of damaged neurons need to be replaced to enable useful locomotion.

Table 8.8 Segment injury—a guide to possible subsequent function

C4	Can use electric chairs with chin control; type with mouthstick; use a 'Possum' environmental control system to turn on lights & open doors
C5	With special devices, he can feed, wash face, comb hair, and help with dressing the upper body. He may be able to push a wheelchair along the flat, if pushing gloves are worn, and there are capstan rims on the wheels. Unable to transfer from wheelchair to toilet
C6	Still needs a strap to aid feeding and washing. Dresses top half of body; helps dress lower half. Can drive with hand controls
C7	Can transfer, dress, feed himself
C8	Independent wheelchair life

Spinal shock A transient physiological loss of function following trauma. There is anaesthesia and flaccid paralysis of all segments and muscles below the level of injury, with hypo- or areflexia. Although the term itself is controversial, most clinicians agree that spinal shock follows a predictable 4-stage pattern (table 8.9) of initial loss of function, followed by gradual return of function and progression to hyperreflexia.

Spinal or neurogenic?

▶NB: *Don't* confuse *spinal shock* with *neurogenic shock*: the latter is BP↓ without tachycardia, caused by impairment of the descending spinal sympathetic pathways, caused by lesions above T6.

Table 8.9 Stages of spinal shock

Stage 1: 0–24h	Areflexia/hyporeflexia Absence of all reflexes including knee and ankle jerks In high lesions, signs may include bradyarrhythmias, AV conduction block, and hypotension
Stage 2: 1–3 days	Hyperreflexia and areflexia Initial reflex return Strong return of cutaneous reflexes, but deep tendon reflexes remain absent
Stage 3: 4–30 days	Hyperreflexia Return of deep tendon reflexes Autonomic dysreflexia may occur during this stage
Stage 4: 1–12 months	Spasticity/hyperreflexia Cutaneous and deep tendon reflexes respond to minimal stimuli Bowel and bladder recovery Resolution of bradyarrhythmias and hypotension in high lesions

Further reading

www.spinal-research.org
www.ninds.nih.gov

Approximately 0.4% of the population in the USA reported paralysis due to spinal cord injury.[60] These numbers are increasing as we continue to improve care for long-term neurological conditions.

Autonomic dysreflexia In those with lesions above the sympathetic outflow (ie above T6) any noxious stimulus may result in sympathetic overactivity below the level of the lesion. There is vasoconstriction and hypertension (potentially life-threatening as may cause seizures/intra-cranial haemorrhage and death). The patient may have a headache, a feeling of anxiety, sweaty/blotchy skin above the lesion with pale, dry skin below the level of lesion. The carotid baroreceptors are stimulated causing reflex vagal bradycardia, but the signals which would normally produce relieving vasodilatation are unable to pass down the cord. The most common cause is bladder distension (eg with a blocked catheter), followed by bowel distension (eg with constipation).[61] Other stimuli which may produce this effect include UTI, calculi, ejaculation, and bladder/colonic irrigation. Ensure good bowel and bladder care. *Treatment:* Sit the patient upright and give **nifedipine** (10mg—bite the capsule) with **glyceryl trinitrate** 0.5mg (not if patient has used sildenafil in the prior 24h).

Bladder dysfunction Genitourinary complications are among the commonest causes for rehospitalization in spinal cord injury patients. Key problems include urinary incontinence, reflex detrusor activity (after acontractility in the initial period of spinal shock), and the presence of residual urine. This predisposes to infection and ureteric reflux. These are major causes of renal failure, morbidity, and mortality. The most common method of bladder drainage is intermittent self-catheterization but no method has shown superiority.[62] *Urinary infection:* Historically used to be a serious cause of mortality (along with infected skin ulceration).[63] It may be prevented by a high fluid intake, ensuring effective bladder emptying, and acidification of the urine (eg **ascorbic acid** 1g/6h PO).

Pressure ulcers Can develop quickly in skin with reduced sensation in patients unable to physically shift their positions. Skin is made more vulnerable when moist, from perspiration or urinary incontinence. Regular skin inspections are essential with good lifting techniques; avoid sliding patients across the bed as this stretches the skin. Healing of an ulcer requires months of pressure-relieving strategies and monitoring for infection.

Bowel dysfunction In lesions below L1, arises from cord compression of the conus and results in reduced peristalsis (and subsequent constipation) and a lax anal sphincter leading to faecal incontinence. Lesions at or above L1 result in an UMN picture with increased anal tone and subsequent retention of faeces and constipation. From the second day of injury, gentle manual evacuation using plenty of lubricant is needed. A flatus tube may be helpful in relieving distension once the ileus of spinal shock has passed. Remember, bowel health affects QOL and increases risk of autonomic dysreflexia—use laxatives wisely. See OHCM p260.

Respiratory function Depends on phrenic nerve involvement (C3, C4, C5). For lesions above C3 the diaphragm loses innervation and no respiratory effort can be made without a ventilator and tracheostomy. Even those with lesions below C5 encounter respiratory complications as their ability to cough forcefully and ventilate the lung bases is inhibited by lack of abdominal musculature. This predisposes patients to repeated pneumonia; a leading cause of death in this patient population. Mucolytics and physiotherapy to assist coughing can help clear respiratory secretions.

Spasticity See p. 566.

Further reading
www.christopherreeve.org

►Sexual counselling is an integral part of rehabilitation. It is important in itself, but we should recognize that sexuality interacts with important determinants of our patients' quality of life eg levels of dependency, aggression, self-esteem, and autonomy. Don't be shy and don't be shocked: for help with discussing sexual issues, see p. 749. ►Given a knowing and patient partner, most people with spinal injury can enjoy a satisfying sex life. In some studies, locomotor impairment and autonomic dysreflexia were more frequently given as causes of reduced sexual pleasure than specific sexual dysfunctions.[64] Bowel and bladder incontinence is a frequent concern, but these can be anticipated if sexual activity is planned. It is equally important to assess the partner's needs and responses to the injury. This takes time. Be aware that sexuality encompasses more than physical attractiveness and intercourse. With spinal cord injury, use of sexual imagery and concentration on body areas that retain sensation have especial importance, as does a certain inventiveness and readiness to experiment.

When helping these patients it is important to distinguish sexual drive and sexual satisfaction from fertility and parenting needs. Both need addressing in a systematic way within the broader contexts of psychosocial, emotional, and relationship aspects. Living with a sci can be tough, there are a whole host of reasons why sexual satisfaction is not met; not just neurogenic.

Sexual health in men The first question will likely be: can I still get an erection? This depends on the site of injury. There are 2 types of erection: psychogenic erections are modulated by impulses from the brain and are the result of audiovisual stimuli or fantasy. Reflexogenic erections are governed by spinal reflexes (s2–s4) and arise from tactile stimuli to the genital area.[65] The latter type is most likely to be preserved in sci, patients with complete sci are unlikely to experience psychogenic erections. Erectile dysfunction is common and a source of distress.[66] In men with lesions between T6 and L5, 75% can expect improvement in erections with use of sildenafil. Fertility issues in men centre around performance and sperm quality, which may be reduced by scrotal hyperthermia, retrograde ejaculation, prostatic fluid stasis, and testicular denervation. Electro-ejaculation and intracytoplasmic sperm injection have useful roles.

Sexual health in women Less affected, largely because, anatomically, a woman can still engage in intercourse. Alternative positioning due to spasticity and additional lubrication may be required. Women can still bear children, but autonomic dysreflexia and the prothrombotic state are serious risks. Only 17% of women with complete lower motor neuron dysfunction affecting the s2–s5 spinal segments can achieve orgasm, compared with 59% of women with other levels and degrees of injury. Evidence suggests the potential for orgasm is there, but patients are disheartened by the lack of sensation.[67]

Talk about sex, it's important!

'Never underestimate the difference you can make' (C Reeve)

Christopher Reeve was an actor who fractured his c1 and c2 after falling from a horse. Made famous on screen through playing the role of Superman, his time after the injury was heroically dedicated to helping establish a foundation to aid sci research. The most recent breakthrough in research is epidural electrical stimulation of the spinal cord. By applying continuous electrical current to the lumbosacral spinal neurons, the spinal cord 'wakes up' and can function at a basic level to allow the repetitive movements which it used to do. This revolutionary treatment enabled a young male with complete motor sci to stand independently while being electrically stimulated in 2011. It was reproduced in 4 more patients in 2014 and is definitely an area of research to keep your eye on.[68,69]

8 Trauma

Personal qualities in therapists Almost as important as exact anatomical lesion. There may be big mood swings from euphoria to despair as the patient accustoms himself to their loss and their new body image.

The occupational therapist (OT) A key person in maximizing the levels of achievement. They can arrange a home visit with a member of the spinal injuries team and a community liaison nurse. The aim is to construct a plan with local services, so that the patient's (and their family's) hopes can be realized to the fullest extent. They can arrange the necessary home modifications, and give invaluable advice about the level of independence which is realistic to strive for. As ever, the aims of the OT extend into augmenting self-esteem, and helping the patient come to terms with loss of role, and loss of confidence, and to mitigate the effects of disability by arranging for as much purposeful activity as possible, in the realms of both work and leisure. They will also be able to make plans for acquiring social skills to assist the patient in their new way of life.

Nursing & physiotherapy • *The chest:* Regular physio with coughing and breathing exercises prevents sputum retention and pneumonia which are likely to follow diaphragmatic partial paralysis (eg C3–4 dislocation). If the lesion is above the T10 segmental level, there is no effective coughing.

- *The straight lift:* (For transferring patients.) 1 attendant supports the head with both hands under the neck so that the head lies on the arms. 3 lifters standing on the same side insert their arms under the patient, 1 at a time, starting at the top. After the lift, withdraw in the reverse order.
- *Posture:* Place joints in a full range of positions. Avoid hyperextensions. Keep the feet flexed at 90° with a pillow between soles and bed-end.
- *Wheelchairs:* The patient should be kept sitting erect; adjust the footplates so that the thighs are supported and there is no undue pressure on the sacrum. ▶Regular relief of pressure on sacral and ischial areas is vital.
- *Standing and walking:* Using a 'tilt table', or the Oswestry standing frame, the tetraplegic patient can become upright. If the injury level is at L2–4, below-knee calipers and crutches enable walking to take place. If the lesion is at T1–8, 'swing to gait' may be possible. The crutches are placed a short distance in front of the feet. The goal is to promote re-establishment of functional connections in neuronal networks and shaping the motor patterns that they generate.[70]
- *Sport:* Consider archery, darts, snooker, table tennis, and swimming for those with paraplegia. Many other sports may also be suitable. There are interesting and important factors to consider such as the optimal heart rate (eg with lesions above T4 there is severely diminished cardiac acceleration, and a maximal rate of ~130bpm) and the reduction in bone density below the lesion.[71]

Spasticity Arises from UMN lesions and is defined as increased muscle tone which tends to develop after the initial phases of spinal shock. Symptoms can manifest as spasms, pain, contractures, or abnormal tone. >80% of SCI patients develop some form of spasticity.[72] ▶Changes in spasticity can herald new changes in the spinal cord (eg post-traumatic syringomyelia). *Treatment:* Intensive physiotherapy with passive stretching exercises to keep muscles supple and exercises to strengthen the spastic and synergistic muscles. Antispastic medications include baclofen, diazepam, and tizanidine. IM botulinum toxin inhibits ACH release, the clinical effects appear ~24 hours afterwards and can last 2–6 months depending on dose.[72] Surgery is reserved for those where severe spasms significantly affect activities of daily living. Orthopaedic surgery targets tendon release or transfers for contractures. Neurosurgical intervention includes ablation of motor nerves and rhizotomy which severs the dorsal sensory roots responsible for spasticity.

Pathological fractures

Definition A # that occurs in diseased or abnormal bone. Disruption of bony structural integrity means that even trivial forces can produce a fracture, so suspect a pathological # if the energy of the trauma is abnormally low for the resulting injury. Common sites include the subtrochanteric femur and the proximal humeral shaft (fig 8.45).

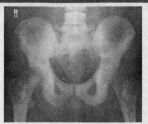

Fig 8.45 Diffuse bony sclerotic lesions, putting the patient at risk from pathological fracture. *Courtesy of The Norfolk and Norwich University Hospitals (NNUH) Radiology Dept.*

Causes The commonest causes are osteoporosis (so-called fragility fractures) and bony metastases (eg from breast or prostate primaries). Rarer causes include osteomalacia, bone infection, primary bone tumour, and osteogenesis imperfecta.

Management If the underlying diagnosis is unclear, then do rigorous directed investigation, eg in a search for a primary cancer. Without treating the bone metastases, the chances of healing are nearly zero. *ΔΔ:* Metastasis from prostate, breast, thyroid, kidney, and bronchus. Rarely GI carcinoma; primary lymphoma; multiple myeloma. ►Remember to image the whole femur if a proximal pathological fracture is identified—the forces through any fixation device could snap any other surrounding infiltrated bone.

Overuse phenomena at work

Activity requiring repetitive actions, particularly those involved with repeated muscle contraction, may lead to chronic symptoms. See also fig 8.46. Sports players, cleaners using heavy equipment, manual labourers (particularly those who use vibrating tools), and musicians can all develop overuse phenomena. Just as with excessive sound protection, employers are duty bound to provide a safe working environment, with well-designed chairs and tools, and limits on vibrating tool use. The cost of these injuries, in terms of suffering and working hours lost, is considerable, and treatment of established symptoms is difficult.

Compensation is a vexed issue, and recent court judgments have gone in favour of employers in some instances, and in favour of patients in others. Some people argue that the condition does not exist as a separate medical entity, emphasizing lack of histopathology. It should be noted that this is not a prerequisite for a disease—and in any case, histopathology *is* sometimes demonstrable. Treatments tried include splinting (may prolong the problem), physiotherapy, β-blockers for relaxation, and the Alexander technique for posture re-education.[14]

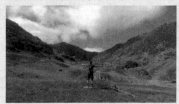

Fig 8.46 Why is the term repetitive strain injury a fallacy? Just because anginal chest pain can be provoked by walking up hills, hill walking does not cause coronary artery stenosis (although the idea for some may be enough to cause a little heart flutter). And so, because use of the arm may provoke the symptoms of an underlying condition (eg carpal tunnel syndrome, OA at the base of the thumb, de Quervain's disease), it does not mean that it is the cause of the underlying condition.

© Nina Hjelde.

14 The *Alexander technique* aims to improve posture and movement. Classes teach gentle lying, sitting, and standing exercises which eliminate unnecessary muscle tension and improve balance. In addition to chronic neck and back pain, evidence suggests patients with Parkinson disease benefit (www.alexandertechnique.com).

9 Emergency medicine

Blair Graham

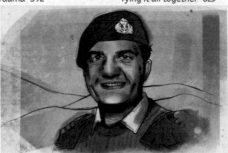

Fig 9.1 Surgeon Captain Rick Jolly OBE (1946–2018)[1] was a British Naval Doctor during the Falklands Conflict in 1982. Following the loss of field hospital tents and equipment during the sinking of the *mv Atlantic Conveyor*, Jolly was tasked to improvise in a disused meat factory—not ideal, but the only place suitable to fulfil the purpose at the time. Throughout the course of the conflict, the hospital, which became affectionately known as the 'red and green life machine' (in recognition of both the Paratroopers and Royal Marines who staffed it), treated over 1000 casualties; 300 of them Argentinian. Only 3 casualties died in the hospital during the course of the conflict—a favourable mortality ratio by any standards, and truly remarkable considering the conditions of the time. Jolly received an OBE for his efforts after the conflict. Perhaps more tellingly, he was also awarded the *Orden De Mayo*, one of Argentina's highest level decorations.

Rick Jolly may not have recognized himself as an emergency physician per se, but in common with the many who flit through civilian emergency departments every 4 or 6 months, that did not limit him. More important than any rank, job title, or postnomials were those attributes he brought to the shores of a desolate and stormy island in the South Atlantic: ingenuity, leadership, humour, team spirit—and above all, recognition of a duty to indiscriminately relieve suffering and save the lives of all who were thrust through the door needing help.

Artwork by Gillian Turner.

With many thanks to Drs Stephanie Bailey, Ffion Barham, Roddy Campbell, Natalie Klanke, Stephanie Rennie, and Jason E Smith for providing invaluable review and feedback on this chapter, and to our junior reader Lema Imam for their contribution to this chapter.

Working as an Emergency Doctor

Think back to when you applied to medical school, and the image of your future self you held in your mind's eye. It is likely that what you'll be doing as an emergency medicine (EM) doctor is not a million miles off that aspirational view. Sure, perspectives might have changed since then, but many junior doctors report that they relish the opportunity to practise as a 'proper doctor' during their first emergency department (ED) job. With this comes responsibility—to apply broad knowledge, make the correct diagnosis, and perform procedures safely for many patients during each shift. A degree of trepidation during the first day of induction is therefore both inevitable and—to a degree—healthy, but irrespective of your intended direction, an ED job should be seen as an opportunity to grow. Most juniors will find themselves well supported by an experienced team. Remember: if in doubt, always (always!) ask for help and advice.

Looking after yourself This is essential during your ED job. While junior doctors fondly reminisce about their time practising clinical EM, the hours, intensity, and work schedule can overwhelm, and many feel reluctant to consider it as a long-term career. This is a shame: at its best, EM is a fresh and dynamic specialty in need of enthusiastic and capable trainees to ensure a bright future.

For this reason, EM is at the vanguard of developments in clinician health and well-being. Some departments have well-being rooms for staff to use where they can practise relaxation and mindfulness (fig 9.2). While it will always be necessary to work weekends and nights in EM, and the tempo will probably always be demanding, the specialty is learning that provision of sustainable careers is essential.

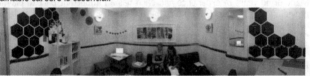

Fig 9.2 Well-being room in the emergency department at Manchester Royal Infirmary.
Courtesy Dr Laura Howard/St Emlyn's.

How to thrive in EM: some tips

(See also Chapter 15.) There are things you can do on an individual level to cope better with a demanding job. Good diet, sleep hygiene, moderation of alcohol intake, and avoidance of drugs are crucial. If you find yourself floundering, the '5 ways to well-being' provides a useful, evidence-based set of recommendations:

1 *Connect*. Don't be an island—working as a member of the wider ED team of doctors, nurses, receptionists, porters, cleaners is not only fun but fosters familiarity, support, and sense of self-worth.

2 *Be active*. Making time for exercise is essential. Actively commute to work, if feasible. You will arrive fresh and de-stress at the end of the day.

3 *Be kind*. Show professional courtesy to colleagues at all times. A little thanks goes a very long way. Remember that if someone is unkind to you, it might be because they are struggling themselves. How can *you* help? Similarly, smile and aim to show compassion to all patients.

4 *Keep learning*. The ED is a great classroom—use the time to meet your own learning objectives. Similarly, learning a new skill or perfecting a hobby away from work is known to be beneficial to personal well-being and will re-energize you.

5 *Notice how you are feeling*. EM will test your emotions. Take stock of how the job is affecting you. ►►If you find yourself struggling, be proactive and seek help from colleagues or your supervisor immediately. Your GP, occupational health department, and the BMA Counselling Service are additional, confidential, sources of help and advice.

Emergency medicine EM formed with the appointment of Maurice Ellis as the first UK casualty consultant in Leeds in 1952. Prior to this, emergency care of the sick and injured was delegated to the most junior surgeons.[2] It seems likely that poor patient care and needless mortality and morbidity resulted.

Things have moved on: EM in the UK now has its own postgraduate training pathway with graduates awarded the *Fellowship of the Royal College of Emergency Medicine* (FRCEM). While EM demands a broad clinical knowledge base, EM physicians are particular specialists in triage, resuscitation, trauma, applied toxicology, and major incidents. Crucially, EM physicians must also facilitate the everyday running of the ED. This skill set lends itself well to practice in other settings such as pre-hospital care, mass gatherings, and disasters/humanitarian crises.

Internationally, EM is recognized as a specialty in the USA, Canada, Australasia, South Africa, and now much of Europe and Asia. Other countries—including many in lower- and middle-income settings—are in the stages of establishing EM as a specialty.

Teams in the Emergency Department (ED)

'A champion team will always beat a team of champions'
John McGrath, British Playwright, 1935–2002

As an ED doctor, you are a small part of a large team consisting of nursing staff, healthcare assistants, radiographers, porters, administrators, and more. Many bring years of experience and each has an important part to play in providing patient care. Give others the time of day: make an effort to learn names, and find out the capabilities of the team. Make sure that you are not the one who is perceived as difficult or undermining. There will be times when you will be required to lead, but good *followership* is just as important.[3]

In critical situations team performance can very literally determine the difference between life and death.[4] ED teams have in the past been compared to sports teams or Formula One pit crews. Such analogies are flawed, since ED teams are usually formed at short notice with little opportunity for practice before a critically ill patient is whisked through the door. But a round of introductions (name, role) and a briefing quickly establish the team, and 'micro-summaries' delivered during an event allow the development of a shared mental model,[5] ensuring everyone is working towards a common objective. The ideal ED team should have a horizontal hierarchy: every member should feel comfortable with raising questions or concerns as they arise. A debrief after the event allows the team to reflect and learn, improving subsequent performance.[6]

Closing the loop

Just because you asked a question doesn't mean it has been heard …

Communication during critical events can be fraught; crucial messages might go unheard or be misinterpreted. Simple misunderstandings are a common source of serious errors, and can often be avoided by using closed loop communication. This involves an explicit acknowledgement from the person receiving the information, thus confirming that the message has been received correctly.[7] This person then 'checks back' to report that the action has been completed.

(Closed loop communication works outside of medicine too, and is even advised by some marriage counsellors!)

The ED is the receiving area of the hospital. In the UK, the public, media, and road signs still refer to the ED as Accident and Emergency (or 'A&E'). The television programme *Casualty* reminds us of the original name afforded to the ED, which probably harks back to Victorian hospital wards where travellers and vagrants ('casuals') could seek medical treatment without appointment (fig 9.3).

Modern EDs are capable of providing care to patients from across the acuity spectrum. With the exception of a few children's hospitals and trauma centres, EDs will see all age groups. In most countries, patients can either self-present to the ED and/or attend by ambulance. The layout of the ED differs from other parts of the hospital, and a walking tour is an essential part of any induction. In the UK, the ED is divided into the following areas:

Triage area This is where patients undergo an initial assessment and set of vital signs, usually by a registered nurse. This will determine the priority afforded to the patient based on the clinical need at the time.

Resuscitation room The area where the sickest patients undergo initial treatment and stabilization. Each resuscitation bay will be equipped to provide intensive therapy support to a ventilated patient. In addition, the resuscitation room is equipped to deliver non-invasive ventilation, massive blood transfusion, selected surgical interventions such as chest drainage and thoracotomy, and usually has its own radiography equipment. Increasingly, this includes a CT scanner.

'Majors' The name given to the area of the department where the majority of non-ambulant patients are assessed and treated.

'Minors' The term traditionally given to the area for lower-priority, ambulant patients. With increasing attendances and patient acuity, it has become a dangerous misnomer. In among the minor illness and injury will be some truly unwell patients waiting (hoping!) to be identified. Remember too that triage (p. 572) is not perfect—could that tingling tooth actually represent an MI?

x-ray Most EDs will have their own x-ray facilities and should have ready access to CT and MRI imaging facilities.

Clinical Decision Unit This is an observation area within the ED. Layout and purpose varies, but generally for patients who are awaiting test results or who require a period of observation before discharge home (eg following a head injury).

Ambulatory care Increasingly, facilities are being developed to allow for the rapid assessment of patients by inpatient teams who may be suitable for discharge post diagnosis (eg by acute medicine). Similarly, frailty teams may provide multidisciplinary assessment for elderly patients to prevent unnecessary inpatient admissions.

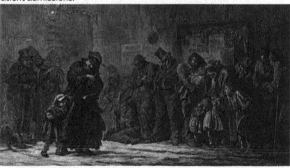

Fig 9.3 Waiting in a queue for admission to the casual ward. Although it doesn't feel like it on a busy Saturday night, waiting room conditions have improved!

Triage

Triage describes the process of prioritizing patients based on clinical need. Triage is an essential function of the ED, and aims to ensure that the sickest patients are seen most promptly. Most EDs will use validated triage systems, such as the *Manchester Triage System*. Patients are assigned categories (number or colour), usually by a nurse. See also pp. 630–1 for pre-hospital triage.

Priority 1 (Red category)—*'immediate'*
These are the sickest patients who must be seen immediately. Examples include uncontrollable major haemorrhage, cardiac arrest, and sight-threatening ocular injury.

Priority 2 (Orange category)—*'very urgent'*
These are patients who should be seen within 10 minutes of their arrival. They might include patients in severe pain or shortness of breath but whose life is not in immediate risk.

Priority 3 (Yellow category)—*'urgent'*
These are intermediate-risk patients, who should be seen within the first hour of arrival. Such patients form the bulk of the 'majors' area workload.

Priority 4 (Green category)—*'standard'*
These are patients with minor illness and injury who can be seen within 2 hours of arrival.

Priority 5 (Blue category)—*'non-urgent'*
These are patients whose care could be delivered in non-urgent settings such as primary care. Many EDs do not use this category as the target 'to be seen time' of 4 hours would lead to a breach! (See BOX 'BREACH!'.)

Triage is not a perfect tool It is also a dynamic process. The assigned triage category may change if a patient deteriorates while waiting, for example. Over-triage is better than under-triage—most systems will accept a degree of the former to minimize the chances of truly sick patients being wrongly under-prioritized.

Triage in mass casualty incidents See p. 630.

Crowding and exit block

Crowding Occurs when the number of patients within the ED exceeds the capacity for which it is able to cope. It is a major problem for hospitals worldwide and is associated with worse patient outcomes, increased length of stay, poor patient experience, and low staff morale.[8]

Exit block Occurs when there is a delay in moving patients from the ED to inpatient wards. Patients stack up in the ED awaiting admission. Ambulances may need diversion elsewhere (adding to delay and danger) and patients with genuine needs may decide they cannot wait any more hours for help—sometimes to their detriment.

Exit block may be exacerbated by internal process delays but also results from inadequate availability of community-based social care for patients with complex care or rehabilitation needs. It has been estimated that exit block affects up to ⅓ of patients and may contribute to increased mortality, wait for surgery, and length of stay.[9]

Further reading
Mackway Jones K (2013). *Emergency Triage* (3rd ED). Manchester: Advanced Life Support Group.

BREACH!

The '4-hour' target stipulates that 95% of patients attending an ED in the UK should be seen, treated, and admitted/discharged within 4 hours. Failure to do so results in a 'breach', which might result in a financial penalty for the hospital. Similar ED performance targets also exist in other countries, such as Canada and Australia.

Performance metrics such as the 4-hour target are controversial. While there are legitimate concerns that time pressure might compromise patient care, the target has served to increase investment in emergency care and allows monitoring of performance.[8]

At an individual level, ensuring your patients are dealt with in 4 hours requires organization and planning—skills that get easier with time. Remember that it is reasonable to allow a patient to breach if there is a genuine need to deliver ongoing clinical care. This may need to be communicated with *grace* to the nurse in charge, often after liaising with a senior doctor.

Another busy shift?

In the middle of an ED shift, you may be forgiven for wondering what is happening outside to prompt such a heave in the number of attendances. It can be tempting to drop your work and shuffle out to the waiting room with your hands held up in defeat and announce to the multitude of bewildered patients; 'We give up … You win!'

Rumours circulate that sunshine means children are out in force at the local playgrounds, or rain means that old ladies will be slipping up on the kerb. Perhaps late on a Friday night you despair at the number of alcohol-related incidents. Factors that have been suggested to correlate with an *increase in the number of ED attendances* include:
• Warm, dry, and sunny weather conditions.
• Local music festivals (despite on-site facilities).
• National sport teams winning at home (sadly, for assault).
• Major natural disasters.
• And yes … Mondays.

Studies have also suggested reduced attendances during major televised sporting events. Trying to predict how busy your shift will be rarely seems to help. Ultimately, the aim of such epidemiological studies is to help in ED staffing and logistics—one clear message remains: ▶▶Don't despair, all of these factors are well beyond your control!

Emergency medicine and warfare

It is an unfortunate truth that progress in EM continues to be driven by warfare. Ambroise Pare's 'wounded man' is a 16th-century depiction of trauma occurring on the medieval battlefield, which features on the crest of the Royal College of Emergency Medicine.

It was Dominique Jean Larrey who established triage during the Napoleonic Wars (p. 630),[10] while introduction of the Thomas splint in WWI reduced mortality for fractured femur by about 60%.[11]

Twenty-first century conflicts have led to advancements in the care of severely wounded patients including haemostatic resuscitation.

Emergency physicians are expected to make many diagnostic and therapeutic decisions every shift. Clinical decision-making is an emerging and fascinating branch of cognitive science, but formal training is currently lacking. What follows is a brief overview of some key concepts. Further reading is advised. See also pp. 790–1.

How do humans make decisions? Economist Daniel Kahneman won a Nobel Prize for work suggesting a dual-processing model for decision-making hard-wired within humans. *System 1* ('fast') is based on pattern recognition and often results in an unconscious decision. The ability to make rapid decisions clearly has an evolutionary benefit (eg when recognizing and evading a hostile predator) and uses minimal cognitive 'bandwidth' but is prone to cognitive biases (see also p. 868). In the clinical context, such biases can lead to misinterpretation of risk, misdiagnosis, and other errors. Inexperienced practitioners are likely to be most vulnerable. *System 2* ('slow') is employed when the problem encountered does not fit a recognized pattern. System 2 thinking represents a conscious, logical effort but uses much more cognitive bandwidth and would be exhausting, if not impossible, to employ all the time in the ED. In reality, clinicians may 'toggle' between the 2 systems (fig 9.4[12]).

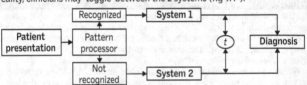

Fig 9.4 Simplified version of dual-processing model for diagnostic decision-making.
Source: data from Crosskerry, P *et al*. Cognitive debiasing 1: origins of bias and theory of debiasing. *BMJ Qual Saf* 2013;22:ii58–ii64.

Rule Out Worst case Scenario (ROWS) Describes a strategy commonly employed in emergency medicine.[13] Assuming that patients who attend the ED are at high risk of serious disease, it seems reasonable to first exclude the riskiest differential diagnoses, as opposed to the most likely. For example, a patient presenting with an episode of acute severe headache may be most likely to have a migraine, but there is smaller possibility of subarachnoid haemorrhage which, if missed, could have fatal consequences. The result is that the patient receives a CT scan and lumbar puncture to rule out this latter diagnosis. While this seems an intuitively safe approach, the patient has been exposed to a protracted hospital stay and investigation which in itself carries risk (eg infection, future malignancy from radiation exposure, post-lumbar puncture headache, etc.). It is important to appreciate that modern EM often errs on the side of caution, but there is often no 'right' answer, and it is up to clinical judgement to seek a comfortable balance between probabilistic and worst-case scenario reasoning.

Exhaustive reasoning Often employed by those arriving in the ED for the first time. Again, thoroughly charting a comprehensive clerking seems like a safe approach, but the result can be a confused problem list and unclear differential diagnoses. Furthermore, this approach is onerous and time-consuming. For this reason, history taking and investigation should always be focused on the problem at hand.

Clinical decision rules (CDRS) Rigorously developed and validated criteria most frequently used to empower clinicians to exclude a diagnosis without the need for extensive investigation. CDRS may also be used to stratify risk of a condition being present. Perhaps the most famous CDR is the *Ottawa ankle rule* (p. 616), which is used to rule out the need for radiography in ankle sprains using simple clinical criteria. CDRS may be employed for excluding pulmonary embolism, deep vein thrombosis, and providing risk assessment in syncope.

Meeting patient expectations

During a typical ED shift you can expect to be confronted by a cross-section of society. One of the privileges of working in the ED is the insight into other people's lives it provides. Nobody comes to the ED because they're having a good day—true colours reveal themselves and such insights can be raw, un-adulterated, and often humbling.

All patients deserve compassionate care. Evidence suggests that patients are more concerned with interpersonal aspects of care than technical skill or prowess (… but maybe the latter is just assumed).[14] Most complaints are re-lated to communication.[15] Smile, show concern, provide updates, and explain the wait. You'll be much better received, and might even receive the occa-sional 'thank you' note.

Studies have also demonstrated that patients struggle to understand and retain discharge instructions.[16] It is well worth taking a few minutes to test understanding (ask the patient to repeat back to you) and, if possible, issue some written information. ▶▶**Safety netting** is essential if sending a patient home. Explicitly inform them what should prompt return or help.

'Inappropriate attendance' A label applied to patients whom staff perceive could be seen in a non-ED setting. No matter how trivial the patient's complaint may seem, always explore their reason for attending the ED. Why are they so concerned that they're prepared to wait for hours to see you? Get to the root of this, and you will often find feelings of frustration transformed to under-standing. Not infrequently, you'll find a shared concern and a serious diagnosis may result. Never berate patients for 'time wasting' and avoid becoming cynical.

'Regular attenders' May rely on ED for 'walk-in' primary care, but often have complex physical and psychosocial needs—and higher mortality than the gen-eral population.[17] Tailored care plans, produced in collaboration with other services, may save resources.

Violence and aggression An unfortunate reality of life in the ED. This does not mean it is acceptable. Recognize and remove yourself from escalating conflict right away, and call for help from colleagues, security and—if necessary—police. ▶▶It is important to recognize *excited delirium*, which can present with extreme aggression and 'super-human' strength. Hyperpyrexia, profuse sweating, and extreme tachycardia are signs. Mortality is high (~10%) and is probably ↑ by physical restraint. Monitor, consider benzodi-azepines, and seek advice.

Making sense of the undifferentiated

Patients seldom present to the ED with a discrete, neatly labelled acute diag-nosis. Instead, they will present with a *symptom* This might be an acutely painful limb, chest pain, abdominal pain, or PV bleeding.

The challenge of emergency medicine lies in *ruling out life-threatening or ser-ious pathology* (this is why a generic framework for primary assessment is so important), providing effective symptomatic relief, and managing risk. Should I do a second troponin assay? Is the patient well enough to go home tonight?

The uncertainty and risk inherent in EM is daunting for all who practise it. As the saying goes, work in the jungle for long enough, and you will surely get bitten by a snake! Fortunately, protocols, guidelines, and clinical decision rules are all designed to make life a little less painful. Colleagues can give advice and act as a sounding board. Judgement, experience, and wisdom build through years of practice—it does get easier!

9 Emergency medicine

Further reading

Croskerry P (2003). The importance of cognitive errors in diagnosis and strategies to minimize them. *Acad Med* 78;8:775–80.

Crosskerry P et al. (2013). Cognitive debiasing 1: origins of bias and theory of debiasing. *BMJ Qual Saf* 22:ii58–64.

Big sick, little sick?

Lifeboat crews must assess casualties on the high seas in appalling conditions, with limited clinical training (fig 9.5). To overcome these challenges, volunteers differentiate the *big sick* patients (who need immediate evacuation and life support) from the *little sick*.[18] The beauty of this paradigm lies in its simplicity—it is exactly what we must first do when assessing our next patient in the ED.

Fig 9.5 Lifeboat.
Artwork by Gillian Turner.

▶▶**The primary survey** Describes the ABCDE that provides a universal framework for the initial management of all sick patients.

A: Airway + O_2. If the patient is talking, the airway is usually patent. Stridor, snoring (stertor), and 'see-saw' breathing all indicate obstruction. Start with a simple jaw thrust, and reassess. If necessary, proceed to using a nasopharyngeal or—if the patient will tolerate it—an oropharyngeal ('Guedel') airway. Apply oxygen and reassess. ▶▶If concerned about airway adequacy, always call for senior help early.

B: Breathing + ventilation. Expose the chest and inspect for external injury and abnormalities. Especially in trauma, firmly palpate the clavicles, sternum, and chest wall to assess for pain and crepitus. Auscultate to assess breath sounds and air entry. Take note of spo_2 and respiratory rate. If respiration is inadequate assist with a bag valve mask (BVM) (fig 9.6). Use the 2-person technique: 1 operator provides airway opening and a mask seal while the other squeezes the bag. Avoid hyperventilation and over-inflation (↑ aspiration risk; ↓ cardiac output).

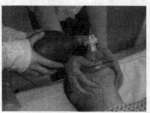

Fig 9.6 2-person BVM technique.
Reproduced with permission from Creed et al., Care of the Acutely Ill Adult (2010), Oxford:OUP.

C: Circulation. Take the patient's hand—is it warm or ice cold, indicating peripheral hypoperfusion? Mucosal condition, capillary refill time, and skin turgor give a general indication of condition and hydration. Take note of pulse and blood pressure. A shock index (pulse/systolic BP) of >0.6 might indicate hypovolaemia and increased need for transfusion.[19] In trauma, examine for abdominal tenderness and ensure femurs are intact. Apply a pelvic sling prior to imaging if a pelvic fracture is likely or suspected.

D: Disability. Take note of the Glasgow Coma Score (GCS) (p. 590). A GCS of <15 is worrying, and <8 indicates the potential loss of protective airway reflexes and need for airway support. The AVPU scale is simple and acceptable for initial assessment (**A**lert; **R**esponds to voice; responds to **P**ain; **U**nresponsive)—a patient who scores 'P' or 'U' is assumed to have a GCS <8. It is also important to note pupillary reflexes, gross evidence of a lateralizing injury (hemiparesis) or spinal cord level. ▶▶Remember that *hypoglycaemia* is an easily reversible cause of neurological derangement.

E: Exposure. Check and maintain body temperature. Examine the patient from head to toe. Exclude rashes, wounds, sores, and other deformities.

Basic life support BLS is the provision of life support—ventilation and external chest compressions, without any equipment. Ensure the scene is safe to approach. In hospital, call for senior help by summoning the cardiac arrest team (2222 via internal phone in the UK) and start BLS in the ratio of 30 chest compressions to 2 rescue breaths).

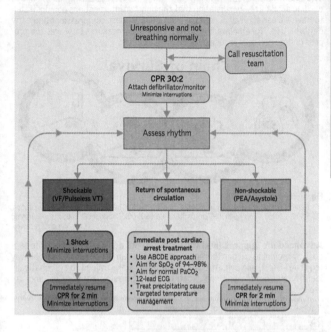

During CPR
- Ensure high quality chest compressions
- Minimize interruptions to compressions
- Give oxygen
- Use waveform capnography
- Continuous compressions when advanced airway in place
- Vascular access (intravenous or intraosseous)
- Give adrenaline every 3-5 min
- Give amiodarone after 3 shocks

Treat Reversible Causes
- Hypoxia
- Hypovolaemia
- Hypo-/hyperkalaemia/metabolic
- Hypothermia
- Thrombosis—coronary or pulmonary
- Tension pneumothorax
- Tamponade—cardiac
- Toxins

Consider
- Ultrasound imaging
- Mechanical chest compressions to facilitate transfer/treatment
- Coronary angiography and percutaneous coronary intervention
- Extracorporeal CPR

Fig 9.8 Adult advanced life support.
Reproduced with the kind permission of the Resuscitation Council (UK).

The chain of survival Highlights the stages crucial to saving life in sudden cardiac arrest. It is worth noting that the only two interventions demonstrated to have a clear survival benefit are high-quality chest compressions and early defibrillation. Nonetheless, the sum of the other measures improves the process of care and may reduce disability in survivors.

Chain of Survival

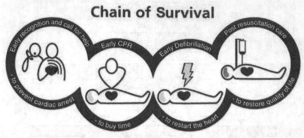

Fig 9.7 Chain of survival.
Reproduced with permission from Nolan, J. *et al.* (2006). The chain of survival. *Resuscitation*, 71(3):270–1. https://doi.org/10.1016/j.resuscitation.2006.09.001. Copyright © 2006 Elsevier Ireland Ltd. All rights reserved.

Advanced life support (ALS) (fig 9.8 p. 577) ALS adds value to basic life support by providing oxygen therapy, ventilation via an ETT or supraglottic airway (eg LMA/i-Gel®), and drug therapy. ALS providers are trained to systematically identify and direct additional treatment for reversible causes ('4Hs' and '4Ts' see table 9.1).

Table 9.1 Reversible causes of cardiac arrest

4Hs	4Ts
Hypoxia	Cardiac Tamponade*
Hypothermia	Tension pneumothorax*
Hyperkalaemia	Toxicity
Hypovolaemia*	Thromboembolism*
*Consider focused ultrasound, if available.	

Adrenaline Advised in current guidelines but controversial: a recent randomized trial recruited over 8000 patients and demonstrated increased overall survival (3.2% vs. 2.4%; NNT=114), but *worse* neurological outcomes in survivors given adrenaline.[26]

Post-resuscitation care Aims to stabilize the patient following ROSC and prevent recurrence of cardiac arrest. Arrange basic investigations (blood gas, ECG, and CXR); consider definitive care (eg percutaneous coronary intervention); and transfer to ICU. Certain patients may undergo *targeted temperature management* (32–36°C for 24h). Prognostication usually occurs after 72h.

Survival to hospital discharge From out-of-hospital cardiac arrest in the UK is 8.6%. This lags behind others (Holland 21%, Norway 25%, and Seattle, USA 20%).[26,27] Public health initiatives now aim to buck the trend by ↑ provision of bystander BLS and availability of public access defibrillators.

Pregnancy Increases risk of haemorrhage, pulmonary embolism, certain cardiac disease (cardiomyopathy, coronary artery dissection), and eclampsia. The uterus must be manually displaced to the left while CPR is ongoing. Reversible causes are identified. If return of spontaneous circulation (ROSC) is not obtained by 4 minutes, a perimortem caesarean section should be considered. This *may* increase chances of mother and fetus surviving.[20]

Hypothermia May induce cardiac arrest or be as a result of the dying process. In the former, *'The patient is not dead until warm and dead'*, and should be aggressively rewarmed. Defibrillation is less effective. Drugs are avoided until temperature >30°c, and double time intervals used until ≥35°c. Warmed IV fluids, irrigation of the peritoneum and bladder are simpler techniques. Heart bypass or ECMO may be considered where facilities exist.

Poisoning With drugs such as *tricyclic antidepressants, calcium channel blockers,* and *beta-blockers* may result in cardiac arrest. Prolonged CPR may be justified (exceptionally, up to 4h!).[21] Make every effort to determine the offending agent, and involve the *Poisons Information Service/Toxbase* for advice on management, and if applicable, management, and if applicable, selecting antidotes. Haemofiltration and/ or haemodialysis is effective at removing some drugs. Seek expert help.

Traumatic cardiac arrest[22] See also p. 650. May be secondary to *hypovolaemia* (blood loss) but also *hypoxia* (head/chest injury, high-level spinal cord transection). Prognosis is better if prior signs of life were witnessed. Secure a definitive airway and deliver 100% oxygen. Tension pneumothoraces are excluded by performance of bilateral finger thoracostomies. The emphasis is then on delivering blood products rapidly (activate the massive transfusion protocol). **Tranexamic** acid (1g IV) may be beneficial (NNT=67, but cheap and readily available). Failure to reach ROSC may be an indication for ED thoracotomy (p. 593). This invasive procedure allows for relief of cardiac tamponade, management of internal chest wounds, and direct pressure on the descending aorta to optimize heart and brain perfusion. A similar protocol for paediatric TCA has recently been proposed.[23]

Chest compressions Must be high quality to maximize chances of successful defibrillation and survival. Place hands in the centre of the chest, and firmly compress to ⅓ (usually 5–6cm in adults) of the depth of the chest at a rate of 100–120 compressions/min. Ensure complete recoil of the chest between compressions (allows ventricular filling). Providing chest compressions is tiring, so rotate rescuers every 2 minutes or sooner (remember to minimize any pauses in chest compressions).[24] Automated devices are useful in prolonged resuscitation attempts and if the patient needs transportation, although no survival benefit has yet been proven from their use.[25]

The identification and relief of acute pain is a raison d'être of EM, yet is often suboptimal. All patients should have a pain assessment within 10 minutes of arriving in the ED, and every effort should be made to relieve a patient's pain as much as is possible. ▶Remember to reassess pain after treatment. The principles of the World Health Organization 'Pain Ladder' apply in the ED, although it is reasonable to start high or take a 'multimodal' approach if the condition demands it.

Non-opiate 'simple' analgesics
Useful for mild pain, and as 'opiate-sparing' adjuncts in severe pain. Oral paracetamol is as effective as IV[28] and doesn't cause delirium or constipation associated with opiates. Likewise, NSAIDS are most effective in acute musculo-skeletal pain and invaluable in renal colic,[29] although avoid in the very old/frail (risks: renal failure and GI bleeding). Consider gastroprotection.

Weak opiates
Weak opiates such as codeine are often used in conjunction with para-cetamol. Although a trial may be reasonable, do not be tempted to continue if they prove non-efficacious in the ED. Side effects are considerable and there is addictive potential.

Morphine
The mainstay of severe pain management in the ED, either intravenously or orally (as morphine sulfate solution). In skilled hands, fentanyl is an alterna-tive and is preferred if analgesia is required during procedural sedation (eg in addition to propofol) (p. 581) due to a short duration of effect.[30] Consider patient-controlled analgesia early on for those with high or ongoing opiate requirements.[31]

Ketamine
An NMDA receptor antagonist which at high doses is a dissociative anaes-thetic. At lower doses, ketamine is an effective analgesic, although more data is probably needed to assess its role in routine use.[32]

Entonox®
A 50:50 mixture of nitrous oxide and oxygen. 2 minutes of inhalation pro-vides effective analgesia although duration of action is extremely short. Contraindications include head injury, pneumothorax, and bowel perforation. Methoxyflurane is an anaesthetic delivered in low doses via a proprietary inhaler (the 'green whistle'). It has been used in Australasia with success for many years and is now being introduced to the UK.

Non-pharmacological pain management
Don't underestimate the value of non-pharmacological pain management. Distraction is especially useful in children, and most adults feel at least a little better after some explanation and kind reassurance. Remember that fractures are likely to remain uncomfortable until adequately immobilized/splinted.

Procedural sedation

▸▸*Procedural sedation should be carried out by those with adequate experience and when staffing and resources permit.*

Procedural sedation provides analgesia and favourable conditions for completion of a procedure. The patient is *not* rendered unconscious and retains the ability to respond to verbal and/or tactile stimuli. If sedation is any deeper, interventions to maintain the airway and cardiovascular stability may be indicated. This is undesirable in a busy ED.

Example indications
• Joint reduction
• Fracture
• Manipulation
• Wound care
• Chest drain placement

Pre-assessment
Includes medical/drug history, fasting status (*ideally* >2h for fluids, at least 4h for solids), and airway assessment. The latter is with good reason: rarely the patient may 'lose' their airway and require endotracheal intubation. Prior informed consent is essential.

Choice of agent
The selection of agent for procedural sedation depends on local factors, operator preference, and patient characteristics, see table 9.2.

Table 9.2 Choice of drug for procedural sedation

Agent	Benefits	Drawbacks
Midazolam	Duration of action ~30min Slow onset—wide therapeutic window Amnesic properties	Prolonged recovery Hypotension Potential for airway compromise
Propofol	Very rapid onset (<30sec) Rapid recovery	Painful injection Hypotension
Ketamine	Maintenance of protective airway reflexes and BP; Analgesia	Emergence phenomena Vomiting Laryngospasm

Post-sedation care
Includes observation until the patient is back to their baseline, and the provision of post-procedure written and verbal advice.

Alternatives
Procedural sedation is a very useful tool, but not without risk. *Is there a viable alternative?* For example, Entonox® to reduce a shoulder, or regional anaesthesia to reduce a fracture?

Further reading
Atkinson P *et al.* (2014). Procedural sedation in the emergency department. *BMJ* 348:g2965.

Shock is a physiological response to a pathological insult that impairs perfusion of vital tissues and organs (eg blood loss, allergen, microbe, pulmonary embolus). See also PHEM p. 634. At the cellular level, oxygenation, the delivery of nutrients, and the extraction of toxic metabolites are all affected. In compensated shock, the body maintains perfusion—eg by increasing heart rate. Shock may progress to a decompensated phase where perfusion becomes critically impaired. The final common pathway of all types of shock is organ failure and death. ▸▸*Get senior help early if you think a patient is shocked.*

Clinical manifestations of shock Include tachypnoea (earliest warning sign), tachycardia, hypotension, and reduced urine output. The brain is exquisitely sensitive to reduced perfusion—altered consciousness or confusion should raise serious concern, especially in a normally well patient. Also remember that 'normal values' are relative—a resting pulse of 90 beats/min in a normally fit and well athlete might represent significant shock. Serial observations reveal trends, which may confirm development of shock.

The foundations of resuscitation medicine lie in the identification and management of shock in its various manifestations. These are:

- *Hypovolaemic shock:* Results from haemorrhage or the loss of fluid into the 3rd space eg occurring due to capillary leak associated with sepsis, pancreatitis, burns, and anaphylaxis.
- *Distributive shock:* Results from profound peripheral vasodilation, which in turn reduces cardiac preload and output. Sepsis and anaphylaxis both cause distributive shock.
- *Cardiogenic shock:* Represents profound failure of the heart to produce adequate cardiac output. Valvular problems, endocarditis, pericardial effusion, and tamponade are causes.
- *Obstructive shock:* Describes a mechanical disruption of the heart or great vessels. Pulmonary embolus and cardiac tamponade are the commonest causes.
- *Neurogenic shock:* A special form of distributive shock which occurs in spinal cord injury: disruption of the autonomic nervous system results in profound vasodilatation and a paradoxical bradycardia.
- ▸*Never diagnose neurogenic shock in trauma until hypovolaemia has been excluded!*

Classifying the severity of shock is accomplished by a thorough assessment and response to initial resuscitative measures. Treatment should address the underlying cause, while supporting circulation (eg via use of blood products, fluids, inotropes, and vasoactive drugs) and specific vital organs (eg aortic balloon pump for cardiogenic shock).

Massive transfusion for hypovolaemic shock

Most healthy adults will tolerate 500–750mL blood loss without developing shock, and will be able to compensate effectively for blood loss of <1.5L. Beyond this, hypovolaemic shock results. Definitive intervention (eg surgery, endoscopy, interventional radiology) 'turns off the tap', but early administration of blood products which include packed red cells, fresh frozen plasma, and platelets (in 1:1:1 ratio) improves mortality. Large volumes of crystalloids is discouraged, as they contribute to haemodilution, acidosis, and impair clot integrity. A bolus of 1g **tranexamic acid** saves lives (NNT=67).[33]

Most hospitals now have a *massive transfusion protocol* which enables all required blood products to be made available quickly in the form of 'shock packs'. Product should be delivered warmed via a rapid infuser, such as the Belmont® device. Large amounts of products may be required (see fig 9.9).

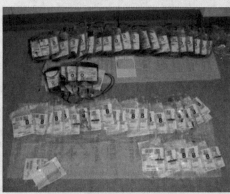

Fig 9.9 Multiple shock packs used in the resuscitation of a single war casualty.
Reproduced courtesy of Major Simon Davies QARANC.

Despite its life-saving potential, massive transfusion is not benign: the potential for mistakes is heightened in the heat of the moment. In addition, allergic and haemolytic reactions, transfusion-associated lung injury (TRALI), and electrolyte abnormalities may all occur (additional calcium may be co-administered with blood). Over-transfusion is a real possibility, and massive transfusion may worsen the systemic inflammatory insult that accompanies major trauma later on.

Further reading

Jansen JO *et al*. (2013). Damage control resuscitation for patients with major trauma. *BMJ* 338:b1778.

Most EDs have dedicated paediatric areas and at least one child-specific resuscitation bay. Larger urban centres may have dedicated paediatric EDs. Ideally, all ED clinicians should be trained in the principles of *Advanced paediatric life support* (APLS), p. 181.

It is not possible to give proper justice to paediatric emergency medicine—now a subspecialty in its own right, but since 20–25% of ED attendances are from children and young people, the 'unwell child' deserves a mention. Most children presenting to the ED will have minor injuries and illness, but some will have serious pathology. See also Paediatrics pp. 178–319.

Paediatric history taking Will often be obtained from carers, but try to take the child's perspective into account if possible. It is useful to ask about prior neonatal care (lung disease), development, immunizations, travel, infectious contacts, and social history including identification of safeguarding concerns. ▶Always be mindful of the potential for *non-accidental* history in any child presenting to ED—never be afraid to escalate concerns, no matter how trivial they may seem.

Principles of assessment of the unwell child Follows the ABCDE schema as with adults (p. 576). Additionally, all generally unwell children should receive a 'top-to-toe' assessment to identify rashes and abnormal bruising. It is important to conduct an ear, nose, and throat exam to exclude otitis media and tonsillitis as causes of fever, and a 'clean catch' urine sample should be obtained in all febrile children to exclude UTI. Although most febrile children will have a benign viral aetiology, it can be difficult to localize the source of infection and exclude serious bacterial infection initially. If in doubt (and especially if any 'red flag' features for sepsis (fig 9.10)), never hesitate to enlist senior help early and—if indicated—administer oxygen, IV antibiotics, and fluid resuscitation. Closely observe those for whom uncertainty exists—as children may deteriorate quickly, with little warning. Common indications for admission include dehydration, inability to feed, supplemental oxygen requirement, and ongoing parental (or professional!) anxiety. ▶Unwell children aged <3 months are at ↑ risk of serious infection. The early presentation may be vague (inconsolability, lethargy, unusual cry). Have a low threshold for admission ± treat for presumed sepsis. Children with significant learning disabilities should also be considered an at-risk population.

▶▶*Never hesitate to escalate concerns about a child you think may be unwell*. Many hospitals will have a paediatric emergency team, whose members would much rather be summoned to manage a problem in its earlier stages.

Some common paediatric presentations to the ED

Bronchiolitis: Viral LRTI caused by RSV that typically affects those <2yr. Symptoms (wheeze, respiratory distress) peak at ~72h. Treatment is supportive with O_2, IV hydration, and—rarely—ventilatory support. See p. 210.

Croup: Viral laryngotracheobronchitis, characterized by its 'barking cough' +/- stridor. Treatment is with O_2, bronchodilators, and steroid. Persistent respiratory distress post treatment requires admission. ΔΔ include foreign body inhalation, epiglottitis, and bacterial tracheitis. See p. 208.

Febrile seizures: Isolated, tonic–clonic seizures lasting <15min. Admit if <18 months old, 1st seizure, atypical features, or diagnostic uncertainty. See p. 232.

▶▶*Non-blanching rashes:* In an unwell child = meningococcal sepsis until proven otherwise. If due to vomiting, the rash is always above the diaphragm.

Vomiting: May be a sign of gastroenteritis but has a broad ΔΔ including urinary tract infection, abdominal pathology, and (rarely) raised ICP or systemic conditions such as diabetic ketoacidosis.

	Green – low risk	Amber – intermediate risk	Red – high risk
Colour (of skin, lips or tongue)	• Normal colour	• Pallor reported by parent/carer	• Pale/mottled/ashen/blue
Activity	• Responds normally to social cues • Content/smiles • Stays awake or awakens quickly • Strong normal cry/not crying	• Not responding normally to social cues • No smile • Wakes only with prolonged stimulation • Decreased activity	• No response to social cues • Appears ill to a healthcare professional • Does not wake or if roused does not stay awake • Weak, high-pitched or continuous cry

Respiratory		• Nasal flaring
		• Tachypnoea:
		  – RR > 50 breaths/minute, age 6–12 months
		  – RR > 40 breaths/minute, age >12 months
		• Oxygen saturation ≤95% in air
		• Crackles in the chest
			• Grunting
			• Tachypnoea: RR > 60 breaths/minute
			• Moderate or severe chest indrawing

Circulation and hydration	• Normal skin and eyes
	• Moist mucous membranes
		• Tachycardia:
		  – >160 beats/minute, age <12 months
		  – >150 beats/minute, age 12–24 months
		  – >140 beats/minute, age 2–5 years
		• CRT >3 seconds
		• Dry mucous membranes
		• Poor feeding in infants
		• Reduced urine output
			• Reduced skin turgor

Other	• None of the amber or red symptoms or signs	• Age 3–6 months, temperature ≥39°C • Fever for ≥5 days • Rigors • Swelling of a limb or joint • Non-weight bearing limb/not using an extremity	• Age < 3 months, temperature ≥38°C* • Non-blanching rash • Bulging fontanelle • Neck stiffness • Status epilepticus • Focal neurological signs • Focal seizures

CRT, capillary refill time; RR, respiratory rate
*Some vaccinations have been found to induce fever in children aged under 3 months

This traffic light table should be used in conjunction with the recommendations in the NICE guideline on fever in under 5s.
See https://www.nice.org.uk/guidance/ng143

Fig 9.10 Any febrile child with >1 red feature is at high risk of serious infection (resuscitate and get help now), and with >1 yellow feature at intermediate risk (investigate and arrange senior review).

Further reading

www.spottingthesickchild.com is a free to access online learning package that teaches assessment of the unwell child.

9 Emergency medicine

Major trauma Major trauma is a disease (not an accident!) characterized by the application of excessive kinetic energy to tissues and organs. The aetiology of trauma is characterized by the *mechanism of injury* (MOI). This is either *blunt* (eg from rapid deceleration of a motor vehicle occupant) or *penetrating* (eg from a stab, gunshot, or shrapnel wound). Deaths from trauma were originally described by Trunkey in 1983 as following the *trimodal distribution* where the 1st peak occurred within minutes due to major neurovascular disruption (rarely treatable). The 2nd peak was attributed to injuries causing airway obstruction and/or haemorrhage; these patients benefit from early intervention. Days–weeks later, the 3rd peak was due to sepsis and organ failure. Improvements in care has greatly diminished this last peak, although frequency of 1st peak/immediate deaths remains similar.[34]

Major trauma forms <3% of ED workload in the UK, but high mortality and morbidity have demanded an improved approach to caring for patients in specialized *Major Trauma Centres* and *Trauma Units* (p. 627). The incidence of trauma is about 20,000 cases per year in England, with 5400 deaths.[35] The burden of trauma is much higher globally, where injuries kill more people than HIV/AIDS, tuberculosis, and malaria combined.[36]

Traditionally, trauma is a disease of males aged 17–45 presumably as a consequence of risk-taking behaviour, occupation, and exposure to violence. In developed settings, older adults are becoming the predominant affected group.[37] The MOI may seem unimpressive (fall from standing) but frailty, comorbid conditions, and impaired physiological response conspire against the patient, injuries may be missed or under-emphasized, and the risk of poor outcome is high.

Major trauma creates a significant work load as a full trauma team is needed to receive the patient: ED, anaesthetics, surgery, orthopaedics, and radiology may be routinely called. Other specialist members include neurosurgery, plastics, cardiothoracics, maxillofacial, and vascular surgery. Continued care is usually a joint effort on ITU or trauma wards. *Intensive rehabilitation* starts early in hospital and continues in the community. Rehabilitation is a priority as eg >50% of young trauma patients report impaired occupational functioning at 5 years post injury.[38]

What we take for granted

A staggering 85% of all RTC-related deaths worldwide in 1998 were from developing countries. It may seem strange that, despite the long-term existence of specialist hospital care, development of pre-hospital services is still in the early phases. To fully appreciate the large-scale cooperation and resources required to set up national ambulance networks, take a moment to reflect on the difficulties pre-hospital services face.

We rarely think about our patient's journey upon their arrival to hospital and take it for granted that our patients will be delivered safely. One of our authors visited Uganda to teach a trauma course. A story about the local service inspired horror and disbelief in equal measure: a villager suffered a serious leg injury and his neighbours enthusiastically facilitated prompt transfer to the local hospital in a pick-up truck. The van sped along the bumpy rural road and arrived hours later, however the patient was not in the back. On re-tracing the journey they discovered the patient in a ditch. It would seem he had been catapulted out of the pick-up by a pothole and died from a simple airway obstruction after being knocked unconscious. It is a sobering thought that this patient died of something so preventable.

▶*Adequate preparation for the trauma patient prevents poor performance.* Traditional ATLS® teaching focuses on the scenario of a lone doctor receiving a trauma patient. Fortunately, these days are largely behind us and trauma is now a team sport. The ED will usually be informed of the impending arrival of a major trauma patient by the ambulance crew, who will convey critical information about the patient(s) and their condition using a format such as the 'ATMIST' handover (see pp. 636-7). This allows the ED team leader to summon the trauma team, allocate roles, pre-alert other facilities (eg theatres, CT scanner), and prepare drugs and blood products if needed.

On arrival The team will receive a formal handover. All team members should listen. Critical problems with airway and haemorrhage are identified at this stage, and the patient is fully undressed so that they can be examined. Cervical spine precautions should be taken, especially for unconscious patients.

Priorities for the trauma team 1 Identify life-threatening injuries 2 Provide life-saving intervention 3 Provide pain relief 4 Expedite transfer to imaging and either surgery or intensive care.

The trauma primary survey Consists of a rapid <c>ABCDE assessment, where <c> stands for catastrophic haemorrhage. Recent wartime experience has taught us that this causes death even before hypoxia, and so application of a haemostatic tourniquet or pelvic binder, where indicated, takes precedence over airway assessment. Adhering to this structure prioritizes the biggest threats to life, and crucially avoids the pitfall of the distracting injury (such as an open fracture) which diverts attention. In modern trauma systems, the *primary survey* aims to identify life-threatening injuries that need immediate intervention: detailed diagnosis is obtained using advanced imaging. Examples of clinically detectable life-threatening injury include external haemorrhage, airway obstruction, massive chest injuries (that impede ventilation), pelvic instability, and long bone fractures. Patients should receive plain film chest x-ray as a routine part of the primary survey ± pelvic x-ray if shocked. The priority then is to transfer the patient for either CT imaging or damage control surgery.

The trauma primary survey may be done by a single practitioner, although it can be useful—and quicker—to delegate roles among the team.

Imaging Following the primary survey, adult patients who are suspected to have multiple injuries and are stable enough should be transferred for a whole-body CT scan. This allows rapid quantification of injuries and information for onward planning of care. *Focused assessment with sonography in trauma (FAST):* Focused abdominal ultrasound cannot rule out major injury and may be of limited practical use in settings where there is ready access to CT.[39] Focused thoracic and cardiac ultrasound can be used to reliably detect pneumothorax and cardiac tamponade in unstable patients.[40] In addition to CT, early MRI may be required in patients with suspected isolated spinal cord injury.

Sources of blood loss in trauma

Think '*one on the floor*' to account for external haemorrhage and '*four more*' to account for the main culprits of occult bleeding. Table 9.3 lists the body cavities that have the potential to harbour life-threatening volumes of blood.

Table 9.3 Sources of blood loss in trauma

Body cavity	Potential capacity (L/blood)
Thorax	2.5L per hemi thorax
Abdomen	5L
Pelvis	3L
Thigh	1-2L each

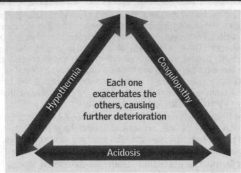

Fig 9.11 The lethal triad.
Reproduced with permission from Baid *et al. Oxford Handbook of Critical Care Nursing* (2016), Oxford: OUP.

The 'lethal triad' Describes the interaction of *hypothermia, coagulopathy,* and *acidosis* in major trauma. Their presence is predictable and associated with high mortality (fig 9.11). The delayed result is systemic inflammatory response syndrome (SIRS) and multiorgan dysfunction that can kill days and weeks after the initial insult has been corrected in severely injured patients.[41]

Hypothermia: Traditionally defined as T° <35°C, but is defined as T° <36°C in trauma since it has been associated with especially poor outcomes.[42] The elderly, intoxicated, burnt, and exposed patients are at increased risk. Hypothermia dampens the CVS compensatory mechanisms against hypovolaemic shock thus worsening tissue hypoxia.

Acidosis: Arises from tissue hypoperfusion and subsequent lactic acid production, further exacerbated by respiratory acidosis arising from hypoventilation (flail chest, opiates/alcohol, COPD). Temperature and pH heavily influence clotting and platelet function; even subtle physiological disruptions can contribute to life-threatening coagulopathies as the patient continues to haemorrhage, which in turn depletes clotting factors and platelets.

Coagulopathy: Develops in ~25% of severely injured patients and is associated with ×4 increase in mortality rates; its presence demands respect.[43] Coagulopathy in trauma was, until recently, thought to arise mainly from haemorrhage and haemodilution from excessive fluid resuscitation; but coagulopathy has been noted to develop within minutes of injury causing reduced tissue perfusion. Note pre-existing medical conditions that alter clotting (liver failure) or oral anti-coagulants (warfarin, DOACs).

▶▶Simple early interventions against hypothermia and haemorrhage control can help stave off this lethal triad. Optimizing the patient's physiological state should be a priority; this starts with basic care on-scene. It is estimated that ~20% of trauma deaths could be prevented with better haemorrhage control.[44] Enthusiastically search for all bleeding points and apply pressure; this includes a pelvic binder for internal haemorrhage. Always assume your patient is becoming cold—this is easy to forget as you sweat from working. Apply blankets, use a Bair Hugger™ and warmed fluids.

Secondary survey

The secondary survey is a thorough head-to-toe examination following completion of ABCDE once the patient is responding to initial resuscitation. It includes taking a more complete history and further imaging (us, angiography, etc.). Continuous re-assessment of ABCDE is still expected. It is often poorly performed and documented in the aftermath of an adrenaline-filled ABCDE assessment. It is especially important in the unconscious patient who is unable to report a finger fracture or testicular rupture.

A mnemonic was proposed to help add focus to this assessment (see MINIBOX):[35]

Mnemonic	Secondary survey
• Has	• Head/skull
• My	• Maxillofacial
• Critical	• Cervical spine
• Care	• Chest
• Assessed	• Abdomen
• Patient's	• Pelvis
• Priorities	• Perineum
• Or	• Orifices (PR/PV)
• Next	• Neurological
• Management	• Musculoskeletal
• Decision?	• Diagnostic tests/ definitive care

Primary traumatic brain injury (TBI) TBI occurs at the time of impact. Secondary injury arises in the minutes, hours, and days following and is a result of ischaemia (eg due to vasospasm), ↑ intracranial pressure (ICP), cerebral oedema, expanding haematomas, seizures, and infection. Emergent management of TBI limits secondary injury.

The severity of TBI can be classified by calculating the Glasgow Coma Scale score (GCS). GCS of >13/15 implies 'mild' injury; 9–13/15 'moderate' injury; and 3–8 'severe' injury. ▶▶*A GCS of <8 implies the loss of protective airway reflexes. Intubation may be required: contact ITU.*

Although classifications are useful for clinicians, the reality is that even 'minor' TBI can result in persistent neuropsychiatric morbidity for patients. For example, 1yr follow-up in one population revealed that 27% had not resumed previous occupation, and 84% had impaired function.[45]

Aetiology: Aetiology of TBI varies by age group: in those aged 15–34, assault is most common, whereas falls predominate in those aged >65yrs.[46] Alcohol ingestion is present in 21% of those that attend ED in the UK, and 68% with a head injury;[47] is it alcohol that is causing vomiting/confusion or is it a serious head injury? This is a common dilemma and the NICE guidance (table 9.4) should be followed irrespective of whether intoxication is assumed, unless senior opinion suggests otherwise. In the latter case, regular neurological observations at least every 15min are essential.[48]

▶▶*It is crucial to avoid hypoxia and hypotension in head injured patients.* It may only take one episode of either to worsen long-term outcome. Always conduct a thorough primary survey—airway obstruction, impaired oxygenation, and control of life-threatening haemorrhage all take precedence over neurosurgical intervention. When conducting the disability assessment, note GCS, pupil size/responsiveness, and any lateralizing neurology. A carefully documented baseline neurological examination is very useful for neurosurgical and ITU colleagues. Exposure should take note of CSF leaks, 'panda eyes' or mastoid bruising, and presence of haemotympanum (all indicate base of skull #). Never forget to check glucose, and take precautions to immobilize the cervical spine ('Collar & Blocks') in all unconscious trauma patients.

Imaging Criteria are provided by the 2014 NICE guidelines, see table 9.4:[49]

- ▶All patients presenting with head injury and reduced GCS, focal deficits, or suspicion of base of skull fracture need a CT head within an hour of injury.
- All patients on warfarin or who have a known coagulopathy should have a CT head within a maximum of 8h. This includes patients on direct oral anticoagulants (eg rivaroxaban). Those on antiplatelets (eg clopidogrel) may also be at increased bleeding risk.[50]
- If CT is abnormal, GCS <15, or significant symptoms or signs discuss with neurosurgery and agree appropriate admission.

Patients without concerning features can be discharged with a head injury advice leaflet. Ensure patients are with a responsible adult for at least 24 hours—all parties must have clear instructions dictating when they should re-present. Likewise, inform that mild post-concussive symptoms (minor mood disturbance, unsteadiness etc.) should resolve within a few days to 2 weeks. The UK Rugby Football Union advises contact sports should be avoided for at least 2 weeks and that players must be symptom free before attempting a graded return to play.

Glasgow Coma Score (GCS)
Eye opening score
4 Spontaneous
3 To voice
2 To pain
Verbal response score
5 Oriented
4 Confused
3 Inappropriate
2 Incomprehensible
Motor response score
6 Obeying commands
5 Lateralizing to pain
4 Withdraws to pain
3 Abnormal flexion
2 Abnormal extension
No response in any category scores 1. Minimum score is therefore 3. Maximum is 15.
A normal GCS is documented as $E4V5M6$=15.

Table 9.4 NICE criteria for imaging in head injury

Urgent CT head if:[49]	And add cervical spine (CT) if:[49] (see p. 522)
• GCS <13 at initial assessment • GCS <15 at 2h post injury • Open or depressed skull or basal skull fracture • Post-traumatic fit • Focal CNS deficit • >1 episode of vomiting	• GCS <13 at initial assessment • Intubation • Definitive diagnosis of c-spine injury is required urgently (eg before surgery) • Other areas are being scanned for head injury or multiregion trauma.
CT head if any LOC/amnesia & • Age >65 years • Dangerous mechanism of injury • Coagulopathy • Retrograde amnesia >½h	The patient is alert and stable, there is a suspicion of c-spine injury and any of the following are present: • Age >65 • Dangerous mechanism of injury • Focal CNS deficit • Paraesthesia in upper or lower limbs

Specific aspects of managing head injury

Physiology of head injury management ICP is raised if >20mmHg. The normal occupants of the cranium are CSF, blood, and brain tissue (90%). The Monro–Kellie doctrine explains how the presence of an intracranial mass can initially be accommodated by displacing venous blood and CSF, but a limit is quickly reached where ICP will ↑ and restrict cerebral perfusion pressure (CPP), thus worsening cerebral ischaemia. Management aims to enhance cerebral perfusion by normalizing ICP and monitoring the mean arterial pressure (MAP) since CPP = MAP − ICP. ▶Target MAP to ~90mmHg to ensure CPP >60mmHg.

Medical management of head injury:
The aim is to prevent secondary brain injury by maintaining physiological parameters:[51]
* *Maintain normal blood pressure:* Aim for systolic BP >100mmHg. Even a single episode of low BP is associated with worse outcomes in severe TBI. Normovolaemia with isotonic solutions are favoured. Avoid volume overload (↑ risk of cerebral oedema) and routine glucose preparations (hyperglycaemia ↑ ischaemia).
* *Maintain normal PO_2 and PCO_2:* Secure the airway (rapid sequence induction p. 670). Aim for normoxia and normocapnia to optimize CPP. Hyperventilation will reduce $PaCO_2$, resulting in cerebral vasoconstriction which in turn ↓ICP, but also leads to cerebral hypoperfusion and may worsen outcomes.
* *Maintain normal ICP:* This is achieved primarily through manipulation of blood pressure, ventilation, and sedation. If at risk of cerebral herniation (eg fixed dilated pupil), administration of hypertonic saline or mannitol may be a life-saving temporizing measure but risks systemic hypotension.
* *Maintain normal blood sugar and temperature:* Some patients may develop hyperpyrexia and need active cooling.
* *Raise head 30°:* Improves jugular venous return. Likewise, avoid tight cervical collars and use tape to secure endotracheal tubes.
* *Control seizures:* Prophylactic antiepileptics may mitigate early seizures, but there is no evidence they reduce occurrence of late seizures.
* *Urgent neurosurgical input:* Mandatory in severe TBI. Evacuation of haematoma may be lifesaving and facilitate excellent recovery in some patients. Decompressive craniectomy may be attempted in patients with uncontrolled ICP but may be associated with poor functional outcomes.[34]

Further reading

Smith J *et al.* (2010). *Head Injuries in Major Trauma* (Oxford Desk Reference). Oxford: Oxford University Press.

A key objective of the primary survey is to identify life-threatening thoracic trauma. ►*Apply high-flow O_2 and arrange an immediate portable chest x-ray.*

Major injuries to the chest may cause hypoxia (direct lung injury; hypoventilation secondary to pain) and circulatory collapse (haemorrhage; obstructive ± cardiogenic shock). There are a finite number of injuries that require identification at this stage—the mnemonic ATOM FC is useful: **A**irway obstruction; **T**ension pneumothorax; **O**pen pneumothorax; **M**assive haemothorax; **F**lail chest; **C**ardiac tamponade (see pp. 644–5 for more details on each of these).

►*Emergency department thoracotomy may be lifesaving in critically unstable patients or those in traumatic cardiac arrest* (see BOX 'Emergency department thoracotomy (EDT)').

Secondary survey

Once the above-mentioned injuries have been excluded or managed, the secondary survey may identify more subtle thoracic injuries:

- *Simple pneumothorax:* Observe for progression to tension pneumothorax. Consider aspiration or drain if large.
- *Simple haemothorax:* (<1500mL blood.) Lacerations in lung or blood vessels tend to be self-limiting and do not require surgery. Large-calibre (36 French) chest tube if haemothorax large enough to visualize on CXR. If not fully evacuated, residual blood can clot and cause lung entrapment or infection.
- *Tracheobronchial tree/aortic disruption:* Tends to cause death at scene and requires urgent surgical intervention. Suspicion based on mechanism of injury and CXR findings (widened mediastinum, altered tracheobronchial anatomy). Missing a diaphragmatic injury can cause insidious respiratory distress or bowel strangulation.
- *Blunt cardiac injury:* Significant injury is quite uncommon as most die on-scene. It may result in life-threatening arrhythmias so consider careful ECG monitoring and us. Troponin rise in blunt injury may indicate cardiac contusion.[52]
- *Oesophageal rupture:* Consider if disproportionally unwell when compared to apparent injury. Typically associated with left pleural effusions and/or pneumomediastinum visible on imaging.
- *Sternal fractures:* Diagnosis is clinical but may be confirmed by x-ray or ultrasound.[53] ECG and chest x-ray exclude blunt cardiac injury.[54]
- *Scapula fractures:* Indicative of high-energy trauma. Look for other potentially life-threatening injuries.[55]
- *Simple rib fractures:* Very common and extremely painful. The diagnosis is clinical based on mechanism of injury and localized tenderness. Bony crepitus may be felt. Chest x-ray is insensitive and cannot be used to exclude (organize CT if multiple fractures or underlying lung injury suspected. Adequate pain relief is imperative. Frail patients, those with uncontrolled pain, multiple rib fractures, or at high risk of respiratory complications require admission for analgesia (including regional anaesthetic techniques), chest physiotherapy, and consideration of operative fixation.[56]

Emergency department thoracotomy (EDT)

EDT[67] aims to allow rapid access to the inner thorax (fig 9.12). Priorities are to 1 Identify and relieve cardiac tamponade 2 Control bleeding points 3 Provide internal cardiac massage (in arrest) 4 Provide compression of the aorta (with a closed fist not a clamp!) to improve cardiac and cerebral blood flow. The complexity of EDT as a procedure lies not only in psychomotor skills, but in simultaneously coordinating a fraught team and organizing definitive care. There is a significant risk of 'needle-stick' injury, both from sharps and the patient's own rib/sternal edges. ▶Always double-glove and use a face shield/goggles—keep all hands not directly involved well out of the way.

Those required to perform EDT should attend training that ideally involves practice on animal or human tissue. In brief summary, the procedure begins with bilateral finger thoracostomies. An incision is then made to 'join up', following the 4th/5th IC space anteriorly. The intercostal muscles are cut using scissors and the sternum divided with a Gigli saw, completing the so-called clamshell incision. The ribs are separated. A generous longitudinal pericardial incision (avoiding the phrenic nerve) then delivers the heart. Clot can be evacuated and any cardiac injury identified. Simple external pressure over cardiac wounds or insertion of a Foley catheter through a wound are preferred temporizing measures prior to definitive surgery.[57]

Success of EDT in penetrating trauma is notable in some case series (eg 18%).[58] There is growing recognition of a role for EDT in the resuscitation of selected blunt trauma patients with cardiac arrest.

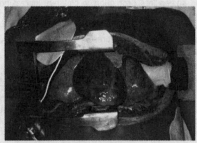

Fig 9.12 Clamshell thoracotomy. The pericardium has been displaced and the gloved hand is compressing the aorta against the vertebral column.
Reproduced with permission from Smith *et al.*, *Major Trauma* (2011), Oxford: OUP.

Abdominal trauma is initially classified by aetiology ('penetrating' or 'blunt'). Early death from abdominal trauma is due to bleeding. Infection, perforation, and abdominal compartment syndrome may occur later. ►Early imaging (CT) and surgical review is essential. Remember that the abdomen extends from nipples to groin anteriorly and to iliac crests posteriorly—although diaphragmatic rupture may also expose abdominal contents to injury in the chest.

Penetrating trauma

High-velocity missiles may cause disproportionate tissue damage as a result of pressure changes caused by cavitation. This has the potential to disrupt entire organs. The path of injury is difficult to predict: the projectile may change course within the body. There is a high risk of infection. Stab injuries are simpler to predict and involve less force. However, beware the seemingly trivial stabbing—eg a sharpened bicycle spoke leaves an innocuous wound but is capable of traversing multiple anatomic regions. Be fastidious in the *search for multiple wounds* (examine back, axillae, and perineum). Most penetrating injuries require prompt laparotomy/laparoscopy if they breach the rectus fascia or peritoneum.[59]

Blunt trauma

Typically occurs from *rapid deceleration* forces or direct blows. Hollow viscus injuries are most common, followed by liver/biliary tract and spleen.[60] Increasingly, patients are managed using non-operative approaches. The ribs afford liver and spleen less protection in children, increasing vulnerability. Retroperitoneal injury may involve kidneys, adrenal glands, pancreas, duodenum, and major vascular structures (aorta, renal, and mesenteric vessels).

►► *Suspect a ruptured spleen* in the presence of shock, abdominal tenderness/distension, left shoulder tip pain, and an overlying rib #.

Unstable patients

Shock; GI, GU, or PR bleeding; evisceration or peritonitis usually warrant laparotomy. If availability and patient status allows, preoperative CT scan is valuable but should not delay transfer to theatre if there is an immediate threat to life and failure to stabilize in the resuscitation room. Activate the massive transfusion protocol if major haemorrhage suspected, and inform theatres of the need for damage control surgery (see BOX 'Damage control surgery (DCS)').

Stable patients

Must still be treated with a high index of suspicion depending on mechanism of injury and clinical symptoms. In particular, CT scanning may miss hollow viscus injury.[61]

Damage control surgery (DCS)

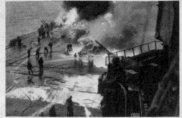

Fig 9.13 Damage control on *USS Saratoga*, 1945.

Damage control has its origins in WWII, where Naval forces quickly learned that prompt firefighting and control of flooding could prevent a stricken ship from sinking, in order for her to be returned to harbour for formal repairs. Thus, both men and machine could return to fight another day (fig 9.13).

The concept has been borrowed to describe the process used to care for a severely injured and unstable trauma patient. Attempting to deliver a definitive surgical procedure to such a patient is likely to worsen their physiological state and reduce survivability. The aim of DCS is to stop bleeding in the minimum time possible. In the first instance, this may involve systematic packing of abdominal and pelvic cavities. The patient receives ongoing resuscitation from an anaesthetic team during the surgery, and is promptly returned to the intensive therapy unit for organ support. Only when the patient is satisfactorily stable are more complex, definitive procedures undertaken.

Major pelvic trauma

Includes *anterior–posterior disruption* (the 'open book' appearance eg from a motorcyclist impacting the fuel tank during rapid deceleration), *lateral compression*, and *vertical shear* (falls from height). The pelvic cavity has a rich blood supply with a capacity of 2–3L. Haemorrhage from fractures can be life-threatening. ▶*Most pelvic bleeding is venous—shock may take time to develop!*

Due to the ring structure of the pelvis, single fractures from falls in the elderly are often stable (see BOX 'The stability of pelvic fractures') and just need a few weeks' rest. In contrast, ≥2 fractures in the pelvis (with 1 above the level of the hip) renders the ring unstable and is serious; >25% have internal injuries.

Signs of pelvic fracture

High-energy mechanism of injury, leg length discrepancy, abdominal distension, loin bruising, perineal or scrotal haematoma, PV bleeding, palpable haematoma or # line on PR/PV exam (rectal injury is common and associated with sepsis risk).

Signs of GU injury

Urethral injury occurs in 15% of males (typically with type B&C fractures, fig 9.14).[62] Extraperitoneal bladder rupture may occur. Check for blood at urethral tip (signifying ruptured urethra), frank or microscopic haematuria, PR exam may help assess bowel integrity and presence of blood, but should not delay imaging. *Seek urology opinion* if suspicion of urethral damage (retrograde urethrography must be performed before catheterization if urethral injury is suspected). Suprapubic catheterization may be necessary.

Reduce blood loss

Place a pelvic splint firmly over the greater trochanters. This is often accomplished in the pre-hospital phase, using a proprietary device (eg SamSplint®) although a bedsheet wrapped and then tied around the pelvis can suffice. Avoid excessive patient handling, and use an orthopaedic 'scoop' stretcher or trauma mattress during transfer to minimize pelvic disruption. ▶▶Check foot pulses and urine output often. Shock in pelvic fracture carries a mortality of 14–55%.[63]

Femoral shaft fractures

Frequently accompany pelvic fractures (esp. if bilateral) and are another potential source of blood loss (1–2L per thigh). *Splinting* (pp. 526–7) is essential to reduce blood loss, prevent soft tissue damage, and provide analgesia.

Associated organ injury?

In all but the frail elderly, pelvic fractures are the result of high-energy trauma. Many unstable fractures will have accompanying internal injuries (30%) with liver (10.2%), small bowel (8.8%), and splenic (5.8%) injuries commonest.[62] For this reason, patients with suspected unstable pelvic fractures should undergo trauma 'Pan-CT' scanning.

Radiology

Only do pelvic x-ray if there is no indication for CT, or if the patient is shocked and it is necessary to rapidly exclude disruption prior to transfer for damage control surgery. Angiography and embolization is increasingly an option for haemorrhage control in addition to surgery, where the pelvis may be temporarily immobilized and can be fixed later when the patient is fit for surgery.

The stability of pelvic fractures

►►*Do not 'rock the pelvis' during primary survey.* If there is concern about pelvic trauma, application of a pelvic splint should be considered and the patient should proceed to diagnostic imaging. Multiple systems exist. Most useful is the Tile classification (fig 9.14).

(a)   (b)   (c)

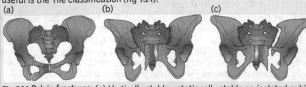

Fig 9.14 Pelvic fractures. (a) Vertically stable, rotationally stable eg isolated pubic rami # or iliac wing fractures. (b) Vertically stable, rotationally unstable eg ipsi-or contralateral ('bucket handle' type) lateral compression #; 'open-book' fracture (look for widening at the sacroiliac (sı) joints and diastasis (=separation) of the pubic symphysis). (c) Vertically unstable, rotationally unstable; eg # through ipsilateral sı joint and pubic rami. Includes Malgaigne's fracture (20% of all pelvic #s, 60% of unstable ones)—disruption of the pelvis anteriorly and posteriorly with displacement of a fragment containing the hip joint. NB: a clue to the presence of vertical instability is superior migration of the pelvic fragment.

Major burns Quite rare in developed settings, but are much commoner in developing settings where naked flames are used to cook, heat, and light homes. Patients require prompt assessment, provision of analgesia, resuscitation, and transfer to specialist care.

First aid *Cooling* is beneficial up to at least 3h post injury and should be started as soon as possible. Remove all burnt clothing and irrigate continuously with cool tap water or sterile saline. This reduces the severity and extent of burns. Cooling should continue for at least 20 minutes.[64] Burns should be kept clean and covered with cling film strips (do not wrap circumferentially). ▶ *Avoid hypothermia* —'cool the burn and warm the patient'.

Burns resuscitation Follows a systematic <c>ABCDE trauma assessment (remember the potential for accompanying injuries—eg from a fall or blast). Involvement of a skilled airway doctor is imperative, especially if there are facial burns, sooty deposits around the mouth, nose, and/or oropharynx. ▶The presence of *stridor* or *hoarseness* is an emergency. Call anaesthetics and ENT—nasal endoscopy may reveal laryngeal swelling. Difficult intubation should be anticipated.

Increased evaporative losses (loss of tissue integrity) and systemic inflammatory response (↑↑ capillary permeability) means that hypovolaemia develops quickly in burns. Monitor urine output and arrange for an arterial and central venous line. Commence IV fluid resuscitation as per the Parkland formula. There is a high risk of secondary infection and sepsis due to loss of skin integrity.[65]

Fluid resuscitation may expedite the development of critical facial and airway oedema in burns—there must be a low threshold for intubation if this develops.

The Parkland formula

24h crystalloid requirement (mL) = 4 × body weight (kg) × TBSA.
Give 50% over 8h, the next 50% over 16h.

Total burn surface area (TBSA) Estimated[66] using the *Lund & Browder Chart* (fig 9.15). Other methods include *Wallace's 'rule of 9s'* and *palmar counting* (patient's palm = ~1% of surface area). The Mersey Burns App (http://merseyburns.com) is a free electronic alternative.[67]

Inhalation injury Results from direct thermal burns to the airways (resulting in sloughing and plugging), localized chemical burns to the airways from acids (eg HCL, HF) found in fire smoke, and systemic toxicity from carbon monoxide, cyanide, and other gases.[68] *Carbon monoxide (co):* Has a half-life of 4h at room air, but this reduces to <60 minutes on 100% O_2. Cell damage may occur after normalization of COHb levels—beware the patient with 'normal' values who has been administered O_2 in the pre-hospital phase. The main effects of co poisoning are neurological (coma, seizures, focal deficits) ±cardiac ischaemia. Cherry-red discolouration of the skin is a postmortem sign; absence does not exclude. Give high-flow O_2 and discuss symptomatic cases with the local hyperbaric medicine unit.

Cyanide Released in the combustion of plastics, paints, and furniture foams and poisoning.[69] *Diagnosis:* Challenging. Consider where there is a history of exposure to smoke accompanied by haemodynamic instability, neurological deficit, and high lactate (>5mmol/L) unexplained by alternative mechanisms. Hydroxocobalamin is probably the best tolerated treatment; sodium thiosulfate is an alternative.

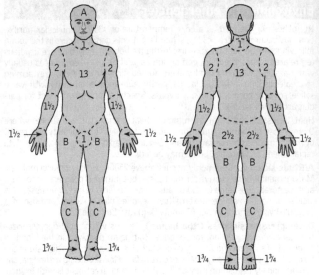

Relative percentage of body surface area affected by growth

Area	Age 0	1	5	10	15	Adult
A: half of head	9½	8½	6½	5½	4½	3½
B: half of thigh	2¾	3¼	4	4¼	4½	4¾
C: half of leg	2½	2½	2¾	3	3¼	3½

Fig 9.15 Lund–Browder chart.

Chemical burns ↑ in incidence due to the use of strong acids as street weapons. 'Acid attacks' result in devastating disfigurement, and may be life-threatening. Immediate irrigation with copious amounts of clean water is imperative (think the need for a fire engine in the pre-hospital setting!). Beware of causing secondary injury to the patient (ensure contaminated water flows away from unaffected areas) and to providers (use apron, heavy rubber gloves, and goggles as a minimum).[70] Diphoterine® is a proprietary chemical buffer which may be applied to chemical burns, potentially reducing severity.[71]

Hydrofluoric acid Commonly used in glass etching. It is rapidly absorbed where fluoride ions bind calcium, causing profound hypocalcaemia. Decontaminate; move to a high dependency area and treat with calcium gluconate (IV/locally around burn site) alongside usual advanced life support.[72] Seek expert advice.

Further reading

Dries DJ, Endorf FW (2013). Inhalation injury: epidemiology, pathology, treatment strategies. *Scan J Trauma Resusc Emerg Med* 21:31.

Enoch S et al. (2009). Emergency and early management of burns and scalds. *bmj* 338:b1037.

Hypothermia Defined as a core temperature of <35°c. Ventricular fibrillation may occur if severe (<32°c)—handle patients gently. Occurs in the young following environmental exposure; in the frail/elderly may be more insidious (eg related to poor heating, comorbidities, and drugs). *Treatment* is usually with passive rewarming (eg blankets, forced air warmer). Active rewarming strategies include lavage of bladder, peritoneum and pleural cavity with warm saline, ECMO, or cardiopulmonary bypass. Special arrangements exist for cardiac arrest (see p. 579).[73]

Heat illness A spectrum from simple heat cramps to heat stroke, where there is loss of thermoregulation (temperature >40°c). Mortality is a result of rhabdomyolysis, renal failure, and seizures. Rapid cooling, fluid/electrolyte replacement, and organ support may be indicated.[74]

Altitude sickness Commonly occurs above 2500m in the non-acclimatized. Management is conservative for mild cases, but if there is progression to high-altitude cerebral oedema (HACE) or pulmonary oedema (HAPE) *rapid descent* is indicated. Acetazolamide, dexamethasone, nifedipine (in HAPE), and use of a portable hyperbaric chamber (Gamow Bag) may buy time.[75]

Decompression sickness ('the bends') Occurs when rapid depressurization, usually during diving, forces gases (nitrogen) dissolved in the blood to come out of solution and form gaseous bubbles. The site of gas deposition determines symptoms, and typically occurs in large joints causing arthralgia. CNS and pulmonary deposition may be life-threatening. Treatment is with oxygen, IV fluids, and rapid transfer for hyperbaric oxygen therapy. *Arterial gas embolism:* A separate decompression illness caused by expansion of gas in the lungs which then enters the systemic circulation. Associated with pneumothorax, pneumomediastinum, and surgical emphysema.[76]

Lightning strike Has an incidence of 30–60/yr and results in an average of 2 deaths/yr in the UK[77] usually either due to arrhythmias or asystole. Recovery from very prolonged resuscitation has been reported. Patients may have burns and other traumatic injuries. Other sequelae include tympanic perforation and neuropsychiatric morbidity.[78]

Expect to see patients who have taken deliberate (or sometimes accidental) overdoses of medicines and/or recreational drugs most shifts. A grasp of basic toxicology is therefore essential. ▶Psychiatric risk, mental capacity, and a physical description must be documented for every patient who has taken a deliberate overdose!

Key questions to ask
• What was taken? At what time?
• Was it a single or staggered ingestion?
• Any co-ingestions, including alcohol or recreational drugs?

▶Consult the *National Poisons Information Service* (NPIS) database *Toxbase®* (www.toxbase.org) for every ingestion. Note information regarding dose-dependent effects, peak concentration (indicating when clinical status will likely be worst), and half-life. Toxbase® provides guidance on management strategies and observation periods. If in doubt, NPIS can be contacted directly by telephone.

Paracetamol overdose Extremely common. The toxic metabolite *N*-acetyl-p-benzoquinone imine (NAPQI) results from depletion of glutathione stores, causing fulminant hepatic necrosis after several days. For a single ingestion, take levels at 4h and administer acetylcysteine (NAC) if levels exceed those on the treatment nomogram.[79] Note that the UK treatment threshold is 100mg/L at 4h in all groups.[80] Refer to the poisons database for details on monitoring and management of complex cases (eg staggered/delayed).

Antidepressant overdose Also occurs commonly. Selective serotonin reuptake inhibitors (SSRIs) may cause prolonged QT syndrome (risk: torsade de pointes), CNS depression, and seizures. The presence of hyper-reflexia and pyrexia should prompt concern regarding serotonin syndrome. This is managed with cooling, fluids, benzodiazepines, and intensive therapy support.[81] Venlafaxine also inhibits noradrenaline reuptake and is more toxic than other SSRIs.[82] Tricyclic antidepressants (TCAs) are very toxic, causing metabolic acidosis, CNS depression, QRS widening (due to sodium channel blockade), and arrhythmias. Treatment is supportive—ITU may be required. Administration of sodium bicarbonate IV is indicated if the QRS is widened.[83]

Recreational drugs Ubiquitous throughout society, and ill effects are frequently encountered in the ED. *Opiates* such as heroin cause itching, miosis, and hypoventilation leading to respiratory arrest. Treatment is with naloxone (IV/IM), usually titrated to the point of adequate respiratory function. Be aware that reversal can be immediate, precipitating agitated behaviour due to withdrawal effects. The half-life of naloxone is shorter than most opiates (~20min) so repeat dosing ± an infusion may be required.[84] Be wary of new synthetic opioids purchased online—these may be extremely potent.[85] *Cocaine* is widely encountered. It is a potent sympathomimetic causing euphoria, hypervigilance, tachycardia, and hypertension. Toxic effects include severe agitation, myocardial infarction and arrhythmias, seizures, and intracranial bleeding. Management is supportive and with benzodiazepines/GTN. *Amphetamine* is another sympathomimetic with similar toxidrome to cocaine. In addition, there is often pyrexia and risk of hyponatraemia, rhabdomyolysis, renal failure, and multiorgan failure. Treatment is with active cooling, fluid resuscitation, benzodiazepines, and ITU support. *Hallucinogenics* include phencyclidine (PCP), psilocybin (mushrooms), and lysergic acid diethylamide (LSD). These drugs cause profound short- and longer-term psychiatric effects, including hallucinosis and psychosis. ℞: supportive; care in a quiet calm environment. Benzodiazepines may be a useful adjunct. *Cannabis* contains the active ingredient tetrahydrocannabinol (THC). Clinical effects include lethargy, psychomotor retardation, postural hypotension, and slurred speech. Supportive treatment usually suffices. Synthetic cannabinoids can have much more profound and prolonged neuropsychiatric effects.

Sepsis Defined as 'the body's overwhelming and life-threatening response to infection that can lead to tissue damage, organ failure, and death'.[86] Sepsis accounts for ~7% of all deaths nationally in the UK, and 27% of ITU admissions.[87] Sepsis is diagnosed if the criteria for systemic inflammatory response syndrome (SIRS) are met (see MINIBOX 'Identifying sepsis') in association with a presumed or confirmed infection.

The key to sepsis management is through early recognition, aggressive initial resuscitation, organ support where indicated, and identification and treatment of the underlying source of infection.

Identifying sepsis
There should be 2 features of SIRS:
• Temperature >38°c or <36°c
• Heart rate >90/min
• Respiratory rate >20/min
• WCC >10 or <4 *and*
• Presumed or documented infection

Although the mortality benefit of goal-directed therapy in itself is debated,[88] the Sepsis Six Care Bundle[89] describes a desirable process of care that should be achieved within 1h of the sepsis criteria being identified in the ED. The beauty of this approach is its simplicity—although don't underestimate the time (and effort!) required to achieve this target in a busy, overcrowded ED!

- *Take blood cultures:* Using aseptic non-touch technique, ideally 2 sets (from 2 sites). Send for MC+S.
- *Measure lactate:* Usually from venous blood gas. Patients with ↑ lactate (>4mmol/L) should have serial measurements—the trend is important in assessing response to treatment.
- *Measure urine output:* Urine output is a sensitive marker of renal perfusion and indicator of responsiveness to fluid resuscitation. Have a low threshold for placing a urinary catheter, especially in severe sepsis or septic shock.
- *Give empiric antibiotics:* Unless you are certain of a source where it may be acceptable to be more specific. Use local antimicrobial policy to guide—be aware that regimens differ for patients who are from nosocomial settings (nursing homes, recent hospital admission, etc.).
- *Give intravenous fluids:* The amount of IV fluid required depends on assessing hydration and haemodynamic instability. It also depends on cardiac function, especially in the elderly/frail. Start with boluses of 250–500mL, assess response (HR, BP, urine output, etc.) and repeat as necessary. Failure to stabilize after 2–3L of crystalloid (less in elderly/frail) may be an indication for vasopressor support. Contact critical care.
- *Maintain normal oxygenation:* Use supplemental O₂ to maintain oxygen saturations at >94% (88–92% in those at risk of type II respiratory failure).

A broad-spectrum antibiotic may be life-saving in the first instance, but a septic screen should be undertaken to find the source and offending organism, and rationalize therapy. Every septic ED patient should receive a urine dip and chest x-ray. Don't forget to consider neurological and skin sources (eg cellulitis, ulcers, and sores). Additional imaging (eg CT in suspected abdominal sepsis) may be required.

Meningococcal sepsis

Suspect in the presence of a new purpuric rash, in profoundly unwell children/teenagers, where there is a positive contact history, or associated signs of meningism (meningitis and meningococcal sepsis do not always coexist!). Usual treatment is either ceftriaxone or cefotaxime, with amoxicillin to cover listeria at the extremes of age.

Neutropenic sepsis

Suspect in all febrile/unwell patients undergoing chemotherapy, on biologic agents, and those who may be functionally neutropenic (eg haematological malignancy). If in doubt, speak to haematology/oncology, but never delay early administration of empiric antibiotics as the patient can deteriorate precipitously.

Transient loss of consciousness

Transient loss of consciousness (TLOC) is a common reason for presentation to the ED (3% of attendances). Rationalize the diagnostic process by considering the 2 main pathological processes of syncope and seizures.[90] The role of the emergency physician is to: 1 Resuscitate and stabilize 2 Differentiate the likely cause of collapse 3 Instigate appropriate investigations, and 4 Undertake a risk assessment to determine need for admission.

Syncope Describes TLOC caused by transient global impairment of cerebral perfusion. Vasovagal syncope is probably most common and usually benign. There should be the presence of *postural factors*, *provocation*, and *prodromal symptoms* (the 'three PS'). There is rapid and complete resolution within minutes. It is important to consider more sinister causes including structural heart disease, pulmonary embolism, arrhythmia, subarachnoid haemorrhage, ruptured aortic aneurysm, stroke/TIA, and ectopic pregnancy, as well as metabolic and toxicological disorders. Good history ± a witness account helps differentiate most cases. *Red flags* for indicating the need for cardiac monitoring and assessment include exertional syncope, chest pain, palpitations, history of heart disease, family history of sudden death, or signs of heart failure, abnormal ECG, anaemia, and electrolyte abnormalities.[91]

All patients with TLOC should receive full observations, a lying/standing blood pressure, and ECG. Order a chest x-ray and arrange echocardiogram if cardiac cause suspected.[92] Blood testing has a low diagnostic yield but may be needed to exclude anaemia, electrolyte disturbance, renal failure, myocardial infarction or a pulmonary embolus.

Clinical decision rules attempt to risk stratify patients, and include the San Francisco Syncope Rule (SFSR).[93]

Seizures Result from an excessive asynchronous discharge of neurons, may cause TLOC and account for 0.6% of attendances.[94] Collateral history is important—witnessed tonic–clonic activity lasting for more than a few seconds following collapse, *lateral* tongue biting, urinary incontinence and a prolonged post-ictal recovery are indicative.[95] Could the seizure have been provoked? Check blood sugar, exclude intracranial event/trauma, systemic upset (meningoencephalitis), and alcohol or drug abuse. Patients with a normal ED workup may be suitable for discharge with a safety net (avoid driving, heavy machinery, and swimming/bathing) and referral to 'first fit' clinic or other ambulatory pathway.[96]

Stroke (*OHCM* p470) Stroke may be ischaemic (80%) or haemorrhagic (20%).[97] It can be devastating for the patient, and since thrombolysis is only effective within a narrow therapeutic window, it is considered a time-critical emergency. Most hospitals will have a *stroke pathway* to expedite imaging and treatment of patients, and allow direct admission to an acute stroke unit.

Thrombolysis in stroke is the subject of controversy, but many centres offer to selected non-haemorrhagic stroke patients within 3–4.5h of symptom onset.[98] Thrombolysis is more effective the quicker it is delivered (most aim for door-to-needle time <60min), so a priority for the emergency doctor is to arrange rapid access to CT scanning and review by a clinician who can assess suitability for, and deliver, thrombolysis.

Acute radiological interventions for stroke show promise but are currently limited to a few specialist hyperacute centres.

Transient ischaemic attack A common cause of acute neurological deficit in the ED. The priority is to exclude any residual symptoms and provide a risk assessment for stroke (ie $ABCD_2$ score),[99] consider the need for neuroimaging, antiplatelet medication, and urgent specialist referral. If there is doubt about the diagnosis, seek a same-day neurology opinion. Patients at high risk of stroke and evidence of 'crescendo' TIA (>2 in 1 week) might warrant admission. Otherwise, patients are typically referred to a stroke clinic, depending on local policy. ▶If discharging a patient following TIA, provide a safety net including advice about features of a stroke (see fig 9.16) and calling for help. This will ensure timely consideration of thrombolysis and minimize morbidity should the worst occur.

Not all acute weakness is stroke! Stroke mimics are commonly encountered in ED (22% of 'stroke' presentations) and include seizures, encephalopathy, syncope, and migraine.[100]

Think stroke—time to act FAST

The onset of stroke symptoms may have less impact than the central crushing chest pain of an acute MI, or bleeding from a traumatic amputation, but are no less devastating. Getting patients and their relatives to promptly recognize and act upon symptoms is a challenge and has been addressed in the UK by a simple public health intervention which compels members of the public to undertake the *Face/Arm/Speech test* and call for an ambulance if any features are present.

The simple test has good sensitivity for the detection of stroke (83%)[101] and seems to have been successful in increasing emergency admissions for stroke symptoms.[102]

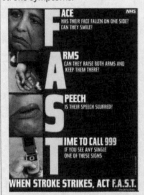

Fig 9.16 NHS FAST campaign.
Reproduced from Department of Health and Social Care. Stroke: Act FAST poster. © Crown Copyright 2012. https://www.gov.uk/government/publications/stroke-act-fast-poster. Contains public sector information licensed under the Open Government Licence v3.0.

The key role of the ED physician in acute headache is to identify and treat life-threatening causes, and provide adequate analgesia. ►Always exclude trauma!

Subarachnoid haemorrhage (SAH) May be aneurysmal or non-aneurysmal and classically presents as a severe, instantaneous 'thunderclap' headache. Maximum intensity is felt at the time of onset. Associations may include vomiting, light aversion, and meningism. Family history, recent coitus, drug use, vigorous exercise, and polycystic kidney disease ↑ likelihood. SAH causes a catecholamine surge which may precipitate cardiac ischaemia ± arrhythmias. Patients may be neurologically 'intact' initially, but the risk of rebleeding and the delayed effects of cerebral vasoconstriction mean that prompt diagnosis is imperative.[103] Sensitivity of CT scan is excellent (98.5%) if undertaken within 6h of headache onset, but decreases thereafter.[104] A lumbar puncture remains necessary in most cases. Disposition is typically to a high dependency setting. Adequate hydration is important. Calcium channel blockers (eg nimodipine) may control cerebral vasospasm.[105]

Meningitis Viral or bacterial. Headache with neck stiffness and light aversion are predominant features. Look for associated malaise, fever, altered mental state and SIRS (p. 602) markers. Brudzinski and Kernig signs are unreliable. If in doubt, treat as for sepsis and give broad-spectrum antibiotics (eg ceftriaxone). Co-administration of dexamethasone improves outcome in bacterial meningitis. If there is behavioural change, confusion, or coma consider *encephalitis* and consider IV aciclovir.[106]

Migraine Classically presents with POUND features (pulsatile, <one day duration, unilateral, nausea, and disabling). Making a diagnosis of new-onset migraine, without first excluding more sinister diagnoses (eg SAH), is difficult in the ED. Known *migraneurs*, on the other hand, may present with an exacerbation of usual symptoms. In these cases, treatment options include NSAIDS, IV fluids (dehydration is a common trigger), and antiemetics. Triptans may be used, especially if the patient presents early in the course of a migraine.[107]

Malignancy Another important cause of headache encountered in the ED. Headaches are subacute, often worse on waking in the morning and on sneezing/defecation (when ICP is naturally highest) and frequently associated with focal neurology (40%), seizures (32.5%), vomiting (27.5%), and speech deficits (15%).[108] Papilloedema may be present but is difficult to exclude using undilated fundoscopy. Have a particularly high index of suspicion in those with a history of (any) cancer. Diagnosis is with CT and/or MRI scanning. Discuss new or progressive diagnoses with neurosurgery and oncology.

Less common but important causes of acute severe headache Include *temporal arteritis* (age >50, unilateral pain over TA, reduced pulsation, history of polymyalgia rheumatica, ipsilateral visual loss (late)),[109] *acute angle-closure glaucoma* (periorbital pain, 'stony hard' red eye, ↓ pupillary response, vomiting, abdominal pain),[110] and *central venous sinus thrombosis* (severe headache ± neurology ± seizures in patient predisposed to hypercoagulability, pregnancy, use of COCP).[111]

Non-life-threatening headaches Have many causes and may still cause great distress. *Cluster headaches* and *trigeminal neuralgia* are such examples. If pain is uncontrolled, admission may still be appropriate, else urgent referral back to GP is indicated. The GP is probably best placed to start and monitor neuropathic pain medication, and arrange referral to a headache clinic.

Further reading
Davenport R (2002). Acute headache in the emergency department. *J Neurol Neurosurg Psychiatry* 72:ii33–7.

Chest pain

Causes both patients and doctors anxiety, and is one of the commonest reasons for ED attendance. A systematic history, examination, and appropriately directed work-up can be used to differentiate major causes of chest pain. Aim to differentiate *pleuritic* from *non-pleuritic* chest pain. The former is sharp, usually well localized, and reliably gets worse with inspiration and coughing.

Acute coronary syndrome (ACS)

Includes *unstable angina (UA)*, *non-ST elevation myocardial infarction (NSTEMI)*, and *ST elevation myocardial infarction (STEMI)*. The classically described symptom complex of crushing central chest pain radiating towards the jaw or left arm is not accurate. Beware of patients who present with vague chest 'discomfort', right arm pain, or epigastric pain that feels like indigestion. Nausea and vomiting may also occur.[112] ▶Think *very* carefully before diagnosing any patient with 'gastritis'/GORD in the ED.

Risk factors of coronary artery disease must be considered. These include diabetes, hypertension, hypercholesterolaemia, smoking, recreational drug use (especially cocaine),[113] and family history. Risk scores such as the Global Registry of Acute Coronary Events (GRACE)[114] and HEART score are helpful to prognosticate those with confirmed ACS.

There may be few signs on clinical examination. Profuse sweating (diaphoresis), bi-basal inspiratory crackles, an S3/S4 'gallop' rhythm, and raised JVP imply acute heart failure. Serial ECG recording may detect dynamic changes as ischaemia evolves. Cardiac *troponin* is sensitive for the detection of myocardial necrosis. Newer high-sensitivity assays are currently being validated and may be capable of doing this as little as 1 hour after the onset of pain. *Management* is with antiplatelet agents, anticoagulation, and revascularization, usually via percutaneous coronary intervention (PCI).[115]

Aortic dissection

(fig 9.17 and table 9.5) An infrequent but potentially devastating diagnosis characterized by a tear to the intimal layer of the vessel. Under pressure, blood enters the tear, leading to the creation of a false lumen. *Classical presentation* is the onset of 'tearing' thoracic back pain, which rapidly reaches peak intensity and may migrate as the dissection progresses. There may be hypertension (49%) and a diastolic murmur (28%). The dissection flap may occlude distal blood flow leading to pulse deficits or differential BP (31%), and neurological deficits (17%).[116] A widened mediastinum, irregular aortic contour, and displacement of intimal calcification are clues on CXR but definitive diagnosis is with contrast enhanced CT. Discuss all cases with cardiothoracic surgery and ITU.[117]

Pericarditis

Has many causes (infectious, autoimmune, neoplastic, post-traumatic, and metabolic) and is characterized by non-exertional pleuritic type pain that is classically relieved by leaning forwards. A friction rub may be heard on auscultation. Diffuse saddle-shaped ST elevation and PR segment depression on the ECG confirm the diagnosis. Non-compromised patients are treated with NSAIDS. The presence of haemodynamic compromise suggests pericardial effusion; arrange urgent echocardiography.[118]

Myocarditis

Causes a spectrum of symptoms from mild chest pain and non-specific ECG changes, to cardiogenic shock and malignant arrhythmias. Mortality is appreciable as there is a long-term risk of dilated cardiomyopathy. Consider in patients with chest pain, ECG changes, and a recent history of viral infection, chemotherapy, or autoimmune disease.[119]

Pulmonary embolus (PE)

Presents with chest pain if the pleura is involved: pain is not necessarily pro-portional to severity (the pulmonary artery has no pain fibres, hence the iso-lated massive 'saddle' embolus may be painless). PE should be entertained in any acutely dyspnoeic, hypoxic, or collapsed patient.[120] The *Well's criteria*[121] help direct investigations—for low-risk patients, a negative D-dimer test effectively 'rules out' the diagnosis. For those with features of DVT, or risk factors (malig-nancy, surgery, immobility >3 days, haemoptysis), imaging is required. Sinus tachycardia (>100) is a sensitive marker of PE. ECG patterns suggestive of right heart strain (right bundle branch block, 'S1Q3T3') are important to appreciate, but are not sensitive nor specific. Sinus tachycardia is common. Investigation is with *CT pulmonary angiography* (CTPA) or *ventilation/perfusion (VQ) scan-ning*. Haemodynamically stable patients receive anticoagulation. If a PE causes cardiac arrest, significant obstructive shock (pp. 582–3), or right heart strain, systemic thrombolysis may be life-saving but is itself associated with significant risks of bleeding.[122]

Other important causes of pleuritic chest pain

Causes include pneumothorax (young, tall, and thin patient with ipsilateral chest pain and shortness of breath), pneumonia, and pleurisy.

Musculoskeletal chest pain

A diagnosis of exclusion in the ED. All of us have tender ribs/costochondral joints if pressed firmly enough! Tenderness is more likely to be benign if it exactly reproduces the presenting symptom, is well localized, and accom-panied by trauma or a lifting/twisting mechanism.

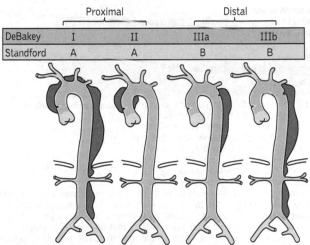

Fig 9.17 Classification schemes of aortic dissection.

Table 9.5 Anatomical characteristics of aortic dissection

Anatomical characteristics	Stanford	DeBakey
Ascending aorta, arch, and descending thoracic/abdominal aorta	Type A	Type I
Ascending aorta only	Type A	Type II
Descending aorta only; limited to the thoracic aorta	Type B	Type IIIa
Descending aorta only; extended to the abdominal aorta	Type B	Type IIIb

Shortness of breath (SOB)

Describes the subjective sensation of dyspnoea and is a common reason for ED attendance. It may be accompanied by signs of increased work of breathing (tachypnoea, use of accessory muscles, inability to complete full sentences) and hypoxia (reduced spo_2, reduced po_2 on blood gases, cyanosis). Enquire about comorbidities, the presence of infective features, cough, wheeze, haemoptysis, and chest pain. In patients with a chronic reason to be dyspnoeic, quantify 'baseline' exercise tolerance and the extent of the acute deterioration. In patients who report predominantly exertional SOB, consider ambulating as able: significant signs and hypoxia may only reveal themselves after a stroll around the department.

Give oxygen to all patients in acute respiratory distress or with a spo_2 of <94%. In those with *confirmed* type 2 respiratory failure (T_2RF = $\uparrow Pco_2$ on a blood gas) it may be acceptable to tolerate spo_2 of 88–92% to avoid excessive co_2 retention. In patients with a normal initial blood gas but a presumed risk of developing T_2RF, assess serial blood gases (eg every 1h initially, after commencement of o_2).[123] Reduced responsiveness and respiratory rate may also indicate co_2 narcosis. Avoid serial arterial blood gases, which are very painful. Venous samples are fine (Pco_2 correlates well with arterial levels). If you must do an arterial stab (eg to determine true po_2 or verify pH), use local anaesthetic (ie subcutaneous bleb 1% lidocaine 3–5min in advance).

Patients with an excessive oxygen requirement (>15L/min via a nonrebreathe mask), profound or progressively worsening respiratory failure, and/or exhaustion require consideration of ventilatory support.

Causes of SOB

May be *respiratory*, *cardiac*, *systemic*, or *psychogenic* in origin.

Respiratory causes for SOB:

Commonly include asthma, exacerbations of COPD, pneumonia, and pulmonary embolus. Less frequent but important causes include pneumothorax, pleural effusion, and malignancy. See table 9.6.

Cardiac failure:

An important differential for acute SOB in the ED.[124] Patients with pulmonary oedema may present in extremis with severe hypoxia, and are typically diaphoretic, peripherally shut down, and hypertensive (catecholamine surge). Bi-basal inspiratory crackles are heard on auscultation, and chest x-ray may reveal diffuse alveolar shadowing, upper lobe diversion, and small pleural effusions.

Causes of heart failure
c—Acute coronary syndrome
H—Hypertension
A—Arrhythmia
M—Acute mechanical cause
P—Pulmonary embolism

Identify and treat the underlying cause. Acute-on-chronic exacerbations may also be precipitated by the increased demands of a hyperdynamic circulation (eg from coexisting sepsis). Management is with supplementary o_2 and nitrates (sublingual → IV). Those with clinical evidence of hypervolaemia (eg peripheral oedema, $\uparrow JVP$) may benefit from diuretics. The use of opiates is contentious, although they may provide an anxiolytic effect. Continuous positive airway pressure (CPAP) is a mode of non-invasive ventilation which aids alveolar recruitment. CPAP can provide excellent short-term resolution of symptoms. Identify and treat the underlying cause.

Systemic:

Causes of apparent SOB not to miss include sepsis (of any source), diabetic ketoacidosis, and salicylate poisoning (hypothalamic-mediated $\uparrow\uparrow RR$).

▸▸Anaphylaxis

May present with wheeze and mimic asthma, but exposure to an allergen ± urticaria/hypotension are clues. Adrenaline saves lives. In adults, give 0.5mL 1:1000 **adrenaline** IM (repeated at 5min) along with fluid resuscitation, steroids (eg **hydrocortisone** 200mg IV), and an H_2 blocker (eg CHLORPHENAMINE 10mg IV).[125] Call for senior (ITU) support if airway swelling, collapse, or deterioration present.

Psychogenic SOB:

A diagnosis of exclusion in the ED, although anxiety will occur in all patients who are acutely breathless. Features of hyperventilation include a sensation of fear and subjective paraesthesias,[126] tachypnoea, normal oxygenation, hypocapnia, and/or carpopedal spasm (due to transient $\downarrow Ca_2^+$). A psychological precipitant or history of panic disorder is supportive. Treatment is with reassurance, controlled breathing, and referral to GP for psychological support. Vital signs should be normal before discharge. ▸Because of the serious potential for life-threatening pathology to mimic a 'panic attack' (eg pulmonary embolus[127]), always seek a senior opinion before making a diagnosis of psychogenic SOB in the ED.

Table 9.6 Differential diagnosis (DDx) for respiratory causes of SOB

DDx	Major features	Get help if ...	Initial RX
Asthma	Prior history Acute onset Wheeze	'Silent chest' Normal or $\uparrow pCO_2$	O_2 Salbutamol Ipratropium Steroids ± Magnesium sulfate IV Salbutamol IV or Theophylline IV Mechanical ventilation
COPD	Prior history Tobacco use Subacute SOB Wheeze Cough ± sputum	T_2RF (pH <7.32, pCO_2 >6), $\downarrow GCS$	Controlled O_2 therapy (SpO_2 88–92%) Nebulized bronchodilators Steroids Consider antibiotics Non-invasive ventilation (BI-PAP)*
Pneumonia	Cough + sputum Fever	Severe hypoxia Unable to match O_2 requirement Exhaustion	O_2 Antibiotics Treat underlying sepsis Severe cases may need ITU and ventilation
Pulmonary embolus**	Pleuritic chest pain Risk factors Haemoptysis Sinus tachycardia	Severe hypoxia Unable to match O_2 requirement Shock	Low-molecular-weight heparin (if profound hypoxia/shock, consider systemic thrombolysis)

* COPD patients can be difficult to wean from mechanical ventilators; BI-PAP may reduce the need for intubation.[128]

** Be aware of the ↑ risk of PE in patients with other lung pathology, esp. COPD exacerbations (25%)[129] and malignancy.

Acute abdominal pain (AP)

AP may be very distressing for patients, and has many potential causes. Short-term priorities are to identify shock, resuscitate if necessary, and provide analgesia. A thorough history, examination, and rational use of investigations will determine who requires admission. ►A lower admission threshold is required for older adults with acute AP, as serious presentations are frequently atypical and mortality increased.[130]

This section is not an exhaustive overview of AP but deals instead with *immediately* life-threatening differential diagnoses that all emergency doctors should consider before discharge or referral.

Abdominal aortic aneurysm

Must always be considered in adults aged >60yrs presenting with acute AP. High-risk features include abdominal, back, flank, and/or groin pain ± syncope and hypotension.[131] ►►Ruptured AAA may mimic the loin-to-groin pain of renal colic.[132] Shock is ominous but may be absent if the haematoma is contained by the retroperitoneum. Prior history is useful (have they had a screening ultrasound?). Clinical examination is of limited value although a pulsatile mass may be detected. Ultrasound can detect the presence of AAA but not rupture[133]—in those who are stable, onward evaluation using CT aortography is required. Management is with analgesia, resuscitation (aim SBP ~100mmHg). Arrange urgent transfer for open or, increasingly, endovascular repair.[134]

Ectopic pregnancy

Must be excluded in all women of childbearing age (ie menarche to menopause) presenting to the ED with abdominal pain or syncope. This is easily accomplished with urinary/serum HCG. If positive, EP must be considered if intrauterine pregnancy is yet to be confirmed. Unilateral pelvic pain and tenderness, with shoulder tip radiation is typical ± vaginal bleeding, but up to 9% may be asymptomatic.[135] Look for signs of shock and resuscitate as necessary while arranging urgent gynaecology review.

Mesenteric ischaemia[136]

May be due to embolus or thrombus and most commonly occurs in the very old, arteriopaths, and those predisposed to emboli formation (eg AF) or hypercoagulability. It may also follow a traumatic insult, or abdominal surgery. Diagnosis is difficult due to non-specific presentation of colicky abdominal pain and few physical features (peritonism may be *absent*). Diarrhoea may occur. Metabolic acidosis with a raised lactate is a helpful clue—but 'normal' lactate does *not* exclude as the liver clears once the bowel has died. Investigation is with CT angiography; resuscitation and urgent surgical consultation is essential.

Bowel obstruction

Most commonly the consequence of adhesions, malignancy, hernia, and complications from inflammatory bowel disease. Bowel ischaemia and perforation are risks if diagnosis is delayed.[137] History is key—colicky pain, constipation, and failure to pass flatus are supportive—progression to bilious vomiting is highly suggestive. Abdominal x-ray may diagnose, but doesn't identify the transition point. Therefore, discuss with radiology and consider opting for CT if the diagnosis seems likely.[138] Treatment is with analgesia, IV fluids, and surgical referral. A nasogastric tube is commonly used to decompress the stomach and is especially important if there is active vomiting.

In the past, perforation commonly occurred as a result of peptic ulcer disease. Incidence has reduced since the widespread adoption of proton pump inhibitors.[139] Other causes include appendicitis, malignancy, diverticulitis, and inflammatory bowel disease. Classical presenting features of peritonism may be absent, esp. in the elderly or comorbid. Patients may be profoundly unwell. Erect chest x-ray is imperfect for the detection of pneumoperitoneum (20% may be missed);[140] CT is therefore preferred.

Gastrointestinal haemorrhage

May originate throughout the GI tract. Fresh blood *usually* indicates lower GI bleeding, although torrential upper GI bleeding (eg from aorto-enteric fistula) may also cause 'fresh' bleeding. Offensive, tarry-black stools ('melaena') ± 'coffee ground vomit' suggests an upper GI source. If shock is present in the context of UGIB, resuscitate and consider the need for emergency endoscopy.[141] Tamponade of oesophageal varices (eg Minnesota tube) may be a life-saving temporizing measure but usually requires intubation.[142] Lower GI bleeding is managed with observation ± surgery.[143]

Other important causes of abdominal pain not to be missed

Include *appendicitis*, *renal colic*, *pancreatitis* (check lipase/amylase for every abdominal pain!), *gallstones/cholecystitis*, *testicular torsion*, and *inflammatory bowel disease* Remember that pneumonia, DKA, PE, and MI may also present with abdominal pain.

Be wary of labelling patients with 'gastroenteritis', 'IBS', and 'constipation'. These are diagnoses of exclusion because of the potential for other serious underlying causes.

A final word

Providing a definitive diagnosis of abdominal pain during a few hours in the ED is challenging. Patients often require admission for extended observation and further imaging. Nonetheless, the emergency doctor can add value by excluding life-threatening causes, providing good analgesia, and 'front-loading' initial investigations.

Most people will have at least one episode of back pain during their life. Fortunately, sinister causes are rare although the socioeconomic fallout from 'simple' musculoskeletal pain is staggering (>£10bn/year in healthcare costs and lost productivity).[144] It is therefore important to treat all patients with back pain seriously and empathetically, while being mindful of the need to exclude serious underlying pathology. See also orthopaedics pp. 478–9, pp. 486–7.

Exclusion of 'red flag' signs and symptoms must be documented for every patient attending the ED with back pain. These include:

• Age <20 or >65 years	• Urinary retention or	• Faecal incontinence
• Foot drop	incontinence	• Motor deficit (any)
• Thoracic pain	• High fever	• Disturbed gait
• Saddle paraesthesia	• Past history of	• Trauma
• Immuno-compromise*	malignancy (any)	• IV drug user.
	• Structural deformity	
	• Night pain	

Source: data from NICE. *cks Back Pain Red Flags* https://cks.nice.org.uk/back-pain-low-without-radiculopathy

Many patients can be discharged provided they have normal neurological and spinal examination, and no red flag features. x-rays are often not required but provision of good analgesia is essential (p. 580) A period of relative rest should not exceed 24–48h—those who mobilize early do better. Early identification of maladaptive coping strategies (depression, hopelessness, anxiety) and referral to GP may reduce chronic pain sequelae.[145] ▶A *safety net* is essential: patients who develop persistent, progressively worsening symptoms or 'red flag' features should be advised to seek further help. Issue written advice if available. Rarely, patients may be so incapacitated from pain and muscle spasm that they require a short stay admission.

Patients with any red flag feature or deficit on examination require senior discussion. Acute motor deficits, sphincter disturbance, or saddle anaesthesia implies a compressive lesion (eg cauda equina syndrome) and requires urgent spinal/neurosurgical consultation. *Imaging* is usually required but modality depends on the presentation. For example, x-ray/CT is suitable for evaluating bony lesions, whereas MRI is required to evaluate soft tissues including cord/nerve root compression, haematomas, and discitis.

Spinal causes of acute low back pain
• Lumbar muscular sprain/strain.
• Osteoarthritis.
• Sciatica (eg from herniated intervertebral disc, spinal stenosis or spondylolisthesis).
• Degenerative disc disease.
• Facet joint arthropathy.
• Inflammatory arthritis (eg ankylosing spondylitis).
• Malignancy (myeloma, metastases, lymphoma).
• Infection (discitis; osteomyelitis).

Non-spinal causes of acute low back pain
• *Gynae:* Endometriosis, PID.
• *Gastrointestinal:* Pancreatitis, cholecystitis, peptic ulceration, IBD.
• *Renal:* Renal colic, pyelonephritis.
• *Infection:* Pneumonia, prostatitis, psoas abscess, shingles.
• *Other:* AAA.

Musculoskeletal problems and 'minor injuries'

Represent a large proportion of ED workload. Such problems may seem trivial at presentation, but a missed diagnosis or improper management can cause significant functional, recreational, and occupational impairment. For this reason, 'minor' injuries represent a significant source of litigation.

Musculoskeletal EM and minor injuries are seldom well taught at undergraduate level, and this is often an area of considerable anxiety for doctors starting in the ED. *Tip:* Learn from senior doctors, emergency nurse practitioners (ENPs), and physiotherapists. See also table 9.7.[146] Attending an ED specific x-ray course is a good idea.

It is often reassuring to know that most departments check x-rays in retrospect, reducing harm from missed injuries. If unsure, another option is to bring patients back to either the ED or fracture clinic for delayed review.

Table 9.7 General principles of orthopaedic examination

Look	Inspect the joint for obvious deformity or redness—compare with the contralateral side
Feel	Identify soft tissue swelling, tenderness, effusions, crepitus, etc. Assess neurovascular status
Move	Ask the patient to move the joint (active motion) and gently compare with passive motion
Function	Undertake an assessment of function—can the patient weight bear in a lower limb injury? Is opposition intact in a thumb injury?

Atraumatic extremity pain

Limb/joint pain without injury must always prompt consideration of *infection (septic arthritis)* and *crystal arthropathy (gout/pseudogout)*, as well as more common benign conditions such as *tenosynovitis*. In children and young people, specific diagnoses such as *transient synovitis ('irritable hip')*, *Perthe disease*, and *traction apophysitis at the knee (ie Osgood–Schlatter disease)* and pelvic girdle are possibilities.

Always record vital signs including a temperature. A baseline x-ray might reveal effusions or signs of arthritis. Inflammatory markers may support a diagnosis, but do not exclude serious pathology if normal. Likewise, uric acid may drop (and therefore normalize) in acute gout. A positive joint aspirate clinches the diagnosis—arrange urgently if there is effusion in a hot, swollen joint.[147] Unless there is evidence of systemic sepsis (pp. 582-3), try to arrange prompt aspiration before administering empiric antibiotics.

Very occasionally, patients may present to the ED with a primary presentation of systemic arthritis. Rarely, atraumatic haemarthrosis may be the primary presentation of a coagulopathy.

▶ *Be wary of extremity pain* out of proportion to history or symptoms. Ask 'What am I missing?', and consider occult fractures (especially in the very old and very young), *compartment syndrome* (may be atraumatic), *limb ischaemia, deep vein thrombosis*, serious soft tissue infections (eg *necrotizing fasciitis*), and referred pain (eg shoulder pain from angina or abdominal pathology).

Hand and wrist injuries Very common. Learn a systematic hand examination. Always document dominance and occupation when evaluating a hand injury and remove jewellery rings early.

Phalangeal and metacarpal fractures Generally treated with analgesia, neighbour strapping, and fracture clinic follow-up. Refer open fractures and injuries with rotational deformity or neurovascular deficit.

Carpal injuries May follow a forceful fall onto outstretched hand (FOOSH) type mechanism. They can be difficult to detect: scrutiny of x-rays is required. *Scaphoid fractures*[148] are of particular concern—disruption of blood supply to the proximal pole may occur due to the distal insertion of the nutrient artery, leading to avascular necrosis later on. Suspect if pain around the 'anatomical snuff box', scaphoid tubercle, or on axial loading of the thumb. Request scaphoid specific x-ray views. Confirmed fractures are placed in a scaphoid plaster and referred to fracture clinic. Those with a negative initial x-ray should be immobilized as a precaution (eg Futura™ splint) and re-imaged (x-ray or CT/MRI) in 7–10 days. Other commoner carpal injuries include *triquetral fracture* (look for a subtle chip of bone on the dorsal aspect of the lateral view), *scapholunate ligament disruption* (the space between the scaphoid and lunate is widened), and *lunate/perilunate dislocation* .

Distal radius fractures Seen daily in most EDs (dorsal angulation = *Colles'* ; volar angulation = *Smith's*). Assess for deformity, integrity of overlying skin, and neurovascular status. Although evidence of long-term benefit is unclear, displaced fractures may be reduced in the ED using sedation, haematoma, or Bier's block.[149] The patient is placed in a below elbow plaster and referred to fracture clinic.

Elbow fractures See BOX 'Can the patient extend their elbow?' and fig 9.18. May affect the supracondylar region (in children), the capitulum, coronoid, olecranon, and radial head. The *'terrible triad'* is the term given to *elbow dislocation, radial head #*, and *lateral collateral ligament injury*.[150] Relocation may be attempted by an experienced practitioner under sedation. As a (very) general rule, non-displaced neurovascular intact injuries can be immobilized and referred to fracture clinic; all others should be seen by orthopaedics in ED. Risks of improperly treated elbow fractures include functional loss and neurovascular deficit.

Shoulder dislocation See fig 9.19. Most commonly the result of *anterior* misplacement of the humeral head from the glenoid fossa. Other possibilities are *posterior* (often resulting from severe trauma, or seizures) and, very infrequently, *inferior* dislocation (luxatio erecta—resulting from forceful abduction). It is important to assess neurovascular status of the limb and identify sensory deficits over the 'badge patch' area of the deltoid (axillary nerve). Reduction may be accomplished with the help of Entonox®, sedation—or even simple relaxation techniques—using a variety of methods.[151] Following repeat x-ray, the arm is placed in a polysling and fracture clinic follow-up arranged.

Rotator cuff injuries Most commonly result from a fall onto outstretched arm in the middle-aged and elderly. Test each of supraspinatus, infraspinatus, and teres minor. Inability to abduct and perform resisted movements may indicate a complete tear which requires surgical repair. Refer to fracture clinic.

Clavicle fractures Common and usually managed conservatively (exceptions: open #, skin tenting, distal #, or neurovascular deficit). ORIF shortens recovery time and may lead to better functional recovery and cosmetic results for some.[152] Injuries to the *acromioclavicular ligament* cause point tenderness over the acromioclavicular joint. Sprains are treated conservatively whereas skin tenting, shoulder droop, or posterior fullness (ie 'grade III–V') injuries may require surgical repair.[153]

See also Orthopaedics p. 470, pp. 476–7 and Trauma p. 530, pp. 538–9.

Can the patient extend their elbow?

If so, the chances of them having a fracture are reduced to <5%. If not, the risk increases to 50% (→x-ray). The 'South West Elbow Extension Test' (SWEET) is an example of a simple clinical decision rule which helps us rationalize the choice of investigation.[154]

Elbow x-rays require specific interpretation. Fractures are frequently occult, but the effusion that results elevates the fat pads which give the appearance of a yacht's spinnaker on the lateral view (the so-called 'Sail sign'). Elevated fat pads may also occur in non-traumatic disease.[155]

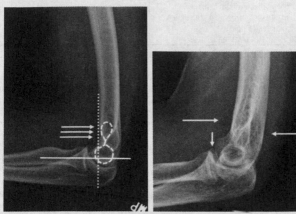

Fig 9.18 (a) Correct bony anatomy of the lateral elbow on x-ray. The anterior humeral line (dotted line) should pass through the anterior third of the capitulum, while the radiocapitellar line (solid line) is drawn through the axis of the radius and bisects the capitulum; (b) Elevated anterior and posterior fat pads arising from a radial head fracture.

Reproduced with permission from Abujudeh, H. (2014). *Emergency Radiology Cases.* Oxford: OUP.

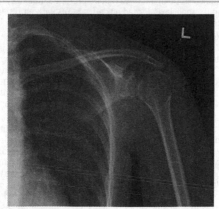

Fig 9.19 Posterior shoulder dislocation is easy to miss on x-ray. The humeral head is locked in internal rotation, giving rise to the 'lightbulb sign'.

Reproduced with permission from Abujudeh, H. (2014). *Emergency Radiology Cases.* Oxford: OUP.

The Ottawa rules Well-recognized clinical decision rules. The ankle/foot rule (OAR)[156] and knee rule (OKR)[157] (see table 9.8) can be used to guide the need for x-ray investigation of injuries to these joints.

Table 9.8 The Ottawa rules

Ottawa ankle rule	Ottowa knee rule
x-ray if any feature:	*x-ray if any feature:*
Bony tenderness at posterior edge or tip of either malleoli (distal 6cm)	Age >55 years
	Isolated patella tenderness
Inability to weight bear* 4 steps in ED	Tenderness at head of fibula
Navicular tenderness	Cannot flex to 90°
Base 5th metatarsal tenderness	Inability to weight bear* 4 steps in ED
* Limping counts as 'weight bearing'.	

Toe phalanx fractures Painful but treated conservatively if non-displaced. Great toe fractures are of more significance and may be initially managed in a cast, pending fracture clinic review.

Metatarsal fractures Managed with immobilization initially; ORIF may be required if displaced. It is important to be vigilant for an injury to the Lisfranc ligament (between 2nd MT and medial cuneiform) or other tarsometatarsal joints as chronic mid–foot instability may result.[158]

Navicular fractures May occur due to stress (eg in athletes) and are at high risk of avascular necrosis. *Management* may be conservative or operative. Similarly, other fractures of the mid-foot require fracture clinic evaluation. Calcaneal fractures are high-energy injuries that typically occur following a fall from height. *Associations* include other limb fractures (24%), spinal fractures (14.5%), chest (21%), and head injury (16%).[159] Most are intra-articular. Size of fracture, displacement, and patient characteristics determine need for repair.

Displaced and dislocated ankle fractures See fig 9.20. Require urgent reduction for pain relief and to protect neurovascular and skin integrity.[160] Following reduction, place in a below-knee plaster backslab, repeat x-ray, and refer to orthopaedics. Open fractures require prompt antibiotics and consideration of tetanus prophylaxis. Closed ankle fractures without displacement or talar shift can be placed in a backslab and referred to fracture clinic.

Knee injuries Difficult to evaluate in the ED as swelling and pain preclude reliable testing for ligamentous stability. True *knee dislocation* is a genuine emergency traditionally associated with high-energy trauma but now also morbid obesity.[161] Conversely, *patellar dislocation* is very common, and reduction easily accomplished. Common fractures include those to the patella (is the quadriceps mechanism intact?), tibial spine, and plateau. Consider immobilizing soft tissue injuries in a splint and arrange for follow-up once swelling has settled.

Hip fractures Occur at the *neck of femur* (NOF) (p. 542) predominantly in the elderly. Good analgesia is essential prior to orthopaedic admission. Regional anaesthesia, such as femoral or fascia iliaca block, may be accomplished in the ED.[162] ►Consider and exclude medical causes for falls, which may have perioperative significance. *Hip dislocation* occurs posteriorly in those with a prosthesis or following high-energy trauma. Reduction may be attempted in the ED, but a good degree of muscle relaxation needs to be achieved during sedation (this leads to a possible ↑ risk of apnoea post procedure, as the painful stimulus is instantly removed).

See also Orthopaedics pp. 488-9, pp. 500-1 and Trauma pp. 540-1, pp. 544-5.

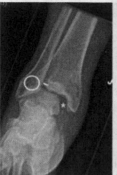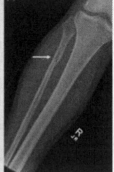

Fig 9.20 Distal fibula fracture with deltoid ligament rupture giving rise to talar shift (asterisk). This case also demonstrates importance of examining proximal and distal joints: there is also a fracture at the fibula head—a *Maisonneuve* injury.

Reproduced with permission from Abujudeh, H. (2014). *Emergency Radiology Cases*. Oxford: OUP.

Bites and stings

From creatures great and small, bites and stings are common presentations to the ED. These may result from indigenous or foreign species (eg in returning travellers), so it is important to have a grasp of key issues such as infection, venom, and toxins.

Animal bites

All animal bites are contaminated.[183] *R:* Irrigate with water ± debride. Do an x-ray if there is query about foreign body involvement (eg tooth fragments), or crush injury. Exclude tendon and neurovascular injury. ▶Avoid primary closure unless essential: even then, loosely appose (allowing for drainage of pus if abscess forms). **Co-amoxiclav 500/125 8h PO for 1wk** is widely accepted for 'high-risk' bites.[184] Aquatic animals may require an alternative regimen; discuss with microbiology.[185] Assess tetanus status (see *OHCM* p437). Bites from macaque monkeys require treatment with valaciclovir to prevent transmission of Herpes virus B, which causes fatal encephalitis.[186] Consider rabies if bitten outside UK (there exists a theoretical risk of rabies transmission from UK bats).[187]

Snake bite

A neglected disease globally.[168] Mortality in low-income countries dwarfs that in developed settings (eg Australia experiences only a few fatalities/yr, but worldwide may be up to 90,000).[169-170] Britain's only poisonous snake, the adder, causes very few deaths. *Pre-hospital care* is supportive (limb immobilization, resuscitation, and transportation—remember to identify the species if possible). Avoid tourniquets. Be prepared to treat respiratory paralysis, hypotension, cardiac arrest, seizures, and disseminated intravascular coagulation.[171] Venom detection kits exist and should be used if there are clinical signs (nausea, reduced GCS, ptosis, weakness, coagulopathy, muscle pain) or abnormal biochemistry. In the UK, give European viper venom antiserum (see *BNF*). Risk of anaphylaxis from antivenoms is appreciable.[172]

If the bite is from a foreign snake, the relevant *antivenom* may be held in London or Liverpool in the UK (available via www.toxbase.org). For adder bites, observe for at least 2h and admit those with evidence of localized swelling or systemic symptoms. Localized pain, swelling, and blistering can occur. Adder toxin continues to damage tissue for 4–5 days so advise rest; and treat with antihistamines to reduce swelling and antibiotics to prevent secondary infection.[173]

Spider

Envenomation in the UK is limited to owners of pets, and those who may inadvertently encounter imported venomous species (eg vets, dockworkers). Recluse spiders may cause tissue necrosis (loxoscelism). Black widow venoms cause lactrodectism leading to muscle rigidity, pain, and vomiting. Funnel web spiders are neurotoxic.[174] Seek specialist opinion. Otherwise, manage as a normal insect bite and give antibiotics if secondary infection develops.

Lesser weever fish stings

Occur if barefoot on UK beaches. These are painful but not serious. Immerse leg for 5–20min in hot water (eg <45°c) to denature the protein-based venom.[175]

Scorpion venom

Causes hypertension (catecholaminergic peripheral vasoconstriction), cardiac and renal failure. Antidotes prepared from animal antisera have variable effectiveness. Treatment is supportive and with benzodiazepines for neuromuscular effects/anxiety.[176] Prazosin is a selective α_1 blocker which may improve haemodynamics by ↓SVR. Lidocaine around the bite may also reduce pain.[177]

Hymenoptera

Includes *hornets*, *wasps*, and *bees*. Single stings are usually trivial; ensure that the stinger is removed and treat symptomatically. Stings from Africanized honey bees or Asian hornets are very painful. Despite much public anxiety, only a few people die from hymenoptera-related anaphylaxis in a year—multiple stings or those from foreign species (eg Africanized honey bee, Asian hornet) ↑ risk. The latter may, very rarely, cause multiple organ failure.[178]

Ticks

Ubiquitous in woodlands and tall grasses and bites may give rise to Lyme disease. If embedded, they can be pulled out or suffocated (eg with lidocaine gel).[179] Symptoms of Lyme disease are non-specific (malaise, myalgia, ocular, and neurologic). Erythema migrans p. 437 is pathognomonic. ℞: Antibiotics (eg doxycycline) are required for symptomatic cases.[180]

A special mention

The beauty of the *Phyllobates* spp. frog belies a sinister secret. More commonly known as the poison dart frog, it is the most toxic vertebrate known to man (fig 9.21). The frog secretes batrachotoxin, which causes irreversible depolarizing neuromuscular blockade and direct cardiac toxicity. There is no specific antidote, although digoxin FAB antibodies (Digibind®) may help.[181] Of note, the toxin is absent in captive frogs, indicating a dietary source (although be aware of patients' exposure to those which may have been recently captured!).

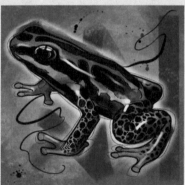

Fig 9.21 Dendrobatidae, the poison dart frog.

Artwork by Gillian Turner.

Children

By far the most common culprits when it comes to foreign body ingestions. They will often be accompanied by a concerned witness and be asymptomatic at presentation. Always consider x-ray, as most commonly ingested items include coins/toys etc. which tend to be radio-opaque. If the x-ray shows a foreign body below level of diaphragm then the patient can go home but advise parents to monitor for signs of obstruction (most pass harmlessly through the GI tract).[182]

▶▶ *Button battery ingestions:* A time-critical emergency. If lodged in the oesophagus, necrosis develops in <1h and oesophageal perforation is possible.[183] Rapid identification (chest and abdominal x-ray) and immediate endoscopic removal, under GA, is required. If distal to the oesophageal sphincter, watchful waiting with serial x-rays may be an option but requires very close observation.[184] Consider chronic oesophageal impaction if presenting fresh haematemesis, poor feeding, FTT, stridor, PUO, or repetitive aspiration pneumonias.

Magnets: Also dangerous: they cause pressure necrosis and perforation if they become attracted either side of a hollow viscus.[185]

Nasal foreign bodies: Very common. What goes in (usually) comes out, but requires reassurance and a patient approach to gain the child's trust. Try asking the parent to occlude the contralateral nostril while making a seal around the child's mouth and administering a short, sharp breath. This method—known as the mother's kiss—is safe, and successful in 6 out of 10 cases.[186]

Aural foreign bodies: May be removed under direct vision. Refer difficult/non-complaint cases to ENT to avoid further trauma: it is easier with an operating microscope. If removal is successful in ED, exclude tympanic membrane injury.

Adults

Infrequently deliberately ingest foreign bodies. An exception to the rule are body packers who ingest packets of illicit drugs in order to smuggle them, typically through customs at a port of entry. The Royal College of Emergency Medicine provides detailed guidance for assessment and management.[187]

Accidental impaction of a fish/chicken bone is a more common scenario. Examine the oropharynx and carefully remove any visible foreign body under direct vision. In the case of a food bolus impaction, try a carbonated drink ± IV/IM hyoscine butylbromide, eg Buscopan® ± GTN may be attempted to dislodge a stubborn food bolus (evidence = poor), otherwise endoscopy is necessary. Always consider underlying causes (eg malignancy).

9 Emergency medicine

Careful evaluation of all wounds is mandatory. Assess size/shape, type (eg laceration vs incision), whether the base is visible, presence of underlying structures, and functional/neurovascular deficits in affected limbs. Most wounds presenting to the ED are minor, but as ever, always exclude the life- or limb-threatening. ▶▶Evaluate stab wounds to the neck or trunk as major trauma—even innocuous wounds may result in significant damage to underlying structures and organs (↑ risk with long, thin implements eg screwdriver). Thoroughly examine all stab victims, including the back, axillae, and perineum for 'missed' wounds.

Complex wounds that are heavily contaminated require debridement; those that involve significant structures or special anatomical areas (eg vermilion border of lip; pinna of ear) may require referral to an appropriate surgeon unless an experienced ED doctor is present.

Otherwise, for wounds that are seen within 6h, thoroughly clean the wound with normal saline or tap water,[188] consider tetanus and infection risk (↑ if soil, manure, or sewerage contamination), and arrange closure. Exclude foreign bodies (eg fragments of glass, wood, or gravel). Grossly contaminated wounds, those on the lower limbs, and occurring in the diabetic or immuno-compromised have ↑ infection risk.[189]

Wound closure There are many options available. Sutures are effective for closing deeper wounds, attaining accurate apposition of certain wounds (eg at vermilion border), and achieving haemostasis. However, suturing takes time and skill, and is less suitable for wounds where tissue viability is poor (eg pre-tibial skin tears in the elderly).[103] Mattress sutures are an option to reduce wound tension. ▶Remember to advise patients to return for removal of sutures—usually a primary care nurse can do this. For many simple lacerations however, cyanoacrylate-based skin glue and/or adhesive sutures (Steri-Strips™) are quick to apply, comfortable for the patient, and give acceptable cosmetic results. Skin staples are very useful for rapidly closing scalp wounds, but should not be used on visible skin.[190]

Self-harm

It is common to manage the wounds of patients who have 'self-harmed' in the ED. These patients are often distressed, and may be embarrassed or ashamed of their actions. Maintain a non-judgemental approach: reprimanding these patients is unkind and may escalate behaviour. Manage the wound, exclude co-ingestion (overdose) of medication or drugs, and undertake a mental state exam/psychiatric risk assessment. Mental health services may not only help manage the underlying issues, but can also advise on strategies to reduce repeat episodes.

By virtue of its open front door, the ED receives all sorts of minor problems which can leave the unfamiliar stumped. What follows are some solutions to the more common calamities encountered in the ED:

'I've hammered my finger, doctor'

This usually causes a subungual haematoma—relieved by expressing the blood through a hole trephined in the nail, using a 19G needle. No force is needed. Simply twiddle the needle vertically on the nail: the cutting edge will make a suitable hole (see fig 8.24).

'I've swallowed a fish bone and it's stuck'

Always examine the throat and tonsils carefully. Often the bone has only grazed the mucosa. Use a good light, and grip the tongue with gauze to move it out of the way before removing any visible bones with forceps. If you fail, refer to ENT.

'My fish hook has barbed my finger'

Infiltrate with lidocaine and push the hook on through the finger, provided no important structures are in its way. Once the barb is through, cut it off. Remove the hook where it entered.

'My tooth has been knocked out'

Send deciduous teeth to the tooth fairy. For permanent teeth, after the patient sucks it clean (do not use water), transport in milk—or reinsert it, stabilizing with finger pressure (or biting). Contact maxillofacial surgery (or see a dentist) for splinting.

Removing a tight ring from a swollen finger

Pass a No. 4 silk suture through the ring from distal to proximal. Wind the distal end around the finger in a distal direction. Then unwind from the proximal end distally (should pull the ring over the coil). Lubrication + compression + traction may also help. If not, use a ring cutter (not for brass/steel).

'I've caught my penis in my zip'

Failing copious lubrication with mineral oil, the most elegant method is to cut out the bridge from the slider or zip with strong wire-cutters. The zip then falls apart and all that is needed is a new zip. (Beware the bridge flying off at speed: hold gauze by it.) What if the trousers are of immense value? Try the Savile Row technique: infiltrate the skin with 1% lidocaine (no adrenaline!); carefully manipulate the prepuce along the side of the slider by an unzipping movement.

'I've got a red eye'

Consider the potential for sight-threatening pathology including perforating ulcers, scleritis, uveitis, acute angle-closure glaucoma, and endophthalmitis. History should include prior eye surgery and use of contact lenses. Always record visual acuity. Corneal abrasions are common and are identified by instilling fluorescein eye drops and examining under uv light where epithelial disruption appears green. Diffuse photo keratitis ('arc eye') occurs as a result of excessive uv light exposure (eg welding, skiing). Treatment is with topical antibiotics ± lubricants.[191] In many localities, patients with ophthalmic problems are referred for same or next-day evaluation by the 'eye casualty' service.

Emergency medicine

Requires a breadth of knowledge, procedural ability, and the personal skills to work effectively at the sharp end of the hospital. To succeed demands a mix of intellect, emotional intelligence, and humility: aspiring to know anything about everything is likely to lead to frustration. Rather, it is necessary to work and learn 'smart'—strive to get the basics right every time, and the rest usually does follow. Indeed, learning something new every day is a great attraction for many who choose to become emergency physicians.

It is important that the specialty continues to flourish, and its practitioners continue to re-educate those who will insist that they are merely a 'jack of all trades' or—should they dare—the 'casualty officers'! Emergency medics are 'expert generalists' with specialist knowledge in the first 10 minutes (or so!) of everything. Where it is delivered well, emergency medicine can improve access to timely healthcare, relieve suffering, reduce disability, and save the lives of many. This is why the specialty is flourishing across the world.

This chapter represents a quick tour through a typical shift, but hopefully gives a flavour of some of what the specialty has to offer. It is important to bear in mind that emergency medicine is only recently established: it is not yet defined by a fixed knowledge base or skill-set, and in many settings finds itself uniquely juxtaposed between the demands of patients and politicians. Subsequently, it is likely to continue its evolution for many years to come.

10 Pre-hospital emergency medicine

Terry
Collingwood

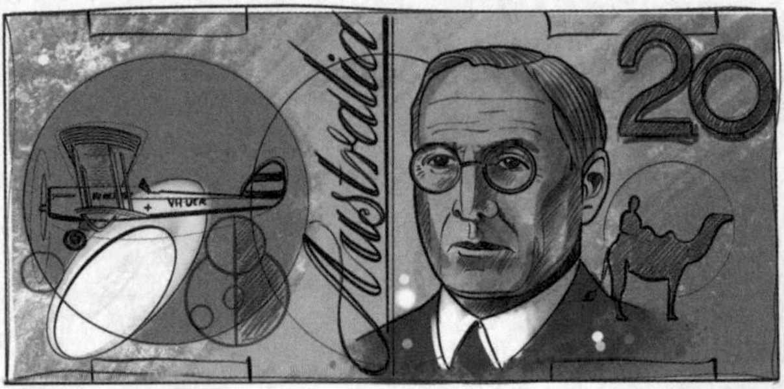

Fig 10.1 The Very Rev John Flynn—founder of the Royal Flying Doctor Service as featured on the Australian $20 banknote.

Artwork by Gillian Turner.

Pre-hospital emergency medicine (PHEM)

PHEM was approved by the GMC in 2010 as a subspecialty of emergency medicine open to doctors in emergency medicine and anaesthetics from ST4 onwards. The specialty focuses on caring for seriously ill or injured patients at the scene of an incident before they reach hospital and during transfer to hospital (fig 10.2). It is a challenging but hugely rewarding specialty requiring team work and quick decision-making. Hazardous working conditions, environmental challenges, and resource limitations must be faced frequently.

Sources

Intercollegiate Board for Training in Pre-hospital Emergency Medicine: http://www.ibtphem.org.uk

Nutbeam T, Boylan B (eds) (2013). *ABC of Prehospital Emergency Medicine*. Chichester: Wiley-Blackwell.

Skinner DV, Driscoll PA (eds) (2013). *ABC of Major Trauma* (4th ed). Chichester: Wiley-Blackwell.

The MIMMS (Major Incident Medical Management and Support) course is essential for any team member of major incidents.

With many thanks to Dr Pete Williams for his kind help and support in the writing and updating of this chapter, and to our junior reader Rachel McDougall for their contribution to this chapter.

Introduction to pre-hospital emergency medicine

In 1917 at Lamboo Station, Western Australia, a 29-year-old stockman named James 'Jimmy' Darcy was grievously wounded when his horse fell during a cattle stampede. His brothers dragged him 46km on a dray to Halls Creek where the postmaster, the only person with any first-aid training, performed a 7-hour operation to repair Darcy's ruptured bladder—using only whiskey and some morphine to sedate his patient, a sharpened pen knife, and instructions via Morse code from Dr Holland 3000km away in Perth. The operation was successful but Jimmy failed to improve. Dr Holland therefore travelled to Halls Creek—2 weeks by cattle boat, car, and horse-drawn buggy—only to find he arrived 24 hours too late. Jimmy had died, not from his injuries but from previously undiagnosed malaria.

Against this background, the Very Rev John Flynn (fig 10.1), Presbyterian Minister, field superintendent of the Australian Inland Mission (AIM), and dedicated servant of the people of the outback, was inspired to provide 'a mantle of safety' to people who, at that time, typically had no access to any medical care. That same year, Flynn received a letter from Lt Clifford Peel, a young airman who later lost his life in WWI. Peel had heard of Flynn's ambitions and outlined to him the potential of a new technology—aviation.

After 10 years of tireless planning, campaigning, and fund raising, in 1928, the AIM Aerial Medical Service, later the *Royal Flying Doctor Service*, was born. Flying De Havilland DH.50 biplanes leased from the newly formed Queensland and Northern Territories Aerial Services Co (QANTAS) for the sum of 2 shillings per mile flown, the new service undertook 50 missions and treated 225 patients during its first year. In those early days they flew with no radio and no navigational aids other than a compass. They followed tracks and telegraph lines and landed at the roughest of air strips, but Flynn's vision had become reality and emergency medicine outside of the hospital was born. It is with Flynn that our story begins.

The essence of pre-hospital emergency medical staff

'Our patients did not choose us. We chose them. We could have chosen another profession, but we did not. We have accepted responsibility for patient care in some of the worst situations: when we are tired or cold; when it is rainy and dark; when we cannot predict what conditions we will encounter. We must either embrace this responsibility or surrender it. We must give to our patients the very best care that we can—not while we are daydreaming, not with unchecked equipment, not with incomplete supplies and not with yesterday's knowledge.'

Source: NAEMT, PHTLS: *Prehospital Trauma Life Support*, 2011: Jones & Bartlett Learning, Burlington, MA. www.jblearning.com.

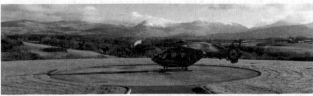

Fig 10.2 In mountainous areas such as Snowdonia (UK), pre-hospital care relies heavily on helicopters to travel longer distances quickly. Landing sites are ideally near the hospital with easy access to the emergency department.

© Nina Hjelde.

Activation of the emergency services

▶▶ The cornerstone of pre-hospital care is forward planning and organization, with prompt activation and distribution of resources when needed. These processes start with the skilled management of 999 calls and appropriate deployment of pre-hospital services. Requests for an emergency ambulance are prioritized into RED (immediately life-threatening), AMBER (urgent), or GREEN (routine). Call-centre staff follow protocols which categorize calls and can provide interim first-aid instructions for bystanders on scene. More complex calls are passed onto PHEM practitioners who are better placed to assess the need for a more advanced response, although immediate dispatch criteria for PHEM practitioners may also be used (see BOX 'Immediate dispatch criteria'[1]).

Immediate dispatch criteria for PHEM practitioners	
• Fall from >20ft	• Explosions/industrial incidents*
• Fall or jumped in front of train	• Amputation above wrist or ankle
• RTA*	• Trapped under vehicle (not motorcycle)
• Ejection from vehicle/another vehicle occupant has died	• Drowning*
	• Shooting/stabbing*
*Need discussion with PHEM team first.	

HEMS Helicopter **E**mergency **M**edical **S**ervices can cover large areas and quickly access locations, bringing skilled PHEM doctors and paramedics to the scene of an incident. HEMS clinicians use standard operating procedures based on evidence-based clinical guidelines to deliver high-level patient care while working in high-pressure environments. Multiagency working is normal and health professionals will work alongside the fire brigade, police, and ambulance crews.

Helicopters may be restricted by appropriate landing sites, fair weather, and daylight hours (although increasingly, transfers of critically ill patients are being performed at night). Arrival by helicopter to a major incident allows a unique overview of the scene and helps identify hazards and patient location. The risks of patient transport must be carefully weighed—short transfers in an urban area may be more appropriate by land ambulance. Air ambulance organizations may also use rapid response cars as an alternative to helicopters. See also table 10.1.

In flight, equipment should be robust with audible alarms and devices that are easily manipulated in poor lighting or turbulence; drugs should be drawn up in advance. Equipment packs should be standardized—there is no opportunity to 'fetch more from the storeroom' at the scene of an incident or in-flight. Checklists to ensure all equipment is stocked and replaced are frequently used.

Table 10.1 Effects and clinical implications of helicopter transfer

Effects of transport[2]	Clinical implications
Vestibular dysfunction	Fatigue, nausea
Temperature changes	Fatigue, coagulopathies
Linear acceleration	Haemodynamic instability Patient positioning affects fractures/injuries Angle of flight affects ICP in head injury (p. 641)
Noise and turbulence	Clot disruption
Poor space and lighting	Limited access to patient/equipment
Altitude	Risk of hypoxia, alterations in acid–base balance Gas volumes increase with altitude (due to decreasing pressure) causing problems in body cavities (bowel, lung, cranium) Endotracheal tube cuffs inflated with saline if flying above 3000ft cabin pressure Consider decompression of gas-filled cavities or equipment prior to flight

The 2007 NCEPOD report *Trauma: Who Cares?* highlighted regional differences in outcome from major trauma within England and the international evidence for improved outcomes when specialized regional trauma centres are used. Following this, in 2011, 26 regional trauma networks began operating throughout England, centred around hospitals designated as *major trauma centres* (MTCs), all of which are in large population centres. 12 MTCs cater for adults and children (of which 4 are in London), 8 accept adults only, and 4 are specialized paediatric centres. The remaining two are collaborative arrangements across multiple hospitals (see fig 10.3). There are no MTCs in Wales—Welsh NHS Trusts commission English MTC services to deliver trauma care to patients who require treatment at an MTC. A project to establish a national network in Scotland is ongoing. The 'Northern Ireland Major Trauma Network' was established in 2016 and work is ongoing to establish an MTC.

'MTCs have all the facilities to provide resuscitation, emergency surgery, and interventional radiology with consultant-led trauma teams 24/7, massive transfusion protocols and immediate access to operating theatres ... and CT/ magnetic resonance imaging. They have dedicated trauma beds, intensive care beds and ... comprehensive rehabilitation services.'[3]

Within London, all patients with major trauma are transferred directly to an MTC. Outside London, lower population density necessitates a network of supporting hospitals designated as *trauma units* which can accept less severely injured patients or allow immediate lifesaving interventions to be made for more severely injured patients prior to onward transfer to an MTC.

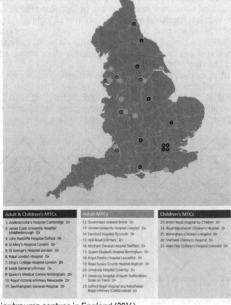

Adult & Children's MTCs
1: Addenbrooke's Hospital Cambridge
2: James Cook University Hospital Middlesbrough
3: John Radcliffe Hospital Oxford
4: St Mary's Hospital London
5: St George's Hospital London
6: Royal London Hospital
7: King's College Hospital London
8: Leeds General Infirmary
9: Queen's Medical Centre Nottingham
10: Royal Victoria Infirmary Newcastle
11: Southampton General Hospital

Adult MTCs
12: Southmead Hospital Bristol
13: Aintree University Hospital Liverpool
14: Derriford Hospital Plymouth
15: Hull Royal Infirmary
16: Northern General Hospital Sheffield
17: Queen Elizabeth Hospital Birmingham
18: Royal Preston Hospital Lancashire
19: Royal Sussex County Hospital Brighton
20: University Hospital Coventry
21: University Hospital of North Staffordshire Stoke on Trent
22: Salford Royal Hospital and Manchester Royal Infirmary (Collaborative)

Children's MTCs
23: Bristol Royal Hospital for Children
24: Royal Manchester Children's Hospital
25: Birmingham Children's Hospital
26: Sheffield Children's Hospital
27: Alder Hey Children's Hospital Liverpool

Fig 10.3 Major trauma centres in England (2016).

▸▸**The number one priority is you** Is the scene safe to approach or should you stand off? Risks in the pre-hospital environment frequently cannot be removed, but efforts should be made to diminish the dangers. Wear *personal protective equipment* (PPE) to protect eyes, ears, head, and hands, plus wear high-visibility clothing. Use life-vests for water rescue and harnesses for rescues involving height. PPE is your responsibility, treat it with respect and include it in training. Donning PPE for chemical protection can be intimidating and difficult—practise regularly! Resuscitators working in PPE quickly become warm and can easily underestimate how cold the immobile patient is becoming—bear this in mind. HARTs (**H**azardous **A**rea **R**esponse **T**eams) are specifically trained for rescue in dangerous environments—prior to this, ambulance crews worked on the edge of incidents, awaiting casualties to be bought to them (see also 'The major incident', pp. 652-3).

Scene safety This is everyone's responsibility and requires continuous re-assessment as conditions can quickly change. A reckless rescuer can become a casualty and a hindrance. Park before the incident at an oblique angle (known as the 'fend off position') and leave hazard lights on.

Always consider the possibility of a CBRN risk (*Chemical, Biological, Radiological, Nuclear*). If suspected, remain upwind/uphill and do not approach a fire or chemical hazard until the fire service have made the area safe. Patient care in CBRN events may be significantly delayed in order to first ensure scene safety.

Communications Liaise with the police (they are in overall command), fire service (for any hazard), and paramedics. Relay number of casualties and severity of injuries to enable the most appropriate medical response.

Read the scene Take the opportunity to get an overview. Once you get hands-on with casualties, situational awareness can be lost. *Read the wreckage:* Try to visualize what has happened as this can aid in anticipating injury patterns. In the first-response scenario, physiology of injuries is developing and anticipation can heighten clinical suspicion leading to earlier identification of occult injuries. Use all available information to identify all casualties eg are there fewer riders than motorbikes?

Assessment of casualties Will commence with triage if there is more than one. A triage tool (see pp. 638-9) can help in drawing order from chaos at this challenging time. Identifying all casualties and determining severity of injury is key. This will feed in to later decisions around prioritization of treatment, methods of extraction, and transport to secondary care.

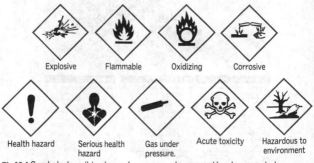

Fig 10.4 Symbols describing hazardous cargo—known as Hazchem symbols.

Hazards to consider

Physical environment Can be significantly more challenging outside the confines of the well-lit, air-conditioned hospital. Adverse weather, poor visibility, water, uneven, steep, or unstable ground, and animals (wild or domestic) can all pose difficulties.

Human factors Present risks which may be difficult to predict; distressed or agitated onlookers or relatives, intoxicated individuals, public disorder, and use of weapons are all potential hazards and a high degree of situational awareness is required.

Type of incident Specific hazards will vary according to the circumstances:

Road traffic collision (RTC): Key dangers include live traffic lanes, unstable wreckage, unactivated airbags, exposed sharp metal edges, glass, and the rescue equipment used. Fire complicates <5% of RTCs and significant burns are rare (<1:500). Hazardous chemicals can be a particular issue (see later).

Electricity: Overhead lines are typically uninsulated and electricity may arc or jump if objects are too close. This can be lethal. Ensure the power is off before approaching.

Rail: An electrified rail can be short-circuited by a bar carried by the fire service or rail authority. Cutting power lines does not stop diesel trains that may operate on the same line. Trains may be stopped by signal lights, red flags, or a series of charges placed on the rail—the noise warns the driver.

Underground/tube/metro: In addition to rail hazards, underground scenarios are complicated by lack of lighting and ventilation, cramped conditions, and difficult access to site.

Hazardous materials May be chemical, biological, radiological (emitting radiation), or nuclear—referred to collectively as CBRN. Some CBRN agents cannot easily be detected by sight or smell; this makes detection of CBRN events challenging. It is therefore recommended that standard precautions are employed for all mass casualty scenarios of unknown cause. Consider also when strange smells or tastes are reported. Public Health England now have an algorithm for diagnosis and early management of chemical incidents that starts with time-critical questions 'Could this be cyanide?', then 'Could this be organophosphates?', followed by other typical chemical culprits.[4]

The fire and rescue services have primacy in ensuring scene safety and in dealing with hazardous materials. New European regulations on classification, labelling, and packaging of substances and mixtures came into force in June 2015[5] (fig 10.4). They are supplemented by hazard warning panels (sometimes called Kemler Plates) which are displayed on vehicles carrying dangerous cargo (fig 10.5).

Decontamination processes are essential for all CBRN events Prompt removal of all clothing followed by a series of rigorous rinsing takes place in specialized decontamination tents. Further casualties can quickly arise if primary cases are not adequately decontaminated. A few chemical agents have particular antidotes. HART will take an active role in organizing safe decontamination.

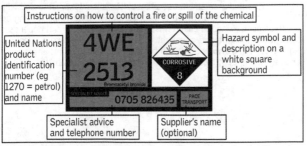

Fig 10.5 The Kemler plate. Understanding the labelling helps you treat spillages.

Triage

(From the French *'trier'* (to sort).) First used in medical terms during the Napoleonic Wars when Napoleon's Chief Surgeon, Baron Dominique-Jean Larrey, recognized that the casualty load far exceeded the limited medical services. His triage system aimed to use resources wisely in order to effectively categorize patients on the battlefield and treat as many injured soldiers as possible. Larrey was a pioneer in trauma surgery and encouraged amputation of limbs to take place immediately after injury, while the body remained in a state of adrenaline-induced vasoconstriction and numbness, rather than weeks later. Speed was of the essence in the absence of analgesia and sedation. His methods famously paid no regard to rank, and officers and soldiers were treated purely on the basis of need.

Distribution of trauma deaths

Classically described as trimodal: *immediate* (eg from aortic deceleration injury, head injury), *early* (from hypoxia and hypovolaemia), and *delayed* (eg from sepsis or multiple organ failure). However, improved resuscitation care has significantly reduced the 'delayed' peak of deaths.

Mass casualty scenarios

The emphasis in triage during mass casualty scenarios aims to deliver the best possible outcome for the greatest numbers of patients. The chart in fig 10.6 is a simple system; its main virtue is speed. It starts by relocating the *'walking wounded'* by asking those who are able to walk towards medical aid, followed by prompt assessment of remaining immobile casualties. Each patient is assigned a colour code (see table 10.2).

When faced with a major incident with an unknown number of casualties, it becomes essential to first identify patients who can be saved. *Resist the temptation to 'stop and treat'* the first patient in distress; if your attention is trapped by a screaming child (demonstrating a patent airway) then a patient needing only a simple airway adjunct might miss a precious window of opportunity (upgrading them from red (will die in minutes) to orange (may die in 1–2h if no treatment). See table 10.2. Approximately 13% of RTC deaths result from an obstructed airway.

The process of mass casualty triage requires a stone heart as some patients may be *'expectant'* ie those who will certainly die in moments. Attempting to treat such a patient may delay in helping those who could be saved. In contrast to a mass casualty incident, if a single expectant patient arrived at hospital, resuscitation attempts would of course be worthwhile. Attempting to 'ignore' expectant patients is understandably difficult amid the chaos of a trauma scene and over-triage is common, especially in children, and this can put pressure on already limited resources

Note that triage is dynamic

It starts with rapid assessment but all casualties should be reassessed when time and resources allow. Triage categories may change while waiting and after treatment. Triage in children is even more specialist, and depends on factors such as height, age, or weight. Once more resources arrive, secondary triage systems (eg *Triage Sort*) can be employed. Senior clinicians may further triage patients by incorporating the GCS, injury severity, and BP.

Triage categories

Table 10.2 Colour categories used in triaging mass casualty incidents

Colour code	Category	Expectancy
	Immediate	Few minutes
	Urgent	1–2h
	Delayed	>4h
	Expectant	Moments
or	Dead	n/a

Use triage labels (table 10.2) to categorize patients into IMMEDIATE (colour-code RED, those who will die in a few minutes if no treatment, eg obstructed airway, tension pneumothorax); URGENT (YELLOW, may die in 1–2h if no treatment, eg hypovolaemia); and DELAYED (GREEN, can wait eg >4h, eg minor fractures). Those who will certainly die are labelled EXPECTANT (BLUE)—to treat them may delay you helping the salvageable, who then die unnecessarily. However, should the expectant patient be your sole casualty (as they would in the ED) then approach them as you would a red patient. Do not forget to label the dead (WHITE or BLACK), otherwise emergency personnel may repeatedly take a doctor to the same victim, so wasting time and resources. Certification of death on scene must be performed by a doctor in the presence of a police officer.

10 PHEM

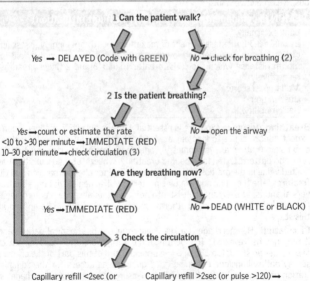

1 **Can the patient walk?**

Yes → DELAYED (Code with GREEN)   No → check for breathing (2)

2 **Is the patient breathing?**

Yes → count or estimate the rate   No → open the airway
<10 to >30 per minute → IMMEDIATE (RED)
10–30 per minute → check circulation (3)

Are they breathing now?

Yes → IMMEDIATE (RED)   No → DEAD (WHITE or BLACK)

3 **Check the circulation**

Capillary refill <2sec (or   Capillary refill >2sec (or pulse >120) →
pulse <120) → URGENT (YELLOW)   IMMEDIATE (RED)

Fig 10.6 The triage sieve. This is a simple system: its main virtue is speed. Once a patient is allocated a triage category, you must move immediately onto the next patient.

Further reading

Gunst M et al. (2010). Changing epidemiology of trauma deaths leads to a bimodal distribution. Proc (Bayl Univ Med Cent) 23:349–54.

Consideration of the mechanism of injury is key to rapid, accurate patient assessment. In the early stages after major trauma, physiological derangement can develop rapidly. Assessing the mechanism of injury informs physical examination and raises suspicion of injuries which may not be immediately apparent.

There are several algorithms in use for guiding the primary survey of patients in the pre-hospital environment. One of the most widely used is the <c>ABC format:

Catastrophic haemorrhage This does not refer to arteriolar oozing but major bleeds which threaten exsanguination within minutes. Such bleeds can be controlled with direct pressure, indirect pressure (eg with a combat application tourniquet (CAT)), or with haemostatic dressings/applications. Some haemorrhage may be incompressible (eg from penetrating trauma).

Airway with c-spine control A patient with quiet breathing and normal phonation has a (currently) patent airway. Reduced GCS is the greatest threat to the airway. Look for facial deformity suggestive of maxillary or mandibular fractures and evidence of airway burns or injuries to the neck/larynx. Penetrating injuries may be subtle. Listen for signs of airway compromise—inspiratory or expiratory stridor or a hoarse or quiet voice. Also take the opportunity to assess and mentally note any features suggestive of difficult intubation (see also p. 671). Mnemonics such as LEMON are available but can be more difficult to use in the pre-hospital environment and do not have high positive predictive value.

LEMON (5 components to assess likely difficult intubation)

- **L**ook externally.
- **E**valuate 3-3-2 rule (assessment of maximum mouth opening by assessing distance between upper and lower incisors, hyoid–mental and thyroid to mouth distance which should be greater than 3, 3 and 2 finger breadths respectively).
- **M**allampati score.
- **O**bstruction.
- **N**eck mobility.

Breathing Adequate exposure is essential. Look in an active manner—don't expect abnormalities to leap out at you. Look for the patient's colour, chest expansion (noting any asymmetry), open/penetrating injuries, respiratory rate, and pattern. Listen for laboured breathing, wheeze, etc. Auscultation has limited value in the pre-hospital environment. Feel for chest expansion and rib fractures—be thorough and examine posteriorly. Tracheal deviation is controversial and is, at best, an inconsistent finding and its absence has zero negative predictive value in pneumothorax. spo_2 monitoring should be applied at this stage.

Circulation Haemorrhage is a key concern in the pre-hospital patient and it may not be 'revealed'. The identification, mitigation, and management of *hypovolaemic shock* (pp. 582-3) is the principal aim of this part of the primary survey and will include obtaining good quality IV/IO access for the administration of drugs and IV fluids as well as measures to control haemorrhage. UK air ambulance services are increasingly carrying blood products. Look for the patient's colour. Capillary refill time may be assessed but may be misleading (eg in a cold patient). Feel the patient's peripheral temperature and their pulse assessing rate and volume. Auscultation of heart sounds is likely to be of limited value.

Further reading

Cook TM, MacDougall-Davis SR (2012). Complications and failure of airway management. *Br J Anaesth* 109(suppl 1):i68–i85.

Leigh-Smith S, Harris T (2005). Tension pneumothorax—time for a re-think? *Emerg Med J* 22:8–16.

Disability and exposure Impaired GCS doesn't just represent severity of illness/injury but is a key threat to airway mandating rapid, definitive airway control if <8 or falling (see RSI section, p. 670). Take care to examine pupils and document. In patients with suspected spinal injury, document peripheral neurological status, especially prior to performing RSI. Don't ever forget glucose—hypoglycaemia might have caused an accident rather than an accident causing head injury. Exposure must be adequate to ensure that injuries are not missed and allow a pelvic binder to be applied directly to skin. However, be aware that rescuers, working hard in heavy PPE, may not notice their patient rapidly becoming hypothermic.

'Golden hours' and 'platinum minutes'? The debate is over

A driving force behind current trauma care systems has been the *'Golden Hour'*—a concept famously coined by Dr Cowley in 1975 who felt that patients should be evacuated to a definitive care facility within the first hour after injury. This approach has since been questioned, as not only is this arbitrary timing lacking in evidence, it also encouraged a culture where speed became the priority. Pre-hospital teams then developed the *'Platinum Ten'* which advised that critically injured patients should be stabilized and evacuated within 10 minutes of the medical team arriving on scene. This was in response to military statistics which showed that most battlefield fatalities occur within 10 minutes of wounding.

However, the pre-hospital environment is unpredictable and obstructive. The two concepts were based on the obsolete debate to *'scoop and run'* or *'stay and play'*. These issues have faded as ambulances and PHEM teams offer more than just a taxi service. Life-saving interventions should be initiated on scene and resuscitation continued during transport. Extrication of the patient must be dictated by scene safety (both for you and your patient), physical barriers, and the patient's condition. Use of the 'Platinum Ten' is more as guidance to encourage efficient decision-making processes and optimizing the patient's situation within the constraints of the working environment. With the rise of trauma centres (see p. 627), value is placed on getting the *right* patient to the *right* place at the *right* time, rather than arbitrarily allocating golden timings. Taking the time to intubate on scene may seem stressful at the time, yet immensely worthwhile when the patient later deteriorates en route. Each trauma patient is unique, facial trauma may only have a few Golden minutes compared to the Golden days of a fractured wrist, yet every patient deserves the same Golden treatment through rapid assessment and efficient evacuation.

10 Pre-hospital emergency medicine

Shock May be obstructive, cardiogenic, distributive or—most commonly in the pre-hospital trauma patient—*hypovolaemic*. Initially shock is subject to compensatory mechanisms such as vasoconstriction and tachycardia in order to maintain vital organ perfusion. If left untreated, this may progress to a de-compensated state, with falling blood pressure, reduced consciousness, and loss of peripheral pulses. Principal sites for blood loss are encapsulated in the phrase *'One on the floor and four more'* —blood lost to outside of the body and then chest, abdomen, pelvis, and long bones (see p. 587). Consequently, as part of the primary survey, a pelvic binder is applied and long bones drawn out to length with traction applied to suspected femur fractures.

Incompressible bleeding sites such as the abdomen require urgent transfer for operative control, the exception being massive haemothorax where a thoracostomy and chest tube may be employed to relieve symptoms. Newer technologies such as REBOA (Resuscitative Endovascular Balloon Occlusion of the Aorta) present an opportunity for pre-hospital control of previously uncontrollable haemorrhage (fig 10.7).

It is standard practice to give tranexamic acid (1g over 10min, followed by 1g over 8h) to all major trauma patients in accordance with the CRASH 2 trial which showed reduced death from major haemorrhage (a recent meta-analysis[5] has demonstrated the importance of giving tranexamic acid quickly with approximately 10% of mortality benefit lost for every 15min delay in administration with all benefit lost at 3h). NB: may cause hypotension if given too quickly + is associated with seizures.

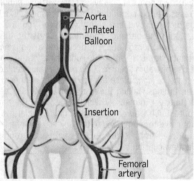

Fig 10.7 REBOA device *in situ*.

Further reading

Bickell WH *et al*. (1994). Immediate versus delayed fluid resuscitation for hypotensive patients with penetrating torso injuries. *N Engl J Med* 331:1105–9.

Brohi K *et al*. (2007). Acute traumatic coagulopathy: initiated by hypoperfusion: modulated through the protein C pathway? *Ann Surg* 245:812–18.

Smith IM *et al*. (2016). Prehospital blood product resuscitation for trauma. *Shock* 46:3–16.

Smith IM *et al*. (2018). RePHILL: protocol for a randomised controlled trial of pre-hospital blood product resuscitation for trauma. *Transfus Med* 28:346–56.

The Birmingham Clinical Trials Unit (RePHILL): www.birmingham.ac.uk/research/activity/mds/trials/bctu/index.aspx

In WWI, Capt Walter Cannon noted poorer outcomes in patients resuscitated to normal blood pressure. He introduced the idea of the *'tenuous clot'* and the concept of *permissive hypotension* (PH). PH gained traction in the 1990s following a seminal paper by Bickell *et al.* which showed a significant reduction in mortality from penetrating thoracic trauma with low-volume resuscitation. In recent times, PH has become the dominant narrative in resuscitation of trauma patients in the acute phase. In principle it makes sense: at the point of injury the patient (in most cases) has a fully functioning clotting cascade, yet with trauma, shock, and vascular damage they may develop *acute traumatic coagulopathy* (ATC). The first clot formed is therefore the 'best' clot and should be preserved. The tradition of siting 2 large-bore cannulas and resuscitating with 2L of crystalloid was thought to lead to an increase in blood pressure, and with this, the risk of rupturing existing clots. In addition, large volumes of crystalloid were thought to dilute the fixed volume of clotting factors and worsen coagulopathy.

However, recent research has cast doubt on the validity of PH as a strategy. Key to this has been a deepening understanding of ATC: once thought to be a consumptive process, worsened by dilution, ATC is now thought to be an inflammatory process. Direct damage, hypoperfusion, and hypoxia affect the vascular endothelium leading to production and activation of protein c which through inhibition of factors va and vIIa inhibits clot formation and (via other mechanisms) promotes fibrinolysis. This inflammatory process is promoted by maintaining the endothelium in a hypoperfused state. PH may therefore promote ATC and worsen patient outcomes.

Evidence around pre-hospital resuscitation is sparse, of poor quality, and often conflicting. The optimum strategy for resuscitation of the pre-hospital trauma patient is not known. Typically, fluids, be they crystalloids or blood/blood products, are given in boluses with reassessment while working to local standard operating procedures (SOPs) for resuscitation. At the time of writing the REPHILL trial, an RCT comparing saline boluses and blood/blood product administration is ongoing and, when published, will help improve the evidence base.

The fire services are unrivalled in their extrication skills and will often take the lead alongside a senior medical officer. Each trauma scene is different and teams must be coordinated and ready to adapt in the face of unexpected challenges. Think about how you would approach a RTC involving a convertible car versus a minivan. Reading the wreckage (see p. 628) helps guide what type of emergency response is needed and where to look for casualties; don't forget to look for patients who may be ejected out of rolled vehicles.

▶▶ **Safety is paramount** Start with simple measures such as making the vehicle safe: turn off ignition, immobilize the battery, swill away any petrol. Be wary of un-deployed airbags. Padding and wedges will stabilize the vehicle. The extrication team works to physically release the patient from the wreck and will work to create space to mobilize the patient safely. Think simple: the easiest way to enter a car is through the door—try this before removing the windscreen or roof! Remove the wreckage from around the casualty; don't try to awkwardly remove a casualty through too small a hole.

The medical team attempts to assess and stabilize the patient. They work in unison with continuous communication as the state of vehicle and patient is closely related. *Rapid extrication* (termed *B-plan*) is required in face of imminent environmental danger (eg fire) or urgent medical concerns (eg airway obstruction). In a more controlled situation (the *A-plan*), greater care can be paid to spinal stabilization, clot preservation, and the avoidance of potential hazards (eg loose wires, glass shards). A sudden shift to B-plan may need to take place if the scene suddenly deteriorates, so always make a solid B-plan before embarking on your A-plan. It can be an intimidating decision; this is the time for clear and confident decisions.

Resist the temptation to set up complex monitoring during the early phases as the many wires/tubes can hinder the extrication processes. Stick to the essentials while the patient remains trapped. Do consider analgesia as this may aid the movement of painful limbs rather than having to spend time dismantling the crushed vehicle. A spinal board[1] is applied as soon possible, often with the patient still partially in the vehicle. Prior to transport away from the scene, carry the patient to a designated medical post ~20 metres from the scene to reassess.

Take care to not disturb aspects of the scene which could be used for evidence (such as tyre marks, paint scrapes) by the accident investigators. For this complex system of extrication and patient management to work, regular joint training between branches of the rescue services is invaluable. The fire service must have an appreciation of basic medical principles and the medical team must be educated in the intricate methods of extrication so as not to hinder each other. The 2 processes cannot function in isolation.

Think about your approach

Minimizing a trauma patient's c-spine movement starts as you enter the scene; if possible, approach the patient in line with their vision to avoid brisk neck movements as the patient strains to see you.

Handover A skill to be honed, and especially important in the pre-hospital environment where treatment moves fast. ATMIST—**A**ge; **T**ime of injury; **M**echanism of injury; **I**njuries; vital **S**igns; **T**reatment—is a useful mnemonic. Always give an ETA to the receiving hospital. *Example handover with succinct information:* 35yr-old female driver of motorcycle. High-speed impact into stationary bus and ejected 9 metres. GCS 3. Tubed and ventilated on scene. Head, facial, and femoral injuries. Peripheral pulses intact. Sats 98%, RR 24, HR 140, BP 95/60. 250mL normal saline given. ETA 16 minutes.

---

1 Spinal boards are now only used as extrication devices. Patients are always transported to hospital on a scoop.

This is a once or never in a career scenario and prior rehearsal through mental modelling and surgical skills courses is essential to be able to perform in this most stressful of situations. The key step will be making the decision to proceed. The decision is difficult and ideally 2 senior clinicians should be involved, eg via telephone. Involvement of other personnel will help to confirm absolute necessity.

Indications

1 Scene so dangerous that patient must be moved immediately eg fire, flooding.
2 If patient is trapped and likely to die before extraction.
3 Other dead people could be amputated to gain access to live casualties.
4 Completion of partial traumatic amputation or removal of unsalvageable limb—most likely indication.

Preparation

Consent is a difficult issue and, in most cases, will not be possible due to patient condition. Discuss plan and mental model with other personnel on scene—preparation, the process itself, and post-procedure exit strategy should be discussed. A kit dump will be established for sedation and the procedure itself. Safety management is essential and should not be overlooked despite the environment: this will include eye protection and other PPE and sharps management. Photographs may be helpful for hospital handover and subsequent learning and clinical governance.

The process

The patient is deeply sedated or undergoes RSI (p. 648). 2 tourniquets are applied and the area cleaned. Operating as distally as possible, a scalpel is used circumferentially for skin and fascia, tuff cut shears for dividing muscle groups and Gigli saw for bone. Be aware that a Gigli saw may spring up once the bone is cut through and steps should be taken to protect against this. Arterial forceps may be used on large bleeding vessels if required. Practice is essential—eg using cadavers. Depending on circumstances, other tools have been studied (eg hydraulic cutting tools used by the fire service, 'jaws of life') but the Gigli saw remains the 1st choice.

This procedure has the potential to cause ongoing distress to those involved including non-medical staff and it is essential to ensure adequate time and space for debriefing. Such events should also be reviewed in the clinical governance framework.

10 PHEM

Further reading

McNicholas MJ *et al.* (2011). 'Time critical' rapid amputation using fire service hydraulic cutting equipment. *Injury* 42:1333–5.

Porter KM (2010). Prehospital amputation. *Emerg Med J* 27:940–2.

Pain Has a huge psychological component which is acutely exacerbated in emergencies when a terrified patient can become very difficult to assess. Physiologically, catecholamines released with pain may further reduce peripheral perfusion and oxygen delivery in hypovolaemic shock. Prompt control of acute pain will not only aid physiological assessment, but will also inspire confidence in the rescuers and thus help to settle a distressed casualty. Your confident approach and calming presence are strong analgesics; do not underestimate these non-pharmacological approaches (fig 10.8).

Beecher noted in 1944 at Anzio[2] that soldiers were indifferent to pain from serious injury. This is unlikely in road crashes; those soldiers were released from war horrors by their injuries, but a crash victim is just beginning their nightmare. So the question is never *why*, but *when* should analgesia be given? In the chaos of pre-hospital scenes, pain is frequently overlooked as rescuers focus on extrication and treatment plans. Unless all hope of life and rescue has been abandoned, the priorities of securing an airway and stabilizing c-spine, and optimizing ABC should come before analgesia.

Assessment of pain can be difficult in impaired GCS; but do not assume that this equates to absence of pain perception. Use visual analogues and pain scoring for rapid assessment, but note that it is the trend in the pain reported that must guide treatment.

Pharmacological approaches to analgesia The options can be mind-boggling, but rather than attempting complex polypharmacy, stick to familiar combinations that work for you. ▶Documentation is key to preventing iatrogenic overdose.

IV paracetamol is frequently used for all patients, especially the elderly trauma patient. Use the plastic 100mL IV bottles and give over 5–10 minutes. PO paracetamol is offered to those who can be discharged from scene.

NSAIDs are excellent for longer-lasting relief of musculoskeletal pain, rarely used in severe injuries, and typically used for those discharged from scene.

Gaseous Nitrous oxide is mixed with 50% O₂ as *Entonox*® in blue cylinders with a white top (store horizontally to prevent gas separation). Fast onset and offset of effect; used while IV access is established or if additional short bursts of analgesia are needed (ie moving injured limb). Do not use in decompression sickness, pneumothorax (may expand with gas absorption), acute head injury, or bowel obstruction.

Opioids Morphine is effective and frequently used. Give 0.1mg/kg (1–10mg) in 2mg aliquots titrated against pain and patient (less needed in elderly). **Fentanyl** is as effective as morphine, easier to titrate due to faster onset of action, and can be given by nasal and buccal routes. Drawbacks of opiates include the impracticality of patiently titrating to pain amid the chaos of an accident scene with variable patient responses to opiates and typical time to maximal effect of 20 minutes. Respiratory depression is avoided with careful titration but **naloxone** should always be available (0.2–0.4mg IV repeated every 2min as necessary). Be careful not to over-administer naloxone as it will reverse analgesic effect. Consider antiemetics, studies have shown that 50mg IV **cyclizine** or 4mg **ondansetron** may be more efficacious than the traditional 10mg metoclopramide.[7]

Ketamine Becoming increasingly popular, especially for use in trauma patients. At sub-anaesthetic doses (0.25–0.5mg/kg IV or IO) ketamine is a potent, short-acting analgesic with rapid onset and amnesic effects. A large therapeutic index and less adverse effects on breathing makes it relatively safe in pre-hospital care. Ketamine in adults can cause profound hallucinations and unpleasant trips or *'emergence phenomenon'*; have **midazolam** 1mg IV available in case the patient becomes difficult to manage (but administration is rarely needed). It can cause tachycardia (usually minimal) and hypertension (but in practice this has little effect on cardiovascular stability or haemorrhage control); do not automatically attribute tachycardia to drug effect—your patient might be shocked.

2 Anzio, 33 miles south of Rome, was a crucial Allied beachhead in recapturing the 'Eternal City' (5/6/1944).

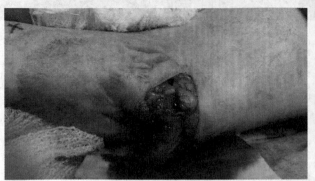

Fig 10.8 ▶▶Photography of a wound will prevent excessive dressing removal which aggravates pain and increases infection risk, but do remember to annotate pictures appropriately as it can be difficult to locate the anatomy.[3]

© Nina Hjelde.

Peripheral nerve blocks Attractive as they can offer excellent analgesia with no sedation, yet this is rarely achievable in the pre-hospital care setting due to time constraints, need for splinting, and multiple injuries requiring opioids.

Procedural sedation Mostly reserved for fracture-dislocation injuries which must be reduced (eg causing neurovascular compromise) on scene. Also consider for painful (extrication of trapped limb) or invasive (chest drain insertion) interventions. A combination of **ketamine** (sedation dose is 0.5–1mg/kg) IV/IO and **midazolam** (1–2mg) can be used with continuous monitoring attached. Only sedate your patient if you are competent in intubation should anaesthesia be induced.

Intranasal (IN) analgesia

IN analgesia has long been used in paediatric emergencies where gaining IV access would cause even more distress. The pre-hospital environment does not lend itself to gaining easy IV access and IN delivery is often used (and can be used for adults too). In hospital, adults tend to be given Entonox® or undergo injections or cannulation just for analgesia, even when resuscitation is not required. Although the majority of studies are in children, interest for IN analgesia in adults is growing, as IN has attractive advantages: rapid onset similar to IV opiates, unskilled delivery technique makes it quickly and ubiquitously available, & higher bioavailability than oral as it passes directly into bloodstream.

IN fentanyl and diamorphine are most commonly used. Dosing can be intimidating since you often need double the IV dose (and sometimes more!) of fentanyl for therapeutic effect, clinicians failing to give proper doses initially halted the popularity of IN techniques. The trick is to use highest concentration available and titrate to pain (as you would do in IV opiates). **Fentanyl** 2mcg/kg and **diamorphine** 0.1mg/kg. Administer half dose into each nostril to maximize absorptive surface area. Reassuringly, naloxone can also be administered IN.[4]

3 Open ankle fracture with dorsalis pedis 'X' marked by paramedics with pen to prove a pulse was present when they assessed patient.
4 http://intranasal.net/Home/default.htm

One of the authors was called to see an elbow fracture as the patient was noted to be tachycardic and hypertensive. While chatting to the patient, she appeared comfortable and the elbow in question was protectively held by her other arm. Cheerfully reassuring her when the pulse was felt at 85, the nurse then diligently checked for a pulse on the painful arm and applied the BP cuff to her other arm; failing to notice the grimace of pain on the patient's face as her self-splinting was temporarily abandoned. The cause of her tachycardia and high BP was now obvious.

We can sometimes be blinded by numbers and forget basic skills. Splinting of soft-tissue injuries will support and protect the injury to help alleviate pain and prevent further damage.

Splinting of limbs This is synonymous with fractures, yet joint immobilization is beneficial in all limb injuries. Splinting aims to immobilize and potentially realign fractured or dislocated bone segments to a neutral position. No limb injury should be transported before splinting takes place (see fig 10.9).

Simple splints can be improvised from clothing; an uninjured leg can splint the injured one. Inflatable jacket splints can be used to immobilize ankle, tibial, and forearm fractures. Femoral shaft fractures can be splinted using a *Kendrick splint* in the pre-hospital environment—once in hospital they may require *Thomas splints* which offer more powerful traction. Pelvic splints (p. 596) are essential for controlling blood loss in addition to providing pain relief. Splint hands by rolling a bandage in the fist with overlying straight fingers. Simple slings can splint an arm to the chest. Pad (eg with blankets) bony prominences to maintain skin integrity (esp. for immobile patients). Splints should cover the joint above and below the fracture site to ensure minimum movement of bone ends.

Reduction Reduction of an injured limb is indicated when faced with deformity which could lead to soft-tissue ischaemia or neurovascular compromise; apply traction to gently restore normal anatomical alignment. Timely reduction of deformity will improve the neurovascular outcomes. Distal perfusion must be evaluated before and continuously after manipulation.

Blood loss Table 10.3[3] shows estimated blood loss caused by long-bone & pelvic fractures.

Table 10.3 Estimated blood loss caused by fractures

Site of fracture	Estimated blood loss (litres)
Humerus	0.5–1.5
Tibia	0.5–1.5
Femur	1–1.25
Pelvis	1–4

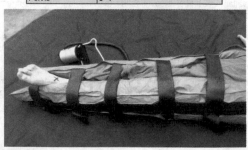

Fig 10.9 Splint fractures distal to the knee in a vacuum splint. The pump pictured functions to suck the air out to create a stiffened splint moulded to the patient's lower limb. Note the dorsal pedis pulse has been marked for palpation both prior to and after the application of the splint.   © Nina Hjelde.

The initial injury Referred to as the *primary injury*. It may result in intracranial bleeding, fracture, or disruption of neurological structures. This damage cannot be undone. The aim of care is to facilitate rapid, safe transfer to definitive care and prevent subsequent, evolving damage to the brain. This further damage is known as *secondary injury* and results from derangement of autoregulation of cerebral blood flow and metabolism. Avoidance of secondary injury essentially calls for normalization of physiology; specifically, avoidance of hypotension (even 1 episode can increase mortality), hypo/hypercarbia, hypo/hyperoxia and hypoglycaemia, and the avoidance of spikes in intracranial pressure (ICP, see later).

Key to assessment of head injury is identification and classification. The Glasgow Coma Scale (GCS) must be calculated for all patients. GCS <8 defines severe head injury. Pupil size and reactivity must also be assessed and recorded.

Provision of an adequate airway is essential for both oxygenation and ventilation (control of carbon dioxide levels). Typically, this will involve stepwise management of the airway with simple manoeuvres and adjuncts until intubation (by rapid sequence induction (RSI), see p. 670) can be achieved. In performing RSI, it is essential to ensure adequate sedation and paralysis both during and after induction to attenuate any increase in ICP. Ketamine, previously thought to increase ICP, is now considered safe in this scenario. The patient should subsequently be carefully ventilated to maintain E_TCO_2 in the target range (see later) and to prevent hypoxia.

Management of circulation can offer a challenge to the pre-hospital practitioner and lead to conflicting aims. A single episode of hypotension doubles the mortality rate of the severely head injured patient and should therefore be treated aggressively. This may conflict with 'permissive hypotension' strategies aimed at protecting a formed clot. By way of compromise a systolic BP of not less than 90mmHg is targeted in the multiply injured patient. Higher targets may be considered in the patient with an isolated severe head injury.

> **Resuscitation goals**
> - spO_2 >97%.
> - Systolic BP >90mmHg.
> - End-tidal CO_2 (E_TCO_2) 4.0–4.5kPa (equivalent to P_aCO_2 4.5–5.0kPa).

In the pre-hospital environment, pathophysiology may develop and change quickly, and head injured patients are no exception. They should therefore be monitored closely with E_TCO_2, continuous spO_2, regular non-invasive blood pressure (NIBP), and assessment of neurological status. Cerebral perfusion pressure (CPP) = MAP − ICP should be maintained in the range 60–70mmHg. In health, ICP is typically <20mmHg but in the head injured patient is assumed to be 30mmHg as it is not measurable. Hence the patient's SBP should be maintained at >90mmHg. Should the patient demonstrate signs of raised ICP (eg pupillary dilation) then this should be managed without delay. *Simple measures* first include treating hypotension, hypoxia, and hypocarbia. If these measures are ineffective then a bolus of hypertonic saline 3%, 3mL/kg may be administered, although evidence for effect is sparse.

Onward transfer should be carried out as soon as can be safely achieved and to the right destination. These patients should go to a facility capable of neurosurgical intervention and with neurointensive care facilities. Head injury is the strongest independent risk factor for cervical spine injury and patients should be immobilized. If a hard collar is used this should be fitted in a manner so as not to impede venous drainage. Packaging within a vacuum mattress has been shown to improve patient comfort and reduce movement compared to the traditional approach of collar and blocks with a spinal board.

Further reading

Hammell CL et al. (2009). Prehospital management of severe traumatic brain injury. *BMJ* 338:b1683.
Nutbeam T et al. (eds) (2013). *ABC of Prehospital Emergency Medicine*. Chichester: Wiley-Blackwell.
Skinner DV et al. (eds) (2013). *ABC of Major Trauma* (4th ed.). Chichester: Wiley-Blackwell.

10 PHEM

Approximately 1000 people suffer spinal cord injuries (SCI) in the UK each year with 50% of these affecting the cervical spine. Young and middle-aged men and older women are most likely to be affected, with road traffic collisions, inter-personal violence, and falls being the major mechanisms of injury. Up to 5% of people suffering polytrauma experience SCI but for each of these a further 5 people may be affected by other spinal injuries such as stable fractures or dislocations. The presence of a head injury is the single biggest predictor of SCI. For more on SCI, see also pp. 558–9, p. 566.

Aims of care

As with head injuries (see p. 641) there is a distinction between the *primary injury* which occurs at the time of the initial insult and *secondary injuries* which occur subsequently. Nothing can be done about the primary injury but further damage may result from hypoxia, hypotension, and careless handling. If the patient has completely severed their spinal cord, this will not be treatable but be aware that because of spinal shock (see BOX 'Neurogenic shock vs spinal shock') it is not possible to assess the extent of SCI in the first 48–72h.

Initial assessment

Initial assessment of the patient with suspected SCI is structured the same as for all pre-hospital trauma patients—that is, SCI is always suspected. After control of catastrophic haemorrhage, the airway is assessed with control of the c-spine by manual inline stabilization (MILS). High-flow oxygen is applied. Jaw thrust and airway adjuncts may be required (especially in the case of reduced GCS) and RSI may be necessary. However, it has been shown that MILS significantly worsens the view obtained on laryngoscopy increasing the chances of failure and requiring a surgical airway. Assess the pattern of breathing—diaphragmatic breathing may be seen with C4–C8 injuries. The risk of SCI can be assessed using the *Canadian c-spine rules* (see BOX 'Canadian c-spine rules').

Circulatory assessment

Circulatory assessment may reveal the signs of *neurogenic shock* —poor perfusion may worsen secondary injury and should therefore be treated aggressively. Give 250mL boluses of crystalloid and assess response. Atropine may also be used. If refractory to these measures then vasopressors may be used. Hypotension should initially be assumed to be the result of hypovolaemia and the usual steps should be taken to treat this, eg pelvic binder. Undertake a focused neurological examination. Assess and document any report of paraesthesia, spinal pain/deformity, respiratory pattern (look for diaphragmatic breathing), priapism, and motor and sensory level. Examine for signs of spinal or neurogenic shock (see BOX 'Neurogenic shock vs spinal shock'). Detailed neuroanatomical knowledge is not required and precise localization of the potential lesion is not warranted and may not be possible in the pre-hospital environment.

Immobilization

Immobilization is essential in these patients (see fig 10.10) but practice has changed in recent years away from the traditional collar, blocks, and spinal board towards methods with greater patient comfort and improved immobilization. A commonly used method is that of a scoop stretcher, head blocks, and vacuum mattress although pragmatism is required, a patient with a pronounced kyphosis may well be injured further by being forced into an unnatural position.

Neurogenic shock vs spinal shock

In the event of sci above the level of T6, loss of sympathetic outflow leads to unopposed parasympathetic effects and *neurogenic shock*. This manifests as bradycardia, hypotension, and vasodilation.

In contrast, *spinal shock* is a flaccid paralysis that occurs in the immediate aftermath of trauma to the spinal cord. This resolves over 48–72 hours and so accurate assessment of the extent of sci in the initial post-injury period can be difficult.

▶Beware of attributing hypotension in the trauma patient to neurogenic shock. Hypotension should be assumed to result from hypovolaemia until proven otherwise.

Canadian C-Spine rules

The person is at *high risk* if they have at least 1 of the following high-risk factors:
- Age 65 years or older.
- Dangerous mechanism of injury (fall from a height of >1 metre or 5 steps, axial load to the head—eg diving, high-speed motor vehicle collision, roll-over motor accident, ejection from a motor vehicle, accident involving motorized recreational vehicles, bicycle collision, horse riding accidents).
- Paraesthesia in the upper or lower limbs.

The person is at *low risk* if they have at least 1 of the following low-risk factors:
- Involved in a minor rear-end motor vehicle collision.
- Comfortable in a sitting position.
- Ambulatory at any time since the injury.
- No midline cervical spine tenderness.
- Delayed onset of neck pain.

The person remains at *low risk* if they are unable to actively rotate their neck 45° to the left and right (the range of the neck can only be assessed safely if the person is at low risk and there are no high-risk factors).

The person has *no risk* if they have 1 of the above-listed low-risk factors and are able to actively rotate their neck 45° to the left and right. See p. 522 for c-spine imaging in the ED.

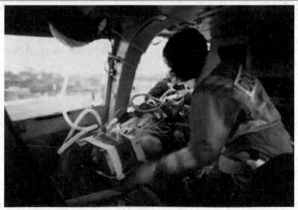

Fig 10.10 Immobilization with tape, blocks, and scoop stretcher.

Further reading

NICE (2016). *Spinal Injury: Assessment and Initial Management* (*NG*41). https://www.nice.org.uk/guidance/ng41/evidence

Nutbeam T *et al.* (eds) (2013). *ABC of Prehospital Emergency Medicine*. Chichester: Wiley-Blackwell.

Skinner DV *et al.* (eds) (2013). *ABC of Major Trauma* (4th ed). Chichester: Wiley–Blackwell.

10 PHEM

Immediately life-threatening respiratory compromise or chest injury will be detected during the primary survey. However, the pre-hospital patient may have rapidly developing physiology or hidden injuries. An open, flexible mind with a degree of suspicion, informed by an assessment of mechanism of injury is a vital tool for the pre-hospital doctor.

The principal life-threatening chest injuries may be remembered using the acronym ATOM FC.

Airway obstruction/disruption Traumatic disruption of the tracheo-bronchial tree may be rapidly fatal. Airway injuries may result from burns, blunt trauma, or penetrating trauma. Inspection may show distorted anatomy or open wounds, sucking/gurgling may be heard. Managing such an airway may be extremely difficult and, if possible, intubation should be undertaken by senior anaesthetic personnel in the presence of a surgical team who can help secure a surgical airway if required.

Tension pneumothorax See BOX 'Tension pneumothorax'.

Open pneumothorax Potentially not problematic in the ventilated patient. Also, if wounds are <⅔ the diameter of the trachea then air will not be drawn through. However, if required, specialist dressings exist eg Russell chest seal. For multiple wounds or large wounds, a self-adhesive defibrillator pad can make a useful alternative.

Massive haemothorax Blood in the thorax >⅓ of the circulating volume *or* >1500mL *or* >200mL/h over 2h. Managed with chest tube insertion and fluid resuscitation which may include blood products/autotransfusion of salvaged blood prior to surgical repair.

Flail chest Fracture of 2 or more contiguous ribs in 2 or more places, typically as a result of blunt trauma. This creates a free-floating segment that moves paradoxically during respiration. Management is supportive with analgesia and ventilatory support if required. Surgical fixation of ribs may be performed in selected cases. Risk of mortality increases significantly if ≥3 ribs fractured, especially in the elderly.

Cardiac tamponade High degree of suspicion required as clinical diagnosis is difficult. Classically described as Beck's triad (muffled heart sounds, distended neck veins, and hypotension)—in the trauma setting, such signs may be impossible to detect. Diagnosis is more likely using ultrasound. R: Needle pericardiocentesis (although this may fail due to clotting blood). Definitive management is surgical.

As with all clinical examinations, assessment of the chest is not a passive process—clinical findings must be actively sought:
• *Look* at the patient for evidence of respiratory distress.
• *Count* the respiratory rate.
• *Look* for chest expansion (is it symmetrical, is it normal?).
• *Examine* the chest thoroughly—including the back looking for evidence of injury (penetrating injuries may be subtle).

In the pre-hospital environment, percussion and auscultation are of more limited value but may indicate gross pathology. As stated earlier, patients in this group may have developing physiology and may change rapidly. Therefore, be prepared to revisit this examination and change your conclusions.

Secondary survey and imaging May detect further injuries such as oesophageal rupture, diaphragmatic rupture, and aortic root disruption—suspect in rapid decelerations. The ascending aorta is mobile whereas the descending is relatively fixed. The junction between the two where the aorta is fixed by the ligamentum arteriosum, around the origin of the left subclavian artery is a point of shear stress and liable to injury.

There is no agreed definition of *tension pneumothorax* and the pathophysiology is often poorly understood. In the *spontaneously ventilating* patient, negative intrapleural pressure in inspiration draws air into the pleura through a one-way defect in either the visceral pleura or chest wall which then cannot escape. This *gradually* leads to increased intrathoracic pressure and mediastinal displacement which impedes ventilation and ultimately leads to *respiratory* arrest.

In contrast, a patient undergoing *positive pressure ventilation* suffers *rapid* accumulation of intrapleural pressure with air being driven through a visceral pleural defect. This leads to rapidly increasing intrathoracic pressure, mediastinal shift, great vessel kinking, and impaired venous return progressing to *cardiac* arrest. Consequently, trauma patients undergoing RSI and ventilation typically have bilateral finger thoracostomies formed after induction to prevent the conversion of an undetected simple pneumothorax to tension. Definitive management involves chest tube insertion and potentially surgical repair.

Thoracic decompression may be necessary in the interim, which may be achieved either by lateral finger thoracostomy or by passing a wide-bore cannula through the chest wall at the 2nd intercostal space, mid-clavicular line. However, in up to 25% of trauma patients, the thickness of the chest wall at this site exceeds 5cm meaning that many cannulas would not reach the pleural space. Specially designed needle decompression devices are longer and avoid this problem. As an alternative, the safe triangle may be used for decompression.

10 PHEM

Further reading
Leigh-Smith S *et al.* (2005). Tension pneumothorax—time for a re-think? *Emerg Med J* 22:8–16.

Certain groups of patients present with particular needs and characteristics. There is no 'one-size-fits-all' approach and so dealing with patients in this group can be intimidating, even for experienced personnel. Knowledge can help restore that most misunderstood of medical attributes—coolness of head in a crisis.

Paediatrics Major paediatric trauma is rare. Children are naturally brave and constructive and will respond to you and work with you if you communicate on their level. Be aware that injured children regress and act younger than they are so if, in your mind, you are finding a child challenging think: could this child have an injury that I have missed? Children are renowned for their ability to compensate and in so doing mask injuries before rapidly deteriorating; therefore, a high degree of suspicion is warranted. The care required by children is broadly the same as for adults (control of haemorrhage, ABC) but some modification is required. One approach to paediatric patients is to address basic needs: reassurance (keeping parents/carers close), warmth, and analgesia. After this, if the child remains distressed then suspect more significant injury and plan for rapid transfer to secondary care. Paediatric airway management is a particular area of difficulty. The airway is anatomically different but can be managed with basic manoeuvres more readily than in adults. Drug and fluid doses can be calculated readily by means of paediatric triage tapes. See fig 10.11.

Pregnant women Undergo a number of relevant physiological changes in pregnancy. The upper airway becomes engorged and friable and laryngoscopy can be impeded by enlarged breasts—the risk of a failed intubation is quoted as 1:300 (compared with 1:2000 for elective anaesthesia). The respiratory rate and tidal volume increase to improve oxygen delivery but compression of the lower thorax by the pregnant uterus reduces functional residual capacity and hence time to desaturation when apnoeic. The pulse rate and stroke volume increase to meet additional circulatory demands and this additional capacity can act to compensate for hypovolaemia. Assessment of the pregnant female is largely the same as for any other adult. Patients should be nursed in a left lateral position or manual displacement of the uterus performed to reduce caval compression. Be aware that the uterus provides a reservoir for occult bleeding but offers some protection to the remaining abdominal viscera. Causes of trauma are the same as for non-pregnant patients but maintain awareness of increased rates of domestic violence seen in pregnancy.

The elderly Vastly improved life expectancy is a great triumph for medicine in the last century. However, the elderly consume comparatively more health resources. Ageing is not a pathological process but comorbidities, organ impairments, and medication usage in the elderly can obscure presentation of injury/disease, render them more vulnerable to injury, and impair recovery. Too often, impairments such as confusion and incontinence are put down to age and elderly people are denied assertive medical care which may be beneficial. Falls are a common cause of trauma in the elderly and can lead to serious injury eg intracranial haemorrhage or c-spine injury. Elder abuse should also be borne in mind. Polypharmacy can lead to injuries occurring (eg sedation), exacerbate injuries (anticoagulants), impair compensatory mechanisms (beta blockade), or impair recovery (steroids). A careful medical and drug history is therefore essential. The elderly are more vulnerable to injury from manual handling (eg skin tearing) and so should be handled with particular care. Functional history can be a useful guide to treatment in so far as it reveals the patient's normal baseline state. Subjective judgements on quality of life should not be made in the pre-hospital environment.

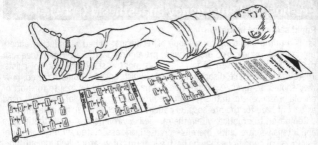

Fig 10.11 The paediatric trauma tape is laid alongside the child. The portion of the tape corresponding to the child's height gives relevant drug doses and other values.

Reproduced with permission from Wallis, L., and Carley, S. (2006). Validation of the Paediatric Triage Tape. *Emergency Medicine Journal*, 23(1):47–50. http://dx.doi.org/10.1136/emj.2005.024893. Copyright © 2006, BMJ Publishing Group Ltd and the British Association for Accident and Emergency Medicine.

10 PHEM

Further reading

Nutbeam T *et al.* (eds) (2013). *ABC of Prehospital Emergency Medicine*. Chichester: Wiley-Blackwell.
Skinner DV *et al.* (eds) (2013). *ABC of Major Trauma* (4th ed). Chichester: Wiley-Blackwell.

Rapid sequence induction

RSI is an umbrella term for a range of techniques aimed at inducing anaesthesia in the unprepared patient while preventing gastric aspiration (see also p. 670). There is no agreed format for RSI and no standard protocol exists. There is considerable disagreement over which agents should be used, how they should be given, what position the patient should be in, use (or not) of cricoid pressure, etc. In this section, we provide an overview of how RSI is used as part of care for the pre-hospital patient, however, it is far from definitive.

Compared to practice within the rarefied environment of anaesthetic bays and intensive care units, there is increased risk associated with pre-hospital RSI. Physical conditions may be hostile in terms of weather, lighting, altitude, and temperature. The location may be remote and/or difficult to access; there may be civil unrest or other deliberately hostile individuals. CBRN hazards may exist. Patients coming under the care of PHEM services are typically critically unwell and therefore more vulnerable when undergoing anaesthesia. In addition, performance of RSI increases scene time—although it may reduce time to interventions in hospital eg progress to CT.

Despite these challenges, RSI is the technique of choice for the trauma patient who is unable to maintain their airway. It should be carried out within a comprehensive governance system and to the same standards as in-hospital anaesthesia with the same monitoring modalities. Techniques used should be simple, robust, and carried out in accordance with challenge–response checklists etc.

Preparation

The indication for RSI should be clearly stated (see MINIBOX). The patient's ultimate destination post RSI should be agreed and plans for anaesthesia and subsequent transfer communicated out to relevant personnel—ambulance crews, incident commander, receiving hospital. This helps to protect against the lull in activity which may occur post procedure and maintain momentum towards definitive care. RSI is performed by a team consisting of a minimum of 3 people—airway (most skilled airway operator available), assistant/cricoid pressure (typically a critical care paramedic), and manual in-line stabilization (MILS). Ensure 360° access, consider lighting (eg move to shade in bright sunlight), and optimize position as far as possible eg on an ambulance trolley at the optimum height. A kit dump is prepared in a convenient position with standardized equipment and pre-drawn drugs. In dangerous environments (eg battlefield, civil unrest), situational awareness is of vital importance and further removal of the patient to a safer environment may be judged to outweigh the risks of delaying RSI. Prior

Indications for RSI
• Airway protection of a patient with reduced or reducing GCS.
• Prevention of secondary brain injury in the head injured patient.
• Protection of the *at-risk* airway—eg burns, facial trauma.
• To support ventilation/ oxygenation in the patient suffering from respiratory failure (asthma, ARDS, chest trauma).
• Patient, crew, and safety in the agitated or combative patient.
• Humanitarian reasons— for a distressed patient or a patient in severe pain.

to RSI, surrounding personnel are requested to remain quiet and not interrupt the intubation process. Challenge–response checklists are used to ensure that all equipment is in place and is working. The anaesthetic plan including backup plans in the event of failed intubation are discussed with the team.

Process

Pre-oxygenation is provided with high-flow oxygen using an appropriate mask. Ventilatory support, if required, should be gentle to avoid gastric distension. For immobilized trauma patients, MILS is applied from anterior position. The collar is then opened and blocks removed. Induction agents (eg **ketamine** 2mg/kg) are given followed by muscle paralysis agent (eg **rocuronium** 1mg/kg). Cricoid pressure may then be applied (and subsequently removed if laryngoscopic view impaired). The endotracheal tube is inserted under direct vision—usually with the use of a gum elastic bougie. Once correct position of the tube is confirmed (chest movement, tube misting, E_Tco_2), it is secured—avoid circumferential ties in head injured patients as these may impair venous drainage. Tube position must be re-verified every time a patient is moved. In the event of thoracic trauma, post-intubation thoracostomies may be formed to eliminate the risk of converting an undiagnosed simple pneumothorax to a tension pneumothorax (see BOX 'Tension pneumothorax', p. 645).

A word on ventilators:

Bag ventilating a patient by hand is conceptually simple but procedurally complex and in the intensity of the pre-hospital environment it is a simple matter to hypo- or hyperventilate a patient. Consider early use of a ventilator for more consistent ventilation/oxygenation and to free up hands.

A word on paediatric RSI:

Children requiring RSI are rare and recognizing that in-hospital paediatric anaesthesia is a subspecialty, pre-hospital RSI in children should only be carried out when more basic techniques have failed to maintain oxygenation and a definitive airway is mandated.

10 PHEM

Further reading

Lockey DJ *et al.* (2017). AAGBI: safer pre-hospital anaesthesia. *Anaesthesia* 72:379–90.

On arrival to a patient in cardiac arrest, a rapid assessment is required as to the potential cause of that arrest—is it medical or traumatic? This decision will be driven by available evidence—physical evidence from the scene, prior health conditions and age of the patient, and history from any relatives or eyewitnesses.

Traumatic cardiac arrest (TCA)

Fundamentally different in pathophysiology from the more familiar medical cardiac arrest. Management is consequently very different. ▶The heart has typically not failed. Key causes of traumatic cardiac arrest are *hypovolaemia* (48% of cases), *hypoxia*, and *obstruction* (*tension pneumothorax* (TPTX) and *tamponade*). These underlying causes are therefore the target for reversal. The other causes of cardiac arrest included in the '4Hs and 4Ts' of ALS are not considered. It is this difference of underlying aetiology that informs the management outlined in the European Resuscitation Council Traumatic Cardiac Arrest algorithm (see fig 10.12). CPR is de-emphasized and on occasions may not actually be done until other potentially more effective interventions have been carried out. TCA management is delivered as a package of interventions known as the HOT bundle but even this may be amended depending on the circumstances of the patient:

Hypovolaemia

Any controllable source of haemorrhage is addressed. External haemorrhage is compressed or tourniquets applied. Internal haemorrhage may be controlled with the application of a pelvic binder, or via resuscitative endovascular balloon occlusion of the aorta (REBOA), if available (see p. 634). Limbs are drawn out to length. IV/IO access is then obtained and fluids given; blood or crystalloid depending on availability and local practice.

Oxygenation

The patient is intubated and 100% oxygen delivered. This does not require large-volume breaths which may increase intrathoracic pressure and thus reduce venous return. The purpose is to deliver adequate oxygen (not restore normal ventilation).

Tension pneumothorax/tamponade

Creation of bilateral thoracostomies and, if clinically indicated (eg in penetrating thoracic trauma), resuscitative clamshell thoracotomy.

In itself, this package of interventions may be sufficient to restore a perfusing rhythm, especially if performed early. At this stage, CPR may be considered an appropriate intervention. The next step is to minimize on-scene time for potentially salvageable patients and rapidly transfer to a place of definitive care, typically a major trauma centre—this process may be summed up as 'HOT and GO'.

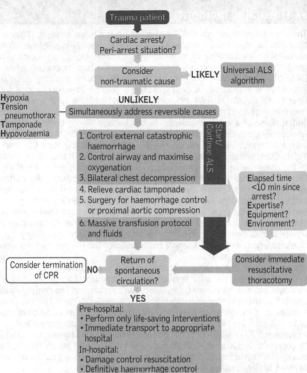

Fig 10.12 Traumatic cardiac arrest algorithm—European Resuscitation Council.
Reproduced with permission from Truhlář, A. *et al.* (2015). European Resuscitation Council Guidelines for Resuscitation 2015: Section 4. Cardiac arrest in special circumstances. *Resuscitation* 95:148–201. https://doi.org/10.1016/j.resuscitation.2015.07.017. Copyright © 2015 European Resuscitation Council. Published by Elsevier Ireland Ltd. All rights reserved.

Keeping records

In the controlled bustle of activity at a pre-hospital scene, the same focus that is applied to provision of care also needs to be applied to recording of care (see MINIBOX). This is vital for safe practice eg on arrival at hospital, a full dose of morphine given on top of an unknown administration in the field can be enough to lead to overdose. Care provision will inevitably come first, but it is vital to create accurate records in retrospect. Widely used pre-prepared sheets avoid delay and confusion. Handover between emergency services is an essential skill which should be practised (see pp. 636–7).

> **Essence of keeping records**
> - Good practice = safe practice.
> - Treat first, then make records.
> - Use well-known formats.

Further reading

Truhlář A, *et al.* (2015). European Resuscitation Council guidelines for resuscitation 2015. *Resuscitation* 95:148–201.

There is no agreed definition of what constitutes a major incident. However, they may be regarded as incidents where the number or type of casualties overwhelms the capacity of local services to treat them. This varies with geography: 5 casualties in a car crash may strain rural resources, while a large city hospital could easily cope. Equally, situations requiring specialist interventions (paediatrics, burns) can quickly overwhelm larger centres too. Operational structures have been introduced to improve joint working between emergency services at major incidents—JESIP (see BOX 'JESIP').

Initial phase of a major incident Will be chaotic. Drawing order from chaos requires discipline, training, and an agreed structure. Within the UK, in accordance with JESIP principles, general management follows the CSCATTT process: Command, Safety, Communications, Assessment, Triage, Treatment & Transport (as taught by the MIMMS course) which guides a highly structured chain of events (fig 10.13).

Flow of *command* is dependent on time of arrival, with responsibility shifting as more senior staff arrive. Overall scene control is police-led, with help from incident commanders representing each emergency service. Each person must report to the scene commander on arrival. Police will also organize bystanders & coordinate media and local authority responses. Organization of the scene must be established early in order to optimize service delivery.

Scene safety: (See p. 628.) Largely the domain of the fire service who work towards mitigating hazards.

Communication: Often a problem at major incidents due to environmental restrictions; although radio use is the primary form of communication, consider written messages and runners in busy times. Codes and call signs must be predetermined and staff should be familiar with radio communication. Good communication allows coordination between services and sensible reassignment of staff after completed tasks. It is a skill to strike a balance between under- and over-communicating!

Assessment: Assessment of the scene and recruitment of the support needed to cope with a major incident is dependent on the first responders acting quickly and having the confidence to declare it; an intimidating call for a junior to make. Seek prompt senior support.

Declaration: Use METHANE—**M**ajor incident declared, **E**xact location, **T**ype of incident, **H**azards (present and future, see p. 629), **A**ccess (remember to consider a safe route in and out), **N**umber, type, and severity of casualties, **E**mergency services now present and those required.

Triage: (See pp. 630–1.) The ambulance first on scene should initiate triage rather than treat the first casualties. It is continuously revised as more staff arrive.

Treatment: Excessive medical intervention must be avoided in the initial stages, only life-saving treatments should be carried out until the scene has been adequately assessed and casualties triaged. Permissible interventions could include placing casualties in the recovery position, simple airway adjuncts, or tourniquets for haemorrhage. The MERIT (formerly 'Mobile Medical Team') consisting of a team of doctors, nurses, and paramedics who perform secondary surveys on casualties in the casualty clearing station (CCS) may be recruited to help with triage and extrication. MERIT members should arrive equipped with kit bags containing limited equipment to support ABC, including rapid sequence intubation and orthopaedic splints. In contrast, HART comprises of medical staff trained to provide life-saving interventions within the hazardous inner cordons to salvageable patients not able to reach the CCS. HART kitbags will carry antidotes. Involvement of voluntary aid organizations, eg Red Cross, is useful for those minimally injured.

Transport: Usually coordinated by the ambulance services, though consider taxis/buses for ambulant patients who require hospital attention to avoid saturating ambulance resources. Secondary triage systems are typically employed to categorize patients prior to transfer. Transport to an on-site morgue must also be considered. Certification of death on-scene in the UK must be in the presence of both a doctor and police officer.

JESIP (Joint Emergency Services Interoperability Principles) was a 2-year project completed in 2014 which set out new methods of emergency service joint working in the event of a major incident. It centres around 5 core principles which govern operations:

1 Co-location of command facilities in a safe zone close to the incident.
2 Communication in clear, plain English.
3 Coordinate efforts by agreeing the lead service and identifying priorities.
4 Jointly understanding risk by sharing information.
5 Shared situational awareness using standardized communication tools eg METHANE (see p. 652).

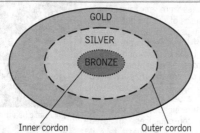

Inner cordon   Outer cordon

Fig 10.13 The outer cordon is defined and patrolled by the police who control access to the scene. The silver area lies within the inner cordon and hosts the incident commanders of each emergency service and the Casualty Clearing Station (ccs); a place of safety close to the incident where MERIT physicians stabilize patients for transport. The bronze area defines the inner area directly surrounding the incident; medical intervention here is limited to triage and extrication.

Peering over the edge

Many lessons in clinical practice will continue to present themselves and your ability to deal with each one grows as you nurture your journey through medicine. Peering over the edge of this precipice can be intimidating for those afraid to look back over their mistakes (that can now be seen so clearly), as the benefit of hindsight is granted through reflection after an event. But only by applying those lessons from past steps can we hope to learn anything. Planning is essential to ensure smooth action which satisfies the public's high expectations of emergency responses in major incidents. The intricate infrastructure required to deal effectively with major incidents is dependent on extensive training and preplanning to facilitate coordinated deployment of the appropriate rescue teams. Effective pre-hospital care also lies in the hands of the public at the very beginning of their desperate dash through emergency care. In response to the July 2005 London bombings, >200 major transport hubs now have emergency dressing packs to equip bystanders and first responders with materials to control catastrophic haemorrhage.

Further reading

Department of Health (2013, updated May 2015). 2010 to 2015 Government Policy: Health Emergency Planning. www.gov.uk/government/publications/2010-to-2015-government-policy-health-emergency-planning

Major incident planning and the required cordons are described well here: Guidance on Emergency Procedures produced by the National Police Improvement Agency (2009).

On the importance of public health

10 Pre-hospital emergency medicine

It is better to encourage prevention than resort to cure. Through public health campaigns (fig 10.14) and continuous health & safety assessments, accidents may now be termed 'preventable occurrences' as we start to recognize all processes are subject to laziness, haste, ignorance, bad design, poor maintenance, false economy, and failure to apply existing knowledge.

Globally, injuries from RTCs rank 10th in the leading causes of deaths but are *the* leading cause in people aged 15–29 years. The majority of these deaths are among vulnerable road users in low- and middle-income countries. Within the UK, the epidemiology of trauma has changed in recent decades. The public are well educated on the dangers involved with driving. Health education posters picturing tragic consequences to loved ones are successful. We almost take it for granted and assume that most mishaps on the road can be avoided if all the rules are followed. No longer is it simply a disease of young men involved in high-energy transfer—the elderly with their greater propensity to suffer injury from

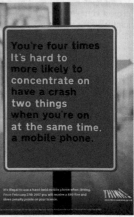

Fig 10.14 Public health advertising.
Reproduced from Department for Transport. THINK! Two things at once poster. © Crown Copyright 2003. https://webarchive.nationalarchives.gov.uk/20090511030049/http://think.dft.gov.uk/think_media/241042/241120/2things.pdf. Contains public sector information licensed under the Open Government Licence v3.0.

low-energy mechanisms have become more prominent. However, injuries related to shooting and stabbing, which disproportionately affect the young, have become considerably more common.

The most dangerous sport?

Each year in the UK, 30,000 people suffer an out-of-hospital cardiac arrest. Despite the recognized benefits of regular exercise, the high incidence of cardiac arrests on the golf course has pushed golf into becoming one of the most lethal sports. This is mainly because golfers are typically males in their 60s who spend their morning hours (most MIs are recorded to happen between 6–11am) walking across large stretches of remote ground. The isolation means that discovery is delayed and access to the patient is limited. In the US, a golf course is the 5th most common place to have a cardiac arrest. *Automatic external defibrillators (AEDs)* have now been enthusiastically introduced across golf clubs as the chance of survival falls by 7–10% for every minute without compressions and defibrillation.

This is an inspiring example of how public health initiatives have been embraced by a population, yet simple interventions such as good hydration, healthy lifestyle choices, and picking a partner who knows CPR remain the best prophylaxis.

▶▶ *How to use an AED*—place 1 pad to the right of the sternum, below the clavicle, and the other in the left mid-axillary line approximately over the position of the V6 ECG electrode. While most pads are labelled left and right (or have a picture indicating position) it does not matter if their positions are switched. Laypeople should follow the AED voice/visual prompts, ensuring that if a shock is indicated nobody is touching the patient.

Our story began with the Rev John Flynn—a man of compassion, vision, humanity, and above all, determination. He established an emergency medical service using infant technology in almost impossibly harsh conditions when no one else had thought of such a thing. Yet, despite his evident ability to conceive of new ideas and his heart for the people of the Australian interior, it was not his genius or his compassion that saw it come to fruition but rather his dedication and commitment. To misquote Calvin Coolidge, it was not education or talent that led to this success, for the world is full of talented failures and highly educated derelicts. The idea had to be harnessed to determination.

Over the intervening decades, the provision of pre-hospital medical care has transformed beyond recognition in terms of capacity, interventions delivered, and technology used, with the highest standards of care delivered to critically ill patients by highly trained and experienced teams of specialist paramedics and doctors. But the fundamental principles remain the same; the reason for our existence is the patient, whoever they may be and whatever their immediate need. To meet this need in the hostile world outside of the hospital we must train, familiarize, check and re-check equipment, develop skills and behaviours, and collectively strain against the limitations of our systems, technologies, and selves. Failure is inevitable, especially in such a challenging environment. On our personal journeys we must be prepared to fail; but then get up and, with humility and openness, try again.

So perhaps that is the lesson? In a profession that rigorously trains us from the start to think, act, and speak like doctors, perhaps now is the time to look behind the carefully constructed professional façade, recognize our individual human frailty, speak openly and honestly about our weaknesses, and support others to do the same. Perhaps then we might develop a lasting resilience in the face of a lifetime spent immersed in others' darkest moments and in so doing, emulate the determination of great people like Flynn, and continue to bring hope where it once seemed remote.

Further reading

Kehoe A *et al.* (2015). The changing face of major trauma in the UK. *Emerg Med J* 32:911–15.

WHO (2014). *Injuries and Violence: The Facts* 2014. http://www.who.int/topics/injuries/en/

WHO (2017). *Global Status Report on Road Safety:* 2017. http://www.who.int/violence_injury_prevention/road_safety_status/report/en/

Other relevant pages Pain relief in
labour (pp. 64–5); resuscitation after
delivery (p. 91); neonatal ITU (pp. 306–7);
ventilating neonates (pp. 308–9).

Online resources www.rcoa.ac.uk,
www.anaesthetists.org, www.niaa.org.uk

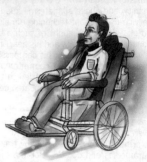

Fig 11.1 'I don't want to just survive, I want
to truly live' were the words voiced by
Robin Cavendish; the longest-lived polio
patient whose survival was dependent on
a ventilator from the age of 28 (in 1958).
His resistance to simply existing on a bed-
bound ventilator inspired him to push the
boundaries of what 'responauts' were
expected to achieve. With the help of his
family and friends, they pioneered a ventilator in a wheelchair which allowed him
to escape the hospital environment. As
you delve further into anaesthetics and
airway management, you'll start to understand the complexities of this feat. Time
spent in intensive care will challenge the
question of how you ensure quality of life,
rather than simply patient survival.

Artwork by Gillian Turner.

Introduction

Anaesthesia evolved from humble origins in 1842 when CW Long gave ether,
but he failed to report this landmark in pain relief. Then, in 1844, Horace Wells
used nitrous oxide for tooth extraction, and in 1846 WTG Morton gave the first
surgical anaesthetic with ether.

Prior to these developments, surgery was limited to quick, simple procedures with obvious benefit (such as amputations) since patients could tolerate
little else. Anaesthesia is now a highly sophisticated specialty in its own right
which enables more complex surgery to take place as the anaesthetist can
provide an optimal surgical environment.

A detailed knowledge of general medicine, physiology, pharmacology, the
physical properties of gases, and the workings of the vast array of anaesthetic equipment are essential in order to practise well. This chapter will
attempt to introduce you to the workings of what goes through the anaesthetic mind when looking after patients, but nothing can replace simply
spending time in theatre and anaesthetic rooms. Note that the UK is one of
the few countries who have anaesthetic rooms, where the patient is anaesthetized in a separate room before moving through to theatre. It is a topic of
debate at the moment over whether this separation should be kept … what
do you think?

With many thanks to our junior reader Matt Heron for their contribution to this chapter.

Reading this book as you're sitting on the bus might just trick your mind into a hypnotic stupor, yet we suspect you would snap back to reality should a needle venture your way. The full triad of: • *muscle relaxation* • *hypnosis* • *analgesia* is required for effective anaesthesia to take place. Should one component be misplaced, situations such as awareness (p. 672), agitation, and pain arise. Anaesthetists are masters at balancing and manipulating this triad to ensure the necessary surgical procedure can take place; just attempting to understand the complex interactions can be hypnotic for any novice.

The first exposure to anaesthetic realms is likely to come in multiple brief interactions around the hospital, rather than a dedicated anaesthetic placement. This reflects the heterogeneous nature of this speciality; don't consider anaesthetists as simply 'gasmen'. Anaesthesia is the largest single hospital speciality in the UK. While the above-mentioned triad remains the fundamental principle behind general anaesthesia (GA) for surgery, the role of the anaesthetist has expanded to encompass not only the provision of ideal operating conditions for surgery, but also:[1]

• Preoperative preparation of surgical patients.
• Resuscitation & stabilization of patients in the ED (see Chapter 9).
• Pain relief in labour & obstetric anaesthesia (see pp. 64–5).
• Intensive care medicine.
• Transport of acutely ill patients.
• Pre-hospital emergency medicine (see Chapter 10).
• Pain medicine including: relief of postoperative pain; acute pain medicine; chronic & cancer pain management.
• Sedation for procedures outside the operating theatre eg different endoscopic procedures, interventional radiology.

Anaesthesia can be really satisfying on your first exposure. Finally! A speciality which works on all those first principles which medical school made you learn. Finally! A speciality which cares about how haemoglobin carries oxygen and what those autonomic nerve receptors are up to. Understanding the basic principles of physiology, pharmacology, and anatomy will make anaesthetics much more tangible. However, despite the detailed knowledge required, it remains an embarrassing mystery that we don't actually know exactly how anaesthetic agents exert their effects. Several theories have been proposed. Perhaps this isn't surprising: we still don't understand consciousness, so how can we comprehend its disappearance?

The first days Theatre can be an intimidating environment. Take great care in wearing appropriate clothing (scrubs, clean shoes, and a theatre cap), in addition to washing your hands regularly. For spinals/epidurals and central lines full surgical scrub is expected. Introduce yourself to the ODP (operating department practitioner) or anaesthetic nurse. Their role is to set up theatre and assist the anaesthetist throughout the operation. They are an invaluable asset to the conduct of safe anaesthesia, often with many years of experience which they are willing to share. Remember to pee before a list, take lunch, and don't just turn up to theatre for the operation—try to see the patients preoperatively too.

Patient safety: the WHO Surgical Safety Checklist The WHO published its surgical checklist in 2008 and worldwide implementation has been associated with a reduction of postoperative complications and mortality.[2, 3] It contains 19 questions which every team member is asked and must respond to (note that there are local variations): • Patient identity • Procedure • Consent • Equipment check • Site marked • Allergies? • Aspiration risk? • Anticipated blood loss >500mL (7mL/kg if a child)? • Have team members introduced themselves by name & role? (This includes students!) • Any patient-specific concerns? • Post-op: have equipment failures been addressed? • Have surgeon & anaesthetist liaised over recovery?

Full checklist: www.who.int/patientsafety/safesurgery

Preoperative care Aims to ensure that patients • Get the right surgery • Are happy and pain free • Are as fit as possible (see the ASA score on p. 659) • Have individualized decisions on type of anaesthesia/analgesia taking into account risks, benefits, and wishes. *It is the anaesthetist's duty to assess suitability for anaesthesia*. It requires an appreciation of the patient's wishes and desires, and pre-morbid state. It requires an understanding of the proposed surgery and the particular anaesthetic techniques to suit both the patient and surgeon.

The preoperative visit Normally takes place the day of surgery and should take place in a private room away from theatre. Take a history as you would normally: have the symptoms, signs, or patient's wishes changed? If so, inform the surgeon. Assess past medical history (PMH) (see MINIBOX 'PMH screen'). Assess cardiovascular and re-spiratory systems, exercise tolerance, existing illnesses—this is important as surgery places a big physiological stress on the body (ask yourself: could this patient's body cope with running a marathon?). Ask about drug history (p. 660) for possible interactions with anaesthetic agents, and allergies—essential since we give many IV drugs which will cause immediate anaphylaxis if not careful. Other specific questions to ask: predict the risk of a diffi-cult airway (p. 671); assess neck movement and ability to open mouth; look at dental hygiene and risk of damage to expensive dental work; past problems with anaesthesia, or recent GA?

PMH screen
• MI or IHD
• Asthma/COPD
• Hypertension
• Rheumatic fever
• Epilepsy
• Liver/renal disease
• Dental problems
• Neck problems
• GI reflux or vomiting
• Past anaesthesia/problems (eg intubation difficulty/PONV)
• Recent GA?

Family history Ask about malignant hyperthermia or suxamethonium apnoea (p. 673); dystrophia myotonica (OHCM p510); porphyria; sickle cell disease (test if needed).

Anaesthetic consent Depends of course on the nature of anaesthetic. Generally, for a GA warn of: danger of dental damage, sore throat, postoperative nausea and vomiting (PONV) (see p. 677), consider the risk of MI/CVA or other specific outcomes (such as postoperative recovery in ITU). See pp. 678-9 for regional anaesthesia (RA).[1]

Tests Be guided by age, history, examination, proposed surgery, and national guidelines. NICE[4] grades the surgery, from grade 1 (eg abscess drainage) to grade 4 (complex+) and beyond: cardiovascular and neurosurgery. NB: tests may not be needed for young fit adults having day surgery.

- *FBC*—anaemia (<120g/L for ♀ and <130 g/L for ♂ should be investigated at least 6 weeks before planned surgery, to give enough time for treatment with oral/IV iron rather than transfusion).
- *U&E*—see MINIBOX 'Check U&E if:' for when to check.
- *Group & save* for all major surgery; *crossmatch* according to local guidelines. Consider autologous transfusion which uses the patient's own blood.
- *LFTs* in jaundice, malignancy, or alcohol abuse.
- *Blood glucose* in diabetic patients (OHCM p588).
- *Clotting studies* in liver disease, DIC, massive blood loss, already on oral anticoagulants or heparin.

Check U&E if:
• On diuretics
• Diabetes
• Burns victim
• Major trauma
• Hepatic/renal disease
• Intestinal obstruction/ileus
• Parenteral nutrition

- *Virology* for HIV, HBₛAg, Hep C, and Hep B.
- *Sickle cell test* in those from Africa, West Indies, or Mediterranean area—and others whose origins are in malarial areas (including most of India). Take con-sent before performing the test, and offer genetic counselling.
- *Thyroid function tests* in those with thyroid disease.

1 The consenting doctor must be capable of performing the procedure or have been specially trained in taking consent. Use only words the patient understands. Make sure his choice is free from pressure from others. A patient may complain if: • He is unaware of what will happen • He has not been offered all options • He was sed-ated at the time of consent • He changed his mind • He was not told a treatment was experimental • A 2nd opinion has been denied • Details of prognosis were glossed over.

- *Pulmonary function tests* ± arterial blood gas for ASA grades 3–4.
- *CXR & ECG*—if known cardiorespiratory disease, pathology, or symptoms.
- *Lateral c-spine x-ray*—consider in rheumatoid arthritis/ankylosing spondylitis/ Down syndrome to check for atlantoaxial instability.

Risk factors associated with perioperative morbidity

- *Age*—the risk of dying doubles every 7 years from the age of 10. Such that the mortality risk at 90 is 5000× greater than the risk at age 10.
- *Sex*—men are 1.7× more likely to die than women of the same age.
- *Socioeconomic status*—the impoverished are 2× as likely to die as the rich.
- *Functional status*—a reflection of the health of the patient at the time of surgery. NB: in most (but not all) studies ASA correlates with morbidity. The *American Society of Anesthesiologists (ASA) score* is:
    1. Normally healthy.
    2. Mild systemic disease, but with no limitation of activity.
    3. Severe systemic disease that limits activity; not incapacitating.
    4. Incapacitating systemic disease which poses a threat to life.
    5. Moribund. Not expected to survive 24h even with operation.
    6. Brain-dead patient whose organs are being removed for donor purposes.
- *Aerobic fitness*—a patient's functional capacity can be measured in metabolic equivalents (METs), where 1 MET equals the resting oxygen consumption of a 40yr-old 70kg male. Ask the patient if they can walk indoors or 100m on level ground (2–3 METs), or climb 2 flights of stairs (4 METs), or participate in strenuous sport (eg singles tennis ~10 METs). When functional capacity is high, the prognosis is excellent, even in the presence of other risk factors. A functional capacity of <4 METs has been associated with poorer outcomes in thoracic surgery, although it has less predictive power with non-cardiac surgery.[3] In the pre-assessment clinic, aerobic fitness can be objectively assessed by cardiopulmonary exercise testing (CPET) which is conducted by monitoring SpO₂, BP, and the ECG of a patient while they exercise against increasing resistance (most commonly on an exercise bike). A mouthpiece measures inspired/expired gases. CPET evaluates the body's ability to deliver O₂ to exercising tissues. O₂ consumption (VO₂), CO₂ production (VCO₂), respiratory exchange ratio (RER), and anaerobic threshold (AT) are all measured. AT is the level of exercise at which the body has to switch from aerobic to anaerobic respiration; <11mL/kg/min suggests a higher risk of post-op cardiorespiratory events or mortality. The results are used to validate the patient's likely tolerance to the physiological stresses of surgery and correlates to post-op survival.
- *Diagnosed myocardial infarction (MI), heart failure, stroke, kidney failure* (creatinine >150μmol/L), *peripheral arterial disease*—multiply long-term mortality risk by 1.5. Angina (without MI) and transient ischaemic attacks increase risk to a lesser degree.
- *Other*—ask about COPD/asthma, diabetes, hypertension, and hypercholesterolaemia as these may contribute to perioperative risk. ►Postoperative chest infections are 6× more likely in smokers (see p. 525 for smoking risk).

Preoperative fasting

Pulmonary aspiration of even 30mL of gastric contents is associated with significant mortality and morbidity; minimize this risk by aiming for an empty stomach. For elective surgery,[5] if there is no GI comorbidity, allow clear fluids (inc. black tea, coffee, or pre-op drinks) up to 2h pre-op (some areas allow 1h for paediatric surgery—check local policy); all other intake (ie food/solids) up to 6h beforehand. Encourage clear fluids up to 2h before surgery to minimize dehydration (which may also subsequently reduce PONV) (see p. 677). In emergency surgery, restrict all oral intake to ≥6h pre-op. Involve the anaesthetist in any decisions if the situation is unclear. Children undergoing elective surgery are allowed formula/cow's milk/solids up to 6h pre-op; breast milk up to 4h pre-op; and clear fluids up to 2h pre-op. Chewing gum may be allowed up to 2h pre-op.

11 Anaesthesia

11 Anaesthesia

Which drugs can you take the morning of surgery?[1]

- *Beta-blockers:* Continue (reduces risk of a labile cardiovascular response).
- *Digoxin:* Continue up to and including morning of surgery. Check for toxicity and check plasma K^+. Suxamethonium ↑ serum K^+ by ~1mmol/L, and can lead to ventricular arrhythmias in the fully digitalized.
- *Statins:* Should be continued, especially in those at high risk of cardiovascular events but discontinue non-statin hypolipidaemic drugs.
- *Bronchodilators:* Continue and consider supplementing with nebulizers.
- *Proton pump inhibitors:* Should be continued.
- *Steroids:* If the patient is on or has recently taken steroids at an equivalent of >10mg prednisolone per day give extra cover for the perioperative period. See BNF for steroid equivalence doses.
- *Anticonvulsants:* Give usual dose up to 1h before surgery. Give drugs IV (or by NGT) post-op, until able to take oral drugs.

Which drugs should you NOT take the morning of surgery?

- *ACE inhibitors:* Many prefer to omit due to risk of perioperative hypotension and kidney injury. ▶Seek advice from the surgeon and anaesthetist.[1]
- *Anticoagulants incl. DOACs:* Know the indication. Timing of stopping/restarting requires • Consideration of the pharmacokinetics of the drug (warfarin requires earlier discontinuation than shorter-acting DOACs) • Risk of bleeding with respect to surgery • Thromboembolic risk for the patient. Check the INR, if needed switch warfarin to heparin preoperatively, leaving sufficient time for the INR to drop to <2. Admit early, and discuss the plan so that all goes smoothly. Avoid epidural/spinal blocks. Beware of regional anaesthesia.
- *Aspirin:* Controversial and dependent on indication and individual procedures, eg patients are given aspirin prior to percutaneous coronary intervention, but may be avoided in non-cardiac surgery due to bleeding risk.
- *Clopidogrel, prasugrel, & ticagrelor:* Stop 5–7 days before surgery. ↑ risk of bleeding/epidural haematoma if neuraxial blockade used.
- *Dual-antiplatelet therapy (DAPT) (often aspirin & clopidogrel/ticagrelor):* In patients already on DAPT for coronary stents, all elective non-cardiac surgery should be postponed until the minimal recommended duration of DAPT (typically 1 year) to minimize risk of stent thrombosis. ▶It is a controversial area so involve the interventional cardiologist (needed anyway if stent thrombosis occurs), surgeon, and anaesthetist if urgent non-cardiac surgery is needed. If possible, defer surgery for at least 6 weeks after bare-metal stents and 6 months after drug-eluting stents.
- *NSAIDs:* Should be discontinued due to renal and antiplatelet effects.
- *Diuretics:* Beware hypokalaemia and hypovolaemia. Check U&E.
- *Insulin:* Continue long-acting (basal) insulin, even when on a sliding scale. See OHCM p.588 for diabetic patients undergoing surgery. Omit oral hypoglycaemics on the morning of surgery.

Which drugs should you consider ceasing earlier?

- *Contraceptive pill & HRT:* Stop 4 weeks before major surgery, restarting at 2wks post-op if mobile due to ↑ risk of VTE. Use heparin thromboprophylaxis + stockings.
- *SSRIs:* Stop 3 weeks prior to certain high-risk CNS procedures due to ↑ bleeding risk but in the majority of patients can be continued.

Common reasons for cancellation[8]

- Insufficient ITU/ward beds, staff, theatre, time or other logistical problems.
- Current respiratory tract infection or exacerbation of other medical illness.
- Patient not in optimum condition, eg poor control of drug therapy (insulin for diabetic patients, digoxin, levothyroxine, phenytoin).
- Recent myocardial infarction (eg within last 3 months).
- U&E imbalance (particularly K^+); anaemia.
- Inadequate preparation (results not available, not cross-matched/fasted).

Definition Sedation is a range of depressed conscious levels from relief of anxiety (minimal sedation) to general anaesthesia (see BOX 'Level of sedation').

Doctors in many specialties may be required to administer sedation. ▶*The doctor giving moderate or deeper sedation must not also be responsible for performing another procedure* (such as manipulation of a dislocated joint). Her sole responsibility is to ensure that the sedation is adequate, and to monitor the patient's airway, breathing, and circulation. Sedation is not a shortcut to avoid formal anaesthesia, and it does not excuse the patient from an appropriate work-up or reasonable fasting (▶risking aspiration of gastric contents, p. 670). Monitoring is mandatory, and must include at least continuous pulse oximetry, end tidal CO_2, ECG, and BP.[7] It is easy for sedation to become general anaesthesia, with its attendant risks (pp. 672-3). The loss of the 'eyelash reflex' (gentle stroking of the upper eyelashes to produce blinking) is a good guide to the onset of general anaesthesia. ▶Remember the need for oxygen and equipment to support ventilation as well as resuscitation equipment when undertaking any form of sedation.

Agents

- *Midazolam:* Initial adult dose 2mg IV over 1min (1mg if elderly). Further 0.5–1mg IV as needed after 2min. Usual range 3.5–7.5mg (elderly max. 3.5mg). SE: psychomotor function ↓.
- *Propofol:* Widely used for sedation, see p. 663. Rapid-acting anaesthetic—but may lead to hypotension and apnoea. In many circumstances (eg manipulation of large joint; painful dressing changes) a *narcotic analgesic* may be used too (eg morphine in 1–2mg aliquots IV, or shorter-acting opioids such as fentanyl) as propofol doesn't have analgesic properties. Typically delivered to effect by anaesthetists as either intermittent small boluses or a target-controlled infusion.
- *Ketamine:* This may be used. It is a dissociative anaesthetic agent which can be used as an induction agent (p. 663), or for procedural sedation (p. 581). It produces deep analgesia with superficial sleep without loss of airway reflexes or hypotension.

Level of sedation

Minimal sedation (anxiolysis) A drug-induced state where the patient is still able to respond to speech. Cognitive function and coordination are impaired but airway, breathing, and cardiovascular systems are unaffected.

Moderate sedation (conscious sedation) Drug-induced reduction of consciousness during which the patient is able to make a purposeful response to voice or *light touch*. Response to pain only indicates deeper sedation. At this level of sedation no airway adjuncts are required, breathing and cardiovascular function should be adequate.

▶*Typically. procedural sedation of patients outside of the operating theatre or ITU is confined to ASA 1 or 2 category patients (see p. 659).*

Deep sedation Drug-induced reduction in consciousness to a point where the patient cannot be easily roused but does respond *purposefully* to painful stimuli (withdrawal is *not* purposeful). At this level, airway intervention may be required (jaw thrust/chin lift). Spontaneous ventilation may become inadequate.

General anaesthesia Drug-induced loss of consciousness during which patients are not able to be roused, even with repeated painful stimulation. Airway typically requires intervention, spontaneous ventilation is frequently inadequate, and cardiovascular function may be impaired.

(Based on American Society of Anesthesiologists Guidelines, 2009.)[7]

Further reading
British Association of Day Surgery: www.daysurgeryuk.net

Induction May be IV or inhalational, usually IV. *A trained & dedicated assistant must be present.*[1]

Intravenous • Establish IV access • Pre-oxygenate, and give co-induction agents (eg an opioid with a fast onset of action to obtund airway responses) • Give a sleep-inducing dose of eg propofol. ►*Beware*: airway stimulation before adequate anaesthesia can have drastic consequences (coughing, breath-holding, laryngospasm). Noise is a stimulus too.

Inhalational • *Either* start with sevoflurane in oxygen according to age and clinical state • *Or* give nitrous oxide: oxygen 60%:40% mixture with a volatile agent eg sevoflurane • Establish IV access as soon as asleep.

Indications for inhalational induction

• At the patient's request • Children • Some patients with partial airway obstruction (actual or potential, eg foreign body, tumour, or abscess), though awake fibre-optic intubation is often used (see p.671).

►► Only once airway control is gained (see p. 666) is it deemed safe to administer muscle relaxants since once the patient is paralysed then there is no option of waking the patient up if you lose control of the airway. The rise of sugammadex has challenged this approach due to its ability to rapidly reverse paralysis from rocuronium when faced with unexpected difficulty in airway management (see p.669).

Some common emergency drugs

Some anaesthetists will draw up emergency drugs in labelled syringes, and put them aside in a clean tray. Here are some common examples in their standard preparations (but note these preparations are simply offered as a guide; always check with the anaesthetist who has drawn them up).

To treat hypotension:
• *Metaraminol* (10mg in each vial, dilute to 20mL with normal saline in 20mL syringe to give 0.5mg/mL).
• *Ephedrine* (30mg in each vial, dilute to 10mL with normal saline in 10mL syringe to give 3mg/mL).

To treat bradycardia:
• *Atropine* (600mcg in each 1mL vial, do not dilute, draw up in small (typically 3mL) syringe to give 600mcg/mL).

Inhalational anaesthetic agents

These are volatile liquids which readily vaporize, permitting administration by inhalation in O_2-enriched air or an O_2/N_2O mix. They help maintain anaesthesia and decrease awareness (by an unclear mechanism). Inhalational agents differ in their levels of respiratory irritation, taste (pungency), odour, and speed of onset–offset.

Sevoflurane A halogenated ether which is well tolerated. It is the agent of choice for inhalation induction of general anaesthesia due to its combination of being minimally irritant, and having relatively fast onset–offset.

Isoflurane A halogenated ether. Theoretically induction should be quick, but isoflurane is an irritant, so coughing, laryngospasm, or breath-holding may complicate the onset of anaesthesia. Opioids can help reduce coughing.

Desflurane Another halogenated ether with a rapid onset of anaesthesia, and quick recovery. It has a low absorption into fat so desflurane is often chosen for surgery in the obese as it provides for the quickest recovery post surgery.[8] However, it is more of a respiratory irritant than sevoflurane, so is typically only used for maintenance rather than induction of anaesthesia. All inhalational agents need to first be vaporized. Desflurane requires a specialized vaporizer to ensure a predictable concentration of anaesthetic is delivered to the patient because its boiling point is close to ambient temperature.

Stopping inhalation reverses all the above-mentioned effects (except for hepatitis resulting from drug metabolism). ►►All can cause malignant hyperthermia (p. 673).

Propofol An emulsion in soybean oil that has become the most commonly used IV anaesthetic agent in the developed world. Its good recovery characteristics and antiemetic effect make it popular, especially in day-case surgery.[9] It is fast acting and its offset of action is due to rapid redistribution, and not metabolism. *Dose examples:* Induction = 2–3mg/kg IVI. Maintenance = 4–12mg/kg/h IVI. ▶Rapid injection can cause cardiovascular depression (↓BP), and respiratory depression can occur when combined with IV narcotics. For procedural sedation: 0.5–1mg/kg IVI over 1–5min. Reduced dose in the elderly, and shocked. *Uses:* It is used in induction and maintenance of GA, and for sedation during regional anaesthesia, short procedures, and as a sedative in ITU. See p. 668 for total intravenous anaesthesia (TIVA). *Problems: Pain on injection* occurs in up to 40% of patients; minimize this by adding lidocaine (eg 2mL of 1%) to the propofol.

Thiopental sodium The other common IV agent.[9] Has in recent years been replaced by propofol as the most popular induction agent. A barbiturate that is typically mixed with water to give a 2.5% solution (ie 25mg/mL). It has a rapid onset of action (arm–brain circulation time about 30sec). Effects last 3–8min, and awakening is due largely to redistribution, not metabolism. *Dose:* 4–5mg/kg IV. *Uses:* Induction of GA; it is also a potent anticonvulsant. *Problems:* Can drop cardiac output by 20%, bronchoconstriction.

Ketamine N-methyl-D-aspartate receptor antagonist.[9] *Dose example:* 1–2mg/kg usually gives 5–10min of surgical anaesthesia. *Uses:* Mainly for paediatric anaesthesia and procedural sedation; it is especially useful in facilitating the positioning of patients for spinal anaesthesia in the setting of painful limb fractures such as a fractured neck of femur (see p. 639 for pre-hospital procedural sedation). Cardiac output is unchanged or increased, producing profound analgesia without compounding shock. Ketamine has potent bronchodilatory properties, so can be considered during intubation in status asthmaticus.[10] *Problems:* Emergence phenomena are troublesome (delirium, hallucinations, nightmares; all made worse if the patient is disturbed during recovery). In the UK, the Home Office classifies it as a class C drug as it is prone to recreational use ('Special-K').

The ideal (but imaginary) *IV* anaesthetic agent

The ideal IV agent would be stable in solution and in the presence of light, be water-soluble, and have a long shelf-life. It would be painless when given IV; non-irritant if injected extravascularly (with a low incidence of thrombosis) with some pain (as a warning) if given intra-arterially.[11] Furthermore:
- It should act rapidly within one arm–brain circulation.
- Recovery should be quick and complete with no hangover effect.
- It should provoke no excitatory phenomena.
- Analgesic properties are advantageous.
- Respiratory and cardiovascular effects should be minimal.
- It should not interact with other anaesthetic agents.
- There should be no hypersensitivity reactions.

The ideal (but imaginary) *inhaled* anaesthetic agent

Inhaled agents have advantages (eg no IV access required, more precise control) and disadvantages (eg claustrophobic) over IV agents. They should:[11]
- Allow rapid recovery.
- Be resistant to any degradation.
- Have no injurious effects on vital tissues.
- Be administrable in a reliable and known concentration.

Muscle relaxants: neuromuscular blockers

These act on the postsynaptic receptors at the NMJ (fig 11.2). There are 2 main types.

Depolarizing agents Suxamethonium (=succinylcholine) is the only one commonly used. It is a partial agonist for acetylcholine (ACh) receptors and causes initial fasciculation through depolarization of the postsynaptic membrane, then paralysis by inhibiting the restoration of normal membrane polarity. Suxamethonium is rapidly inactivated by plasma cholinesterases. *Dose:* 1–1.5mg/kg (total body weight). *IV uses:* It has been the most popular paralytic agent in rapid sequence inductions (RSI) due to its rapid onset (30–60sec), and short duration (3–5min) but popularity has started to wane with the increasing use of rocuronium. The rapid onset lessens the time between induction and intubation—decreasing the risk of aspiration and potential hypoxia. The short duration means that if intubation is impossible, the patient regains muscle tone, and starts protecting their own airway again. *Side effects:* ↑K⁺ (enough to raise the plasma K⁺ by ∼0.5–1.0mmol/L). ↑ intraocular pressure (eg increases risk of vitreous extrusion). 30% of patients get postoperative muscle pains. Repeated doses of suxamethonium may lead to bradycardia—more common in children—treat with atropine. ▶Beware suxamethonium apnoea (p.673).

Non-depolarizing agents These drugs are competitive antagonists of ACh—that is, they compete with ACh at the NMJ—but without producing initial depolarization (so no fasciculations). Their action can be reversed by anticholinesterases (eg neostigmine) which lead to an increase in the amount of ACh available at the NMJ. They are used during anaesthesia to facilitate intermittent positive-pressure ventilation (IPPV) and surgery. Examples include: *Rocuronium:* Lasts 20min. Typically given at dose of 0.6mg/kg although in RSI has been used at doses of 0.9–1.2mg/kg to produce intubating conditions within 60sec. It can cause anaphylaxis (rate =5.9/100,000). Historically, rocuronium has not been used for RSI due to its duration of action. The availability of *sugammadex* (a reversal agent for rocuronium) is allowing this to change. At doses of 16mg/kg (given 3–5min post rocuronium) sugammadex is able to reverse rocuronium faster than the time taken for suxamethonium to wear off.[12] Given its lower side effect profile, RSI with rocuronium could be considered an attractive alternative to RSI with suxamethonium (see p.670 for RSI). *Atracurium:* Lasts ∼25min. Metabolism is by *Hoffman elimination* (spontaneous molecular breakdown), so it is the drug of choice in renal and liver failure. *Dose:* 0.5mg/kg IV.

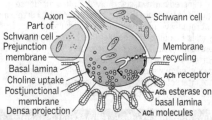

Fig 11.2 When an action potential arrives at the nerve terminal, acetylcholine (ACh) is released from the presynaptic membrane (via exocytosis of vesicles). The ACh then diffuses across the synaptic cleft and binds to postsynaptic nicotinic receptors. This opens ionophore channels (linked to the receptor) and allows an influx of Na cations. Membrane depolarization ensues which facilitates signal progression and results in muscle contraction. Hydrolysis of ACh (by acetylcholinesterase while ACh is bound to the receptor) causes termination of the endplate potential, bringing the trigger to contraction to an end.

11 Anaesthesia

Autonomic learning ...

The autonomic nervous system (ANS, fig 11.3, table 11.1) is primitive, but not simple. It responds sensitively to intraoperative stress and many of the drugs used in anaesthesia (eg atropine, β-blockers) have a further effect on this system.

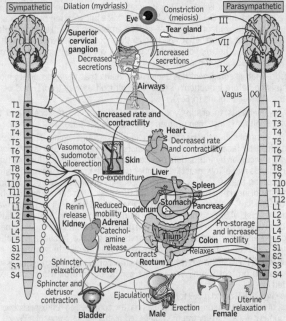

Fig 11.3 The autonomic nervous system.

11 Anaesthesia

Table 11.1 Autonomic nervous system neurotransmitters and receptor types

Sympathetic			
Site		**Neurotransmitter**	**Receptor type**
Pre-ganglionic	All	ACh	NAChR
	Adrenal gland[1]	ACh	NAChR
Post-ganglionic	Sweat glands	ACh[2]	MAChR[2]
	All other	NA	NAR
Parasympathetic			
Site		**Neurotransmitter**	**Receptor type**
Pre-ganglionic	All	ACh	NAChR
Post-ganglionic	All	ACh	MAChR

Key: ACh = acetylcholine; NAChR = nicotinic acetylcholine receptor; MAChR = muscarinic acetylcholine receptor; NA = noradrenaline; NAR = noradrenaline receptor

1 The sympathetic fibres that innervate the adrenal gland are pre-ganglionic

2 This is the main oddity: sweat glands have MAChRs in the sympathetic system

NB: there are a number of other (co-)transmitters in the autonomic system (such as ATP to adenosine receptors). The gut also has a large independent neuronal network.

Anaesthetics is often compared to aviation: the majority of time is spent planning and practising for an event which is usually quite unremarkable. Yet when it goes wrong, the consequences can be disastrous. Just like in commercial flights, when the pilot notices an engine error on ground, the flight is delayed until this is fixed. This is what the preoperative checks are for. However, in conflict, the air forces have no choice but to attempt the mission; even in the face of identified problems. The emergency theatre list will often feel like this. An anaesthetist will frequently encounter patients who will be difficult to anaesthetize; you must ensure that you are armed with the correct skills to face any consequence.

▶Ensure that all equipment has been checked and that the appropriate monitoring is on before induction. Assess for a difficult airway (p. 671) and be familiar with rescue plans (p. 669).

▶▶2 key elements to ensure you have control over are IV access and the airway. If either is lost then problems can quickly escalate.

Airway control sounds very easy, but can be very challenging. The airway is maintained by facemask ± airway adjuncts, by inserting a SAD (supraglottic airway device), or by intubation. Novices should start with holding the mask with 2 hands and a jaw thrust (remember to lift the face into the mask, rather than pushing the mask down into the face and causing airway obstruction), do not be disheartened if you can't hold the mask with 1 hand on your first try. Use airway adjuncts (such as oropharyngeal or nasopharyngeal airways to assist this).[2] After administering IV induction agents (p. 663), ventilation can be provided by bag–mask ventilation until the patient is adequately paralysed and anaesthetized to facilitate laryngoscopy and tracheal intubation. Paralysis with neuromuscular blocking agents helps facilitate intubation.

Intubation Passing an ET tube through the cords into the trachea is the only way to protect the airway against aspiration (p. 670). Most commonly needed in:
- (See figs 11.4–11.6 and p. 669 for the technique.)
- Risk of vomiting/aspiration (▶▶p. 670) of gastric contents: eg reflux oesophagitis, abdominal disease, major trauma, non-fasted, hiatus hernia, pregnant >15wks.
- An inaccessible or shared airway (eg as in head and neck surgery).

Supraglottic airway devices (SAD)
SADs were developed from the concept that facemasks could be redesigned to fit over the laryngeal opening; but it is still not counted as a definitive airway (as there is no tracheal cuff to protect against aspiration). Advantages over simply holding a facemask are that it frees up the anaesthetist's hands for other tasks and it enables monitoring of expired/inspired gasses. The absence of a laryngoscope leads to less airway/dental trauma during insertion and lower levels of skill required for insertion (subsequently often used in cardiac arrests where a skilled intubator is not present). 1st-generation SADs include laryngeal mask airway (LMA), although 2nd-generation devices (igel™, LMA Proseal™, LMA Supreme™) are rising in popularity due to additional features such as bite-block and oesophageal suction ports.

So when can you use a SAD? SAD is used in >50% of elective UK surgery. Increasingly patients who used to be intubated, are receiving a SAD for airway control due to the many advantages listed previously. They are typically advocated in surgery <1 hour, in ASA 1 or 2 patients (see p. 659) with low risk of aspiration. It is inappropriate for abdominal surgery due to the required ventilatory pressures. There remains a risk of laryngospasm if stimulated during inadequate anaesthesia.

2 Note that airway adjuncts (eg oropharyngeal or nasopharyngeal) may produce vomiting or laryngospasm at light levels of anaesthesia.

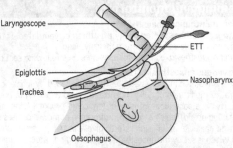

Fig 11.4 The anatomy of intubation. The fact that our airways are located right next to the entry point for food doesn't seem like the most logical design, yet it is what keeps anaesthetists in a job. Managing an airway starts with very basic manoeuvres where you simply prevent the tongue flopping backwards, all the way to difficult intubating conditions. A cross section of the airway anatomy demonstrates where the endotracheal tube sits. Note that the cuff is inflated inferior to the vocal cords and thus protects the airway from aspiration of gastric contents.

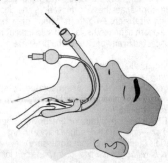

Fig 11.5 Supraglottic airway device in place. Note that although the SMA maintains airway patency, it does not fully seal the airway from the oesophagus and subsequently there is still a risk of gastric aspiration as it sits above the glottis. Hence this family of airways are called 'supraglottic airway devices' (SADs).

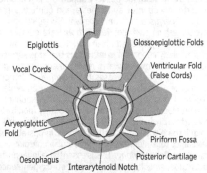

Fig 11.6 View at laryngoscopy. Laryngoscopy is a skill you learn in the anaesthetic room, yet what we advise is a sound knowledge of the view you expect to see as you hope to guide your endotracheal tube through the vocal cords to inflate the cuff just beyond the cords.

Options for maintaining anaesthesia

1 *Volatile agent.* Either spontaneously breathing or ventilated. If the patient is ventilated, muscle relaxants are generally used.

2 *IV infusion anaesthesia*, eg propofol ± opiates. See following section on TIVA.

Total intravenous anaesthesia (TIVA)

Historically, the maintenance of anaesthesia was provided by inhalational agents as perioperative monitoring of gas concentrations and adjusting to patient needs was easier. TIVA is a continuous infusion of (typically) propofol & remifentanil (an ultrashort-acting opioid) which is delivered through a pump which uses pharmacokinetic data to calculate an infusion rate to give a target concentration (blood or effect site) which is set by the anaesthetist depending on surgery, stimulation, etc. It is especially useful for patients with a history of PONV (p. 677) or operations on the airway (eg tracheal stent) as there are no inhalational agents involved. TIVA is associated with a higher risk of awareness, if not monitored appropriately (see BOX 'Gauging depth of general anaesthesia').[13]

Gauging depth of general anaesthesia

Whatever the technique, the dose and concentration of each drug is adjusted according to the level of anaesthesia achieved vs the desired level (determined by monitoring vital signs—eg HR, BP, signs of sympathetic stimulation). Inappropriate depth of anaesthesia (and subsequent risk of awareness, p. 672) should be suspected in any patient in the presence of:

- ↑HR[s] and/or ↑BP.[s]
- Eye signs: lacrimation,[s] dilated pupils.[s]
- Movement or laryngospasm.
- Note that many of these responses are mediated by autonomic sympathetic drive (=[s], see p. 665), and *all* should be picked up with appropriate and continual clinical monitoring.

Other measures Bispectral index (BIS) or entropy EEG monitoring can help assess the depth of GA—and can also reduce PONV and anaesthetic consumption. Evoked potentials (auditory and somatosensory) have also been used.

▶*No single method is reliably accurate, and these cannot replace the vigilance and clinical suspicion of the anaesthetist.*

Monitoring during anaesthesia

Clinical monitoring supplemented by (not substituted by) a range of monitors of the patient and the anaesthetic delivery apparatus is mandatory.[14] The process begins prior to induction of anaesthesia and continues throughout. ▶*A warm, pink, and well-perfused patient is the aim.* Sweating and lacrimation invariably indicate something is wrong: *Respiration:* Rate, depth. *BP:* Intra-arterial in long/high-risk cases may be sited after induction (also allows ABG analysis). *Temperature:* Particularly important in infants, as the large surface area to body mass may lead to hypothermia. A warm environment, warming blankets, and warm IV fluids, are important in long cases. *Pulse oximetry:* Computes HR and arterial O_2 saturation. *ECG:* Reveals rate, arrhythmias, and ischaemia. *Oesophageal Doppler monitoring:* Doppler probe positioned in the oesophagus of an intubated patient can provide estimates of cardiac output by monitoring the flow in the descending aorta. It helps differentiate hypovolaemia from ↓ cardiac function. Insert when large blood loss is anticipated, or in unstable patients. Other methods of cardiac output monitoring include pulse contour analysis with an intra-arterial catheter. *Capnography:* This is essential: a low end-tidal CO_2 warns of a displaced ET tube, emboli, and more. Inspired oxygen concentration and end-tidal volatile agent concentration should also be monitored. Also monitor urine output, neuromuscular status, and ventilator pressures. Alarms should be set to appropriate levels prior to the case.

Difficult Airway Society (DAS) guidelines

If unable to intubate?

Prior to induction you must know the plan should intubation fail: PLAN A (eg tracheal tube); PLAN B (supraglottic airway device p. 666); PLAN C (bag–mask ventilation/wake patient if able); and PLAN D (needle/surgical cricothyroidectomy) before you start (see fig 11.7).[15] There are national failed intubation guidelines: www.das.uk.com Difficult Airway Society ►Adequate oxygenation is top priority: • Get senior help; *can't intubate, can't ventilate* is an emergency • Do not repeat the dose of suxamethonium: allow the relaxant to wear off while maintaining oxygenation. This scenario is vitally important and all junior anaesthetists must demonstrate that they can deal with this in a simulated setting before they are allowed to give anaesthetics without immediate senior supervision.

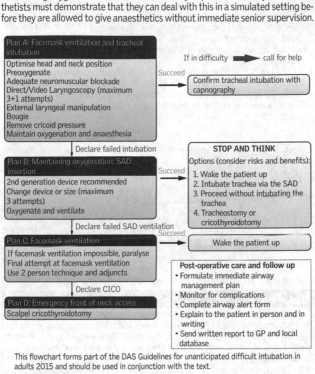

This flowchart forms part of the DAS Guidelines for unanticipated difficult intubation in adults 2015 and should be used in conjunction with the text.

Fig 11.7 Management of unanticipated difficult tracheal intubation in adults.

Reproduced from Frerk, C. et al. (2015). Difficult Airway Society 2015 guidelines for management of unanticipated difficult intubation in adults, *BJA: British Journal of Anaesthesia*, Volume 115, Issue 6, December 2015, Pages 827–848, https://doi.org/10.1093/bja/aev371.

11 Anaesthesia

Rapid sequence induction (RSI) This is the method of endotracheal intubation used in the emergency setting when the airway of an acutely unwell patient is threatened and the subsequent risk of aspiration is high (see also p. 648). ▶As patients are unlikely to be fasted, it relies on prompt induction and paralysis in order to minimize risk of aspiration. If haemodynamically unstable, take the time to resuscitate your patient to optimize their ability to cope with anaesthesia.

RSI: a quick overview
• Skilled assistant, tipping trolley, suction
• NGT and IV access
• Pre-oxygenate
• IV induction
• Fast-acting muscle relaxant
• Cricoid pressure
• ET intubation

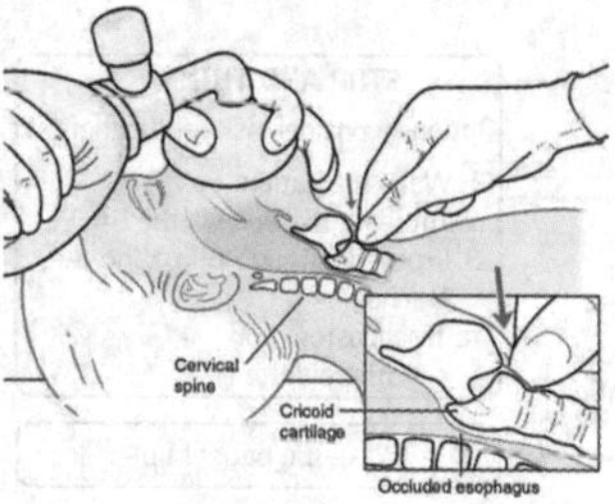

- Pre-oxygenate with 100% O_2 for 3min to provide an O_2 reservoir in the lungs for use during the period of induced apnoea.
- *Apply cricoid pressure* (fig 11.8) and give induction agent (eg propofol) then immediately give muscle relaxant (eg suxamethonium). Wait 60sec for muscle relaxant to work (patients will often twitch before relaxing).
- The trachea is then intubated and cuff inflated, cricoid pressure may be released once the anaesthetist is satisfied with ETT position and capnography has been confirmed, and a volatile agent added to maintain anaesthesia.
- Give a longer-acting muscle relaxant (ie non-depolarizing) when suxamethonium wears off.

Fig 11.8 You may be asked to apply cricothyroid pressure during an RSI. Apply firm backward pressure (aim for force of 10–30N) on the cricoid cartilage (used because it is a full ring of cartilage which can be pushed down) to occlude the oesophagus in an attempt to stop gastric reflux to the larynx. It is a skill to practise as poor placement of fingers will fail to occlude the oesophagus and pressure on the larynx may make intubation more difficult. Possible risks include disruption of cervical spine injuries and oesophageal injury. There is controversy over whether this pressure actually prevents aspiration.

Reproduced with permission of Goodman & Green 'Current Procedures Pediatrics' ©McGraw Hill.

11 Anaesthesia

Aspiration

Aspiration of foreign material into the respiratory tract can occur at any time around anaesthesia. It is unlikely to occur if a tracheal tube is *in situ* but may occur with supraglottic airway device (p. 666). ▶Aspiration is a much greater risk in emergency surgery, pregnancy, diabetes, and with a hiatus hernia, causing fatality in ~1 in 70,000 of all anaesthetics. It can be the result of passive regurgitation, or of active vomiting in the presence of reduced airway reflexes. If suspected (direct visualization at laryngoscopy, coughing, vomiting, laryngospasm, bronchospasm, SaO_2↓, tachypnoea, wheeze and crepitations on auscultation), then immediately do the following:
▶▶ Apply cricoid pressure (unless actively vomiting; risks oesophageal rupture).
▶▶ Use suction to clear the mouth of debris.
▶▶ Endotracheal intubation, use soft catheters to suction the upper airway.
▶▶ Refrain from ventilating while undertaking these procedures, providing oxygenation levels are acceptable (to prevent dispersion of aspirate).
▶▶ Empty the stomach with an NGT at the first available opportunity.
▶▶ Put the patient head down and in the left lateral position.
▶▶ Cancel surgery, unless it is for an emergency.
▶▶ Consider ongoing ventilatory support to ensure adequate oxygenation.
▶▶ Arrange a CXR. Further investigation may be needed eg bronchoscopy.

Preparation is the key. Assess the mouth/neck preoperatively.

Prediction of difficult intubation May be possible with assessment of the Mallampati classification (fig 11.9), thyromental and sternomental distances; these subjective predictive tests vary between users and should simply be employed as a guide.[16] Be prepared for a difficult airway even if the prediction has been for an easy intubation and vice versa.

Difficult intubation
• Obese
• Short neck
• Limited neck movement
• Receding chin/mandible
• Protruding teeth.
• Limited mouth opening

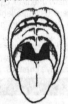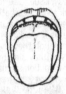

Fig 11.9 The Mallampati Test (with Samsoon and Young's modification). Examine the patient's oropharynx with the patient opening their mouth maximally and protruding their tongue without phonation. Class 1: soft palate and uvula visible. Class 2: uvula tip masked by base of tongue. Class 3: only soft palate visible. Class 4: soft palate not visible. When used alone it correctly predicts 50% of difficult laryngoscopies and has a false +ve rate of >90%.

Reproduced from Allman and Wilson, *Oxford Handbook of Anaesthesia*, 2016, with permission from OUP.

Technique Endotracheal tube (ETT) sizes (mm internal diameter, ID):

Adult ID: ♂ = 8.5mm, ♀ = 7.5mm *Children ID:* = [age in years/4] + 4.0mm
Length for child: Oral = [age /2] + 12.5cm. *Nasal* = [age/2] + 14.5cm

- Lubricate the tube, and check that its cuff and the laryngoscope work.
- Position the patient with neck flexed and head extended using a pillow.
- Hold the laryngoscope in the left hand; open the mouth with the right.
- Slide the blade down the right side of the tongue into the vallecula (area between tongue and epiglottis), guarding the lip and teeth with the fingers of your right hand. ▶*Do not lever on the teeth; you may damage them.*
- Lift the laryngoscope blade upwards and away from yourself.
- Lift the epiglottis from view: the cords should become visible. When they are, insert the tube with your right hand (anatomy—fig 11.6).
- Once the cuff of the ET tube is beyond the cords, remove the laryngoscope; ask the assistant to inflate the cuff to prevent air leak.
- Attach to the circuit. Gently inflate lungs. Watch the chest move. Do both sides move equally? Is the abdomen moving and not the chest (seen if oesophagus intubated)?
- Confirm placement with capnography, which detects CO_2.
- Auscultate both sides of the chest. Is air entry equal? Fix the tube with a tie.
- ▶*Remember: if in doubt, take it out.* Failure to intubate is not a cause of death, failure to oxygenate is! It is safer to reintubate than to risk leaving a tube in the oesophagus. Tubes may slip down a main bronchus (usually right). If so, withdraw until both sides of the chest move equally and air entry is equal (so avoiding collapse in the unventilated lung, or pneumothorax on the overventilated side).

If difficult intubation is predicted Use of video laryngoscope or awake fibreoptic laryngoscopy is recommended to guide ETT placement. Give mild sedation (see p. 661), an anticholinergic (to reduce secretions), and local anaesthesia to the nasal cavity and pharynx (not just for comfort, they will gag and cough too much without it; this distress could lead to loss of airway). Deep anaesthesia is only initiated once ET intubation confirmed (by vision and capnography).

If unable to intubate? See p. 669.

The most important cause of mortality and morbidity attributable to anaesthesia is associated with inadequate airway management. *Patients do not die from failure to intubate, they die from failure to ventilate.* The majority of cases are due to unexpected difficulty or poor preparation for patients with predicted difficulty. ▶Predicting barriers to rescue techniques (eg in obese patients it will be difficult to access the cricothyroid membrane) are just as important as planning for difficult intubation.[17]

Continuous monitoring of the patient under your care is essential. ▶▶Always call for help early while turning FiO$_2$ to 100%. First look for anaesthetic issues (airway issues are lethal faster), then surgical, and finally medical causes. Check for anaesthetic issues by starting from the patient (eg tube kinking/displacement), circuit (is it the correct one?), back to the anaesthetic machine (is it working properly?). Don't forget that you can touch your patient even though they are initially hidden by surgical drapes. Feel the pulses and skin; are they clammy? You should ideally always listen to a patient's chest after induction so that you can recognize acute intraoperative changes.

How to approach any perioperative problem

Ask yourself these questions when any problem arises:
• Anaesthetic:
  • Presence of hypoxia/hypercapnia?
  • Correct gas flow/volatile settings?
  • Is monitoring on properly?
  • Risk of awareness/pain?
  • Malignant hyperthermia?
• Surgical:
  • Reflex bradycardia following ocular/cervical/peritoneal stimulation?
  • Haemorrhage (may be hidden)?
• Medical:
  • Underlying disease (pulmonary/cardiac)?
  • Undiagnosed disease (phaechromocytoma)?
  • Biochemistry/haematology?

If unable to intubate? See p. 669 for the DAS guidelines.

Atelectasis and pneumonia Atelectasis is best seen on CT (not CXR). Starts within minutes of induction, and is partly caused by using 100% O$_2$. *R:* Good pain relief aids coughing. Arrange physiotherapy + antibiotics.

Tension pneumothorax Can arise when ventilating a patient with an undiagnosed spontaneous pneumothorax, emphysematous/bullous lung disease, or asthma (although all patients do have the risk of developing a pneumothorax during positive pressure ventilation). Risk is increased during use of nitrous oxide as this gas is less soluble than o$_2$ and quickly fills any gas filled space. Signs include hypoxia, 'silent chest' on auscultation, high airway pressures with difficulties in ventilation, ↑HR/↓BP. *Treatment:* Large-bore cannula in 2nd IC, mid-clavicular line followed by appropriate placement of a chest drain.

Awareness This is most distressing for patients and can lead to post-traumatic stress disorder. The patient can become aware of events during the operation; ~^{1}/$_2$ recollect conversations between theatre staff, ~^{1}/$_4$ feel the presence of the ETT, ~^{1}/$_3$ experience pain. *Incidence:* ~1:19,600 anaesthetics. It is more frequently reported in cardiac and obstetric surgery as they typically undergo lighter anaesthesia. Paralysis makes diagnosis difficult and relies on close monitoring (p. 668) for signs of physiological distress. Residual paralysis during emergence from anaesthesia can be perceived by patients as awareness.[18]

Wheeze First needs to be identified by pulmonary auscultation—it's easy to forget a patient exists under the drapes while your attention is held by focusing on the monitors. ΔΔ: Bronchospasm (see following topic); cardiac failure/pulmonary oedema, endobronchial (likely right bronchus) or oesophageal intubation, obstructed or displaced ETT, aspiration.

Bronchospasm If intubated, check tube position (carina stimulation may be the cause: withdraw tube slightly). Check for pneumothorax. Ventilate with 100% O_2. ↑ concentration of volatile agent if he is 'light'—most volatiles (esp. sevoflurane) are good bronchodilators. **Salbutamol** 250mcg IV ± **aminophylline** 250mg IV. **Magnesium sulfate** 2g IV may help. Give **hydrocortisone** 100mg IV. ▸▸**Anaphylaxis** See OHCM p795.

▸▸**Malignant hyperthermia** Rare, autosomal dominant, life-threatening condition triggered by exposure to suxamethonium or volatile anaesthetics. Suspect when there is unexpected ↑O_2 consumption, ↑CO_2, and ↑HR. Rapid temperature rise (>2°c/h) may be a late sign. *Treatment:* Hyperventilate with 100% O_2; maintain anaesthesia with IV agent; abandon surgery; muscle relaxant with *non-depolarizing muscle relaxant*. Give **dantrolene 2.5mg/kg IV** as initial bolus. Check for ↑K^+, arrhythmias; acidosis; myoglobinaemia; coagulopathy; ↑creatinine kinase. Take to ITU.[19]

Damage to teeth Occurs in around 1:4500 GA and is a risk even when the anaesthetist uses the appropriate technique with care. Dental damage is the leading cause for litigation against anaesthetists so ensure that your patient's dental hygiene is well documented in the preoperative assessment. Give patient information leaflets: 'Damage to teeth, lips and tongue'.[20] www.rcoa.ac.uk

Suxamethonium apnoea Rare. Abnormal cholinesterase leads to prolonged drug effect lasting 2–24h. Ventilate & sedate until relaxant effect wears off. Fresh frozen plasma (for plasma cholinesterase activity) can be offered but mostly this condition is self-limiting. Risk of awareness (p. 672).

Aspiration See p. 670.

Laryngospasm Reflex closure of the vocal cords resulting in partial or complete airway obstruction and potentially negative pressure pulmonary oedema. Frequently due to laryngeal stimulation (airway devices/secretion) but can also follow surgical stimulation (which is why the surgeons should always check with the anaesthetist before starting to ensure an adequate level of anaesthesia has been reached). Treat with 100% O_2, high PEEP, and a firm jaw-thrust. Deepening anaesthesia (±paralysis), intubation, and ventilation may be required.

Intraoperative hypoxia Review the delivered gas mixtures, ventilation settings (are they appropriate for your patient? Are you achieving parameters of tidal volumes, RR, and airway pressures that should be expected? ↑ airway pressures—think laryngospasm, bronchospasm), poor O_2 delivery (systemic hypoperfusion, emboli), or ↑O_2 demand (sepsis, malignant hyperthermia). Hypoxia can be multifactorial and time-consuming to diagnose; especially if associated with equipment. The priority is to provide adequate oxygenation and ventilation. ↑FIO_2 to 100% then examine the patient and equipment methodically.

Intraoperative hypotension Common and not always requiring immediate treatment. For example, induction agents will typically cause hypotension which is well tolerated in young and fit patients—the surgical stimulus will increase the BP without the need for vasopressors. Always double check any seemingly erroneous NIBP measurements as the BP cuff might have loosened etc. and always feel the pulse! Patients at risk of significant hypotension include those with pre-existing fluid deficits (eg D&V, haemorrhage, dehydration), sepsis, trauma, heart disease, any surgery associated with blood loss and obstructing venous return to the heart (eg mediastinal/hepatic surgery). ΔΔ: Haemorrhage (ask the surgeons if they suspect any occult loss), ↑ intrathoracic pressure (eg tension pneumothorax), anaphylaxis, and exacerbation of pre-existing CVS disease.

What to do at the end of anaesthesia

- Change inspired gasses to 100% O_2 then stop anaesthetic drug infusions. (Although it has been suggested that hyperoxia can be damaging.)[21]
- After ascertaining that adequate spontaneous reversal has occurred (use a peripheral nerve stimulator), reverse any residual muscle paralysis with **neostigmine** (~2.5mg in adults) + an anticholinergic to prevent muscarinic side effects (↓HR, salivation) eg **neostigmine** (2.5mg)/**glycopyrronium** (0.5mg).
- The process of extubation can be intimidating to watch the first time as patients often appear uncomfortable and distressed. Don't worry: they never remember this stage. It is important to ensure that the patient can obey commands and demonstrate muscle tone before you remove the ETT; extubating too early while the patient is in a very light plane of anaesthesia can result in challenging airway compromise (eg laryngospasm), see fig 11.10.
- Experienced anaesthetists will sometimes perform 'deep extubation' when the coughing/gagging associated with awake extubation is undesirable for the type of surgery (eg neurosurgery).
- If no problems, transfer to recovery, but be ready to reassess at any time

Low-risk patients

Tend to be well and fasted with uncomplicated airways. They typically undergo *awake extubation*. Once spontaneously breathing with adequate ventilation, inspect mouth and oropharynx under direct vision and suction as appropriate. Insert a bite block (e.g. rolled gauze). Remove ET tube by applying positive pressure, deflate the cuff and remove tube. Then administer oxygen by facemask for as much and for as long as necessary to counteract hypoxia due to diffusion hypoxia, respiratory depression, or ventilation/perfusion mismatch.[3]

At-risk patients

Include patients with multiple risk factors where the ability to oxygenate post extubation is uncertain and reintubation would be potentially challenging. The decision here is between immediate or delayed extubation (eg in ITU) using more advanced techniques.

Shivering

Be aware that shivering increases O_2 consumption 5-fold, although it is not a cause of clinically significant hypoxaemia since that in itself will ameliorate the shivering. Not always due to hypothermia. Treatment options include tramadol, nefopam.[22]

Recovery

- Patients will stay here until safe for transfer to the ward (alert and orientated, pain and nausea controlled, anaesthetist and surgeon satisfied).
- Look for hypoventilation (?inadequate reversal—check with nerve stimulator; narcosis—reverse opiates with naloxone *cautiously* to minimize pain; check for airway obstruction). Ensure adequate analgesia.
- Monitor temperature, HR, & BP; return the patient to the ward when you are satisfied with their cardiovascular and respiratory status and pain relief.
- Give clear instructions on postoperative fluid regimens, blood transfusions, oxygen therapy, pain relief, and physiotherapy.

11 Anaesthesia

Enhanced recovery after surgery (ERAS)

Aims to improve the physiological disruption and psychological distress of surgery. A notable difference in the preoperative assessment now is encouraging the patient to drink up to 2h prior to surgery. Key principles include the preoperative optimization of medical comorbidities, carbohydrate drinks 2h prior to surgery to avoid the metabolic state associated with fasting, careful intraoperative fluid management with use of minimally invasive surgical techniques when appropriate. Postoperative care focuses on early mobilization and prompt return to normal nutrition; this includes vigorous treatment of pain. There should be clear discharge instructions with an aim to get the patient home early, if not on the same day. ERAS programmes are effective in reducing length of hospital stays and complication rates in surgery.[23,24]

Prehabilitation

The value of optimizing patients before major surgery is increasingly recognized. Prehabilitation is the process of enhancing the functional capacity of an individual before surgery to enable him to better withstand the physiological stressors. The aim is to improve postoperative outcomes. Prehabilitation programmes typically last 4–8 weeks and include a tailored exercise programme, nutritional advice, psychological support, and optimization of any existing medical concerns.[25]

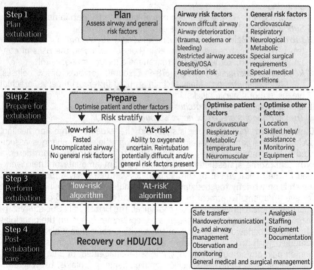

Fig 11.10 DAS extubation guidelines: basic algorithm.

Reproduced with permission from Popat, M. *et al*. (2012), Difficult Airway Society Guidelines for the management of tracheal extubation. *Anaesthesia*, 67: 318–340. doi:10.1111/j.1365-2044.2012.07075.x. Anaesthesia © 2012 The Association of Anaesthetists of Great Britain and Ireland.

---

3 For a short duration (<5min) while very soluble nitrous oxide is diffusing out of the circulation into the alveoli, the concentration of O_2 in alveolar gas will be falling (diffusion hypoxia).

Analgesia promotes well-being, sleep, and facilitates recovery or, in the case of palliative medicine (*OHCM* p532), the easeful passage into oblivion. Pain relief also aids physiotherapy (allowing coughing and mobility), preventing pneumonia. Pain also exacerbates hypo/hyperventilation, hypertension, and tachycardia, and can lead to urinary retention.

Methods of analgesia (See *OHCM* p574 and *OHCM* p532.)

1 *Oral:* Try paracetamol 1g/6h—then:
- NSAIDs: **naproxen** 250mg–500mg/12h (remember danger of GI bleed; cover with PPI; caution in asthma). Effects on renal function are minimal if pre-op U&E is normal[28] but be cautious if hypovolaemic.
- **Tramadol** 50–100mg/4–6h PO/IV. Fewer SE than morphine, but less potent.
- *Opioids* eg codeine, morphine sulfate solution. NB: most are poorly absorbed from the gut.
- *Neuropathic agents* eg gabapentin for neuropathic pain associated with complex regional pain syndrome (CRPS, p.529) or diabetic/vascular neuralgia. See *BNF* section 4.8.1.

2 *Sublingual:* **Buprenorphine** (an uncommonly used synthetic opiate; 'controlled' drug): 0.4mg/6h sublingually, or buccal fentanyl drops/lozenges.

3 *Inhalational:* Nitrous oxide/oxygen (Entonox®), useful for labour pains, changing dressings, and physiotherapy.

4 *Intramuscular:* Rarely used—eg **morphine** 10mg IM; **pethidine** 100mg IM.

5 *Subcutaneous:* Used in palliative care eg diamorphine.

6 *Intravenous:* Boluses or continuous infusion. Patient-controlled analgesia (PCA). The patient can give themselves boluses, avoiding the risks of continuous infusion. Remember to programme a maximum dose limit.

7 *Regional anaesthesia (RA):* (pp. 678–9) Epidurals (opiates, or LA, boluses, or continuous infusion). Many techniques used (intercostal nerve, brachial plexus, femoral nerve blocks).

8 *Transcutaneous opioid patches.*

9 *Transcutaneous electrical nerve stimulation (TENS).*

Chronic pain Pain that persists beyond the expected time for healing, such that the continuous pain causes pathophysiological changes associated with complex disease processes rather than pain simply considered a symptom. Some anaesthetists dedicate significant amounts of their workload to the management of chronic pain; it is an extremely important topic which is only briefly touched upon here. No single treatment will be effective for every patient. Treatment may be broadly categorized into 3 categories—pharmacological, physical, and psychological. The British Pain Society recommends individualized pain management programmes based on the principles of cognitive behavioural therapy for those with chronic pain which cannot be remedied with drug and physical treatments alone. These consist of education on pain physiology, psychology, and self-management of pain problems.[27] Pharmacological treatments include simple analgesia, opioids, tricyclic antidepressants, neuropathic pain medicines (eg gabapentin), and regional anaesthetic techniques. Interventions which may help certain patients include acupuncture and hypnosis.

Pain in the pre-hospital environment See pp. 638–9 & pp. 648–9 for analgesia in the pre-hospital environment.

Further reading

Pergolizzi Jr JV *et al.* (2014). The WHO pain ladder: do we need another step? *Pract Pain Manage* 14. http://www.practicalpainmanagement.com/resources/who-pain-ladder-do-we-need-another-step
SIGN (2013). *Management of Chronic Pain* (SIGN 136). Edinburgh: SIGN.

Postoperative nausea and vomiting (PONV)

PONV is one of the most unpleasant side effects imposed by anaesthesia. Scoring systems such as the Apfel score[28] allow risk to be quantified. 1 point is scored for each of: • Female sex • History of PONV/motion sickness • Non-smoker • Opiates planned postoperatively. Scores of 0 = 10% vs 4 points = 78% probability.

Control symptoms to optimize patient comfort and minimize post-op complications. PONV is the most common cause of delayed discharge after surgery.

- Electrolyte imbalance and dehydration.
- Pulmonary aspiration.
- Wound dehiscence or bleeding.
- Damage to site of surgery (direct, eg ENT, or indirect, eg neurosurgery).
- Inability to take oral medication.

The exact mechanisms of action for all the factors involved (see MINIBOX 'PONV risk factors') are unknown, though the central mechanisms behind the vomiting reflex are somewhat better understood. It is initiated in the vomiting centre of the medulla (fig 11.11), which itself receives input from higher centres, the chemoreceptor trigger zone (CTZ), afferent somatic and visceral fibres, and the vestibular apparatus of the middle & inner ear. Of these, the CTZ in the area postrema (located in the floor of the 4th ventricle) is probably the most important as it is exposed to drugs not crossing the blood–brain barrier.

PONV risk factors
Patient factors:
• Female (3× risk)
• Previous history
• Obesity
• Motion sickness
• Preoperative anxiety
Anaesthetic agents:
• Opioids
• Nitrous oxide (N_2O)
• Etomidate/ketamine
• Volatile agents
NB: total IV anaesthesia with propofol ↓ PONV
Surgery type:
• GI/GU/Gynae
• Neurosurgery
• Middle ear
• Ophthalmic
Post-op factors:
• Dehydration
• Hypotension
• Hypoxia
• Early oral intake

11 Anaesthesia

For specific antiemetics see OHCM p251. Neurokinin 1 (NK1) receptor antagonists, eg **aprepitant** (80mg PO, given 3h prior to anaesthesia), are a new class of antiemetics which appear more effective than 5-HT3 antagonists (eg ondansetron). Non-pharmacological approaches such as P6 acupuncture point stimulation are effective[29] and ginger may help.

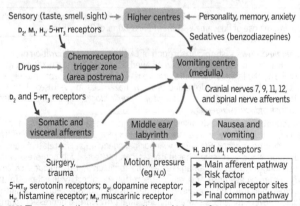

Fig 11.11 The neural pathways, receptor sites, and triggers for PONV.

Further reading

PONV calculator: http://daysurgeryuk.net/en/resources/ponv-calculator/

RA is broadly split into peripheral nerve blocks (PNBs) (table 11.2) or neuraxial anaesthesia. The aim is to reduce nerve conduction of painful impulses to higher centres, where the perception of pain occurs. It is used either alone or to supplement general anaesthesia (GA) by providing prolonged and effective post-operative analgesia. Regional anaesthesia is especially useful for operations on the lower limbs and abdomen where avoidance of a GA is desirable due to medical comorbidities (notably cardiac & pulmonary). ▶Regional techniques may still lead to loss of airway and so require the same resuscitation facilities as for a GA.

Continual regional anaesthesia Involves placement of a catheter near the nerve to allow continuous delivery of local anaesthetic, as compared to a single dose.

Locating peripheral nerves Requires sound knowledge of anatomical landmarks. Historically, nerves were located by direct nerve stimulation with the needle (invoking a sensory or motor response), but visualization with US or use of peripheral nerve stimulators is now common to minimize nerve trauma and maximize success rates.[30]

Types of local anaesthetic (LA) agents

1 **Lidocaine:** max. dose in healthy adult=3mg/kg IBW. A rapid onset of action with a relatively short duration. 1% or 2% frequently used to infiltrate the skin prior to line insertion.
2 **Prilocaine** ($t\frac{1}{2}$=2h): moderate onset. Dose is 3–5mg/kg IBW. Max. 400mg.
3 **Bupivacaine** ($t\frac{1}{2}$=3h): slow onset and prolonged duration. More cardiotoxic than others. Dose for local infiltration is 2mg/kg IBW to a max of 150mg.
4 **Levobupivacaine** (isomer of bupivacaine) is less cardiotoxic. Dose for local infiltration or peripheral nerve block: 2mg/kg (max. 150mg). Use <150mg (use 5–7.5mg/mL solution) for epidural; <15mg for intrathecal.
5 **Ropivacaine** ($t\frac{1}{2}$=1.8h): Dose: 3mg/kg IBW. Less cardiotoxic than bupivacaine. Less motor block when used epidurally.
6 **Tetracaine** ($t\frac{1}{2}$=1h): Slow onset. High toxicity. Eye drops for topical anaesthesia, and now topically (Ametop®) as an alternative to EMLA®. Also available as a gel (combined with adrenaline & lidocaine) for open wounds.

NB: 0.5% solution=5mg/mL. 1% solution=10mg/mL. So for a 70kg man, the maximum dose of lidocaine is 20mL of 1% or 10mL of 2% solution.

Adrenaline slows systemic absorption of LA (thus increases duration of LA effect) + alters maximum dose of LA allowed. It is useful in areas of increased vascularity (eg intercostal blocks) where risk of systemic absorption is higher. Systemic effects from adrenaline are esp. hazardous in CVS disease or ↑BP. ▶Adrenaline is contraindicated in digital or penile blocks, and around the nose/ears (risk of local ischaemia).

Complications *Failure* is user and procedure dependent, always have a backup which is likely to be GA. *Nerve injury* is rare and tends to settle within weeks if it does occur. *Bleeding:* ▶Abnormal coagulation is a relative contraindication since even small haematomas can cause enough compression to cause long-term nerve damage, especially for neuraxial techniques. LA *toxicity:* From excess dose, too rapid absorption, or direct IV injection. Initial features: perioral tingling; numb tongue; anxiety; lightheadedness; tinnitus. Signs of severe toxicity: seizures; apnoea; direct myocardial depression; coma. ▶▶Stop injection of LA ▶Call for help and follow national protocol which guides the use of lipid emulsion (Intralipid®).[31] This may work by binding to the LA and thus reducing the amount of free LA in the circulation. If in circulatory arrest manage with standard ALS protocols plus Intralipid®. Recovery from LA-induced cardiac arrest may take >1h. *Seizures:* Benzodiazepines/propofol/thiopental in small incremental doses.

11 Anaesthesia

Table 11.2 Specific peripheral blocks and their uses

Block type	Examples of use
Cervical plexus	Carotid endarterectomy
Interscalene (brachial plexus)	Shoulder surgery (good prolonged post-op analgesia)
Axillary block	Hand/forearm surgery
Lumbosacral plexus (psoas compartment block)	Hip surgery (combined with a sciatic nerve block)
Ilioinguinal–iliohypogastric nerve	Inguinal hernia repair
Femoral nerve (see 'Further reading')	Femoral fracture, knee surgery (when combined with a sciatic block)
Sciatic nerve	Surgery below the knee
Popliteal & saphenous nerves	Ankle or foot surgery

►Ensure that the anaesthetized area is positioned and protected sufficiently both intra- and postoperatively to avoid injury.

Transversus abdominal plane (TAP) nerve block

This block is frequently used as part of the analgesic regimen for any surgery on the lower abdomen involving the anterior abdominal wall. **Anatomy** The anterior abdominal wall comprises of 3 key muscle layers: external oblique (EO) (most superficial), internal oblique (IO), and transversus abdominis (TA) muscle (most internal). Sensory innervation is composed of the anterior rami of T7–L1. **Target** Aim to deliver the LA to lie in the plane between IO and TA since this is where the sensory nerves travel through to reach the abdominal wall. Place the US probe midway between the costal margin and iliac crest; the needle should pierce the skin just above the iliac crest through the triangle of Petit (figs 11.12 & 11.13). In this lateral position, the EO muscle is still present as fascia so you will feel 2 'pops' as the needle passes through EO and IO to enable LA injection (volume is more important than concentration to encourage spread to as many nerves as possible) between IO and TA. A catheter is often left for continuous analgesia.

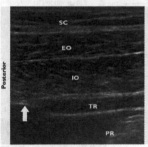

Fig 11.12 US is an essential piece of equipment for siting a TAP block.

Reproduced from Warman *et al*, *Regional Anaesthesia, Stimulation, and Ultrasound Techniques* (2014) with permission from OUP.

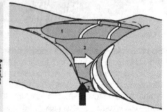

Fig 11.13 Diagram to indicate the markings of the lumbar triangle of Petit. 1 rectus abdominis muscle; 2 external oblique muscle; 3 latissimus dorsi muscle; 4 iliac crest; white arrow, inferior costal margin; black arrow, lumbar triangle of Petit.

Reproduced from Warman *et al*, *Regional Anaesthesia, Stimulation, and Ultrasound Techniques* (2014) with permission from OUP.

Further reading

Bogacz A *et al.* (2012). Femoral nerve block – a guide for medical students and junior doctors. *Scot Univ Med J* 1:185–91.

New York School of Regional Anaesthesia: www.nysora.com

11 Anaesthesia

Spinal and epidural anaesthesia are the 2 key neuraxial techniques. The spinal cord terminates at ~L1 in adults (L3 in children). Ideally, injection should take place at level L3/L4. Take great care above this as research suggests that we are poor at judging vertebral levels through palpation—most clinicians overestimate the height. Palpate the iliac crests with your fingertips and your thumbs should meet in the middle over L4/L5 space (Tuffier's line). See p. 477 for surface anatomy of the back. USS is increasingly used to improve accuracy of level location.

General considerations for safety

Imperative in all RA techniques, but especially in neuraxial blocks as haemodynamic compromise can happen quickly even if it's in the right place; have full monitoring on and IV access with fluids running before you start. Have quick access to resuscitation equipment (see pp. 678–9 for LA toxicity). A trained assistant should be present. Position the patient upright on the bed with their legs resting on a stool in front (the left lateral position is possible in special circumstances). Coaching the patient into proper positioning will greatly enhance chances for success! (Shoulders and hips square with the bed, back curled 'like an angry cat' with the lumbar portion pushed back towards the anaesthetist). Be kind and acknowledge this position is uncomfortable for the labouring woman or the elderly with a hip fracture. All neuraxial blocks require a full surgical scrub and sterile field using 0.5% chlorhexidine to clean the back (not 2% as fears over neurotoxicity).[32] Infiltrate the skin with 2% lidocaine (typically 2–5mL, but more if pain reported by the patient).

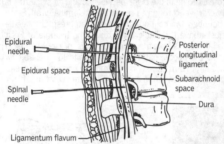

Epidural needle

Epidural space

Spinal needle

Ligamentum flavum

Posterior longitudinal ligament

Subarachnoid space

Dura

Fig 11.14 Subarachnoid and epidural spaces.
Reproduced from Allman et al. Oxford Handbook of Anaesthesia (2016), with permission from OUP.

So which layers does the needle pass through?

(fig 11.14) Both epidural and spinal needles pass through: skin, subcutaneous fat, supraspinous ligament, interspinous ligament, ligamentum flavum, epidural space (epidural needle stops here), dura mater, arachnoid mater, subarachnoid space (spinal needle stops here). The epidural space lies outside the meninges and contains nerve roots, venous plexus, fat, and lymphatics. The subarachnoid space is the space between pia mater and arachnoid mater and contains cerebrospinal fluid (CSF).

Spinal anaesthesia

Anaesthetic into the **subarachnoid space** (fig 11.15). The aim is to anaesthetize the spinal roots passing through here.

A small total drug concentration is required—producing sympathetic blockade (vasodilation, ↓BP), sensory blockade (numbness) and finally motor blockade (↓ or absence of lower limb power).

Complications of spinal anaesthesia: • Total spinal block (↓BP, ↓HR, anxiety, apnoea, LOC) • Headache • Urinary retention • Permanent neurological damage (very rare).

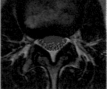

Fig 11.15 Approximation of the subarachnoid space in red on this T2-weighted MRI. Note spinal nerve roots.
Courtesy of Norwich Radiology Department.

Epidural anaesthesia
This is anaesthetic into the *epidural space* (fig 11.16). Insertion of indwelling catheter allows prolonged instillation of LA and/or opiates. Larger volumes of LA are required than with spinal anaesthesia as the epidural space is bigger. Opioids enhance sensory and not motor block. Lumbar most common site, but cervical/thoracic possible (requires greater skill).

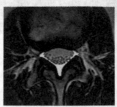

Fig 11.16 Approximation of the extradural space in yellow on this T2-weighted MRI.

Courtesy of Norwich Radiology Department.

Complications of epidural anaesthesia
Dural puncture: <1%. CSF leak may not be obvious; hence the importance of test dose. Push oral fluids, with caffeine. Nurse flat. Give analgesics for headache, laxatives to prevent constipation/straining. Blood patch is usually necessary if headache lasts >24–48h, most patients benefit after the 1st blood patch, nearly all after the 2nd.[33] *Vessel puncture and inadvertent injection:* Treat with ABC remembering: O_2, IVI, pressor drugs, atropine if bradycardia (due to block of sympathetic outflow to heart T2–4). *Hypoventilation:* Motor block of intercostals; may need control of ventilation. *'Total spinal':* ie injection of a large epidural dose into the CSF. Marked hypotension. Apnoea. Loss of consciousness. Treatment: ABC resuscitation and 100% O_2. Treat ↓BP. ▶▶*Death will occur from asphyxia if treatment is not prompt. Epidural haematoma or abscess:* Aim for early diagnosis to prevent permanent CNS damage. ▶▶Get emergency neurological review and MRI. *Other:* Patchy or unilateral block. Nerve root damage.

Benefits of epidural anaesthesia
See pp. 64–5 for obstetric epidurals. Epidurals are frequently sited in the awake patient prior to major abdominal surgery to provide effective intra- and postoperative analgesia. Early recovery of mobilization, gut function, and sleep patterns have demonstrated benefits (see p. 675). Epidurals facilitate analgesia on movement and at rest, attenuation of the surgical stress response as the sympathetic nerve supply from the surgical site is blocked, and subsequent reduced incidence of ileus. The latter may be associated with a lower opiate requirement. Overall there are reduced pulmonary, cardiovascular, and thromboembolic complications too when epidural analgesia is used.[34]

GA or RA?
This depends on type of surgery (can the surgical site be fully anaesthetized by RA?), patient preference, and comorbidities (note that RA typically offers more haemodynamic stability and less pulmonary complications). The options include RA with no sedation, RA with sedation to improve tolerance, and RA supplemented with GA (such as a shoulder block during arthroscopy under GA to reduce the stress response and post-op pain). Abdominal, pelvic, and lower limb surgery are ideal for regional techniques (eg hernia repair, THR). There is no demonstrated difference in 30-day mortality between RA/GA in hip fracture surgery.[35] In day-case surgery the priority is to avoid delays in discharge home—epidurals are inappropriate as analgesic onset is too slow; spinals should be done early on the list to ensure full neurological recovery by the end of the day.

Absolute contraindications to all neuraxial anaesthesia:
1 Anticoagulant states (the risk is pressure damage to cord from bleed—there is an extensive local vertebral venous plexus).
2 Local sepsis (risk of introducing infection to CSF).
3 Shock or hypovolaemic states (effective reduction in circulating volume due to vasodilatation).
4 Raised intracranial pressure (→coning).
5 Unwilling or uncooperative patient.
6 Fixed output states (eg mitral and aortic stenosis).

11 Anaesthesia

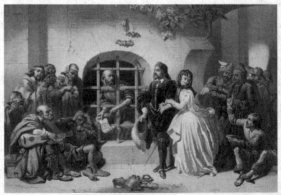

Fig 12.1 The lunatic asylum: Salomon de Caus incarcerated in the mental asylum of Bicêtre.

With many thanks to Lorna Hobbs and Jayne Kavangh, our specialist readers for the Gender identity section, and junior reader Paul Hanna for their contribution to this chapter.

In 1656, King Louis XIV founded the Pitié-Salpêtrière Hospital in Paris. It was built for the treatment of 'prostitutes and the mentally defective'. On the eve of the Revolution, it had become the world's largest hospital, housing over 10,000 patients (plus 300 prisoners). Up until this point, the only place a person suffering from mental health difficulties could seek help outside of their community was the church, eg the Priory of the Order of St Mary of Bethlem (now the Royal Bethlem Hospital, previously 'Bedlam Hospital'). While these places were rat-infested, bureaucratic, and expensive, it was the start of something new: treating mental health difficulties as illness not criminality (or evil—see p. 684).

Almost 200 years later, The Lunacy Act, 1845 was passed in the UK. This explicitly changed the status of those with mental health difficulties to patients who required treatment. This Act of Parliament coincided with the development of alienism, now known as psychiatry, as a medical specialty. At the same time, the Age of Enlightenment helped shift attitudes towards 'lunatics' and it was accepted that compassionate treatment would aid in the rehabilitation of 'the victim'. Slowly, mental health difficulties were seen as something which could be treated, perhaps even cured.

The lunatic asylum, as a place where patients could be kept to protect the public, and themselves, from danger, was commonplace. Patients were routinely physically restrained in dark, poorly ventilated rooms without access to outside spaces, choice, or visits from their family. In 1797, Bicêtre Hospital's governor first freed patients of their chains and banned physical punishment. He allowed patients to move freely around hospital grounds and replaced the 'dark dungeons' with sunny, airy rooms. With this, he aimed to treat each patient's 'excessive exposure to social and psychological stresses'—or as we would think of it today, their holistic needs.

Over time, these asylums became regulated with government inspections, written regulations, and the need for a resident qualified doctor. Often universities took a role in management and treatment, and through this, the focus changed to more recognizably therapeutic activities for patients including writing, group activity, and art, alongside more traditional medical interventions such as psychopharmacology, psychotherapy, and ECT. But asylums were still problematic places and by the beginning of the 20th century there was serious overcrowding, underfunding, and abuse. This led to deinstitutionalization: long-stay psychiatric hospitals were replaced with less isolated community mental health services. Patients were cared for at home, clinics and general hospitals and these large institutions were closed down (or sold off and repackaged as luxury flats).

The role of the asylum is a complex one. Initially they were considered progressive and empowering, a place for people with mental health difficulties to be treated, not imprisoned. With this, they became overloaded and impractical, albeit with good intentions, and now the name itself—or its synonyms 'loony bin', 'funny farm', 'madhouse', etc.—is tainted. However, at their best, asylums were an attempt to find a way to help people when there wasn't an understanding of what was happening or a language to explain what was wanted. It may be that 200 years from now, we will look back at some of the current treatments or approaches across psychiatry (or all of medicine) and wonder why we offered such crude systems of help.

Mental illness In the 1400s, people held the impression that physical illnesses were natural and mental illnesses were supernatural. As this became entrenched in society, it was found necessary to legally define what comprised witchcraft, possession, and insanity. The book, *Malleus Maleficarum* (or the *Witches' Hammer*) was written in 1489 and quickly became the authority for witch identification. It was so popular that 10 editions were produced over the next 150 years. Thomas Szasz[1] describes this as the 'scapegoat theory of witchcraft'—the human tendency to try to master human problems and social conflicts, often through organized persecution (fig 12.2).

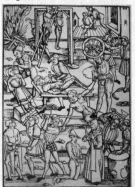

It was Johann Weyer, a Dutch doctor, occultist, and demonologist who challenged this belief. Born in 1515 (2015 marks his 500th anniversary), he described 'melancholy' in women accused of practising witchcraft and became the 'founder of modern psychiatry'. It wasn't well received. The political philosopher Jean Bodin wrote that he 'should stick to examining urine rather than intruding into the lofty territories of theology and jurisprudence'.

Weyer, in his book *De Praestigiis Daemonum*, said that these 'witches'—shunned and punished by society'—actually had 'disorders of the senses'. From this approach, he illustrated several different 'melancholies', including those *melancholics* who 'fear death, and yet sometimes they choose death by committing suicide'. He theorized that when the 'melancholic humour seizes control of the brain it alters the mind'. Where society saw a supernatural

Fig 12.2 Punishments for witchcraft in 16th-century Germany.
Woodcut from Tengler's *Laienspiegel*, 1508.

evil, Weyer saw suffering. It is this legacy that we should continue to explore.

Empathy As well as showing empathy, we should give our patients respect and protect their dignity—not the dignity that they deserve but the dignity that confirms to our patients that, mad, bad, or rambling, they are just as human as their doctors despite their suffering. Let patients:
- Decide on modes of address, 'Mr Pettifer' may be preferred to 'John, dear'. Dignity entails giving choices, and then respecting them.
- Know who we are (eg wear a name badge). But don't label patients ('Go and see the new schizophrenic on Amber ward'). If you put a patient in a box the next thing you'll do is put a lid on it and stop thinking.
- Participate in their treatment plans; explain about common side effects.
- Choose whether to see students or take part in research.
- Have personal and private space to keep their belongings, and to have a space to be in whether alone, or with visitors.
- Wear their own clothes. Clothe them decently if they have none.
- Know what to do if a crisis develops. It's a great help to know that you will be seen in 4 hours rather than be left to stagnate all weekend.

People claimed that Weyer 'must be a wizard in league with the devil to have shown such sympathy with witches'. But these 7 points are congruent with NICE and Human Rights law which lay out the right to life, freedom from inhuman or degrading treatment and torture, respect for privacy, the right to a fair hearing, and freedom of expression. Some of these rights are inalienable and irrevocable. Hopefully things have moved forward in the last 500 years.

1 Thomas Szasz is a psychiatrist who is best known as a strong critic of the moral and scientific foundations of psychiatry (often called an anti-psychiatrist). He has described Weyer as the founder of a system which 'confines and silences troublesome individuals'. It is interesting to read Szasz's arguments regarding psychiatry and its place in the modern world, but perhaps wait until after you have finished the chapter …

12 Psychiatry

Suspending judgement We want our patients to achieve insight. Our judging does not help this. Judgement turns patients away from us. We cannot expect them to be honest with us if they know we are judging them.

- The good listener is not silent, but reflective—a mirror not a message. Mirrors do not judge but they enable self-judgement. If a mirror is a reflective listener, a silent listener would be a void rather than a message. This is about 'active listening'.
- Unless some criminal act is underway, it really does not matter what we think about our patients. What matters is how the patient thinks about him- or herself and their near-ones—and how these thoughts can be transformed.
- If we judge people they will not trust us. No trust ≈ no therapeutic alliance.
- If we judge, patients will leave us for others perhaps less well qualified.
- There is no evidence that judging improves outcomes. Worse outcomes are likely if the patient feels alienated.
- Patients know if we think negatively of them. They may internalize this, and assume that things will always be bad because they themselves are bad.

Despite these bullets, there is a problem that won't go away. If we find ourselves talking to perpetrators rather than victims, we may not be wise to suspend judgement forever. If a crime is afoot putting others at risk, you may need to break confidentiality. Discuss this with a colleague.

Whenever you think the time may have come to judge, check with yourself that it is not from outrage or disgust, and not through the exercise of pride or from a position of power that you are judging—but reluctantly, and from duty. Unless we exercise judgement, it might be thought, we may be condoning evil. 'For evil to flourish in the world, all that is required is for the good to remain silent.' What human duties do doctors have which trump anything that goes on in the consulting room? We must be human first, and physician-scientists second. Or as Weyer pleaded, 'let the judgement of the physicians be consulted—physicians are renowned for their understanding of natural objects and the properties thereof'.

Recovery Quite a few doctors hope to *make* patients better by taking responsibility for ordering their internal world and the credit when things go well. In psychiatry this approach is wrong. Mental health is about people (not patients) taking responsibility for themselves and their programme of change. The psychiatrist knows that their job is done, not when the patient is cured but when they become self-actuating, insightful, and interact with the world in creative (not necessarily satisfactory) ways.

'Why am I as I am? To understand that of any person, his whole life, from birth must be reviewed. All of our experiences fuse into our personality. Everything that ever happened to us is an ingredient.'

Malcolm X, *The Autobiography of Malcolm X*

On starting psychiatry you may feel unskilled. A medical problem will come as a relief—you know what to do. Do not be discouraged: you already have plenty of skills (which you will take for granted) to build on. Anyone who has sat an important exam knows what anxiety is like, and anyone who has passed one knows how to master anxiety, at least to some extent. We have all survived periods of being 'down'. While not the same as clinical anxiety or depression, these experiences allow us to develop the psychiatric skills of respect and empathy and a curiosity to ask how we have recovered and how others might too.

The first element is *time*. Simply waiting for time to go by is an important psychotherapeutic principle. (Voltaire teasingly remarked that the role of the doctor is to amuse the patient until nature effects a cure.) Of course, there are instances when waiting for time to go by leads to fatal consequences. But this does not prevent the principle from being useful.

Another skill which we are all able to use is *listening*. One of the central tenets of psychiatry is that it helps our patients just to be listened to. Just as we all are helped by talking and sharing our problems, so this may in itself be of immense help to our patients, especially if they have been isolated, and feel alone—which is a very common experience.

Both spontaneous improvement and relapse are common occurrences in psychiatry as many mental disorders go through a relapsing/remitting course. To understand this, we need to have *humility*, an essential psychiatric skill. Our current understanding of mental illness and the mind (not the brain) remains limited. While psychopharmacology and therapy can significantly benefit some patients, to consider them a 'cure' is naive. Often the best management is to support each individual through a difficult time, reducing the duration of their illness while trying to minimize the harm done to their health, relationships, and life. Every management plan should be *holistic,* including psychological therapy and social support alongside biological therapy. Looking through the admissions register of any acute psychiatric ward is likely to show that the same people keep on being readmitted. In one sense, this is a failure of the processes of psychiatry, but in another sense each (carefully planned) discharge is a success, and a complex infrastructure often exists for maintaining the patient in the community. These include group support meetings, group therapy sessions, and social trips out of the hospital. For those with a chronic condition, the concept of 'recovery' is important—rather than removing symptoms this can mean living well, with purpose and meaning, in spite of their symptoms.

So taking time, listening, and thinking holistically are our chief skills, and with these simple devices much can be done to rebuild the bridges between the patient and their outside world. These skills are simple compared with highly elaborate skills such as psychoanalysis and psychopharmacology for which psychiatry is famous. The point of bringing them to the fore is so that the newcomer to psychiatry need not feel that there is a great weight of theoretical work to get through before they start doing psychiatry. You can engage in the central process of psychiatry from day 1. In fact, with the exception of specific knowledge about conditions and treatments, the skills that make a good psychiatrist are not specific to psychiatry. Rather they are they skills that define a good communicator, and a caring, empathic, and effective doctor.

Talking and listening

Taking a history sounds like an active, inquisitorial process, with lists of questions, and the tone of our page on this process (see p. 688) and mental state examination (see p. 690) seems to perpetuate this error. It isn't a question of *taking* anything. It's more about *receiving* the history, and allowing it to unfold. If you only ask questions, you will get only answers as replies.

As the history unfolds, sit back and listen. This sounds easy, but during a busy or difficult day you will find your mind wandering (or galloping away)—over the last patient, the next patient, or some aspect of your own life. You may find yourself worrying about having to 'section' this patient or see the relatives afterwards. By an act of Zen, banish extraneous thought, and concentrate totally on the person in front of you—as if your life depended on it. Concentrate on the whole person—the language, the words, the non-verbal cues, and get drawn into their world. Initially don't even think of applying diagnostic labels. Open your mind and let everything flood in. Listening is hard. We wish we did it better. We all need to practise it more. Listening enables patients to start to trust us. Depressed patients often believe they will never get better. To believe that they can get better, patients need to trust us, and this trust often starts the therapeutic process. In general, the more we listen, the more we are trusted. Our patients' trust can be one of our chief motivations, at best inspiring us to pursue their benefit with all vigour.

Avoid interruptions and seeming to be too purposeful, at least for the first few minutes. Expect periods of silence. If prompts are needed try 'and then how did you feel?' or just 'and then … '; or repeat the last words the patient spoke. Don't be anxious if the patient is not covering major areas in the history. Lead on to these later, as the interview unfolds. Early in your career you will have to ask the relevant questions (p. 688) in a rather bald way (if the information is not forthcoming during the initial unstructured minutes), but it is important to go through this stage as a prelude to gaining information by less intrusive methods. Always keep in mind the chief aims of making a diagnosis, defining problems, and establishing a therapeutic relationship.

Even if we all listen the same way, what we will hear will depend on our own expectations, anxieties, and past experience. Listening, not judging. So often when we listen, the fact that we are also judging leaks out in an unconscious disapproving gaze—and our patient clams up.

The first meeting …

The mnemonic FIRST can help when you meet a new patient:

Frank conversation about why they came in today. What changed? Let the patient tell you about their problems in their own words—validate their concerns. Consider the sense of fear and isolation they may feel in this new environment.

Individualize your care for every patient through active listening, empathy, and appropriate questioning. Everyone should have a say in their own treatment.

Reach out to the patient's family and friends for collateral information and for support; get them to think about the strengths and skills in your patient.

Use Somatic symptoms to engage that person—many find it easier to talk about physical symptoms than emotional ones (partly due to the stigma attached to mental health).

Tease out which psychiatric symptoms are important. Keep a high index of suspicion to rule out medical conditions without medicalizing the situation.

Introduce yourself; explain how long the assessment may take. Describe its aim; emphasize that 'this is a safe place to talk'. Find out how they came to be referred, and what their expectations are. If they deny any problems or are reluctant to start talking, don't hurry. It is important to take what they say seriously and include the content that they bring to the consultation. Try asking 'How are you?', 'What has been happening to you?', 'Does anyone else think there is a problem?' These are beautiful questions because they don't impose categories. Hearing what your patient brings unprompted, will often tell you plenty. Listen, without interrupting, noting relevant information but also give eye contact and establish a rapport. Don't make judgements, challenges, or interpretations at this point, just gather information.

Presenting symptoms Agree a problem list with the patient early on, and check it is comprehensive, eg by asking 'If we were able to deal with all these, would things then be all right?' Then take each problem in turn and find out about onset, duration, effects on life and family; events coinciding with onset; solutions tried; reasons why they failed. Next enquire about mood and beliefs during the last weeks (this differs from the mental state examination (p. 690), which is the mental state at the time of interview). Specifically check for suicidal thoughts, plans, or actions—the more specific these are, the greater the danger. Discussing suicide does not increase the danger. Once you have a thorough understanding of the patient's perspective of their problems, you might need to ask specific questions about particular symptoms to help you reach a diagnosis. At this point 'soft' skills are no longer adequate and a structured approach to history taking is needed, requiring specific knowledge about which symptoms support a particular diagnosis. Specific examples are given in the box 'Specific questions to ask'.

The present Find out about their current situation. Housing, finance, work, relationships: Where do they live? With whom? Do they work? How is their home and work life? Are they facing any danger, threat, police action? How do they spend their time? Has this changed because of their symptoms? Relationships are often very important in mental disorder and changes in these can result in a presentation to mental health services.

Birth and development Particularly for younger patients, but helpful for everyone to consider how they have developed. Ask about school, further education, and employment history. What were their significant relationships (sexual and friendships) and relationship style(s)? Think about social life: play and hobbies. Have they always been shy and lonely, or do they make friends easily? In life, what stress have they had and how have they coped with it?

Premorbid personality Before all this happened, how were they? Happy-go-lucky or driven, tense or laid-back, social or antisocial? How would others describe them? Impulsive, fussy, irritable, shy? Talk to whoever accompanies them, to illumine premorbid personality and their view of current problems.

Relevant past history Including *psychiatric* admissions, treatments and previous psychiatry contact; *medical,* particularly anything that might have a neurological impact, eg opiate analgesia, or cause stress, eg illness; *family* members with mental illness, consider making a genogram going back to grandparents; *forensic* contact; and *substance (mis)use* including alcohol.

Lastly examine the *mental state* (p. 690). At this point you may have enough information to make a confident diagnosis, or decide that labelling is unwise. Often, the patient's problems are complex and do not fit neatly into a diagnostic category at this point. A differential diagnosis, impression, or formulation may be a more appropriate way to summarize the case.

Ask yourself '*Why did they get ill in this way, at this time?*' and '*What are the consequences of the illness?*'

Specific questions to ask

Some direct questions to try:
- *Depression*—are you low/depressed? Is life worth living? Can anything give you pleasure? Energy levels? Sleep and appetite? Can you concentrate? Are you feeling guilty? Is your confidence low? Have you lost your libido? Are you preoccupied with guilt, regret, and/or hopelessness? Suicidal thoughts?
- *Mania*—have you felt you have more energy than normal (despite not sleeping)? Is it too much? Can you focus on things? Are you having difficulty settling? Are you spending more than usual? Are you more interested in sex (with different, inappropriate people)?
- *Psychosis* (persecutory beliefs, delusions, hallucinations)—has anything odd or unusual been happening recently? If they have odd ideas ask how did these occur? What actions do you feel you need to take? Ask about thoughts: Might your thoughts be being interfered with? Do you feel anyone is controlling you? Is anyone putting thoughts into your head? Do other people access or hear your thoughts? Is anyone harming you? Any plots against you? Do you hear voices when there's no one nearby? What do they say? Telling you off? Do you see things that others cannot see?
- *Drug and alcohol use*—what do you take? How much, how often, and for how long? How much do you spend on all this? Is it impacting on you the next day? Has your use changed recently (up or down)? Withdrawal signs?
- *Obsessions*—any odd thoughts? Recurring, intrusive worries? Note compulsive behaviour, eg excessive hand-washing.
- *Anxiety*—any worries/anxieties? Are you always worried or does it happen in discrete episodes ('attacks')? What causes this? What physical symptoms do you get? How do you manage your anxiety?
- *Eating disorders* (often not volunteered, and important)—what are you currently eating? How do you feel about your weight? Are you dieting?
- *Suicide*—have you ever felt so low that you have considered harming yourself? Have you ever actually harmed yourself? What stopped you harming yourself any more than this? Have you made any detailed suicide plans? Have you bought tablets for that purpose?
- *Risk*—are you wanting to harm anyone? Yourself? Have you stopped caring about yourself (dressing, washing, eating, drinking)?

12 Psychiatry

Differential diagnosis vs formulation

Differential diagnosis A limited list of 3 or 4 possible diagnoses with one selected as the most relevant (or likely) working diagnosis. It is sometimes helpful to mention other less likely possibilities you have considered and excluded if this has been brought up by the patient or referrer, eg 'The patient reported feeling "psychotic" but she did not have any first-rank symptoms and her presentation was more in keeping with a diagnosis of PTSD'.

Formulation Aims to contextualize the patient's symptoms in a broader, personalized way by identifying the '3 P's'(**P**redisposing, **P**recipitating, and **P**erpetuating factors) for the current presentation. Every formulation should include a statement on why that person has become ill at this point in time.

After an assessment, psychiatrists will often write a formulation and/or a differential diagnosis list. While both can contain similar information—summarized assessment, key symptoms, and relevant background information—the formulation focuses on a prediction of how a patient might react to a new situation or psychotherapy whereas the differential diagnosis is aimed at categorizing the illness into a diagnostic label. Together both of these are important in guiding us towards a suitable management plan which will include investigations and treatment options.

The mental state examination (MSE) is a structured and formalized approach to describing someone's state of mind at the time of interview and recording these under standard headings. It is obtained through a doctor's observation of a patient's mental processes, communication, and behaviour. Data is collected by a combination of direct and indirect means: unstructured observation during history taking, focused systematic questioning, and formalized testing. The MSE and psychiatric history together should provide evidence regarding current mental health, and if mental illness is present, judgement about its type, severity, and any risks to patient and others. The MSE should be recorded and presented in a standardized format under the following headings:

Appearance The majority of the MSE is focused on the patient's internal experiences; however, direct observation of the appearance, behaviour, and manner yields important information regarding mental state. For example, a patient may deny psychotic symptoms but appear to react to internal stimuli.
• Overall impression • Physical condition • Suitability of dress • Cleanliness.

Behaviour A general observation of activity and arousal levels and specific observations of the patient's eye contact, gait, and any abnormal movements.
• Appropriateness of behaviour, eg aggressive, agitated, overfamiliar • Eye contact • Distractibility • Abnormal involuntary movement • Rapport.

Speech Content of speech (what the patient says) is the main source of our history and MSE. The form of speech (how they say it) can reveal abnormal thinking processes. It is helpful to record a patient's description of significant symptoms exactly and any abnormal phrases or sentences verbatim.
• Rate, rhythm, volume, and tone • Coherence • Relevance • Quantity and fluency • Abnormal associations, clang, and punning • Flight of ideas.

Mood There is a distinction between mood (the emotional state over a long period) and affect (our emotional state at a certain point). The common analogy is: 'affect is the weather, whereas mood is a climate'. Any disturbance should be probed for severity, duration, and ubiquity and for associations with other pathological (biological or psychotic) features.
• Subjective (patient's) and objective (doctor's) assessment of mood in full • Anxiety and panic symptoms • Obsessional thoughts ('ruminations').

Perception Perceptual experiences can be a distorted internal perception of a real external object (altered perception, eg illusions) or without an external object (false perceptions, eg hallucinations).
• (Pseudo) Hallucinations in any modality • Depersonalization.

Thought As in speech form describes the structure and process of thought and content is the meaning and experience.
• Formal thought disorder • Delusions • Overvalued ideas • Preoccupations • Obsessive thoughts, ideas, and impulses.

Risk and suicidal ideation Thoughts of suicide, deliberate self-harm, or harm to others are included to stress their importance and act as a reminder to ask:
• Intent • Plan (active and imagined) • Lethality of plan • Urge to act upon these • Reasons for/against • Other dangers (to themselves or others).

Cognition Consciousness ranges from fully alert to clouded for a variety of reasons (organic, iatrogenic, psychiatric) and may fluctuate.
• Attention and concentration • Orientation to time, place, and person • Level of comprehension • Short-term memory (memory can also be tested formally).

Insight In physical illness, patients recognize their symptoms as 'anomalous' and seek a diagnosis and treatment. In contrast, many psychiatric illnesses impair insight so a patient reacts differently to their difficulties and cause (denial or failure to recognize problem). This reduces help-seeking behaviour.

Asking a patient whether they think they have a mental disorder, and what they think should be done, often establishes the divergence between the patient's and the clinician's perspective, if there is one.

What is a mental state?

Drugs, psychotherapy, and behavioural methods are the main tools available to the clinician for significantly improving a person's mental state. However, we cannot tell if these methods are actually helping when we can't access a patient's mental state, which is why the MSE on p. 690 is so important.

If you think you can access mental states just by applying the formulaic regimen on p. 690, you will often fail, as any trip into the mind of another is not just a voyage without maps, it is ultimately a creative and metaphysical enterprise. A true description of mental state entails valid knowledge about current emotions plus reactions to those emotions. So often it's non-verbal behaviour that allows valid judgement about mental state: don't rely on words alone—those capricious (but indispensable) tokens of disguise and deception.

Non-verbal behaviour

Why are we annoyed when we blush, yet love it when our friends do so? Part of the answer to this question is that non-verbal communication is less well controlled than verbal behaviour. This is why its study can yield valuable insights into our patients' minds, particularly when analysis of their spoken words has been not particularly revealing. For example, if a patient who consistently denies being depressed sits hugging himself in an attitude of self-pity, remaining in a glum silence for long periods of the interview, and when he does speak, using a monotonous slow whisper unadorned even by a flicker of a gesticulation or eye contact—we are likely to believe what we see and not what our patient would seem to be telling us.

All of these aspects of behaviour can be commented on as part of the MSE:

Items of non-verbal behaviour
- Gaze and mutual gaze
- Facial expression
- Smiling, blushing
- Body attitude (eg 'defensive').

Signs of auditory hallucinations
- Inexplicable laughter
- Silent and distracted while listening to 'voices' (but could be an 'absence' seizure, p. 232)
- Random, meaningless gestures.

Signs of a depressed mood
- Hunched, self-hugging posture
- Little eye contact.

Dress
('The apparel oft proclaims the man')[1]
- Hairstyle
- Make-up
- Ornament (ear-rings, tattoos, piercings).

Anxious behaviour
- Fidgeting, trembling
- Nail-biting
- Shuffling feet
- Squirming in the chair
- Sits on edge of chair.

- Downcast eyes; tears
- Slow thought, speech, and movement.

Predicting the future Surely we should be able to predict what will happen. In draughts (chequers), games are won or lost by using rules of thumb (heuristics). In 2007, for the first time, there was sufficient computing power to replace these rules of thumb by *perfect knowledge*. In draughts, there are >500 billion billion play-positions (500,995,484,682,338,672,639), and each has been analysed to decide what the next best move is. Well-programmed computers are right every time. When we ask psychiatrists to do a risk assessment we want them to be right every time too. It is vital that they are. We blame them if they are wrong. But this isn't rational. Psychiatrists do best using rules of thumb combined with validated risk assessment tools *(imperfect knowledge)*, such as the violence risk appraisal guide.[2] Forensic risk-assessment models all stress risk factors, but often disregard the other side of the equation: protective factors. Mediating and moderating effects must also be considered.[3] We need to involve patients in risk assessment and management. This may increase validity,[4] but it also adds unpredictability.

This is a common problem: the courts, the GP, or the relatives want to know 'Will he be violent again if he takes the medication?' A great deal—a person's freedom, no less, may depend on our answers. But risk is not dichotomous despite often being treated as such and nor is it fixed—within any individual, it will change over time, circumstance, and intervention. Every assessment of risk has two parts. The initial part can be weighed up using an objective (actuarial) approach, while the second is a more subjective decision based on pragmatic pressures. We consider the extent of the risk then we estimate the tolerability of that risk. Often professionals within a team cannot reach a consensus about the overall risk, reflecting the different priorities, biases, and experience each individual has.

Approaches to risk assessment These have broadly been grouped into 'actuarial' versus 'clinical' approaches. The *actuarial approach* provides us with clues to broad populations at risk, but informs us inadequately on the individual. The *clinical approach* has been characterized as providing an individualized and contextualized assessment, but purely clinical perspectives are vulnerable to poor inter-rater reliability and influence of political considerations. Defensive psychiatry will always prefer false positives over false negatives.

Risk assessment provides useful information regarding management but can also impact our relationship with a patient and their engagement and concordance with treatment. Several key principles underpin risk assessment:

- *Risk cannot be eliminated* so a more achievable aim is risk minimization: anticipating problems, lowering stress, and reducing or stopping harm.
- *A patient's risk fluctuates* as it is perpetually influenced by their perception, experience, and interaction with the world. Risk assessment is a dynamic process; risk management plans should be continually evaluated and amended.
- The best way to reduce risk is to *engage a patient* in a positive therapeutic relationship. This is strengthened with support, engagement, and listening.
- *Continued skills development* through ongoing training, reflection, and clinical supervision will increase the effectiveness of clinical work and practice.

Risk factors Regression analysis shows that 4 factors are paramount: 1 Previous violence 2 Substance abuse 3 Lack of empathy 4 Stress.[5] But risk factors are based on population studies and do not necessarily allow practitioners to identify risks in a particular individual. When in doubt, use a formal risk assessment tool. Some of the advantages of these tools derive simply from having a well-structured approach, others from combining specific kinds of risk factors (static and dynamic).[6]

Focusing on risk The emphasis on extreme but fortunately rare events such as suicide or murder, takes attention away from the much more common risks of self-neglect, discrimination and abuse, and disenfranchisement from society.

Confidentiality

'And about whatever I may see or hear in treatment, or even without treatment, in the life of human beings, I will remain silent, holding such things to be unutterable.'   Hippocratic Oath

As today, patients in ancient times shared deeply personal information with doctors on the assumption that their details would not be revealed to others. Without this trust, patients may withhold facts that would help the doctor make an accurate diagnosis. Patients have a right to expect that all material about their assessment, symptoms, and mental state will be kept confidential. This must be genuine if we expect patients to speak freely and establish a trusting therapeutic alliance between them and their doctor. In the absence of this assurance, patients will be reluctant to disclose their inner world which limits the care they can receive.

Being clear from the start about the nature of the confidentiality, its scope, and its limits is essential. For every encounter, but most importantly the first, you should be prepared to spend a few minutes explaining:
• Who you will share the information with: the multidisciplinary team, referrer, GP, patient's family.
• Who you will approach for collateral and what you will say for this request.
• In what circumstances you will break confidentiality.

Breaking confidentiality Information should not be disclosed to a relative, solicitor, or police officer without express consent being given by the patient, except in exceptional circumstances. If the risk to someone is so serious that it outweighs the patient's privacy then you must inform the appropriate person or authority without delay. If you make this decision, you should always document your judgement and reasons. You should feel able to justify this decision to whoever asks (patient, relative, or court).

Examples of this include:
• Where disclosure will prevent a serious crime (risk of serious harm or death).
• A patient who continues to drive, against medical advice. There is a duty to inform the medical adviser of the Driver and Vehicle Licensing Agency (DVLA).

If you are unsure whether a disclosure is justified, consult with a professional body (BMA or your protection organization) and/or seek advice from a senior colleague. Do this without delay; don't avoid a decision.

Tarasoff vs Regents of the University of California (1976)

NB: although this case has no legal bearing in the UK, it is often quoted when considering when to break confidentiality.

Prosenjit Poddar attended the University of California as a graduate where he met Tatiana Tarasoff. After she rebuffed his advances, he stalked her, developing a wish for revenge. Poddar sought help from Dr Lawrence Moore, a psychologist, and confided his intent to kill Tarasoff. Poddar was diagnosed with paranoid schizophrenia but not detained. Neither Tarasoff nor her parents received any warning of the threat. Poddar befriended Tarasoff's brother, even moving in with him, and over 6 months later he killed Tarasoff.

The Supreme Court of California decided all mental health professionals have a 'duty to protect' anyone being threatened with physical harm by a patient. The professional may perform this duty by notifying the police, warning the individual, and/or taking other reasonable steps to protect the intended target. This decision was reached despite one member of the Supreme Court, Justice Clark, dissenting 'the very practice of psychiatry depends upon the reputation in the community that the psychiatrist will not tell'. As a final statement, the Court stated 'protective privilege ends where public peril begins'.

12 Psychiatry

'Good psychiatry begins with a responsible Doctor undressing the patient and carrying out a proper physical examination.'

Donald Winnicott, paediatrician and psychoanalyst

A thorough physical examination is a fundamental part of the psychiatric assessment to identify a physical illness imitating a mental disorder, occurring alongside a mental disorder, or due to an existing mental disorder (or its treatment).

If a physical disorder is present, it may be the primary cause of, or a contributing factor to, the psychiatric symptoms (table 12.1). For example, a treatable UTI in an elderly patient may result in disinhibited behaviour. Physical symptoms can be a direct result of a mental health problem, eg bradycardia in anorexia nervosa (table 12.2). Deterioration may result from self-neglect in severe mental illness such as depression or due to psychiatric drug side effects, eg antipsychotic-induced parkinsonism. Poor mental health can increase the risk of physical health problems just as poor physical health can negatively affect mental health. A baseline set of physical findings allows medication to be commenced safely and quickly, and allows for early detection of new physical conditions.

But often the physical examination is brief in order to 'medically clear' the patient before the real assessment is started or deferred and never completed. If a patient is acutely unwell, labile in mood, or expressing conflicting delusions, it makes sense to avoid causing unnecessary distress, but minimal investigations can be completed and properly documented.

As in all of medicine, a routine physical examination should document any abnormal signs, or their absence if important, record the baseline physical state, and make plans for anything which needs further investigation.

Table 12.1 Physical causes of psychiatric symptoms

'Psychiatric' symptom	Examples of physical causes
Mood changes (depression/mania)	Multiple sclerosis, stroke, diabetes mellitus, brain tumour, hypothyroidism
Insomnia	Sleep apnoea, hyperthyroidism, gastro-oesophageal reflux disease (GORD), pain
Confusion/disorientation	Renal failure, cerebral arteritis, sepsis
Personality change	Multiple sclerosis, mass lesion, SLE
Hallucinations	Migraine, substance misuse, encephalitis, seizures
Behavioural change	Lyme disease, vascular infarct, Parkinson disease, subdural haematoma, mass lesion
Psychosis	Sensory loss, syphilis, dementia, Wilson disease
Irritability	Vitamin B_{12} deficiency, drug withdrawal (eg analgesics), substance misuse/withdrawal

Medically unexplained symptoms (p. 803) These need careful management. All new symptoms need an initial assessment which will include a focused history, examination, and investigation. However, this needs to be balanced with 'over-investigating' physical symptoms without considering a psychological component. For example, a patient may have real unexplained pain, which they focus on. This attention (to the exclusion of other alleviating factors such as work, hobbies, etc.) amplifies their experience, increasing their subjective pain and leading to low mood and further focus on the pain. A vicious circle can result which may also trigger other symptoms (physical and psychological).

Occasionally a patient may 'cry wolf' so often (eg with central chest pain) that it becomes necessary to reduce unnecessary repeated investigations and prevent behavioural reinforcement. This should be done in a thoughtful, holistic, and safe manner—not in the middle of the night with a new patient!

Table 12.2 Some physical signs in psychiatric illness and possible cause

General appearance	
Parkinsonian facies	Antipsychotic drug treatment
	Depression (psychomotor retardation)
Abnormal pupil size	Opiate use
Argyll–Robertson pupil	Neurosyphilis
Enlarged parotids ('hamster face')	Bulimia nervosa (secondary to vomiting)
Hypersalivation	Clozapine treatment
Goitre	Thyroid disease
Multiple forearm scars	Borderline (emotionally unstable) personality disorder
Needle tracks/phlebitis	IV drug use
Gynaecomastia	Antipsychotic drug treatment
	Alcoholic liver disease
Russell's sign (knuckle callus)	Bulimia nervosa (secondary to inducing vomiting)
Lanugo hair	Anorexia nervosa
Piloerection ('goose flesh')	Opiate withdrawal
Excessive thinness	Anorexia nervosa
Cardiovascular	
Rapid/irregular pulse	Anxiety disorder
	Drug/alcohol withdrawal
	Hyperthyroidism
Slow pulse	Hypothyroidism, anorexia nervosa
Abdominal	
Enlarged liver	Alcoholic liver disease
	Hepatitis
Multiple surgical scars ('chequer-board' abdomen)	Somatization disorder
Multiple self-inflicted scars	Borderline (emotionally unstable) personality disorder
Neurological	
Resting tremor	Increased sympathetic drive (anxiety, drug/alcohol misuse)
	Antipsychotic drug treatment
	Lithium treatment
Involuntary movements	Antipsychotic drug treatment
	Tic disorder
	Huntingtons/Sydenham chorea
Abnormal posturing	Antipsychotic-induced dystonia
	Catatonia
Broad-based gait	Cerebellar disease (alcohol, lithium toxicity)
Festinant (shuffling) gait	Parkinsonism (Parkinson disease or drug-induced parkinsonism)

12 Psychiatry

Reproduced from Semple and Smyth, *Oxford Handbook of Psychiatry* (2013) with permission from OUP.

'And I said, "You're not seein' things like how I'm seein' things. I'm seein' things that I don't wanna see. I see the devil sit right before me. Fire in his eyes as he spoke to me.' 'Awfully Deep', Roots Manuva

It is important to decide if a patient has delusions, hallucinations (that the patient believes are real), or a major thought disorder, because if present, the diagnosis must be schizophrenia, an affective disorder, an organic disorder, or a paranoid state (or a culturally determined visionary or spiritual experience), and not a neurosis or a personality disorder.

Patients may be reluctant to reveal odd ideas. Ask gently: 'Have you ever had any thoughts which might now seem odd; perhaps that there is a conspiracy against you, or that you are controlled by outside voices or the radio?'

Delusions Delusions are beliefs held unshakably, irrespective of counter-argument, that are unexpected and out of keeping with the patient's cultural background. If the belief arrives fully formed, and with no antecedent events or experiences to account for it, it is said to be *primary,* and is suggestive of schizophrenia. Such delusions appear 'out of the blue' as a fully formed idea (delusional intuition) or form around a real perception given a delusional interpretation (delusional perception), as illustrated by the patient who, on seeing the traffic lights go green knew that he had been sent to rid his town of capitalism. Especially relevant if these involve persecution and loss of control.[7] A careful history may reveal the delusions are *secondary* based on the patient's current affect or preoccupations (eg fear, hope, stress) in an understandable manner.

Delusions can be mood congruent in affective psychosis, eg a depressed person who believes that he is literally rotting away (nihilistic delusion), or the manic patient who believes she is the Queen of England (grandiose delusion). In schizophrenia, delusions are often mood incongruent, with horrific beliefs discussed without commensurate distress.

Specific delusions Those most associated with psychosis (eg mania, schizophrenia) are:
- Persecution: the most common type of delusions. A theme of being followed, spied on, and conspired against with a belief that the persecutors intend to cause harm. Often described by patients as a feeling of 'paranoia'.[2]
- Infestation: a belief that the skin is infested with parasites causing itching (formication), eg in organic states and cocaine use (*Ekbom syndrome*).
- Religious: eg on visiting Jerusalem, a person becomes overwhelmed and develops religious themed delusions. Shown to affect people of all backgrounds: Jews, Christians, and Muslims (*Jerusalem syndrome*).
- Delusional misidentification: a person believes that those close to them have been replaced by an exact double (*Capgras syndrome*) or that a single person is impersonating multiple familiar people (*Fregoli syndrome*).
- Jealousy: firm belief that a sexual partner is unfaithful made without proof; whether actual infidelity occurred is immaterial (*Othello syndrome*).
- Love: belief that a celebrity, high-status individual, or stranger is in love with them, and secretly sending messages or signs (*de Clérambault syndrome*).
- Communicated: an already psychotic person transmits their beliefs to another, usually subservient close relative, who now shares them (*folie à deux*).

Ideas of reference Coincidental or innocuous events which are interpreted to have great personal significance, eg a TV news broadcast making direct references to the patient, or other people on the train talking (or thinking) about them. Associated with social phobia, psychosis, or stress. Often accompanied by *delusions of reference* —with bizarre, unfeasible interpretations, eg a dog's bark carries coded message. Differ from overvalued ideas: understandable and reasonable beliefs which dominate a patient's life to detriment of functioning.

2 Paranoia really means: mental illness where an organized system of delusional beliefs of any variety, not just persecution, is the most prominent feature.

What is descriptive psychopathology?

Psychopathology is the '*systematic study of abnormal experience, cognition and behaviour; the study of the products of a disordered mind*'.[1] Descriptive psychopathology attempts to describe, and in so doing understand, the experiences in mental illness. It does this through observation of behaviour, empathic exploration of subjective experience, and classification of these into categorical symptoms. This forms the basis of all clinical psychiatry. These general qualifiers describe terms used in this chapter:

- *Subjective* and *objective*—subjective signs are reported by the patient; objective signs are seen by an external observer.
- *Primary* and *secondary*—primary symptoms arise directly from disordered mental states, and cannot be fully understood (although we can still empathize with the subjective experience); secondary symptoms occur as an understandable reaction to another condition, eg depression, drug use.
- *Congruent* and *incongruent*—a subjective impression regarding the 'appropriateness' of a patient's experience, affect, or behaviour. If this fits with the apparent mental state, it is congruent; if not, it is incongruent, eg a patient talking pleasantly while describing a traumatic experience has an incongruent affect.
- *Form* and *content*—every abnormal symptom has both form—the type of experience (eg primary delusion, hallucination) attributable to the underlying mental illness, and content—the composition of the symptom which is richly illustrative of the patient's internal world.
- *Structural* and *functional:* often used in neurology/neuropsychiatry to distinguish syndromes which have abnormal investigation findings (eg Huntington's) from those without (eg conversion paralysis). In the past, brain disorders with observable structural abnormalities on postmortem (eg dementia) were compared to those without (eg schizophrenia); however, modern imaging has shown observable brain changes in many disorders formerly called functional.
- *Endogenous* and *reactive*—rarely used today, it was thought that some conditions arose spontaneously from within (endogenous) whereas others arose in response to external events.

What's it like having hallucinations? Try virtual reality to find out

Doctors often get hung up on hallucinations, without acquiring any real knowledge of what it's like to have them. For doctors who have never experienced hallucinations, Professor Yellowlees has devised a virtual reality experience on *Second Life*[3]: a complex, unruly 3D world where people get sucked into virtual clinics … Floors can fall away, leaving us walking riskily on stones above clouds. The eyes of a portrait flash 'shitface' as we pass, and a politician on an in-world TV might move in a single breath from platitudes to shouting 'Go and kill yourself, you wretch!' When it gets to the stage of our reflection in a mirror bleeding its eyes out before expiring, most of us switch off.[9] But our patients cannot quit so easily. Virtual reality is just one way of sensitizing us to their difficulties: other ways include blogs, painting (figs 12.3–12.5 p. 699), and arts (eg Shakespeare's Ophelia effect).[10] Consideration of the 'patient experience' is an essential part of medicine and never more so than in psychiatry where there is often a stigma attached to the diagnosis and discrimination to those having to manage their symptoms.

3 Example YouTube video: https://www.youtube.com/watch?v=s33Y5nI5Wbc

Hallucinations Occur in any sensory modality (visual, auditory, olfactory, proprioceptive) without any external stimulus. The main characteristics of a hallucination are that they are felt to occur in the external world alongside other objects, have the same qualities as everything else (eg colouring, density), and cannot be consciously manipulated or stopped. To the person experiencing them, these experiences are real. fMRI imaging studies show similar areas of brain activity are seen when 'hearing' an auditory hallucination or real voices.

Most hallucinations start as simple, brief experiences in a single modality, with only some going on to change over time into a more complex, multiple sensory experience. A patient reporting hearing a sudden voice giving them a specific instruction should be followed up carefully—with consideration to any secondary gain given from a mental health diagnosis (eg avoiding blame).

Auditory hallucinations Can be elementary (eg hissing, whistling) or complex (eg voices, music). The subjective experience can vary depending on the hallucination: a pleasant, friendly, known voice offering support or an aggressive, unfamiliar voice (or voices) criticizing. Patients can experience both. These hallucinations must be felt to originate from outside the body and out of conscious control. Experiences include: *thoughts spoken aloud,* heard either as they are thought (*gedankenlautwerden*) or just after (*écho de la penseé*); *second-person hallucinations,* a voice talking directly to the person or giving them instructions (eg 'you are being followed; run away'); *third-person hallucinations,* voices heard arguing or giving a running commentary (eg 'He is going off to sleep') just before, simultaneously, or after the person's actions.

Visual hallucinations Much more common in eye pathology and epilepsy than psychosis. Not to be confused with an illusion, an involuntary misperception of a real stimulus transformed or distorted often brought on by tiredness or emotion; affective component, eg fearful mood = scary images.

Non-pathological hallucinations Experiences we all have, eg feeling your leg vibrate with a text message before remembering the phone is plugged in elsewhere. These are common and do not indicate pathology: 2–4% of the general population experience auditory hallucinations, but only ~30% of these have a mental illness (more likely if associated with distressing delusions).⁷ *Hypnagogic and hypnopompic hallucinations* eg hearing a voice calling our name when going (hypnagogic = **g**oing) to sleep or waking up. A *pseudohallucination* is one in which the person knows the stimulus is in the mind (eg a voice heard within themselves, rather than over the left shoulder)—these may also be a sign that a genuine hallucination is waning. *Panoramic memories* are seen with near-death and out-of-body experiences alongside complex hallucinatory phenomena (all have proved to be unsubstantiated, so far …).⁴ *Extracampine hallucinations* or 'concrete awareness' occur outside the sensory field (eg 'right behind me') as a non-specific feeling which can be associated with epilepsy, psychosis, but also when anxious (eg at home, alone). *Pareidolia* where an ill-defined, random stimulus is given significance, occurring without conscious effort (eg seeing a rabbit shape in clouds).

Organic disorders Present as tactile or visual hallucinations without any auditory input. Seen in alcohol withdrawal or Charles Bonnet syndrome (p. 355).

Obsessional thoughts Sometimes hard to distinguish from hallucinations. Often both are 'odd' and cause distress. If a person recognizes a 'voice' or their unusual thoughts as their own, then they more likely have obsessive thoughts or pseudohallucinations. If they experience a voice as external to themselves (auditory hallucination) or a thought as being 'put into their head' by an external agency (thought insertion) they may have a psychotic illness.

4 AWARE II study (awareness during resuscitation) used hidden targets on shelves only visible from above to test this. For updates on this study, follow its author on Twitter: @SamParniaMDPhD.

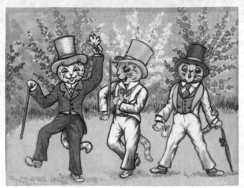

Fig 12.3 Three cats performing a song and dance act. Gouache by Louis Wain, 1925/1939.

Wellcome Collection.

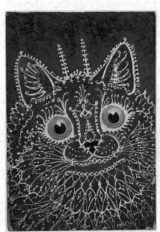

Fig 12.4 A cat in 'gothic' style. Gouache by Louis Wain, 1925/1939.

Wellcome Collection.

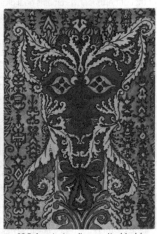

Fig 12.5 A cat standing on its hind legs, formed by patterns supposed to be in the 'Early Greek' style. Gouache by Louis Wain, 1925/1939. Wellcome Collection.

Figs 12.3–12.5 Wain's cat paintings. Thought to show a progressive schizophrenic illness. ♠※ Louis Wain (5 August 1860–4 July 1939) was an English artist known for his drawings of anthropomorphized cats. He developed schizophrenia (perhaps related to the parasite *Toxoplasma gondii* found in cats' faeces) and, in 1924, he was committed to a pauper ward. Later after appeals from the rich and famous, including HG Wells, and the personal intervention of Prime Minister Ramsey MacDonald he was transferred to the Bethlem Royal Hospital. He remained in hospital for the rest of his life.

These paintings, arranged by Dr Walter Maclay, a psychiatrist treating Wain, show a series of different styles thought by Maclay to demonstrate Wain's deteriorating mental state. This is a controversial claim, as it is unclear of the chronological order of the paintings; however, it is clear that Wain's paintings move between charming and psychedelic and aptly illustrate the different views of the world as seen by an artist with schizophrenia. For the full range of Wain's cat variations see: bristolunipsychiatrysoc.wordpress.com/2014/08/18/psychiatry-in-public-louis-wain/

Conventional thought processes 4 broad characteristics: 1 *Thought stream:* Speed, quality, and quantity of thinking; how is something being thought about? 2 *Thought content:* Substance of thinking: what is being thought about? 3 *Thought form:* Formation and coherence of thinking: how are separate thoughts linked to one another? 4 *Thought possession:* Who created thoughts: are these considered by the person to be their own thoughts?

Major thought disorder Most healthy thinking shows constancy, organization, and continuity—a thought (or speech) begins, continues, and reaches a goal in a logical manner without veering off track or leaping between disconnected points. Without this, bizarre thoughts, or incongruent transition from one idea to another, occur (*mania*—flight of ideas, p. 716; *schizophrenia*, pp. 704-5).

Disorders of thought stream Flight of ideas is subjective quickening of thoughts so most are not carried to completion before being overtaken. Meaningful connections between ideas are kept although often linked by distracting environmental cues or from words themselves spoken aloud (eg puns, rhymes, and clang associations). Retardation of thinking is a slowing of the train of thought although it remains goal directed. The opposite is pressure of speech.

Disorders of thought content Delusions and overvalued ideas (p. 696).

Disorders of thought form Main features of a formal thought disorder (FTD) include: • Derailment: a break in the linked association of sequential thoughts or change in track of thoughts—neither patient nor observer understands the connection • Omission: all or part of a thought is absent without a reason • Fusion: thoughts are fused together • Substitution: an inappropriate or illogical thought replaces another as though slotted into a space.

'Loosening of association' occurs where normal thought structure breaks down resulting in confused, illogical answers which no exploration can explain. The more questions asked, the less clear things become. Here, answers show: • Circumstantiality: laborious detail given no matter how inconsequential or insignificant it is but without losing track of the question • Overinclusion: inability to maintain the boundaries of a topic or restrict thoughts to the limits of a topic • Tangential thinking: talking past or around the point as thoughts diverge from the topic. Also called *knight's move thinking*—the pattern of movement a knight in chess makes • Talking past the point: getting close to the discussion point, but then skirting around it and never actually reaching it • Verbigeration (also called *word salad* or *schizophasia*) speech is reduced to a senseless repetition of sounds and phrases. Different to neologisms (made up words/phrases or normal words used in idiosyncratic ways eg *foothat* to mean *shoe*) and metonyms (word approximations, eg *menu* to mean *meal*).

Disorders of thought possession Most of us never question the belief that: 1 We have ultimate control of our thoughts 2 Our thoughts are our own 3 These thoughts are not being externally manipulated. An *obsession* (or rumination) is a thought which endures and dominates thinking even though the person knows that it is unhelpful and irrelevant. These cannot be dismissed or controlled which often results in anxiety and distress (see OCD, p. 720). *Thought alienation* (or thought interference) is the subjective experience of one's own thoughts being under the control of an outside agency. Often described as: 1 Thought insertion: foreign thoughts placed into one's mind 2 Thought withdrawal: thoughts suddenly disappearing—having been taken by an external force 3 Thought broadcast: thoughts being transmitted to everyone around—as though being played on a radio. These are considered to be a first-rank symptom of schizophrenia (pp. 704-5)—pathological when present.

Diagnostic classification systems are used throughout medicine to categorize and collate conditions. The purpose of this classification: • Enhance reliability • Facilitate communication (and reduce confusion) • Aid research • Formulate management plan • Medico-legal issues. Having a universally recognized 'depression' diagnosis means that a patient can move from China to France to the UK and all clinicians involved would reach the same diagnosis and treatment.

Unfortunately, there is no single handbook for diagnosing mental illness. There are two classification systems used today: the American Psychiatric Association's *Diagnostic and Statistical Manual of Mental Disorders* (DSM-5, as it's in its 5th edition), and the WHO's *International Statistical Classification of Diseases and Related Health Problems* (ICD-11, for the 11th edition, released June 2018). Why are there these two separate, but similar, systems? The ICD is global, multidisciplinary, and multilingual. It is written by authors from 193 WHO countries, distributed at low cost (free online: https://icd.who.int/browse11/l-m/en/), and aims to help countries reduce the disease burden of mental disorders (table 12.3). The DSM is approved and produced by an American professional association for American psychiatrists. It generates money for that association through book sales, related products, and copyright.

Table 12.3 Hierarchical categories used in ICD-11

06 Mental, behavioural, or neurodevelopmental disorders:	
Neurodevelopmental disorders	Disruptive behaviour or dissocial disorders
Schizophrenia or other primary psychotic disorders	Personality disorders and related traits
Catatonia	Paraphilic disorders
Mood disorders	Factitious disorders
Anxiety or fear-related disorders	Neurocognitive disorders
Obsessive-compulsive or related disorders	Mental or behavioural disorders associated with pregnancy, childbirth, or the puerperium
Elimination disorders	Sleep/wake disorders
Disorders of bodily distress or bodily experience	Sexual dysfunctions
Disorders due to substance use or addictive behaviours	Gender incongruence
Impulse control disorders	

Multiaxial classification The DSM previously used this (dropped in DSM-5)
- *Axis I—clinical disorder* with acute symptoms which require immediate intervention, eg major depressive episode, anorexia nervosa.
- *Axis II—personality disorders and mental retardation:* Lifelong and permanent difficulties arising in childhood, which may affect treatment (ICD multiaxial version splits this into two axes, making the total axes into six).
- *Axis III—general medical conditions:* Conditions which may influence or impact on a mental health problem, eg diabetes can exacerbate depression by causing fatigue and altering which antidepressant is initially prescribed.
- *Axis IV—psychosocial and environmental problems:* Life problems and acute psychosocial stressors affecting well-being, eg homelessness, bereavement.
- *Axis V—global assessment of functioning (GAF):* Using an established scale of 0–100 to quantify a patient's ability to socially, occupationally, and psychologically function in daily life. 100 is superior functioning; generally <50 indicates severe symptoms. (Google 'GAF+scale' for full copy.)

Strengths and weaknesses Both manuals allow for common and universal diagnosis. Through revisions they remain relevant and clinically useful. Critics argue they promote a medicalization of living (eg patients have anorexia so they are 'ill' and need 'treatment'). Categories reflect societal norms—so homosexuality was considered a 'deviant sexual behaviour' in DSM until 1973.

12 Psychiatry

12 Psychiatry

Since the 1980s, most UK inpatients with psychosis have had the focus of their care moved from hospital to the community. The aim has been to save money and improve care. But has community care failed, or have there been successes? 5 questions keep recurring, each (ominously) prefixed by a 'surely ...'

1 *Surely hospitals will always be needed for severely mentally ill people?* In general, the problem is not the severity of the mental illness but its social context which determines if community care is appropriate. Patients aren't always admitted to hospital because they aren't able to manage life in the community, sometimes a community is unable to manage the person. Clinic appointments are inadequate for chaotic, disorganized individuals. Assertive community management is demonstrated to reduce hospital admissions.

2 *Surely community care, if it is done properly, will be more expensive than hospital care, where resources can be concentrated?* Not so—at least not necessarily so. Some concentration of resources *can* take place in the community in day hospitals and mental illness hostels. It is also true that the 'bed and breakfast' element of inpatient care is expensive, if the running and maintenance costs associated with deploying inpatient psychiatric services are taken into account. In most studies, costs of each type of service doesn't differ much, and sometimes good community care turns out cheaper.[13,14]

3 *Surely there will be more homicides and suicides if disturbed patients are not kept in hospital?* Offending by the mentally ill is of great public concern (60 homicides/year in England). A cohort study, however, found rates of violent offending are low and the strongest association with offending was previous offending. Psychiatric variables were less important, with diagnosis and number of previous admissions showing no significant association. Substance misuse and sexual abuse are associated with increased offending risk.[15]

4 *Surely if inpatient psychiatric beds are not available, however good the daytime team is in the community, some patients will still need somewhere to go at night?* The implication is that the skills available in bed-and-breakfast accommodation may be inadequate at times of day when there is no other support, other than the ED. Studies that have looked at this have certainly found an increase in non-hospital residential care in those selected for community care, and this increase may be as much as 280% over 5 years. In the UK, new proposals guarantee 24-hour open access to skilled help, but it is not known what pressures this will put services under.

5 *Surely community care will involve a huge bureaucracy in pursuit of the unattainable goal of 100% safety?* This will be so if every patient has a lengthy care plan and repeated risk assessments. Concern for safety may also spawn a non-therapeutic custodial relationship.

Advantages reported for community care are: better social functioning, satisfaction with life, employment, and drug compliance—but in randomized studies in the UK these advantages are not always manifest. Furthermore, trends have been repeatedly found indicating that the longer studies go on for, the harder it is to maintain the initial advantages of community care. If teams and patients don't keep up their enthusiasm during a trial, it will be even harder once the trial period ends and regular life sets in.

Assertive community care and case management is one way out of this impasse (here a key-worker has direct responsibility for care plans). This set-up helps ensure more people remain in contact with psychiatric services; this inevitably increases hospital admission rates.[16,17] When combined with family therapy and social skills training results are good.[18]

How to use the full range of psychiatric services

Current UK community psychiatric services can be categorized as follows:
- Intensivist teams: crisis and home treatment, eg with 24h phone helpline.
- Support and recovery teams—community mental health teams (CMHT); assertive outreach; rehabilitation.
- Drug and alcohol teams: part of a wide range of substance abuse services.
- Inreach mental health services—residential care, acute hospital liaison, primary care liaison teams (PCL)—integrated CPNs/psychiatrists with GP practices/hospitals with good links into secondary community services.
- IAPT services (improved access to psychological therapies)—offer a wide range of community-based therapies eg, CBT (p.754), group therapy, etc.

Typically all these services are multidisciplinary (to a varying degree) with nurses, OTs, physios, psychologists, psychiatrists, and social workers.

Many of these community services are supported by 3rd-sector (voluntary) organizations, eg MIND, Alzheimer's society, and other local organizations and charities that provide drop-in centres, group or individual therapy, homecare, advocacy, educational information, etc.

PWD (patients with dementia) use more or less specialist residential or nursing homes; social services input is very important as is close working with local councils, and health authorities. Integrated care has theoretical advantages—eg for a schizophrenic patient who is a substance abuser.[11,12]

12 Psychiatry

Schizophrenia A common chronic relapsing condition often presenting in early adulthood with *psychotic symptoms* (hallucinations, delusions); *disorganization symptoms* (incongruous mood, abnormal speech and thought); negative symptoms (apathy, ↓ motivation, withdrawal, self-neglect, blunted mood); and, sometimes, *cognitive impairment*.[19,20] It has major implications for patients, work, and families. *Incidence:* ~0.15:1000/yr. *Prevalence:* ~1%.

Psychosis, distorted thinking and perception, eg delusions and hallucinations, is a common symptom: **1** Affective psychoses (depression, bipolar disorder) **2** Transient psychotic disorders (usually substance misuse) **3** Psychosis due to a medical disorder (eg brain tumour) and **4** Schizophrenia-like non-affective disorders (brief psychotic disorder; delusional disorder; schizophreniform disorder).[21] When diagnosing schizophrenia look for:

1 *Thought insertion:* 'He is putting ideas into my head.' *Thought broadcasting:* 'People overhear my thoughts.' *Thought withdrawal:* 'Thoughts are being taken out of my head' (seen objectively as a patient suddenly stopping mid-sentence), or repeating of thoughts.
2 Delusions that thoughts, feelings, impulses, or actions are influenced or even controlled by external forces. Also includes delusional perceptions (p. 696).
3 Hallucinatory voices giving a running commentary on a patient's behaviour, or discussing the patient among themselves.
4 Persistent delusions of other kinds that are culturally inappropriate and completely impossible ('Ryan Reynolds has put a transmitter in my brain').
5 Persistent hallucinations in any modality (somatic, visual, tactile) which occur every day for weeks on end.
6 Breaks or interpolations in the train of thought, resulting in incoherence or irrelevant speech—*knight's move thoughts* that change direction, flying off at tangents, with odd logic, or neologisms (made-up words).
7 Catatonic behaviour described as 'strange, purposeless behaviour', such as sudden excitement, posturing, or waxy flexibility, negativism, mutism, echopraxia (involuntary imitation of the movements).
8 Negative symptoms (apathy, paucity of speech, blunting or incongruity of affect, eg laughing at bad news) usually resulting in social withdrawal.

(1–5 are co-extensive with Schneider's 1st-rank symptoms of schizophrenia.)

Diagnostic guidelines for schizophrenia The main criterion is at least 1 very clear symptom (and usually 2 or more if less clear-cut) belonging to any of the groups 1–4 just listed, or symptoms from at least 2 of groups 5–8. Because many people have brief psychosis-like symptoms, *do not diagnose schizophrenia unless symptoms last for ≥6 months *and* symptoms are present much of the time for at least 1 month, *and* there is marked impairment in work or home functioning. Also, 'rule out' other causes of psychosis (eg bipolar disorder, drugs/alcohol, cns tumours, head injury).

Schizophrenia was considered to have different subtypes: *Paranoid*[5] (commonest subtype, here hallucinations and/or delusions are prominent). *Hebephrenic* (age of onset 15–25yrs, poor prognosis, fluctuating affect prominent with fleeting fragmented delusions and hallucinations). *Catatonic* (characterized by stupor, posturing, waxy flexibility, and negativism). In *simple* and *residual* types, negative symptoms predominate.

Prodromal symptoms Precede most first episodes of psychosis by up to 18 months (sometimes just a few days). It is characterized by a gradual deterioration in functioning—sometimes conceptualized as 'altered life trajectory'.

---

5 In ICD-11 all subtypes of Schizophrenia have been removed. It is replaced by a dimensional model which focuses on assessment of different symptoms groups: positive, negative, depressive, manic, psychomotor, and cognitive.

Changes include: • Transient and/or attenuated (lower intensity) psychotic symptoms • Odd (out of character) thoughts, beliefs and behaviours • Concentration problems • Altered affect • Social withdrawal • Reduced interest in daily activities.

Other 'schizophrenia' disorders *Schizoaffective* causes confusion as it's either (or both) a variant of schizophrenia and affective (mood) disorders. It is given when a patient experiences symptoms of both a mood disorder (mania or depression) and schizophrenia at the same time (within days) and of the same intensity without another medical disorder or substance misuse cause. Treatment is managing both conditions: often an antipsychotic and mood stabilizer. Lifetime prevalence is ~0.5%.

Schizotypal is a personality disorder (see pp. 744–5) which may represent a partial expression of schizophrenia. Usually treated without medication.

Schizophreniform is given to those disorders that fail to meet the threshold for schizophrenia (usually duration of psychosis) but have some symptoms of schizophrenia and deterioration in functioning. Treated with antipsychotics.

Genes and environment

Many genes implicated in schizophrenia also increase risk of bipolar disorder.[22-34] [International Schizophrenia Consortium] Some are susceptibility genes (needing environmental triggers). Genome-wide studies point to a gene coding for myosin on chromosome 22 and a region of >450 gene variants, in the major histocompatibility complex (MHC) region on 6p. The dysbindin gene on chromosome 6 is important too. Early use of cannabis is a trigger: those with vv homozygosity of the catechol-o-methyl-transferase gene (COMT; risk ↑ ×10 compared with MM variants). The timing of triggers is important.[35] Those starting cannabis at 15yrs old are 3× more likely to develop schizophreniform psychosis.[36,37]

Is schizophrenia a neurodevelopmental disorder?

People with schizophrenia may suffer unusual neurodevelopment either through inheriting genes and/or some insult to the brain that impairs its development. This leads to subtle cognitive and behavioural effects in childhood[38] and then psychosis at or just after adolescence. Relevant prenatal/obstetric events: early rupture of membranes, gestational age <37 weeks, incubator use, winter births.[39]

MRI Shows differences in the brains of those with schizophrenia (and their 1st-degree relatives[40]): eg larger lateral ventricles, reduced frontal lobe and parahippocampal gyrus. Reduced (particularly on left) temporal lobe, hippocampus (subserves memory/emotion), and amygdala (involved in expression of emotion). MRI has shown diffuse reduction in cortical grey matter associated with poor premorbid function.[41] NB: use of psychotics may also cause brain shrinkage—eg up to 20%.[42] However, schizophrenia also has an onset later in life, particularly women over 30.[43] It has been estimated that about 40% of people who develop schizophrenia have a developmental problem, but the majority are not remarkably different from the general population and have no cognitive deficits. So what are the other pathways that lead to psychosis?

Social factors Being brought up in cities increases the risk of schizophrenia (UK incidence is particularly high in London), and there are higher levels of schizophrenia in migrant groups such as Asians and African-Caribbeans (possible mechanisms through social adversity, racial discrimination, social isolation).[44] The associated 'stress' on the brain has been suggested to affect the morphology of the brain via hormonal influences as well as the stress of being psychotic resulting in high cortisol levels causing further brain changes.

Psychosis and schizophrenia Some believe that the term 'schizophrenia' has outlived its usefulness as it implies that everyone with schizophrenia has the same pathology and all need antipsychotics. A more nuanced approach is to avoid diagnostic labels, and treat the first episode as 'psychosis' (see p. 707).

Patients require a range of management interventions but the first step is to determine what it is that you, and the patient, want to focus on treating (and the methods used to do this). *Frequent symptoms:* Lack of insight,[97%] auditory hallucinations,[74%] ideas of reference,[70%] paranoia,[66%] flat affect,[66%] persecutory delusions.[62%] *Frequent behaviours:* Social withdrawal,[74%] anhedonia (inability to feel pleasure),[50%] apathy,[56%] lack of conversation,[54%] psychomotor retardation,[48%] overactivity,[41%] self-neglect,[30%] posturing ± odd movements.[25%]

Medication Once a diagnosis is made of psychosis (or schizophrenia), then antipsychotic medication should be commenced (see p. 708). Don't dawdle! Delaying antipsychotics worsens negative symptoms.[45] but managing schizophrenia is much more than drugs; it requires an individualized *care plan* that includes psychosocial interventions and *support for families.*[46] If concordance with medication is an issue, depots (long-lasting injections) are useful.

Psychological interventions Given the adverse effects of antipsychotic drugs, psychological interventions should be recommended in all management plans to promote *quick recovery* and *relapse prevention.* There is strong evidence to support early use of cbt, general or targeted on auditory hallucinations ('hearing voices'), and other interventions aimed at reducing the impact of symptoms on the patient's life, limit relapses, and promote early detection of another episode. Towards the end of an acute episode, focus on treating residual symptoms, eg difficult thoughts, voices, negative symptoms. If there is concurrent substance misuse (high prevalence), abstinence improves overall prognosis—in fact, there is a better prognosis at 18 months than if a patient had never had a substance misuse problem at all.

Other interventions include *working with family*—address carers' issues (embarrassment, self-blame, and shame are prevalent).[47] Family therapy may have a role[48] and support groups.[6] *Social support:* Particular social circumstances may result in alterations in dopamine that ↑ relapse likelihood. Addressing housing, benefits, and social skills training are just as important as being concordant with medication. Supported employment can be helpful.

Referral to an Early Intervention Service (see box 'Early Intervention Services (eis)') should be considered. They offer these interventions under a single dynamic team.

Aftercare Coordinated via an allocated key worker and a multidisciplinary team (to look at biological, psychological, social, and risk issues). It is performed through the Care Programme Approach (cpa).

Prognosis Better if: sudden onset; no negative symptoms; supportive home; ♀ sex (better social integration[49]); later onset of illness; no cns ventricular enlargement; no family history.

Overall, only 10% ever have one episode. With treatment, ≤7% need intensive input/hospital admission for more than 2 years after *first* admission. 28% go over 2 years without needing further hospital admission. Recovery at 15 years (measured by global assessment of function >60) in 40% of patients. *Suicide rates:* Incidence of 10% during acute phase, then 4% in chronic phase.

6 eg Rethink (http://www.rethink.org/) and Mind (http://www.mind.org.uk/) are UK mental health charities.

Psychosis: 'a break from reality'

Psychosis is a mental disorder causing a person to perceive, believe, or interpret things differently. In its florid form, it is the archetype of the layman's 'madness' But, the *usual* picture is less obvious: the patient may be sitting alone, quietly attending to his or her voices. Psychosis interferes with the ability to function and can be very debilitating. If hallucinations, delusions, or a thought disorder (defined on p. 696) are present, the cause could be schizophrenia (or related disorders), a disorder of affect (mania, p. 716, or depression, p. 710, or both), or be organic (eg head injury drug-induced—a transient psychosis).

So the term psychosis is not in itself a diagnosis, but is a useful term to employ, while the underlying diagnosis is being formulated. Beware labelling people; remember that even during the best of times, only a thin veil separates us from insanity.

Early Intervention Services (EIS)

The principal aim of an EIS is to provide a service to identify, assess, treat, and support people experiencing their first psychotic episode. Their aim during the formative stages of the condition is: 1 Reduction of an individual's duration of untreated psychosis 2 Provision of the most effective possible care at an early stage to maximize the chance of recovery 3 Increase likelihood of return to education or employment 4 Prevent loss-of-life trajectory.

The EIS model has clinicians with a small caseload working with patients in a proactive manner, meeting in a patient's home, workplace (or school), and local community rather than clinic. EIS provide holistic care to reflect patients' needs and priorities using a multidisciplinary team. Dates and times of these appointments are often not fixed in frequency or duration. Because of this flexibility EIS are better able to reflect the needs of this complex group and react quickly to changes in their mental state or acute difficulties. EIS will often receive referrals from psychiatric services, other statutory and non-statutory services (eg housing providers, probation, drug services).

EIS model is of low-threshold for discussion, referral, and acceptance of patients. Usual exception criteria are limited to location, organic (including substance-induced) psychosis, and previous EIS care of over 2 years. Most teams offer an initial assessment period (eg up to 8 weeks) to engage the person and ascertain suitability for the service with liaison with the referrer, and other services as required. If accepted, EIS work intensively with the patient, and their support network, for 3 years, even if they are admitted.

This is a model which has been shown to have good outcomes: halving likelihood of admission (especially detention under the Mental Health Act), lowering rates of negative symptoms, reducing suicide risk (from 15% to 1%), limiting duration of episode, and increasing early relapse detection. Employment rate for 18–35s in an EIS is 35% (12% for people in standard mental health care) and social functioning has been shown to improve.

EIS is not without critics. Accusations include selectively cited findings to support early intervention, focus on short-term improvements without longer-term follow-up, and more 'spin' than research in published literature. An analysis of published abstracts showed implied positive results in 75%, whereas examination of primary measures found only 13% positive results.[50]

Advice and monitoring Before starting an antipsychotic ask about personal/family history of diabetes, hypertension, and cardiovascular disease. Give advice on diet, weight control, and exercise. Perform BP, weight, fasting blood glucose, lipid profile, FBC, ECG if on clozapine. Additional 6-monthly monitoring of LFT, U&E, prolactin, weight, HbA1C is recommended.[51]

Antipsychotic medication All show a degree of D2 antagonism—responsible for antipsychotic efficacy. Historically divided into *typical* (neuroleptic) or *atypical* based on side effect profile. However, a more helpful way to consider these is into 'generations' based on when they were first commonly used.

First generation (FGA) are D2 antagonists which also cause extrapyramidal side effects (EPSE). Side effects are often what make people stop their tablets. Examples include: chlorpromazine, haloperidol. *Second generation* (SGA) are 5HT2A and D2 antagonists; associated with lower risk of EPSE but more metabolic side effects: weight gain, hyperglycaemia, and dyslipidaemia. Examples include amisulpride, olanzapine, quetiapine, risperidone, zotepine. *Third generation* (TGA) are dopamine partial agonists. Only licensed TGA is aripiprazole.

Comparing efficacy SGA relieve psychotic symptoms as effectively as FGA[52,53] and may lower relapse rates. NICE considers oral SGA 'the choice of first-line treatment for those with newly diagnosed schizophrenia' ☞ However, CATIE and CUTLASS trials suggest there is not enough evidence to favour either. SGA and TGA are much more costly than FGA—with additional pressure from pharmaceutical companies promoting non-generic medication and funding research designed to produce biased findings. Risperidone was top when psychiatrists were asked 'If you become psychotic, what would you want?'[54] n=543 Except for clozapine (see next paragraph) there is no clear advantage within any generation of one medication over another, so side effects, and long-term compliance are important in tailoring treatment to the individual patient. Most unwanted effects are dose related, so 'start low, increase slow'.

Clozapine Remains the most popular medication of treatment-resistant schizophrenia with clear utility despite its risks (agranulocytosis risk ≤0.8% in 1st year of treatment: specialist monitoring is needed). Associated ↓ suicide risk.

Treating EPSE: Above all else, try to reach the lowest tolerated dose of antipsychotic to encourage concordance • Parkinsonism: ↓ dose, change to SGA, or try procyclidine • Acute dystonia can occur within hours of starting antipsychotics. Treat with procyclidine IM/IV—may take up to 30 minutes to work; discouraged due to anticholinergic side effects • Akathisia (subjective sense of psychomotor restlessness) occurs within hours to weeks of starting antipsychotics, it may be very distressing; so use lowest possible dose or change to SGA—treatment may be needed with propranolol ± cyproheptadine • Tardive dyskinesia (chewing, grimaces, choreoathetosis) may be irreversible; but try tetrabenazine.

Main lifestyle issues • Hunger after taking medication (~3 hours): consider bedtime dose • Increased thirst: suggest water or sugar-free alternatives • Smoking induces metabolism and thus reduces antipsychotic plasma levels: higher doses and review dose if they quit smoking • Include targeted health promotion: 3 key areas are diet, physical exercise, and smoking cessation.

Failure to respond A number of interventions, not limited to medication, should have been completed before 'treatment failure' is confirmed. Within this, all medication must have been given at an adequate dose with verified compliance, cross-tapered to a new drug;[55] and clozapine considered and/or attempted. At this stage, combination therapy[56] is often tried, eg olanzapine with either amisulpride or risperidone, or quetiapine with risperidone. In theory, by acting on different receptors benefit may occur.[57] But often it doesn't go according to plan, and safety issues are opaque.

Common side effects of antipsychotic medication

Extrapyramidal side effects Drug-induced movement disorders which include: tremor, slurred speech, akathisia (motor restlessness), dystonia (continuous spasms and muscle contractions). These are rare with quetiapine[58] and clozapine; uncommon with aripiprazole and zotepine; but can occur at high doses with amisulpride, olanzapine, and risperidone.

Hyperprolactinaemia Aripiprazole, clozapine, and quetiapine have no or minimal effect on serum prolactin, olanzapine does at higher doses.[59]

Sexual dysfunction All SGA can cause sexual dysfunction, eg erectile dysfunction, ↓ libido, ↓ arousal, anorgasmia, eg from ↑ prolactin (check level)[60] and ↓ semen volume/viscosity;[61] retrograde ejaculation (α1-receptor antagonism, eg with risperidone).[62] In one study, ~30% had stopped their drugs at some point owing to sexual side effects.[63] So ask about sex (p. 749); few will volunteer this information. Even drug-free patients with schizophrenia have reduced libido so it's not a dose-related side effect.[64]

Weight gain Common. This causes ↓ compliance, ↑ risk of cardiovascular events and diabetes (greatest with olanzapine and clozapine, moderate with risperidone and zotepine; least with amisulpride and aripiprazole).[65]

Diabetes mellitus Prevalence in schizophrenia is twice the expected rate;[66] antipsychotics further increase risk (esp. clozapine and olanzapine).

Cardiovascular effects Olanzapine and risperidone ↑ risk of stroke in the elderly when used to treat behavioural symptoms of dementia.[67] Postural hypotension is common (α1 adrenoreceptor blockade), especially in the first 3 months of starting. Long QTc on ECG; fatal myocarditis and cardiomyopathy (clozapine).

Daytime drowsiness ~40% of those on clozapine (30% if on olanzapine or risperidone; 15% if on amisulpride or quetiapine).

Seizure threshold All antipsychotic medications decrease seizure threshold.

Special patient groups Elderly, children, and adolescents may get more side effects. In breastfeeding, most SGA enter breast milk. Trials of use in pregnancy are few; weigh up potential benefits against harm to mother, fetus, and neonate. Advise against breastfeeding.

'I don't want to go on with the tablets ...'

Take the time to talk with your patient and understand their reasoning for stopping. There are lots of reasons why people want to stop and some may be due to misunderstanding or incomplete information. Relapse is not always a disaster, and drug side effects can be difficult to deal with (or embarrassing to talk about). We tend to be over-impressed by positive symptoms (eg hallucinations) which respond better to drugs than negative symptoms.[68]

Ultimately, respect the patient's decision (unless there is genuine risk of stopping medication and an admission needs to be considered). It is better to work with a patient to safely withdraw medication with careful monitoring than refuse to discuss it and have them manage their own stopping in secret. If they feel listened to and understood, the therapeutic relationship can be strengthened.

In any year, 40% of us experience intense feelings of low mood, unhappiness, and disappointment which resolve without clinical intervention. But clinical depression is different from depressive symptoms. Worldwide, 5.8% of men and 9.5% of women will experience a depressive episode in a 12-month period, around 121 million people. It ranks 4th as a cause of disability worldwide and accounts for 5–10% of consultations in primary care in the UK.

Diagnosis Symptoms must be present every or nearly every day without significant changes throughout the day, for over 2 weeks and represent a change from normal personality without alcohol/drugs, medical disorders, or bereavement. There must be at least 2 *core symptoms:*

- Depressed mood for most of the day, every day. Little variation in mood despite changes in time, circumstances, or activity. There may be diurnal mood variation (worse in mornings and improving as day proceeds).
- Anhedonia: loss of interest or pleasure in daily life especially in things previously enjoyed; this change can be a subjective or observed change.
- Fatigue: a lack of energy which goes beyond poor sleep and pervades life.

Plus 2 or more *typical symptoms* (the first 5 are 'biological' symptoms):

- Poor appetite with marked weight loss (>5% of body weight in the past month) without dieting. Rarely, there is increased appetite and weight gain.
- Disrupted sleep: initial insomnia or early waking (3+ hours earlier than usual).
- Psychomotor retardation (limited spontaneous movement or sluggish thought processes) or agitation (subjective feeling of restlessness).
- Decreased libido (sexual drive) and other appetites.
- Evidence of (or subjective feelings of) reduced ability to concentrate.
- Feelings of worthlessness, inappropriate guilt (which may be delusional), or self-reproach. Not just about current illness but also past decisions or events.
- Recurrent thoughts of death, suicide ideation, or suicide attempts. These may be passive 'I wish I could disappear' or active 'My plan to overdose is …'.

Classification of a depressive episode Based on number and severity of these features; helps to determine management, treatment, and prognosis.

Aetiology Likely due to the interaction between biological, psychological, and social factors in any individual with risk factors for these. *Biological* • Point estimate of heritability for major depression is 37% • Twin studies show 60% more concordance for depression in monozygotic twins than dizygotic twins • Monoamine theory of depression: ↓ monoamine (eg 5-HT, noradrenaline, dopamine) function may cause depression. Antidepressants ↑ monoamines • Endocrinology ♀:♂ >1:1; dexamethasone suppression test is abnormal in ⅓ • Structural brain change: ventricular enlargement and raised sucal prominence. *Psychological* • Personality traits: neuroticism (high 'N' in Five Factor Model[7]) suggests mood lability, autonomic hyperarousal, and negative biases in attention and processing • Low self-esteem is considered a risk factor but is debatable if cause or symptom • Childhood experiences may ↑ sensitivity to events. *Social* • Disruption due to life events (birth, job loss, divorce, illness) in 60% of cases • Stress associated with poor social environment and social isolation can precipitate and perpetuate depression; social drift to lower social class.

Differentials • Psychiatric disorders: bipolar disorder, schizophrenia, anorexia nervosa, anxiety • Substance misuse • Dementia • Sleep disorders • Neurological disorders • Physical illness • Medication SE (eg β-blockers).

Depression is often missed or ignored when patients (♂ > ♀) dismiss depressive symptoms as temporary or due to a physical illness. An avoidance of psychiatric labels (often due to the stigma attached to these diagnoses) obstructs help-seeking behaviour. If professionals and patients collude to ignore depression or focus on physical causes then serious symptoms are untreated.

7 Collectively known as OCEAN: openness, conscientiousness, extraversion, agreeableness, and neuroticism.

Criteria for severity in depression (ICD-10)

The categories in table 12.4 should only be used for a single (first) depressive episode. Further depressive episodes should be classified as a recurrent depressive disorder. Categorization guides management and prognosis.

Additional classification includes with/without:
• Somatic symptoms (biological features of depression).
• Psychotic symptoms (mood-congruent delusions or hallucinations).
• Manic episodes (suggestive of bipolar not unipolar depression).

Table 12.4 Severity of depression

	Typical symptoms	Other core symptoms
Mild	2	2
Moderate	2	3+
Severe	3	4+

'Normal depression': adjustment disorder and bereavement

It is important to differentiate reactions to stress, life events, and bereavement from a depressive episode, in order to determine prognosis and treatment. Adjustment disorders are proof that stress can cause psychopathology (also: extraordinarily severe responses such as acute stress reaction and post-traumatic stress disorder, see p353). In adjustment disorder there is 'subjective distress and emotional disturbance, usually interfering with social functioning and performance ... [which] would not have arisen without the stressor' (ICD-10). For example, abnormally excessive reactions to life stressors such as a fire or flood, divorce, financial difficulties, or physical illness. In normal adaptive reactions to stress, functioning is less impaired. If there is an adjustment disorder without criteria met for major depression then antidepressants are not useful.

In bereavement there is an assumed period of grief, low mood, and adaptation, which has been summarized in the Kubler–Ross model. These 'stages' are no longer considered to occur in a defined order—so someone can start in, and move to, any stage (or revisit a stage multiple times) during the bereavement process:

Denial: Shutting out reality to cope with overwhelming difficult feelings.

Anger: Can be angry with themselves, or with others, or at a higher power.

Bargaining: Hoping to avoid or undo grief through negotiation or promises.

Depression: Disconnect from people in an attempt to avoid further trauma.

Acceptance: Coming to terms with inevitable situation; create calm mind-set.

If someone becomes stuck in a stage and unable to resolve their grief then additional support is needed from a GP or psychiatrist. If mood symptoms deepen and affect appetite, energy, and sleep then it may be depression.

NB: grief can be about many things, not just death, eg divorce or incarceration, and can be experienced by the patient given a terminal prognosis.

12 Psychiatry

Medication improves mood and ↑ synaptic availability of noradrenaline or serotonin (5HT). So, medication and therapy (p. 752) should be part of a holistic approach. Think about how you manage your own mood. Increasing activity is important: exercising, engaging in productive activity, socializing. Improve sleep, relaxation, and 'self-soothing' (being kind to oneself) techniques. Work out what each patient wants and support them to move in that direction. Inactivity, drugs, alcohol, daytime TV, and isolation will perpetuate a problem.

Mild depression Suggest low-intensity psychological interventions focused on sleep hygiene, anxiety management (mindfulness), and problem-solving techniques. These include individual guided self-help (books, websites, and apps, eg Headspace), computerized CBT, and structured group-based physical activity programmes. Unless the symptoms persist beyond 8 weeks or previous history of depression, antidepressants should not be routinely used.

Moderate depression Use a combination of an antidepressant and a high-intensity psychological intervention (8–12 sessions CBT or interpersonal therapy). The Improving Access to Psychological Therapies (IAPT) programme has been created to meet this need—it offers a realistic and routine first-line treatment across the NHS.[8] For a first episode of depression, a generic selective serotonin reuptake inhibitor (SSRI) is recommended (see p. 714).

Severe depression Includes psychotic depression, high risk of suicide, and atypical depression. These need a rapid specialist mental health assessment with a consideration of inpatient admission (using the MHA if necessary) or ECT (see BOX 'Electroconvulsive therapy (ECT)').

Recurrent depression 50–85% of people who have had one episode of moderate or severe depression will have further episodes and may require maintenance treatment to reduce relapse risk. Intervene quickly and early for any recurrence. If a medication has worked before it has a very good chance of working again, so this should always be first line. Continuing antidepressants lowers the odds of relapse by ~65%, halving absolute risk.[69] CBT can be offered to manage residual symptoms. Psychoeducation around the relapsing nature of the condition is essential. Normalize reoccurrence—many conditions carry a risk of this (eg basal cell carcinoma).

Lifestyle changes Many people want to avoid medication or therapy. If safe to do so, positive suggestions should include: exercise (in wild nature), tai chi, yoga, social interaction, psychotherapy, reading clubs, meditation, poetry (reading/writing). For some, rest from work—always plan a phased return.

Follow-up All patients should be reviewed regularly, frequently at first and then less often, to consider their current symptomatology and level of functioning. Investigate their response to any interventions, adherence to treatments, and adverse effects—direct questioning and probing may be required to elicit 'embarrassing' or assumed unconnected complaints. Alongside this, consider: comorbid conditions associated with depression (eg alcohol or drug misuse), suicide risk, and safeguarding concerns (children or vulnerable adults). Include psychoeducation on depression and recovery—promotion of lifestyle changes (using identified stressors and supports) with ongoing reviews and reflection to highlight gains and maintain positive changes.

St John's wort (*Hypericum perforatum*) Widely available as a (non-prescribed) herbal remedy for depression. A Cochrane review states superiority to placebo and equivalent to antidepressants in major depression with fewer side effects (½ that of SSRIs). However, use should not be encouraged: it upregulates the CYP3A4 cytochrome (within liver's P450 system), affecting drug metabolism, eg reducing efficiency of oral contraceptive pill. In addition, different preparations have varying amounts of active ingredient. Always ask if it is being taken.

8 Also developed for under 18s: Children and Young People's IAPT (or CYP-IAPT).

Severe depression

When there is persistent low mood or anhedonia for >2 weeks, and ≥4 of the following 7 markers of severe depression, there is a high risk of suicide:

Suicide plan or ideas of self-harm.
Unexplained guilt or worthlessness.
Inability to function (eg psycho-motor retardation or agitation).
Concentration impaired.
Impaired appetite.
Decreased sleep/early waking.
Energy low/unaccountable fatigue.

Enquire about these whenever depression is possible. Ask the patient sensitively but directly whether they think about suicide and how often.

Sometimes, in severe depression, antidepressants need to be prescribed as a matter of urgency, eg if suicide is likely or if a parent's functioning is so impaired they cannot look after their family.

Over-diagnosing severe depression is undesirable. Patients' lives can become medicalized and drugs, with significant SE, are needlessly given. In some areas of the UK prescriptions for antidepressants tripled from 1993 to 2007 without clear benefits for patients. In primary care there isn't the luxury of an hour-long assessment to differentiate clinical depression from its alternatives. NICE and QOF recommend using the PHQ-9 diagnostic tool to help prevent this.

12 Psychiatry

Electroconvulsive therapy (ECT)

ECT is a very effective treatment for depression, particularly severe depressive episodes which have not responded to medication. However, the public perception of it as barbaric, coercive, or dangerous makes it controversial. Sadly, there is often a gross misunderstanding of ECT based on a belief that treatment hasn't changed since 1950s or films ('One Flew Over the Cuckoo's Nest' shows a lobotomy not ECT). The reality of ECT (fig 12.7) is less scary than the perception (fig 12.6).

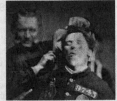

Fig 12.6 Patient at the West Riding Lunatic Asylum, Wakefield, Yorkshire; attributed to Henry Clarke. Number 17, young man restrained by two warders.

Wellcome Collection.

Mechanism There is MRI evidence for the idea that ECT interrupts the hyperconnectivity between the various areas of the brain that maintain depression.[70]

Indications NICE recommends ECT is used to gain rapid improvement of severe symptoms after an adequate trial of other treatments has proven ineffective and/or when the condition is considered to be potentially life-threatening, in patients with: • A prolonged or severe manic episode • Severe depression • Catatonia.

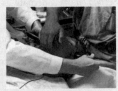

Fig 12.7 Modern ECT.
Courtesy of University of Michigan.

Emergency ECT is possible, but rarely used—the success rate is good (80%).[71] Carry on antidepressants when ECT ends: this *may* prevent recurrences.[72] *Typical course length*: 6–12 sessions (2 per week).

Contraindications Mainly to the general anaesthesia. There are no absolute contraindications to ECT itself; no consent (p. 772; involve relatives, but they cannot consent for an adult). **Cautions** Recent subdural/subarachnoid bleed, stroke, MI, arrhythmia, CNS vascular anomalies.

Side effects Memory loss: short-term retrograde amnesia (usually resolves completely), confusion, headaches, and clumsiness; common anaesthetic SE.

There is good evidence that antidepressants are helpful in major depression and in particular preventing relapse, but their limitations shouldn't be ignored. It can feel perplexing prescribing antidepressants; often more like trial and error to work out what works well in one person but may not help another. In this context, the basic approach to prescription should be:

- Discuss choice of drug and non-pharmacological therapy. CBT is known to be as effective as antidepressants in mild to moderate depression.[73] Combined use is better than either treatment alone.[74,75]
- Discuss side effects. Warn patient that there may be an initial worsening of symptoms in the first weeks so persevere before therapeutic effects are seen. Remember to monitor closely during this time for increased suicidality. Not all side effects are undesirable (SSRI may help premature ejaculation).
- Assess formally after (at least) 4 weeks. If effective continue for at least 6 months after recovery; if stopped too soon 50% of patients relapse.[76]
- If there is a minor/low response, titrate the dose up looking for additional response. Switching is better than augmenting although commonly doctors will combine medication if there has been a partial recovery on one drug.
- If no response after 4 weeks or poor tolerability, switch to an alternative class of antidepressant. Do not continue to increase the dose; there is little evidence for dose response except tricyclics, venlafaxine, and escitalopram.[9]

NICE guidance Full guideline on depression concluded that antidepressants have largely equal efficacy and that choice should mainly depend on: • Side effect profile • People's preference • Previous experience of treatments • Propensity of discontinuation symptoms • Safety in overdose • Interactions • Cost.

SSRIs are recommended as first choice due to favourable risk–benefit ratios. Neither escitalopram nor the 'dual action' antidepressants (eg venlafaxine, duloxetine), were judged to have any clinically important advantages. *First line:* A generic SSRI should be commenced with low starting dose which can be titrated up. Advise that full effect may take up to 6 weeks (initial positive effects most likely due to placebo) and effective dose will be continued for at least 6 months after recovery. Fluoxetine (only antidepressant licensed for <18s), citalopram (or escitalopram), or sertraline (best in IHD) are all good choices in terms of safety, efficacy, and tolerability. Monitor FBC (anaemia due to GI bleeding and avoid concurrent NSAIDs) and U&E (hyponatraemia) in any SSRI. With citalopram there may be dose-dependent prolongation of QTc interval so check ECG (if unnoticed, torsades de pointes). Discuss potential adverse effects and risks of discontinuation/withdrawal symptoms—including sexual side effects (often an unspoken reason why medication is stopped).

Second line: An alternate SSRI from first line (all are very different molecules).

Third line: In no particular order, mirtazapine (noradrenergic and specific serotonergic antidepressant: NaSSA), or venlafaxine (serotonin and noradrenaline reuptake inhibitor: SNRI) are all acceptable. Mirtazapine can cause drowsiness at low doses, which may be helpful to aid sleep when given as an evening dose, and can lead to weight gain. Venlafaxine may be more effective for patients who are anxious, but requires a baseline BP and ECG and monitoring for any cardiovascular side effects.

Fourth line: The Star* D trial essentially showed that if a medication is ineffective, keep switching until you find one that works. Lithium is effective as an adjunctive therapy but has significant toxicity problems. Consider older antidepressants • Tricyclics (TCAs): nortriptyline, clomipramine • Monoamine oxidase inhibitors (MAOIs): moclobemide, phenelzine • Serotonin agonist and reuptake inhibitor (SARI): trazodone. Whatever is used, review regularly.

9 Escitalopram is the active enantiomer of citalopram. While some studies show an increased efficacy, others question if there is any appreciable difference—and if this was a means to re-patent, and therefore sell at a high price, an older drug (citalopram) which was about to become available in a cheaper generic form.

12 Psychiatry

Swapping antidepressants: how to cross-taper

When an antidepressant has been unsuccessful at an adequate dose, or is poorly tolerated, changing the drug is appropriate. Avoid abrupt withdrawal when swapping antidepressants; cross-tapering is preferred (see table 12.5[77]). Speed of cross-tapering is best judged by patient tolerability. NB: co-administration of some antidepressants is absolutely contraindicated, see 'Cautions'—dangers include precipitating the *serotonin syndrome*[78] (restlessness; diaphoresis, ie excessive sweating; tremor; shivering; myoclonus; confusion; convulsions; death).

Cautions When swapping from MAOIs to any other antidepressant, withdraw and wait for 2 weeks (the time taken for monoamine oxidase to be replenished); for moclobemide wait 24h. Do not co-administer clomipramine and SSRIs or venlafaxine. Beware of fluoxetine interactions (may still occur for 5 weeks after stopping, due to long half-life).

Table 12.5 Example of cross-tapering based on the Maudsley regimen

	Week 1	Week 2	Week 3	Week 4
Withdrawing amitriptyline from 150mg/24h	100mg/24h	50mg/24h	25mg/24h	Nil
Introducing sertraline	25mg/24h	50mg/24h	75mg/24h	100mg/24h

Antidepressant medication effects and side effects

Eight pharmacological actions are known, and over 20 antidepressants exist. How do all they lead to a similar response? Why is there a delay? Two theories: the *neurotransmitter receptor hypothesis* postulates that a change in receptor sensitivity by desensitization and down-regulation of different receptors (not just ↑ neurotransmitter at the synapse) leads to clinical effects after a few weeks. The *monoamine hypothesis of antidepressants on gene expression* suggests the effect of increased neurotransmitter at the synapse initiates a sequence of events to give the antidepressant response. This includes up- and down-regulation of various genes with subsequent varying expression of receptors and critical proteins.[79]

The associated side effects, cautions, and contraindications for all antidepressant medications are too numerous to list here. Use the *British National Formulary* (*BNF*) or Maudsley Prescription Guidelines (http://maudsley-prescribing-guidelines.co.uk/) for up-to-date information and current recommendations regarding prescribing dosages.

Prevalence Lifetime: 1.5% ♀=♂; peak prevalence is between 15–19♀ and 20–24♂.

Signs of mania *Mood:* Irritability,[80%] euphoria,[71%] lability.[69%] *Cognition:* Grandiosity,[78%] distractibility/poor concentration,[71%] flight of ideas/racing thoughts,[71%] confusion,[25%] lack of insight. *Behaviour:* Rapid speech,[98%] hyperactivity,[87%] ↓ sleep,[81%] hypersexuality,[57%] extravagance.[55%] *Psychotic symptoms:* Delusions,[48%] hallucinations.[15%] This elevated mood must be present for at least a week (or shorter but requiring admission) to be considered mania. Any impairment must be severe enough to limit function.

Less severe states are termed *hypomania* with characteristic symptoms of mania except for psychotic symptoms, impairment in daily functioning, or need for inpatient treatment. If depression alternates with mania, the term *bipolar affective disorder* is used (the term 'manic-depressive' is still used colloquially but not clinically). During mood swings, risk of suicide is high. Cyclical mood swings with subclinical features are termed *cyclothymia*. A patient's ability to manage their symptoms (ie degree of 'impairment') is partially socially defined—a single mother of twin toddlers may have a harder time 'coping' than a wealthy, childless married woman.

Causes *Medication:* Steroids, illicit substances (amphetamines, cocaine), antidepressants. *Physical:* Infection, stroke, neoplasm, epilepsy, multiple sclerosis, and metabolic disturbances (esp. hyperthyroidism).

Assessment *Ask about:* Infections, drug use, and past or family history of psychiatric disorders. *Do:* CT of the head, EEG, and screen for drugs/toxins.[80]

Treating acute mania *Assess:* Psychotic symptoms (p. 696, p. 698); cycling speed; suicide risk. For acute moderate/severe mania: any SGA (SE: weight ↑; glucose ↑), or semisodium valproate (eg Depakote*). NB: some people are most fulfilled and creative when manic[10] and don't want to change; others recognize, in retrospect, that use of mental health law (a last resort) was a turning point.

Prophylaxis Those who have bipolar affective disorder after successful treatment of the manic or depressive episode should have a mood stabilizer for longer-term control. If compliance is good, and U&E, ECG, and T4 normal, give lithium carbonate. Adjust dose to give a plasma level of ~0.6–1mmol/L Li+, by day 7, ~12h post-dose. Elderly show ↑ sensitivity to Li+ neurotoxicity.[81]
• Check Li+ levels weekly (~12h post-dose) until the dose has been constant for 4 weeks; then monthly for 6 months; then 3-monthly, if stable; more often if on diuretic, NSAIDs, ACE inhibitor (all ↑ Li+), low-salt diet, or if pregnant.
• If Li+ levels are progressively rising, suspect progressive nephrotoxicity.
• U&E + TSH 6-monthly; Li+ SE: hypothyroidism; nephrogenic diabetes insipidus.

►Avoid changing brands [Li+↓↑]. ►Ensure you can reach them urgently if Li+ >1.4mmol/L. ►Toxic signs: vision ↓; D&V; K+↓; ataxia; tremor; dysarthria; coma.

Psychosocial interventions Target the emotional consequences of having a cycling disorder with periods of acute illness, stigma, fear of recurrence ('I'm having a good time but am I happy, or *too* happy?') and other problems arising from illness (eg manic overspending, hypersexualized behaviour, etc.). Key elements include psychoeducation, CBT, and support groups.

Risk of suicide Higher if: • Previous suicide attempt • Family history of suicide • Early onset of bipolar disorder • Extent of depressive symptoms (eg hopelessness) • Increasingly bad affective signs • Mixed affective states • Rapid cycling • Abuse of alcohol or drugs.[82] Lithium reduces risk of suicide. If contraindicated, olanzapine and fluoxetine may be better than lamotrigine. ►But don't only rely on medication: CBT (p. 754) is of great value in helping people (who retain some insight) to ride their cycles without falling off.[83]

10 A counter argument from the periodically depressed poet Thomas Krampf: 'one can have a vision but no vision is worth anything if one is too sick to implement it'—and many writers have found their creativity flourish more when treatment is underway. M Berlin 2008 *Poets on Prozac*, Baltimore.

Bipolar disorder and pregnancy

There is an increased risk of perinatal psychiatric illness in women with bipolar disorder so regular discussions about contraception and the importance of seeking advice early if she is thinking about pregnancy (or unexpectedly pregnant) are essential. >50% of pregnancies are unplanned. Remember this, when considering medication in any woman of childbearing potential. NICE recommends that sodium valproate should **not** be used in this group if avoidable, due to its particular teratogenic and developmental effects.

Lithium is considered to be the most teratogenic medication in bipolar disorder with an increased risk to lithium-exposed babies being up to 12% (compared to 4% in control group). Particular concerns about Ebstein anomaly (see p. 846), floppy baby syndrome, and thyroid abnormalities.

For these women, frequent reviews and close contact is essential during the perinatal period. Stopping medication when pregnant carries a risk of relapse, with studies showing women who stop medication are over twice as likely to have symptom recurrence compared to those who continue. If a woman decides to stop (and there is no strong evidence for either choice) immediately commencing prophylactic medication postpartum should be considered—with advice about breastfeeding. Other interventions include reducing stress, and promoting good sleep (especially in late pregnancy and first months after birth).

When lithium does not give good control

Note that abrupt cessation of lithium precipitates acute mania in up to 50% of patients. Discontinuation should be gradual over 2–4 weeks.

Anticonvulsants Consider semisodium valproate or carbamazepine as 2nd line. The most specific indication may be in rapid cyclers (≥4 acute mood swings/year). Lamotrigine is a mood stabilizer and as good as citalopram in bipolar depressive states.[84] Gabapentin and topiramate are potential mood stabilizers.

Antipsychotics Olanzapine has a role.[85] In one meta-analysis, there was no difference in overall efficacy of treatment between haloperidol and olanzapine or risperidone. Some evidence suggests that haloperidol could be less effective than aripiprazole.[86]

Combination treatments (Often tried.) Lithium plus carbamazepine may be synergistic.[87] If mania persists despite long-term treatment with lithium, adding in another antimanic such as an antipsychotic or valproate is a rational strategy. Lithium (or valproate) plus a 2nd-generation antipsychotic, eg risperidone or olanzapine, may help if unresponsive to monotherapy.[88,89]

Antidepressants with lithium Lithium (or an alternative mood stabilizer) reduces risk of mood fluctuations from mania to depression in people with bipolar affective disorder. For depression occurring during lithium treatment, antidepressants can be used: SSRIs and venlafaxine are considered the most effective. Avoid tricyclics as they seem most likely to cause iatrogenic mania. Also consider antipsychotics such as quetiapine. Taper from 2 to 6 months after remission to minimize manic relapse.[90]

Consider monoamine oxidase inhibitors for anergic (=lacking in energy) bipolar depression.[91] ECT also has a role (p. 713),[92] and meta-analyses support use of omega 3 oils (only for when mood is low).[93]

Anxiety is a normal response to threat or danger and part of the usual human experience, but it can become a mental health problem if the response is exaggerated, lasts more than 3 weeks, and interferes with daily life. Anxiety disorders ($\varphi:\sigma\approx2:1$) can cause suffering and cost the UK $\gtrsim$£5 billion/yr. **Neurosis** Refers to *maladaptive psychological symptoms not due to organic causes or psychosis, and usually precipitated by stress.* Apart from generalized anxiety and depression, symptoms include: fatigue,[27%] insomnia,[25%] irritability,[22%] worry,[20%] obsessions, compulsions, and somatization—all more intense than the stress precipitating them would warrant. Symptoms are not just part of a patient's normal personality, but they may be an exaggeration of personality: a 'worrier' may become even more so, ie develop an anxiety neurosis, as a result of job loss. The *type* of neurosis is defined by the chief symptom (eg anxiety, obsessional, depressive). Before diagnosing anxiety, consider carefully if there is underlying depression needing antidepressants.[94]

Symptoms of anxiety *Cognitive:* Agitation; feelings of impending doom; poor concentration; difficulty in getting to sleep (insomnia); excessive concern about self and bodily functions; repetitive thoughts and activities (p.720). *Somatic:* Tension; trembling; a sense of collapse; 'goose flesh'; 'butterflies in the stomach'; hyperventilation (so tinnitus, tetany, tingling, chest pains); headaches; sweating; palpitations; nausea; 'lump in the throat' unrelated to swallowing (globus hystericus). *Behaviours:* (Not strictly symptoms but these actions in response to anxiety reinforce the anxiety state.) Reassurance seeking (from partner, doctor, etc.); avoidance; dependence on person or object. *Children's symptoms:* Thumb-sucking; nail-biting; bed-wetting.

Causes Genetic predisposition; stress (work, noise, hostile home), events (losing or gaining a spouse or job; moving house). Others: *Faulty learning* or *secondary gain* (a husband 'forced' to stay at home with agoraphobic wife).

Treatment *Symptom control:* Listening is a good way to ↓ anxiety. Explain that headaches are not from a tumour, and that palpitations are harmless. Anything done to enrich patients' relationship with others may well help. Anxiety management teaches that anxiety feels bad (even life-threatening) but it does not cause physical damage and that if left, it will resolve with time.

- *Regular (non-obsessive!) exercise:* Beneficial effects appear to equal meditation or relaxation. Acute anxiety responds better than chronic anxiety.
- *Meditation:* Intensive but time-limited group stress reduction intervention based on 'mindfulness meditation' can have long-term beneficial effects.[95]
- *Progressive relaxation training:* A type of behavioural therapy (see: p.756).Teach deep breathing using the diaphragm (see box 'Deep breathing exercise'), and relaxation of muscle groups (see p.757). Practise is essential. CDs aid learning; in some contexts, eg stress, relaxation is not as good as cognitive restructuring.
- *Cognitive behavioural therapy and relaxation:* (p.754) Appear to be the best specific measures[96] with 50–60% recovering over 6 months.[97] N=404
- *Behavioural therapy* with a graded exposure to anxiety-provoking stimuli.
- *Hypnosis:* Initially the therapist induces progressively deeper trances eg using guided fantasy and concentration on bodily sensations, eg breathing. Later, some patients will be able to induce their own trances. It can strongly reduce anxiety, and is useful, eg medical contexts (eg post-op).[98]
- *Medication:* NICE recommend medication or CBT—equal efficacy but no evidence of synergy (strangely): see box 'Treating anxiety with medication'

Prognosis General anxiety disorder (GAD) often gets better by ~50yrs although is frequently replaced by somatization.[99]

Deep breathing exercise

▶Try this yourself. You never know when an ability to calm yourself down and avoid becoming overwhelmed with stress may come in use.

We all tend to breathe faster and/or too deeply than normal when stressed or anxious. This can make us feel light headed, which in turn, increases our anxiety, so we breathe even faster, feel dizzier and become more anxious …

This exercise should take around 5 minutes. It is recommend you practise this every day at a time when not anxious. In a stressful situation, or when you feel your stress rising, having a well-rehearsed technique is very helpful.

1 Breathe slowly and deeply in through your nose, and out through your mouth in a steady rhythm.
2 Try to make your breath out twice as long as your breath in. It is often helpful to count slowly 'one, two' as you breathe in, and 'one, two, three, four' as you breathe out. This increases vagal tone, slowing heart rate.
3 Fill up the whole of your lungs with air, without forcing. Imagine you're filling up a bottle, so that your lungs fill from the bottom
4 Focus on mainly using your diaphragm ('lower chest muscles') to breathe. When we become anxious we tend to forget to use this muscle and favour the muscles at the top of the chest and shoulders. These create shorter, shallow breaths. Diaphragmatic breathing pulls the lungs downwards which expands the airways to allow air to flow in.
5 Relax your shoulders and upper chest muscles when you breathe. With each breath out, consciously try to relax those muscles until you are mainly using your diaphragm to breathe.

(If this is unclear, you can check if you are using your diaphragm by feeling just below your sternum at the top of your abdomen. If you cough, you can feel the diaphragm push out here. When you hold your hand here you should feel it move in and out as you breathe using your diaphragm.)

Treating anxiety with medication

Based on NICE guidelines, published in January 2011:
• Consider 1st-line treatment with a SSRI (as best tolerated). Use the ones you are familiar with, the evidence doesn't strongly favour one over another. Also consider SNRI (venlafaxine or duloxetine) or tricyclic antidepressants, MAOI (phenelzine) as 2nd- or 3rd-line treatments.
• Benzodiazepines are often used 1st line but patients can build up a tolerance to them, and they can be hard to stop. People with a history of harmful drug and alcohol use are likely to over-rely on them. Generally they are not a long-term solution to an anxiety disorder and are best used sparingly and infrequently for acute distress and agitation. If trials of several other medications have failed then long-term use of a benzodiazepine isn't unreasonable.
• Pregabalin can be used as a monotherapy or in conjunction with an antidepressant.
• Antipsychotics (eg quetiapine) are generally reserved for acute distress or sometimes used to augment antidepressant therapy, eg in OCD.
• β-blockers can improve the somatic symptoms of anxiety such as tremulousness, sweating, etc. and can be useful, eg for those who give public speeches. However, they do not improve cognitive anxiety—and can in fact be detrimental as people feel anxious but do not look it—which can affect relationships adversely.

12 Psychiatry

Obsessive–compulsive disorder (ocd) Compulsions are senseless, repeated rituals. Obsessions are stereotyped, purposeless words, ideas, or phrases that come into the mind. They are perceived by the patient as intrusive, nonsensical (unlike delusional beliefs), and, although out of character, as originating from themselves (unlike hallucinations or thought insertion). The compulsions are normally a way to reduce the distress of the obsession. They are often resisted by the patient, but if chronic, the patient may have given up resisting them.

2–3% of people will experience ocd during their lifetime with 7% of British adults reporting 'obsessions' in any week and 4% reporting 'compulsions'. However, it often takes 10–15 years for people to seek professional help.

An example of non-verbal compulsive behaviour is the rambler who can never do a long walk because every few paces he wonders if he has really locked the car, and has to return repeatedly to ensure that this has, in fact, been done. Cleaning (eg hand-washing), counting, and dressing rituals are other examples. *Pathophysiology:* cns imaging implicates the orbitofrontal cortex[100] and the caudate nucleus. Successful treatment is reflected by some normalization of metabolism in these areas.[101] *Treatment:* cbt (p. 754). **Clomipramine** (start with 25mg/day po) or ssris (eg **fluoxetine**, start with 20mg/day po) really can help (even if patients are not depressed): see p. 714.

What's it like to have ocd? 'That afternoon, I found that when I got home from school, I couldn't get around the house or do normal things without performing rituals to cancel out bad thoughts over and over again. It was weird and I didn't want to do it, but if I didn't I would feel a lot of anxiety and panic like something was very wrong. I kept having to enter and re-enter through the front door. I ended up spending about three or four hours in the bathroom because I couldn't get out of there because every time I tried to do the perfect ritual, my body would itch or something else would go wrong and I had to redo the rituals over again. After a few hours, I wanted to get out of there bad, I felt like a prisoner in my own bathroom!'[102]

Phobic disorders Phobias describe a group of disorders in which anxiety is experienced only, or predominantly, in certain well-defined situations that are not dangerous. As a result, these situations are avoided or endured with dread. They become a disorder when they cause marked distress and/ or significantly impair a person's ability to function. Phobias are much more common in women than men, affecting about 22 in 1000($\female$) compared with 13 in 1000 ($\male$) in Britain. Phobias are labelled according to specific circumstance:

- Agoraphobia (*agora*, Greek for market place): cluster of phobias: fear of crowds, travel (usually alone on trains or buses) or events away from home.
- Social phobias: where we might be minutely observed, eg small dinner parties; characterized by a fear of scrutiny by other people. Symptoms may include blushing, shaking hands, nausea, or the urgent need to go to the toilet.
- Simple phobia: numerous phobias restricted to specific situations eg dentists (odontophobia), spiders (arachnophobia, p. 756), clowns (coulrophobia).[11]
- There may also be a free-floating 'fear of fear', or fear of disgracing oneself by uncontrollable screaming.

Elicit the *exact* phobic stimulus. It may be specific, eg travelling by car, not bicycle. Why are some situations avoided? If deluded ('I'm being followed/ persecuted'), paranoia rather than phobia is likely. For panic attacks, try cbt[103] (p. 754), ± ssri, tca, pregabalin, clonazepam (paroxetine has a short half-life and the worst discontinuation symptoms of ssri).[104,105]

---

11 For an exhaustive list of phobias see: http://phobialist.com/. It includes every phobia from Agateophobia (fear of insanity) to Zemmiphobia (fear of the great mole rat).

'There are some experiences and intimations which scar too deeply to permit of healing, and leave only such an added sensitiveness that memory reinspires all the original horror.' HP Lovecraft; *At the Mountains of Madness*

A reaction to a stressful event is to be expected (and worrying if absent). An *acute stress reaction* is a transient condition (lasting hours to days). There is an immediate dissociation ('daze'), followed by mixed emotions including anxiety, anger, and confusion. These usually resolve without psychiatric intervention (although talking to friends and family often helps). If these symptoms become *chronic*, adjustment disorder (within 1 month) or PTSD (within 6 months) should be considered; symptoms may be delayed for years in some.

Post-traumatic stress disorder (PTSD) Develops after an exceptionally stressful, life-threatening, or catastrophic event or situation. Common symptoms include re-experiencing the event in vivid nightmares or flashbacks (often with autonomic arousal: ↑ pulse; ↑BP; ↑ sweating) often precipitating anxiety or panic attacks, avoidance of things associated with the event, hypervigilance (increased startle reaction), sleep disturbance, and poor concentration. Depression, emotional numbing, drug or alcohol misuse, and anger are also common comorbid conditions. In children, re-experiencing symptoms may take the form of re-enacting the experience, repetitive play, or frightening dreams without recognizable content. There is often denial or suppression of memory for the traumatic event. Intentional acts of violence are more likely than natural events or accidents to result in PTSD. The risk of developing PTSD after a traumatic event is 8% for men and 20% for women.

Pathophysiology: MRI implicates the anterior cingulate area, with failure to inhibit amygdala activation ± ↓ amygdala threshold to fearful stimuli.[106,107]

Treatment: Immediate debriefing does more harm than good. Evidence strongly supports trauma-focused treatments, specifically CBT and *eye movement desensitization and reprocessing* (EMDR). EMDR uses a patient's voluntary rapid, rhythmic eye movements to reduce the anxiety associated with traumatic thoughts/images and thereby process the emotions attached to these experiences. While this approach is 'unique', there is enough evidence to suggest that it is effective (and NICE approved). That said, the mechanism for EMDR has not been explained and it has been shown that eye movements are not actually an essential part of the intervention. Other interventions include hypnotherapy (to help control arousal) and stress management. After the 2004 Indian Ocean tsunamis, psychopathology was as common as physical injury; WHO advised practical outreach help, and to avoid mental health labels (different culture to NICE's medicalizing approach to PTSD).[108]

Medication is 2nd line to therapy, however it can be used in combination or if a patient is too distressed to use psychological therapy. If used, SSRIs (paroxetine) are licensed; also consider TCAs (amitriptyline), mirtazapine, MAOIS (phenelzine), and 2nd-generation antipsychotics (p. 708); warn of SE and discontinuation phenomena (p. 724).[109, 110, 111]

Prognosis: Dependent on initial symptoms and their severity; usually 50% will recover within 1 year. Recovery improved by lack of maladaptive coping strategies (eg denial), single traumatic event, and no ongoing secondary problems (eg disfigurement, legal action, acquired disability).

Prevention: Rehearse teamwork—and techniques of stress inoculation (by exposure), and desensitization (by helping real casualties, eg if preparing for war). Keeping combatants in tight-knit groups cemented by the ties of mutual interdependency is recommended by military strategists. NB: morphine use at the time of injury may be protective. www.killology.com

Depersonalization This is an unpleasant state of disturbed perception in which people, or the self, or parts of the body are experienced as being changed ('as if made of cotton wool'), becoming unreal, remote, or automatized ('replaced by robots'). There is insight into its subjective nature, so it is not a psychosis, but the patient may think they are going mad. Depersonalization may be primary, or part of another neurosis. CNS imaging shows that it is associated with functional abnormalities in the sensory cortex in areas where visual, auditory, and somatosensory (cross-modal) data integrate.[112]

Derealization These are psychosensory feelings (akin to depersonalization) of detachment or estrangement from our surroundings. Objects appear altered: buildings may metamorphose in size and colour. The patient acknowledges the unreality of these ideas, but is made uneasy by them.

Dissociation (Formerly *hysteria*.) *Example of mass hysteria spread by TV*—Pokémon-induced 'seizures': see '*the Pokémon contagion*'.[113] ℞: Behavioural therapy (p. 756 ± antidepressants) if patient really wants to change.

Types of dissociation: Amnesia is the commonest type: see BOX 'Is this amnesia dissociative?' *Depersonalization*: feeling of being detached from one's body or ideas, as if one were an outsider, observing the self; '*I'm in a dream*' or '*I'm an automaton*' (unrelated to drugs/alcohol) eg from stress.

Dissociative identity disorder: the patient has multiple personalities which interact in complex ways. It is present in 3% of acute psychiatric inpatients.

Fugue: inability to recall one's past ± loss of identity or formation of a new identity, associated with unexpected, purposeful travel (lasts hours to months, and for which there is no 'me' ie the person is no longer themselves).

Follow-up (~6yrs) shows that ~5% of those referred to a CNS hospital who had hysteria/dissociation diagnosed turned out to have organic illness.

Treatment Exploring life stresses may help. Be ready to recognize psychological components of physical illness, and get expert psychiatric help, while leaving the door open for new diagnoses.

Seeking a physical cause Why do some doctors preferentially diagnose somatic illness? Why, when confronted by unexplained symptoms, do we often subconsciously try to fit them to a physical ailment? The reason is usually that prescribing a pill is easier than changing, or regulating, intrapsychic events. The patient and the doctor may collude with this approach, and then get angry when it yields nothing. Alternatively, some doctors are so used to diagnosing psychopathology that they are all too prone to launch into treating someone's depression and malaise, rather than their endocarditis or brucellosis. There is no single correct approach. We all make errors: the point is to find out in which direction you tend to make errors, then allow for this in your work.

Some patients are naively keen to name their condition, eg 'fibromyalgia', or 'somatization disorder'. Being able to name a disease or a condition is to start to control it. But it's only a start. In time, having named a condition may not prove all that helpful—and neither may be seeing a string of experts. This paves the way for a cognitive shift that may allow progress—even healing—to come about. As one patient said: 'I stopped focusing on the specific diagnoses years ago, and switched to finding the best ways to increase my overall wellness. I use what I learned about my fibromyalgia to inform my choices, and have figured out what works best for me ... Experts are just people, and are sometimes wrong ...'

Is this amnesia dissociative?

Hypnotic phenomena share features with conversion (hysterical) symptoms, eg lack of concern, involuntariness with implicit knowledge, and a compliant tone (la belle indifférence—a relative lack of concern about the nature or implications of symptoms). Theories of consciousness postulate an altered relationship between self-awareness and the supervisory attentional system in both conditions (frontal and cingulate cortices are implicated).[114] Most subside spontaneously, but if they do not it is important to refer early to a psychiatrist, before associated behaviour becomes habitual.

Things to consider with a dissociative experience include:
- Has a physical cause been carefully discounted? (Drugs, epilepsy, etc.)
- Is the patient young? Beware making the first diagnosis if >40yrs old.
- Have the symptoms been provoked by stress? Ask the family.
- Do related symptoms 'make sense' (eg aphonia in a news-reader)?
- What is the pattern of amnesia? If for distant *and* near memories, then dissociation is more likely (vs organic causes) than if the amnesia is for shorter-term memory.
- Indifference to major handicap is of little diagnostic use.
- Is malingering likely? The answer is usually 'No', except in prisons and the military (when secondary gain is easy to identify).
- Is there a dissociative personality?

The dissociative experiences scale (DES) screens for this: a 28-item visual analogue scale about the proportion of time spent on dissociative experiences (not those from drugs/alcohol) going from the normal, eg being so absorbed in TV that we are unaware of events around us, to severe forms, eg of having no memory of cardinal personal events, or feeling that our body belongs to another. In dissociative disorders, typical DES scores are ≥30; most others score nearer 0.[115]

12 Psychiatry

Withdrawing benzodiazepines ▶*The withdrawal syndrome may well be worse than the condition for which the drug was originally prescribed.* So try to avoid benzodiazepine use, eg relaxation techniques for anxiety, or, for insomnia, a dull (text)book, sexual intercourse, and avoiding night-time coffee may facilitate sleep (see p. 739). If not, limit hypnotics to alternate nights.

The 'Z' drugs: zaleplon, zolpidem, and zopiclone are commonly prescribed, although this is not advised because tolerance develops with long-term use. Of those on benzodiazepines for 6 months, 30% experience withdrawal symptoms when treatment is stopped, and some will do so after only a few weeks of treatment. Symptoms appear sooner with rapidly eliminated benzodiazepines (eg lorazepam vs diazepam or chlordiazepoxide). It is not possible to predict which patients will become dependent, but 'passive dependent' or neurotic personality is partly predictive. Symptoms often start with anxiety or psychotic symptoms 1–2 weeks after withdrawal, followed by many months of gradually decreasing symptoms, such as insomnia, panic, and depression. Irritability and feelings of unreality and depersonalization (p. 722) are common; hallucinations less so. Multiple sclerosis may be misdiagnosed as there may be diplopia, paraesthesiae, fasciculation, and ataxia. Gut symptoms include D&V, abdominal pain, and dysphagia. There may also be palpitations, flushing, and hyperventilation symptoms. The problem is not so much how to stop benzodiazepine treatment, but how to avoid being manipulated into prescribing them unnecessarily. This is addressed in 'Manipulative patients and boundary setting', p. 868.

How to withdraw: • Augment the patient's will to give up (stress disadvantages of continuous treatment) • Withdrawal is harder for short-acting benzodiazepines, so change to diazepam • Agree a contract to prescribe a weekly supply, and not to add to this if it is used up early • Withdraw by ~2mg/week of diazepam. Warn to expect withdrawal symptoms, and not to be alarmed.

Withdrawing antidepressants All antidepressants may cause a *discontinuation syndrome.* Distinguish between this and *withdrawal symptoms* (implies addiction). Patients often worry that they will get hooked on medication which can affect compliance. Discontinuation symptoms are explained by the theory of *receptor rebound,* eg an antidepressant with potent anticholinergic effects may be associated with diarrhoea on withdrawal,[116] ~30% get the syndrome and it may mimic the original symptoms of the illness (don't confuse withdrawal for relapse.).[117] Withdrawal is best over ≥4 weeks unless fluoxetine is co-prescribed (it has a long t½, so no withdrawal regimen is needed, and it also helps reduce symptoms). For antidepressant cross-tapering, see p. 715.

Discontinuation symptoms: • Onset is within ~5 days of stopping, sometimes after cross-tapering or missing doses. Usually mild and self-limiting but can be prolonged and severe. Some symptoms are more likely with certain drugs. ▶Consider stopping alcohol before starting withdrawal, and starting meditation and an exercise programme.[118,119] *SSRIS:* Common: • 'Flu-like symptoms; headaches; nasty shock-like sensations;[120] dizziness; insomnia; tears; irritability; vivid dreams. *Rare:* • Movement disorders; poor concentration/memory; delirium. *The most troublesome is:* paroxetine (short half-life). *MAOIS: Common:* • Agitation; irritability; ataxia; movement disorders; insomnia; ↓ cognition; altered speech. Rare: • Hallucinations; paranoid delusions. *The most troublesome:* tranylcypromine (metabolized it has amphetamine-like properties so may have real withdrawal). *TCAS: Common:* • 'Flu symptoms; insomnia. *Rare:* • Movement disorders; mania; arrhythmias. *The most troublesome:* imipramine.

▶Warn the patient about these symptoms. If they expect to feel worse before they feel better, then their reaction will be more measured. They will also tell you if there is something unexpected happening. Ask them to tell family and friends 'I won't be myself for a while' but assure them this is transient.

Gender identity

Although many transgender*/non-binary* (TGNB) people are not distressed and don't need psychological or medical support, others do. Where needed, support is available for people to explore their gender identity* and help alleviate gender-based distress. We need to be aware and sensitive to all our patients' needs, including those of our TGNB patients. **From pathology to human diversity** Until recently, being transgender was considered a 'mental disorder' in the ICD/DSM. Now, consensus among healthcare professionals is that experiencing a gender different from the one assigned at birth (on basis of biological sex) is not a disorder, but rather, a natural variation in human experience. ICD-11 removed Gender Identity Disorders and introduced Gender Incongruence in its new chapter 'Conditions related to sexual health'. **Aetiology** There is considerable variability in gender-diverse identity development, including age of onset, gender expression, sexual orientation, comorbid conditions (eg ASC), and desire for gender-affirming interventions, which may reflect different causal pathways.[121] Looking for causes of transgender identities can be problematic, as it assumes *cause* is followed by 'solution' (or cure). Underlying this assumption is the idea that a transgender identity is pathological and less preferable than a cisgender* identity which can impact resilience and mental health. **Health and mental health** Discrimination towards transgender individuals leads to unjust prejudicial judgements from others, eroding sense of self and putting significant strain on mental health. The Minority Stress Model helps explain why LGBTQ+ individuals have higher rates of anxiety, depression, suicidality, DSH, and substance use than their cisgender/straight peers.[122] All healthcare professionals have a duty, under the Equalities Act 2010, to work to reduce stigma and prejudice towards LGBTQ+ people. **Gender affirming interventions** Aimed at alleviating gender-based distress and/or helping align a person's body with their gender identity. Those chosen will vary widely. Specialist teams (gic.nhs.uk, gids.nhs.uk) can support the following interventions: • *Psychological support* to explore gender identity, role, and expression; impact of prejudice on mental health; external/internalized transphobia; Improve body image and promote resilience • *Hormone blockers* pause puberty (development of secondary sex characteristics) in young people to allow time and space (without distress of a changing body) to explore gender identity • *Hormone treatment* testosterone/oestrogen to masculinize/feminize the body • *Surgery* including breast/chest, genitalia, facial features, and body contouring.

Many TGNB people choose not to medically transition,* and may seek other forms of support or ways to change their gender expression (wpath.org): • Online or in-person *social support and advocacy groups* (tranzwiki.net) • *Socially transitioning** to align gender expression, role, name, and pronouns with gender identity • *Non-medical interventions* eg chest binding and 'packing' (transgender men), or chest padding and hair removal (transgender women).

Terminology

- **Gender identity:** a person's sense of themself as male, female, a combination of both, neither, or another gender. Originally coined by Robert J. Stoller in 1964.
- **Gender dysphoria:** when a person experiences discomfort or distress due to a mismatch between their gender identity and the one assigned at birth. A clinical diagnosis in the DSM-5.
- **Gender expression:** how a person expresses their gender (through clothing, social behaviour, posture, mannerisms, speech etc).
- **Transgender (or trans):** an umbrella term for people whose gender is not the same as the one assigned at birth.

- **Non-binary:** people who identify outside of the traditional male/female binary.
- **Binary:** people who identify within the traditional male/female binary.
- **Cisgender (or cis):** someone whose gender identity is the same as the one they were assigned at birth.
- **Transitioning:** the steps a person may take to live in the gender they identify as.
- **Social transition:** may include changing gender expression, role, name, and pronouns.
- **Medical transition:** may include hormone blockers, sex hormones, and surgeries.

*See 'Terminology' Box for definitions.

Suicide can be simply defined as an intentional self-inflicted death. It is the most common cause of death in men under 35 (in 2014, 78% of deaths by suicide were men <45). In the UK, it is the 3rd ranked category to 'years of potential life lost' after coronary heart disease and cancer. The most common method of suicide in the UK was 'hanging' (56% and 40% of all 6233 suicides)—previously the most common method by women was overdose ('poisoning').

Understanding suicide For some, suicide may feel like the only solution to a life of unyielding mental distress or unbearable social situations—the only viable way to end torment. It can be a form of protest, a way of avoiding shame, ameliorating physical pain (assisted suicide) while keeping honour/autonomy.

Risk Increased with mental illness: bipolar disorder, depression, EUPD, anorexia, substance abuse, and with past self-harm and suicide attempts. See BOX 'Demographics of suicide' for further suicide risk demographics.

Assessment Think of a target with 3 concentric rings.[12]

The inner ring is the circumstances of the act: what happened that day; were things normal to start with? When did the feelings and events leading up to the act start? Get descriptions of these in detail. Was there any last act (eg a suicide note)? What happened after the act? Who called for help? Was what followed what they expected? How do they feel about it now? Embarrassed, guilty, regretful (because they attempted suicide or because it didn't succeed)? *The middle ring* is the background to the act: how things have been over the preceding months. Might the attempt have been made at any time over the last months? What relationships were important over this time? Have they planned for these? Hoarding tablets (by not taking medication they may precipitate mood changes), researching methods, looking at pro-suicide websites. *The outer ring* is the relevant family and personal history (p. 688). Remember to include strengths and positives as well as negatives. Use the patient's own words and descriptions—it is much more powerful to use these later to suggest coping strategies and demonstrates that you really did listen.

Now ... come to the *bullseye*, the intention lying behind the act, and the present feelings and intentions. Does the attempt reflect a wish to die (a grave, not-to-be-ignored sign); was it sending a message or to change circumstances? Ask: 'If you were to leave hospital today, how would you cope?' Examine the mental state (p. 690): is there any mental illness? Ask 'what has changed?' *Summary:* • Any plans? What? When? Where? • Are means available? • Other attempts? Seriousness? • Preparations (writing a will, giving things away).

Before arranging hospital admission, ask what this is for. Is it only to make you feel less anxious or to gain something that cannot be gained outside hospital. Ask: *why will discharge be safer in a few weeks rather than now?*

After the assessment, there are 4 stages in trying to help survivors
- Agree a contract offering help, by negotiation. Discuss confidentiality, then if possible, talk with the support network (ie family, friends) as to how problems are to be tackled. Patients may want to 'go it alone' but is this helpful?
- Treat any comorbid conditions: depression, anxiety, substance misuse.
- Problem-solving therapy helps by pointing out how the patient coped with past problems[123] [N=1094] The aim is to engender a greater ability to cope in the future and to help with immediate personal or social problems.
- Follow-up, either alone or with the family, with *preventive strategies*.[124] *Promote access to:* Samaritans and doctors; online help (Facebook is addressing this). *Limit access* to lethal means (guns, stored tablets, rope for a noose). *Shift position* from an unstable position (drugs, alcohol, abuse, violence, criminal action) to a stable one (job, community support, caring relationships etc.). Social support if needed.

12 Use clinical judgement and assessment tools.

(margin) 12 Psychiatry

Demographics of suicide

A knowledge of risks associated with certain demographics helps inform decisions made about service planning and public health interventions. However, these are based on general trends, treat each individual on their own terms:

• *Sex:* In Britain, completed suicides have a ratio of 3♂:1♀ (between 25–34 this increases 4♂:1♀). These differences are less marked in Asia. Attempted ('unsuccessful') suicides have a ratio of 1♂:3♀ suggesting overall rates are equal. The WHO noted men tend to choose more violent mechanisms (eg hanging and firearms), whereas women favour less violent acts (eg poison).
• *Age:* Highest rates (20% of all suicides) are in the elderly with 2♂:1♀.
• *Marital status:* Risks highest in widow > divorced > single > married.
• *Occupation:* Higher in unemployed and retired, within employment highest rates in unskilled workers, followed by professionals (access to lethal drugs or guns — vets four times expected rate, pharmacists and farmers two times). High rates among prisoners, especially those on remand. Students, contrary to assumption, show risk similar to general population age group.
• *Ethnicity:* Rates among immigrants closely reflect those of their countries of origin, although added pressure from other factors (eg occupation, refugee status). In the UK, place of birth rather than ethnicity is recorded so research is harder. In a London study those of African–Caribbean origin had relatively low suicide rates and young Indian women relatively high rates.
• *Seasonal:* Worldwide, suicide rates are highest in spring and summer.

NB: comparing global suicide trends is complex as economic and political changes impact differently. In many countries, until recently unexplained deaths were not classified as suicide due to cultural pressures and stigma. Changes over time (ie ↑ suicide rates) may reflect societal acceptance.

Managing threats of suicide

A psychiatrist can become enmeshed in a web of suicide threats, and may wrongly assume that because someone threatens suicide, they should be admitted to hospital (compulsorily if necessary) so that they can be kept under surveillance, and suicide prevented. This reasoning has 3 faults. The first is the idea that it is possible to prevent suicide by admission. There is no such thing as constant surveillance. Second, admission may achieve nothing if it removes the person from the circumstances they need to learn to cope with. Third, we must distinguish between suicide gestures, which have the object of influencing others' behaviour, and a genuine wish to die.

Before death, many suicide victims see a GP, and it is wise to be alert to undercurrents of suicide which only sometimes surface during consultations. Ask *unambiguously* about suicide plans (p. 692). On deciding that a threat is more manipulative than genuine, very experienced therapists may influence the person's use of suicide behaviour by forcing him to face the reality of his suicide talk, eg by asking: 'When will you kill yourself?' 'How will you do it?' 'Who will discover the corpse?' 'What sort of funeral do you want? Cremation, burial, with or without flowers?' 'Who will come?'

See BOX 'Demographics of suicide' for risk factors for suicide; they may be of no help in individual cases, so aim to think dynamically of risks and protective factors (eg family support), with suicide occurring after key events that accumulate risk.

▶*Take all suicide threats seriously*—but emphasis differs depending into which group the patient falls. Aim to form a *contract* with the patient, eg:
• The therapist will listen and help if the patient agrees to be frank, and to tell the therapist of any suicide thoughts or plans.
• Agreement about which problems are to be tackled is made explicit.
• Agree the type of change to aim for and who will be involved in treatment (eg family, friends, GP). Agree the timing and place of sessions.
• An agreement to collaborate with the therapist, and to do any homework.

Suicide and deliberate self-harm (DSH) are not on a continuum. DSH is 'self-poisoning or injury, irrespective of the apparent purpose of the act' whereas suicide is 'intentionally taking of one's life'. NICE states 'DSH is an expression of personal distress, not an illness, and there are many varied reasons for it'.

▶DSH may be 'a cry for help' but *every non-fatal event may be fatal next time*.

Prevalence The UK has one of the highest rates of self-harm in Europe: 0.4%. Of those who have engaged in DSH, 15% repeat the act within 1 year and 25% within 4 years. In a school survey of 15–16-year-olds:[125] DSH lifetime act was 10%, with 7% in previous year. 4♀:1♂ (thoughts of DSH 2.5♀:1♂). WHO estimates 50% of 13–19-year-olds experience suicidal ideation at some point in adolescence. Overdose makes up 90% of referred cases (although it is estimated only 50% of overdoses present to hospital) followed by laceration (8%).

Why do people self-harm? Communicating a message, or gaining power by escalating conflict, often after an argument with a partner. Emotional immaturity, inability to cope with stress, weak religious ties, and availability of drugs (psychotropics and alcohol are popular poisons) are important. For many, DSH offers a release from psychological pain (emotions and worries), re-placing these feelings with physical pain. A maladaptive coping strategy with long-term consequences—but in the short term often feels effective (patients report feeling 'alive') and can become addictive due to its immediate effect.

Risk factors *Witnessed DSH:* Family history of DSH (likely environmental and genetic factors), learned behaviour/'copycat' DSH from friends or celebrities—exacerbated by social media (eg tumblr #dsh). *Biological:* Reduced endorphin response to emotional arousal (eg traumatic brain damage), abnormalities in serotonin release (mechanism unknown). *Developmental:* Poor early care (neglect), physical, emotional, and sexual abuse, parental separation. *Peer relations:* Conflicts, bullying, poor interpersonal skills. *Psychological:* Identity problems (eg cultural, sexual orientation, poor body image), low self-esteem. *Antisocial behaviour:* Conduct disorder, impulsivity, substance misuse.

DSH occurs equally across all socioeconomic groups in adolescence. In adults higher rates occur in lower socioeconomic groups.

Management Before a psychiatric intervention, prioritize treating physical effects of DSH. NICE includes a telling statement 'adequate anaesthesia and/or analgesia should be offered to people who have self-injured throughout the process of suturing or other painful treatments'. During this, issues of capacity (p.773), informed consent, and when to override these should be considered.

All patients need a psychiatric assessment. Most hospitals will offer a specialist approach in <18s (eg admission and assessment by a CAMHS professional trained to engage this group); some offer this for >65s (increased risk of completed suicide). Waiting for a specialist should be balanced with delay.

Focus assessment on: **1** Initial risk management—immediate risk of suicide; need for admission **2** Ongoing risks with subsequent DSH **3** Relevant psychiatric, medical and social issues. Try to create a positive therapeutic relationship.

Discharge against medical advice If a person with DSH states a desire to leave before this assessment has been completed, decide if there is diminished capacity and/or the presence of a significant mental illness. If so, referral for urgent mental health assessment is needed. Take time to explain the situation and discuss their options, try to understand why they wish to leave (eg do they have a child due home from school?). Offer food/drink (never underestimate what 'a nice cup of tea' can accomplish). If that fails, you may have to take appropriate measures to prevent a person leaving this 'safe' environment.

Prognosis ~10% of DSH patients require psychiatric admission (mainly depression or alcohol misuse), 1/3 need psychiatric follow-up in community; remainder need help to understand and cope with their psychosocial stressors.

12 Psychiatry

Crisis intervention

Occupying the interval between the spilling of our lives and their congealing into history, crisis intervention recognizes that moments of maximum change are times of greatest therapeutic opportunity (fig 12.8).[126] Debate these questions:

- What events have led to these difficulties? Thoughts/actions in the last days.
- What is the patient's mental state *now* (p. 690)? Depressed? Suicidal? Psychotic?
- In the past how have they been able to combat stress and to resolve crises?
- What solutions to this crisis have been tried? How have they failed?
- Who are the significant people in their life? Can you rely on any of them?

Therapeutic strategy

- If he has been very badly affected by the crisis, you may insist on postponing all normal obligations/responsibilities to allow concentrated contact ('intensive care') in a therapeutic environment (eg a hospital or crisis unit).

- Take practical steps to safeguard patient's commitments (eg transport of children to other family).

- Choose the best way of lowering arousal (time spent talking is often preferable to administering anxiolytics, which may only

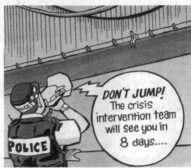

Fig 12.8 Crisis intervention teams must be responsive, immediate, accessible, and available 24/7—anywhere.

delay the natural process of adaptation). If the patient is shocked, stunned, or mute, take time to establish normal channels of communication.

- As soon as the person is receptive, promote a sense of hope about the outcome of the crisis. If there is no hope (a mother, consumed by grief, after losing all her children in a fire), then this too must be addressed.

- The next step is to encourage creative thinking about ways whereby the patient might solve the problems. Start by helping them think through the consequences of all options open to them. Then help compartmentalize their proposed solutions into small, easily executed items of behaviour.

As the immediate crisis passes, and the patient has reasonable psychological functioning, it will be necessary to put them back in charge of their own life. A period of counselling is likely to be appropriate (p. 762). Making a contract about therapy is important in encouraging the patient to transfer from the 'sick role' to a self-dependent, adult role.

Crisis intervention often focuses on loss of face, loss of identity, or loss of faith—in oneself, in one's religion, one's goals, or one's roots.

Meta-analyses suggest that crisis intervention is a viable part of home-care, and can be used during the acute phase of any mental illness.[127]

▶*All home-care packages for severe mental illness need crisis management plans.* Where implemented, this keeps the vulnerable in contact with staff (NNT ≈ 13 over 1 year) *and* reduces family burden (NNT ≈ 3), *and* is a more satisfying form of care for patients and families. It is also said to be cheaper. In one trial,[128] availability of a crisis-resolution team reduced admission rates from 59% to 22% at 8 weeks—and was highly cost-effective.

There is a widespread misconception that psychiatry has no *genuine* emergencies. It's true that psychiatrists won't descend onto a ward in a flurry of bleeps blaring, ABGs rushing off, and everyone shouting 'Stat!'. Psychiatrists often work without a larger team as immediate back-up, expected to make decisions, start treatments, and manage problems alone. Help is often available over a telephone or via discussion the next day so 'holding the anxiety' of the patient, family, and your own is a skill that is often developed through training. That said, overnight on-calls can be lonely and, even in quieter periods, sleep can be prevented as past choices are considered, self-checked, and doubted.

When there are acute situations, a psychiatrist should act as doctor first. That means keeping up to date and confident in essential examination techniques and basic life support. Knowing their limits is equally important: when to call for help and how to do this—familiarize yourself with local protocols, crash team contact numbers, and where important equipment is kept (and if it's missing then follow this up and request a replacement—better to ask early than need something on a dark and lonely 2am call out and discover it absent).

> *'At a cardiac arrest, the first procedure is to take your own pulse.'*
> Laws of the House of God, House of God, Samuel Shem

When arriving at a crisis, don't forget first principles: find out who requested you attend, ask them what has happened, what their main concerns are, what they have already done, and what they expect you to do (ie what's your role?).

▶ Whatever else is happening, keep safety a priority: yours, staff and patient's.

Severe behavioural disturbances Can be due to a variety of causes: *Organic:* Delirium (p. 732), brain injury, intellectual disability (p. 742). *Intoxication:* Drugs and alcohol. *Psychiatric:* Psychosis, anxiety, mania. *Personality:* Antisocial personality disorder (p. 744-5), frustration—or a combination of any of these. If there are concerns about safety then manage the danger first (see p. 731) before attempting an assessment. When safe to do so, consider triggers, diagnosis, and management. If there is no psychiatric or physical reason for the behaviour then have a low threshold to involve hospital security and/or police.

Intoxication It is unhelpful to try to engage a patient in a meaningful assessment while they are intoxicated. If you have ever had a conversation with a very drunk friend you will have experienced slurred speech, unfinished sentences, and misplaced melancholy. Better to allow them to 'sober up' before assessing. However, it is important to ensure their medical needs are still cared for and not ignored. Agree a plan with ED staff and a time you will return.

Self-harming behaviour It is tempting to not respond to these behaviours in an effort to avoid reinforcing them, however it is essential that appropriate medical care is given promptly. Try to manage your frustrations in these cases. If in doubt, liaise with medical colleagues, eg consult Toxbase® (www.toxbase.org) in overdose, and delay a full assessment until medically safe to do so.

Safeguarding Everyone working with vulnerable patients has a duty to keep them safe. Safeguarding is often applied to <18s but can equally relate to older adults or those who lack capacity. Concerns can be direct (ie reported abuse, domestic violence) or indirect (admitting a single father means children will need to have someone to look after them). Ask about risks and dependants. Discuss any concerns with nominated safeguarding team. A safeguarding lead should always be available.

Neuroleptic malignant syndrome Uncommon life-threatening neuroleptic (antipsychotic)-induced disorder which requires immediate treatment. *Symptoms:* Fever, muscle rigidity, delirium, and autonomic instability. Markedly raised serum creatine kinase. *Management:* Stop the causative factor, use supportive measures, treat rhabdomyolysis, and admit. *Mortality:* 10-20%

A person can be violent as a result of psychiatric illness, substance misuse, personality disorder, or physical illness. Or it may be the result of adverse ward environments: overcrowding, noise, alienation, and nowhere to go (no blue skies or green fields). This is the danger if sequestration on the ward is the result of withdrawal of privileges for 'bad behaviour'.

- Recognize early warning signs: tachypnoea, clenched fists, shouting, chanting, restlessness, repetitive movements, pacing, gesticulations. Your own intuition may be helpful here. At the first hint of violence, get help. If alone, make sure you are nearer the door than the patient.
- Do not be alone with a patient you do not feel safe with; have a low tolerance to request security/police if needed (although be aware that this can intimidate a patient or cause them to become more aggressive).
- Try and take them out of a crowded area if that is appropriate and possible—consider the other patients and bystanders.
- Try calming and talking with the patient. Do not touch him or her. Use your body language to reassure: sitting back (closer to door than the patient), open palms, attentive. Listen to their concerns without judgement:
  ▶▶De-escalation ▶▶Time-out ▶▶Placement, as appropriate.
- Get his or her consent. If they do not consent to treatment, emergency treatment can still be given to save life, or if serious deterioration.
- Use minimum force possible.
  (Source: data from Maudsley *Prescribing Guidelines*.)

Rapid tranquillization
This is the use of medication in controlling behaviour. It should only be used as a last resort when non-pharmacological methods of behaviour control have failed. Below is offered as a guide only. Consult your local protocols.

↓

- Offer *oral* treatment. If the patient is prescribed a regular antipsychotic, **lorazepam** 1–2mg or **promethazine** 25–50mg avoids risks associated with combining antipsychotics. Oral options if not already on regular oral or depot antipsychotic (**olanzapine** 10mg, **quetiapine** 100–200mg, **risperidone** 1–?mg, or **haloperidol** 5mg). Avoid using more than 1 antipsychotic to avoid QT prolongation (rapid tranquillization predisposes to arrhythmias).
- Repeat after 45–60min. Monotherapy with buccal **midazolam** 10–20mg may avoid the need for IM drugs (unlicensed).

↓

If 2 doses fail or sooner if the patient is placing themselves or others at significant risk—consider IM treatment. Consider the patient's legal status and consider consulting a senior colleague. Options:

- **Lorazepam** 1–2mg IM (dilute with equal volume of water for injections). Have flumazenil to hand ∴ respiratory depression. Be cautious if very young or elderly, and those with pre-existing brain damage or impulse control problems, as disinhibition reactions are more likely.
- **Promethazine** 50mg IM is useful in a benzodiazepine-tolerant patient. Promethazine has slow onset, but is often effective. Dilution is not needed before IM injection. It may be repeated up to 100mg/day. Wait 1–2h to assess response. It is an extremely weak dopamine antagonist.
- **Olanzapine** 10mg IM; don't combine olanzapine with IM benzodiazepine.
- **Haloperidol** 5mg is last-choice as incidence of acute dystonia is high; ensure IM procyclidine is to hand. Repeat after 30–60min if insufficient effect.

↓

Seek expert advice from consultant or senior clinical pharmacist on call. ▶▶Monitor vital signs every 5–10min for 1h, and then half-hourly until ambulatory (if he refuses, observe for signs of pyrexia, hypotension, oversedation, and well-being). If unconscious, monitor oximetry. A nurse must accompany until ambulatory. Monitor ECG, U&E, & FBC if high-dose IM antipsychotics used.

Acute confusion state (ACS) or delirium is an organic reaction which can be differentiated from chronic conditions, such as dementia. Patients in ACS have a fluctuating, impaired consciousness with onset over hours or days, or a rapid deterioration in pre-existing cognitive function, with associated behavioural changes which include:

- *Cognitive function:* Worsened concentration, slow responses, confusion, and disorientation in time (doesn't know day or year).
- *Perception:* Visual or auditory hallucinations.
- *Physical function:* Reduced mobility, reduced movement, restlessness, agitation, changes in appetite, sleep disturbance. Often these behaviours are fluctuating: varying between quiet or drowsy with occasional agitated outbursts so that you are called when they are 'disrupting the ward'.
- *Social behaviour:* Lack of cooperation with reasonable requests, withdrawal, or alterations in communication, mood, and/or attitude. As part of their ACS, patients may become delusional (usually poorly developed delusions), eg accusing staff of plotting against them.

ACS can be hyperactive (agitated and upset), hypoactive (drowsy and withdrawn), or mixed. On a busy ward, it is the hyperactive ACS patients who cause disruption and gain attention while those hypoactive ACS are not noticed.

It is most often seen in those patients with prior vulnerabilities such as postoperative patients, the elderly, and the very young, and therefore common on surgical and medical wards (10–20%). ACS can have serious consequences (such as increased risk of dementia and/or death) and, for people in hospital, may increase their length of stay in hospital and their risk of new admission to long-term care. If there is no past psychiatric history, and in the setting of a physical illness or after surgery, an ACS is particularly likely.

Differential diagnosis Withdrawal from alcohol/drugs, mania, post-ictal or if agitated, consider psychosis or anxiety. All are readily distinguished on history-taking. Always consider dementia (which usually has an insidious onset and occurs in clear consciousness ie without drowsiness, etc.)

Causes See table 12.6; almost anything with a neurological/systemic effect can result in an ACS. Most often the cause is: infection; drugs (benzodiazepines, opiates, anticonvulsants, digoxin, L-dopa); U&E↑↓; hypoglycaemia; ↓p$_a$O$_2$; alcohol withdrawal; trauma; surgery (esp. if pre-op Na↑↓ or sensory loss).

Investigations U&E, FBC, blood gases, glucose, cultures (blood, MSU), LFT, ECG, CT, CXR, LP. If a cause is not identified, consult a neurologist urgently.

Management Should consider a holistic approach:
- Find the precipitating cause and treat this, and other exacerbating factors.
- Optimize supportive surroundings and nursing care (see BOX 'Interventions to limit acute confusional states').
- Avoid sedation unless there is extreme agitation, risk, or needed for investigations to take place. Give antipsychotics in first instance as benzodiazepines tend to worsen delirium with exception of alcohol withdrawal.
- If needed, consider **haloperidol** 1–10mg/24h or **olanzapine** 2.5–10mg/24h (smallest dose possible, esp. if elderly). Monitor BP. Wait 20min to judge IM effects (side effects: BP↑↓, stroke, insomnia, dyspepsia).
- Regular clinical review and follow-up.

Interventions to limit acute confusional states

Because ACS is a common occurrence, it is often thought of as an unavoidable adverse effect to admission. However, pre-emptive steps can be taken:

- Avoid moving people within and between wards unless absolutely necessary.
- Manage disorientation by providing appropriate lighting, clear signage, and a clock (consider providing a 24-hour clock in critical care) and a calendar.
- Talk to the person to re-orientate them by explaining where they are, who they are, and what your role is; explanation of what is happening and why.
- Introduce cognitively stimulating activities: talking, reminiscence work, and facilitating regular visits from family and friends.
- Address dehydration and nutritional needs by ensuring adequate fluid intake to prevent dehydration and by encouraging the person to drink and eat.
- Address infection by looking for and treating infection, avoiding unnecessary catheterization, and implementing infection control procedures.
- Address immobility or limited mobility by encouraging people to mobilize soon after surgery.
- Carry out a medication review for people taking multiple drugs, taking into account both the type and number of medications.
- Address sensory impairment by resolving any reversible cause, eg impacted ear wax, and ensuring hearing and visual aids are available to and used by people who need them, and that they are in good working order.
- Promote good sleep patterns and sleep hygiene by avoiding nursing or medical procedures during sleeping hours, if possible scheduling medication rounds to avoid disturbing sleep.

Table 12.6 Causes of acute and chronic confusion

	Acute (delirium)	Chronic (dementia)
Degenerative		★Alzheimer's; Huntington's (OHCM p702); ★Lewy-body (OHCM p486), CJD & Pick's (p. 854)
Other CNS	Cerebral tumour or abscess; subdural haematoma; epilepsy; acute post-trauma psychosis	Tumours; subdural haematoma; multiple sclerosis; Parkinson's; normal pressure hydrocephalus
Infective★	Many, eg meningoencephalitis; septicaemia; cerebral malaria; trypanosomiasis	Late syphilis; chronic or sub-acute encephalitis; CNS cysticercosis; cryptococcosis; HIV
Vascular	Stroke (or TIA); hypertensive encephalopathy; SLE	Thromboembolic multi-infarct (arteriosclerotic) dementia
Metabolic	★U&E↑↓; ★hypoxia; ★liver and kidney failure; non-metastatic cancer; porphyria; ★alcohol withdrawal	Liver and kidney failure; non-metastatic or metastatic cancer
Endocrine	Addisonian or hyperthyroid crisis; diabetic pre-coma; hypoglycaemia; hypo/hyperparathyroidism	T4↓; Addison's; hypoglycaemia; hypopituitarism; hypo-/hyperparathyroidism[129]
Toxic	★Alcohol; many drugs (check datasheet/statement of product characteristics); lead; arsenic; mercury	★'Alcohol dementia'; barbiturate abuse; too much manganese or carbon disulfide
Deficiency	Thiamine; vitamin B₁₂; folate; nicotinic acid	Thiamine; vitamin B₁₂; folate; nicotinic acid

★ denotes a leading cause.

Dementia is a syndrome of progressive and global intellectual deterioration without impairment of consciousness. Memory loss is often the first symptom noted although progression to other deficits will continue including:

- *Behaviour*—restless, repetitive, and purposeless activity; rigid, fixed routines.
- *Personality changes*—sexual disinhibition; social gaffes; shoplifting; blunting.
- *Speech*—syntax errors; dysphasia; mutism.
- *Thinking*—slow, muddled; poor memory (with confabulation); no insight.
- *Perception*—illusions, hallucinations (often visual).
- *Mood*—irritable, depressed, emotional incontinence (labile mood and crying).

Remember the **4A's** *of Alzheimer's*: **A**mnesia, **A**phasia, **A**gnosia, **A**praxia.

Dementia incidence is 6% of those ≥65 years old. For a diagnosis to be made, there should be significant impairment of normal function with other differentials, in particular normal ageing, delirium, and depression, ruled out.

Irreversible causes of dementia include: Alzheimer disease,[62%] vascular,[15%] mixed,[10%] Lewy body,[4%] fronto-temporal.[2%] Reversible causes[15%] include: subdural haematoma, hydrocephalus, hypothyroidism.

Investigations

Full history of function and decline; a collateral history from friends/relatives; FBC; vitamin B_{12}; folate (MCV↑ suggests alcoholism, or ↓B_{12} or folate); ESR (malignancy); U&E, LFT, γGT, Ca^{2+} (renal/hepatic failure, alcoholism, malignancy, endocrinopathy (Ca^{2+} ↑ or ↓). TSH (hypothyroidism); serology: syphilis (*OHCM* p412) ± HIV (only if suspected by history); CT/MRI excludes tumours, hydrocephalus, subdural, stroke, etc.

Management

▶*Involve the patient in their own therapy.*
- Full assessment, including functional and social needs for the patient and consider the needs of carers and any risk factors.
- Exclude the treatable and manage exacerbating factors eg medical illness, depression (SSRI), insomnia (hypnotics), agitation (antipsychotics).
- Psychological work: patient and carer; there may be a time when the patient no longer recognizes those closest to them and may need institutionalized care.
- Cognitive enhancement: acetylcholinesterase inhibitors and/or antioxidants.
- Supportive work: promote independence; help with functional (mobility, self-care) and social (financial, accommodation) issues.
- Relative support: carer's allowance, holiday, admissions, and support groups.

Alzheimer disease (as an example of dementia)

Presentation: In *mild Alzheimer disease* there is amnesia and spatial disorientation. In *moderate Alzheimer disease* (some years later), personality disintegration, eg with aggression or depression, and focal parietal signs, eg dysphasia and apraxia. Parkinsonism may occur. Patient may use their mouth to examine objects (hyperorality). In *severe Alzheimer disease*, neurovegetative changes with apathy (or ceaselessly active—akathisia), wasting, incontinence, ±seizures/spasticity.

Mean survival: 7 years from clinical (overt) onset; 5–15 years from diagnosis.

Pharmacological treatment: Increase CNS acetylcholine by inhibiting the enzyme causing its breakdown (donepezil; rivastigmine; galantamine). **Memantine**, a NMDA (*N*-methyl-D-aspartate) receptor antagonist, may help moderate to severe Alzheimer disease. Cautions: creatinine ↑; epilepsy; bradycardia with ACE inhibitor. SE: confusion, headache, hallucinations, and tiredness; rarer: vomiting, anxiety, hypertonia, and cystitis, ↑ libido. Dose: initially 5mg each morning; ↑ in steps of 5mg at intervals of 1 week to 10mg/12h.

Prevention/protection: Looking after cardiovascular health, attaining higher educational level before the illness ('cognitive reserve'), statins (relative risk 0.29); antioxidants.[138][n=1364]

Cognitive function tests

For mild memory impairment the TYM test (Test Your Memory) is widely available The most commonly known measure for cognitive impairment is the Mini-Mental State Examination. It is a sensitive, valid, and reliable 30-point questionnaire which includes checks for registration, attention and calculation, recall, language, ability to follow simple commands, and orientation. However, it cannot be freely used in clinical settings for copyright reasons. This has led to researchers looking for alternative strategies in assessing cognition eg the abbreviated mental test:

The following questions are put to the patient. Each question correctly answered scores 1 point. A score of 7–8 or less suggests cognitive impairment at the time of testing, although further and more formal tests are necessary to confirm a diagnosis of dementia.

1 Patient's age?
2 Time (to the nearest hour)?
3 Address for recall at end of test (eg 42 West Street)
4 Current year?
5 Identification of this place (eg hospital).
6 Identification of two persons (doctor, nurse, etc.).
7 Date of birth?
8 Year of First World War?
9 Name of present monarch?
10 Count backwards from 20 to 1.

Clearly this test is very culturally specific, and while it can be updated (eg changing monarch to prime minister) this will impact its validity.

The MOCA (Montreal Cognitive Assessment: 30-points) and the Addenbrooke's Cognitive Examination revised (ACE-R: 100-points) are also widely used. The AMT is a screening tool mostly used in acute medical settings.

Frontal lobe function tests

The frontal assessment battery (FAB) is a bedside test to help discriminate frontotemporal type dementia from others. The maximum score is 18, higher scores indicating better performance.

1 Similarities (conceptualization).
2 Lexical fluency (mental flexibility).
3 Motor series 'Luria' test (programming).
4 Conflicting instructions (sensitivity to interference).
5 Go–No-Go (inhibitory control).
6 Prehension behaviour (environmental autonomy).

For further information see:
https://emedicine.medscape.com/article/1135866-clinical#b4

12 Psychiatry

Many issues in child psychiatry overlap with aspects of adult psychiatry, and also with paediatrics. The psychiatry of intentional overdose is a good example. Many of these patients will be in the last phases of childhood, and it is unclear which service will suit them best. As ever, take a holistic view of the young person and tailor a care plan which takes these facets into account.

Child and Adolescent Mental Health (CAMH) services are organized into 4 tiers to provide help to children, young people, and their support network

- T1: professionals whose main training and role is not CAMH eg GP, teacher.
- T2: CAMH specialists working in teams in community eg psychologist.
- T3: multidisciplinary CAMH team in a specialized service for more severe, complex, or persistent disorders eg CAMH psychiatrist, nurse, OT.
- T4: essential tertiary services such as intensive community treatment services, day units, and inpatient units eg eating disorders or secure ward.

Depression in children and adolescents Remembering back to our own teenage years, it's no surprise that many adolescences face major mental health challenges as they change and start to develop their adult identity: body, dress, responsibilities, and sexuality. Add to this pressure from school (exams!), peers (sex, drugs, and socializing), parents, urban stress, and the media ('fizzy drinks make teenagers more violent'[13]). It's a lot to manage.

Depression affects around 3% of children and 5.6% of adolescents. The stress–vulnerability model is helpful to consider aetiology: vulnerability (genes, endocrine) interact with stress to cause depression at times of life stress.

Clinical features Often more subtle and less constant than in adults:
- Mood changes: grumpy or irritable rather than very 'sad'; anhedonia.
- Thought changes: loss of self-esteem, confidence, and concentration.
- Physical changes: reduced energy, sleep, appetite; self-harming behaviour.

But the result is an impairment of functioning: missing school and social life.

Assessment One-to-one interviewing is often difficult as adolescents are not very talkative so it's important to pick up on non-verbal communication, use silences to give space, and non-judgemental language. Collateral from parents and school is helpful, as are objective rating scales. Always ask the patient directly about alcohol and drug use, bullying, abuse, and suicidal thoughts. Offer them the opportunity to discuss these issues initially in private.

Treatment Mild depression is best managed in tier 1/2 services with up to 4 weeks of 'watchful waiting' followed by simple non-directive supportive therapy or guided self-help; if unresponsive then refer to CAMH specialists. For moderate/severe depression, newest NICE guidance suggests an antidepressant (only fluoxetine is licensed in under 18s) and psychological therapy may be started concurrently, without an initial trial of psychological therapy (previously NICE suggested therapy alone for at least 3 months). There is little clear evidence to favour one psychological therapy over another. Antidepressant use should be 'cautiously' in children aged 5–11. If combined treatment is not effective within a further 6 sessions, review the formulation in a MDT.

Also consider addressing sources of distress (eg bullying) and removing opportunities for self-harm (eg no paracetamol at home). Improve sense of belongingness, especially if they feel like an outsider (eg sexuality, substance abuse).[131] If criminality and gang culture involved, peer mentorship may help.[132] *Specific drugs to avoid if <18yrs old, if possible (BNF):* Citalopram, paroxetine, sertraline. Also tricyclics, venlafaxine, and fluvoxamine.[133,134]

Recovery 10% at 3 months, 50% at 1 year, and 80% at 2 years. Treatment shortens the illness duration. Even after recovery 3% risk of completed suicide over next 10 years. Follow-up monitoring is essential.

13 Chris Smyth, *The Times*, asks (www.thetimes.co.uk/tto/health/news/article3204986.ece) and NHS choices answers (www.nhs.uk/news/2011/10October/Pages/fizzy-drinks-teenage-violence.aspx). Spoiler: 'No.'

12 Psychiatry

Child and adolescent psychiatry: psychosis

Psychotic symptoms do not mean psychosis or 'schizophrenia'. In fact, around 3 out of every 100 young people will experience a psychotic episode and many more will have transient psychotic symptoms. There can be many reasons for this: sleeplessness, drugs, music ('earworms'), or cultural norms (eg ghosts[139]). In young children, fantasy play involving imaginary friends and a blurring of reality and fact is an important stage of neurotypical development. However, 5% of adults with schizophrenia report onset of psychosis before 16 years and 20% before the age of 20, so all new symptoms should be fully assessed.

In many centres, early-onset schizophrenia is diagnosed with the same criteria as adults as it seems to be continuous with later-onset forms (eg more males affected). A sustained psychosis is considered to be >4 weeks.

Assessment As with any new patient, take a full history to understand that individual's difficulties at that time. Obtain collateral information from carers and school—especially about recent changes. Complete a MSE (p. 690) and physical examination and consider screening investigations (urine drug screen).

Symptoms Adolescents occasionally present with non-specific psychotic symptoms, such as odd beliefs, mistrust of others, and magical thinking. These overvalued ideas lead to a decline in interpersonal and school functioning. Whether this represents the prodromal phase of a severe psychotic disorder is difficult to answer prospectively. However, frank psychosis develops in up to 40% of affected patients within 12 months of symptom onset. A positive family history of psychosis and marked impairment of functioning with evolving psychosis-like symptoms are considered to be risk factors for psychotic illness.

▶ Some hallucinations are more serious and should receive urgent attention:
- Those which are imperative ('kill your sister') or exciting strong emotions.
- Those heard unambiguously outside the head.
- Those referring to ideas that the person feels are not their own.
- Multiple voices talking at once, and especially voices talking to each other.

Sometimes hallucinations resist diagnosis. This is not in itself a problem as the diagnosis will sooner or later become clear. Check whether these odd ideas are likely to indicate an increased risk of serious outcome eg suicide.[136,137]

Causes of odd ideas • Substance abuse • Psychosis (schizophrenia) • Anxiety • Depression • Hypomania • Head injury • Epileptic aura • SLE • Anti-NMDA receptor antibody encephalitis • Alice-in-Wonderland syndrome (OHCM p694).

Management Early intervention (see p. 707) helps, and may reduce chances of later chronic illness, so prompt referral is essential.[138] Every treatment plan should include a named worker and incorporate antipsychotics (if indicated) in conjunction with psychoeducational work, psychotherapy (individual CBT and family interventions), and social components. Newer antipsychotics (p. 708) are rarely specifically licensed for children, but their use in well-monitored environments is encouraging.[139] If a clear diagnosis of psychosis cannot be made, NICE advise regular monitoring for changes in symptoms and functioning for up to 3 years in CAMH or by the patient's GP.

Compliance is especially challenging in adolescents. Keep the young person engaged in their treatment by establishing a good rapport, encouraging insight, and education about relapse prevention. Even with the best of care, often adolescents want to experiment with non-compliance. It may be better to shift from optimal care to harm minimization in order to keep engagement.

Prognosis Spontaneous improvement of psychotic-like symptoms occurs in the majority of children. In one follow-up study, many developed chronic mood disorders; <50% met diagnostic criteria for a major disorder (schizoaffective, bipolar, depression). In those not developing a mood or psychotic disorder, disruptive behaviour disorders are very common.[140]

12 Psychiatry

Attachment The powerful emotional bond between baby and caregiver. Babies need someone to protect, care, and look after their emotional and physical needs. Sensitive care giving helps a child learn to understand the world and their place in it. They establish a fundamental understanding of love and trust, which allows a child to develop emotional regulation, awareness of others' feelings, and promotes healthy relationships. Attachment fails if a child is abused, neglected (eg drug addiction), or abandoned physically or psychologically (primary care-giver with severe mental illness eg postnatal depression, psychosis). Without secure attachment, a child is at risk of forming emotional, social, and behavioural problems lasting into adulthood.

Reactive attachment disorders can be diagnosed before 5 years old. These fall into 2 categories: a child is *inhibited* (extremely withdrawn, emotionally detached, and hypervigilant) or *disinhibited* (seeking comfort from anyone, even strangers, and extremely dependent and immature). Most have anger, an undeveloped conscience, and control issues. Treatment combines psychological therapy (family and play therapy) and parenting skills education.

Behavioural disorders 30–40% of all CAMH referrals will be for a disruptive <18-year-old; within these referrals oppositional defiant disorder (ODD): 5–10% children; and conduct disorder: 2–9%. Many behaviours eg changing appearance, withdrawing (a little) from family, emotional lability, experimentation (drugs, alcohol), and selfies might seem bizarre to parents but are a normal part of adolescence. Even fighting, lying, and stealing are seen in varying degrees in most 'normal' children over the course of development.

Conduct disorder (CD) This costs £100,000 more per person aged 10–28 than average. The lifetime cost of a 1-year cohort of CD children is £5.2 billion. The overriding feature is an intense, repetitive, and persistent pattern which significantly deviates from age-related, socially acceptable norms. These cause significant impairment of the child as judged by parents, teachers, or others. Isolated acts of aggression, destruction, theft, or fire setting may be sufficiently severe to warrant concern in their own right. *Diagnosis:* CD core symptoms are: 1 Defiance of will of authority (usually police) 2 Aggression 3 Antisocial behaviour (eg property damage, vandalism, theft, truancy). 3 acts must have been exhibited in the last 12 months with at least 1 present in the last 6 months in multiple places (school, home, community). *Oppositional defiant disorder* is considered a subsection of CD with an enduring pattern of negative, hostile, and defiant behaviour without serious violation of societal norms or rights of others. It may only be present in one environment and is more evident in interactions with familiar adults or peers. *Treatment:* 3 empirically supported treatments: 1 Parent training programmes (eg 'Triple P' or Webster Stratton courses) 2 Individual cognitive therapy for older children 3 Multisystemic therapy (eg with young person, family, school, criminal justice system). *Prognosis:* Most children with CD will not progress to antisocial personality disorder (although 40% of those with an adult PD met criteria for childhood CD). CD infers higher risk of other mental health problems, substance misuse, criminal activity, and early death often by violent and sudden means.

School refusal This is different from truancy (intentional non-attendance at school). It is a severe difficulty in attending school, often amounting to prolonged absence with parental knowledge, due to emotional upset and excessive fearfulness, and somatic complaints. *Setting:* Emotional overprotection; high social class; neurotic parents; schoolwork of high standard. In truancy, the reverse is true. *Treatment:* Liaise with head teacher, parents, and an educational psychologist. Escort by an education welfare officer aids prompt return. Other methods: educational-support therapy, CBT, and parent-teacher interventions.[141] In the past, hypnosis has been used. Often anxiety (eg separation-anxiety or phobias) ± depression need treatment too.[142]

Not falling asleep Try plenty of daytime activity (each hour of sitting ↑ sleep latency by 3min).[143] Insist on a routine wind-down 1 hour before bed→warm bath for 10min→a story→then straight into a darkened bedroom.[Gurney method]

Waking at 3am *(Ready to play or wanting entry to parent's bed)* Most don't appreciate these visitations, refuse to play, and buy earplugs to lessen the impact of tantrum (or let the child into the bed). Try extinguishing the behaviour by attending to the child ever more distantly: cuddle in bed→cuddle on bed→sitting on child's bed→voice from doorway→distant voice. Some accept this as part of normal development (I was awake today at 6:20am thanks to my 3-year-old!). In any case, avoid hypnotics (unless there is extreme concern).

Other sleep disturbances Hunger/colic (infants); poor routines (preschool); worry (adolescence). Bedroom TV may be to blame. Try behavioural therapy before hypnotics. Day-time sleepiness: Causes: night sleep ↓; depression; sleep apnoea (*OHCM* p194); narcolepsy;[14] encephalitis lethargicans (rare in children): suspect this whenever sleepiness occurs with extrapyramidal effects, oculogyric crises, myoclonus, inversion of diurnal rhythms, obsessions, and mood change. Possible causes: influenza; 'flu vaccination; measles; Q fever; mycoplasma. MRI: subcortical involvement.

Sleepwalking & parasomnias[15] The young are by far the best somnambulists (sleepwalkers) although the old may emulate them, eg if stress is augmented by excess alcohol or caffeine use, and lack of stage IV sleep—our deepest sleep. Any psychic event associated with sleep may be termed a parasomnia. *Parasomnias comprise:* • *Arousal disorders* (sleepwalking; night terrors; 'confusional arousal') • *Sleep–wake transition disorders* (rhythmic head-banging disorder) • *REM sleep parasomnias* REM sleep-associated nightmares, sleep paralysis, hallucinations, and REM sleep behaviour disorder. • *Others.*[15]

It is common to observe movement in children during sleep: it is their *repetitive* nature which allows the diagnosis of rhythmic movement disorder. The movement may be body-rocking, leg-rolling, or head-banging (this 'jactatio capitis' may lead to subdurals, fractures, eye injuries, and false accusations of abuse). Tongue-biting may suggest epilepsy. But do not try to be too obsessive in differentiating parasomnias from nocturnal epilepsy. EEG: rhythmic slow anterior activity; video polysomnography: sleep-related violent behaviour, sudden awakening and dyskinetic or dystonic movements, and complex behaviours ± enuresis.[144] *Antiparasomniacs:* Bedtime clonazepam; amitriptyline; carbamazepine. Self-hypnosis or waking ¼h before the expected event.[145]

Sleep hygiene Teaches patients to sleep without medication. SLEEP summarizes the non-pharmacological treatment of uncomplicated sleep disturbances: • schedule—consider a patient's sleep–wake schedule. Consistency is key to normalizing sleep. Keep sleep to night-times only • Limit caffeinated or alcoholic drinks and nicotine (nocturnal withdrawal) well before bedtime • Eliminate factors that create a 'hostile' sleep environment: noise, excessive light, and poor ventilation and temperature control (cooler is better) • Exercise performed during the day (but not immediately before going to bed) is an effective antidote to the psychic stress and physical tension that often contribute to insomnia. Helpful exercise routines enhances overall health and restrict day-time sleeping • Psychotherapy (CBT) for insomnia has demonstrated efficacy and may simultaneously improve associated anxiety and/or depression.

14 In narcolepsy we succumb to irresistible attacks of inappropriate sleep ± vivid hallucinations, cataplexy (sudden hypotonia), and sleep paralysis. Mutations lead to loss of hypothalamic hypocretin-containing neurons, via autoimmune destruction. HLA DR₂+ve. ℞: 1 **Methylphenidate** 10–15mg PO after breakfast and lunch) may cause dependence and psychosis 2 **Modafinil** (~200mg/d po, before noon); SE: anxiety, aggression, dry mouth, euphoria, insomnia, BP↑, dyskinesia, alk phos↑ 3 Gamma-hydroxybutyrate (GHB).

15 Sleep-related dissociative disorder, sleep enuresis, exploding head syndrome, hypnagogic or hypno-pompic hallucinations, catathrenia (end-inspiratory apnoea + groaning), sleep-related eating disorders, drug-induced parasomnias, myoclonus nocturnus, nocturnal bruxism, ie teeth grinding.

ASDs are *the* lifelong pervasive developmental disorders of our times. *Prevalence*: ≥1:200[146] ♂:♀ ≈ 4:1. Managing autism is challenging, however ASDs are a range of conditions along a severity spectrum. The core symptoms are:

1 Persistent deficits in social communication and social interaction across multiple contexts (NB: previously split into language and social interaction).
2 Restricted, repetitive patterns of behaviour, interests, or activities.

These must have been present in the early developmental period, although may not have become problematic until social demands exceed limited capacities. When manifested, these symptoms cause clinically significant impairment in functioning (social, occupational, etc.). These difficulties are not due to another condition, intellectual disability, or global developmental delay.

Cause Unknown; genes (on chromosome 11p12 ± neurexin) play a part.[147] If one child is affected, risk of next sibling being affected is ~5–10%. There is associated epilepsy in 30%. No association with MMR vaccine (p. 256).[148]

Diagnosis Requires a specialist team often made up of doctor (psychiatrist/paediatrician), psychologist, and speech and language therapist. There is no individual test so assessment includes a detailed history, collateral from school, and observation across different settings. Often a team will be trained to use diagnostic instruments such as the Autism Diagnostic Observation Schedule (ADOS) or developmental, dimensional, and diagnostic interview (3di) to produce a formalized framework for diagnosis, including severity.

Clinical features Fall into 3 broad areas. These are usually observed by the child's carers or teachers prior to referral as being 'different' than others.

1. *Impaired reciprocal social interaction:*
• Unawareness of the existence and feelings of others (treating people as furniture; being oblivious to others' distress or need for privacy).
• Abnormal response to being hurt: he doesn't come for comfort; or makes a stereotyped response, eg just saying 'Kiss it better, kiss it better, kiss it …'
• Impaired imitation (eg does not wave 'bye-bye' or copies/echoes without understanding, eg waves on passing a door when no one is in fact leaving).
• Repetitive play: eg solitary, or using others as mechanical aids.
• Bad at making friends (lack of empathy). If he tries at all, the effort will lack the social conventions, eg reading the phone directory to uninterested peers.

2. *Impaired imagination (part of abnormal communication):*
• Little babbling, few facial expressions, or no gestures in infancy.
• Avoids mutual gaze; no smiles when making a social approach; does not greet his parents; stiffens when held.
• Does not act adult roles; no interest in stories; no fantasy/pretend play.
• Odd speech, eg echolalia (repetitions); odd use of words and pronouns.
• Difficulty in initiating or sustaining reciprocal roles in conversations.

3. *Poor range of activities and interests:*
• Stereotyped movements (hand-flicking, spinning, head-banging).
• Preoccupation with parts of objects (sniffing or repetitive feeling of a textured object, spinning wheels of toys) or unusual attachments (eg to coal).
• Marked distress over minor or trivial changes (eg a vase's place).
• Insists on following routines in precise detail.
• Narrow fixations, eg lining up objects, or amassing facts about weather.

Management *Early intensive behavioural intervention:* ± *speech therapy*[149] ± *special schooling* starting at 3 years can ↑IQ in >60% and enhance motor, social, and living skills.[150] *Parent training:* ↑ ASD knowledge, enhances parent–child interaction, and ↓ parental maternal depression.[146] *Support:* eg National Autism Society. *Social skills training:* This can help. *Drugs* have a small role: risperidone (aggression), melatonin (sleep), and SSRIs (repetitive behaviour).[151] *Diet:* Eliminating gluten is popular but unproven.[152] *Benefits:* eg Disability Living Allowance.

Attention deficit hyperactivity disorder (ADHD)

Attention deficit hyperactivity disorder (ADHD) The most common neurobehavioural disorder of childhood. It has prevalence of 3–5% in Western nations.[153] 80% of cases are genetically inherited. The core diagnostic criteria are: *impulsivity, inattention, hyperactivity* (see MINIBOX) across settings. *There is no diagnostic test* (but positron emission tomography may show ↓ function of frontal lobes and nearby connections). Most parents first note hyperactivity at the toddler stage, but most locomotor hyperactivity at this stage abates with time, so the diagnosis is usually delayed until school entry or later. *Differentials:* These include: age-appropriate behaviour, low (or high) IQ, hearing impairment, and behavioural disorders. *Associations:* Conduct disorder (p. 738) or other disruptive behaviour disorders (eg ODD p. 738).[154] Young people with ADHD are at risk of being victims of assaults, as well as suicide and self-harm.[155] Signs often attenuate during adolescence, but may persist into mid-adulthood—evidence suggests by 18 years ⅓ have no symptoms, ⅓ have symptoms which don't need medication, and ⅓ still need medication. *Diagnosis:* This is made through careful history taking from young person and collateral from parent and teachers, observation at school

Inattention

Often unable to:
- Listen/attend closely to detail (∴ carelessness)
- To sustain attention in play activities
- Follow instructions
- Finish homework (when not due to defiance)
- Organize tasks needing sustained application
- Loses/forgets things

Hyperactivity:
- Squirming/fidgeting
- 'On the go all the time'
- Talks incessantly
- Climbs over everything
- Restless
- No quiet hobbies

Impulsivity:
- Blurts out answers
- Interrupts others
- Cannot take turns
- Intrudes on others
- Poor road safety

and clinic, rating scales (eg Conner's), and screen for comorbidity and organic causes. *Treatment:* [156]NICE Diagnosis and treatment ought to be initiated by a specialist (eg psychiatrist/paediatrician). Following diagnosis, time for explanation is required; offer a booklet to parents, give advice on positive parenting and behavioural techniques. In moderate ADHD impairment, parent training/education programmes are recommended. Older children may also benefit from CBT. If non-drug treatments fail, the 1st-line treatment is methylphenidate available as immediate release (eg Ritalin®) lasting 4 hours or modified release lasting up to 12 hours. Longer-lasting medications are better tolerated and allow a child to last an entire school day. It is recommended that medication is not given at weekends/holidays as it reduces appetite and therefore can suppress growth. Atomoxetine, an alternative drug, takes up to 6 weeks to reach full efficacy but appears to show lasting effect even on withdrawal (maybe due to its gradual effect rather than the on/off effect in methylphenidate). Severe ADHD in school-age children: methylphenidate and atomoxetine are 1st-line treatments so ensure referral. Evidence for long-term use is uncertain,[157,158] but 70% of young people show symptomatic improvement on medication. Caution is required when prescribing methylphenidate (a controlled drug) due to its street value as a drug of misuse (as it is an amphetamine, similar to speed). Check for substance misuse.

Does ADHD exist?

ADHD 'overdiagnosis' is a controversial topic with some claiming that doctors are medicalizing normal childhood activity and undermining parents in order to increase pharmaceutical profits (mainly in the US). However, those who have treated a child who is initially unable to sit still and focus in school before treatment and then, on medication, has improved grades and demonstrably social functioning feel justified in continuing to use the label ADHD.

12 Psychiatry

12 Psychiatry

Definition Below-average general intellectual functioning which originated during the development period and is associated with impairment in adaptive behaviour (Heber 1981). Be aware: *people with an intellectual disability are at an increased risk of developing physical and mental illnesses*.

Four subtypes: *Mild:* (IQ 50–70.) Accounts for 80% of people with intellectual disabilities. There is useful development of language, and intellectual difficulty only emerges as schooling gets under way. Most can lead an independent life. *Moderate:* (IQ 35–49.) Most can talk and find their way about. *Severe:* (IQ 20–34.) Limited social activity is possible. *Profound:* (IQ <20.) Simple speech may be unachievable. Special schooling and medical services are needed, as is adequate care and counselling for the families involved. In the UK, lack of resources and ambiguous community responsibilities are big problems.[159] *Further information:* ask MENCAP (www.mencap.org.uk).[160]

Epidemiology 27 per 1000 (80% have IQ 50–70). People with intellectual difficulties are at ↑ risk for mental illness compared to the general population.

The patient *Physical:* Sensory and motor disabilities, epilepsy, incontinence. *Psychiatric:* All psychiatric disorders can occur but the *presentation* is modified by low intelligence. In the *diagnosis* of psychiatric disorder, emphasis is given to the behavioural manifestation of the disorder.

Causes *Physical causes:* Found in 55–75% of severely intellectually disabled individuals. *Chromosomal abnormalities:* Down syndrome, fragile x syndrome (Martin–Bell syndrome, p. 852). *Antenatal causes:* Infections, alcohol, hypoxia, nutritional growth retardation, hypothyroidism. *Perinatal causes:* Cerebral palsy. *Postnatal causes:* Injury, infections, impoverished environment.

Forensic issues Arson and sexual offences, eg exhibitionism (♂) or, more rarely, 'public disrobing' (♀).[161] Care is needed in questioning a person with an intellectual disability about an alleged offence, due to increased suggestibility and risk of making false confessions. Treatment may centre on issues of accepting that the offence took place, the taking responsibility for offences, accepting the intention of the offending behaviour, and on victim awareness.[162] Behavioural approaches might focus on masturbatory satiation, covert sensitization, and stimulus control procedures.[163]

Assessing a person with an intellectual disability • Cause(s) of the intellectual disability • Associated medical conditions • Intellectual and social skills development • Psychological and social functioning • Dialogue with and support for carers.

Care of people with an intellectual disability • Prevention and early detection is the aim—as is care in generic eg NHS services (minimized specialist care) unless there are complex physical, emotional, and behavioural issues.[164] • Regular assessment of attainments and disabilities • Advice, support, and help for families—eg teaching parents how to be better 'tutors' can help[165] • Arrange special needs teaching at school and training/occupation • Housing and social support to enable self-care • Medical, nursing, and other services, as outpatients, day patients, or inpatients • Psychiatric and psychological services usually from a community-based multidisciplinary team.

Treatment of psychiatric disorders • Side effects of medication may not be apparent as a person with an intellectual disability may not be able to draw attention to them • Antipsychotics can lower seizure threshold and patients with intellectual disability are more likely to get seizures • Behavioural therapy is widely used.

Human rights for those with intellectual disability

The following 14 *specific* rights must be taken in the context of *general* psychiatric rights: • To have a professional skilled in dealing with your condition • To receive treatment based on sound evidence • To have treatment in a setting which is decent, humane, and non-abusive • Regimens must promote a fulfilling social life • Active participation in all decisions taken about care.

1 Ensure full assessment within the context of joint strategic needs assessment by Social Services, GPs, and other professionals fully trained in 'partnership working'.
2 Include the person in all decisions affecting him or her.
3 Promote enriching activity to counter idle humdrum impoverished living.
4 Listen to concerns of both the person and their carer.
5 Derive personalized care plans via dialogue with the person and carer(s).
6 Explain what the options are, ideally in terms that he/she understands.
7 Help him or her decide from a defined list of genuine choices.
8 Don't hurry through consultations 'to get back to normal people'; spend *more* time; go *slowly*. Not being able to give a good history doesn't mean you can skip this bit: it means you must use other methods to get the information. For example, discussions with carers eg 'The Cardiff Healthcheck for People with a Learning Disability' a questionnaire looking at all aspects of health completed by carers prior to annual review, or by your own direct observation of the patient.
9 Don't be pleased because they are not complaining of anything. No reported symptoms and no complaints about circumstances does not let you off the hook! You may need to insist to carers that a nasty but apparently painless ulcer be treated—or that a fire-escape be unblocked.
10 Check for physical illnesses which may otherwise go unreported and screen for those with associations eg hypothyroidism in Down syndrome.
11 Watch for neglect/abuse from well-meaning, under-trained, over-worked staff (who may desperately crave your support and encouragement).[188]
12 Don't reach too readily for drugs to curb behaviour. Consider all options.
13 Be aware of local authority *'Protection of Vulnerable Adults'* protocols.
14 No tokenism! (Paying lip service to the other points without intending change.)

12 Psychiatry

There's such a lot of different Annes in me. I sometimes think that is why I'm such a troublesome person. If I was just the one Anne it would be ever so much more comfortable, but then it wouldn't be half so interesting.'

LM Montgomery, *Anne of Green Gables*

Personality is a mix of lasting characteristics which make us who we are: easygoing or anxious; optimistic or pessimistic; placid or histrionic. This spectrum of distinct traits overlap and are describable in terms of a few independent dimensions (eg introvert/extrovert). Those with abnormal personalities occupy an extreme in the spectrum. Abnormal personality only matters if it is maladaptive, causing suffering either to its possessor or his associates—called a *personality disorder*. In general, psychological symptoms which are part of a personality disorder are harder to treat than those arising from other causes.

But personality can change and develop as we learn and adapt (consider the naïve medical student morphing into confident consultant) so is it really fixed? Many consider this a controversial diagnosis. Critics claim it is used to medicalize anyone having difficulties coping with life or as a final resort when symptoms do not easily fit any other diagnosis. At worst, a diagnosis of blame.

Personality disorders are characterized by long-lasting rigid patterns of thought, affect, and behaviour. The attitudes of people with a disorder usually exaggerate part of their personality and result in behaviour at odds with 'normal' expectations. These conditions must not be attributable to brain damage or another psychiatric disorder. They all meet the following criteria:

1 Markedly disharmonious attitudes and behaviour, involving usually several areas of functioning, eg affectivity, arousal, impulse control, relationships.
2 Prevailing, chronic, abnormal behaviour patterns, not limited to discrete episodes, which are pervasive and clearly maladaptive.
3 Present in a broad range of personal and social situations.
4 Manifestations appear <18 years old and continue into adulthood.
5 There is considerable personal distress caused by these patterns of behaviour (although this may only become apparent later in the course).
6 Associated (usually but not invariably) with significant problems in occupational and social performance.

Classification Classification of personality disorders is categorical whereas personality is dimensional. Table 12.7 is provided to give a summary and should be used to understand features rather than form a diagnosis.

▶ Remember everyone has a personality but not every personality, no matter how distinct it may be, is disordered. Avoid labels and engage with the person.

Management Scant evidence that psychiatry helps those with a personality disorder diagnosis—essentially treating someone with a problem integrating into society not a mental illness. However, these disorders are associated with higher rates of premature death (including suicide) and other mental illnesses. In general: • Treat the individual • Reflect their goals • Help manage crises • Treat comorbid conditions • Consider patient/professional relationship.

Medication plays no part in treating a personality disorder (can be used for comorbid condition) so talking therapies are recommended: • Dialectical behavioural therapy (DBT) combines individual and group therapy using mindfulness, CBT, and Eastern philosophy • Therapeutic communities • Mentalization.

Prognosis Generally poor. As mentioned, people diagnosed with a personality disorder have higher rates of morbidity and mortality, worse outcomes for associated mental and physical illnesses, and lowered quality of life markers. Taking this in account, the prevalence of personality disorders (particularly borderline and antisocial) declines with age. This may be as older adults tend to be less impulsive and aggressive or maybe just better at hiding these traits.

Personality disorder clusters Research suggests that personality disorders tend to fall into three groups, according to their emotional 'flavour' (historically and anecdotally labelled as 'mad, bad, and sad'):
• Cluster A: *odd or eccentric.*
• Cluster B: *dramatic or emotional.*
• Cluster C: *anxious or avoidant.*

Table 12.7 Personality disorder clusters
In ICD-11, these clusters have been replaced by 'Prominent personality traits or patterns' rather than named disorders. These traits include: Negative affectivity, Detachment, Dissociality, Disinhibition, Anankastia, and Borderline pattern. ICD-11 further classifies these into mild/moderate/severe. We continue to use the ICD-10 here as these changes have not been widely adopted yet—in clinical life or assessments.

	ICD-10	Gender bias	Description
A	Paranoid	Male	Suspicious, preoccupied with conspiratorial explanations, distrusts others, holds grudges
	Schizoid	Male	Emotionally 'cold', lacks interest in others, rich fantasy world, excessive introspection
B	Dissocial (*in DSM-5:* Antisocial)	Male	Aggressive, easily frustrated, callous lack of concern for others, irresponsible, impulsive, unable to maintain relationships, criminal activity, lack of guilt, conduct disorder (<18yrs)
	Emotionally unstable (2 types)	Female	*Borderline:* feeling of 'emptiness', unclear identity, intense and unstable relationships, unpredictable affect, threats or acts of self-harm, impulsivity, pseudohallucinations
Impulsive: inability to control anger or plan, unpredictable affect and behaviour
	Histrionic	Male	Over-dramatize, self-centred, shallow affect, labile mood, seeks attention and excitement, manipulative behaviour, seductive
	(*DSM-5 only*) Narcissistic	Male	High self-importance, lacks empathy, takes advantage, grandiose, needs admiration
C	Anankastic (obsessive–compulsive)	Male	Worries and doubts, orderliness and control, perfectionism, sensitive to criticism, rigidity, indecisiveness, pedantry, judgemental
	Anxious	Equal	Extremely anxious and tense, self-conscious, insecure, fearful of negative evaluation by others, timid, desires to be liked
	Dependent	Female	Passive, clingy, submissive, excess need for care, feels helpless when not in relationship, feels hopeless and incompetent

12 Psychiatry

►You may well recognize some aspects of your own personality in these descriptions. This doesn't (necessarily) mean a personality disorder. Some of these characteristics may even be helpful in some areas of your life (eg anankastic renal physicians triple check U&Es and narcissistic surgeons operate successfully where others might waver). Disorder arises when there is disruption to the person's life (whether they see it or not).

Anorexia nervosa ►The most fatal of all mental illnesses (~20%, if severe). There is a compulsive need to control eating and body shape. Weight loss becomes an overvalued idea, ie belief in being 'fat' even when weight is very low. Males with anorexia tend to want high muscle mass rather than thinness. In both of these, ideal body shapes are 'achieved' by food refusal (initially diet restriction) combined with over-exercising, induced vomiting, and laxative abuse. Many also have episodes of binge eating, followed by remorse, vomiting, and concealment. Low self-worth is common in all. *Diagnostic criteria:* 1 Weight <85% of predicted (taking into account height, sex, and ethnicity), or BMI ≤17.5kg/m² 2 Intense fear of gaining weight, or becoming fat, with persistent behaviour that interferes with weight gain 3 Feeling fat when thin.

NB: endocrine change (♀: amenorrhoea, ♂: ↓ libido) have been removed in DSM-5. *Epidemiology:* ♀:♂ ≥ 4:1.[167] Men are likely to be undiagnosed as anorexia isn't investigated. Typical age of onset is mid-adolescence—but can start at any age. *Prevalence:* 0.7% in teenage girls and no restriction to a particular ethnic group. *Incidence in primary care:* 20:100,000 ♀ aged 10–39. *Cause:* The exact cause of eating disorders is unknown.[168] The evidence for risk factors includes: *biological:* genetics (55% concordance in MZ twin studies); serotonin dysregulation; *psychological:* depression; anxiety; obsessive compulsive features; perfectionism;[169] low self-esteem; absent sense of identity; *developmental:* adverse life events and difficulties (most commonly in close family/friend relationships); dietary/feeding problems in early life; parents preoccupied with food (ie parent with own eating disorder). There is scant evidence that the chief problem is psychosexual immaturity (antecedent sexual abuse is not a *specific* risk factor); *sociocultural:* substance abuse; negative body images due to media exposure; image-aware activities (eg ballet);[170] past teasing or criticism for fatness.[171] *Signs:* Most due to starvation or vomiting. *General:* fatigue, ↓ cognition, altered sleep cycle, sensitivity to cold, dizziness. *Gastrointestinal:* constipation, fullness after eating. *Reproductive:* psychosexual problems, subfertility, amenorrhoea. *Haematological:* ↓WCC, anaemia, ↓ platelets. *Endocrine/metabolic:* glucose↑↓, ↓K⁺, ↓PO₄³⁻, ↑ bicarbonate, ↑LFT, ↑ amylase, ↑T3/T4, ↓TSH, ↓LH/oestrogen, ↑GH, ↑ cortisol, ↑CCK, ↓ renal function, osteoporosis. *Cardiovascular:* ↓BP; prolonged QT; arrhythmias. *Neurological:* ↓ visuospatial ability, ↓ visual memory, ↑ speed of information processing, peripheral neuropathy. *Dental:* caries. *Dermatological:* dry skin, brittle hair, lanugo hair (fine downy hair all over body).

SCOFF questionnaire: (Can be used for screening.) Do you ever make yourself sick because you feel too full? Do you worry you've lost control over eating? Have you recently lost more than one stone in 3 months? Do you believe you are FAT when others say you are thin? Does FOOD dominate your life? 1 point for every 'yes'; >2 indicates a likely anorexia nervosa or bulimia

ΔΔ: Depression, Crohn's/coeliac disease, hypothalamic tumours.

Red flags—risk ↑↑ if ✏️BMI <13 or below 2nd centile ✏️Wt loss >1kg/wk ✏️T°: <34.5° ✏️Vascular: BP <80/50; pulse <40; saO₂ <92%; limbs blue and cold ✏️Muscles: unable to get up without using arms for leverage ✏️Skin: purpura ✏️Blood (mmol/L): K⁺ <2.5; Na⁺ <130; ↓PO₄³⁻ <0.5. ECG: long QT; flat T waves.

Treatment: Aim to restore nutritional balance eg weight gain of 0.5–1kg (~3500–7000 extra calories/week); final BMI 20–25. Treat complications of starvation. Explore comorbidity. Involve family/carers: difficult family dynamics are often a prominent feature; address this appropriately (avoiding blame) and include family in treatment and as a resource needed to help manage the condition. Address factors maintaining the illness. Patients initially coming into services will often be in denial—do not allow them to disengage.

Severe anorexia (BMI <15kg/m², rapid weight loss + evidence of system failure) requires urgent referral to eating disorder unit (EDU), medical unit (MU), or paediatric medical wards not used elsewhere. Refeeding is considered 'treatment' under the Mental Health Act 1983/Children Act 1989, and it may be needed if insight is lacking. In *moderate anorexia* (BMI 15–17.5, no evidence of system failure) routine referral to local eating disorder service or EDU if available. In *mild anorexia* (BMI >17.5) focus on building a trusting relationship, acknowledging problem, and change. If no response in 8 weeks, consider referral to secondary care. Psychological interventions include CBT (p. 754), interpersonal, supportive, or family therapy (±parent-to-parent consultations[16]). In <18s consider family therapy.[172] Limited evidence base for pharmacological treatment; mainly to treat comorbid conditions. Olanzapine may help stimulate appetite (unlicensed use). Fluoxetine has been used (need to monitor QT interval). *Prognosis:* $1/3$ recover completely, $1/3$ improve, and $1/3$ develop a chronic eating disorder. 5% die (mostly from suicide or direct medical complications eg $\downarrow$K$^+$ and prolonged QT interval predisposing to arrhythmias). Median time between diagnosis and death is ~11 years.[173] Mortality is higher if: aged 20–29 at presentation, delayed access to treatment, bingeing, and vomiting.

Refeeding syndrome Potentially fatal condition from $\downarrow$PO$_4^{3-}$, due to rapid initiation of food after >10 days of undernutrition. *Signs:* Rhabdomyolysis, respiratory or cardiac failure, $\downarrow$BP, arrhythmias, seizures, and sudden death. *Treatment:* Consult a dietician to develop a plan of slow refeeding with careful increase in calories. Monitor serum PO$_4^{3-}$ (stop refeeding if falling), also glucose $\uparrow$, K$^+\downarrow$, and Mg$^{2+}\uparrow$. Milk is often used initially (high in PO$_4^{3-}$ and well tolerated); correct metabolic imbalances (PO route). Prescribe thiamine, vitamin B complex strong, and multivitamin. Over 4–7 days increase dietary intake.

Bulimia (binge eating disorder)

Definition 1 Recurrent episodes of binge eating characterized by uncontrolled overeating 2 Preoccupation with control of body weight 3 Regular use of mechanisms to overcome the fattening effects of binges eg starvation, vomit-induction, laxatives, over-exercise 4 BMI >17.5.[174]

Epidemiology $\female$:$\male$ $\approx$ 9:1. Prevalence ($\uparrow$ in developed countries) $\approx$ 0.5–1.0% in young women. No social class differences. In Britain, young Asian women are at $\uparrow$ risk.[175] Homosexuality/bisexuality may be a specific risk factor for bulimia in males (asexuality is more typical in $\male$ anorexia nervosa).[176]

Cause/associations Urbanization (*not* a risk factor for anorexia); premorbid obesity. Commoner in female relatives of anorexics (?shared familial liability). Genetic contribution of 54–83%. **Natural history** *Age of onset:* ~18yrs.

Symptoms Fatigue, lethargy, feeling bloated, constipation, abdominal pain, oesophagitis, gastric dilatation with risk of gastric rupture, heart conduction abnormalities, cardiomyopathy (if laxative use), tetany, occasional swelling of hands and feet, irregular menstruation, erosion of dental enamel, enlarged parotid glands, calluses on the back of the hands (Russell's sign, from tooth marks during induction of vomiting), oedema (use of laxatives and diuretics), metabolic alkalosis, hypochloraemia, $\downarrow$K$^+$, metabolic acidosis (if laxative use), less commonly: $\downarrow$Na$^+$, $\downarrow$Ca^{2+}, $\downarrow$PO$_4^{3-}$, $\downarrow$Mg^{2+}, abnormal EEG, abnormal menstrual cycle, blunted response of TSH and GH to thyroid-releasing hormone.

Treatment Mild symptoms: support, self-help books, and food diary (similar to anorexia). Referral to EDU in case of no response, moderate/severe symptoms, and to a medical unit if medical complications.[177] Antidepressants are recommended to $\downarrow$ binges and purging. 1st line: SSRIs—specifically **fluoxetine** (effective dose higher than for depression: 60mg); CBT can help (p.754).[178]

Prognosis In 2–10yrs, 50% improve, 20% show no change.[179]

---

16 Parents describe parent-to-parent consultations as an intense emotional experience that helps them to feel less alone, to feel empowered to progress, and to reflect on changes in family interactions.

The historic division between 'organic' (physical) and 'non-organic' (mental) conditions reinforced a mind/body split limiting treatment of common conditions, including psychosexual difficulties. Now sexual dysfunction is agreed to involve an interaction between physical and psychological factors.

Sexual dysfunction is hard to define because defining what is 'normal' is complex and has changed over time. As always, if there are persistent impairments in functioning, response, or enjoyment then this should be considered an area to explore by questioning.

Sexual history Early experiences; present practices; any hints pointing towards transsexualism, commercial sex work, or drug abuse? Orientation to either or both sexes. Difficulties with other partners? When did you meet? What attracted you to each other?

Common triggers for sexual problems[17] *Psychological:* Relationship problems; life stressors; anxiety/depression; low self-esteem; sexual performance anxiety; excessive self-monitoring of arousal; feelings of guilt about sex; fear of pregnancy or sexually transmitted infections (STIs); body changes, eg following surgery; lack of knowledge about sexuality/'normal' sexual responses; previous significant negative sexual experience (especially rape or childhood sexual abuse issues). *Environmental:* (Fear of) interruptions (eg from children, parents); physical discomfort. *Physical:* Use of drugs or alcohol; medication side effects; pain or discomfort due to illness or injury; feeling tired or 'run down'; recent childbirth. *Factors related to the partner:* Sexual attractiveness (gender, physical characteristics); evidence of disinterest, constant criticism, inconsideration, and inability to cope with difficulties (esp. sexual); sexual inexperience/poor technique; preference for sexual activities that are unappealing to the partner.

Prescribed medication Hypotensives (erectile dysfunction, ED); SSRIs (delayed ejaculation); β-blockers, finasteride, OCP (see p. 148), and phenothiazines (loss of libido). *Other causes of ED:* Diabetes, cord pathology, ↑ prolactin, drugs, and alcohol.

Psychosexual therapeutic interventions There is much more to helping people with sexual difficulties than *couple therapy.* Often the problem is not specifically sexual, and sexual difficulties may recede once other aspects of the relationship improve. Specific sexual dysfunctions are considered using a modernized *Masters & Johnson* approach with a model of sexual response entailing excitation, plateau, orgasm, and resolution. But this is just one approach to one problem, behavioural therapy is not suited to dealing with forbidden or disturbing sexual feelings, fantasies, and urges. For this, experiential psychotherapy and psychodynamic approaches are valid alternatives.[180] Also, we should not focus on performance of acts at the expense of promoting the quality of erotic connection.

In any therapy the following concepts need to be understood:
- Never assume that a patient is too old or too ill for sexual issues to be relevant.
  ▶Assume that everyone has a sex life, perhaps in fantasy only (fantasy is always found to be an important component of sexuality).[181]
- Treat sexual problems holistically—eg there may be relevant medical, drug, or other psychopathologies (depression is common).
- Psychological approaches are always important, whatever is offered by way of physical props or drugs such as sildenafil. Men randomized to receive group therapy *plus* sildenafil had more successful intercourse than those receiving only sildenafil. Group psychotherapy also significantly improves erectile dysfunction compared to sildenafil alone.[182]
- Psychological events have physical sequelae, and physical events have psychological sequelae.

17 'Problems' means that these issues cause difficulty for the person. For example, fetishism and fetishistic transvestism were removed from ICD-11 because, if they don't cause distress or harm, they are not considered mental disorders. However, frotteuristic disorder has been newly added.

Sexual issues are easier to talk about when an overt part of consultations (contraception, fertility, and sexual diseases). More commonly they are a covert part of other emotional or behavioural problems. We may find sexual dialogue embarrassing and avoid it—with unpredictable or fatal consequences, eg distress caused by abuse[183] or confusion from emotions relating to sexuality.

Language is important. It may be medical ('coitus'); slang ('screwing'); or socially acceptable ('having sex'). It is not advisable to use slang—it's unprofessional, makes some people confused or uncomfortable, and can make you appear very outdated. Most will expect socially acceptable language; slang may shock and may put up barriers. Occasional mirroring of patient's words can gain rapport but use verbal or non-verbal cues to check if words are acceptable. If in doubt, ask. If you aren't afraid to talk about sex they won't be.

- Ambiguity is a frequent pitfall. Make sure that you both know what the other is talking about! If a new phrase or ambiguous euphemism crops up (slang changes all the time), ask for an explanation right away (a little gentle helping on your part usually overcomes any embarrassment).
- Don't *assume* sexual knowledge. People are often exposed to graphic sexual content on the Internet at a young age, however don't confuse this with understanding. Sex can be confusing and mysterious. There are still many myths, and it is just as hard as it ever was for someone to admit that they don't know something. Sex education in schools is uneven, and may be useless or non-existent (teachers may be too embarrassed to do it).[184]
- Don't assume a sexual orientation. It may be best to let these issues surface gradually rather than asking directly early on. Imply that it is safe to reveal feelings that are confused or non-standard. Your patient may be boxed in by societal, religious, or family views of what sexuality should be, so that suicide can seem the only way out.[185] Through your dialogue you may be able to show that there are other options, and that 'there is no straight way through this world for any of us'.[186] If orientation is causing distress, point out that there is more to a person than sexuality—roles they are good at may include being a friend, colleague, parent, or child—as well as lover, now or in the future. 'You don't need to have sex just to settle the issue of sexuality; feelings can be explored without sex acts, which can be left until you feel ready'. In helping gay people decide when to 'come out', eg to parents, explain that reactions can be unpredictable.[187] 'How well do you know your parents?'; 'How have they dealt with religious or sexual issues with your brothers and sisters?'; 'Are you economically dependent on them?'; 'Do you have social support outside the home?'[188]
- Don't appear embarrassed. It is easier for people to open up if they think that you aren't going to blush, tell them off, or, worst of all, laugh. Don't act shocked and don't judge; give the wrong impression and they will stop being honest with you—see p. 685 for further discussion of this vital point.
- Act as if you have plenty of time to listen—this is a hard conversation for anyone to have, don't make them finish prematurely or feel rushed.

The more you practise talking about sex, the easier it gets. If you avoid it, it will remain a problem to you. Also, your patients may learn communication techniques, helpful in their lives as a whole, augmenting self-esteem, enabling sexual negotiation (useful in negotiating safer sexual practices with partners).[189] Also, you may lay the foundation for honest sexual dialogue between this person and their family, improving everyone's communication.

Asking about sexual abuse Have you been in any relationships that made you feel uncomfortable? Has anyone touched you in a way that made you feel embarrassed? I am wondering if anyone has hurt you in a sexual way?

Confidentiality People need to know that you will only ever breach this if they, or someone else, is in serious danger[190] (see p. 693).

Baby blues A transient, self-limiting condition seen in up to 75% of new mothers, most often 3–5 days after delivery. She is tearful, anxious, and irritable, commonly lasting for 1–2 days, but may persist for up to 2 weeks. Reassurance from midwifery with increased social/family support is normally enough. If symptoms fail to resolve, psychiatric review should be completed.

Postnatal depression The risk of major depression after pregnancy is greater in those with a history of postpartum depression (50%) or unipolar/bipolar depression (25%) compared to 10% without psychiatric history. Other factors include unplanned pregnancy, lack of support, marital problems, social circumstances, sleep deprivation, and hormonal changes.[191]

Natural history: Although most postnatal depression resolves in ≤6 months, don't put off treatment, and just hope for the best. *Consider these facts:*
- For the patient, 6 months is a long, long time.
- For the infant, 6 months is more than a long time: it's literally an age.
- Suicide is always awful but the worst outcomes in postpartum mental health are universally devastating.
- Postnatal depression impairs infant cognitive and social skills.[192,193]

Management of postnatal depression: ▶*Have a low threshold for referring to multidisciplinary teams in mother-and-baby units.* Screen for depression (table 12.8) to avoid missing major depression. Pregnancy and motherhood is often reported as a time of unclouded joy. But what if she is not delighted? Instead, *she* is unaccountably sad, spends the nights crying, and her exhausted days are filled with a sense of foreboding. The place to start to pre-empt these feelings is in the antenatal clinic. ▶Involve fathers;[194] explain: 'When the baby comes you'll need help and rest—don't think you can do it all yourself: become a team—eg taking turns in getting the baby off to sleep.'[195] In the puerperium give permission for the new mother to tell her woe. When this is revealed, counselling, and input from a health visitor and a psychiatrist/GP is wise, as is close follow-up. You may need to arrange emergency admission under the Mental Health Act: but the point of being prepared for postnatal depression is to avoid things getting this bad. *Pharmacology:* short-term, antidepressant medication is as good as CBT. All antidepressants are excreted in breast milk, but tricyclics and SSRIs are rarely detectable by standard tests, *except for fluoxetine which shows significantly higher levels.* Observe babies for possible SE; it may be best to stop breastfeeding if large doses are used. In severe cases, where the patient is not eating/drinking or is strongly suicidal, ECT should be considered. The quicker the mother's symptoms can be brought under control, the less the disruption to the mother and baby bond.

Postpartum psychosis ▶*Any suspicion of postpartum psychosis should trigger an emergency referral to a specialist team.* Peak onset at 2 weeks postpartum, this is a psychotic episode with prominent affective symptoms (depression or mania) occurring with rapidly fluctuating symptoms, mood lability, insomnia, and disorientation. Previous postpartum psychosis has 30% recurrence risk (~40% risk of postnatal depression). Other factors include single parenthood, reduced social support, and previous mental illness. *Prevention:* High-risk patients need an individualized care plan with antenatal specialist perinatal mental health input. *New cases:* Early detection is essential. Due to the risks to self and baby—infanticide is a rare (1 in 50,000) but serious risk—hospitalization is often necessary. A combination of medication to target affective symptoms (mood stabilizer, antidepressant, or ECT) and psychotic symptoms (2nd-generation antipsychotic and long-acting benzodiazepine) combined with therapy, reassurance, and emotional support (with and for family) is best practice. At discharge, a referral to local mental health services and health visitors will be needed.

Table 12.8 Edinburgh postnatal depression scale (EPDS)[191,196]

1 *I've been able to laugh & see the funny side of things:*	As much as always could
	Not quite so much now
	Definitely not so much
	Now not at all
2 *I've looked forward with enjoyment to things:*	As much as I ever did
	Rather less than before
	Definitely less than before
	Hardly at all
3★*I've blamed myself unnecessarily when things went wrong:*	Yes, most of the time
	Yes, some of the time
	Not very often
	No, never
4 *I've been anxious or worried for no good reason:*	No, not at all
	Hardly ever
	Yes, sometimes
	Yes, very often
5 *I've felt scared/panicky for no very good reason:*	Yes, quite a lot
	Yes, sometimes
	No, not much
	No, not at all
6★*Things have been getting on top of me:*	Yes, most of the time I haven't been able to cope at all
	Yes, sometimes I haven't been coping as well as usual
	No, most of the time I have coped quite well
	No, I have been coping as well as ever
7★*I've been so unhappy that it is difficult to sleep:*	Yes, most of the time
	Yes, sometimes
	Not very often
	No, not at all
8★*I've felt sad or miserable:*	Yes, most of the time
	Yes, quite often
	Not very often
	No, not at all
9★*I've been so unhappy that I've been crying:*	Yes, most of the time
	Yes, quite often
	Only occasionally
	No, never
10★*Thoughts of harming myself have occurred to me:*	Yes, quite often
	Sometimes
	Hardly ever
Instructions *Underline what comes closest to how you have felt in the last 7 days*	Never

12 Psychiatry

Ask to score answers 0, 1, 2, or 3 according to increased severity; some (★in table 12.8) are reverse scored (3, 2, 1, 0). Add scores for 1–10 for the total. Let her complete the scale herself, eg at the 6-week check-up, unless literary difficulty. ►A score of 12/30 has a sensitivity of 77% for postnatal depression (specificity: 93%).

Validity Validity for the EPDS is limited with a suggestion that face-to-face detection is still the best determinant of postnatal depression.

When Hollywood wants to show psychotherapy (or psychiatry), they show an older, bearded, white man (Freud, fig 12.9), with a patient on his couch, asking 'How was the relationship with your mother?'—this is not modern psychotherapy.

> *Psychotherapy denotes treatment of mental disorders and behavioural disturbances using ... support, suggestion, persuasion, re-education, re-assurance, and insight in order to alter maladaptive patterns of coping, and to encourage personality growth.* _{Dorland's Medical Dictionary}

Today's psychotherapy can be active, dynamic, and used to treat a range of different conditions. It has a strong evidence base and hardly ever uses a chaise longue.

Therapy is of great importance in psychiatry—and of great importance in therapy is communication. The first step in communication is to open a channel. The vital role that listening plays has already been highlighted (p. 687). So is 'just being nice to patients' in the course of one's medical activities an example of therapy at work? The answer is 'no'—not because being nice is therapeutically neutral, but because one's attention is not focused on planning change through the systematic use of interpersonal techniques.

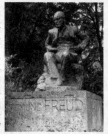

Fig 12.9 Sigmund Freud. Pictured as an older, bearded, white man.
© Gil Myers.

This section is a highly selective glimpse at different types of therapy, in an attempt to show the range of skills needed, and to whet your appetite. It's unlikely you will be given an opportunity, and it would be unsafe, to try out the more advanced techniques without appropriate supervision.

Medicine has 3 great branches: prevention, curing by technical means, and healing—and psychotherapy is the embodiment of healing: a holistic approach in which systematic human dialogue becomes a humanizing enterprise for the relief of suffering and the advancement of self-esteem. Questions such as 'What is the meaning of my life' and 'What is significant?' are answered in a different way after exposure to a gifted therapist. Changes occur in cognition, feelings, and behaviour. This is why therapy is dangerous and exciting: it changes people. Hence the need for supervision and ongoing training and self-awareness on the part of the therapist.

The *types of psychotherapies* may be classified first in terms of *who is involved* in the treatment sessions: an individual, a couple, a family, or a whole group; and secondly they may be classified by their *content and methods* used: analytic, interpersonal, cognitive, or behavioural.

Cognitive therapies (p. 754) Focus on thoughts and assumptions, promoting the theory that we respond to our interpretation of events, not to raw events alone. If this is the case, cognitive change is required to produce emotional and behavioural change.

Behavioural therapies (p. 756) Aim to alter behaviour first, with the theory that if these change then our thoughts and emotions will also evolve.

Psychodynamic therapies (p. 758) Also called psychoanalytical therapies, are concerned with the origin and meaning of symptoms, not necessarily the 'presenting complaint'. They are based on the view that vulnerability comes from early experiences and unresolved issues, often from childhood.

Group therapies (p. 764) As the name suggests, are delivered to a group rather than an individual. Group interactions change the therapeutic environment and provide an alternative space to explore interpersonal relationships.

Play and art therapies (p. 766) Demonstrate the variety of approaches to therapist-patient communication within the field of psychotherapy.

Which psychotherapy is most successful? See p. 753.

Westen's dictum Beware making false dichotomies into supported and unsupported therapies. Randomized trial methodologies don't suit all therapies.[197][198] What follows does not entirely avoid the trap Westen alludes to. Also be aware of many different variations on a theme, eg CAT (cognitive and analytic therapy) and DBT (dialectical behaviour therapy).[18]

Principal recommendations and levels of evidence

- Psychological therapy should be routinely considered as an option when assessing mental health problems.[19] B Evidence shows benefits over no treatment for a wide range of mental health difficulties.
- Patients who are adjusting to life events, illnesses, disabilities, or losses may benefit from brief therapies such as counselling.B Evidence of counselling effectiveness in mixed anxiety/depression, most effective when used with specified client groups eg postnatal mothers, bereaved groups.
- Post-traumatic stress symptoms (p723) are helped by psychological therapy, with most evidence for trauma-focused cognitive behavioural methods. Routine debriefing following traumatic events is not recommended.A Studies have shown that playing *Tetris* reduces likelihood of developing ongoing stress sequelae.
- Depression (p. 710) may be helped (but is often not cured) by cognitive therapy or interpersonal therapy (IPT). A number of other brief structured therapies for depression may be of benefit, eg psychodynamic therapy and counselling.A
- Anxiety disorders (p. 718) including agoraphobia, panic disorder, social phobia, obsessive–compulsive disorders, generalized anxiety disorders are likely to benefit from cognitive behaviour therapy (CBT).A
- Psychological intervention should be considered for somatic complaints with a psychological component, including gastrointestinal and gynaecological problems, with most evidence for CBT for improving functioning in the treatment of chronic pain and chronic fatigue.C
- Eating disorders (pp. 746-7) can be treated with psychological therapy. Best evidence in bulimia nervosa is for CBT, IPT, and family therapy for teenagers. Treatment usually includes psychoeducational methods. There is little strong evidence on the best therapy type for anorexia nervosa.C Early onset of anorexia may indicate family therapy, and later onset, broadly based individual therapy but the evidence is weak.
- Structured psychological therapies delivered by skilled practitioners can contribute to the longer-term treatment of personality disorders (pp. 744-5). A number of therapy approaches have shown some success with personality disorders, including DBT, psychoanalytic day hospital programme, and therapeutic communities.

18 CAT is a collaborative programme for looking at the way a person thinks, feels, and acts, and the events and relationships that underlie these experiences (often from childhood or earlier in life). It combines understandings from cognitive psychotherapies and psychoanalytic approaches into an integrated whole.

19 A Based on a consistent finding in a majority of studies in high-quality systematic reviews or evidence from high-quality studies. B Based on ≥1 high-quality trial, a weak or inconsistent finding in high-quality reviews, or a consistent finding in reviews that don't meet all the high-quality criteria. C Based on evidence from single studies that don't meet all the criteria of 'high quality'.

12 Psychiatry

CBT helps change unhelpful thoughts (cognitions) and actions (behaviours) which can occur during times of distress. Altering these changes how we feel about the world, other people, and ourselves. It focuses on the here-and-now problems, tackling the current state of mind rather than exploring past causes of distress or developmental experiences. It is not a quick fix. A therapist is like a personal trainer who can advise and encourage—but cannot 'do' it for the patient. CBT needs a patient to actively participate in their own recovery.

Key concepts The 'hot cross bun' model (fig 12.10) illustrates the many interactions between thoughts, feelings, behaviours, and body sensations. Any situation will trigger a set of internal and external reactions. These can result in a negative experience creating a vicious cycle which maintains or increases avoidant or negative patterns.

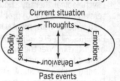

Fig 12.10 Hot cross bun diagram.

Beck suggests that a person who habitually uses depressed or anxious *cognitive distortions* (see BOX 'Cognitive distortions') will be more likely to become distressed when faced with minor problems. These mechanisms lead to distortions within the cognitive triad of the self, the world, and the future.
- In CBT, the patient first learns to identify cognitive distortions from present or recent experiences with the guided use of daily diaries and questioning.
- The patient records such ideas and then learns to examine the evidence for and against them and experiment, testing out these beliefs in real life.
- The patient is encouraged to restart the pleasurable activities that were given up at the onset of difficulties (even if they don't enjoy them … yet!).
- In this way, cognitive restructuring takes place when the patient is able to identify, evaluate, and change the distorted thoughts and associated behaviour.

Technique • Grounded history of the nature of the difficulties • Assessment tools or questionnaires used • Treatment usually takes place on a weekly basis for 5–20 sessions, each lasting 30–60 minutes • A *treatment plan* is formulated with clear goals and objectives and progress is monitored • Each session breaks difficulties into different areas of thoughts, feelings, and behaviours, and helps the patient analyse these to determine effect and consider change • Between sessions, the patient is expected to do 'homework' (practise these changes in their everyday life) and report back the effect in the next session.

Refresher courses CBT teaches skills which can be applied straightaway to a current problem and later to new issues. There is always a risk that these skills will need updating or encouraging (especially if they haven't been practised recently). A short refresher course of a few sessions is encouraged and efficient.

Indications[19] *General:* • The patient prefers a psychological intervention, either alone or in addition to medication • The target problems for CBT (extreme, unhelpful thinking; reduced activity; avoidant or unhelpful behaviours) are present • No improvement or only partial improvement has occurred on medication • Side effects prevent a sufficient dose of medication from being taken over an adequate period. *Specific:* • Depression • Generalized anxiety or panic disorder • Phobias • OCD • PTSD • Hypochondriasis • Bulimia.

Caution • Severe depression • Poor concentration • Difficulties talking about feelings • Patient focused on childhood events • Poor motivation to change.

Modalities CBT is efficient in a variety of different forms • Individual therapy with one-to-one therapy sessions • Group CBT (see p. 764) • Bibliotherapy self-help books as recommended by 'Reading Well Books on Prescription' scheme • Computerized CBT (CCBT) with (free) online resources such as MoodGym, an interactive website to prevent depression and FearFighter, an online program treating panic/phobia (Trusts must pay a fee, then doctors can 'prescribe' it).

Cognitive distortions

Main cognitive distortions in cognitive theory:
- *All-or-nothing thinking:* Seeing everything as binary: black/white, true/false, good/bad, etc. Thinking in these terms is called dichotomous reasoning and often forces negativity as things are rarely wholly positive.
- *Arbitrary inference:* Quickly drawing conclusions (usually negative or of failure) with little or no evidence to support them.
- *Disqualifying the positive:* Ignoring or undermining any positive statements/events/relationships.
- *Emotional reasoning:* Assuming that (negative) emotions reflect the way things truly are: 'I feel it, therefore it must be true.'
- *Jumping to conclusions:* Reaching a negative conclusion from insufficient (if any) evidence. This utilizes *mind reading*, concluding that someone is thinking negatively from their behaviour and then reacting to this assumption without checking with them and *fortune telling*, predicting a negative outcome and acting as though this prediction was an established fact.
- *Magnification and minimization:* Exaggerating any perceived failure/weakness and diminishing any success/strength. Also called the 'binocular trick'. An extreme example of this is *catastrophizing*, assigning the greatest emphasis to the most terrible possible outcome, however unlikely.
- *Mental filtering:* Concentrating on a negative element in a situation to the exclusion of everything else.
- *Overgeneralization:* Drawing global conclusions about worth/performance on the basis of insufficient (often only a single) negative experience. In its extreme form, this is *(mis)labelling*—attributing a person's whole character based on a single action/behaviour which may have been due to error.
- *Personalization:* Attaching personal responsibility, and usually guilt, for an event over which there was no control. Also *blaming* (opposite of personalization) is holding other people responsible for distress (often emotional) caused even if it was out of their control.
- *Selective abstraction:* Dwelling on insignificant (negative) detail while ignoring more important features or stimuli.

: 10 **key facts about** CBT

change: your thoughts and actions.
Homework: practice makes perfect.
Action: don't just talk, do!
Need: pinpoint the problem.
Goals: move towards them.
Evidence: shows CBT can work.
view: events from another angle.
I can do it: self-help approach.
Experience: test out your beliefs.
write it down: to remember progress.

▶From the Royal College of Psychiatrists' excellent leaflet on CBT (Google: RCPSYCH+CBT). This is a very useful resource for patient information leaflets on many different therapies, disorders, and treatments. Highly recommended.

Behavioural therapy aims to change a person's behaviour using one of several techniques depending on the condition. It is most often used as part of CBT (see p756) but can be used independently.

Relaxation training *Indication:* Mild/moderate anxiety. *Technique:* • A system of exercises (p759) and regular breathing (p721) to progressively relax individual muscle groups • Link the relaxed state with pleasant, imagined scenes so that relaxation can be induced by recalling the imagined scene.

Systematic desensitization *Indications:* Phobic disorders. *Technique:* Patients form a hierarchy of fears about the phobic stimulus. Therapy uses graded exposure (least fearsome first) to real or imagined stimuli,[Joseph][Wolpe][200] while patients perform relaxation techniques until anxiety is extinguished. It is ethically less controversial than flooding[201] as progress up the hierarchy is only when patients are completely comfortable with the current level; eg fig 12.11 can be preceded by an almost neutral image, such as ψ.[202]

Fig 12.11 (See text.)
© JML.

Response prevention *Indications:* Obsessions. *Technique:* • Involves exposure to an anxiety-provoking stimulus (eg a toilet seat for patients fearing contamination) • The patient is subsequently prevented from carrying out the usual compulsive behaviour or ritual until the urge to do so has passed.

Exposure/flooding/implosion *Indication:* Phobias. *Technique:* • The anxiety-provoking object or situation is presented *in vivo* or in imagination (prolonged *in vivo* in flooding) • Implosion involves imagined exposure to stimuli in a non-graded manner • The patient then stays with the anxiety-provoking stimuli until there is habituation (ie she becomes accustomed to the anxiety by frequent exposure), and the avoidance response is extinguished.

Thought stopping *Indications:* • Obsessional thoughts occurring without compulsive rituals • Undesired sexually deviant thoughts. *Technique:* The patient is asked to ruminate and then taught to stop negative anticipatory thoughts or obsessional thoughts before they gather enough momentum by arranging a sudden intrusion eg snapping an elastic band on the wrist.

Aversion therapy/covert sensitization ⚡ *Indications:* • Alcohol dependence syndrome (disulfiram used to induce nausea if alcohol is consumed) • Sexual deviations. *Technique:* • Aversive therapy involves producing an unpleasant sensation in the patient in association with an aversive or noxious stimulus (eg electric shocks, chemically induced nausea, pain) with the aim of eliminating unwanted behaviour • Covert sensitization involves the use of aversive stimuli in imagination (eg the approach of a policeman to arrest him/her for his/her undesirable behaviour). *Cautions:* • Punishment procedures are generally ineffective unless patients are taught more appropriate behaviours.

Social skills training *Indications:* Patients with social deficits due to a psychiatric disorder. *Technique:* • Aims to modify a patient's social behaviour in order to help overcome difficulties in forming/maintaining relationships • Video is used to define and rate elements of a patient's behaviour in standard social encounters • The patient is then taught more appropriate behaviour by a combination of direct instruction, modelling, video-feedback, and role play.

Token economy *Indications:* • Children • Intellectual disability • Addictive disorders • Chronic psychiatric disorders. *Technique:* Positive reinforcement improves behaviour: tokens are given when desirable behaviour is displayed. These can later be exchanged for goods or privileges. *Problems:* • Patients become mercenary as they only behave well in exchange for tokens • Poorly prepares people for a world where rewards are subtle and delayed.

Modelling and role play *Technique:* The acquisition of new behaviours by the process of imitation. *Indications:* Lack of social skills and assertiveness.

12 Psychiatry

Muscle group relaxation exercise

►Try this yourself. Experimental learning or 'learning through reflection on doing' helps us to remember things more efficiently than just reading it.

Preparation In a quiet, comfortable place, sit down (a reclining chair is great for this), loosen any tight clothing, close your eyes, and let your whole body go loose. Some people like to lie down—the danger with this is that this will precipitate sleep (which is nice but not the point of the exercise). Assume a passive attitude: tune out all other thoughts and focus on yourself and on achieving relaxation in specific body muscles.

Tension Apply muscle tension to a specific part of the body. Focus on just the target muscle group, eg left hand. Practice allows you to isolate just that group rather than surrounding muscles (eg shoulder or arm). Take a slow, deep breath and squeeze the muscles as hard as you can, eg make a fist, for the count of 5 seconds. Make the muscle tension deliberate, yet gentle. This may cause slight shaking or discomfort but should never cause pain. The intention is to really feel the tension in that muscle group.

Relaxation After the count of 5, quickly relax the tensed muscles, allowing it to become limp and loose. Exhale slowly as the tightness dissipates. Make a conscious effort to notice the difference between states; observe the feelings of relaxation compared to tension in that muscle group.

Systematic order To avoid confusion, start at your toes and work up (or vice versa). Focus on each muscle group in turn and repeat the exercise, at each group deliberately focus on those muscles and the difference between tension and relaxation.

Example muscle group exercises

For each limb complete the 3 muscle groups and then repeat, starting at the distal point, on the other limb.

Foot	Curl toes downward
Lower leg & foot	Tighten calf muscle by pulling toes towards body
Entire leg	Squeeze thigh muscles while doing above
Hand	Clench fist
Entire arm	Tighten biceps by drawing forearm up towards shoulder and 'make a muscle', while clenching fist
Buttocks	Tighten by pulling your buttocks together
Stomach	Suck your stomach in
Chest	Tighten by taking a deep breath
Neck & shoulders	Raise shoulders up to touch bottom of ears
Mouth	Open mouth wide enough to stretch the jaw hinges
Eyes	Clench eyelids tightly shut
Forehead	Raise eyebrows as far as possible

12 Psychiatry

12 Psychiatry

Key concepts 1 *The unconscious:* Individual dynamic psychotherapy is based on the premise that a person's behaviour is influenced by unconscious factors (thoughts, feelings, fantasies). Evidence for the existence of unconscious activity include • Dreams • Artistic and scientific creativity • Hysterical symptoms (p. 722) • Abreaction[20] • Parapraxes, a 'slip of the tongue' (often called a Freudian slip: 'saying one thing, but meaning your mother').

2 *Psychological defences:* Our immune system protects our physical integrity, and our psychological vulnerabilities are shielded by psychological defences. In both cases, overactive defences can lead to trouble eg: *Psychotic defences:* • Delusional projection/paranoia • Denial • Distortion. *Immature defences:* • Projection[21] • Schizoid/autistic fantasy • Dissociation • Acting out • Hypochondriasis • Passive aggression. *Neurotic defences:* • Repression • Displacement[22] • Reaction formation[23] • Intellectualization. *Mature defences:* • Altruism • Humour • Suppression • Anticipation • Sublimation.[24] [203]

3 *Transference and countertransference:* The past patterns (transfers) our present reactions to people. If we have trusted our parents, we will be likely to trust our doctors, teachers, and friends. The intense psychotherapeutic relationship brings these assumptions to the fore where they can be examined, understood, and learned from. We in turn have unconscious reactions to patients based on our past, ie countertransference. Errors from this arise when we react as though our patient were a significant person in our early life[204] (if our mother was an alcoholic we may be oversolicitous or rejecting with alcoholics). *Our reactions are also a key to our patient's feelings:* if a patient makes us feel rejected (as alcoholics often do), perhaps that person themself was rejected as a child and turned to the bottle in compensation.

Assessing suitability *Psychological understandibility:* The patient's difficulties must be understandable in psychological terms. *Psychological mindedness:* The capacity to think about problems in psychological terms. *Motivation:* There must be motivation for insight and change. *Intelligence and verbal fluency:* The ability to communicate thoughts and feelings through talking. *Introspectiveness:* The ability to reflect and think about their feelings. *Dreams:* The capacity to remember dreams. *Ego strength:* The ability to tolerate frustrating or distressful feelings without engaging in impulsive behaviour. *Capacity to form relationships:* There should be a history of at least one sustained relationship in the past or present.

Specific indications • Dissociative/conversion disorders • Depression • Psychosomatic disorders • Relationship problems • Grief.

Technique The therapist provides a secure *frame*—a regular time and place and her own consistency and acceptingness. The patient *narrates* vignettes about himself and his life (~3/session). The therapist *listens* carefully, to the stories and to her reactions to them. She then makes *linking hypotheses*, or *interpretations* that offer *meaning*. Previously inexplicable behaviour begins to make sense. Meanwhile, the patient forms a close relationship with the therapist based on *empathy*, *genuineness*, and *non-possessive warmth* (shown experimentally to be key factors) and sometimes *challenge*. These may be novel experiences for the patient that can be *internalized* as he *works through* difficulties safely. Reactions to *ending* will bring up past unprocessed losses.

Psychodynamic therapy can be *time-limited* (brief dynamic psychotherapy)—suitable for circumscribed problems (eg unmourned grief) or *open-ended* (eg if there are severe personality disorders or complex needs).[NB=1053] In depression, 16 sessions seem to be no better than eight.[207]

---

20 *Abreaction:* cathartic reliving of buried traumas; repressed terrors are made conscious and *tamed*.[205]
21 *Projecting* our own undesirable impulses to another, so pretending that the subjective is objective.
22 *Displacement:* redirection of an undesired intense emotion towards someone neutral and harmless.
23 *Reaction formation:* doing the opposite of true desires (eg training to be a pilot to cover up fear of flying).
24 In sport, for example, we *sublimate* (and make safe) brutal urges into rituals of formal competition.

Cautions: when dynamic psychotherapy might not be right

1 Repeated admissions, many suicide attempts, repeated risk-taking, and severe somatization suggest insufficient ego strength for psychotherapy.
2 A history of repeated failed ventures or dropping out of relationships.
3 In general, patients with acute psychosis are less amenable.
4 Severely depressed patients may be too slowed up and too unresponsive.
5 Over-sedation may hinder capacity to access feelings (?reduce doses).
6 Patients who are actively abusing alcohol or illicit drugs are problematic.
7 No real motivation to change or grossly unreal expectations of therapy.

What used to be called family therapy is now better known as systemic practice, which is an evolving body of ideas and techniques focusing on a person's difficulties within the context of the people and culture that surround them. Therapy is based on the assumption that most people have the resources and potential for resolving life's difficulties.

A family can be described in terms of dimensions. Research interviews have given rise to a measure of 'expressed emotion' (EE) which is associated with severity of chronic illness in many disorders (eg schizophrenia, anorexia nervosa, cystic fibrosis). Therapists work in partnership with families and others, not on them. Family therapy practice is sensitive to diverse family forms and relationships, beliefs, and cultures. Families do not necessarily mean just those related by genetics and can include step-parents, half-siblings, etc.

Family therapy sessions

Family therapists tend to adopt an approach which does not blame individuals, favour adults over children, or take sides. Family therapists tend to be more interested in the maintenance and/or solving of problems rather than in trying to identify a single cause. The therapist should be inclusive and considerate of the needs of each member of the family (not putting anyone above or below the others). The focus is on getting the family to discuss the problems that are putting a strain on their relationships. The therapist helps the family recognize and build on each person's strengths and relational resources in ways that respect their experiences, invite engagement, and support recovery. Everyone is given an opportunity to contribute so that the family explores ways forward which will work for them as a unit.

Deciding which family members attend each session will vary depending on a family's therapy goals and availability (eg elder sibling away at university may join during holidays). A family therapist may offer supplemental individual sessions before or between regular family sessions. This is particularly helpful for those wanting to consider how best to express their thoughts and feelings with the wider family. When parents and children are involved, the therapists may meet with parents separately to work on themes or topics they feel are inappropriate to discuss in front of their children (eg sex, drugs, and death).

Although some family therapists work individually, most will collaborate with a co-therapist or a larger team. Often co-therapists observe family interactions during therapy via a one-way screen ('team behind the screen'). They can observe how the family therapist and family interact. They will then be in a position to share reflections and explore possibilities to help resolve issues. Many families find this approach to complex issues very helpful.

Family therapy models

- Systemic—focus on family beliefs, patterns, and meanings with no objective truth—everyone has their own 'truth' which is subjective.
- Structural—focus on a family's hierarchies and rules; if these are broken a 'problem' individual is blamed. Family structure is viewed by Minuchin[208] as an invisible set of functional demands that organize family interactions. These patterns are self-regulating in a way that attempts to return a family to its habitual mode and minimize anxiety. The therapist actively tries to highlight behaviours and re-organize structures within the family.
- Solution focused—focus on the family, setting, the task, and their goals; the therapist helps the family to collaborate to reach these.
- Narrative—focus on family 'scripts' which are ways to live; problems emerge when individuals deviate from the 'dominant family narrative'; the therapist helps the family to develop a new encompassing narrative.
- Transactional—focus on the problem actually serving a purpose (eg difficult child prevents parents divorcing) and interplay between family members ('transactions'); family given tasks by therapist to challenge these roles.

Dimensions of family functioning

The McMaster Model of Family Functioning has 6 dimensions of family life. A family therapist can observe and consider all of these, and their relation to each other, in order to understand how a family behaves:

* *Problem-solving:* Can the family act together to solve everyday emotional and practical problems? Can they identify a problem, develop, agree, and enact solutions, and evaluate their performance? Success may be dependent upon functioning in other dimensions.
* *Congruence of verbal and non-verbal communications:* Are communications clear and direct or are there hidden agendas or hidden meanings? Do people listen to one another?
* *Roles:* Who is in charge and how are executive decisions made? Who provides for the family? Who is concerned for the child's education and emotional development? Families may function most effectively when roles are appropriately allocated and responsibilities explicit.
* *Affective involvement:* Relationships in families tend to exist on a continuum from overinvolved (enmeshed) to disinvolved (disengaged). Empathic involvement is ideal. This depends on development, as greater involvement is needed for babies than adolescents. Enmeshment may lead a child to be so anxious about a parent that they feel unable to leave them, and avoid school as a consequence.
* *Affective responsiveness:* How do individual family members respond emotionally to one another both by degree and quality? Welfare feelings would include love, tenderness, and sympathy. Emergency feelings would include fear, anger, and disappointment.
* *Behavioural control:* How is discipline maintained? Is there negotiation? Is it flexible? Chaotic? Absent (depends on quality of communication)?

Dysfunctional family patterns

* *Triangulation:* When parents are in conflict, each demands the child sides with them. When the child sides with one, they are automatically considered to be attacking the other. The child is paralysed in a no-win state where every movement is a perceived attack on a parent.
* *Scapegoating:* When an individual is singled out by the family as the sole cause of the family troubles. This serves to temporarily bury conflicts that the family fear will overwhelm them.
* *High expressed emotion:* Derived from a family interview: reflects hostility, emotional over-involvement, critical comments, and contact time.

'A problem shared is a problem halved.' Old English proverb.

Counselling is defined as 'provision of professional assistance and guidance in resolving personal or psychological problems'; counselling is, in essence, 2 people talking together in order to find a solution to a stressful situation or problem. It has existed in many forms for years (family, priests, teachers) but more recently has been professionalized, diversified, and accepted into modern medicine as a legitimate management option for treating psychological needs.

There are a myriad of different modalities of counselling, those focused on career, bereavement, or pre-conception, and in a variety of approaches: email, telephone, or face to face. Counselling remains distinct from other types of therapy and should never be considered to be psychotherapy-lite or diet-CBT. As with all therapies, counselling is not advice-giving or persuasion orientated to the therapist's point of view. Proper counsellors are trained, registered (eg www.bacp.co.uk), and self-reflective.

Indications • Current problems and stresses (eg experiencing acute psychological distress in response to life events or relationship problems) • Brief anxiety disorders, especially when anxiolytic drugs not required.

Technique Aim for adult relationships between patient, family, and therapist, eg with a contract vis-à-vis duties, frequency, and duration of therapy, and what is expected of the client (homework) • Listening, understanding, and reflecting • Note how past stress has been coped with • Producing an agreed full list of problems • Redefining problems in terms of attainable goals • Use of therapeutic contracts to negotiate small behaviour changes, eg learning anxiety-reducing techniques, and carrying out rewards • Talking out (not acting out) anger in safe but cathartic ways • Reassurance: the therapist must give overt reassurance and also, by demeanour, reassure the patient that whatever he reveals (eg incest or baby battering), he will not be condemned.

Not all counselling is non-directive: problem-solving models of counselling are sometimes directive, and may be appropriate if you know the client well.

Caution • 'Giving expert advice': patients may need medical, legal, or financial advice. It may be best if this comes from a specialist agency not involved in the counselling • Patients with personality disorder, where the problems are too deep seated to be changed by counselling. Here there must be an awareness of the need to refer such patients for more formal psychotherapy.

Counselling has long been a central activity in primary care. Many UK general practices employ or have access to counsellors. This huge growth reflects the fact that people love to be listened to, and that a GP may not have the time or inclination to satisfy this need. It is hard to prove the effectiveness of counselling, especially as skills and training vary markedly. This does not mean it is ineffective. Some psychiatrists also offer an 'advisory' service for counsellors.

There are 3 facets to *counselling in general practice:*

1 In some patients, problem-solving strategies are used, with the counsellor using a non-directive approach.
2 In fostering coping strategies, the therapist helps the patient to make the most of the position they are in (eg afflicted by a chronic disease).
3 In cognitive therapy, we concentrate on elucidating negative thinking, and help patients learn how to intervene in negative cycles of thinking.

Randomized trial evidence Counselling and CBT within primary care are both more effective in treating depression than usual GP care in the short term. But in 1 study, there was no difference[25][209] in outcome after 1 year[210][211]$_{N=197}$

25 'No difference' may indicate that too few counselling sessions were offered, that GPs involved were already effective counsellors, or maybe more focused counselling would be more effective.

Supportive psychotherapy

Supportive psychotherapy is an attempt by a therapist to help patients deal with their emotional distress and reinforce health patterns of behaviour through a pragmatic combination of psychodynamic, interpersonal, and CBT approaches. Unlike some therapies, the therapist engages in an encouraging and supportive relationship (not a passive conduit) who comforts, reassures, and listens attentively and sympathetically.

Techniques include:
- Listening to what the patient is saying, picking up verbal and non-verbal cues. Ensure a reasonably full account of the situation and problems.
- Reassurance: relieve fears, boost self-confidence, and promote hope.
- Explain to a patient why they are experiencing certain symptoms.
- Guidance and suggestion with regard to a particular problem.
- Expression of feelings eg anger and despair within a supportive setting.

Although supportive psychotherapy is not currently included in NICE guidance as the primary therapy for most conditions, it can be useful in engaging patients and introducing therapeutic modalities eg CBT. It also has been shown to be beneficial in crisis intervention and in bulimia nervosa.

Brief solution-focused therapy

Brief solution-focused therapy[212] Makes use of a structured approach to draw on people's resilience, and motivate problem-solving. It centres conversations on solutions, not problems. 'If it works, do more of it. If it doesn't work do something different. No problem happens all the time.' In this therapy the therapist may use various questioning techniques:

'Miracle' question Help the patient think about how the future will be different without the problem and set positive goals: 'If you woke up and a miracle had occurred overnight, how would you know? How would life be different?'

Exception question Search with the patient for possible times when the identified problem is less severe or absent. Then encourage them to identify these occurrences and ask 'What happened that was different?'

Spectograms These allow a patient to quantify, measure, and track their own experience, in a non-threatening way. 'On a scale of 0 to 10, how much would you like your miracle to happen?' 'What would have to happen/What would you have to do to make your score move from 3 to 4?'

Coping questions Elicit information about a patient's positive approach that may have gone unnoticed. Even the most hopeless story can have examples of coping which can be shown: 'Things have been really difficult for you, yet you get up each morning and get organized for work. How do you do that?'

Problem-free talk Create a judgement-free zone where patients can discuss what is going well and what areas of their life are problem-free, without minimizing the real problems they have.

Groups are interactive microcosms in which the patient can be confronted by the effect his behaviour and beliefs have on others, and be protected during his first attempts to change. Group therapy involves 1 or more therapists working with several people at the same time. The therapy delivered can be of any type (CBT, interpersonal, etc.), however, usually this name is given to psychodynamic therapy where the group itself and communication within the group are used to explore interpersonal relationships and develop new ways of interacting, thus promoting change through observation and experimenting.

General indications We know that the most suitable patients are:

1 Those who enter into the group voluntarily, not as a result of pressure from relatives or therapists.
2 Those who have a high expectation from the group, and do not view it as inferior to individual therapy.
3 Those who have adequate verbal and conceptual skills. See also psychodynamic psychotherapy (see p. 758).

Specific indications • Personality disorders • Addictions,[213] drug and alcohol dependence (12-step models are all group therapies) • Victims of childhood sexual abuse • People with difficulties in socialization • Major medical illnesses—eg breast cancer.[214]$_{N=50}$

Contraindications Those who are unlikely to benefit include those with severe depression, acute schizophrenia, hypochondriacs, or extreme schizoid personality (cold, aloof, hypersensitive introverts). Group therapy is contraindicated for extreme antisocial behaviour and perpetrators of abuse (especially paedophilia) as the group itself can condone or normalize past thoughts or actions rather than weaken them.

Technique The group selection procedure should be completed by an experienced psychotherapist. Each group is limited to 6–8 members, balanced for sex, and avoiding mixing extremes of age. A decision is made beforehand if the group is to be 'closed', or whether it will accept new patients during its life. The therapist will usually take on a co-therapist of the opposite gender.

The life of the group (~18 months) will develop through a number of phases ('forming → storming → norming → performing'). First there is a settling-in period when members are on their best behaviour, seeking to be loved by the therapist, and looking to them for directive counselling (which is rarely provided). Next is the stage of conflict, as each person strives to find their place in the group other than through dependency on the leader. Frustration, anger, and other negative feelings are helpful by testing the group's trustworthiness. Learning that expressing negative feelings need not lead to rejection is a vital prelude to the next stage: intimacy, in which the group starts working together.

Typically the therapist steers the group away from outside crises and searches for antecedent causes towards the here and now—eg asking 'Who do you feel closest to in the group?' or 'Who in the group is most like you?' The therapist avoids sacrificing spontaneity, and learns to use what the group gives eg 'You seem very angry that John stormed out just now'. Unanswerable questions, especially those beginning 'Why?' are ignored in favour of interaction, observation, and learning. Special methods used to augment this process include written summaries of group activities, video, and psychodrama.

Yalom's therapeutic factors

Irvin Yalom, an American existential psychiatrist, developed a number of therapeutic factors essential to positive group work and group therapy:

- *Universality*—recognition of shared experiences and feelings among group members to remove individual sense of isolation, validate experiences, and raise self-esteem.
- *Altruism*—group members help each other. By doing this an individual will experience giving something to another person which helps develop own self-esteem, adaptive coping styles, and interpersonal skills.
- *Instillation of hope*—in a mixed group with members at various stages of development or recovery, members are inspired and encouraged by another member who has overcome the problems with which they are still struggling.
- *Imparting information*—not a true psychotherapeutic process, however members usefully learn factual or practical information from other members in the group (but not the therapist).
- *Corrective recapitulation of the primary family experience*—members often unconsciously identify the therapist and other members with their own parents and family. Group interpretations help group gain an understanding of the impact of their experiences on their personality, and learn to avoid unconsciously repeating unhelpful past behaviour patterns in current relationships.
- *Development of socializing techniques*—the group setting provides a safe and supportive environment for members to take risks by extending their repertoire of interpersonal behaviour and improving their social skills.
- *Imitative behaviour*—group members develop social skills through a modelling process, observing and imitating the therapist and other members.
- *Cohesiveness*—all members feel a sense of belonging, acceptance, and validation from being in the group.
- *Existential factors*—learning that one has to take responsibility for one's own life and the consequences of one's decisions.
- *Catharsis*—relief from emotional distress through the free and uninhibited expression of emotion. When members tell their story to a supportive audience, they can obtain relief from chronic feelings of shame and guilt.
- *Interpersonal learning*—self-awareness through feedback given by the group on the member's behaviour and impact on others.

Therapeutic communities, and the example of substance misuse

Therapeutic communities (TCs) are a popular treatment for the rehabilitation of IV drug users and dealing with personality disorders—in both the USA and Europe. The rationale is that the benefits of peer-feedback (group therapy) can be magnified in the microcosm of a therapeutic community. Also these communities provide a safe environment for those with complex needs.

In trials of residential therapy vs therapeutic communities the latter can come out better vis-à-vis staying off drugs and not reoffending (eg if the 'residential' arm of the trial is prison).[215] Life in a community is more beneficial (vis-à-vis reoffending or reusing drugs) if it is for 12 months compared with 6 months. After the time in the community, aim to give continuing aftercare.[216] However, there is little evidence that TCs offer major benefits compared with other residential treatment, or that one type of TC is better than another.

European TCs adapt the early harsh behaviourism found in the USA by concentrating more on milieu-therapy and social learning emphasizing dialogue and understanding. Either professionals or ex-addicts can provide input.[217]

►Never underestimate a child's capacity for insight: *don't expect children's methods of communicating insight to mesh with adults.*

Play therapy Children often communicate their experiences and reactions to events through their actions (fig 12.12). This therapy allows them to express emotions through play and also to develop an understanding of themselves and others, resolve psychosocial challenges, and gain acceptance of their experiences and feelings. This builds toward social integration and emotional regulation.

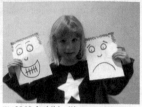
Fig 12.12 A child with an emotion.
© Gil Myers.

Play therapy is often divided into directive or non-directive play. In directive play, the therapist offers more structure and guidance in order to lead the play toward an identified difficulty to work through. Non-directive play therapy encourages a child to play freely without intrusion and in so doing recognize and solve problems. Non-directive play is more comparable to psychodynamic therapy than the behaviourist/CBT approach offered by directive play.

Technique (non-directive) Play, rather than talk, may be the medium for communication between child and therapist.[217]

The basic 10 rules are:

1 Take time early on to make friends with the child. *Don't rush.*
2 Accept the child on their own terms—*exactly as he or she is.*
3 Avoid questioning, praising, or blaming. Be *totally permissive.*
4 *Don't say 'Don't',* and only restrain to prevent serious imminent harm.
5 Show the child that he or she is free to express *any* feeling openly.
6 The responsibility for making choices is *always* the child's *alone.*
7 Follow *wherever* the child leads: avoid directing the conversation.
8 Use *whatever he/she gives you.* Reflect his or her feelings back to him.
9 Encourage the child to move from acting-out their feelings in the real world, to *expressing them freely* in words and play.
10 Prepare the parents for change in the child.

Play therapy is usually used with children aged 3–11 although more frequently with those children who are less verbal or who use play more. Compared to control groups, play therapy treatment groups show an improvement by 0.8 standard deviations.[219] Play therapy appeared equally effective across age and gender. Using parents in play therapy produced the largest effects.

Evidence Evidence on 'activity-based interventions' (broader than play therapy) is mixed: no effect on war-torn children,[220] but good effects on social functioning after sexual abuse,[221] neglect,[222] and in autism.[223]

Play as a diagnostic tool Play can be used in diagnosis, however this is separate from play therapy. Here, the therapist observes the child's play: choice of toys, situations, and actions, and their interactions with others, and considers the underlying reasons for these behaviours and their impact on the child's life. Rich evidence can be drawn from seeing a child explore an environment at their own rate, even when they know they are being watched. For example, school observations in ADHD assessments can highlight differences in playtime routines: does she play football with the rest of the class or sit alone in the corner? And if she does play can she take turns in goal (waiting for the ball to come) or is she always chasing after it impulsively? These are observations which are missed in a foreign, clinical environment.

12 Psychiatry

Art therapy

Art therapy is the use of art materials for self-expression and reflection in the presence of a trained art therapist. No previous experience or skill in art is needed as the art therapist is not primarily concerned with making an aesthetic or diagnostic assessment of the client's work. It is not an art lesson or recreational activity. The chief aim is to effect change and growth in self-esteem through use of art materials in a safe and facilitating environment. Patients stop being patients, and take the initiative in externalizing pain and problems through self-expression.[224]

As ever, the relationship between therapist and client is vital, but art therapy differs from other psychotherapies as it is a 3-way process between client, therapist, and artefact. The therapist's evaluating of the art establishes the intellectual, spiritual, cultural, and emotional status of clients in ways that are helpful to those who find it hard to express thoughts and feelings verbally.[225] It can be a mistake for therapists to interpret the art: leave this to the client.[226]

Art therapists have a good understanding of art processes with sound therapeutic knowledge. They work with individuals and groups of all ages across a range of issues: mental health (in anorexia and dementia, art therapy can improve interactive and coping skills[227]), learning disabilities, palliative care (coping with a cancer diagnosis), disaster zones,[226] and in prisons.

NICE says to always consider non-drug treatments for depression. In a trial with artists-in-residence (a ceramicist, a poet, and a painter), there was a reduction in anxiety, an increase in self-esteem, and fewer consultations from 'heartsink' patients.[228] Art therapy also helps coping in the context of cancer.[229]

Art therapy myths

Edited list from: *Top 10 Art Therapy Myths* on Art Therapy Spot blog:[230]

Art therapy is only for children and not for adults. Children are usually receptive to art therapy because it appeals to their innate curiosity and desire to create. But art therapy can be beneficial to adults of all ages. Art has the ability to express what (even adults) do not always have the words for. Art may bypass purely intellectual thought, and shed light onto the unconscious.

The art therapist knows patients' secrets just by looking at their art work. Art therapists do have a foundation training in interpreting art. However, this understanding helps them ask questions, rather than supply answers. The meaning of the artwork is always derived directly from the patient.

Art therapy is like going to an art class. During art therapy you learn to draw, paint, or sculpt. The goal of art therapy is not to 'teach' art skills. Some art therapists may instruct clients in how to use various art materials so that the client has the freedom to then create whatever they desire.

An art therapist cannot be your primary therapist, but must be an adjunct therapist. An art therapist can be the primary therapist or be part of a treatment team, made up of psychiatrists, psychologists, social workers, etc.

Sessions are awkward for patients because the art therapist just stares at them in silence as they draw. Most art therapists are directly engaged during sessions. Everyone will have their own personal style within the therapeutic relationship. Some create art alongside their clients or some ask clients to create art outside of sessions and bring this in to share and discuss.

Patients have to make art during every art therapy session. There may be sessions when the client decides to just talk or engage in a different type of therapy experience—eg guided meditations, dream work, or more body-centred work such as breathing exercises. Some sessions may be devoted to 'problem-solving' skills such as creating daily schedules.

AC	approved clinician	MCA	Mental Capacity Act 2005
AMHP	approved mental health professional	MHAC	Mental Health Act Commission
CPA	care programme approach	MHRT	Mental Health Review Tribunal
CTO	community treatment order	NHSFT	NHS foundation trust
ECHR	European Convention on Human Rights	CCG	clinical commissioning group
ECT	electroconvulsive therapy	RC	responsible clinician
GSCC	General Social Care Council	RMO	responsible medical officer
IMCA	independent mental capacity advocate	SCT	supervised community treatment
IMHA	independent mental health advocate	SOAD	Second Opinion Appointed Doctor
LSSA	local social services authority		

'I want freedom for the full expression of my personality.' Mahatma Gandhi

The Mental Health Act (MHA), enacted in 1983 and amended in 2007, is the law which allows people with a 'mental disorder' to be admitted to hospital, detained, and treated without their consent. A person is detained in the interests of their own health or safety or with a view to the protection of other persons. The law only applies in England and Wales; Scotland and Ireland have their own laws about compulsory treatment with mental disorders.

Under this Act, there are a set of guiding principles to be considered when making decisions:

- Purpose principle: the MHA must be used to minimize the undesirable effects of mental disorder by maximizing the safety and well-being (mental and physical) of patients, promoting recovery, and protecting others from harm.
- Least restrictive principle: people taking action without a patient's consent must attempt to keep to a minimum the restrictions they impose on the patient's liberty.
- Respect principle: people taking decisions under the MHA must recognize and respect each patient including their race, religion, culture, age, etc.
- Participation principle: patients must be involved in their care as much as is practicable. The involvement of family and friends is encouraged.
- Effectiveness, efficiency, and equity principle: this refers to the most appropriate use of resources to meet the needs of patients.

Procedures governing use of compulsory powers (2007)

Stage 1—preliminary examination: Decisions to begin assessment and initial treatment of a patient under compulsory powers must be based on a preliminary opinion by two doctors and an AMHP that a patient needs further assessment or urgent treatment by specialist mental health services and, without this, might be at risk of serious harm or pose a risk of serious harm to others.

Stage 2—formal assessment/initial treatment under compulsory powers: A patient will be given a full assessment of his or her health and social care needs and receive a formal care plan; the initial period of assessment and treatment under compulsory powers is up to 28 days; after that, continuing use of compulsory powers must be authorized by a new independent decision making body, the Mental Health Tribunal, which gets advice from independent experts as well as taking evidence from the clinical team, the patient ± his or her representatives, and other agencies, as appropriate.

Stage 3—care and treatment order: The Tribunal (or the Court in the case of mentally disordered offenders) can make a care and treatment order to authorize the care and treatment specified in a care plan recommended by the clinical team. This must be designed to give therapeutic benefit to the patient, or to manage behaviour associated with the mental disorder that might lead to serious harm to other people. The first 2 orders can be up to 6 months each; subsequent orders may be for periods of up to 12 months.

Mental Health Act 2007 amendments

Significant amendments were made in 2007 to the Mental Health Act (1983):
- A single definition of 'mental disorder' is used throughout, replacing the previous 4 subcategories, which included mental impairment and psychopathic disorder. Dependence on alcohol or drugs is not considered to be a disorder in the amended MHA.
- Community treatment orders were introduced (see BOX 'Community treatment orders').
- A new 'treatability' test to ensure that compulsory treatment is of therapeutic benefit. So any prolonged detention should include 'medical treatment the purpose of which is to alleviate, or prevent a worsening of, the disorder or one or more of its symptoms or manifestations'.
- People diagnosed with severe antisocial personality disorders are now within the scope of mental health law and can be detained even if they have committed no crime, if they are deemed a danger to themselves or others.
- Age-appropriate services are expected: children protected from admission to adult wards (section 140) and under 18s treated in a suitable environment for their age.
- Widening professional roles to allow non-medical staff (such as psychologists, nurses, etc.) to be Responsible Clinicians and non-social workers to be approved mental health professionals (AMHPs).
- ECT (see p. 713) cannot be given when there is capacitous refusal, other than in emergency ie if immediately necessary to save life or immediately necessary to prevent a serious deterioration.
- Patients may be transferred from one place of safety to another. The hope is that patients detained by police on section 136 will be quickly transferred from a police cell to a more therapeutic environment (see pp. 770-1).

Community treatment orders

In the 2007 amendment, community treatment orders (CTOs) were introduced which allow for compulsory treatment in the community. A patient under section 3 can be discharged from hospital to receive treatment which can be provided outside hospital but they remain subject to a power of recall if specific conditions are not met (outlined when CTO is made) or the risk of harm to patient or others necessitates immediate return to hospital.

CTOs are authorized by the Responsible Clinician and AMHP using the same criteria as for a section 3 application. CTOs have a similar duration and renewal period as section 3 orders.

12 Psychiatry

A patient who makes the capacious choice to come into hospital cannot be held under the Mental Health Act (MHA). They are a 'voluntary' patient. If they are held using the MHA they are called 'involuntary' or, more colloquially, 'sectioned' as a section of the MHA is used (for 2007 law, see p. 772).

▶ If voluntary means have failed, before compulsion may be used, it must be demonstrated that: 1 A patient has a mental disorder and 2 needs detention for assessment/treatment of it, or 3 admission is to protect him/herself or others.

The main sections used for compulsory detention in hospital are section 2: admission for assessment, section 3: admission for treatment, section 4: emergency admission, and section 5(2): emergency detention of an inpatient.

Section 2: admission for assessment (for ≤28 days)
• The period of assessment (and treatment) is up to 28 days.
• The AMHP makes the application on the recommendation of two doctors, one of whom is 'section 12 approved' under the MHA (in practice a psychiatric consultant or registrar) and ideally knows the patient in a professional capacity. The other doctor should be from a different Trust. If not possible, the Code of Practice recommends the second doctor should be an 'approved' doctor.
• It is the site manager's responsibility to read patients' rights, part of which is the right to appeal. Patient's appeals must be sent within 14 days to the Mental Health Tribunal (composed of a doctor, lay person, and lawyer).

Section 3: admission for treatment (for ≤6 months)
• The exact mental disorder must be stated and the appropriate treatment should be available and specified. A patient can be compelled to have certain treatments under a section 3.
• Two doctors must sign the appropriate forms and know why treatment in the community is contraindicated. They must have seen the patient within 24 hours. They must state that treatment is likely to benefit the patient, or prevent deterioration; or that it is necessary for the health or safety of the patient or the protection of others.
• Detention is renewable for a further 6 months (annually thereafter).

Section 4: emergency treatment (for ≤72 hours)
• Admission to hospital must be an urgent necessity.
• May be used if admission under section 2 would cause undesirable delay (admission must follow the recommendation rapidly).
• An AMHP, or the nearest relative although this is rare, makes the application after recommendation from one doctor (usually here the patient's GP).
• The patient must be seen within 72 hours by a second doctor, usually on arrival in hospital by the duty psychiatrist, at which point the decision is made: conversion to a section 2 (or 3), voluntary admission, or discharge. This section should not be allowed to lapse.

Section 5(2): detention of a patient already in hospital (≤72 hours)
• Any doctor looking after the patient (although officially only the doctor in charge or their delegated deputy can complete this section).
• Plan where the patient is to go before the 72 hours has elapsed eg by liaising with psychiatrists for a formal MHA assessment.
• A patient in an ED is not in a ward, so cannot be detained under this section. Common law is all that is available, to provide temporary restraint 'on a lunatic who has run amok and is a manifest danger either to himself or to others' while awaiting an assessment by a psychiatrist.

12 Psychiatry

Nurses' holding powers: section 5(4) (for ≤6 hours)

- Any authorized nurse may forcibly detain a voluntary 'mental' patient who is taking his own discharge against advice, if such a discharge would be likely to involve serious harm to the patient (eg suicide) or others.
- During the 6 hours the nurse must find the necessary personnel to sign a section 5(2) application or allow the patient's discharge.

Sections 7 and 8: guardianship (for 6 months)

- A guardian, usually a social worker, acts in the best interest of someone with a 'mental disorder', to ensure their welfare or protect other people. They help someone live as independently as possible within the community.
- Application is made by an AMHP or 'nearest relative' and also needs two medical recommendations. It can be renewed after 6 months.
- Under section 8, a guardian can require the patient to live in a specified place, to attend for treatment and allow authorized persons access to the residence. Guardianship does not allow treatment to be given without a person's consent.

Section 17: leave of absence from hospital

- While detained in hospital, it is against the law for a patient to leave without permission.
- Under section 17, the responsible clinician agrees to a time-limited leave of absence. Often for family visits or a trial visit home prior to discharge. Sometimes, a member of staff might escort a patient on leave.

Section 117: aftercare & the Care Programme Approach (CPA)

- Section 117 requires provision of after-care for patients who have been detained on the 'long sections' (3, 37, 47, or 48).
- The CPA is not part of the Act but stipulates that no patient should be discharged without planned aftercare: the systematic assessment of health and social needs, an agreed care plan, the allocation of a keyworker, and regular reviews of progress.

Police powers—'place of safety' orders

A 'place of safety' is a nominated safe space where a person can be kept safe and assessed. Every ED should have a designated room for this as well as every police station (for over 18s only) and the police will have a list of these. Colloquially these spaces are called a '136 suite', as this is their main function, although often all 'psychiatric referrals' are assessed there as they offer more privacy.

Section 135 Allows the police to force entry into someone's premises to allow an assessment under the MHA to be made, or to bring them to a 'place of safety'. A warrant from a Magistrates' Court is required before this power can be used. The police must be accompanied by an AMHP and/or a doctor.

Section 136 Allows police to arrest a person 'in a place to which the public have access' who they believe to be suffering from a mental disorder in order to convey them directly to a 'place of safety'. People can be held under section 136 for up to 24 hours, during which time they should be seen by a doctor and by an AMHP who can choose to complete a MHA assessment, admit them informally or discharge them from the section.

Consent to treatment comes in Part 4 of the MHA; it applies to:
• Treatments for mental disorders.
• All formal patients unless detained under sections 4, 5, 35, 135, and 136. The Act doesn't apply to those subject to Guardianship or Supervised Discharge, who have the right to refuse treatment, except in emergencies.

Where a person is deemed to have given their consent to treatment under section 57 or section 58, the person can withdraw that consent at any time. The treatment must then stop and the appropriate procedures followed, unless discontinuing treatment would cause 'serious suffering' to the patient, in which case continued treatment *may* be justified.

Section 57: treatments requiring consent and a 2nd opinion
Some treatments are deemed so restricting that patients cannot automatically have them even if they do consent. Also:
• Three people (one doctor and two others who cannot be doctors) must certify that the person concerned is capable of understanding the nature, purpose, and likely effects of the treatment and has consented to it (*competence*). They are appointed by the Mental Health Act Commission.
• Treatments falling into this category are destruction of brain tissue, or functioning and implantation of hormones to reduce male sex drive.

Section 58: treatments requiring consent or a 2nd opinion
Applies to people who are detained under certain sections without consent, or where the person is not able to consent, eg to ECT or drugs for a mental disorder if 3 months since the person first had the drugs during their current period of detention under the Act.
• In the first 3 months the treatment can be given without consent. The 3-month period starts from when drugs are first given.
• If the person is capable of understanding the nature, purpose, and effects of the treatment and consents to it, the Responsible Medical Officer (RMO) must certify that understanding and consent are present. If the person is capable of understanding the nature, purpose, and likely effects of the treatment and doesn't consent to it, or has ↓ capacity so cannot consent, then a doctor is appointed by the Mental Health Act Commission to give a 2nd opinion. She must consult two professionals involved in the patient's treatment; one must be a nurse.
• The certificates must state the treatment plan in precise terms, eg the number of ECT treatments. If the plan changes, new certificates are required.
• The provisions of section 58 don't prevent urgent treatment (section 62).

Section 62: urgent treatment
The requirements of section 57 and section 58 need not be followed for urgent treatment to save the patient's life or to:
• Prevent serious deterioration, so long as the treatment is not irreversible.
• Alleviate serious suffering (if the treatment isn't irreversible or hazardous).
• Prevent the patient behaving violently or endangering self or others, so long as the treatment is neither irreversible nor hazardous, and is not excessive.

Capacity

Capacity entails being able to grasp and retain information relevant to a decision, and to weigh it as part of a process of making that decision.[231] Mental Capacity Act 2005

Mental Capacity Act (2005) This has 5 statutory principles:

1 A person must be assumed to have capacity unless it is established that they lack capacity.

2 A person is not to be treated as unable to make a decision unless all practicable steps to help him to do so have been taken without success.

3 A person is not to be treated as unable to make a decision merely because he makes an unwise decision.

4 An act done, or decision made, under this Act for or on behalf of a person who lacks capacity must be done, or made, in his best interests.

5 Before the act is done, or the decision is made, regard must be had to whether the purpose for which it is needed can be as effectively achieved in a way that is less restrictive of the person's rights and freedom of action.

In order to decide that someone lacks capacity they must be unable to do any (or all) of the following, in regard to a particular decision at that point in time:

• Understand the information given to them, ensuring it is appropriately presented (eg in a language they understand) about the decision.

• Weigh up the information, considering both pros and cons of any decision in an environment free from inappropriate external influence (eg a relative pressuring them to choose one decision through emotional or physical force).

• Retain that information while they make the decision.

• Communicate their decision (in any means possible: talking, sign language, written, or by any other means).

We mustn't assume that because a patient lacks capacity today for one issue that they will lack capacity on all issues. We must plan for changes in capacity.[232]

However old the person is, it is capacity which matters not age. Parents' wishes are *not* supreme so long as that young person has capacity. If we make a decision on behalf of a patient, we must have a 'reasonable belief' that capacity is lacking and that the act is in their best interests.

Medicolegal issues: use of common law in clinical situations

Deliberate self-harm Adapted from Feldman 2000:[233] *'A 30-year-old man is brought to ED after an overdose. There is no history available and the patient refuses to say anything, other than he wants to be left alone to die. He refuses to give blood for a drug level and is refusing any treatment.,* What should we do? Should we assume he has full capacity? If so, he may die—but autonomy is maintained. Or should the clinician act in the patient's best interests (the doctrine of necessity) as part of their duty of care?

Most people who self-harm are depressed—but this does not prove incapacity. However, in the acute setting, Feldman asserts that 'there are usually good grounds for reasonable doubt with respect to the patient's capacity to make a fully informed and reasoned choice, and to proceed with whatever action is necessary to save his life under the common law'.

Restraint The MHA is an *enabling act* (it needn't be used in all valid situations). Its use gives certain legal safeguards for patients and staff. *'A 40-year-old woman with alcohol problems was admitted 2 days ago with a head injury. She has fluctuating levels of confusion, agitation. She is now trying to leave the ward.'*

Here, due to refusal or lack of capacity, the transient nature of the disturbance, and the need for intervention, common law is applicable. If stronger measures are needed, or the situation persists, it is wise to use the MHA to detain a patient with delirium; however, it is not commonly used.

12 Psychiatry

Relevant pages elsewhere ▶*Every page in all chapters and* OHCM. This is why
this contents list is oddly starved of clinical topics See pp. 778–81.

*With many thanks to Dr Roz Clift our specialist reader, and Joshua Getty our junior reader, for their contribu-
tion to this chapter. Thanks also to Dr Chantal Simon, author of the Oxford Handbook of General Practice, for
permission to use content (as acknowledged) from the OHGP.*

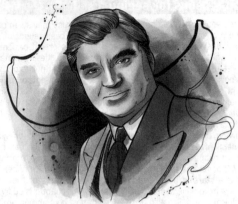

Fig 13.1 In the month he turned 14, Nye Bevan started work underground as a coal miner in the Ty-tryst Colliery, just as his father and brothers had done before him. Schooling had been tough and he fought both an intense stammer and hatred of an unsympathetic headmaster. Against this background, Bevan found solace in the local Workmen's library absorbing as much learning as he could. He became involved in local and Union politics and was elected to Parliament aged 31. As an MP he relentlessly championed the cause of the poor and unemployed, and in 1948 oversaw the founding of the National Health Service (NHS) which allowed people to receive free medical treatment—an idea that seemingly germinated as he cared for his dying father and reflected on the help received from the local Tredegar Medical Aid Society. The NHS is arguably the most significant and lasting reform in the history of UK politics and Bevan's vision has stood the test of time and change. It remains a uniquely powerful engine of social justice.

Artwork by Gillian Turner.

An introduction to general practice

General practice is often the first point of access to healthcare. In the UK it forms the cornerstone of primary care and over 97% of the UK population are registered with a GP.

Scope of general practice Patients have an average of 6 consultations with their GP every year in the UK, yet only 1 in 20 consultations results in a referral to secondary care. Everything else is dealt with within the primary care setting. To do this, GPs must:
• Have a working knowledge of the whole breadth of medicine.
• Maintain ongoing relationships with their patients—they are the only doctors to remain with their patients through sickness and health.
• Take responsibility for people's care across many disease episodes and over many years.
• Be able to deal with undifferentiated illness and the widest range of patients, presentations, and conditions.
• Focus on patients' response to illness, rather than the illness itself—taking into account personality, family, and the effect of these on the presentation of symptoms.
• Be able to draw on a far wider range of resources than are taught in medical school, including intuition, communication skills, and business skills.
• Coordinate care across organizations both within and between health and social care.

The first time you work as a doctor in general practice may seem daunting. Many of the problems you encounter will not have been taught at medical school and almost never encountered on the wards or out-patient clinics. Patients will want you to confidently diagnose and effortlessly manage their problems, yet there will be many times when you will not know what to do—this is normal considering the myriad of possible presentations. Having a management plan at your fingertips and being confident in diagnosis comes with experience. If you are unsure how to manage a patient don't be afraid to ask, however trivial it may seem. You should have a supervisor available for any immediate advice or to discuss cases at the end of surgery.

The following topics are commonly encountered problems or symptoms seen in general practice. More detailed information on each can be found in the relevant chapter in this, or other handbooks (eg the *Oxford Handbook of Clinical Medicine* and the *Oxford Handbook of General Practice*). The following list is a starting point—each page in all chapters of this book and *OHCM* are relevant to general practice, and is why this chapter is oddly starved of meaty clinical topics. See also pp. 194–5, 'Signposting common problems'.

Fever in children Assessing under 5s with a fever is something you will do often. Most children with a fever have a self-limiting viral illness. It is important to exclude the possibility of underlying serious infection. Bacteraemia occurs in 4% of febrile children so a thorough history and examination (including ENT ± urine dip) are required to determine the source. See pp. 192–3.

Acute respiratory and ENT problems *URTI/common cold—children:* Fever, nasal congestion, and cough. A fever of 38–39°C is common in pre-school children. >38°C if <6 months, or >39°C if >6 months especially if cold or shutdown peripheries indicates higher risk for serious illness (see pp. 192–3). Always document observations (p. 192 details normal ranges for age). Respiratory distress should prompt admission. ℞: fluid, rest, paracetamol or ibuprofen (as antipyretic or analgesia). *URTI/common cold—older children & adults:* Most will self-diagnose. *Symptoms:* rapidly developing symptoms of sore throat, nasal congestion/discharge, ± cough, hoarse voice, and general malaise. There may be low-grade fever. Examine to exclude complications and consider differential diagnosis (eg lower respiratory tract infection, influenza, sinusitis, or otitis media). Consider those most at risk of complications (elderly, chronic lung disease, pregnancy, immunocompromised). ℞: most symptoms peak at 2–3 days and resolve by 7 days. There is no curative treatment. Rest, fluids, and simple painkillers if needed.

Chest infection/LRTI/pneumonia (adults): Cough ± sputum ± pleuritic chest pain ± fever/systemically unwell with chest signs (decreased air entry, coarse crackles, pleural rub). Document CRB-65 score and decide if admission required (≥2). If patient can be managed at home start oral antibiotics (**amoxicillin** 500mg TDS or **clarithromycin** 500mg BD if penicillin allergic). Give worsening advice and review/reassess if deteriorating (*OHCM* p166).

Bronchiolitis: Very common in under 1s. Wet cough, raised respiratory rate, bilateral crepitations, and reduced feeding (see p. 210).

Croup: Barking cough ± inspiratory stridor (see p. 208).

Acute sore throat/tonsillitis: (pp. 414–15) Often viral and self-limiting. Symptoms resolve in 40% within 3 days. Use the FeverPAIN score to try and differentiate streptococcal infection and those requiring antibiotics from viral causes.

Otitis media: Middle ear inflammation with pain and fever often after a viral URTI. The TM is bulging and red. Resolves in 60% within 24h but antibiotics may be needed (pp. 394–5).

Otitis externa: Pain, discharge, itch, and tragal tenderness due to inflammation of the skin of the meatus (p. 392).

Hayfever: Rhinitis ± conjunctivitis ± wheeze due to an allergic reaction to pollen—*trees* (spring), *grass/weeds* (summer). ℞: antihistamines, steroid nasal spray, topical eye drops (eg nedocromil) may help.

Sinusitis: Frontal headache/facial pain typically worse on bending forwards ± nasal discharge/congestion ± fever. 80% resolve in 14 days without antibiotics, intranasal steroid sprays may help (pp. 406-7).

Vertigo: Patients may say they feel dizzy but this is ambiguous. Explore what they mean. Some may feel light-headed (consider an alternative diagnosis), others will describe the room spinning. Common disorders causing vertigo include BPPV, acute vestibular neuronitis/labyrinthitis, and Ménière disease. Treatment depends on cause (pp. 404-5)—but is often multifactorial.

Skin problems *Eczema:* Dry, red, inflamed, itchy skin often in antecubital or popliteal fossae and on hands, common in children. ℞: regular emollient (moisturizer), with topical steroid if required for flare-ups (see p. 446). Treat any infected eczema with antibiotics.

Fungal skin rashes: Body—aka ringworm: red/pink ring-shaped lesions with red scaly border and central clear area. *Groin*—red/brown skin lesions in inguinal folds and/or perineum (may not be central clearing)—also seen in submammary and abdominal folds. *Feet*—aka athlete's foot/tinea pedis. Scaly, itchy, white inter-digital skin. ℞: hygiene advice + topical antifungal (eg 1% clotrimazole—in combination with hydrocortisone if marked inflammation) (see p. 448).

Nappy rash: Red skin in nappy area sparing skin folds ± satellite spots beyond the main rash. ℞: nappy free periods + frequent changes + antifungal cream (eg 1% clotrimazole) applied before barrier cream (eg Sudocrem®) (p. 292).

Warts and verrucae: Small nodules with hyperkeratotic or filiform surface. Will resolve spontaneously without treatment or scarring (may take up to 2 years). Consider topical treatment if painful, unsightly, or persisting (see p. 448).

Acne: Comedones (white and black heads), papules, and pustules on face and upper trunk. See p. 450.

Molluscum: Pink papules with a depressed central punctum. Common in children. Treatment not recommended—they resolve spontaneously without scarring (p. 448).

Solar (actinic) keratosis: Crumbly, yellow-white scaly crusts (feels like sandpaper) on sun-exposed skin. See p. 440 for treatment options.

Basal cell carcinoma (BCC): Commonest skin cancer. Pearly raised edge with telangiectasia ± central ulceration. Causes local destruction if not treated. Excision is often treatment of choice (p. 440).

Mole check: Patients will often ask for a mole check—either as a primary consultation or a 'while I'm here' additional request. Use the ABCDEF criteria to identify suspicious pigmented lesions and refer urgently if criteria met (p. 442).

Anxiety and depression Commonly seen and managed in general practice. *Diagnosis:* Depressed mood and loss of interest (anhedonia) ± lack of energy every day for >2 weeks + 2 or more 'typical/biological' symptoms (p. 710). Assess suicide risk (p. 713). Learn to differentiate reactions to stress, life events, and bereavement from a depressive episode. Management depends on severity but is usually a combination of antidepressant and psychological intervention (CBT/counselling).

Headaches A good history is the key to differentiating *tension, chronic* and *medication overuse* headaches (common) from *migraine* and *cluster headaches* (disabling but treatable) and rare but sinister headaches (eg space-occupying lesions, subarachnoid haemorrhage, meningitis/encephalitis, or venous sinus thrombosis). Chronic progressive headaches can indicate raised ICP (worse on waking, lying, bending forward, or coughing). Treatment depends on type of headache. See *OHCM* p456.

Musculoskeletal problems *Low back pain:* Extremely common and often self-limiting. 90% can be attributed to lower back strain or degenerative disease. Associated sciatica is common. The goal is to rule out rare but serious pathology. For 'red flag' symptoms see pp. 486–7. Advise on self-help measures and try to avoid opiate analgesia.

Osteoarthritis: The commonest joint condition with pain and crepitation on movement + background ache at rest. Worse with prolonged activity. ℞: exercises to improve muscle strength. Weight loss if overweight. Paracetamol ± topical NSAID; intra-articular steroid injections. Consider joint replacement (hips or knees) for severe OA which has a significant impact on quality of life (p. 498).

Carpal tunnel: A common cause of hand pain and tingling (esp. at night) due to compression of the median nerve as it passes under the flexor retinaculum. Tingling or pain is felt in the thumb, index + middle finger. Wrist splint, steroid injection, and surgery are all options (see p. 513 & p. 555).

Trigger finger: A flexor tendon nodule ± swollen tendon sheath causes a finger or thumb to become locked in the flexed position (+ has to be flicked straight) (p. 477). Steroid injections help, surgery may be needed.

Ganglia: Smooth cystic swellings from joint capsules or tendon sheaths, often found at the wrist. Treatment is not needed unless causing pain or pressure (p. 476).

Osteoporosis: Reduced bone density secondary to age or to a specific cause (eg early menopause, steroid use). May be picked up incidentally on x-ray (poorly mineralized bone). *Diagnosis:* DXA bone densitometry score of −2.5 or worse. ℞: bisphosphonates (alendronic acid) are 1st line. *OHCM* pp682–3.

Gastrointestinal and genitourinary *Gastroenteritis:* Diarrhoea (>×3 in 24/h) (± sudden-onset vomiting) is the main symptom of gastroenteritis. There may be associated malaise, low-grade fever, and blood/mucus in the stool. ▶▶Diarrhoea may be an early sign of any septic illness. Send stool sample if any blood/mucus, recent travel, or if persisting >7 days. Document frequency of stools/vomiting. *Management:* children p220; adults *OHCM* pp258–9.

Constipation: Definitions vary. Consider present if ≤2 bowel movements per week. Try to identify and address the cause eg opiates, dehydration, poor diet, hypothyroid. Consider/exclude major pathology (the threshold for investigation should reduce with rising age). Consider worrying symptoms eg weight loss, PR bleeding, iron deficiency anaemia. ℞: increase fluid + healthy diet advice. Bulk-forming laxative eg ispaghula is 1st line (*OHCM* p260).

Haemorrhoids/piles: May cause pain (if prolapsing through the anus) or bright red bleeding on tissue/dripping into the pan. Never ascribe rectal bleeding to piles without examination or investigation. Internal piles are not palpable on PR examination. Tenesmus, weight loss, and change in bowel habit should prompt thoughts of other pathology. ℞: increase fluid and fibre. Consider stool softener (bulk forming). Topical analgesia ± steroid (short-term use if topical steroid). Consider surgical referral if medical options not effective.

Irritable bowel syndrome: Accounts for a mixed group of abdominal symptoms for which no pathological cause can be found. IBS results in recurrent abdominal pain or discomfort associated with (at least 2 of) relief by passing stool, altered stool form, and altered (or alternating) bowel frequency. Bloating, distention, and mucus PR are also common. *Examination:* generalized abdominal tenderness is common (*OHCM* pp266–7). Commonly seen with chronic pain overlap syndromes (fibromyalgia, chronic fatigue, chronic pelvic pain).

Urinary tract infection: Cystitis is common in women and may cause frequency, dysuria, urgency, suprapubic pain, polyuria, and haematuria. If ≥3 symptoms, treat empirically. Use dipstick if <3 symptoms. ℞: 3 days of nitrofurantoin (if eGFR >30) or trimethoprim (resistance increasing). Men need treatment for 7 days + MSU ± urology investigations if recurrent or upper UTI (consider prostatitis). *Acute pyelonephritis* causes fever, rigor, vomiting, loin pain ± associated cystitis symptoms. Consider hospital admission. Avoid nitrofurantoin if systemically unwell as it does not achieve effective concentrations in the blood. Diagnosis and management of UTI is different for pregnant women and catheterized patients. See OHCM pp296–7.

Vulvovaginal thrush: Vulva and vagina may be red, sore, and fissured ± itch ± discharge (classically white curds). ℞: **clotrimazole pessary** 500mg + cream for vulva is as effective as oral **fluconazole** 150mg PO single dose (CI in pregnancy). Pregnant women need a longer course of pessaries/cream (7 days).

Incontinence (female): Stress urinary incontinence is the involuntary leakage of urine on effort, exertion, or raised intra-abdominal pressure (coughing/sneezing) due to urethral sphincter weakness. *Urge incontinence* is involuntary leakage of urine with a strong desire to pass urine due to underlying detrusor overactivity (overactive bladder). There may be mixed (urge and stress) symptoms. Discuss sensitively—some women wait many years before seeking help. For assessment and management see p.158.

Lower urinary tract symptoms (males): Irritative symptoms include urgency, nocturia, dysuria, frequency. *Obstructive* symptoms include hesitancy, poor stream, and terminal dribble. Often due to benign prostatic hyperplasia (BPH). Other causes = prostate tumour/cancer ►►(>exclude!), urethral stricture, bladder neck obstruction. ℞: BPH: Lifestyle—avoid caffeine/alcohol; relax when voiding, void twice in a row, 'holding on'. Drugs—α-blockers eg **tamsulosin** 400mg/day are 1st line; surgery eg transurethral resection of prostate (TURP). See OHCM p642.

Contraception The options may initially seem vast yet women will often know what type of contraception they want. It is worth briefly discussing options (especially long-acting methods) as these may not be known. If starting a contraceptive pill ensure you cover when to start, missed pill rule + ensure there are no contraindications and that the patient is not pregnant. Is emergency contraception required? See p.148, pp.154–5.

Miscellaneous *Styes:* Infection or abscess in an eyelid eyelash follicle (=*stye*) or meibomian gland (=*chalazion*). ℞: warm compresses (p.338).

Conjunctivitis: Watery, itchy, gritty eyes with red and inflamed conjunctiva. Acuity and pupil responses are unaffected. ℞: symptomatic relief, hygiene measures ± topical antibiotics (p.336). Red painful eyes ± reduced VA is not conjunctivitis and should prompt urgent ophthalmology review.

Blepharitis: Eye lid/lash inflammation causing burning or itching (p.338).

Ear wax: Causes muffled hearing/fullness. Olive oil ear drops (2 drops BD for 1–2 weeks) will often clear wax. Microsuction/ irrigation may be needed.

Sleep problems: Insomnia is common. Good sleep hygiene is key. Consider hypnotic drugs (eg zopiclone) only if daytime impairment is severe. Treatment should not continue for >2 weeks. Consider CBT if chronic insomnia (>4 weeks).

Chronic disease management Chronic disease accounts for over half of all GP appointments. Chronic diseases may be managed by the practice's nursing team who undertake annual reviews and implement changes to management eg asthma/COPD reviews. See also pp.800–1.

General practice is the most efficient and cost-effective way of providing patient care. Over 90% of patient contacts in the NHS are dealt with in general practice which operates on 8.1% of the total NHS budget. The main roles performed by GPs include:[1]

- *Consultations.* Face-to-face, phone consultations, or visits (to housebound patients). The average person will see a GP 6 times a year. Consultations are used to manage pre-existing conditions or make effective diagnosis of a new problem and may lead to a combination of advice, a prescription, treatment, or referral to a specialist. The cost of a GP consultation in the UK is ~£23. The average cost of an emergency department attendance is £108.[2]
- *Prescriptions.* The NHS spends >£10 billion on prescription drugs each year, the vast majority are prescribed by GPs.
- *Treatments.* GPs provide advice and treatment for many illnesses and may also perform minor surgery and soft tissue and joint injections.
- *Referrals.* GPs are seen as gatekeepers to other NHS services. Patients are usually referred to specialists only after seeing a GP, which helps ensure cost-effective care.
- *Screening and immunization.* Most practices run screening programmes (eg to detect cervical cancer) and undertake immunization for both adults and children.
- *Management of long-term conditions.* 18 million patients in the UK are estimated to suffer from a chronic health condition, with the majority being managed in the community by GPs and practice nurses. This is set to increase due to an ageing population with complex health conditions.
- *Health promotion.* GPs provide information to *promote* health and allow patients to understand their illness and enable self-care.

Differences between GPs and specialists

The increasing sophistication, complexity, and subspecialization of hospital-based medicine also highlights the need for high-quality generalists who deal with undifferentiated problems and 'illness'. Research by Marinker[3] (see table 13.1) encapsulates neatly the contrast in roles between GPs and specialists. GPs have shown the intellectual framework within which they operate is different from, complementary to, but no less demanding than that of specialists.

Table 13.1 Contrasts between GPs and specialists

GPs	Specialists
Exclude the presence of serious disease	Confirm the presence of serious disease
Tolerate uncertainty—managing patients with undifferentiated symptoms	Reduce uncertainty—investigating until a diagnosis is reached
Explore probability seeing patients from a population with a relatively low incidence of serious disease	Explore possibility seeing a pre-selected population of patients with a relatively high incidence of serious disease
Marginalize danger—recognizing and acting on danger signs even when a diagnosis is not certain	Marginalize error—ensuring accurate diagnosis and treatment

To perform their roles well, GPs must show empathy for their patients, engage and commit to involve themselves in every aspect of patient care, and appreciate the limits of their skills and expertise.*

---

* The material in the section 'Differences between GPs and specialists' has been adapted from the *Oxford Handbook of General Practice* 4th edition by Simon *et al*, and has been reproduced by permission of Oxford University Press.

Pressures of primary care

There are many pressures unique to general practice. Dealing effectively with these is important in order to improve job satisfaction and prevent adverse effects on clinical work and home life. Generally, pressures ease with experience and managing them is addressed in training.

Time The standard GP appointment is just 10 minutes long in the UK. How can you deal with everything that needs to be done for a patient in that time? GPs are often interrupted during surgeries and have a myriad of business management tasks and clinical administrative tasks to do, in addition to their face-to-face clinical work. Time management is a key skill and stressor.

Isolation GPs spend a lot of time working alone seeing patients. In smaller practices they may be the only doctor working in the practice.

Dealing with uncertainty Few GPs work in settings where investigations can be accessed immediately. GPs must therefore manage uncertainty regarding symptoms or diagnosis and use time (eg follow-up appointments) to guide further management.

Managing long-term relationships with patients Marriages fail but GPs have to see patients on an ongoing basis, often for years or decades—whether they get on with them personally or not. Relationship management (including setting boundaries) is very important for GPs and can cause considerable stress; it is a skill that is not taught at medical school. General practice is a patient-centred discipline and GPs need to be accepting of patients' subjective health beliefs, family and cultural influences. The opinion of a clinician is no longer sacrosanct—in part due to availability of information via the Internet but also as patients become consumers of healthcare with increasing expectations.

Switching emotions GPs see 15–30 patients in a single surgery. Each appointment is just 10 minutes long and anybody can come with any problem. It is not uncommon to deal with a patient who has acute chest pain, immediately followed by a patient who is suicidal. Switching emotions and maintaining empathy over such diverse and often conflicting situations so quickly can be very demanding.

Managing patient demand vs budget restraint As gatekeepers GPs have a constant conflict between being criticized for not referring or prescribing appropriately, but being criticized and financially penalized if arbitrary targets are exceeded.

Constant reorganization The pace of change in primary care has been immense. Keeping up with those changes and ticking every box required to maintain practice income is a major stressor.

Interventions and solutions These apply to us all, not just GPs!
- *Improve your working conditions:* eg develop a specialist clinical or academic interest within or outside the practice. Learn to decline extra commitments. GPs with higher stress levels do not necessarily have low morale, but there is a close correlation between levels of job satisfaction and morale—job satisfaction seems to protect against stress.
- *Look at your own behaviour and attitudes:* Stop being a perfectionist; resist the desire to control everything; don't judge your mistakes too harshly.
- *Look after your own health and fitness:* Set aside time for rest and relaxation; make time for regular meals and exercise.
- *Allow time for yourself and your family:* Do not allow work to invade family time. Consider changes in working arrangements if it does.
- *Don't be too proud to ask for help:* As well as formal channels for seeking help, there are several informal doctor self-help organizations and counselling services for those in need (see p. 878).

Analysis of the healthcare systems of 11 Westernized countries by The Commonwealth Fund⁴ found the UK ranks 1st overall as the best, safest, and most affordable healthcare system. The UK also spends the 4th lowest per head on healthcare—9.9% GDP compared to 16.6% in the USA, which as the most expensive in the world consistently underperforms relative to other countries (most notably in its absence of universal health insurance coverage).

A good primary care system underpins a good healthcare system. Health systems that are orientated towards primary care are associated with better health for the population, lower costs of care, higher satisfaction of the population with its health services, and lower medication use. Specific features of the healthcare system that help to achieve this are universal access to services, equitable distribution of resources across a population, a high percentage of physicians who are primary care physicians/family doctors (and who have earnings equitable to specialists), and a system that attempts to achieve a higher level of performance (through first-contact, comprehensive, coordinated, family-centred care).[5]

First contact Primary care is the 1st contact with health services. This is not just a routine appointment with a GP, but encompasses a wide spectrum of services: 1 *General practice* 2 *Out-of-hours GP* 3 *Phone advice* (NHS 111) 4 *Walk-in centres* 5 *Emergency department* 6 *Pharmacies.*

The cornerstone of primary care is the responsibility that individuals and families have for their own physical and mental well-being. ►*75% of health problems are taken care of outside formal health systems.* Only 25% of patients who experience symptoms cross the threshold to consult a GP and of those, only 5% are subsequently referred to hospital. Unless individuals and families act on their own initiative to promote their health, no amount of medical care is going to make them healthy. In assessing how good a community is at primary healthcare, one needs to look not just at medical care, but also at social, political, and cultural aspects.

GPs with extended roles (GPwER) *(Previously GPs with special interests—GPwSI)* GPs can develop special interests to enhance their skills and improve management of workload between primary and secondary care (by reducing and enhancing referrals to consultants). The GPwSI framework was originally designed to run outside GP practices but newer models allow GPs to offer extended roles within their day job (hence the change of name). Typical roles are in diabetes, dermatology, cardiology, women's health, and palliative medicine. They deliver a service beyond that of the GP eg in requesting specialist investigations, starting treatment, or undertaking advanced procedures. Although GPwERs reduce waiting times, the chief issue for patients is not the wait to see a specialist but the thoroughness of the consultation and the expertise of the clinician.

Intermediate care This type of care lies between traditional primary care and secondary care. It integrates facilities from many areas to address complex health needs which do not require use of hospital services. There is a trend for more secondary care services to transfer to the community. Examples include pre-admission assessment units; early and supported discharge schemes; community hospitals; stroke rehabilitation units; hospital-at-home schemes (eg providing dialysis or parenteral nutrition). It is one of the mechanisms by which health and social services mesh to allow patients to receive the most appropriate care. The main advantages are: 1 Care close to home 2 Best use of new technology eg near-patient testing 3 Cost-effective use of resources 4 Less rigidly demarcated professional roles 5 Creative integration of working practices.*

---

* The material in the section 'Primary care models' has been adapted from the *Oxford Handbook of General Practice* 4th edition by Simon *et al*, and has been reproduced by permission of Oxford University Press.

Simple self-care constitutes the health activities which we do on our own and within a family eg brushing our teeth, or taking paracetamol for a headache or fever. Empowered self-care is what can happen when health-care professionals work together with the patient and other services. Empowered self-care is a key strategy for primary care, both for disease prevention and chronic disease management.

Chronic disease management Most patients with diabetes will spend at most a few hours face-to-face with a healthcare professional over the course of a year. For the rest of the time they must manage the disease themselves and need to be given the resources and education to do this. Self-management plans are commonplace in primary care. They encourage an interactive partnership between the clinician and the patient to support self-management of chronic conditions. An example is the provision of standby 'rescue' medication to those with COPD, along with instructions on when to start these for an exacerbation. Self-management plans are commonly used in diabetes, asthma, and COPD.

Disease prevention A 'stages of change'⁶ approach can be used to help patients change their behaviour and address addictions, lifestyle modification, and disease prevention. This model shows that a change in behaviour usually occurs gradually through identifiable stages:
• *Precontemplation:* Patients are uninterested, unaware, or unwilling to make a change (eg a patient may feel 'immune' to the problems caused by smoking or high cholesterol).
• *Contemplation:* Patients may assess barriers as well as benefits to change. Giving up an enjoyed activity may cause a sense of loss despite the perceived gain.
• *Preparation:* Patients prepare to make a specific change eg trying a low-fat diet or decreasing their alcohol intake.
• *Action:* This demonstrates a desire for lifestyle change; however, glossing over the previous stages may show that action itself is not enough.
• *Maintenance and relapse prevention:* Involves incorporating the new behaviour in the long term.

Motivational interviewing⁷ In all scenarios, motivational interviewing techniques can be helpful in empowering patients. It encourages both the doctor and the patient to discuss the gains and losses of changing behaviour in a non-judgemental manner (as opposed to the doctor telling the patient what to do). Compare *'You need to stop smoking, it's bad for you,'* with *'Have you ever thought about giving up? What do you think is stopping you?'*

Barriers to self-care
• *Patient factors:* Patients may be blinkered ('It will never happen to me'); we like to rebel ('I know it's bad, but I like it'); there may be a lack of motivation ('I can't be bothered to change'—the path of least resistance). All of these can be influenced by those who are rendered helpless and hopeless by unemployment, poverty, and family strife. Others may have difficulty accessing care eg the homeless, refugees, drug abusers, ethnic minority groups, and patients living in rural areas without public transport.
• *Healthcare professional factors: Time:* it takes time to educate people regarding self-care (eg why antibiotics aren't required for a viral illness). *Motivation:* health education may be seen as repetitive and boring. *Money:* health promotion requires personnel and resources.
• *Society factors: Responsibility lies with the GP:* pharmacists, schools, and the media suggest GP appointments for minor ailments in order to 'cover their backs'; *pressure from business* (eg tobacco advertising); there are also those who want to monopolize and medicalize health.

The primary care team incorporates a broad range of professionals who undertake a wide variety of activities. Each team member should understand and acknowledge the skills, knowledge, and role of others within the team, and should also recognize and include the patient, carer, or their representative as an essential member of the team.

General practitioner GP *principals/partners* are independent contractors, usually within a partnership, who provide primary healthcare services (± additional services). These GPs are self-employed and run the practice as a business, with responsibility for staff, premises, and equipment. Pay depends on income and expenditure. *Salaried GPs* are employed by a practice or other organization under an agreed contract and salary. They may not want the commitment or managerial tasks associated with being a partner. *Locum GPs* are self-employed GPs providing medical cover to different practices on a regular or intermittent arrangement. *FY2 doctors* and *GP registrars* are qualified doctors in training programmes undertaking a rotation within a GP surgery.

Practice nurses These are nurses caring for patients within a GP practice. Activities include: • *Tests:* Audiometry; ECGs; spirometry • *Advice:* Contraception; diet; lifestyle; travel • *Treatment:* Dressings; injections • *Prevention:* Vaccinations; BP; cervical smears • *Chronic disease management:* Diabetes, asthma, COPD, etc.

Nurse practitioners Registered nurses who have acquired expert knowledge and clinical competencies for expanded practice, and who work autonomously in carefully delegated roles. Within general practice they triage patients, diagnose, and initiate treatment. Patient satisfaction is high and no increase in adverse outcomes has been found.

Paramedics Increasingly employed by GP practices to undertake acute home visits, routine reviews of housebound patients with frailty/chronic diseases, and also minor illness clinics.

Physician associates Support doctors in the diagnosis and management of patients. They may run triage/acute illness clinics, manage and undertake chronic disease reviews & other roles, under the supervision of a GP.

District nurses Provide nursing care to those who are housebound (eg frail elderly patients, or those who are terminally ill or disabled). Activities include dressing leg ulcers, changing urinary catheters, administering drugs and injections; providing emotional support to patients and their families; caring for those who wish to die at home; identifying social care issues and liaising with other services. *Community matrons/advanced care nurse practitioners* have case-loads of vulnerable patients eg who have >1 chronic disease. They provide home care (*active case management*) with the aim of reducing emergency admissions to hospital.

Community midwives Provide advice, care, and support for pregnant women and their babies in the antenatal and postnatal period (including home deliveries). They provide parenting support and care for the newborn in the early postnatal period.

Health visitors Have nursing and midwifery backgrounds, plus health visiting qualifications. Most of their work is focused on families with children <5yrs old. They promote good health and prevent illness by offering practical help and advice (eg on breastfeeding; prevention of accidents; and safeguarding).

Clinical pharmacists and physiotherapists Increasingly working in primary care, as are *social prescribers* (see p. 817).

Practice managers Non-clinicians who lead on finance; employment law; tax; risk assessment/reduction; health & safety, statutory and eg CQC requirements.

The term *primary care* is used (in the UK and North America) to describe primary medical care to individuals (eg family/general practice). *Primary healthcare* is a broader term which describes an approach to health policy and services.

The World Health Organization's (WHO) *Alma Ata* declaration[8] (as follows) describes an ideal model of primary healthcare and was adopted at the International Conference on Primary Health Care held in Alma Ata, Kazakhstan in 1978.

Primary care should '*be made universally accessible to individuals and families in the community, by means acceptable to them, through their full participation, and at the cost that the community and country can afford to maintain in the spirit of self-reliance … [and] addresses the main health problems in the community, providing promotive, preventative, curative and rehabilitative services accordingly'*.

There is huge inequality in access to, and provision of, healthcare services between and within countries, as well as vast differences in the health status of individuals. How can these issues be addressed? Is it possible to provide primary healthcare for all?

The ultimate goal of primary healthcare is better health for all. Outlined here are some of the basic principles identified in the Alma Ata Declaration, which should be incorporated into national policies in order to help develop and sustain primary healthcare as part of a comprehensive health system:[9]

* *Accessibility (equitable distribution of healthcare).* Health services must be provided equally to all people irrespective of economic status, race, or location. This concept helps shift accessibility of services from cities to rural areas.
* *Community participation.* Meaningful involvement of the community in planning and maintaining their health services. This grass-roots approach allows sustainability due to local ownership.
* *Health promotion.* Developing skills and understanding of health education, immunization, nutrition, sanitation, maternal and child health, and prevention/control of endemic diseases.
* *Use of appropriate technology.* Use of technology that is cost-effective and feasible eg refrigerators for vaccine cold storage.
* *A 'multi-sectional approach'.* Recognition that health cannot be improved by intervention within just the health sector and that other sectors are equally important, including: agriculture (eg food security); education; communication; housing; access to safe water and basic sanitation.

Critics argue that the declaration is too broad, does not have clear targets, and is generally not attainable, yet the approach has seen significant health gains in some of the world's poorest and politically unstable communities.

Targeted, selective, and cost-effective approaches have also been shown to save lives, such as UNICEF's GOBI–FFF program: Growth monitoring; Oral rehydration therapy for diarrhoea; Breastfeeding; Immunizations; Family planning; Female education; and Food Supplementation.

The consultation is the central act of general practice. It is something that has been studied extensively and various models on how to undertake a consultation exist (see pp. 788–9). The key to a good consultation is the successful exchange of information. There is no 'correct' way to perform a consultation and approaches vary depending on individual preference and style, and according to the patient and situation.

Potential barriers to effective communication There are many! Lack of time, language problems, differing age, gender, ethnic or social background of doctor and patient, 'sensitive' issues to address, 'hidden' or differing agendas, lack of trust between patient and doctor.

Patient centredness An approach where the doctor focuses on what the patient thinks and feels is important to the problems they bring. The patient's views are considered and integrated into the diagnosis and decision-making process. This is a shift in value from the traditional doctor-centred consultation where the patient is passive and the doctor decides on what to discuss and do. It is easy for the patient's own needs to get crowded out of a busy surgery. Depressed patients, for example, frequently hold back information they would like to discuss, as the doctor seems too busy. This concern about 'not worrying the doctor' can be counterproductive. So, every so often try saying 'Take your time—I'm not in any hurry. Let's try to get to the bottom of what's going on … [pause]'.

Consulting in a patient-centred way seems to improve patient satisfaction and may improve health outcomes. It consists of 6 interactive components:[10]

1 *Exploring both the disease and the illness experience:* Integrating the history, physical examination, and investigations with understanding of the unique experience of the patient's illness (their feelings, ideas, effect on day-to-day life and expectations). See fig 13.2.

2 *Understanding the whole person:* Awareness of the multiple aspects of a person's life, family, employment, social support, and the context in which they live (eg cultural issues, community).

3 *Finding common ground regarding management:* Identifying the problem and priorities and establishing the goals of treatment.

4 *Incorporating prevention and health promotion.*

5 *Enhancing the doctor–patient relationship:* At each consultation try to build on the relationship. Include compassion, trust, and a sharing of power and healing.

6 *Being realistic:* About time and the wise use of resources.

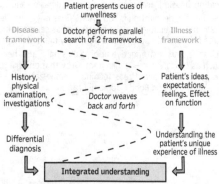

Fig 13.2 The patient-centred process.
Reproduced from Simon *et al. Oxford Handbook of General Practice* (2014) with permission from OUP.

13 General practice

Time and the consultation

Consultation times have risen by 40% in the last 20 years (now on average ~12min). Short consultations are riskier than longer ones (eg less time to look things up and less time for safety netting; 'If x, y, or z develops, you need to come back ...'). ►Does heavy demand produce short consultations, or do short consultations produce heavy demand by failing to meet patients' needs?

The consultation time influences the degree of patient satisfaction, and may influence the consultation rate, with lower return visit rates for longer consultations (not shown in all studies), lower rates of prescription issue (esp. antibiotics), and more preventive activities. Running late is stressful for doctors (and patients). Factors which increase (↑) or decrease (↓) consultation rates (apart from season, distance to the GP, and sex—women consult more than men):

- Social deprivation (↑) and morbidity (↑).
- Increasing requirements to monitor almost all diseases and drugs eg DMARDs for rheumatoid arthritis, diabetes reviews, etc. (↑).
- Low frequency of contact associates with ↑ educational status, paid employment in the health sector, + expectations of GP not to care for minor illness.
- The cheaper the housing (council tax band[UK]) the higher the consultation rate.
- List size, and having personal lists (consultation rate ↓ by 7%—ie patients are encouraged to consult with only 1 doctor decreases overall attendance).
- Not prescribing for minor ailments—see p. 802 (?↓).
- New patients (for their 1st year with a new GP), and patients >65yrs (↑).

There is some evidence for the Howie hypothesis that consultation duration is a valid and measurable marker of quality (effectiveness, safety, equity, and holistic patient experience). However, extending consultation times does not *automatically* increase health and satisfaction.[11]

13 General practice

Consultation models can provide a useful framework for consulting in a structured or organized way, and can help develop consultation skills. As we learn to consult, they can give orientation to a consultation and a 'checklist' of things to do. Consultation models don't need to be followed from start to finish—pick areas from different models that work well for you. There are many different consultation models and the following list outlines just a few.

(Bio)Medical model *Traditional/hospital model:* History-taking→examination→investigations→diagnosis→treatment→review. While being thorough, it is time-consuming, doctor centred, and disease focused.

Balint *The Doctor, His Patient and the Illness (1955):*
A philosophy rather than a consultation model.[12] Balint was a psychoanalyst who aimed to help GPs better understand the psychological aspect of practice.
• Psychological problems are often manifested physically.
• Doctors have feelings. Those feelings have a role in the consultation.
• Doctors need to be trained to be more sensitive to what is going on in a patient's mind during a consultation.

Byrne & Long *Doctors talking to patients (1976):*
Analysis of taped consultations led to a compilation of 6 areas covered in a consultation:[13]
1 The doctor establishes a relationship with the patient.
2 The doctor attempts to/actually discover the reason for attendance.
3 The doctor conducts a verbal or physical examination, or both.
4 The doctor, or the doctor and the patient, or the patient (in that order of probability) considers the condition.
5 The doctor (and occasionally the patient) details treatment or further investigation.
6 The consultation is terminated—usually by the doctor.

This model was the first to include the tasks of introduction and finishing. It also involves the patient and introduces the notion of 'illness'.

The Stott & Davis model *Exceptional potential of the consultation (1979):*
4 tasks that can take place in any consultation:[14]
1 Management of presenting problems.
2 Management of continuing problems.
3 Modification of help-seeking behaviour eg advise self-treating minor illness.
4 Opportunistic health promotion.

Like Byrne & Long it does not actually tell us *how* to carry out the consultation.

Pendleton et al. *The doctor's tasks (1984):*
This model involves exploring the patient's detailed thoughts, including their ideas, anxieties, and expectations, and identifying the effects of the illness.[15]
1 Define the reason for attending: the nature and history; aetiology; the patient's ideas, concerns, and expectations; the effects of the problem.
2 Consider other problems: eg continuing problems and at-risk factors.
3 The doctor and patient choose an appropriate action for each problem (negotiation between doctor and patient).
4 The doctor and patient achieve a shared understanding of the problem.
5 The patient is involved in management of the problem and encouraged to accept appropriate responsibility.
6 The doctor aims to establish and maintain a relationship with the patient.

This model is the essence of patient centredness (see p. 786).*

* This material in the section 'Consultation models' has been adapted from the *Oxford Handbook of General Practice* 4th edition by Simon *et al*, and has been reproduced by permission of Oxford University Press.

Neighbour *The Inner Consultation (1987):*

The doctor works in 2 different ways throughout the consultation, as *The Organizer* and *The Responder*.[16] Each consultation comprises 5 activities:

1 *Connecting* is the process of establishing rapport.
2 *Summarizing* marks the point at which the patient's reasons for attending, hopes, feelings, concerns, and expectations have been well-enough explored, acknowledged, and summarized for the consultation to progress.
3 *Handing over* follows the doctor's assessment and diagnosis of the presenting problems and entails an explained, negotiated, and agreed management plan.
4 *Safety netting* allows the doctor the security of knowing that she has prepared, or could prepare for, contingency plans to deal with an unexpected event and some departures from the intended management plan (p. 876).
5 *Housekeeping* allows the GP to deal with any internal stresses and strains.

This model thoughtfully redefines the tasks of a consultation, but it is fairly complex.

Kurtz & Silverman *The Calgary–Cambridge Model (1996, update 2003):* (fig 13.3) A comprehensive (and daunting) list of 55 consultation skills is contained within a framework that emphasizes patient-centred communication.[17]

• *Initiating the session:* establishing initial rapport and identifying the reason for the consultation.
• *Gathering information:* exploring problems; understanding the patient's perspective; providing structure to the consultation.
• *Building the relationship:* developing rapport; involving the patient.
• *Explanation and planning:* providing the correct amount and type of information; aiding recall and understanding; achieving a shared understanding (by incorporating the patient's perspective); sharing decision-making.
• *Closing the session.*

It is a useful teaching tool and allows structured analysis of a consultation, but possibly too much to remember!

THE CALGARY-CAMBRIDGE GUIDE: A GUIDE TO THE MEDICAL INTERVIEW

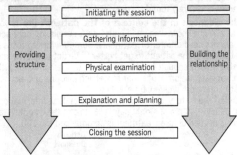

Fig 13.3 The Calgary–Cambridge model.
Reproduced with permission from Kurtz, S. *et al.* (2003). Marrying content and process in clinical method teaching: enhancing the Calgary-Cambridge guides. *Academic Medicine*, 78(8):802–809. Copyright © 2003, Association of American Medical Colleges.

Further reading
Bevington B (2013). *Talking with Patients: A Consultation Handbook* (6th ed). London: KSS Deanery.

Doctors are called on to make decisions about every patient they meet: few are curable at once, so making a plan for what to do for the best is the secret of success at the bedside. The aim here is to explain this secret, to enable you to flourish in the clinical world, and to keep you out of trouble.

Let us look at the steps of the history, physical, or mental examination, and investigations.

By the end of taking the *history*, you need to have acquired 3 things:
1 Rapport with the patient.
2 A diagnosis or differential diagnosis.
3 The placement of the diagnosis in the context of the patient's life.

Rapport Consultations are shorter when rapport is good. The patient is confident that he or she is getting the full attention of the doctor, and these patients are more understanding, and more forgiving when things go wrong. Doctors are far from infallible, so we need to have confidence that the patient will feel able to come back if things are not right, tell us what has happened, agree on an adjustment of the treatment, and, by giving feedback, improve our clinical acumen.

Diagnosis Studies have shown that skilled physicians have made a provisional diagnosis soon after the consultation starts, and they spend the rest of the history in confirming or excluding it. What happens if you are not skilled, and you have no hint as to the diagnosis? You need to get more information.
- Pursue the main symptom: 'Tell me more about the headache …'
- Elicit other symptoms—eg change of weight or appetite, fevers, fatigue, unexplained lumps, itching, jaundice, or anything else odd?
- Get help from a colleague or even a diagnostic support system.
- Check you still have rapport with the patient. Are you searching for a physical diagnosis when a psychological diagnosis would be more appropriate? Here you might ask questions such as 'How is your mood?' 'What would your wife or partner say is wrong?' 'Would they say you are depressed?' 'What would have to change for you to feel better?'

▶Do not proceed to the physical examination until you have a working diagnosis: the answer is rarely found there (<10%).

Placing the diagnosis in the context of the patient's life If you do not do this, you will not know what will count as a cure, and, more specifically, different patients need different treatments. Some factors to focus on might be: the motivation of the patient to get better ('I've got to get my knee better so that I stay strong enough to lift my wife onto the commode'); their general health; social situation; drugs (not forgetting nicotine and alcohol); is help available at home; work (yes/no; type)?

At the end of the history, occasionally there is enough information to start treatment. Usually you may be only, say, 70% sure of the diagnosis, and more information is needed before treatment is commenced (fig 13.4).

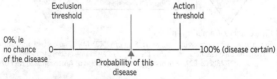

Fig 13.4 Probability of the disease after taking a history.

It is time for the physical *examination*. This aims to gain evidence to confirm or exclude the hypothesis, to define the extent of some process, or to assess the progress of known disease. At each step, ask 'What do I need to know?' Following the examination the diagram may look like this (fig 13.5):

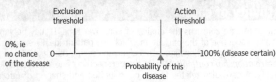

Fig 13.5 Probability of the disease after physical examination.

Investigations If the action threshold has not been crossed, further information is needed. Action thresholds vary from doctor to doctor, and from disease to disease. When the treatment is dangerous, the action threshold will be high (eg leukaemia). In self-limiting illnesses, eg pharyngitis, the action threshold will be lower. Note that 'action' may be that, in agreement with such a patient, only symptomatic treatment is needed, and future episodes could be managed without medical input. Similarly, it may be important to move the probability of a serious but unlikely disease beyond the exclusion threshold.

Once the probability of a disease passes the action threshold, treatment can commence, if the patient wishes (fig 13.6).

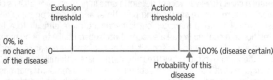

Fig 13.6 Passing the action threshold.

Supposing neither the action threshold nor the exclusion threshold is exceeded, then more information is needed eg from pathology, imaging, or the passage of time. Time itself is an investigation: it may reveal sinister causes or the benign nature of the disease. To use time this way, you need to be reasonably sure that immediate treatment is not required.

If there is still not enough certainty to initiate management, get further information eg from books, the Internet, colleagues, further tests—or you may feel it appropriate to refer the patient. Or go round the process again, starting with the history—from a different viewpoint.

Once above the action threshold, it is time to decide what to do for the best. This is a decision shared by the doctor and the patient. It entails informed consent and consideration of:[18]
- The probability of the diagnosis.
- The likelihood of the different possible outcomes.
- The costs and side effects of treatment.
- The hope and values of those affected, particularly the patient.
- What is possible, considering the skills, resources, and time available.

Finally, tell your patient how they will know if they are on the path to improvement or relapse, and if so, at what point to seek help (fig 13.7; record this in the notes)—eg 'If your peak flow falls by 40%, start this prescription for prednisolone, and come and see me'.

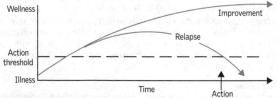

Fig 13.7 Pathway to improvement or relapse.

Continuity of care concerns the quality of care over time. It may be viewed from the perspective of the patient, in which the patient ideally experiences a continuous caring relationship with a clinician ('seeing the GP you know and trust' = *relationship continuity*). From the perspective of healthcare workers, continuity of care also relates to the coordination and sharing of information between different health professionals eg timely access to notes, case management, or multidisciplinary team working (= *management continuity*).

Should we actively encourage patients to see the same GP? Do certain patients (eg those with chronic or multiple health problems) have a greater need for continuity? A 2010 King's Fund report[19] found relationship continuity is highly valued by patients and clinicians. The balance of evidence suggests it leads to more satisfied patients and staff, reduces costs, and improves health outcomes.

The importance of continuity of care Continuity of care has been identified as an assumed strength of general practice around the world. The patient and doctor build a relationship of trust and the GP accepts overall responsibility for coordinating care. However, recent developments in primary care such as changing work patterns (more GPs working part time) and a focus on rapid access suggest that relationship management is becoming more difficult to achieve. Good relationship continuity can also contribute substantially to good management continuity. A GP's clinical responsibility as coordinator of care can include helping patients understand their treatment, navigate unfamiliar services, and remain engaged with their care. Practice nurses and community matrons are also increasingly coordinating care, which is highly valued by their patients.

Patients' experiences of continuity Continuity becomes increasingly important for patients as they develop multiple health or complex problems, or become more socially or psychologically vulnerable; however, relationship continuity is also valued in other circumstances. Patients actually play a large part in securing continuity and this requires good negotiating skills, especially when access is difficult. Patients are often faced with making a choice between seeing the clinician of their choice or the need for an urgent appointment with anyone who is available. Those less confident or with poor language skills may need support in securing continuity.

Clinicians' perspectives on continuity GPs advocate the importance of continuity of care and consider access arrangements (particularly what happens at the front desk) as crucial to securing this. Quality of consultations (including sufficient time) helps cement 'committed' relationships. Management continuity is also important but GPs' attempts to coordinate care with professionals outside the practice can be a source of frustration.

Despite professional recognition for continuity of care there is little practical guidance on how to achieve it.

Tips for good practice *For relationship continuity:* Encourage patients to establish a relationship with a particular professional; support patients to maintain these relationships: • By providing patients with information on availability • That staff know who a preferred GP is • That sufficient capacity exists for same-day and advance appointments • That results, documents, and medication requests/reviews to go to the usual GP.

For management continuity: • Make full use of IT systems and electronic communications • Ensure timely availability of relevant clinical communication—particularly from hospitals • Arrange personal contact with other professionals, including meetings and informal discussions • Ensure proactive follow-up after significant events.

Further reading
Freeman G *et al.* (2010). *Continuity of Care and the Patient Experience*. London: The King's Fund.

13 General practice

Primary care This is about risk and uncertainty, but sometimes unnecessary risks cause ourselves and our patients unnecessary harm. Defence organization records suggest that ~½ of all successful negligence claims reflect poor clinical judgement on the doctor's part; the other ½ represent avoidable mishaps which would be susceptible to risk management approaches—often failures in simple administrative systems, communication failures, inadequate records, or lack of training.

Risk management Means taking steps to minimize risk and keep ourselves and others as safe as possible. There are 4 stages:
 1 Identify the risk—through analysis of complaints and comments from GPs, other practice staff, or patients; through significant event analysis/audit or by using defence organization material to identify common pitfalls.
 2 Assess frequency and severity of the risk.
 3 Take steps to reduce or eliminate the risk.
 4 Check the risk has been eliminated.

Categories of risk relevant to general practice:
• Clinical care eg prescribing errors • Non-clinical risks to patient safety eg security and fire hazards • Organizational risks eg failure to safeguard confidential information or unlicensed use of computer software • Financial risks eg employment of a new staff member.

Key safety issues for primary care:
• *Diagnosis:* 28% of reported errors.
• *Prescribing:* 1 in 5 prescriptions contains a prescribing error; 1 in 530 prescriptions contains a serious error; 9% of hospital admissions are due to potentially avoidable problems with prescribed drugs. 4% of drugs are incorrectly dispensed each year.
• *Communication:* poor communication is a major cause of complaints; 28% of patients have discrepancies between the drugs prescribed at hospital discharge and those they receive in the community.
• *Organizational change:* in industry, better teamwork, communication, and leadership decreases adverse incidents.

In each case, consider:
• *Organizational and management factors:* financial resources/constraints; practice policies; organization.
• *Work environment factors:* staffing levels; skill mix; work load; equipment.
• *Team factors:* team structure; communication; supervision.
• *Individual (staff) factors:* knowledge, skills; competence; health.
• *Task factors:* availability/use of protocols/guidelines; availability of results.
• *Patient factors:* condition (complexity and seriousness); language and communication; personality and social factors.

On average, 20 NHS prescription items are issued per person per year in England at a total cost of £9204 million.[20] GPs account for 75% of NHS annual prescribing costs (~10% of the total cost of the NHS), although many of these 'GP drugs' will have been initiated in hospital. Unused prescriptions cost the NHS an estimated £300 million each year. There are various causes to medication wastage, including patient recovery, changing regimens, and non-adherence.

Compliance, adherence, and concordance

Compliance is the extent to which a patient follows a health professional's advice in taking a treatment.[21] It suggests that the doctor knows best and patients who lapse are foolish. Patients may actively decide not to take a prescribed medication and in doing so commonly fail to confide this to their doctor. This concept has been replaced as it implies a submissive uninvolved patient.

Adherence is the extent to which a patient's behaviour corresponds with agreed recommendations from a healthcare provider. Non-adherence may limit the benefit of a medicine and result in deteriorating health. It should not be seen as the patient's problem—it is often due to a failure to fully agree on the prescription in the first place. Failure to adhere can be common in chronic disease, especially when patients do not feel ill and treatment may be abandoned.

The term *concordance* has evolved as a process by which prescribing is based on partnership. This agreement is between the patient and healthcare professional and is reached after negotiation that respects the beliefs and wishes of the patient in determining whether, when, and how their medicine is taken. Patients are more likely to commit to treatment and adhere to a decision they have actively made. The degree to which a patient may want to be involved in decision-making is variable and patients will often ask the doctor's opinion and defer to it. In some instances a patient may make a decision which is not recommended by the doctor. As long as the doctor believes the patient has understood the issues or risks, and there are no ethical concerns, the patient's decision can usually be supported. The major advantage in a concordant consultation is that the patient's views and decisions will be elicited and respected, allowing any subsequent problem to be discussed. See fig 13.8.

Concordance is a liberating concept, promoting egalitarianism in medicine. ►*There is no healthier ideal.* Are you nodding in the direction of concordance while still covertly believing in compliance? Then let us put the boot on the other foot and await the time *you* are monitored for compliance with some guideline: we predict that concordance will now seem more rational and desirable!

Predictors of non-adherence
• Low literacy • Homelessness • Depression • Psychiatric disease • Substance abuse • Lack of insight into illness • Lack of belief in benefit of treatment • Cultural incongruency with medication • Belief that the drug is not important or is harmful • Complexity of medication regimen • Weariness of taking medications • Inconvenience of medication regimen • Side effects or fear of side effects • Inadequate follow-up.[22]

Improving adherence

Assessment	Assess all medications—can any be stopped?
Individualization	Individualize the regimen eg tailor timing to suit routine
Documentation	Provide written communication eg why a medicine is prescribed/what it is treating + eg common SEs
Education	Tailor education to the needs of the individual
Supervision	Provide continuing supervision—are all meds being taken?[23]

Prescribing: cost-effectiveness

Formularies Aim is to make prescribing more cost-effective, by compiling an agreed list of favoured drugs. This voluntary restriction can work in tandem with compulsory NHS restricted lists, and lead to substantial savings.

Computer software Can flag up more cost-effective prescribing solutions, which can be swapped with one click, if the GP so desires (eg valaciclovir→aciclovir).

Generic prescribing Using generic names when prescribing is one of the simplest ways to reduce cost (eg prescribing **desogestrel** 75mcg/day, instead of using a brand name eg Cerazette®). All drugs have a chemical name, a generic name, and a proprietary or brand name. When a new drug is brought to market, the company that developed the drug will derive income from prescriptions—whether the generic or brand name is prescribed—while the patent is still valid. Once the patent expires, any company can manufacture and market the drug. At this point, if drugs are prescribed generically, the pharmacist can decide which brand to supply and market forces drive the price down.

Advantages of generic prescribing:
- *Cost:* generic prescribing is usually cheaper.
- *Clarity:* there can be several brand names for the same drug. Using generic names allows everyone to be clear which drug is being used.
- *Convenience:* pharmacists do not stock all brand names and may have to order a supply whereas generic preparations of all commonly used drugs are available.

NB: reasons not to prescribe generic drugs include: • Drugs with a low therapeutic index (where small differences in plasma concentration may be significant eg lithium, phenytoin) • Modified-release formulations, where pharmacokinetic properties are not standardized eg diltiazem, sulfasalazine, nifedipine, aminophylline • Formulations containing ≥2 drugs eg inhalers.

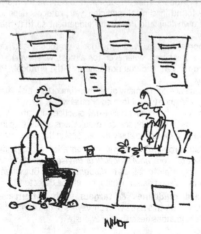

"I'd prescribe the drug, but considering the side effects, you're better off with the disease."

Fig 13.8 There is some truth in this humour: consider the elderly gentleman with clinically insignificant prostate cancer and the side effects of hormone therapy—one of many possible examples.

With permission from CartoonStock.com.

►There is nothing better (for the doctor and the patient) than doing a job for the love of it—and not many people love targets set by other people—so the target has to entail great benefits to outweigh its unintended consequences.

►Beware accepting a protocol without knowing if it will affect your sympathy and time to communicate.

►Is the protocol independently validated? What is its *hidden objective* eg cost-containment, conformity, self-advertisement, empire-building, or care?

►Reject protocols that don't specify conflicts of interest: most protocols (87%) are written by people with financial links to drug companies or public bodies wishing to curtail expense.[24]

If a protocol says that you must do 9 things to Mrs James who has diabetes, both of you may be irritated by the time you reach item 5: the doctor is running out of time, and the patient is running out of goodwill. She is worrying about her husband's dementia, having long since stopped worrying about her own illnesses. Sympathy is a flower which has often withered before the end of morning surgery.

Guidelines are seen as friendly, if flexible, allowing for the frailties of clinical science as it meets bedside reality; they can also be interactive, if computer programming is skilful. *Protocols*, however, particularly if they have been handed down from some supposedly higher authority, have a reputation for being strict, sinister, and stultifying instruments for thought control.

How well do these stereotypes stand up in practice? It is known that doctors working in highly regulated environments with strict protocols perform suboptimally.[25] It is also worth noting that very few laws define their own exceptions. You could say that patients have a right to be asked if they want to participate in a protocol, and if so, that it should be done properly. Herein lies the paradox of protocols. They are designed to remove the many indefensible inconsistencies found in clinical medicine, yet protocols depend on the individual doctor's own flair and instinctive judgement so that they are applied in the best way.

The best approach is to welcome good protocols, and develop meta-protocols to be answered whenever (or almost whenever) such protocols are not adhered to. Why did you not adhere to the protocol? Please tick the appropriate box:

• My own convenience eg too many other more important tasks to do.
• My patient's preference (well informed or otherwise).
• Evidence is shaky and may not apply to my practice population.
• Inefficient use of resources eg scarce consultations are used up in follow-up.
• My instinct warned me not to apply the protocol in this case.[1]

To get round the problems of non-implementation of guidelines, some NHS CCGs sent in visitors from *pharmaceutical advisers* who had trained in outreach visiting (it is unfair to call them *thought-police*). But when this has been evaluated in randomized trials, no impact could be detected.[28]

Can we square guidelines & targets with patient-centred care? Answer: *No*; discussing this issue with purveyors of guidelines is a good way to reveal the hidden agendas described previously.

---

1 Understandably, many GPs don't follow protocols despite high awareness of them: other reasons include the fact that precise targets (eg for BP control) are always arbitrary, and should allow for some variation. Be prepared to defend your deviation from a guideline should it ever be questioned.

There is great variability in individual GPs' referral statistics, which leads purveyors of government strategy to the error of saying 'Why is there a 4-fold difference in referral rates between GPs? Such variation is insupportable; some doctors must be referring too much ...' An advance is made when this issue is reframed as: *'There is information contained in this variability'*. This information can guide service development.

Referral rates Understanding the intricacies of purchasing healthcare depends on understanding referral patterns. If high-referring GPs refer needlessly, then the proportion of their referrals resulting in further action will be smaller than that of practices with low-referring GPs. Usually, this is not the case. Those with high referral rates have high rates of intervention. If I refer an ever-increasing number of my patients to an elderly care clinic, must a time come when admissions level off? The idea of a 'levelling-off effect' is important. If the consultant is 'correct', and the GP's expectation as to the outcome of referral are uniform (probably never true), then when a levelling-off effect is observed, it may be true that the *average* referral rate is optimal, and that low-referrers are under-treating, and high-referrers are wasting money. In fact, levelling-off effects are rarely seen, except in general surgery. If the consultant is over-enthusiastic, and overstates treatment benefits, then the lower referrers are to be applauded for limiting the excesses of the consultant.

Appropriateness of referrals ►*In general, only agree that a referral is inappropriate if the patient, the GP, and the consultant concur on its lack of utility.* Each of these parties has different motivations—eg reassurance/explanation, medicolegal, as well as providing therapy. Despite the rhetoric, secondary care can be preoccupied by its own agendas and may have little interest in the unique needs of referred patients. Overall, referral rates are no more variable than admission rates, even in populations with similar morbidity. The reason may be that there is still a great deal of uncertainty underlying very many clinical decisions. We don't know who *exactly* should have a knee replacement or cholecystectomy, etc.

►There is no known relationship between high or low referral rates and quality of care. Here are 3 cautions in interpreting referrals:

1 Don't accept GP list size as a denominator (it takes no account of differing workloads in a practice). Consultations/yr is a better denominator.

2 If a GP has a special interest, this will influence referral patterns. More knowledge may lead to more referrals as partial knowledge leads to greater, not less, uncertainty. For example, after a while all GPs with a special interest in dermatology will have been tricked by melanomas masquerading as seborrhoeic warts—so their referrals will be higher than GPs who have less experience.

3 Years of data are needed to compare referrals to rarely used specialties.

Referral incentive schemes Are a complex and uncertain way to influence referrals. Local educational interventions with secondary care specialists and structured referral sheets can impact on referral rates. 'In-house' 2nd opinions and other primary care based alternatives to out-patient referral are promising. In 2013–14 >100 million out-patient appointments were scheduled by hospitals in England, an increase of 8.2% on the previous year.

Telephone consultations are increasingly used to try and manage workload and reduce unnecessary face-to-face consultations. There has been a 63% increase in the number of telephone consultations in the last 5 years.[27]

Routine calls Most GP surgeries offer telephone consultations to discuss conditions that do not require an examination, such as self-limiting minor illness, to answer patient queries to follow up chronic disease eg hypertension or diabetes control, or to discuss results of investigations.

The main drawback of telephone consultations is the inability to examine a patient and a lack of visual cues to aid communication. Be alert to verbal cues such as distress or hesitation and ask the patient about their ideas and concerns. Invite them to ask questions and only give advice once you have sufficient information on which to base your judgement. ►If examination is needed, arrange to see the patient.

Emergency calls Nearly all calls for emergency care are made by telephone. In many instances an emergency ambulance is more appropriate and should be called. If giving advice, make it simple and use language the patient can understand and ask them to repeat what you've told them. Give specific safety netting advice should symptoms change and inform the patient how to access further help if needed. Appear helpful, keep calm and friendly—worried callers often appear abrupt or demanding. ► If in any doubt about the problem or how to manage it, arrange to see the patient or ensure an ambulance has been called.

Telephone triage Phone triage seems a tempting way to reduce the need for precious appointments, however research suggests phone triage actually increases workload. Patients who had phone consultations with either a GP or nurse were 75% or 88% more likely to need a 2nd consultation, compared to 50% if the 1st contact was face-to-face.[28] Much of the work in general practice can be managed on the telephone but many patients also need to be seen. Telephone triage is not a substitute for meeting demand.

GP video consultations There is increasing use of private and NHS video consultations via a PC or smartphone which allow patients to video call a GP. This is convenient for patients and gives visual information that is lacking in telephone calls. Critics argue that organizations offering this service are 'cherry picking' younger healthier patients to the exclusion of others and this risks destabilizing 'traditional' general practice.

Email consulting

Email has been used relatively little to consult with patients. Successful use depends on a clear understanding of its role:
- Establish turnaround time for messages (do not use for urgent matters).
- Warn that email is not secure and confidentiality cannot be assumed.
- Retain copies of email communication with patients in their notes.
- Request patients to put their name and DOB in the email for identification.
- Ask patients to be concise and to put the category of request in the subject line for appropriate filtering (eg prescription; appointment; advice).
- Append messages with standardized text containing the GP's full name, contact information, and reminders about security and alternative forms of communication for emergencies.

Further reading

Campbell JL *et al.* (2014) Telephone triage for management of same-day consultation requests in general practice (the ESTEEM trial): a cluster-randomised controlled trial and cost-consequence analysis. *Lancet* 384:1859–68.

Glory or drudge? We may dread home visits as requests filter in through a busy morning surgery, while patients are waiting to be seen, results are waiting to be filed, phone calls and referrals are waiting to be made, and letters are waiting to be read and actioned. But when we are *doing* home visits, we might rather like them. We are less interrupted, and the possibilities of practising holistically are much enhanced because we see the family in their own context. Home visits are greatly valued by patients and are a good way to avoid unnecessary 999 calls.

Who should be visited? Home visits provide the best way to assess those who are acutely or chronically housebound. This includes those who are terminally ill or who are truly housebound and for whom travel to a GP surgery would cause unacceptable discomfort or deterioration.[29] Home visits are not usually required to assess those who are able to travel by car to a doctor's surgery. This includes the elderly with poor mobility or general malaise; adults with common problems such as most cases of back pain or abdominal pain; and children with common symptoms such as fever, diarrhoea, and vomiting. It is not the doctor's job to arrange transport for these patients, which is usually readily available from family, friends, or taxi firms. Clinical effectiveness and efficiency of care must take precedence over patient convenience.

It is the doctor's decision whether a patient can be expected to attend the surgery. GPs are only obliged to visit if they feel it would be inappropriate for the patient to attend surgery. General practice is not an emergency service—there is not the infrastructure or workforce to try and attend patients who may be suffering from a serious medical emergency in the middle of a pre-booked surgery. In such circumstances it is unlikely that a GP could contribute beyond the care of a paramedic and an ambulance should be called.

The doctor's bag

In order to undertake home visits you will need your own doctor's bag, which should include the following:

Equipment Stethoscope; auroscope; ophthalmoscope; patella hammer; BP monitor; thermometer; pulse oximeter; peak flow monitor; urine dipstix; capillary glucose machine; needles; syringes; gloves/lubricating jelly; specimen bottles; sharps box.

Drugs Keep in date (check regularly) and consider carrying the following (exact contents will vary according to your location and circumstances): adrenaline; analgesia (opiate and NSAID); antibiotics (including benzylpenicillin + water for injection); antiemetic; antihistamine; aspirin; diuretic; GlucoGel*; glycerin suppositories; GTN spray; lorazepam/diazepam; naloxone; prednisolone; salbutamol inhaler. NB: if you carry controlled drugs, your bag must be lockable and a record of drug use kept.

Other items *BNF;* headed notepaper; prescription pad; smartphone with street map app + list of useful numbers eg pharmacy, ambulance, local hospitals.

The predominant disease pattern in the developed world is one of chronic or long-term illness. In the UK, over 40% of adults (43% ♀;41% ♂) report a long-term illness. Chronic disease is more prevalent in older people and in poorer social classes. People with chronic disease are intensive users of health services accounting for over 50% of all GP appointments; 65% of out-patient appointments; and 77% of hospital bed days.

Although details of chronic illness management depend on the type of illness, people with chronic diseases of all types have much in common with each other. They all have similar concerns and problems, and must deal not only with their disease(s) but also its impact on their lives and emotions.

Common patient concerns

- Finding and using health services and other community resources.
- Knowing how to recognize and respond to changes in a chronic disease.
- Dealing with problems and emergencies.
- Making decisions about when to seek help.
- Using medicines and treatments effectively.
- Knowing how to manage stress or depression that is associated with chronic illness.
- Coping with fatigue, pain, and sleep problems.
- Getting enough exercise.
- Maintaining good nutrition.
- Working with their doctor(s) and other healthcare providers.
- Talking about their illness with family and friends.
- Managing work, family, and social activities.

Examples of chronic disease
• Diabetes
• COPD
• Cancer
• Heart failure
• Stroke
• Rheumatoid arthritis
• Chronic pain
• Renal disease
• Mental health problems
• Dementia

Effective chronic disease management Common elements include:

Involvement of the whole family: Chronic diseases do not only affect the patient but everyone in a family.

Collaboration: Between patients, carers, and healthcare providers.

Personalized written care plan: Taking into account the patient and carers' views and using current evidence for disease management.

Tailored education in self-management: A patient with diabetes spends only 3h/year with a health professional—the other 8757h they manage their own condition. Helping patients with chronic disease understand and take responsibility for their condition is vital.

Planned follow-up: Planned reviews and follow-up according to the patient's care plan, disease registers, and recall systems is important.

Monitoring of outcome and adherence to treatment: Use of disease/treatment markers (eg HbA1c in diabetes or CRP/ESR in rheumatoid arthritis); monitoring of concordance (eg checking repeat prescription use).

Tools and protocols for stepped care: Provide a framework for using limited resources to greatest effect; step professional care in intensity—start with limited professional input and systematic monitoring; and select subsequent treatment according to the patient's progress, clinical need, and guidelines.

Targeted use of specialist services: For those patients who cannot be managed in primary care alone.

Monitoring of process: Continually monitor management through clinical governance mechanisms.

Depression and chronic disease

Depression is 2–3 times more common in patients with a chronic physical health problem than in people who have good physical health. A chronic physical health problem can both cause and exacerbate depression and treating depression in these patients has the potential to increase their quality of life and life expectancy.[30] Depression is associated with:

• ↑ mortality, ↑ morbidity, ↑ disability, and poorer quality of life.
• ↑ presence of smoking and a sedentary lifestyle.
• Poorer chronic disease outcome measures (eg HbA1c).
• ↑ use of services and healthcare costs.
• Poor concordance with medication and management plans.

The presence of a physical illness can complicate the recognition and assessment of depression, because some symptoms are common to both.

Further assessment and management p. 710.

Frailty

Frailty is a clinically recognized state of increased vulnerability resulting from ageing and a decline in physical and psychological reserves.[31] From aged 85, 25–50% of people will display some degree of frailty. Frailty varies in severity and is not static. There may be both gradual and episodic deterioration. It is not an inevitable part of ageing and is not the same as multimorbidity or disability. Those with long-term conditions or disability may be frail, but some patient's only long-term condition may be frailty. Frail older people are the highest users of health and social care.

Those with frailty are at risk of dramatic deterioration in health after an apparently minor event (eg infection, fall, surgical procedure, or new medication). The presence of 1 or more *frailty syndromes* should raise suspicion that a person has frailty (and may have more serious underlying disease):
• Falls • Immobility/sudden change in mobility • Delirium/acute confusion or worsening of pre-existing memory loss • New or worsening incontinence • Susceptibility to side effects of medication. These syndromes may affect a person's ability to manage at home and remain independent, with resultant impact on quality of life and significant cost implications.

Assessing frailty: • *Gait speed*: taking >5 seconds to cover 4 metres • *Timed up-and-go test* >10 seconds to get up from a chair, walk 3 metres, turn, and sit down • PRISMA-7 questionnaire (scores >3 =frailty). GP practices are required to identify patients >65 with moderate–severe frailty. The Electronic Frailty Index (eFI) is an automated tool which uses pre-existing electronic GP health records to do this.

Management and prevention: Management of frailty involves a comprehensive review of medical, functional, psychological, and social needs, including referral to geriatric medicine/older people's mental health if significant complexity. Medication reviews (eg using STOPP START criteria), falls review/management, and personalized care plans (eg respect form) should be completed.

NICE advises on mid-life lifestyle changes to help delay or prevent the onset of dementia and frailty.[32] NB: there is no evidence that routine population screening for frailty improves health outcomes.*

Further reading

NICE (2009). *Depression in Adults with a Chronic Physical Health Problem* (CG91). London: NICE. https://www.nice.org.uk/guidance/cg91

* The material in the BOX 'Frailty' has been adapted from the *Oxford Handbook of General Practice* 4th edition by Simon *et al*, and has been reproduced by permission of Oxford University Press.

GPs may not want to spend much time on minor conditions (minor for whom …?), but this may become unavoidable if a prescription is issued for each consultation on minor illness (rather pointless if all the patient wanted was reassurance). This reinforces attendance, as a proportion of patients will come to assume that a prescription is necessary. GPs rate a fifth of their consultations as being for minor illness (upper respiratory problems, presumed viral infections, mild gastroenteritis, and childhood rashes for example). In some studies, 80% are likely to receive a prescription (but this number may be falling), and >10% are asked to return for a further consultation. Why does this great investment of time and money occur? Desire to please, genuine concern, defensive medicine, prescribing as a way to end a consultation, and therapeutic uncertainty all play a part.

Positive correlations with low prescribing rates include a young doctor, practising in affluent areas, and longer consultation times. Not everyone wants to reduce prescribing, but advice is available for those who do.

- Encourage *belief in one's own health* and innate powers of recuperation. '*The art of medicine is amusing the patient while nature cures the disease*' (Voltaire).
- Using a *resource* which gives information (eg NHS website).
- Using *self-medication* (eg paracetamol for fever).
- Using the *larder* (eg lemon and honey for sore throats).
- Using *time* (eg cough—follow-up if symptoms persist or worsen).
- *Using deferred prescribing:* 'He'll get over it in a few days; but here is a prescription if I am wrong: it's good for his body to learn to deal with these infections, but if this doesn't happen, this is plan B.'
- Using *pharmacists*, or a more experienced member of the family eg granny.
- *Pre-empting requests* for antibiotics (eg for sore throat): 'I'll need to examine your throat to see if you need an antibiotic, but first let me ask you some questions … From what you say, it sounds as if you are going to get over this on your own, but let me have a look to see.' [GP inspects to exclude tonsillitis.] 'Yes, I think you'll get over this on your own. Is that all right?'

Empowering patients Any illness, minor or otherwise, is an opportunity to empower patients. Use the time to enable patients to improve their ability to:
- Cope with life and to understand their illness.
- Cope with and manage specific minor illnesses.
- Feel able to keep themselves healthy.
- Feel confident on handling health issues.
- Be confident about their ability to help themselves or their family.

We know that time spent this way improves patient satisfaction and clinical outcome (although simply extending consultation times in the hope that this will happen is not enough).

Medically unexplained symptoms (MUS)

MUS are physical symptoms for which no organic cause can be demonstrated. GPs deal with MUS in 25% of consultations (costing the NHS £3.1billion/yr). MUS cause disability as severe as that originating from pathology. ⅓ of patients will have a concurrent psychiatric diagnosis—usually anxiety or depression.

Risk factors for developing MUS • ♀>♂ • Physical illness/trauma • Stressful life events (enquire about a history of psychological or sexual past abuse, including in childhood) • Media campaigns for specific diseases.

Classification 3 types of complaint (there are common overlaps):
- Pain of a specific location eg back pain, headache, fibromyalgia
- Functional disturbance in a particular organ eg IBS, palpitations
- Fatigue/exhaustion eg chronic fatigue syndrome

Underlying mechanism 2 mechanisms seem to underpin MUS:
- *Enhanced sense of bodily awareness:* A tendency to notice and amplify normal physical sensations such as heartbeat. Over-awareness increases anxiety and in turn makes the sensation more likely.
- *Misattribution of symptoms:* Rather than normalizing symptoms, patients attribute somatic explanations (eg a headache is due to a brain tumour rather than stress).

Assessment Consider in any patient with physical symptoms for >3 months that affects functioning but cannot be readily explained. Perform your assessment without prejudice—patients have the same chance as developing serious new illness. *Ask:*
- What are the *symptoms*? Are there signs on examination (rule out red flags)?
- What type of *impairment* do they cause?
- What are the patient's *concerns* and what would they like you to do?
- Does the patient have low mood or anxiety?
- Are there any other social/psychological factors triggering symptoms?

Investigation Review the notes carefully before requesting investigations (which usually clarify the diagnosis and reassure the patient and GP). In patients with MUS, 50% are not reassured following negative investigations. False-positive results lead to ↑ anxiety and further investigation. Colluding with the patient ↑ illness behaviour. ►Try to find a balance between appropriate investigation and risk of harm through over-investigation.

Management 4 key areas:
1 *Connecting:* Go back to the beginning, listen to the patient, acknowledge suffering, use existing knowledge of the patient.
2 *Summarizing:* Allow the patient to summarize problems, recap your understanding of the problem to the patient, and show an interest.
3 *Hand over:* Develop a shared action plan with realistic goals to improve functioning and provide reassurance about long-term outcome.
4 *Safety-netting:* Share uncertainty. Inform patients about red flags indicating serious disease; offer access should symptoms change.

Regular appointments (eg once a fortnight) might be helpful, as might a brief examination at each visit to check for signs of disease. Suggest increasing physical activity levels or voluntary work. Avoid referral unless a clear indication.

Treatment Amitriptyline 10mg ON (unlicensed) may help. Start with a low dose as response is not dose dependent. Explain it is not being used for depression. CBT allows patients to change their thinking and cope more effectively.

4–10% of patients will have an alternative organic explanation.*

Further reading

RCGP/Royal College of Psychiatrists/Trailblazers/National Mental Health Development Unit (2011). *Guidance for Health Professionals on* MUS. www.rcgp.org.uk

* The material in the section 'Medically unexplained symptoms (MUS)' has been adapted from the *Oxford Handbook of General Practice* 4th edition by Simon *et al*, and has been reproduced by permission of Oxford University Press.

137 million working days were lost to sickness in the UK in 2016 costing >£100 billion. The most common reasons for sickness absence were:
• Minor illness eg coughs and colds (34 million days lost).
• Musculoskeletal problems (31 million days lost).
• Stress, depression, and/or anxiety (16 million days lost).[33]

Sickness absence ↑ with age; ♀ have higher rates than ♂. The longer someone is not working, the less likely they are to return to work. ▶Someone who has been off work for >6 months has an 80% chance of being off work for 5 years.

Returning to work can help recovery, improves physical/mental health and well-being, and decreases social exclusion/poverty. In contrast, long periods out of work can contribute to:
• Higher GP consultation rates, medication use, and hospital admissions.
• ×2–3 increased risk of poor general health, mental health problems, and excess mortality.

The role of the GP When someone of working age presents with a problem that affects their ability to work, record a brief occupational history:
• Address the underlying health problem and any personal, psychological, organizational, or social factors preventing a return to work.
• Where possible, suggest adjustments to enable a return to work (eg amended duties or hours, or a phased return via the option of 'may be fit to work' on the Med 3 form—see BOX 'Forms for certifying incapacity to work').
• Liaise with the employee's occupational health service for prolonged absences.

Time off work for emergencies In many cases, patients have the legal right to take time off work to deal with an emergency involving someone who depends on them, but they may only be absent for as long as it takes to deal with the immediate emergency. Employers do not have to pay for time taken off.

Dependants: Include spouse or partner, children, parents, or anyone living with the patient as part of their family, or others who rely wholly on the patient for help.

Emergencies: Include situations in which a dependant is ill and needs help; goes into labour; is involved in an accident or assaulted; needs the patient to arrange their longer-term care; needs the patient to deal with an unexpected disruption or breakdown in care (such as childminder or carer failing to turn up); needs to make funeral arrangements/attend the funeral.

Postoperative time off work Table 13.2 lists expected time off work for uncomplicated procedures. These are not hard and fast rules—alter them to fit individual circumstances (eg someone performing manual labour may need longer).*

Table 13.2 Expected time off work for uncomplicated procedures

Operation	Minimum expected (wks)	Maximum expected if no complications (wks)
Angiography/angioplasty	<1	4
Appendicectomy	1	3
Arthroscopy (knee)	1	4
Cataract surgery	<1	2
Cholecystectomy	2	12
Colposcopy/cystoscopy/laparoscopy	<1	<1
CABG or valve surgery	6	12
ERPC or TOP	<1	<1
Femoral–popliteal grafts	4	12
Haemorrhoidectomy	2	4
Hysterectomy	2	8
Inguinal or femoral hernia	1	6
Laparotomy	6	12
Mastectomy	2	12
Total hip/knee replacement	6	26
Transurethral resection of prostate	2	8

Certifying fitness to work (UK)

Individuals must self-certify for the first 7 calendar days of illness/incapacity, then sickness certification from a doctor is needed until the patient is able to return to work, or a Work Capability Assessment is carried out (see later).

Statutory Sick Pay (SSP) Applies to anyone who is in work (not self-employed), is unwell for 4 full days or more in a row (including non-working days), and earns on average at least £113/week before tax. SSP applies to the first 28 weeks of illness. The GP assesses if the patient is fit to do his/her *own* job.

Work Capability Assessment (WCA) This is carried out by assessors contracted to work for the Department for Work and Pensions (DWP). It is not diagnosis dependent and assesses a variety of different mental/physical health dimensions for ability to work. The WCA establishes if a person is:

- Fit for work.
- Unfit for work but fit for 'work-related activity' (termed the *Work-Related Activity Group* who are expected to meet strict work-related conditions to continue receiving benefits including eg attending activities and interviews).
- Unfit for work or work-related activity (the *Support Group*) eg those with severe disability or illness.

The WCA is undertaken within the first 13 weeks of any claim for Employment Support Allowance (ESA) or Universal Credit (p. 810) and applies to:

- Everyone after 28 weeks of illness/incapacity.
- Those who do not qualify for SSP from the start of their illness/incapacity.

Forms for certifying incapacity to work

SC1 Self-certification form for people not eligible to claim SSP who wish to claim ESA/Universal Credit. It certifies the first 7 days of illness.

SC2 As SC1 but for people who can claim SSP.

Med 3: Statement of Fitness for Work Completed by a GP or hospital doctor who knows the patient. It certifies periods of incapacity likely to be ≥7 days. Most are now computer issued.

During the first 6 months of incapacity a Med 3 can only be issued for a maximum period of 3 months. On the form there are 2 options:

- The patient is unfit for work.
- The patient may be fit for work—this allows the GP to recommend circumstances under which the patient may be able to return to work eg with amended duties or reduced hours.

The form gives space for the GP to record the patient's functional limitations. This is designed to allow the employer to make adjustments to facilitate the employee's return to work.

The statement of Fitness for Work may be issued:

- On the day of assessment (telephone consultations are acceptable).
- On a date after your assessment if you think it would have been reasonable to backdate and issue a Statement from the day of your assessment.
- After consideration of a report about the patient from another doctor or registered healthcare professional.

Only 1 Statement can be issued per patient per period of sickness. If mislaid, reissue and mark 'duplicate'.

Mat B1 Signed by a doctor or midwife. It is provided once to pregnant women within 20 weeks of estimated delivery date and enables her to claim statutory maternity pay and other benefits.[*]

Further reading

Department for Work and Pensions (2013, updated 2015). *Getting the Most Out of the Fit Note: GP Guidance.* https://www.gov.uk/government/publications/fit-note-guidance-for-gps

[*] The material in the sections 'Time off work' & 'Certifying fitness to work (UK)' has been adapted from the *Oxford Handbook of General Practice* 4th edition by Simon *et al*, and has been reproduced by permission of Oxford University Press.

13 General practice

For UK drivers, the DVLA provides detailed condition-specific guidance about fitness to drive, which is regularly updated.[34] It is the responsibility of the driver to inform the DVLA if required. It is the responsibility of doctors to advise patients about medical conditions (and drugs/alcohol) which may affect their ability to drive. The guidance in table 13.3 applies to group 1 (car and motorcycle) drivers:

Table 13.3 Guide to DVLA 'Fitness to Drive'

Cardiovascular	Guidance
Acute coronary syndromes	Don't drive for 4 weeks. If successful angioplasty and no further revascularization planned can drive after 1 week
Angioplasty or pacemaker	Don't drive for 1 week post procedure
Angina	If symptoms at the wheel, at rest, or with emotion, don't drive until symptoms controlled
CABG	Don't drive for at least 4 weeks
Arrhythmias	Must not drive if arrhythmia has/is likely to cause incapacity. Driving may resume after underlying cause identified and arrhythmia controlled for ≥4 weeks
Ablation	If successful can resume driving after 2 days
Hypertension	Continue driving unless malignant hypertension (= ≥180/≥110 + evidence of progressive organ damage)
AAA ≥6.5cm	Must not drive. If 6–6.4cm: inform DVLA; needs annual review
Stroke	Resume driving after 1 month if satisfactory clinical recovery and no neurological/visual/cognitive deficit. May need to inform DVLA
TIA	Single = no driving for 1 month; multiple = 3 months

Diabetes	Guidance
Insulin controlled	Must inform DVLA. If meets medical standard a 1, 2, or 3yr licence is issued. Drivers must have adequate awareness of hypoglycaemia, must not have had >1 episode of hypoglycaemia requiring the assistance of another person in the last 12 months, and must monitor blood glucose levels 'appropriately'. Vision must conform to standard
Tablets causing hypoglycaemia	(eg sulfonylurea); OK to drive if regular review of DM and has not had >1 episode of hypoglycaemia requiring the assistance of another person in the last 12 months. No need to inform DVLA

CNS disorders	Guidance
Epilepsy	Inform DVLA. Licence revoked until 1 year after last seizure (special rules apply if fits only occur in sleep). If withdrawing medication, stop driving during period of withdrawal and for 6 months afterwards
Likely first fit/ isolated seizure	Don't drive for 6 months. If clinical factors/investigations suggest seizure risk ≥20%/yr = 12 months off driving
Loss of consciousness	*Typical vasovagal syncope:* No driving restrictions if solitary episode which occurred while standing
Loss of consciousness	*Likely cardiovascular or unexplained cause:* Inform DVLA and stop driving. If no cause found = 6 months off driving. If cause found and treated = 4wks off driving
Chronic neurological disease	eg Parkinson disease, MS, dementia, MND. Inform DVLA. Licensing depends on clinical condition
Sleep apnoea	Inform DVLA. May restart if symptoms controlled
Traumatic brain injury	Inform DVLA. Usually 6–12 months off driving

13 General practice

	Guidance
Acute psychoses	Inform DVLA. Licence revoked. Restored if well and stable for ≥3 months, regained insight, compliant with treatment, and free from adverse drug effects which would impair driving. Specialist report required
Drug or alcohol misuse or dependency	6months—1yr off driving which must be free of misuse or dependence on alcohol, cannabis, amphetamines, ecstasy, ketamine, other psychoactive substances (eg LSD), opiates (heroin, morphine, & methadone), cocaine, or benzodiazepines. DVLA arranges assessment prior to re-licensing

Fitness to drive

Vision
- *Visual acuity* (± corrected with glasses/contacts) must allow reading a 79mm-high number plate at 20.5 metres (~ at least 6/12 on Snellen chart).
- *Visual fields:* binocular field of vision must be 1200 (extending 500 to left and right). This means homonymous or bitemporal defects are usually not allowed to drive.
- *Monocular vision* is allowed if acuity standards are met and after clinical advice of successful adaptation to the condition.
- *Diplopia* isn't allowed unless controlled by glasses or an *eye-patch*.
- *Diabetic retinopathy:* if visual acuity and visual field standards are met it is ok to drive.

Drug driving
Many drugs affect alertness and driving ability, so warn patients not to drive until they are sure of side effects, not to drive if feeling unwell, and not to drive within 48h of a general anaesthetic.

It is an offence to drive while impaired through drug use—whether non-medical or due to legitimate use.

Prescription medication: Newer legislation covers specified controlled drugs that have a high liability to be abused. These include benzodiazepines, methadone, morphine, and other opiate-based drugs (eg codeine and tramadol). Patients may drive if prescribed these medications so long as it does not cause them to feel impaired. There is a statutory 'medical defence' for patients taking legally obtained medication in accordance with prescription instructions if found to be above specified levels.[35]

Recreational drugs: It is illegal to drive with commonly abused drugs above a specified blood level including cannabis (THC), cocaine, MDMA (Ecstasy), LSD, methylamphetamine, and heroin/diamorphine.

Old age
DVLA says: 'progressive loss of memory, impairment in concentration and reaction time with possible loss of confidence, suggest consideration be given to cease driving.' This is vague, as when reapplying for a licence (every 3yrs after 70) a driver simply signs to say 'no medical disability is present'.

Further reading
Department for Transport (2014). *Drug Driving and Medicine: Advice for Healthcare Professionals.* https://www.gov.uk/government/publications/drug-driving-and-medicine-advice-for-healthcare-professionals

DVLA (2018). Assessing Fitness to Drive – A Guide for Medical Professionals. https://www.gov.uk/government/publications/assessing-fitness-to-drive-a-guide-for-medical-professionals

Each year >1 billion people travel by air. Air travel is increasingly accessible to all and health professionals may be asked to assess a patient's fitness to fly.[36] Most patients are able to fly safely and the following guidelines (from the UK Civil Aviation Authority) address the most common issues that may affect fitness to fly. Most in-flight medical emergencies occur when a passenger's individual medical condition is unknown to the airline and it is therefore essential that the airline is given adequate details in advance. Key information required:
• The nature of the condition and its severity/stability • Medication being taken • Mobility issues. • Patients should carry any medication in their hand luggage.

Physiology of flight The 'cabin altitude' in commercial aircraft should not exceed 8000ft and is typically between 5000–7500ft. This results in a decrease in the partial pressure of alveolar oxygen, but due to the shape of the oxyhaemoglobin dissociation curve, this only results in a fall of arterial oxygen to ~90% and is well tolerated by healthy travellers. Those with medical conditions associated with hypoxia or reduced oxygen carrying capacity (eg anaemia, respiratory/cardiac conditions) may not tolerate the reduction in barometric pressure without support.

Cardiovascular disease The majority of patients with cardiac conditions can travel safely. For contraindications to fly and indications for oxygen see BOXES 'Cardiovascular indications for oxygen' and 'Cardiovascular contraindications'. *Angina:* Can fly if stable. *MI:* May travel after 7–10 days if no complications. *CABG:* (+ Other chest/thoracic surgery.) May travel 10–14 days after surgery. *Angioplasty/stent:* May be fit after 3 days (individual assessment essential). *Symptomatic valvular heart disease:* Relative contraindication (individual assessment required). *Treated hypertension:* OK to fly. *Pacemaker/ICD:* May travel once stable. *CVA:* Advised to wait 10 days (within 3 days if stable).

Diabetes Air travel should not pose significant problems if diabetes is well controlled. *Insulin-treated diabetes:* Patients must carry adequate equipment and all insulin in hand baggage. Temperatures in the hold may degrade insulin (+ there is the potential for lost luggage). Insulin can be satisfactorily carried in a cool bag for long sectors. Individual regimens should be discussed. *General guidelines:* if travelling east (shorter day): fewer units of intermediate or long-acting insulin may be required. If travelling west (and day extended by >2 hours): supplemental short-acting or intermediate-acting insulin may be required. Those controlled with medication should not have a problem.

Haematological *Anaemia:* Hb ≥80g/L may travel without problems, assuming there is no coexisting cardiovascular/respiratory disease. If Hb <75g/L, special assessment is required (flying may be restricted). *Sickle cell anaemia:* Patients may need supplemental O_2 (+ delay travel for ~10 days following a sickling crisis). *Sickle cell trait:* Should not pose a problem. For air travel and DVT see OHCM p579.

Pregnancy Delivery in flight, or flight diversion is undesirable. For this reason, most airlines do not allow travel after 36 weeks for a single pregnancy and 32 weeks for multiple pregnancy. Most airlines require a certificate >28 weeks confirming estimated due date and that the pregnancy is progressing normally. Babies <2 days old should not fly (preferably wait until >7 days).

Respiratory If able to walk 50 metres at a normal pace or climb 1 flight of stairs without severe dyspnoea, it is likely they will tolerate flying. Those with significant disease may require O_2. *Asthma:* Ensure all medication is carried in hand baggage. Consider giving a rescue course of oral steroids. *COPD:* Supplemental O_2 may be required (some airlines charge for this; some allow passengers to carry their own O_2). *Bronchiectasis/cystic fibrosis:* Appropriate antibiotic therapy, adequate hydration, and O_2 may be required. ► *Pneumothorax:* Contraindicated until 2 weeks after successful drainage with full expansion of the lung. *Respiratory infection:* Postpone travel until infection has resolved and exercise tolerance is satisfactory.

Psychiatric illness Air travel should not be a problem for the majority of individuals. Patients should not travel if they have disturbed or unpredictable behaviour that could disrupt the flight.

Ear problems Flying with otitis media or sinusitis may result in pain and perforation of the tympanic membrane. Patients are advised not to fly until symptoms resolve.

Surgery Patients should not travel <10 days after surgery to the chest, abdomen, or middle ear. *Laparoscopy* or *colonoscopy* patients may travel after >24h; *neurosurgery* patients may travel after >7 days.

Fractures Flying should be delayed 24h (if flight <2h) or 48h (for flights >2h) after application of a plaster cast. If needing to fly sooner, the airline will usually require the cast to be split along its full length.

Cardiovascular indications for medical oxygen during commercial airline flight

- Use of oxygen at baseline altitude.
- CHF NYHA class III–IV or baseline P_aO_2 <70mmHg.
- Angina Canadian Cardiovascular Society class III–IV.
- Cyanotic congenital heart disease.
- Primary pulmonary hypertension.
- Other CVD associated with known baseline hypoxaemia.

Cardiovascular contraindications to commercial airline flight

- Uncomplicated MI within 7 days.
- Complicated MI within 4–6 weeks.
- Unstable angina.
- Decompensated congestive heart failure.
- Uncontrolled hypertension.
- CABG within 10 days.
- CVA within 3 days.
- Uncontrolled cardiac arrhythmia.
- Severe symptomatic valvular heart disease.
- Respiratory contraindication = pneumothorax is an absolute contraindication to air travel as trapped air may expand and result in a tension pneumothorax (see p. 645).

Further reading
UK Civil Aviation Authority. *Assessing Fitness to Fly. Guidance for Health Professionals.* www.caa.co.uk

Universal Credit Both unemployed and working people can claim Universal Credit to supplement low income. It is a single monthly payment which replaces previous benefits including • Income Support • Child Tax Credit • Working Tax Credit • Income-based Jobseeker's Allowance • Housing Benefit • Income-related Employment and Support Allowance.

Low-income benefits not replaced by Universal Credit
• *Contributions-based Jobseeker's Allowance:* A non-income assessed benefit paid for ≤26wks to people ≥19yrs and under state pension age who are unemployed or working <16h/wk, capable and available for work, and have paid sufficient National Insurance in 1 of the 2 complete tax years before the start of the year the claim is made.
• *Local authority payments:* Council Tax Benefit, Community Care Grants, and Crisis Loans for general living expenses have been replaced with payments from local authorities.
• *Short-term advances:* Provided by the Department for Work and Pensions if financial hardship because of issues with benefit payments.
• *Automatic health benefits:* People claiming low-income benefits can claim free NHS prescriptions, dentistry, eye tests/glasses, etc.

Who can claim Universal Credit? Adults resident in the UK: • >18yrs and under state pension age • Not in full-time education • Who have accepted a Claimant Commitment (see later). *Capital rules:* People with savings/capital ≥ £16,000 cannot claim. Payments are reduced for those with savings/capital £6000–£16,000.

Amount paid: Payments are a standard allowance plus elements for:
• *Age:* whether >25yrs and single/has a partner.
• *Children:* 1 rate for first child; lower rate for additional children.
• *Childcare costs:* up to 70% of childcare costs (criteria apply).
• *Inability to work:* higher rates for those in the support group.
• *Carer status:* if caring for a severely disabled person for >35h/wk.
• *Housing:* if paying rent or a mortgage.

Benefits cap: Amount of benefit usually cannot exceed £500/wk if a lone parent or part of a couple, or £350/wk if single. Certain benefits are excluded when calculating the cap (eg Cold Weather Payments, free school meals). The cap does not apply in certain circumstances (eg if anyone in the household is claiming Attendance Allowance, Disability Living Allowance, Personal Independence Payments, or either partner is unfit for work after Work Capability Assessment).

Claimant commitment: Claimants may be placed into 1 of 4 groups:
• *No work-related requirements:* no need to seek work if earning over individual threshold (national minimum wage if working 35h/wk); responsible for a child <1yr; over state pension age; carer; pregnant and <11wks prior to EDD; <15wks postnatal; aged 16–21yrs with no parental support and in full-time non-advanced education.
• *Work-focused interview requirement:* regular interviews with job coach to get support with preparing for work in the future (but no obligation to seek work). If responsible for a child aged 1–5yrs or lone/nominated foster carer for a foster child aged <16yrs.
• *Work preparation requirement:* claimants must undertake activities to prepare for work eg attend training, work experience, interviews.
• *All work-related requirements:* apply to everyone else—individuals must seek and be available to work.

Volunteering: People claiming Universal Credit can do voluntary work for a maximum of half the hours they are expected to seek work for.

UK benefits for disability and illness

Employment and Support Allowance

Eligibility
- Age ≥16yrs and under state pension age.
- Not entitled to Statutory Sick Pay (p. 805).
- Unable to work due to sickness or disability—SC1 certification for the 1st 7 days then Med3 certification until work capability assessment (p. 805).
- Sufficient National Insurance contributions.
- Unable to work and claiming ESA for <1yr.

Disability Living Allowance (DLA) (for children <16yrs)

Eligibility NB: DLA is being replaced by Personal Independence Payment (PIP) for disabled people aged 16–64yrs.
- Only available now if <16yrs at time of application.
- Disability >3 months and expected to last >6 months more.
- *Mobility component:* Help needed to get about outdoors. 2 levels + age restrictions apply.
- *Care component:* Help needed with personal care. 3 levels. If terminal illness, highest rate is automatically awarded.

Personal Independence Payment

Eligibility
- Age 16–65yrs.
- Disability requiring assistance present >3 months and expected to last >9 months more. 2 payment components:
- *Daily Living Component:* Paid at the standard or enhanced rate depending on criteria scored (enhanced rate automatically paid if terminal illness).
- *Mobility component:* Paid at standard or enhanced rate.

Attendance Allowance (AA)

Eligibility
- Disability >3 months and expected to last >6 months more.
- ≥65yrs and not permanently in hospital/local authority accommodation.
- Needs attention/supervision.
- Lower and higher rates—higher rate if 24h care required or terminal illness.

Carer's Allowance

Eligibility
- Aged ≥16yrs.
- Spends >35h/wk caring for a person with a disability who is getting AA *or* Constant Attendance Allowance *or* National Insurance contributions PIP *or* middle/higher rate of care component of DLA.
- Earning <£116/wk after tax and allowable expenses.
- Not in full-time education.
- Other benefits (eg state pension) may affect eligibility.

DS1500

Eligibility
- A DS1500 form can be completed for anyone with a terminal illness whose death can 'reasonably be expected within the next 6 months'. The form allows fast-track processing of claims for the benefits listed previously. The patient does not wait the 3-month qualifying period for PIP/DLA etc. and automatically qualifies for the enhanced or highest rate.
- If a person lives longer than 6 months they can continue claiming and will usually be reviewed at 3 years.*

*The material in the section 'UK benefits for disability and illness' has been adapted from the *Oxford Handbook of General Practice* 4th edition by Simon *et al*, and has been reproduced by permission of OUP.

13 General practice

Medical certificate for cause of death The doctor who attended the deceased during the last illness is required to issue a *'medical certificate of cause of death'* (MCCD). The cause of death listed in part Ia should reflect what ultimately led to the patient's death. If this was a sequence of events then part Ib ± Ic should also be completed. Avoid using modes of death and organ failure for Ia (eg cardiac arrest or heart failure). Include any comorbidity in part II that may have contributed to the death but did not lead directly to it.

If the cause of death is not clear or requires clarification, contact the coroner's office[2] and do not issue the MCCD unless instructed to do so (p. 813).

There is no obligation to see/examine a body before issuing the MCCD, however cremation regulations *do* require the body to be examined after death.

Death in the community 1 in 4 deaths occur at home.

Expected deaths: You may need to visit and verify death. Advise the family to contact the undertakers for the deceased to be removed and ensure the patient's own GP is notified. For deaths occurring out of hours (OOH) at home or in residential homes, the OOH GP or district nurse may visit to verify death.

Unexpected and/or 'sudden' death: The death should be reported to the coroner. If any suspicious circumstances, or circumstances of death are unknown/unclear the police should be called.

Cremation Cremation Regulations (2008) require 2 doctors to complete a certificate to establish identity and that the cause of death is not suspicious before a person can be cremated. There are 2 parts:

- *Cremation 4:* completed by the patient's usual medical attendant—usually his/her GP if death occurs in the community.
- *Cremation 5:* completed by another doctor who must have held full GMC registration for 5yrs and is not connected with the patient in any way nor directly connected with the doctor who issued cremation form 4.

▶Pacemakers and radioactive implants must be removed prior to cremation.

Medical Examiner ▶The death certification process is currently under review and due to change in the near future. All deaths will be scrutinized by a Medical Examiner (Medical Reviewer in Scotland)—a qualified doctor who will have access to the patient's notes, discuss the death with relatives, and provide guidance to doctors on completing the MCCD. They will work closely with the coroner and registrar services and feedback statistical information to allow for future healthcare planning.

Stillbirths and neonatal deaths If a baby is born dead after the 24th week of pregnancy a medical certificate of stillbirth is issued. Any pregnancy loss before the 24th week is not registered as a stillbirth. Any infant that has breathed or shown any signs of life, irrespective of gestation, but who dies within the first 28 days of life should be certified using the Neonatal Death Certificate.

2 The role of the Procurator Fiscal in Scotland is broadly similar to that of the coronial service elsewhere in the UK. Although covered by different legislation the same basic roles and rules apply.

Deaths that must be reported to the coroner

Examples of deaths that should be referred to the coroner (NB: this list is not exhaustive and is for guidance; if in doubt check with the coroner's office):

- The cause of death is unknown.
- The deceased was not seen by the certifying doctor either after death or within 14 days before death.
- The death was violent, unnatural, or suspicious.
- The death may be due to an accident (whenever it occurred).
- The death may be due to self-neglect or neglect by others.
- The death may be due to an industrial disease or related to employment.
- All deaths of children/young people under 18, even if due to natural causes.
- The death occurred during an operation or before recovery from the effects of anaesthetic; or the death may be related to an abortion.
- The death may be suicide or might have been contributed to by the actions of the deceased (eg history of drug abuse or overdose).
- If there is an allegation of medical mismanagement or the death may be related to a medical treatment or procedure.
- The death occurred during or shortly after detention in police or prison custody; or while detained under the Mental Health Act.
- Some coroners require notification of all deaths which occurred within 24 hours of admission to hospital.

On discussion with the coroner or coroner's officer, if the cause of death is agreed, you will be instructed to complete the MCCD and must indicate that the coroner has been informed. The coroner may decide that further information is required either through postmortem, an inquiry, or both. In this instance the reporting doctor need not complete the MCCD.

When to consider making a Do Not Attempt CPR (DNACPR) decision

GMC guidance[37] If cardiac or respiratory arrest is an expected part of the dying process and CPR will not be successful, making and recording an advance decision not to attempt CPR will help to ensure that the patient dies in a dignified and peaceful manner. In cases in which CPR might be successful, it might still not be seen as clinically appropriate. When considering whether to attempt CPR, you should consider the benefits, burdens, and risks of treatment if CPR is successful. If such treatment is unlikely to be clinically appropriate, you may conclude that CPR should not be attempted. Some patients with capacity to make their own decisions may wish to refuse CPR; or in the case of patients who lack capacity it may be judged that attempting CPR would not be of overall benefit to them.

General principles[38] •The circumstances of cardiopulmonary arrest must be anticipated • When CPR would fail, it should not be offered as a treatment option • Appropriate and sensitive communication and the provision of information are an essential part of good patient care • Quality of life judgements should not be part of the decision-making process • Where no advance decision about CPR has been made there should be an initial presumption in favour of providing CPR.

Responsibility for making a decision Rests with the senior clinician with clinical responsibility for the patient (eg consultant/GP). DNACPR decisions should be made in consultation with the patient, relatives, and other members of the care team, usually as part of the RESPECT process. Junior doctors without full GMC licence to practise (FY1) should not make this decision.

A DNACPR or RESPECT form Should be completed and used to communicate this information to those involved in the patient's care. It is important that all relevant healthcare and social care professionals are informed of a DNACPR decision.

The WHO definition of health as *'a state of complete physical, mental and social well-being and not merely the absence of disease or infirmity'* was formulated in 1948 and has never been adapted. At the time it was groundbreaking in its breadth and ambition. It overcame the negative definition of health as 'absence of disease' and included physical, mental, and social domains.

The requirement for 'complete' health, however, would leave most of us unhealthy most of the time. Some argue that this contributes to the medicalization of society and lowers thresholds for intervention for conditions that were not previously defined as health problems. Disease patterns have changed: chronic disease previously led to early death, but is now burgeoning worldwide. People live with chronic disease for decades and ageing with chronic disease has become the norm. Are all these people definitively ill?

The WHO definition also minimizes the role of human capacity to cope autonomously with life's ever-changing physical, emotional, and social challenges and to be able to live with fulfilment and a feeling of well-being.

Redefining health is an ambitious and complex goal. There is support for moving towards a dynamic concept of health based on restoring integrity, equilibrium, & well-being through self-management—the ability to 'adapt and to self-manage' in the face of social, physical, and emotional challenges.[39]

Why does health matter? If health is the goal of healthcare, then knowing what health is and how to measure it is important. If the new definition is correct, we must consider how we can build and sustain human capacity to adapt and cope. The French physician, Georges Canguilhem, in his 1943 book, *The Normal and the Pathological*, rejected the idea that there were normal or abnormal states of health. Health is not a fixed entity—it varies for every individual, depending on their circumstances and health is the ability to adapt to one's environment. Health is defined not by the doctor, but by the person, according to his or her functional needs. The role of the doctor is to help the individual adapt to their unique prevailing conditions.

'The beauty of Canguilhem's definition of health—of normality—is that it includes the animate and inanimate environment, as well as the physical, mental, and social dimensions of human life. It puts the individual patient, not the doctor, in a position of self-determining authority to define his or her health needs. The doctor becomes a partner in delivering those needs.'[40]

▶*How do you move a Western post-industrial population from a low level of health to a higher level of health?*

Future determinants of health are thought to rest on:
- Controlling climate change and reducing health inequalities (human health cannot be separated from the 'health' of our planetary biodiversity—we live an interdependent existence with the living and inanimate world).
- Decline in tobacco consumption in all age groups.
- Better health services with more effective, more acceptable treatments.
- Fewer under-doctored areas and more GPs in deprived areas.
- Education capable of influencing behaviour to ↓ exposure to risk factors.
- Better protection of the environment and better housing.
- More patient-centred healthcare, so that patients are not passive recipients of care, but well-educated partners living with disease.

The inverse care law and distributive justice

'Availability of good medical care varies inversely with the need for it in the population served. This operates more completely where medical care is exposed to market forces ... The market distribution of medical care exaggerates maldistribution of medical resources.'

There is much evidence in support of this famous thesis formulated by Tudor Hart.[41] Premature death and long-term limiting illness are both strongly associated with deprivation. It is not just availability of care but access to services that matters: those who need healthcare the least use services more, and more effectively, than those with the greatest need. Distributive justice is the fair distribution of health resources, based on the premise that all are equal in terms of healthcare provision. Ideally, sufficient healthcare would be provided to all, but the health budget doesn't allow for this. So, resources should preferably be distributed in relation to need, within a society that has equal access. In the UK, medical care does exist in deprived areas, but this does not ensure that services are accessed, or that they are of good quality.

Social class and inequalities in health

With the introduction of the British NHS and its ideal of each according to need and equal access, we assumed that differences in the health of different social classes would be abolished. The reverse has happened![42 The Black Report: Inequalities in Health]

Do health inequalities matter as long as overall health is improving? Yes, because justice matters too. It is the lack of justice which led to the NHS—which would have been the best invention of the 20th century, if only it *had* removed inequalities.

Mortality rates are higher in social class V (unskilled manual) vs class I (professional). This is true for stillbirths, perinatal deaths, infant deaths, deaths in men aged 15–64 and women aged 20–59, and for deaths due to lung cancer, heart disease, and stroke. Poor people living in North London live ~17yrs less than rich people in Chelsea.

Within occupations, the effect of social class is seen in a 'purer' way than when groups of many occupations are compared: in a study of >17,000 Whitehall civil servants there was a >3-fold difference in mortality from all causes of death (except genitourinary disease) comparing those in high grades with those in low grades. Similarly in the army, there is a 5-fold difference in mortality from heart disease between highest and lowest ranks.

Illness makes us descend the social scale, but this effect is probably not big enough to account for the observed differences between classes. Cognitive ability can partly explain socioeconomic inequalities in health ('intelligent people look after themselves'—has some truth). However, it is more likely that differences are due to *smoking, education, diet, poverty, stress*, and *overcrowding*.

Social, psychological, and physical factors These are inter-related components which interact and play a significant role in the context of health, disease, and illness. Health is not purely a biological process but a combination of biological, psychological, and social factors.

The traditional biomedical model Assumes that all illness can be traced back to a single disorder of a *part* of the body and that all symptoms are due to disease within the body.

Problems with the biomedical model:
- Symptoms are common—something we all experience on a daily basis and most of the time recognize as being within the limits of normal experience.
- All disease does not cause symptoms—much disease or pathology is asymptomatic (hence the need for screening programmes).
- Another problem is that patients are seen as 'passive victims' of disease, yet some diseases are closely related to behaviour (eg smoking; obesity), and so a proportion of diseases are caused in part by the patient. Similarly, patients are not 'passive recipients' of treatment. For treatment to succeed, the patient needs to be an 'active partner' eg at its most extreme, medication will not work if it is not taken.
- The biomedical model also assumes people have 2 parts to their existence—the 'physical' and 'mental'—and that these aspects are separate and unrelated (this is reflected in the separation between 'physical' and 'mental' health services).
- The biomedical model cannot explain functional (non-organic) illness, which affects up to 20% of our patients. This group of disorders includes medically unexplained symptoms (p. 803), fibromyalgia, irritable bowel syndrome, and chronic fatigue syndrome.

▶*Does illness arise from a disease which affects only a part of the whole body, or from a problem at the level of the whole person within their situation?* In relation to illness, the reductionist biomedical model assumes there must always be a disorder of a part of the whole, and does not consider that the whole person may be ill without any specific part of the person being abnormal.

The biopsychosocial model This model first recognized the complex nature of illness, specifically the importance of biological, psychological, and social factors that contribute to illness—acknowledging the importance of factors other than disease.

A holistic approach This approach to illness acknowledges objective scientific explanations of physiology, but also admits that people have inner experiences that are subjective, mystical (and, for some, religious), which may affect their health and health beliefs. It can help in understanding the problems faced by patients and emphasizes that in most illnesses there are many factors that may contribute to a person's experience. It predicts that in some people illness may arise without any disorder within the person (functional illnesses).

▶The key for us is to try and understand our patients as a biopsychosocial 'whole', and develop skills to transform holistic understanding into practical measures. We must show tolerance and understanding of our patients' experiences, beliefs, values, and expectations. Empower your patient to value themselves by listening to their concerns, consider their mind–body connection, and take account of their emotional state. The whole-person approach strives to create health as well as treat illness.

Further reading
Wade DT (2009). *Holistic Health Care: What is it, and how can we achieve it?* http://www.ouh.nhs.uk/oce/research-education/documents/HolisticHealthCare on 11-15.pdf

The role of the GP as patient advocate

In order to act as advocates for our patients, an RCGP report 'The 2022 GP: A Vision for General Practice in the Future NHS'[43] states that a GP will:

- Act as 'gatekeeper' and 'navigator' to specialist services. This ensures effective resource utilization (eg referring appropriately, and referring to the most appropriate specialty), and coordination of care between different specialties or services.
- Retain his ability to be an independent advocate for patients and to meet professional obligations as a doctor first, irrespective of contractual arrangements or commissioning responsibilities eg pressure not to refer x or prescribe y.

And herein lies the complexity and value of general practice: GPs must balance being gatekeeper and steward (of finite resources), while being able to advocate freely for patients and enable them to access services they need.

What does it mean to be a patient's advocate and navigator? GPs must support and represent a patient's best interests to ensure they receive the best and most appropriate health and social care. It means helping patients make choices concerning their own care, and coordinating this across an increasingly complicated health and social care system. In order to do this, GPs need to know the make-up of their practice population and understand the context of their patients and families. This includes socioeconomic factors, ethnic and religious groupings, types of housing, and unemployment rates.

Social prescribing

Social prescribing enables GPs, nurses, and other health professionals to refer patients to a range of local, non-clinical services. It seeks to address people's needs in a holistic way, recognizing that health is determined by a range of social, economic, and environmental factors. It aims to support people in taking greater control of their own health.

Social prescribing schemes typically involve a variety of activities which are often provided by voluntary or community sector organizations eg voluntary befriending schemes, arts activities, group learning, cookery, or gardening. Those who benefit include people with mild or long-term mental health problems, vulnerable groups, those who are socially isolated, or who frequently attend primary care.

Evidence suggests social prescribing can lead to a range of positive health and well-being outcomes with improvements in quality of life and emotional well-being, and decreased anxiety. It may also lead to a reduction in the use of NHS services and highlights the role of the voluntary sector to help reduce pressure on NHS services. Social prescribing also contributes to broader government objectives in relation to volunteering, learning, and employment.[44]

Primary prevention (preventing occurrence) This means taking action to reduce the incidence of disease or health problems either through universal measures that reduce lifestyle risks and their causes, or by targeting high-risk groups. Examples include vaccination, pre-conception folic acid, or screening for hypertension.

Why is it important? Primary prevention aims to reduce the overall burden of disease and improve health outcomes (and reduce the cost of treating disease). Prevention in childhood provides the greatest benefits, but it is valuable at any point in life. 80% of cases of heart disease, stroke, and T2DM and 40% of cancers could be avoided if common lifestyle risk factors were eliminated. Lifestyle risk factors are known to cluster in the population, which has a dramatic effect on life expectancy. Addressing this clustering (and its socioeconomic determinants) is likely to reduce inequalities and improve overall population health.

Examples of current UK prevention programmes for health
• Health checks for those aged 40–74yrs (which aim to prevent cardiovascular disease and diabetes).
• Cancer screening: >90% of cervical cancer screening is done within primary care.
• Chlamydia screening for those aged 16–24yrs.
• Antenatal screening and care.
• Healthy child programme.
• Newborn bloodspot screening.
• Newborn hearing screening.
• Diabetic retinopathy screening.
• Renal, hypertension, and cholesterol monitoring for those with diabetes.
• Abdominal aortic aneurysm screening.
• PSA informed choice programme.
• Alcohol screening.
• Smoking screening/cessation.
• HIV screening for new patients.
• Dementia screening.

How to do it Supporting individuals to change behaviour eg through brief advice during a consultation (*Have you ever thought about giving up smoking? What do you think is stopping you?*—see 'Motivational interviewing' p.783); or through systematic community interventions or national 'stop smoking' initiatives.

Secondary prevention (screening for 1st stages) Secondary prevention is systematically detecting the early stages of disease and intervening before symptoms develop—eg cervical cytology to screen for cervical cancer, mammograms to detect breast cancer, or treating hypertension/prescribing statins to those with cardiovascular disease. Successful secondary prevention improves life expectancy and reduces complications of disease.

Why is it important? Secondary prevention interventions are highly cost-effective. In areas where the 'inverse care law' applies (p. 815), those in greatest need are likely to receive benefit. Identifying those at risk and intervening is one of the most effective ways in which GPs can reduce the widening gaps in life expectancy and health outcomes. However, there is substantial variation between practices in the implementation of secondary prevention—only a minority of patients receive all recommended interventions.

How to do it; Secondary prevention largely involves the systematic application of standard interventions and includes use of disease registers, systematic screening, and control of eg hypertension and diabetes.

Tertiary prevention (preventing complications) Aims to reduce the impact of the disease by identifying and treating disease-related complications eg retinal photography in diabetes. Where the condition is not reversible, tertiary prevention promotes quality of life through active rehabilitation.

Further reading

The King's Fund (2015). *Transforming our Health Care System: Ten Priorities for Commissioners.* http://www.kingsfund.org.uk/sites/files/kf/field/field_publication_file/10PrioritiesFinal2.pdf

Barriers to prevention

Genetic barriers Not everyone responds to preventive measures. Some of us, because of our genes, are 'immune' to the benefits of exercise, for example. As genetic advances occur, our habitual blanket advice of 'take more exercise' looks increasingly old fashioned. What we should really do is get to know our patients psychologically and genetically, and tailor advice such as 'for you, diet advice is more important than exercise'.

Cognitive barriers When, if ever, we contemplate cataclysmic but preventable ill health in ourselves, we may either believe that '*It won't happen to me*' or we deliberately dare fate to *make* it happen to us. Some people are proud to announce that '... I eat everything, as much butter and fried foods as I can ... I smoke 40–60 cigarettes a day ... To eat cornflakes, you've got to have sugar on them, otherwise there is no point in eating them ... As long as you keep smoking cigarettes, and drink plenty of whisky, you'll go on for ever'.

Psychological barriers All of us at times are prone to promote our own destruction as keenly as we promote our own survival. Knowing that alcohol may bring about our own destruction gives the substance a certain appeal, when we are in certain frames of mind—particularly if we do not know the sordid details of what death by alcohol entails. It provides an alluring means of escape without entailing too headlong a rush into the seductive arms of death. Gambling and taking risks are all part of this ethos.

Logistic barriers A general practice needs to be highly organized to be in a state of perpetual readiness to answer questions like 'Who has not had their BP checked?' or 'Who has not turned up to their request to attend for screening?' or 'Who has stopped sending in for their repeat prescriptions for antihypertensives?' Screen pop-ups enable the GP to consider opportunistic preventative activities. The price of this is that patient-centred activities are crowded out, and that, with many preventive activities offered, no guidance on prioritizing individual intervention is forthcoming.

Another example of logistical barriers is providing a sequence of working fridges in the distribution of vaccines to rural developing areas.

Political barriers It is not unknown for governments to back out of preventive obligations as if influenced by groups who would lose if prevention were successful. Some countries are keener to buy tanks than vaccines.

Ethical barriers If child benefits were available only to those children who had their MMR vaccine, more mumps would be prevented (an unpopular approach!).

Financial barriers The NHS has limited financial resources and cost must be considered for any new activity (eg the introduction of a new vaccine in which children born before a certain date are not eligible).

Motivation barriers Changing from a crisis-led work pattern to strategic prevention is one way that GP practices can lead the way. Chronic disease clinics and IT templates ensure that the meticulous tasks on which all good prevention depends can be systematically followed by healthcare workers (eg by ensuring all areas in a diabetes annual review are covered).

13 General practice

Screening entails systematic testing of a population or a subgroup for signs of illness—which may be of established disease (pre-symptomatic eg breast cancers) or symptomatic (eg unreported hearing loss in the elderly).

Wilson and Junger were the first to define criteria (in 1968) to guide the selection of conditions that would be suitable for screening. These help ensure a screening programme is viable, effective, and appropriate:[3]

Modified Wilson criteria for screening (1–10 spells IATROGENIC)

1 The condition screened for should be an Important one.
2 There should be an Acceptable treatment for the disease.
3 Diagnostic and Treatment facilities should be available.
4 A Recognizable latent or early symptomatic stage is required.
5 Opinions on who to treat as patients must be agreed.
6 The test must be of *high discriminatory power* (below), *valid* (measuring what it purports to measure, not surrogate markers which might not correlate with reality), and be *reproducible*—with safety Guaranteed (see BOX 'Problems with screening').
7 The Examination must be acceptable to the patient.
8 The untreated Natural history of the disease must be known.
9 A simple Inexpensive test should be all that is required.
10 Screening must be Continuous (ie not a 'one-off' affair).

Informed consent: Rees' rule Before offering screening, we have a duty to quantify for patients the chance of being disadvantaged by it as well as the chances of benefit eg anxiety while waiting for a false-positive result to be sorted out may be devastating; or there may be complications of subsequent tests (eg bleeding after biopsy after an abnormal cervical smear).[4] We are all guilty of exaggerating benefits and avoiding discussion of controversial areas with patients. All tests have false-positive and false-negative rates, as summarized in table 13.4.

Table 13.4   Performance of screening tests

		Patients with condition	Patients without condition
TEST RESULT	Subjects appear to have the condition	True +ve (A)	False +ve (B)
	Subjects appear not to have the condition	False –ve (C)	True –ve (D)

Sensitivity: How reliably is the test +ve in the disease? A/A+C.
Specificity: How reliably is the test –ve in health? D/D+B.

Partly effective screening:
Cervical smears (if >25yrs, p. 164-5)
Mammography (after menopause)
Finding smokers (+quitting advice)
Faecal occult bloods (colorectal ca)
Abdominal aortic aneurysm
Chlamydia screening for <25s.

Unproven/ineffective screening:
Mental test score (dementia, p. 735)
Urine dip (diabetes; kidney disease)
Antenatal procedures (pp. 16-7)
PSA screening for prostate ca (detects too many harmless cancers?) ●✱
Elderly visiting to detect disease.[5]

Why screen in primary care? If screening is to be done at all, it makes economic sense to do it in primary care. In the UK, ≥1 million people see GPs each weekday, providing great facilities for opportunistic 'case-finding' (90% of patients consult over a 5yr period). Private clinics do limited work, but there is no evidence that their multiphasic biochemical analyses are effective procedures, and NHS resources are wasted chasing false-positive results.

3 ►For an excellent critique of the Wilson criteria, see Gray J (2004) *Br J Gen Pract* 501:292–8.
4 There is evidence that some screening causes morbidity (mortality awareness and hypochondriasis ↑)—so why is screening promoted? Because it is easier for governments to be optimistic than to be rigorous?
5 In one study (n=43,000 patients >75yrs old) neither in-depth assessment nor a targeted approach focused on those with ≥3 problems offered gains in survival or quality of life.[45]

Problems with screening

Take a healthy person, screen them, turn them into a patient, and then kill them. From a report on cervical screening: 'By offering screening to 250,000 we have helped a few, harmed thousands, disappointed many, used £1.5m each year, and kept a few lawyers in work.' Typical problems are:

- Those most at risk do not present for screening, thus increasing the gap between the healthy and the unhealthy—the *inverse care law* (p. 815).
- The 'worried well' overload services by seeking repeat screening.
- Services for investigating those testing positive are inadequate.
- Those who are false positives suffer stress while awaiting investigation, and remain anxious about their health despite reassurance.
- A negative result may be regarded as a licence to take risks and signs of interval disease (arising between screenings) may be ignored by patients who assume they are in the all clear.
- True positives, though treated, may begin to see themselves as of lower worth than hitherto.

▶Remember: with some screening programmes of dubious value, *it may be healthier not to know.*

Health education presumes that people are rational and want to promote their own survival. It begs the question: what should we live for? Unless an individual has an optimistic answer, health education will fail. For 60% of UK people, death is an attractive option compared with doing more exercise.[46] Alcohol and drugs—anything that achieves oblivion as soon as possible—is an ever more popular approach to life, despite years of health education. So society needs to ask itself 2 questions:

1 *Are we making it easy for people to make wise health choices?*
—and, more importantly,
2 *Are we making it easy for people to find something worth living for?*

In city after city, country after country, the answer is *No* and *No*. Britain is the worst place to live in the developed world, based on UNICEF measures of childhood well-being,[47] so there is a long way to go before we get to the starting line where most people are amenable to health education.

Health education messages These must be *specific* and *direct* eg in getting people to accept help for alcohol misuse, it is of little use saying:
• 'If you don't stop drinking you'll get these diseases ...' (~25% may respond).
• Saying 'Accepting help is good for you because of these benefits ...' (~50% will respond).
• 'If you don't accept help, you've had it' brings the biggest response.

Optimum messages must be specific about dates, times, and places of help. Well-chosen images and a degree of 'fear' in the message helps: in enlisting patients for tetanus vaccine a 'low-fear' message gets a 30% response, while more fear can double this. Graphic images depicting the effects of smoking are mandatory on UK cigarette packets (evidence is rather flimsy) and it is possible that too high a level of fear is counter-productive. A gruesome film about the worst effects of dental caries produces petrified immobility, not self-help or trips to dentists. A better approach is *professional teaching*. Compared with parents, teacher-based oral health education has a better effect on oral health.[48]

Changing attitudes The following paradigm holds sway: *knowledge → attitudes → intentions → behaviour*. As Chinese thought reformers knew so well, attitude changes depend on a high level of emotional involvement. In questions of belief, as in so many other questions, emotion trumps reason: *'people don't demand that a thing be reasonable if their emotions are touched. Lovers aren't reasonable, are they?* Graham Greene p115 The End of the Affair Only resort to applying reason to attitudes if emotions are too hot to handle. NB: the arrows in the earlier model may be reversed—if our behaviour is inconsistent with our ideas (cognitive dissonance), it is often our ideas, not our behaviour which change.

Objective feedback Giving standard written advice about physical activity helps promote exercise. But to make big strides, it helps to give quantifiable feedback—ie a pedometer. This sort of feedback also improves quality of life.

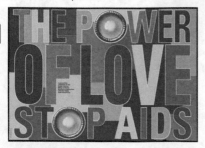

Fig 13.9 HIV/AIDS posters promoting safer sex through the use of condoms advanced beyond the simple messages of who is at risk and how HIV is transmitted by explaining how to prevent infection.
Wellcome Collection.

Health education: who should do it?

Traditional approaches Leaflets and multimedia programmes can increase knowledge and change behaviour eg using graphic artists to provide emotionally charged, slick messages. See fig 13.10.

Peer-to-peer methods Leaflets are authoritative, but this authority is itself a problem. Risk-takers are unlikely to listen to the prim and proper. So peer education has been developed as a tool to reach certain groups, and evidence suggests that this is promising. Peers may be better than authority figures

Online education and training Online education and training for patients in the form of 'self-help' is increasing in provision and popularity. These include online cognitive behavioural therapy websites such as *MoodGym*, which provides free information and skills training to help cope with depression, and *Living Life to the Full*, a life skills course for people feeling distressed. Other examples include self-help modules for the management of symptoms of irritable bowel syndrome.

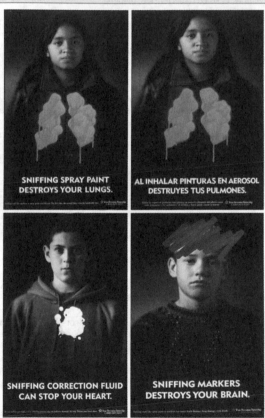

Fig 13.10 These bilingual posters, produced by the Texas Prevention Partnership, contributed to a campaign against inhalant misuse. Use of inhalants fell by more than 32% in elementary schools and by ~20% in high schools.[40]

With permission from SYNERGIES, dba National Inhalant Prevention Coalition, www.inhalants.org.

Cardiovascular disease (CVD) is a significant cause of mortality and morbidity and accounts for ~⅓ of all UK deaths. However, deaths from CVD have fallen in the UK since the late 1970s—due to better intervention and treatment, and greater preventative measures.

Goals of CVD risk assessment and management

- To reduce the risk of developing cardiovascular disease, which includes coronary heart disease (angina and MI), stroke and TIA, and peripheral arterial disease (ie all diseases caused by atherosclerosis).
- To improve quality of life and life expectancy.

Risk factors for developing CVD

Non-modifiable: ↑ age; ♂>♀; family history; ethnicity (eg South Asian > European). *Modifiable:* Smoking; low HDL-cholesterol/high non-HDL-c; sedentary lifestyle; unhealthy diet; excess alcohol; obesity.

Comorbidities (↑ risk): Hypertension; diabetes; CKD; dyslipidaemia; AF; RA/SLE; severe mental health problems.

Other factors: CVD risk is strongly associated with low income and social deprivation.

▶Targeting and modifying risk factors and optimizing treatment of comorbidities reduce the risk of developing CVD.

Strategies for preventing CVD

Primary prevention: eg NHS *Health Check Programme*—those aged 40–74 without CVD are invited every 5 years for a free health check, including CVD risk assessment (although evidence suggests general health checks do not have an effect on overall total mortality or mortality due to CVD).[50]

Secondary prevention: People who already have CVD can benefit from risk factor modification and cardiac rehabilitation (if appropriate).

Assessing risk

CVD risk assessment tools assess the risk of developing cardiovascular disease eg QRISK®3. This computer-based program uses details of age, sex, ethnicity, postcode, smoking status, selected medical and family history, blood pressure, BMI, and cholesterol/HDL ratio to determine a percentage risk of developing a heart attack or stroke over the next 10 years. NB: the calculator is not valid in those with a diagnosis of coronary heart disease (including angina or MI) or stroke/TIA, or if >85yrs.

The QRISK®3 score is expressed as a percentage (eg 14% risk of developing CVD within the next 10 years). Remember the risk score is an estimate. Everyone is at risk—low risk does not mean no risk.

Management of risk

CVD risk <10%: Although risk is low, advice can be given on reducing risk within relevant lifestyle factors or optimizing relevant comorbidities.

CVD risk >10%: As well as advising on lifestyle factors and optimizing treatment of relevant comorbidities, NICE recommend offering lipid-modifying therapy (eg **atorvastatin** 20mg OD; if no CI) to reduce risk. This can be delayed if lifestyle interventions are likely to reduce risk to <10%. Discuss the benefits and risks of starting a statin.

Lifestyle advice: Stop smoking; weight loss if overweight; eat a healthy diet; keep alcohol within recommended limits; encourage physical activity.

Further reading

NICE (2014). *Clinical Knowledge Summaries: CVD Risk Assessment and Management* (revised 2019). http://cks.nice.org.uk/lipid-modification-cvd-prevention

NICE (2014). *Lipid Modification: Cardiovascular Risk Assessment and the Modification of Blood Lipids for the Primary and Secondary Prevention of Cardiovascular Disease* (cg181) (updated 2016). London: NICE.

In the UK, smoking prevalence has fallen by 10% since 2000 when 26.8% of adults smoked (compared with current levels of 15.5%). The smoking in public places ban in 2007 is estimated to have helped ≥400,000 people quit.ⁿⁱᶜᵉ

Epidemiologists say that ~50% of smokers will die of smoking if they don't quit, losing ~25 years. Stopping smoking diminishes excess risk from tobacco, so that after 10–15yrs the risk of lung cancer approaches that of lifelong non-smokers. A similar but quicker decrease of excess risk (halved in 1st year) is found for deaths from coronary disease and, to a lesser extent, risk of stroke.[52]

▶60% *of smokers want to give up*, and help with this achieves better outcomes.

Advantages of stopping smoking
- Less cancer—smoking accounts for ~29% of all cancer deaths.
- Less chronic lung disease (COPD, recurrent chest infection, asthma exacerbation).
- Less cardiovascular disease (CHD, CVA, and peripheral arterial disease).
- Fewer problems in pregnancy—less pre-eclampsia, IUGR, preterm delivery, neonatal and late fetal death.
- Less risk from passive smoking (cot deaths, lung disease, lung cancers).
- Return of the sense of taste and smell—and relative wealth.

To quit
1 Ask about smoking in all consultations (not just where relevant; be subtle; patients won't listen if agendas clash). Greet *any* success with enthusiasm!
2 Advise according to need. Ensure that advice is congruent with beliefs.
3 Motivate patients by getting *them* to list the advantages of quitting.
4 Assist in practical ways eg negotiate a commitment to a 'quit date' when there will be few stresses; agree on jettisoning all smoking junk (cigarettes, ash trays, lighters, matches) in advance. Inform friends of new change.
5 Arrange follow-up. Texting patients (get consent) to send messages of encouragement (can ↑ quitting from 13% to 28%).[53]

Pharmaceutical aids to smoking cessation (BNF 4.10)

Nicotine replacement therapy (NRT): Increases the chance of quitting by ×1.5. All preparations are equally effective. Start with higher doses for heavy smokers. Continue treatment for 3 months and tail off gradually over 2 weeks before stopping (except gum which can be stopped abruptly). *Contraindications:* immediately post-MI, stroke, or TIA; and if arrhythmia.

Nicotine withdrawal symptoms
• Urges to smoke (70%)
• ↑ appetite (70%) mean 3–4kg weight ↑
• Depression (60%)
• Restlessness (60%)
• Poor concentration (60%)
• Irritability/aggression (50%)
• Night-time awakening (25%)
• Light headedness (10%)

Varenicline (eg Champix®): Smokers (>18yrs) start taking the tablets 1wk before the intended quit day (0.5mg OD for 3 days; then 0.5mg BD for 4 days; then 1mg BD for 11wks; 1mg OD if renal impairment/elderly). Cessation rate increased ×2. If the patient has stopped smoking after 12wks consider a further 12wk course to ↓ risk of relapse. *Caution* in psychiatric disease. Advise to stop if agitated, depressed, or suicidal.

Bupropion (eg Zyban®): Smokers (>18yrs old) start taking the tablets 1–2wks before an intended quit date (150mg for 6 days then 150mg BD for 7–9wks). Cessation rate increased ×2. *Contraindications:* epilepsy, or ↑ risk of seizures, eating disorders, bipolar disorder.

▶ Prescribe *only* for smokers who commit to a target stop date. Initially prescribe enough to last 2wks after stop date. Only offer a further prescription if the patient demonstrates a continuing commitment to stop smoking. If unsuccessful the NHS will not fund another attempt for ≥6 months.

The problem isn't alcohol, it's life—lives in which sobriety poses insuperable problems: consciousness of futility, debt, responsibility, and social inhibitions. Alcohol obliterates all these. UK alcohol-specific deaths = >7000/yr.[14]

With the toll that excess alcohol takes in terms of personal misery and cost to the NHS (>£3.5 billion/yr[UK]), the need to reduce alcohol use and its root causes should be almost top of the government's social policy goals. But a powerful industry ensures that alcohol is cheaper (relatively) and more readily available than ever before—so that its use on an individually moderate scale arouses little comment. It is assumed to be safe, provided one is not actually an alcoholic. ▶Alcohol risks and benefits should be viewed as a spectrum.

Prevalence of excess alcohol and recommended limits

- To help keep health risks associated with alcohol to a low level, the recommended 'low-risk' guidelines are for men and women to drink ≤14 units/week. 14u = ×6 175mL glasses of 13% wine; ×6 pints of 4% beer or ×14 25mL shots of 40% spirit. 7% regularly drink over this amount.
- Alcohol and pregnancy (see p. 7).
- *Binge* drinking = >6u for ♂ or ♀ in 1 episode (affects 21% ♂; 9% ♀).
- *Hazardous/harmful/problem* drinking is excess intake causing potential or actual harm, but without dependence (affects 32% ♂; 15% ♀).
- Alcohol *abuse* implies that repeated drinking harms a person's work or social life.
- *Addiction/dependency* implies (see also BOX 'Dependence syndrome' p. 829):
  - *Increased tolerance* to alcohol.
  - Narrow drinking repertoire.
  - Failure of abstinence.
  - *Withdrawal*—sweats, nausea, or tremor.
  - Priority to maintain alcohol intake.
  - Often aware of compulsion to drink.

Assessment History usually shows a gradual deterioration in function, as alcohol dependence overtakes work, relationships, financial stability, and health as the patient's primary concern. An early warning sign is that the patient's drinking habits are excessive within their own social context.

Screening questions A simple short tool to highlight at-risk drinking is the CAGE questionnaire (see BOX 'Alcohol screening tool'). It does not assess dependence or abuse.

Withdrawal signs (Delirium tremens.) Pulse ↑; BP↓; tremor; fits; visual or tactile hallucinations eg of insects crawling under the skin (formication).

Management Does the patient want to change? If so, be optimistic. Should *abstinence* or *controlled intake* be the aim? If the former, remarkable recovery of organs is possible.

Refer for specialist management ± self-help/group therapy (eg Alcoholics Anonymous). Specialists may prescribe: **Disulfiram** 200mg/24h PO, which causes vomiting if alcohol is taken; **Naltrexone** 25–50mg/24h PO (an opioid receptor antagonist) which reduces the pleasure that alcohol brings (and craving on withdrawal) and can halve relapse rates. CI: hepatitis; liver failure; monitor LFT; or **Acamprosate** which can improve abstinence rates. CI: pregnancy; severe liver failure; creatinine >120μmol/L; dose example: 666mg/8h PO if >60kg and <65yrs old.

Alcohol & organ damage *Liver:* (Normal in 50% of alcoholics.) *Fatty liver:* acute, reversible; hepatitis; 80% progress to cirrhosis (*liver failure* in 10%). *Cirrhosis:* 5yr survival 48% if alcohol intake continues (if it stops, 77%). *CNS:* Poor memory/cognition; cortical/cerebellar atrophy; retrobulbar neuropathy; fits; falls; accidents; neuropathy; Korsakoff's/Wernicke's encephalopathy (*OHCM* p714); ▶▶Urgent parenteral vitamins are needed.

Further reading
NICE (2011). *Alcohol Use Disorders: Diagnosis, Assessment and Management of Harmful Drinking and Alcohol Dependence* (CG115). London: NICE.

NICE (2010). *Alcohol Use Disorders: Preventing the Development of Hazardous and Harmful Drinking* (PH24). London: NICE.

Gastrointestinal: D&V; peptic ulcer; erosions; varices ± bleeding; pancreatitis.
Heart: Arrhythmias; BP↑; cardiomyopathy.
Skeleton: Heavy drinking disrupts calcium metabolism (osteoporosis risk ↑).
Sperm: Fertility ↓; sperm motility ↓.
Malignancy: GI & breast.
Marrow: Hb↓; MCV↑.
Social: Alcohol is related to violent crime and suicide.

Alcohol and drug levels Regular heavy drinking *induces* hepatic enzymes; binging *inhibits* enzymes. Be alert with phenytoin, warfarin, tolbutamide, etc.

Homelessness: Common; help with housing & rent, problem-solving, communication, drink refusal, and goal setting *can* help this desperate problem.

Alcohol screening tool

CAGE questionnaire

1 Have you ever felt you should **C**ut down on your drinking?
2 Have people **A**nnoyed you by criticizing your drinking?
3 Have you ever felt bad or **G**uilty about your drinking?
4 Have you ever had a drink first thing in the morning to steady your nerves or to get rid of a hangover (**E**ye opener)?

A total score of *2 or greater* is considered clinically significant (sensitivity of 93% and a specificity of 76% for the identification of problem drinking). However, CAGE is less sensitive for identifying those not alcohol-dependent but still 'at-risk' drinkers. A patient's demographics have been found to limit its performance. Some studies show a sensitivity as low as 50% in adult white women and just 40% in at-risk groups aged 60+.

Helping people to cut down alcohol intake

▶Time interventions for when motivation is maximal eg before pregnancy.
• Take more non-alcoholic drinks; reduce the sip frequency of alcoholic drinks.
• Don't drink alone or with habitual drinkers; sip, don't gulp.
• Don't buy yourself a drink when it is your turn to buy a round of drinks.
• Go out to the pub later (but some pubs now open all night).
• Take 'days of rest' when no alcohol is used.

Agree goals to maintaining ↓ drinking

• An alcohol diary helps get facts right.
• Teach how to estimate alcohol intake (u/week).
• Give feedback—eg if GGT (γ-glutamyl transpeptidase) falls are discussed, there is much lower mortality, morbidity, and hospitalization.
• Enlist family support; suggest a system of 'rewards' for sobriety.
• Community alcohol teams/treatment units may be required if dependency.

▶*Primary care is a good setting for prevention*: intervention leads to less alcohol consumption by ~15%, reducing the proportion of heavy drinkers by 20%—at one-twentieth the cost of specialist services. There is no evidence that GP intervention has to include more time-consuming advice such as compressed cognitive/behavioural strategies. Simple advice works fine as judged by falling GGT levels.[55]

'I hurt myself today. To see if I still feel. I focus on the pain. The only thing that's real. The needle tears a hole. The old familiar sting. Try to kill it all away. But I remember everything.' 'Hurt', Johnny Cash (originally by Nine Inch Nails)

Assessment of drug misuse The most frequently abused drugs are cannabis, amphetamine, ecstasy, and cocaine. 14% of ♂ and 8% of ♀ aged 16–59 report taking illicit drugs in the last year. 3 factors appear important: availability, vulnerable personality, and social pressures—particularly from peers.

Suspect drug addiction if: • Arrests for theft (to buy drugs) • Odd transient behaviour eg visual hallucinations, elation, mania • Unexplained nasal discharge (cocaine sniffing or opiate withdrawal) • Withdrawal symptoms (eg red eyes, shaking) • Injection stigmata: marked veins; abscesses; hepatitis; HIV • Repeated requests for analgesics—only opiates acceptable ± no clear medical indication; prescription requests which are too frequent.

Clinical presentation *Acute intoxication:* Administration of a psychoactive substance resulting in disturbances of level of consciousness, cognition, perception, affect, or behaviour. *Harmful use:* A pattern of psychoactive substance use that is causing actual damage to mental or physical health or social functioning. *Dependence syndrome* (see BOX 'Dependence syndrome') is a cluster of physiological, behavioural, and cognitive phenomena where the use of a substance takes on a much higher priority than other behaviours which once had greater value. There is evidence that returning to a substance after abstinence leads to a more rapid dependence than occurs with non-dependent individuals.

Take a history of drug use/behaviour: Reason for consulting now; willingness to change; current and past usage; knowledge of risks; unsafe sex?

Take a medical and psychiatric history: Complications of drug abuse; alcohol use; overdose (accidental/deliberate). Consider urine toxicology to confirm drug misuse.

Management of drug misuse Aims to reduce drug-related morbidity and mortality; decrease risk of infectious diseases, and decrease criminal activity used to finance drug habits. The GP and primary care team have a vital role in:
• Identifying drug misusers.
• Assessing health/willingness to modify drug behaviour (see stages of change model in BOX 'Self-care and empowered self-care' p. 783).

Education • Advise on safer routes of administration (eg smoking); discourage IM/SC administration.
• Specific risks of drugs (eg psychosis with amphetamines).
• Safe injecting, overdose prevention (naloxone auto-injector), and basic first-aid training.
• Safe sexual practices/condom use.
• Discuss driving and drug misuse (see p. 807).
• Test for blood-borne diseases + offer hepatitis B immunization.

Treatment of dependence
• The aims of treatment are best met by specialist services and substitute maintenance prescribing eg with methadone for heroin abuse.
• Set conditions for acceptable behaviour and treatment withdrawal. Agree on the pharmacy to be used and involve the pharmacist.
• Review regularly.
• Report patients who start treatment for drug abuse to the national drug treatment monitoring system.

13 General practice

Opiate detoxification and methadone maintenance Carried out ideally as part of a regimen in which a contract is made with the patient eg in a specialist clinic or in primary care, provided GP has a special interest.

Methadone prescribing should be used as part of the transition to abstinence. Physiologically, methadone use is still opiate addiction—the difference being it is free (eliminating a need for crime to fund the next fix) and taken orally (no injection-related issues). In reality, many patients cannot commit to abstinence so methadone maintenance is used as an alternative which is safer to both addict and society. *Daily observed methadone dosing:* This is the norm (NB: monthly supplies are not necessarily abused). Cocaine use by patients on methadone is a big problem, and is associated with a poorer prognosis. **Buprenorphine** is a synthetic partial opioid agonist and is an alternative to methadone. **Naltrexone** is an opioid antagonist which blocks the euphoric effect of opiates and is used in former addicts to prevent relapse.

Psychological support: Tailor to specific needs (residential or out-patient care, in groups or 1-to-1). Counselling, motivational therapy, cognitive therapy (p. 754), Alcoholics Anonymous, '12 steps programme', and family therapy (p. 760) are all valuable ways to address triggers, motivation to change, and relapse prevention. Counsel about HIV & hepatitis C risk, needle exchange, and safe sex.

Dependence syndrome

A central descriptive characteristic of the dependence syndrome is the desire (often strong, sometimes overpowering) to take a substance (which may or may not have been medically prescribed). Requires 3 or more of the following:

1 A strong desire or sense of compulsion to take the substance (craving).
2 Difficulty in controlling substance use (onset, termination, level of use).
3 A physiological withdrawal state when reducing or ceasing substance use (or using the same (or closely related) substance to avoid withdrawal).
4 Tolerance: increased doses are required to produce the original effect.
5 Progressive neglect of alternative pleasures or interests.
6 Persisting use despite clear evidence of harmful consequences.

The prevalence of obesity (BMI >30kg/m$_2$): USA 39%, UK 27%, Japan 3.6%. Obesity is the commonest disorder of childhood and adolescence.

BMI is the best measure of obesity (see MINIBOX 'Body mass index (BMI)'). Waist circumference (measured midway between lower ribs and iliac crest) is an alternative measure of body fat correlated with CHD risk, DM, ↑BP, and ↑ lipids.

Body mass index (BMI)	
BMI = weight in kg/(height in m)^2	
18.5–24.9	Healthy weight
25–29.9	Overweight
30–34.9	Obesity I (>27.5 if Asian)
35–39.9	Obesity II
>40	Obesity III (morbid obesity)

Health risks of obesity
- *Greatly increased risk*: (RR >3.) Mortality (BMI >30); T2DM; gallbladder disease; dyslipidaemia; insulin resistance; breathlessness; sleep apnoea.
- *Moderately increased risk*: (RR 2–3.) CHD (5–6% of deaths are due to obesity); ↑BP; OA (knees); hyperuricaemia/gout.
- *Slightly increased risk*: (RR 1–2.) Cancer (breast, endometrial, oesophageal, colon); reproductive hormonal abnormalities; impaired fertility; PCOS; low back pain; stress incontinence; anaesthetic/surgical risks; suicide; bullying.

Causes • Physical inactivity • Cultural factors • Low education • Polygenic genetic predisposition • Smoking cessation • Childbirth (especially if not breastfeeding) • Drugs eg steroids, antipsychotics (olanzapine), contraceptives (depot-injections), insulin • Endocrine causes (rare; eg hypothyroidism, Cushing's, PCOS).

Typical needs Women: 2000kcal/day; men: 2500 kcal/day; most eat ≥10% more. Once weight goes up, physical activity lessens, and weight increases further.

Management Prevention begins in childhood with healthy patterns of exercise/diet. In obese adults, the main problem is maintaining lost weight.

Initial assessment: Assess willingness to change (see 'stages of change' model in BOX 'Self-care and empowered self-care' p.783), eating behaviour and diet, physical activity, psychological distress, and social and family factors affecting diet. Measure BMI and waist circumference. Check BP, blood glucose/HbA1c (for undiagnosed diabetes), and lipid profile.

Advice: Whether willing to change or not, provide advice on risks of obesity and benefits of healthy eating and physical exercise. Tailor your advice to the individual and if unwilling to change reinforce at each encounter.

Diet: Advise a weight loss diet for any patient who is overweight or obese and is willing to change:
- *Low-calorie diets:* All obese people lose weight on low-energy intake. Aim for weight loss of 0.5–1kg/week using a reduction of ~600kcal/day with a target BMI of 25, in steps of 5–10% of original weight. There is no health benefit of weight loss below this. If simple diet sheets are not effective, refer to a dietician. 500kcal/day reduction without any change of activity leads to ~0.45kg of weight loss/wk. Easy!

Drug therapy: Orlistat (120mg TDS with food) is the only drug licensed for treatment of obesity in the UK. It acts by ↓ fat absorption. Consider a 3-month trial if supervised diet/exercise has failed and BMI >30 (or >27 if comorbidity). Continue after 3 months only if weight ↓ is ≥5% initial body weight.

Group and behavioural therapy: Group activities (eg Weight Watchers®) have a higher success rate in producing and maintaining weight loss. Behavioural therapy together with low-calorie diets is also effective.

Surgery: Consider if BMI >40 (>35 if comorbidity) and non-surgical measures have failed. Laparoscopic adjustable gastric banding, sleeve gastrectomy, and gastric bypass are all options (OHCM p626).*

Further reading
SIGN (2010). *Management of Obesity*. Edinburgh: SIGN.

Insomnia Describes a perception of disturbed or inadequate sleep. ~1:4 of the UK population (♀>♂) are thought to suffer in varying degrees. *Prevalence:* Increases with age (1:2 if >65yrs old). It can adversely affect quality of life, concentration and memory, performance of daytime tasks, and cause relationship problems. 10% of traffic accidents are thought to be related to tiredness. Causes are numerous—common examples include:

• *Minor, self-limiting:* Travel, stress, shift work, small children, arousal.
• *Psychological:* ~½ have mental health problems: depression, anxiety, mania, grief, alcoholism.
• *Physical:* Drugs (eg steroids), pain, pruritus, tinnitus, sweats (eg menopause), nocturia, obstructive sleep apnoea.

What counts as 'a good night's sleep'? • <30min to fall asleep • Maintenance of sleep for 6–8h • <3 brief awakenings/night • Feeling well and refreshed on waking.

Management Careful evaluation. Many do not have a sleep problem themselves, but a relative feels there is a problem (eg the retired milkman who continues to wake at 4am). Others have unrealistic expectations: 'I need 12h sleep a night'. Reassurance may be all that is required. For genuine problems:

• *Eliminate physical problems preventing sleep:* eg treat asthma/eczema; give long-acting painkillers to last the night.
• *Treat psychiatric problems:* eg depression, anxiety.
• *Sleep hygiene:* see BOX 'Principles of "sleep hygiene"'.
• *Relaxation techniques:* eg self-help CDs.
• *Consider drug treatment:* Last resort: 'only when insomnia is severe, disabling, or subjecting the individual to extreme distress'.

Drug treatment Zolpidem (5–10mg nocte), zopiclone (3.75–7.5mg nocte), benzodiazepines (eg **temazepam** 10mg nocte), and low-dose amitriptyline (10–30mg nocte) are all commonly prescribed for patients with insomnia. *Side effects:* Amnesia and daytime sleepiness. Most hypnotics affect daytime performance and may cause falls in the elderly. Warn about the effect on driving/operating machinery. Up to 40% of people with insomnia are thought to self-medicate with over-the-counter hypnotics that are available without prescription (eg sedative antihistamines).

▶Concerns about the use of benzodiazepines/z-drugs are that many people develop tolerance to their effects, gain little therapeutic benefit from long-term use, become dependent on them (both physically and psychologically), and suffer a withdrawal syndrome when they stop taking them. The Committee on Safety of Medicines recommend that the use of benzodiazepines for the treatment of insomnia should be restricted to severe insomnia and that treatment should be at the lowest dose possible and not be continued beyond 4 weeks.

▶▶Beware the temporary resident who has 'forgotten' his/her night sedation.

Principles of 'sleep hygiene'

• Don't go to bed until you feel sleepy.
• Avoid daytime naps.
• Reserve a room for sleep only (if possible), do not eat, read, work, or watch TV in it.
• Avoid caffeine, alcohol, and nicotine.
• Take regular exercise, but avoid late night hard exercise (sex is ok).
• Don't stay in bed if you're not asleep.
• Establish a regular bedtime routine.
• Make sure the bed is comfortable and avoid extremes of noise or temperature.
• Have a warm bath at bedtime.
• Monitor your sleep with a sleep diary (length and quality of sleep).
• Rise at the same time every morning regardless of how long you've slept.*

---

* The material in the sections 'Obesity' & 'Managing sleep problems' has been adapted from the *Oxford Handbook of General Practice* 4th edition by Simon *et al*, and has been reproduced by permission of Oxford University Press.

Recommended amounts of activity Adults: ≥30min/day of moderate intensity exercise ≥5 days/wk; children ≥1h/day moderate intensity exercise every day. In the UK, 60% of adults are not active enough to benefit their health.

Health benefits of exercise *There is decreased risk of:* DM—through ↑ insulin sensitivity; CVD—physically inactive people have ×2 ↑ risk of CHD and ×3 ↑ risk of stroke; osteoporosis—exercise ↓ risk of hip fractures by ½; cancer— ↓ risk of colon cancer; obesity.

Exercise is a useful treatment for BP—can delay onset of hypertension and ↓BP by 10mmHg; MI; COPD; DM; hypercholesterolaemia—↑HDL and ↓LDL; arthritis and back pain; mental health problems—↓ depression and anxiety. *In the elderly:* Exercise maintains functional capacity; ↓ levels of disability and risk of falls/hip fracture; and improves quality of sleep.

Effective interventions
- *Practical advice*: Enquire about activity levels and remind of the benefits of exercise; reinforce with leaflets/posters around the surgery. Assess willingness to change and suggest moderate exercise (eg walking/cycling) that can be incorporated into daily life (eg to work/school). Apps can help eg 'Couch to 5k' or 7-minute workouts. Congratulate any success!
- *Healthcare*: Counselling is as effective as more structured exercise sessions. Specialist rehabilitation schemes are available for specific conditions (eg post MI; COPD). Exercise schemes operate in some areas eg supervised gym exercise accessed via 'GP prescription'. Many sports facilities offer special sessions for pregnant women, the over 50s, and people with disability.*

Healthy eating

The ideal diet should include a variety of foods. Advise patients to avoid snacking between meals.
- *Use starchy food* (eg bread, pasta, rice, potatoes) as the main energy source.
- *Eat plenty of fruit and vegetables*—>5 portions of fruit and vegetables/day.
- *Eat plenty of fibre*—good sources are high-fibre breakfast cereals, beans, pulses, wholemeal bread, potatoes (with skins), pasta, rice, oats, fruit/veg.
- *Eat fish* at least ×2/wk, including 1 portion (max. ×2 if pregnant) of oily fish (eg mackerel, herring, salmon).
- *Choose lean meat*—remove excess fat/poultry skin and pour off fat after cooking; use unsaturated oil to cook; boil/steam/bake in preference to frying. Use less cooked or processed red meat—consider substituting meat with vegetable protein (eg pulses; soya). Avoid fatty meats (eg sausages; salami).
- *Use skimmed milks* and low-fat yoghurts/spreads/cheese.
- *Avoid adding salt*—aim for <6g of salt/day. Avoid processed foods, crisps, and salted nuts.
- *Avoid adding sugar* and cut down on sweets, biscuits, and desserts.
- *Drink at least 2–3l of fluid daily*—preferably not tea, coffee, or alcohol. Drinking a large glass of water with meals can reduce the urge to overeat.

Malnutrition 50% ♂; 25% ♀ >85yrs are unable to cook a meal alone. ►Malnutrition is common among the elderly. *Risk factors:* Low income; living alone; mental health problems; dementia; recent bereavement; gastric surgery; malabsorption; ↑ metabolism; difficulty eating/swallowing (eg MND; CVA); chronic disease (eg IBD; IBS; cancer; CCF; COPD).

Management of malnutrition: Encourage to eat more and consider using nutritional, vitamin, and mineral supplements on dietician advice. Consider referral to social services if an inability to prepare meals/shop, or OT referral if difficulty with utensils.*

---

* The material in the sections 'Exercise' & 'Healthy eating' has been adapted from the *Oxford Handbook of General Practice* 4th edition by Simon *et al*, and has been reproduced by permission of Oxford University Press.

Alternative/holistic medicine

We need to know about alternative medicine to understand our patients' undeclared distress, which use of these treatments is so often a sign of. We can also advise on the safety of various therapies. We must also learn from therapists about patient-centred care.

Some alternative therapies are the orthodoxies of a different time (eg *herbalism*) or place (the *Ayurvedic medicine* of India), some are mainly diagnostic (*iridology*), some therapeutic (*aromatherapy*). Some doctors are suspicious of unorthodox medicine, and feel that its practitioners should not be 'let loose' on patients. But in many places the law is that, however unorthodox a practitioner may be, he or she cannot be convicted of unethical practice in the absence of clear harm. Many people (~5 million/yr in the UK) consult alternative practitioners, often as a supplement to orthodox treatment. Some will feel unable to tell their doctor about trips to alternative therapists, unless asked.

Modern medicine is criticized for sacrificing humanity to technology, and with little benefit for many people. In contrast to the orthodox doctor, alternative therapists are seen as taking time to listen, laying on hands rather than instruments, and giving medicines free (not always!) from side effects.

Acupuncture Can treat many ailments and is increasingly used in orthodox practice for pain relief (recommended by NICE in treatment of non-specific low back pain), control of nausea, and treatment of addiction. 2 predominant theories as to how it works are: 1 By causing muscle relaxation through trigger point stimulation and 2 Through endorphin release. In some circumstances, a combination of the 2 mechanisms is likely to make it effective (eg back pain). For migraines, endorphin release is the likely predominant mechanism.

Aromatherapy The use of essential plant oils (from flowers, herbs, or trees), either inhaled or massaged via the skin, with the aim of improving physical, mental, and spiritual well-being. It is often used to help treat anxiety, nausea, sleep, and pain.

Homeopathy This is based on the idea that 'like cures like' and uses highly diluted substances which practitioners claim can cause the body to heal itself. The principles on which it is based are 'scientifically implausible' and randomized trials show no greater efficacy than placebo.

Manipulative therapies (osteopathy; chiropracty) These are widely used and may help musculoskeletal problems. Evidence is lacking for benefit in treating headaches/migraines, digestive disorders, depression, and infant colic.

Yoga An ancient Indian discipline with physical, mental, and spiritual components that aim to achieve a state of spiritual insight and tranquillity. RCTs show yoga can produce worthwhile benefit to physical and mental well-being.

Herbal medicines Are those with active ingredients made from plants. Evidence for their effectiveness is generally limited, and use is largely based on tradition rather than scientific research. The traditional herbal registration (THR) marking means compliance with safety and manufacturing quality standards (but does not necessarily mean it is safe to use).[56] Herbal medicine may cause harm (eg black cohosh and hepatotoxicity) or interact with other medication (eg St John's wort).

Reflexology This is a type of massage where pressure applied to the feet is thought to stimulate corresponding organs in the body and start a healing process via energy pathways. There is no evidence to support its use for any medical condition.[57]

Integrative medicine This is a patient-centred, interdisciplinary, non-hierarchical mix of conventional and complementary solutions to case management of patients with complex problems eg chronic low back or neck pain.[58]

Intimate partner violence (IPV) Defined as any incident or pattern of incidents of controlling, coercive, or threatening behaviour, violence, or abuse between those aged ≥16yrs who are/have been intimate partners or family members, regardless of gender or sexuality. This can encompass, but is not limited to, the following types of abuse: • Psychological • Sexual • Financial • Physical • Emotional.

Controlling behaviour: Acts designed to make people subordinate/dependent by isolating them from sources of support, exploiting their resources/capacity for personal gain, depriving them of means needed for independence, resistance ± escape, and regulating their everyday behaviour.

Coercive behaviour: Act/pattern of acts of assault, threats, humiliation, and intimidation or other abuse used to harm, punish, or frighten victims.

Prevalence Although men may be the victims of IPV, ~80% of reported violence is against women by male partners. IPV affects 1 in 4 women and is the most common form of inter-personal crime: 60%—current partner; 21%—former partner; half suffer >1 attack; 1 in 3 have been attacked repeatedly.

Effects High incidence of psychiatric disorders, particularly depression and self-damaging behaviours eg drug/alcohol abuse, suicide.

Factors preventing the victim leaving the abusive situation
- Loss of self-esteem makes the victim think they are to blame.
- Disruption of the family and children's relationship with partner.
- Loss of intimate relationship with the partner.
- Fear of partner.
- Fall in income.
- Risk of homelessness.
- Fear of the unknown.

Presentation General practice is often the first place in which victims seek formal help, but only 1 in 4 actually reveals the true nature of the problem. Without appropriate intervention, violence continues and often increases in severity and frequency. By the time injuries are visible, violence may be a long-established pattern. On average, victims will be assaulted 35 times before reporting it to police.

Guidelines for care
- Consider the possibility of IPV—ask directly ▶30% of IPV starts in pregnancy. Use screening tools eg HARK (see BOX 'HARK screening questions for IPV').
- Emphasize confidentiality.
- Accurate, clear documentation, over time, at successive consultations may provide cumulative evidence of abuse and is essential for use as evidence in court, should the need arise.
- Assess the present situation—gather as much information as possible.
- Provide information; offer help to make contact with other agencies.[6]
- Devise a safety plan eg give the phone number of a local refuge; advise to keep some money and important financial and legal documents hidden in a safe place in case of emergency; help plan an escape route in case of emergency.

▶Do not pressurize the victim into any course of action. If the patient decides to return to the violent situation, she or he will not forget information and support given. In time this might give them the confidence and back-up needed to break out of the situation.

▶▶If children are likely to be at risk you have a duty to inform social services or the police, preferably with the patient's consent.

6 Women's Aid 0808 2000 247 www.womensaid.org.uk; police domestic violence units.

HARK screening questions for IPV

The majority of women experiencing IPV do not spontaneously disclose it to a clinician. A short screening tool can accurately and quickly identify a high proportion of women affected. The acronym HARK denotes 4 short questions which represent different components of intimate partner violence:

Humiliation: within the last year, have you been *humiliated* or emotionally abused in other ways by your partner or your ex-partner?

Afraid: within the last year, have you been *afraid* of your partner or ex-partner?

Rape: within the last year, have you been *raped* or forced to have any kind of sexual activity by your partner or ex-partner?

Kick: within the last year, have you been *kicked*, hit, slapped, or otherwise physically hurt by your partner or ex-partner?

A score of ≥1 will identify 81% of women affected by IPV and may help women disclose IPV in general practice, allowing for appropriate specialist help.[59]

Elder abuse

This is a single or repeated act or lack of appropriate action, occurring within any relationship where there is an expectation of trust, which causes harm or distress to an older person. Prevalence is 4% (↑ with age; ♀:♂≈ 2:1). Older people often do not report abuse. Forms of abuse:
- *Physical*—eg cuts, bruises, unexplained fractures, burns.
- *Psychological*—eg unusual behaviour, unexplained fear, appears helpless or withdrawn.
- *Financial*—eg removal of funds by carers, new will in favour of carer.
- *Sexual*—eg vaginal or anal bleeding, genital infections.
- *Neglect*—eg malnourished, dehydrated, poor personal hygiene, late requests for medical attention.

Signs Inconsistent story from patient and carer; inconsistences on examination; fear in presence of carer; frequent attendance at ED; frequent requests for GP visits; carer avoiding GP.

Management Talk through the situation with the patient, carer, and other services involved in care. Assess the level of risk. Consider admission to a place of safety—contact social services and/or police as necessary; seek advice from Action on Elder Abuse.[7]

Adult safeguarding An adult (>18yrs) at risk of harm:
- May be in receipt of community care services by reason of mental/other disability, age, or illness, and
- May be unable to take care of him/herself, or
- Is unable to protect him/herself from serious harm/exploitation.

If suspected, contact local social services adult safeguarding lead (with consent if the patient is able to give consent).

13 General practice

7 Action on Elder Abuse 0808 808 8141 www.elderabuse.org.uk

GPS as managers GP partners have dual roles as both clinicians and managers of small businesses. As such they must cooperate with their partners and practice manager to run the business side of the practice and work with primary healthcare team members to cover all areas of clinical work.

Management This is the process of designing and maintaining an environment in which individuals work together efficiently to accomplish selected aims. This requires technical skill (knowledge specific to the business of the organization), interpersonal skills (ability to work with others), conceptual skills (to see the 'big picture'), and problem-solving skills. There are a number of managerial functions:

1 *Planning:* Selecting aims & objectives, and the actions to achieve them.
2 *Organizing:* Defining roles—ensuring all tasks necessary to accomplish goals are assigned to those people who can do them best.
3 *Staffing:* Ensuring all positions in the organizational structure are filled with people able to fulfil those roles.
4 *Leading:* Influencing people so they contribute to organization and group goals.
5 *Controlling:* Measuring and correcting individual and organizational performance to ensure events conform to plans.

Management and teamwork Key features contributing to successful teamwork are:
* *Communication:* Information sharing, feedback, and grievance airing.
* *Clear team roles:* Especially with regard to responsibility and accountability.
* *Sympathetic leadership:* A weak leader may allow the team to drift but an autocratic leader may be too directive and diminish the status of others, thus reducing the effectiveness of the team.
* *Clear decision-making process:* Especially if there are differences of opinion.
* *Pooling:* Knowledge, experience, skills, and responsibility for outcome.
* *Specialization of function:* Team members must understand and respect the role and importance of other team members.
* *Delegation:* Work of the team is split between members and each member leaves the others to carry out functions delegated to them.
* *Group work:* Team members share and are committed to a common, agreed purpose or goal which directs their actions.*

* The material in the section 'GPS as managers' has been adapted from the *Oxford Handbook of General Practice* 4th edition by Simon *et al*, and has been reproduced by permission of Oxford University Press.

13 General practice

Commissioning

The *Health and Social Care Bill* (2011) laid the foundations for groups of GPs and other clinical professionals to group together in *Clinical Commissioning Groups* (CCGs) to take on formal responsibility for commissioning the majority of NHS services in England, working in partnership with other health professionals, hospital and mental health trusts, local communities, and local authorities.

Aims of commissioning • To design improved patient pathways • To enable more efficient use of funds so that savings can be used to provide better patient services • To enable improved community and hospital services that better meet the needs of patients.

CCGs Every GP practice in England must be part of a CCG. The CCG governing body has decision-making powers, which meets in public and publishes minutes of meetings. The board is comprised of: • ≥2 lay members (1 championing public and patient involvement and 1 overseeing governance) • 1 registered nurse, and • 1 secondary care doctor (neither employed by a local provider).

Principles of commissioning These are the same whichever organization is undertaking it. *Planning:* Assessing needs of the local population and resources available. *Contracting:* Commissioning services for local patients. *Monitoring:* Monitoring delivery of the service and ensuring the service is kept on track. *Revision:* Revising the needs of the CCG and arrangements with providers.

As we move away from providing care in expensive high-technology hospitals, more is expected of primary care, with implications for capital expenditure, acquiring new skills, and local access to procedures needing expensive equipment eg endoscopy or ultrasound. Whole specialisms such as dermatology and day-case surgery may move out of the secondary sphere, as the distinction between primary and secondary care becomes redundant. Similar distinctions separating health and social care may also become redundant as more care is provided in people's homes and the community. Greater priority is also required to prevent ill health by working with local authorities and other agencies to tackle the wider determinants of health and well-being.

How are these developments to be structured? What are the dangers and opportunities?

Market-led models Well-capitalized companies take over running general practices, after winning provider contracts from CCGs. Such companies create free-standing clinics, or run a chain of GP surgeries. GPs become salaried employees of the company providing services. However, there are clear problems with corporate healthcare: the USA is the most expensive healthcare system in the world yet it consistently underperforms relative to other countries (eg on access, efficiency, and equity), and fails to achieve better health outcomes.[4]

Federated GP-led models General practices club together to consolidate services. This flexible model can rapidly adapt to local priorities, causes the least disruption to existing services, and maintains continuity of care. Under this model GPs develop special interests and 'portfolio careers' playing to their strengths in both the clinical and administrative spheres in an increasingly complex health environment—in which they both commission and provide care.

Various kinds of federated GP models exist, from informal alliances to limited companies owned and run by GPs. One thing held in common is that they are part of the NHS family, and share core NHS values of inclusivity, fairness, and distributive justice. The primary motive for their creation is to maintain general practice-based primary care—and the system whereby patients can see the doctor of their choice near where they live.

Primary Care Networks These were introduced in 2019 and consist of groups of general practices (of between 30,000 & 50,000 patients) working together, along with a range of integrated community teams, to provide proactive, coordinated care + address population health/health inequalities. PCNs will bring general practices together to work at scale and provide a wider set of staff roles than might be feasible in individual practices eg first contact physiotherapy, clinical pharmacists, extended hours, and social prescribing. Requirements include delivery of structured medication reviews, enhanced health in care homes, supporting early cancer diagnosis, and cardiovascular disease case-finding.

Health and Social Care Alliances Aim to develop fully integrated health and social care systems which reflect the fact that more and more people require long-term support from both NHS and social care services. This means CCGs, hospital trusts, mental health trusts, and county councils working together as a single health and care organization, pooling budgets, and providing 'joined-up' services.

Conflicts of interest If a GP federation is a for-profit organization (with funds flowing from the NHS) and if the doctors are sitting on boards deciding on which services are to be commissioned, there is a conflict of interest. The NHS is establishing procedures to minimize risk from this possibility—but nevertheless, probity is a vital issue, for doctors as well as other NHS staff.

13. General practice

Patient participation groups (PPGs) ▸Working *with* your patients is as important as working *for* them.

PPGs meet with healthcare professionals and managers to improve services to patients and discuss some of the following:

• Harmonizing the 'consumer's' and the 'provider's' aims.
• Feedback to aid planning, implementation, and evaluation of services eg undertaking a patient survey to assess satisfaction with services.
• Identifying unmet needs (eg as a result of comments in survey feedback).
• Improving links between the practice and other (eg voluntary/charity) services.
• Health promotion in the light of local beliefs.
• Pressurizing government institutions over inadequate services.
• Dealing with complaints (less adversarial than with formal methods—and independent of the NHS and doctors—hence reasonably credible).

Due to lack of interest, or to there being no clear leader or task, up to 25% of groups close over time. The complaint that participation mechanisms lead to tokenism (ie the democratic ideal has been exercised, but what has been created is just a platform for validating the status quo) does not turn out to be true if a group has power over funds which it has raised. Here, our experience is that analysis may be penetrating and decision swift, in a way that makes even the best-run health authorities/trusts look pedestrian.

Another role for PPGs is to have dialogues with CCGs on proposed changes to services—eg whether practices are to be amalgamated or services withdrawn or replaced by provision via non-NHS private companies. CCGs have a responsibility to consult, and PPGs have a valid role in bringing CCGs to account.[60]

The Patients Association This group represents and furthers the interests of patients by giving assistance, advice, and information. It aims to promote understanding between patients and the medical world. patients-association.org.uk

Contact is a charity providing guidance and information to families with disabled children. contact.org.uk

Self-help organizations Many thousands of groups have been set up worldwide for sufferers of specific rare or common diseases. They offer information, companionship, comfort, and a lifeline to patients and their families eg for sharing support and treatments. A danger is that they share nightmares as well eg unnecessarily graphic descriptions of their children dying, causing unneeded despondency. They raise funds for research, providing a 'welcome alternative to the expensive services of professionals'.

Groups as a way out of passive dependency If people learn in groups they take more control of their lives and they are more optimistic about being able to change things in their lives (such as their weight); self-esteem improves—and also objective measures of health (such as HbA1c).

Expert patients

The term expert patient was coined to denote a well-informed patient in full possession of the facts about his or her case, and contributing to decisions in a valid way. Doctors often fear the expert patient, as so much time has to be spent investigating whether their viewpoints really are valid. This may lead to lack of harmony in the consulting room.

The inherent contradictions and strengths in the idea of expert patients are revealed through *reductio ad absurdum* ('argument to absurdity'—a logical technique beloved of Socrates).[81] Imagine a urologist consulting his GP about whether to have a radical prostatectomy or radiotherapy for his newly diagnosed prostate cancer. The GP might say to himself: 'Why on earth is he consulting me? He knows far more about the options than I do.' But let us imagine that his GP is, in fact, Socrates, who proceeds to ask various questions to reveal his inner fears (incontinence, erectile problems), and what he hopes to achieve by the various treatments on offer (to live long enough to see his disabled son through school). Socrates-the-GP is not adding any new facts. He is twisting the kaleidoscope, so that new patterns come into view. When a coherent pattern emerges he shows the urologist the door—saying 'Let me know what you decide'. The urologist sincerely thanks him. The man who leaves such a consultation is not the same as the one who entered. ▸ *The expert patient has met a different sort of expert.*

Greater patient involvement in health issues and in the decisions relating to patients' own illnesses may lead to greater satisfaction, and better health. The more the patient knows about his or her own set of diseases, the better he or she will be able to decide what treatments to opt for. Expert patients (who are confident and assertive) are said to live longer, be healthier, and have a better quality of life,[82] and are exemplars of what health is all about (in chronic disease, health is not the absence of decay but an optimum, dynamic adaptation to it).

Nonetheless, there is a group of expert patients who tend to be middle-class know-alls who consult at great length about various maladies, arriving with sheaves of Internet printouts about treatments you have never heard of. Don't reject these patients out of hand. And don't assume any sort of superiority or inferiority. Just give your advice as best you can. You may get better results than Socrates—whose last attempt at *reductio ad absurdum* (during his famous trial) ended fatally when he was forced to drink hemlock. He was right—but it didn't do him much good. And so with you: you don't always have to be right. And by not insisting on this you may live to consult another day.

13 General practice

14 Eponymous syndromes

Andrew Baldwin

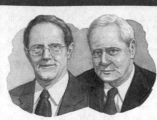

Fig 14.1 We like eponyms. What better way to achieve immortality and recognition than have your name live on. The true origin of eponymous discoveries is often contentious: Professor of Statistics Stephen Stigler in *Stigler's Law of Eponomy* asserts that 'No scientific discovery is named after its original discoverer' and credits sociologist RK Merton as the first to formulate *Stigler's Law*—thus deliberately making it exemplify itself. Eponyms sound far more glamorous than histologically driven disease titles, the names of which often evolve as more becomes known. While the golden age of eponyms may be behind us, we hope those that remain will carry on forever.

Alphabetical list of eponymous syndromes

See also *OHCM* p694–717. Biographical details sourced from www.whonamedit.com.

Alport syndrome A group of inherited, progressive, haematuric nephropathies which may also affect the cochlea (sensorineural deafness) and eye (lenticonus; dot-and-fleck retinopathy). Associated with mutations in genes encoding the α3, 4, or 5 chains of collagen IV, the major constituent of the basement membrane. *R:* No effective treatment is available. Those with end-stage renal disease usually undergo transplantation.[1,2] *Arthur C Alport, 1880–1959 (South African physician)*

Asperger syndrome Characterized by poor social skills, difficulty interpreting emotions, and restricted intense interests, but with normal language and IQ. Once a discrete disorder, the diagnosis was recategorized in DSM-5 as a form of autism spectrum disorder. *Hans Asperger, 1906–1980 (Austrian paediatrician)*

Bardet–Biedl syndrome Autosomal recessive A rare multisystem disorder of underlying ciliary dysfunction and a key genetic cause of chronic renal failure in children.[3] *Features:* Renal failure (dysfunction of renal tubule cilia), GU tract malformations, obesity, cognitive impairment, poor visual acuity, and limb deformities. ♂:♀≈1.3:1. *Georges L Bardet, 1885–1970 (French physician); Artur Biedl, 1869–1933 (Hungarian pathologist)*

Batten disease *(neuronal ceroid lipofuscinoses)* A group of severe neurodegenerative diseases. Neuronal loss occurs due to increased apoptosis and altered autophagy from defects in the CLN genes (pathogenesis unknown). *Features:* Visual loss, seizures, loss of motor and cognitive function, and early death. *Tests:* Molecular testing for CLN1-3 mutations.[4] *Frederick E Batten, 1865–1918 (British neurologist)*

Becker muscular dystrophy x-linked recessive There are mutations in the dystrophin gene (xp21), but unlike Duchenne (p. 846, where there is near-total loss of dystrophin) there is 'semifunctional' dystrophin, with later onset, milder symptoms, and slower progression. Cardiac involvement is the main factor influencing survival. *Tests:* ↑CK, mm biopsy, genetic tests. *R:* Supportive (exercise programmes; physio; managing complications). *Peter E Becker, 1908–2000 (German physician)*

Beckwith–Wiedemann syndrome An overgrowth syndrome of complex genetic cause characterized by macrosomia, macroglossia, hemihyperplasia, and abdominal wall defects. There is predisposition to embryonal tumours (esp. Wilm's, p. 229) in ~10%.[5] *J Bruce Beckwith b1933 (American pathologist); Hans-Rudolf Wiedemann 1915–2006 (German paediatrician)*

Bourneville disease *(tuberous sclerosis complex) (epiloia)* =EPIlepsy, LOw Intelligence + Adenoma sebaceum, see fig 14.2) Autosomal dominant A multiorgan disorder resulting in hamartomatous lesions that affect virtually every organ system. The main complication is epilepsy or developmental delay from 'tubers' within the brain. *Cause:* Mutation of tumour suppressor genes TSC1 (loci on 9q34, making *harmatin*) or TSC2 (16p13 makes *tuberin*; mutations here are worst). *Prognosis:* Highly variable. *Diagnosis:* See BOX 'Diagnosing tuberous sclerosis (Bourneville disease)' and table 14.1. *Désiré-Magloire Bourneville, 1840–1909 (French neurologist)*

Johnnie Walker or Dandy–Walker?

We are surrounded by eponyms commemorating the Great and the Good, from the Nobel Prize and the Ryder Cup, to Jack Daniels and Johnnie Walker. Medical eponyms are pickled in something almost as intoxicating: the hidden recesses of our own minds. We store away the bizarre, the fearsome, and the mundane—and then, years later, as if playing some game of snap, we match these features with the person sitting in front of us, and say: 'Dandy–Walker!' or 'Prader–Willi!' But as the years go by we may wonder more and more about the people behind the eponyms. We might read about these quacks and geniuses—yet it is always rather unsatisfying. History shows us everything except the one thing we want to see: the spark that made these eponymous characters truly original.

Diagnosing tuberous sclerosis (Bourneville disease)

Clinical diagnostic criteria (table 14.1)

Definite diagnosis: 2 major features, or 1 major and 2 minor features.[6]

Possible diagnosis: Either 1 major, 1 major + 1 minor, or ≥2 minor features.[6]

Genetic criteria: Identification of a pathogenic mutation of TSC1 or TSC2 is sufficient to make a definite diagnosis. However, a negative result does not exclude diagnosis as ~15% have no mutation identified by conventional testing.[6]

Table 14.1 Major and minor features of Bourneville disease

Major features		Minor features	
1	Hypomelanotic (ashleaf) macules (≥3)	1	'Confetti' skin lesions
2	Angiofibromas (≥3) (fig 14.2)	2	Dental enamel pits (≥3)
3	Ungual fibromas (≥2) (fig 14.3)	3	Intraoral fibromas (≥2)
4	Shagreen patch (sacral plaque, like shark skin)	4	Retinal achromic patch
5	Multiple retinal hamartomas	5	Multiple renal cysts
6	Cortical dysplasias* (≥3)	6	Non-renal hamartomas
7	Subependymal nodules* (≥2)		
8	Subependymal giant cell astrocytomas*		
9	Cardiac rhabdomyoma		
10	Lymphangioleiomyomatosis		
11	Angiomyolipomas		
*=brain lesions.			

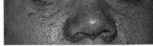

Fig 14.2 Angiofibromas (adenoma sebaceum).

© DermNet New Zealand, reproduced with permission.

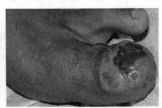

Fig 14.3 Ungual fibroma.

Reproduced from Lewis-Jones, *Paediatric Dermatology* (2010), with permission from OUP.

Briquet syndrome Renamed *somatic symptom disorder* in DSM-5: chronic, multiple, medically unexplained (but unfeigned) symptoms, affecting any body part. Psychological cause. Onset <30yrs (see BOX 'Helping people with Briquet syndrome'). *Paul Briquet, 1796–1881 (French physician)*

Buchanan syndrome A single artery arises from normally formed ventricles (the *truncus arteriosus* fails to divide into the pulmonary trunk and aorta). There is cyanosis from birth. R: Surgical correction. *A Buchanan; described 1864*

Capgras syndrome *(delusional misidentification syndrome)* The patient believes a person has been replaced by an exact clone, who is an impostor. *Cause:* Psychosis; head injury; dementia. *Jean Marie Joseph Capgras, 1873–1950 (French psychiatrist)*

Castleman disease *(CD; angiofollicular lymph node hyperplasia)* A lymphoproliferative disorder comprising 3 distinct diseases which share a similar microscopic appearance: 1 *Unicentric CD* with a solitary enlarged lymph node 2 *Human herpesvirus-8 multicentric CD* 3 *Idiopathic (HHV-8 negative) multicentric CD Symptoms:* Localized lymphadenopathy + systemic symptoms in multicentric disease eg flu-like symptoms, neuropathy. R: Depends on subtype.[7] *Benjamin Castleman, 1906–1982 (US pathologist)*

Chédiak–Higashi syndrome Autosomal recessive Hypopigmentation (skin, eyes, hair), prolonged bleeding, recurrent infection, abnormal NK cell function. Morbidity results from frequent infections or lymphoproliferation into organs.[8] *Cause:* 1q43 mutation (CHS1/LYST gene). Fatal in 90% by 10yrs of age without marrow transplant.[9] *Otokata Higashi, 1902–1981 (Japanese paediatrician); Alexander M Chédiak, 1903–1993 (Cuban physician)*

Conradi–Hünermann syndrome *(chondrodysplasia punctata)* A group of skeletal dysplasia disorders characterized by skeletal abnormalities (shortening of limbs, x-ray epiphyseal stippling, cataracts, and skin lesions (ichthyosis, alopecia). *Cause:* Genetic (most are x-linked dominant; severity is variable); warfarin teratogenicity.[10] *Erich Conradi, 1882–1968; Carl Hünermann, 1904–1978 (German physicians)*

Cornelia de Lange syndrome A multisystem malformation syndrome causing characteristic facial dysmorphism in association with growth retardation, IQ↓, and upper limb anomalies. ~50% are due to NIPBL gene mutation. There is wide clinical variability.[11] *Cornelia Catharina de Lange, 1871–1950 (Dutch paediatrician)*

Corrigan syndrome Congenital aortic regurgitation (AR). Corrigan's pulse is the collapsing pulse of AR. *Sir Dominic John Corrigan, 1802–1880 (Irish physician)*

Cotard delusion *(nihilistic delusions)* The patient may state he is already dead and demand burial, deny his existence, or believe his insides are rotting away. *Cause:* Psychotic depression (especially elderly patients), alcohol, syphilis, parietal lobe lesion, or just being born. *Jules Cotard 1840–1889 (French neurologist)*

Crigler–Najjar syndrome 2 rare syndromes of inherited unconjugated hyperbilirubinaemia presenting in the 1st days of life with jaundice ± CNS signs. *Cause:* Mutation in UGT enzyme activity causing absent (type 1) or impaired (type 2; mild) ability to excrete bilirubin. R: T1: Liver transplant before irreversible kernicterus (pp. 294–5). *John F Crigler, b1919; Victor A Najjar, 1914–2002 (US paediatricians)*

Dandy–Walker syndrome Congenital obstruction of the foramina of Luschka and Magendi leads to progressive head enlargement, congested scalp veins, bulging fontanelle, separation of cranial sutures, papilloedema, and bradycardia (fig 14.4). R: CSF shunt. *Walter E Dandy, 1886–1946 (US neurosurgeon); Arthur E Walker, 1907–1995 (US neurologist)*

De Clérambault syndrome *(erotomania)* The patient (usually female) is persistently deluded that a person of higher social status is in love with them (eg a politician or celebrity). Stalking is one manifestation. There may be a persecutory delusional belief that individuals are conspiring to keep them apart. *Enduring Love,* Ian McEwan *Gaëtan Gatian de Clérambault, 1872–1934 (French psychiatrist)*

Diamond–Blackfan anaemia *(erythrogenesis imperfecta)* An inherited red cell aplasia. *Features:* ↓ marrow erythroid production (→normochromic macrocytic anaemia); growth retardation; ~30–50% have craniofacial, upper limb, heart, and urinary malformations. 25% due to mutations in RPS19 gene on 19q13.[12] R: Steroids ± bone marrow transplant; or stem-cell transplant from donor embryo (PGD confirms HLA matching).[13] *Louis K Diamond, 1902–1999; Kenneth D Blackfan, 1883–1941 (US paediatricians)*

Helping people with Briquet syndrome (somatic symptoms)

- Give time—don't dismiss these patients as just the 'worried well'.[14]
- Explore with the patient the factors perpetuating the illness (disordered physiology, misinformation, unfounded fears, misinterpretation of sensations, unhelpful 'coping' behaviour, social stressors).
- Agree a management plan which focuses on each issue and makes sense to the patient's holistic view of him- or herself.
- Treat any depression (p. 712); consider cognitive therapy; make the patient feel understood; broaden the agenda, negotiating a new understanding of symptoms including psychosocial factors.[15]

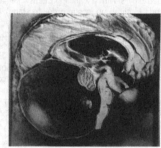

Fig 14.4 Dandy–Walker dilatation of the 4th ventricle. The large cyst is actually an enlarged 4th ventricle and not separate from it. The 3rd and lateral ventricles are much enlarged, secondarily.

Courtesy of Professor Ralph Józefowicz.

DiGeorge syndrome A severe form of the chromosome 22q11.2 deletion syndromes. *Signs:* Congenital heart disease, abnormal facies, cleft palate, underactive parathyroids (∴ Ca^{2+}↓), thymus hypoplasia, ↓ T-cell-immunity and cognitive/behavioural problems.

Angelo Mari DiGeorge, 1921–2009 (US paediatrician)

Di Guglielmo disease *(acute erythroid leukaemia)* An M6 subtype of acute myeloid leukaemia (AML) characterized by invasion of pathological dysplastic RBCs into the liver, spleen, lymph nodes, kidneys, & heart. 3 stages: erythromyelosis, erythroleukaemia, & AML. R: chemotherapy ± bone marrow transplant.[16]

Giovanni Di Guglielmo, 1886–1961 (Italian haematologist)

Duchenne muscular dystrophy $_{recessive}^{x-linked}$ Mutations in dystrophin gene (xp21.2) result in near-total loss of dystrophin (muscles get replaced by fibroadipose tissue). *Presentation:* Boys aged 1–6yrs, with a waddling, clumsy gait, and classic Gower's manoeuvre (using hands to climb up legs in order to stand). No abnormality is noted at birth. Selective wasting causes calf pseudohypertrophy. Mean age of wheelchair use =9–12yrs. There is respiratory impairment and infections; cardiomyopathy and orthopaedic complications (tendon contractures, scoliosis, osteoporosis). *Prevalence:* 1:3600–6000 ♂ births. *Creatine kinase:* This is ↑; ►measure in all boys not walking by 1½yrs. *Muscle biopsy:* Abnormal fibres surrounded by fat and fibrous tissue. R: Interdisciplinary management and coordinated clinical care. Aim to maintain walking (eg using orthoses). Prednisolone slows decline in muscle strength in the short term.[17] A disease-modifying agent (AVI-4658) is under development.[18] Gene therapy may be an option. *Prognosis:* Mechanical ventilation improves longevity (median age of death =31yrs). *Carrier* ♀: ~10% show some disease manifestation. *Prenatal screening* is available.[20]

Guillaume Benjamin Amand Duchenne de Boulogne, 1806–1875 (French neurologist)

Ebstein anomaly A congenital defect with downward displacement of the tricuspid valve (±deformed leaflets) atrializing the right ventricle causing right-sided heart failure. There may be no symptoms, or cyanosis, clubbing, arrhythmias, systolic, and diastolic murmurs. It can be associated with other cardiac malformations. *Tests:* Echo; ECG: tall P waves, ↑PR interval; right bundle branch block. *Prognosis:* Varies according to severity.

Wilhelm Ebstein, 1836–1912 (German physician)

Edward syndrome *(trisomy 18)* The 2nd commonest trisomy (Down's is 1st, p. 16) causing extensive and characteristic congenital malformations (see fig 14.5). There is severe psychomotor and growth retardation in the 5–10% who survive beyond the first year of life. *Prevalence:* 1:~7000 live births (80% ♀).[19]

John Hilton Edwards, 1928–2007 (British physician)

Ehlers–Danlos syndrome (EDS) A clinically diverse condition with skin fragility (figs 14.6 & 14.7), ligament laxity, short stature, spinal deformity, vascular fragility, and (rarely) retinal detachment. *9 sub-types:* Hypermobility (type III) is the most common and probably synonymous with joint hypermobility syndrome. Vascular rupture is a major concern in type IV. $Δ$: Primarily clinical; genetic testing (via skin biopsy).[20]

Edvard L Ehlers 1863–1937 (Danish dermatologist); Henri-Alexandre Danlos 1844–1912 (French physician)

Eisenmenger syndrome Refers to any congenital heart defect with a left-to-right shunt (eg large septal defects) in which the development of pulmonary hypertension leads to subsequent shunt reversal. *Victor Eisenmenger, 1864–1932 (Austrian physician)*

Erb's palsy Caused by damage to the brachial plexus (usually C5/C6 nerves) from birth trauma. See p. 74 & p. 556. *Wilhelm Heinrich Erb, 1840–1921 (German neurologist)*

Fallot's tetrad *(OHCM p157)* 1 Ventricular septal defect (VSD). 2 Pulmonary stenosis 3 Right ventricular hypertrophy 4 The aorta overriding the VSD (accepting right heart blood). It is the commonest cyanotic congenital heart disorder (10%; 3–6/10,000). *Signs:* Severity depends on degree of pulmonary stenosis. Cyanosis, dyspnoea, faints, clubbing, thrills, harsh systolic murmur at left sternal base. *Tests:* Echo shows anatomy & degree of stenosis. Cardiac CT/MRI helps plan surgery. R: Surgical repair entails VSD closure and correcting pulmonary stenosis, eg before 1yr. *Prognosis:* Without surgery, mortality rate is ~95%. After repair 85% survive to 35yrs. *Etienne-Louis Arthur Fallot, 1850–1911 (French physician)*

x-linked muscular dystrophies

1 Duchenne muscular dystrophy (severe).
2 Becker muscular dystrophy (later presentation; much slower progression).
3 Emery–Dreifuss muscular dystrophy (benign; early contractures).
4 McLeod neuroacanthocytosis syndrome.
5 Scapuloperoneal (rare).

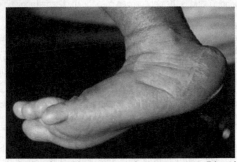

Fig 14.5 Rockerbottom feet with prominent calcaneus, as seen in Edward syndrome. Other features: microcephaly, microphthalmia, micrognathia, microstomia, rigidity with limb flexion, odd low-set ears, receding chin, proptosis, cleft lip/palate ± umbilical/inguinal herniae, short sternum (makes nipples look widely separated). The fingers cannot be extended + 2nd and 5th fingers overlap 3rd and 4th.

Reproduced from eMedicine.com, 2007. Available at: www.emedicine.com/ped/topic652.htm with permission.

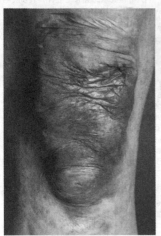

Fig 14.6 Skin on the knee in EDS. The skin is weak, fragile, and easily bruised or torn, with wide atrophic scars as thin as cigarette paper. Look for piezogenic papules (easily compressible outpouchings of fat through defects in the dermis on the sides of the feet).

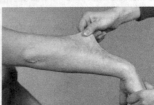

Fig 14.7 Elastic skin in EDS. Bennett's paradox: the woman at a drag ball is the true impostor for, unlike everyone else, she is what she seems. So with EDS, which doesn't behave like a connective tissue disease *because it really is one* (a true disease of collagen). Other 'connective tissue diseases' are really diseases of something else.

Fanconi anaemia >99% are auto-somal recessive Defective stem cell repair and chromosomal fragility leads to progressive marrow failure and aplastic anaemia. There is increased risk of acute myelogenous leukaemia and solid tumours. Congenital anomalies (present in ~75%) include absent radii, thumb hypoplasia, syndactyly, missing carpal bones, skin pigmentation, microsomy, microcephaly, strabismus, cryptorchidism, ↓IQ, deafness, and short stature. 15 causative genes have been identified. *R:* Stem cell transplant has increased survival (~80% with well-matched donors), and is the only proven cure for the haematopoietic manifestations of FA. Gene therapy trials are in progress.[21]   *Guido Fanconi, 1892–1979 (Swiss paediatrician)*

Galeazzi fracture Distal radial shaft fracture with associated dislocation of the distal radioulnar joint (fig 14.8).   *Ricardo Galeazzi, 1866–1952 (Italian orthopaedic surgeon)*

Ganser symptom A patient gives repeated wrong but 'approximate answers' to questions eg 'How many legs does a horse have?'—'3'; 'What colour is snow?'—'Black'. The nature of the answer reveals an understanding of the question posed. *Ganser syndrome* has varying definitions and includes approximate answering + clouding of consciousness, hallucinations, and conversion symptoms. It may be organic, psychiatric, or factitious (a form of malingering in those feigning mental illness).[22]   *Sigbert Josef Maria Ganser, 1853–1931 (German psychiatrist)*

Gaucher disease Autosomal recessive The commonest lysosomal storage disease, characterized by deposition of glucocerebroside in cells of the macrophage-monocyte system. Three subtypes are defined based on the presence or absence of CNS signs: 1 *Non-neuronopathic* presents with painless splenomegaly, anaemia, thrombocytopenia, & skeletal disease. 2 *Acute neuronopathic* (rare) characterized by rapid and progressive neurodegeneration, organomegaly, and death in infancy (usually by aspiration and respiratory compromise). 3 *Chronic neuronopathic* appears like type 1 *plus* with progressive slowing of oculomotor horizontal saccades ± learning disability, epilepsy, or dementia. 75% present before the age of 20 but severity varies widely for types 1 & 3. *Δ:* Measure acid β-glucosidase activity in peripheral WBCs. *R:* Enzyme replacement therapy (eg **imiglucerase**); glucosylceramide synthase inhibitors.[23]   *Philippe Charles Ernest Gaucher, 1854–1918 (French dermatologist)*

Hand–Schüller–Christian syndrome *(HSC; Langerhans' cell histiocytosis (LCH); histiocytosis X)* The group of disorders now known as *LCH* were initially divided into a number of diseases (including *HSC*), depending on the site and severity. Monoclonal Langerhans-like cells are pathognomonic of this destructive, infiltrative disease in which bone, liver, skin, and spleen show lytic foci of eosinophils, plasma cells, and histiocytes. Patients with *HSC* (=25% with multifocal *LCH*) often present with recurrent episodes of otitis media and mastoiditis or with polyuria and polydipsia. Other signs: see MINIBOX 'Signs of HSC'. *R:* Bone surgery, steroids, cytotoxics, and radiotherapy may induce remissions.   *Alfred Hand Jr, 1868–1949*

Signs of HSC
• Diabetes insipidus*
• Exophthalmos*
• Lytic bone lesions*
• Failure to thrive; dyspnoea
• Scalp lumps/skin erosions
• Eczema-like rash/pustules
• Cord compression ± fits
• Ear discharge, stomatitis
• Honeycomb lung
• Hepatosplenomegaly
• Lymphadenopathy
• ↑T°; anaemia; ↓ platelets
*Classic triad; seen in 10%

(US paediatrician); Artur Schüller, 1874–1957 (Austrian neurologist); Henry A Christian, 1876–1951 (US physician)

Hartnup disease Autosomal recessive Increased GI & urinary loss of neutral amino acids causes pellagra-like photosensitive skin rash, cerebellar ataxia, and aminoaciduria. Causative gene: SLC6A19. *R:* High-protein diet; avoid sun exposure if symptomatic; **Nicotinamide** if niacin-deficient.[24]   *Baron et al. (1956) described this disorder in the Hartnup family of London*

Hunter syndrome *(mucopolysaccharidosis II)* X-linked recessive (NB: all other MPSs are AR). Iduronate 2 sulfatase deficiency results in glycosaminoglycan accumulation in the lysosomes of organs and tissues. *Types:* MPS IIA (severe)—developmental delay, deafness, short stature, unusual face, joint contractures. Slow systemic somatic and neurological progression leads to death aged 10–15 years. MPS IIB —mild. *Δ:* Enzyme analysis for IDS. *R:* None is curative. Enzyme replacement (idursulfase); bone marrow transplant.[25]   *Charles A Hunter, 1873–1955 (Scottish–Canadian physician)*

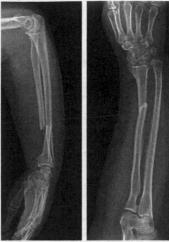

Fig 14.8 x-rays of a Galeazzi fracture show a short oblique fracture of the distal radius with distal ulnar dislocation from disruption of the distal radioulnar joint.

Reproduced with permission from Abujudeh, H. (2014). *Emergency Radiology Cases*. Oxford: OUP.

Huntington disease Autosomal dominant A progressive neurodegenerative disorder with spiny neuron loss in the neostriatum due to excessive CAG repeats in the huntingtin gene (chromosome 4). Normally, there are <28 repeats. 29–35 CAG repeats means no signs but they may pass Huntington's to their children. 36–39 CAG repeats mean ↓ penetrance. If >40 CAG repeats there is full penetrance (+ anticipation). Symptoms usually do not appear until adulthood (~30–50yrs). *Early findings:* ↓ auditory & visual reaction times, then mild chorea (flitting, jerky movements), odd extraocular movements, ↑ reflexes, ↓ rapid alternating movements. Unpredictable motor impairment is found until chorea starts. *Late signs:* Personality change, self-neglect, apathy, clumsiness, fidgeting, fleeting grimaces, dementia, and progression to death 10–30yrs from diagnosis. ℞· None prevents progression. Ethical dilemmas surround testing, as symptoms may only start after completing a family. *George Huntington, 1850–1916 (US physician)*

Hunt syndrome *(pyridoxine (vitamin B₆)-dependent seizure; PDS)* Classic PDS: intractable neonatal seizures resistant to conventional anticonvulsants respond rapidly to parenteral pyridoxine. *James Ramsay Hunt, 1872–1937 (US neurologist)*

Hurler syndrome Autosomal recessive A severe form of *mucopolysaccharidosis type 1*, a lysosomal storage disorder caused by deficiency of α-L-iduronidase with resultant inability to break down dermatan sulfate (DS) & heparan sulfate (HS) (essential for normal growth). There is accumulation of mucopolysaccharides in urine, cartilage, periosteum, tendons, valves, meninges, & eyes. After briefly normal growth, there is physical and mental decline, hydrocephalus, thick skin, hirsutism, and CCF. *Cause:* IDUA gene mutation (chromosome 4). *Tests:* Metachromatic Reilly bodies in lymphocytes; ↑ urinary DS/HS. ℞· Multidisciplinary approach; enzyme replacement. Death is often ≤10yrs.[26] *Gertrud Hurler, 1889–1965 (German paediatrician)*

Hutchinson's triad *(congenital syphilis)* VIIIth nerve deafness + interstitial keratitis + notched, pointed incisors. *Sir Jonathan Hutchinson, 1828–1913 (British surgeon)*

Ivemark syndrome The association of asplenia with visceroatrial heterotaxia (abnormal organ position; AKA situs ambiguus). *Björn Ivemark, 1925–2005 (Swedish pathologist)*

Kartagener syndrome Autosomal recessive Primary ciliary dyskinesia (inflexible, poorly beating cilia) *associated with* situs inversus/dextrocardia. Clearance of mucus & bacteria is poor, hence chronic sinusitis and bronchiectasis. ♂ infertility, ♀ salpingitis, and otitis media are common. ℞· Antibiotics, continuous or intermittent, for airway infections; immunization.[27] *Manes Kartagener, 1897–1975 (Swiss physician)*

Kawasaki disease A febrile vasculitic syndrome causing coronary aneurysms. *Cause:* Unknown. *Median age:* 18–24 months. 3 phases: 1 *Acute febrile:* Lasts 1–2wks; the child has fever ≥5 days + major signs (see BOX 'Diagnostic criteria for Kawasaki disease' & fig 14.9). 2 *Subacute:* Lasts from remission of fever to weeks 4–6. Hallmarks of this phase include the development of coronary artery aneurysms (& the risk for MI/sudden death), desquamation of the digits, thrombocytosis, irritability, and conjunctival injection. 3 *Convalescent:* Resolution of clinical signs + normalization of inflammatory markers (weeks 6–12). *Tests:* ESR & CRP ↑; α1-antitrypsin ↑; platelets ↑; echocardiogram; MRA accurately defines aneurysms. ℞· Immunoglobulin 2g/kg as a single IVI dose (further dose IVIG + prednisolone if non-responsive to initial dose; aspirin (80–100mg/kg/day) reduced once afebrile for 48–72h to 3–5mg/kg/day for 6–8 wks.[28] *Prognosis:* Good with prompt treatment. Mortality ~1%. *Tomisaku Kawasaki, b1925 (Japanese paediatrician)*

Klinefelter syndrome *(47, XXY karyotype)* The chief genetic cause of male hypogonadism presenting with gynaecomastia and infertility. *Associations:* Psychosocial issues, mild learning disability, autoimmune disease, osteoporosis, ↓ sexual maturation. ℞· Androgen therapy; mastectomy. Lifespan is normal, but arm span may exceed body length. *Harry Fitch Klinefelter Jr, 1912–1990 (US physician)*

Klippel–Feil syndrome Autosomal recessive or dominant Congenital fusion of cervical vertebrae ± neurological symptoms. The clinical triad seen in 50% is short neck, low posterior hairline, and limited neck movement. *Mirror movements* (synkinesia) may occur (=*voluntary* movements in one limb cause the same *involuntary* movement in the other). *Maurice Klippel, 1858–1942; Andre Feil, 1884–1955 (French neurologists)*

Diagnostic criteria for Kawasaki disease

Fever for ≥5 days + at least 4 of the following:[29] *
  1 Bilateral non-exudative conjunctivitis.
  2 Cervical lymphadenopathy (often unilateral, firm, tender nodes).
  3 Pharyngeal injection, dry fissured lips, strawberry tongue. No mouth ulcers.
  4 Polymorphous rash (especially on the trunk).
  5 Changes in extremities: arthralgia, palmar erythema or later, ►swelling of the hands/feet ± skin desquamation.

*Kawasaki disease may be diagnosed with <4 of these features if coronary artery aneurysms (CAAs) are present. Fever is often high (>40°C) and can persist for ≥2 weeks if untreated. CAAs develop in 20–25% of untreated patients.
►Incomplete forms exist, so get expert help *today* while wrestling with this difficult, important diagnosis. There is paradoxical data that incomplete or atypical forms are *more* likely to have complications such as CAA.

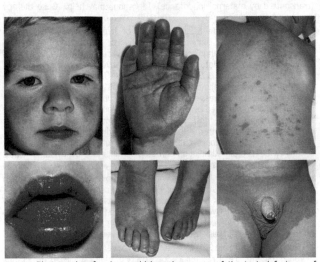

Fig 14.9 Photographs of a 4-year-old boy show some of the typical features of Kawasaki disease including (from top left–right), bilateral non-exudative conjunctivitis; erythematous and oedematous hands and (below) feet; an erythematous truncal rash; dry, fissured, erythematous lips with a 'strawberry' tongue; and a desquamating perineal rash.

Kugelberg–Welander *(spinal muscular atrophy type 3)* Autosomal recessive Weakness and hypotonia from loss of LMN in the spinal cord & brainstem nuclei. Usually manifests >18 months old. *Erik KH Kugelberg, 1913–1983; Lisa Welander, 1909–2001 (Swedish neurologists)*

Landouzy–Dejerine *(facioscapulohumeral) muscular dystrophy* Autosomal dominant Distinct and slowly progressive (asymmetrical) regional weakness appears at 12–14yrs of age. There is shoulder weakness, winged scapulae, difficulty in closing the eyes, sucking, blowing, and whistling. Extraocular and pharyngeal muscles are spared. *Associations:* Foot drop (anterior tibialis weakness); high-frequency hearing loss. *Joseph J Dejerine, 1849–1917 (French neurologist); Louis TJ Landouzy, 1845–1917 (French physician)*

Laurence–Moon syndrome Autosomal recessive Retinitis pigmentosa, obesity, polydactyly, hypogenitalism, ↓IQ, ↓ body hair, azoospermia (♂), learning disability, speech delay, and renal abnormalities (calyceal clubbing, cysts, or diverticula; end-stage renal failure in 15%). It is distinct from Bardet–Biedl syndrome, p. 842 (no polydactyly). *John Z Laurence, 1829–1870; Robert C Moon, 1844–1914 (British ophthalmologists)*

Leber hereditary optic neuropathy Bilateral, painless, irreversible blindness occurring in young adults (♂:♀=4:1), caused by mutations in mitochondrial DNA (transmitted by maternal inheritance). Idebenone may help.[30] Gene therapy may be a future option. *Theodor Karl Gustav von Leber, 1840–1917 (German ophthalmologist)*

Lesch–Nyhan syndrome X-linked recessive Deficiency of hypoxanthine-guanine phosphoribosyl transferase (HPRT) causes 3 problems: 1 *Uric acid overproduction:* Hyperuricaemia (orange crystals in the nappy) causing renal stones ± renal failure, and gout. 2 *CNS:* Motor delay, IQ↓ (eg <65), severe generalized dystonia ± choreoathetosis and fits. 3 *Behavioural problems:* Cognitive impairment, persistent and severe self-injurious behaviour (lip/foot biting, head banging, face scratching). Smiling aggression to others may occur. Δ: Measurement of HPRT enzyme activity (confirmed by identifying a mutation in the HPRT gene). Nearly all cases are in males. *Prognosis:* Death is usually before 40yrs, from renal failure or infection. Sudden death may occur. ℞: Good hydration (urine flow ↑); allopurinol prevents urate stones, but not CNS signs. Protective devices to prevent self-injury. Deep brain stimulation can stop self-injurious behaviour and help dystonia.[31] Milder variants exist. *Michael Lesch, 1939–2008; William L Nyhan, b1926 (US physicians)*

Lewy body dementia Dementia with intracytoplasmic neuronal inclusion bodies (fig 14.10) in brainstem/cortex + fluctuating cognitive impairment, parkinsonism, hallucinations, & visuoperceptual deficits. ℞: Cholinesterase inhibitors (eg rivastigmine). Overlap with Alzheimer and Parkinson diseases makes treatment hard as antiparkinsonian agents can precipitate delusions, and antipsychotics worsen parkinsonism.[32] *Friedrich H Lewy, 1885–1950 (German neurologist)*

Li–Fraumeni syndrome Autosomal dominant A familial cancer predisposition syndrome in which patients are at risk for a wide variety of malignancies. It devastates families, but fascinates geneticists due to germ-line mutations of the tumour suppressor gene TP53; see BOX 'Li–Fraumeni syndrome, p53, and the guardian of the genome'. *Frederick P Li, b1940; Joseph F Fraumeni, Jr, b1933 (US physicians)*

Martin–Bell *(fragile x)* **syndrome** X-linked semi dominant The leading monogenic cause of cognitive impairment (♂ 1:4000; ♀ 1:8000). *Cause:* The FMR1 gene (fragile x mental retardation-1) on xq27 includes a CGG-repeat that lengthens as it is passed from generation to generation. Once the repeat exceeds a threshold length (>200), no fragile x protein is made, and disease results. *Signs:* Delayed speech & language; delayed motor milestones (secondary to hypotonia). ↓IQ, hyperactivity, emotional and behavioural problems, anxiety, mood swings, autism, and tactile defensiveness (little eye contact; no hugging). 15% have seizure disorders. *Physical features:* A long narrow face, large ears, prominent jaw, big testes (♂). *Tests:* Molecular genetic testing of FMR1 gene. Prenatal screening is possible. ℞: Improvement in general behaviour has been shown with minocycline.[33] Sertraline may help language development in those with coexisting ASD.[34] *James P Martin, 1893–1984 (British physician); Julia Bell 1879–1979 (British geneticist)*

Fig 14.10 Lewy body (arrow). NB: there are no generally accepted biomarkers to distinguish dementia with Lewy bodies (DLB) from other dementias. Think of DLB whenever there is progressive anxiety, depression, apathy, agitation, sleep disorder with psychosis, and memory disorders.

The best imaging candidate may be striatal dopamine transporter system scintigraphy using FP-CIT SPECT.[35]

Courtesy of Kondi Wong and the National Human Genome Research Institute.

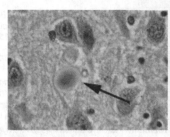

Li–Fraumeni syndrome, p53, and the guardian of the genome

TP53 is a tumour-suppressor gene that codes for p53, a protein that regulates the cell cycle (chromosome 17p13.1; encoding nuclear phosphoprotein—a transcription factor allowing passage through the cell cycle). In Li–Fraumeni syndrome, as only one allele is affected, development is normal until a spontaneous mutation affects the other allele. Somatic mutation of p53 occurs at both alleles in 50–80% of spontaneous human cancers. Cells with a p53 mutation do not pause in G1 (a phase in which DNA repair takes place, and faulty DNA purged), but proceed straight to S1 (DNA replication), which is why p53 protein is known as the 'guardian of the genome'. Examples of cancers caused this way include early-onset breast cancer, brain tumours, sarcomas, leukaemia, lymphoma, melanoma, & adrenal cortex carcinoma.[36]

Note that tumours are associated with >1 syndrome, eg adrenal cortex tumours are associated with familial cancer syndromes such as the Beckwith-Wiedemann and Li–Fraumeni syndromes, the Carney complex, multiple endocrine neoplasia type 1, congenital adrenal hyperplasia, and the McCune-Albright syndrome (p. 854).[37]

In a retrospective study of 200 cancer-affected carriers of TP53 germline mutations, 15% developed a 2nd cancer, 4% a 3rd cancer, and 2% a 4th cancer. In some populations (eg in South Brazil), there is a high prevalence of otherwise rare mutations in p53, partly explaining high rates of colon and other cancers (eg fatal stomach cancer in children as young as 12).[38]

McCune–Albright syndrome ≥2 of: 1 Polyostotic fibrous dysplasia of bone 2 Café-au-lait pigmentation 3 Autonomous endocrine hyperfunction (eg precocious puberty). See fig 14.11 and BOX 'McCune–Albright syndrome'.
Donovan J McCune, 1902–1976; Fuller Albright, 1900–1969 (US physicians)

Monteggia fracture Fracture of the proximal ⅓ of ulna, with dislocation of the radial head (IV types).
Giovanni Battista Monteggia, 1762–1815 (Italian surgeon)

Morquio syndrome *(mucopolysaccharidosis IV)* Autosomal recessive Lysosomal storage disease caused by GALNS gene mutation *(type A)* or β-galactosidase gene mutation *(type B)*. Overlapping clinical features of short stature and skeletal dysplasia, with no CNS involvement & normal IQ.
Luis Morquio, 1867–1935 (Uruguayan paediatrician)

Niemann–Pick disease *(sphingomyelinase deficiency)* Autosomal recessive A neurovisceral lysosomal lipid storage disorder. *Type A:* Early-onset, rapidly progressive neurodegenerative course, systemic disease, and death in early childhood. *Type B:* Traditionally non-neuronopathic, milder, with later onset and variable severity (often detected by hepatosplenomegaly or lung symptoms). *Δ:* Sphingomyelinase activity in peripheral blood white cells; targeted gene mutation analysis.[39]
Albert Niemann, 1880–1921 (German paediatrician); Ludwick Pick, 1868–1944 (German pathologist)

Noonan syndrome Autosomal dominant A multisystem disorder characterized by short stature, characteristic facial features (ptosis, down-slanting eyes, low-set ears), congenital heart defects (in 50%, most commonly hypertrophic cardiomyopathy and pulmonary stenosis), ± chest and spine deformities, webbed neck, clotting disorders, and learning disability. *Cause:* Mutations in genes that are part of the RAS/RAF/MEK/ERK signalling pathway (a regulator of cell growth) have been identified.[40] *Prevalence:* 1:2500.
Jacqueline Anne Noonan, b1928 (US paediatric cardiologist)

Ondine's curse *(congenital central hypoventilation syndrome)* Autonomic dysfunction causes central alveolar hypoventilation and apnoea (especially during sleep). There is variable requirement for ventilatory support. *Cause:* PHOX2B gene mutation. Ondine was a nymph who sacrificed her immortality by falling in love with a prince who promised to honour her with every waking breath. When the prince lost interest, Ondine uttered her curse: 'for as long as you are awake, you shall breathe. But should you ever fall asleep, that breath will desert you'.

Othello syndrome *(delusional jealousy)* A lover has a fixed belief that their partner is being sexually unfaithful. They may go to great lengths to provide delusional 'evidence' to back up this belief (engaging a spy; examining underwear). *Associations:* Alcohol, schizophrenia, depression, frontal lobe dysfunction, dementia. ▶Get psychiatric help: jealousy is the most deadly of all the passions and there is a significant association with violence. In Shakespeare's play, Othello murdered his wife as a result of a false belief that she had been unfaithful (but he was deceived rather than deluded—so did
Othello actually have the Othello syndrome?).41 Othello, 1603–∞ (Described in 1955 by John Todd, British psychiatrist)

Patau syndrome *(trisomy 13)* Cleft lip & palate (± other midline facial defects), microcephaly, neural tube defects, omphalocele, hernias, cardiac defects (seen in 80%, eg patent ductus arteriosus, VSD ± dextrocardia). Hands show flexion contractures ± polydactyly. *Median survival:* <3 days; 5% survive >6 months. *Prevalence:* 1 in 7500 births.[42]
Klaus Patau, 1908–1975 (German-born US geneticist)

Pick disease Early-onset progressive *frontotemporal dementia.* 15:100,000 aged 45–64yrs. *Signs:* Before cognitive loss, look for: personality change, social disinhibition, emotional blunting, impaired insight, dietary changes, perseverative behaviours (eg drinking from an empty cup). *Tests:* MRI. *R:* AChEIs unlikely to be beneficial.
Arnold Pick, 1851–1924 (Czech neurologist & psychiatrist)

Pierre Robin syndrome *(PR sequence)* A sequence of events due to a small mandible (± cleft palate), causing posterior tongue displacement and airway obstruction + poor neonatal feeding. *R:* Prevent the tongue slipping back by prone positioning; surgery if severe airway compromise.
Pierre Robin, 1867–1950 (French dentist)

McCune–Albright syndrome

In McCune–Albright syndrome (MAS), multiple pathologic fractures may be prominent early in the history and often predominate on one side of the body. Deformities and pain further complicate the picture (pain can be relieved by bisphosphonates). The craniofacial fibrous dysplasia may encroach on the optic nerve, causing visual problems.

Precocious puberty in MAS is gonadotropin independent and does not respond to GNRH agonists (but they may be used as adjuncts to treatment). The largely experimental treatment for precocious puberty includes aromatase inhibitors for females (which block the effects of oestrogen), and anti-androgen (eg spironolactone) + aromatase inhibitors for males.

Precocious puberty is not the only endocrinopathy: hyperthyroidism, acromegaly, and Cushing's also occur.

The cause is a sporadic mutation of the GNAS1 gene coding the α subunit of the stimulatory guanine-nucleotide binding protein, G-protein, which activates adenylate cyclase and increases intracellular cyclic AMP.[43]

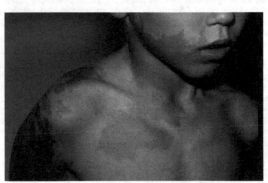

Fig 14.11 Hyperpigmented café-au-lait macules (which frequently predominate on one side of the body without crossing the midline) in a child with McCune–Albright syndrome.

Reproduced with permission from Warrell, D. *et al.* (2010). *Oxford Textbook of Medicine*. Oxford: OUP.

14 Eponymous syndromes

Pompe disease *(glycogen storage disease-II acid maltase deficiency)* Autosomal recessive
Glycogen accumulation in lysosomes due to ↓ lysosomal α1,4-glucosidase activity. 3 forms. 1 *Early (infantile, classic):* Progressive and rapidly fatal if untreated. There is left ventricular outflow obstruction, respiratory distress, & hypotonia 2 *Juvenile (non-classic):* Delayed motor milestones, weakness, & hypotonia 3 *Adult:* Proximal weakness ± respiratory symptoms. Glycogen accumulates in heart, muscle, liver, CNS, & kidneys. *R:* Alglucosidase alfa (enzyme replacement therapy) prolongs life and can reverse cardiomyopathy.
Joannes Cassianus Pompe, 1901–1945 (Dutch pathologist)

Prader–Willi syndrome (PWS) *Cause:* Loss of paternal contribution of the proximal part of the long arm of chromosome 15. *Prevalence:* 1:25,000. *Signs: Infancy:* hypotonia, poor feeding, genital hypoplasia, delayed motor milestones. *Childhood:* hyperphagia with progressive obesity; food seeking behaviour (eg shoplifting food, eating spoiled foods); short stature; behavioural problems, eg obsessive–compulsive traits; psychosis in 5–10%; ↓IQ. *Δ:* Chromosomal analysis. *R:* Growth hormone if growth failure. Intranasal oxytocin may reduce appetite + improve socialization, anxiety, and repetitive behaviours.[44]
Andrea Prader, 1919–2001; Heinrich Willi, 1900–1971 (Swiss paediatricians)

Ramsay Hunt syndrome *(herpes zoster oticus)* This is herpes zoster infection of the facial nerve. Often in the elderly, severe otalgia precedes VII cranial nerve palsy (± VII, IX, V, VI in order of frequency). Zoster vesicles appear around the ear, in the deep meatus (± soft palate & tongue, fig 14.12). There may be vertigo, tinnitus, or deafness. *R:* Aciclovir + prednisolone.
James Ramsay Hunt, 1872–1937 (US neurologist)

Rett syndrome A neurodegenerative disorder occurring almost exclusively in females. After initially normal perinatal development there is neurological regression. 4 stages: 1 *Developmental arrest:* (6–18 months.) Developmental delay, hand wringing, ↓head growth 2 *Rapid regression:* (1–4yrs.) Loss of acquired skills, hand sterotypies, autistic behaviour, seizures, breathing irregularities 3 *Pseudostationary:* (2–10yrs.) Some improvement in behaviour/communication 4 *Late motor deterioration:* (>10yrs.) Slow motor regression. *Cause:* Various mutations in MECP$_2$ gene located on the X chromosome.[45]
Andreas Rett, 1924–1997 (Austrian paediatrician)

Reye syndrome Acute encephalopathy and liver failure occurs days after a febrile viral illness (eg URTI, varicella, influenza). Aspirin intake is a risk factor and there was a dramatic decline in incidence of the disease following its association (now exceedingly rare). *Tests:* Transaminases ↑; blood ammonia ↑ (correlates with survival); INR↑; glucose ↓ (none are specific). Liver biopsy: swollen, pleomorphic mitochondria (ATP↓, gluconeogenesis & ureagenesis↓). *CT:* Cerebral oedema; but may be normal. *ΔΔ:* Inborn errors of metabolism. *Prognosis:* Mortality <20%; full recovery in >60%.[46]
Ralph Douglas Kenneth Reye, 1912–1977 (Australian pathologist)

Silver–Russell syndrome A clinical and genetically heterogeneous congenital disorder, characterized by severe intrauterine and postnatal growth retardation, dysmorphic facial features, small stature, and relative macrocephaly. *Cause:* Genetic and epigenetic alteration can be detected in most cases, including hypomethylation in the chromosome 11p15 imprinting centre, and maternal uniparental disomy (inheritance of both alleles from the mother) of chromosome 7. *Prognosis:* Relatively good. Growth hormone improves linear growth.
Henry K. Silver, 1918–1991 (US paediatrician); Alexander Russell, 1914–2003 (British paediatrician)

Prader–Willi syndrome (PWS), imprinting, and epigenetics

Chromosome 15q11–q13 is a critical region for PWS, which results from loss of expression of *paternally* expressed genes at this site. Angelman syndrome, a rare disorder characterized by severe physical and intellectual disability, seizures, and frequent laughter, occurs from loss of *maternally* expressed genes at the same locus. But how do our genes know where they come from?

PWS was the first human disorder attributed to genomic imprinting, where certain genes can be expressed in a parent-specific manner. Normally, we inherit 2 copies of a gene, 1 from each parent, and both copies shape how we develop. In genomic imprinting, 1 copy of a gene is inactivated. If the remaining functional gene is defective, this may cause disease. The processes whereby genes can be activated or deactivated are referred to as epigenetic. In general, methylation of the DNA in a gene will cause that gene to be inactivated whereas acetylation of histones (simple proteins around which DNA is coiled) can activate inactive genes. Such changes, known as imprints, appear prior to germ cell (sperm or oocyte) maturation, and hence in the embryo.[47] Silver–Russell syndrome and Beckwith–Wiedemann syndrome are other examples of imprinting disorders.[1]

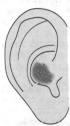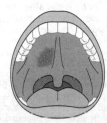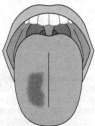

Fig 14.12 Shingles is generally a disease of sensory nerves; however, Ramsay Hunt syndrome is distinctive in that there is a motor component causing facial paralysis. The rash of herpetic blisters is in the distribution of the *nervus intermedius* (part of the facial nerve) and may include the anterior ⅔ of the tongue, the soft palate, the external auditory canal, and auricle.

1 Our thanks to Dr Guy Bradley-Smith for his advice on this section.

Still's disease *(systemic-onset juvenile idiopathic arthritis/SJIA)* Accounts for ~10% of all JIA and presents with *systemic* upset and spiking fevers that typically occur around the same time once or twice each day. There is arthralgia and generalized myalgia. Fever spikes are usually accompanied by a salmon-pink macular (often linear) rash on the trunk and limbs. There may be hepatosplenomegaly & lymphadenopathy (esp. axillary). Serositis causes chest pain or shortness of breath (± pleural and pericardial effusions).[48] *Other subgroups:* Juvenile ankylosing spondylitis; psoriatic arthritis; ulcerative colitis-associated arthritis; juvenile-onset rheumatoid arthritis—here Rh factor is +ve, and systemic upset is rarer. There is also *adult-onset Still's disease. Tests:* WCC↑; ESR↑; CRP↑ (≈ poor response); Hb↓; ferritin↑; LFT↑; albumin↓; echo. *R:* The goal is to prevent joint damage & loss of function and control pain. A multidisciplinary approach is used and includes physiotherapists, OTs, dieticians, & counsellors. Medication is aimed at inducing remission. NSAIDs may be adequate for patients with low disease activity. Systemic corticosteroids (eg prednisolone) have a short-term role. Methotrexate is used in those with ongoing active disease. Abatacept, adalimumab, etanercept, and tocilizumab are recommended as immunomodulators if inadequate response to, or intolerance of conventional DMARDs.[49] *Sir George Frederick Still, 1868–1941 (British paediatrician)*

Sydenham chorea *(St Vitus dance)* A neurological manifestation of acute rheumatic fever and the chief cause of chorea in children. It may be the *only* feature, appearing up to 6 months after clinical signs of strep infection have abated. *Pathogenesis:* Thought to involve molecular mimicry with *Streptococcus*-induced antibodies cross-reacting with antigens of the basal ganglia. *Motor signs:* Involuntary purposeless movement, worsened by stress and disappearing on sleep, with clumsiness, grimacing, a darting lizard's tongue and unclear speech. *Non-motor features:* Include obsessions, compulsions, attention deficit, ↓ verbal fluency, ↓ executive function.[50] The term PANDAS (Paediatric Autoimmune Neuropsychiatric Disorder Associated with *Streptococcus*) denotes a putative subset of obsessive–compulsive disorder and Tourette syndrome that bears some resemblance to Sydenham chorea. *ΔΔ:* Wilson disease, juvenile Huntington's, thyrotoxicosis, SLE, polycythaemia, Na+↓, hypoparathyroidism, kernicterus, phenytoin, neuroleptics, hereditary chorea. *R:* Spontaneous remission occurs in the majority. Sodium valproate can help control chorea. Despite treating active and recurrent strep infections vigorously, chorea may persist. *Thomas Sydenham, 1624–1689 (British physician)*

Syme amputation Amputation of the foot through the articulation of the ankle with removal of the malleoli. *James Syme, 1799–1870 (Scottish surgeon)*

Tay–Sachs disease Autosomal recessive *Type I GM2 gangliosidosis* affecting ~1:4000 Ashkenazi Jewish births (1:320,000 in the general population). Decreased lysosomal hexosaminidase A enzyme activity results in accumulation of gangliosides in neurons and progressive neurodegeneration. Low levels of enzyme are detectable in carriers. Children are normal until ~6 months old, when developmental delay, photophobia, hyperacusis, and irritability occur. There is progression to uncontrolled seizures, spasticity, blindness, and dementia. Death occurs at ~3–5yrs, typically from pneumonia. *Δ:* HEX A enzyme activity; DNA analysis. *Ophthalmoscopy:* Cherry-red spot at macula. The condition is now rare due to genetic screening, prenatal diagnosis (made by amniocentesis), & preimplantation genetic diagnosis. *Warren Tay 1843–1927 (British ophthalmologist); Bernard Sachs, 1858–1944 (US neurologist)*

Tolosa–Hunt syndrome Painful ophthalmoplegia and ipsilateral ocular motor nerve palsies, from non-specific granulomatous inflammation in the cavernous sinus or superior orbital fissure. The cause is unknown. MRI may show inflammatory changes. Corticosteroids are the treatment of choice, but may not resolve ophthalmoparesis. *Eduardo Tolosa 1900–1981 (Spanish neurosurgeon); William E Hunt, 1921–1999 (US neurosurgeon)*

Treacher Collins syndrome *(mandibulofacial dysostosis)* ^{Autosomal dominant} Craniofacial deformities with characteristic flattening of malar bones, hypoplastic zygoma, micrognathia, cleft palate, oblique palpebral fissures, external ear anomalies, and conductive hearing loss. *Cause:* TCOF1 gene mutations. *Reconstructive surgery* is an option.

Edward Treacher Collins, 1862–1932 (British ophthalmologist)

Turner syndrome 45,X0 monosomy in 40–60% or mosaic pattern in remaining karyotypes, eg 45,X/46,XX or 45,X/47,XXX. *Prevalence:* 1:2000 girls. *Signs: Newborn:* lymphoedema of the hands & feet; cardiac and renal abnormalities (coarctation of aorta; absent kidney). *Infancy:* short stature, webbed neck, behavioural difficulties, recurrent otitis media, and hearing loss. *Adolescence:* gonadal dysgenesis (streak ovary) results in absent or incomplete puberty, amenorrhoea, and impaired growth. Δ: Chromosomal analysis. *Association:* Autoimmune disease (screen for thyroid disorders, diabetes, & coeliac disease). ℞: Recombinant human growth hormone is used to treat short stature. Supplemental oestrogen (started ~12yrs) initiates pubertal development and prevents osteoporosis. Treatment is progressed to maintenance with larger oestrogen doses cycled with progesterone (eg as COCP). Surveillance and screening of cardiac, renal, ENT, & autoimmune problems. Psychological support. Almost all affected women are infertile but pregnancy with donor embryos is possible.[51]

Henry Turner, 1892–1970 (US endocrinologist)

Ulysses syndrome After the Trojan war, Ulysses decided to come home, but it took him 10 years and many perilous and perhaps pointless adventures before he returned to his starting place. Similarly, our patients with Ulysses syndrome find themselves caught in a web of further investigations, referrals, and sometimes treatment before finally being recognized as healthy, which they were in the first place. It is a side effect of unnecessary and inappropriate investigations or wrong interpretation of results. NB: the term is also applied to the effects of chronic extreme stress on migrant populations with resultant somatoform symptoms.

Described by Mercer Rang, 1933–2003 (British paediatric orthopaedic surgeon)

Von Gierke syndrome *(type 1a glycogen storage disease; GSD1A)* ^{Autosomal recessive} Glucose-6-phosphatase deficiency blocks the final steps of glycogenolysis and gluconeogenesis causing clinically significant end-organ disease. Δ: Mutation analysis of G6PC gene. *Signs:* Hepatomegaly (glycogen & fat accumulation), renomegaly, growth retardation, hypoglycaemia, hyperuricaemia, failure to thrive, dyslipidaemia, xanthomata over joints and buttocks, and platelet dysfunction. ℞: Diet therapy to prevent hypoglycaemia. *Complications:* Hepatic adenoma; hepatocellular cancer; kidney disease.[52]

Edgar Otto Conrad von Gierke, 1877–1945 (German pathologist)

Werner syndrome *(WS; progeria)* ^{Autosomal recessive} The commonest premature ageing syndrome. *Signs:* Lack of pubertal growth spurt & scleroderma; prematurely aged appearance (20–30yrs old) + typical associated problems: loss or greying of hair, cataracts, dyslipidaemia, diabetes, atherosclerosis, and ↑ malignancy. The complex molecular and cellular phenotypes of WS involve features of genomic instability and accelerated replicative senescence. The gene involved (WRN) has been cloned and its gene product (WRNP) is a helicase. Helicases play important roles in a variety of DNA transactions, including DNA replication, transcription, repair, and recombination, and in WS unwinding of DNA pairs is disordered.[53] ℞: None specific; treat related problems.

CW Otto Werner, 1879–1936 (German physician)

Wiskott–Aldrich syndrome *(WAS)* ^{X-linked recessive} A severe primary immunodeficiency (p. 244) with eczema, recurrent infections, thrombocytopenia, autoimmune disorders, IgA nephropathy ± haematopoietic neoplasia. Platelets are too few and too small. Without marrow transplant, most die before adulthood. Prenatal diagnosis is possible. ℞: Antibiotics ± IV immunoglobulin for infections. Haematopoietic stem cell transplant is 1st-choice therapy. Gene therapy is awaited.

Alfred Wiskott, 1898–1978 (German paediatrician); Robert A Aldrich, 1917–1998 (US paediatrician)

The 9th edition of this book claimed to be the first medical book to take the health of its readers seriously—on the grounds that the health of one person (a patient) must not be bought at the expense of another (their doctor). It is an unsettling paradox that when we study and practise medicine, our own health may be forgotten. This new chapter aims to support and resource you, and if needed, allow you to reclaim yourself.

Medicine is challenging and stressful. Healthcare environments are emotional places to work. Your every day is often a patient's or relative's worst ever day and this can take its toll. While the majority of doctors derive satisfaction from their work, it is important to recognize increasing burnout, stress, and dissatisfaction, which for some translates into mental illness, depression, or anxiety.[1] If you are feeling drained, isolated, dehumanized or are experiencing hurt or insecurity, remember that your identity as a doctor does not take precedence over your identity as a human. Before we attempt to heal others we should, if needed, take care of our own healing. By concentrating on our physical, psychological, and emotional well-being, we can be more empowered and better capable of helping our patients.

You will have bad days, and at times medicine may not seem worthwhile, yet among the valleys there should also be peaks of satisfaction and fulfilment. Remember and cherish the mountaintop experiences, but also remember that very little grows on the summit. Finding out what can lead you through adversity is the art of living. We hope this chapter helps.

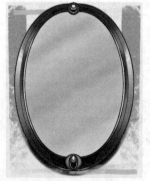

Fig 15.1 Throughout this book, at the start of each chapter, we have included inspiring stories of people or inventions that have changed and shaped healthcare. Our hope is that these stories can inspire you to achieve things that may at present seem beyond your perceived ability or possibility.

For this reason, at the start of this chapter, we include a mirror. Imagine a reflection of yourself. You are the inspiration: to your patients or colleagues, to family or friends. It may be because of who you are and how you treat others; it may be through advances that you bring—to your hospital, surgery, or specialty. Be the inspiration, and be encouraged.

Artwork by Gillian Turner.

With many thanks to our junior readers Grace Castronovo and Eliot Hurn for their contribution to this chapter.

Quis custodiet ipsos custodes? ('Who watches the watchmen?') Juvenal

Doctors have a higher than average incidence of suicide and alcoholism, and we must all be prepared to face, and try to prevent, these and other health risks of our professional and private lives. Our own illnesses are invaluable in allowing us to understand our patients, what makes people go to the doctor (or avoid going to the doctor), and the barriers we may erect to resist advice.

If the time comes when our health seriously reduces our ability to work, we must be able to recognize this and take appropriate action. The following may indicate that this point is approaching:

• Drinking alcohol before ward rounds, surgeries, or patient contact.
• The minimizing of every contact with patients, so that the doctor does the bare minimum which will suffice.
• Inability to concentrate on the matter in hand. Your thoughts are entirely taken up with the workload ahead or with other problems in your life.
• Excessive irritability with those around you at work or outside work.
• Inability to take time off without feeling guilty.
• Feelings of excessive shame or anger when reviewing past debacles. ►To avoid mistakes it would be necessary for us all to give up medicine.
• Emotional exhaustion—eg knowing that you should be feeling pleased or cross with yourself or others, but on consulting your heart you draw a blank.
• Prospective studies suggest that introversion, masochism, and isolation are important risk factors for doctors' impairment.

The first step in countering these unfavourable states of mind is to recognize that one is present. The next step is to confide in someone you trust (fig 15.2). Give your mind time to rejuvenate itself.

If these steps fail, various psychotherapeutic approaches may be relevant, eg cognitive behavioural therapy (p. 754), or you might try prescribing the symptom. For example, if you are plagued by recurring thoughts about how poorly you treated a patient, set time aside to deliberately ruminate on the affair, avoiding distractions. This is the first step in gaining control. You initiate the thought, rather than the thought initiating itself. The next step is to interpose some neutral topic, once the 'bad' series of thoughts is under way. After repeated practice, the mind automatically flows into the neutral channel once the bad thoughts begin, and the cycle of shame

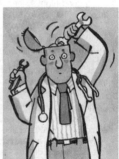

Fig 15.2 Hands-off! Don't get too drawn into treating your own mental health without consulting a colleague.

and rumination is broken. ►In addition ... learn from the experience!

If no progress is made, the time has come to consult an expert, such as your GP or the Practitioner Health Programme (see p. 878). If you think you need to consult a doctor, then do so, in privacy. Avoid 'corridor consultations' with colleagues. Other than for minor ailments, avoid self-diagnosis and management. Treat yourself as you would expect a patient with the same condition to be treated—and have a confidential consultation with a trusted health professional.

If you are the expert that another doctor has approached, do not be deceived by this honour into thinking that you must treat your new patient in any special way. Special treatment leads to special mistakes, and it is far better for doctor–patients to tread well-worn paths of referral, investigation, and treatment than to try illusory short cuts.

Every person's experience with stress is different. What is common is that we all have stresses in our lives—whether it is money, relationships, work, or something else. Stress is something many of us find hard to talk about. Stress is generally assessed with the General Health Questionnaire (GHQ). Higher scores imply likelihood of depression and anxiety difficulties. Burnout (p. 863) is different than 'simple stress', with work-related instead of physical symptoms.

Engaging in reflection can help you manage stress. Acknowledge your emotions about difficult patients or challenging clinical scenarios—reflection is a valuable part of practice and is different from rumination (repetitively going over a thought or problem without completion). Consider joining a Balint group or engaging in Schwartz rounds.

While everyone has different ways to manage stress, here are 10 elements—5 things to do and 5 things not to do—to incorporate into your daily life in order to manage and reduce stress:

Do

1 Set (achievable) goals to feel more in control. Choose a realistic target but one that is important and map out how to achieve it. Positive steps forward help us feel more in charge and reduce stress.

2 Have a heathy diet with green vegetables (folate), oily fish (omega-3), whole grains (complex carbohydrates), and berries (vitamin c). All increase serotonin and boost mood.

3 Get a good night's sleep. Aim for 7–9 hours most nights. We can get into an unhealthy cycle: stress reduces sleep and tiredness increases stress. Find what works for you to sleep better. But avoid too much sleep as that can have a similar negative impact.

4 Do something you enjoy which raises your heart rate. Physical activity releases endorphins which relieve tension.

5 Socialize with people who you love and who support you. Stress can make us isolate and shut down.

Do not

1 Do not touch your phone for a couple of nights or a whole day each week. Social media can be stressful—it's easy to compare yourself unfavourably against a filtered version of someone else's life. Switch screens off once you're home or at least don't check work emails. Avoid using screens before bed which disrupts sleep.

2 Do not asssociate with stressful people—reduce the amount of time you spend with them or end the relationship. You don't have be friends with everyone you meet.

3 Do not use too much caffeine and sugar as mood boosters. Your blood sugar will soon come crashing down again, bringing your stress back with it.

4 Do not say 'yes' to everything. You can easily become overworked and stressed. Learn to say 'no', set healthy work limits, and delegate more by dividing jobs and sharing projects.

5 Do not ignore your feelings. It's easy to accept stress as part of life. Chronic stress can be damaging, resulting in an increased risk of IHD, a weakened immune system, and faster ageing processes.

☺ Burnout (running beyond empty)

Definition Falling performance and personal accomplishments, emotional exhaustion, negative affect, poor leadership, and depersonalization brought on by months or years of overexposure to emotionally demanding situations at work, on the battlefield, or at home (see MINIBOX and fig 15.3).

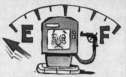

Fig 15.3 Have you felt this way?

Measurement The Five Minute Speech Sample and the Maslach Burnout Inventory.[3]

Risk factors

For doctors: Lack of hobbies, lack of physical activity, and lack of enough time for vacations and religious activities are all important.[4] Pressure of work, conflict with colleagues,[5] less personal relationships with patients, overly formal hierarchies, & suboptimal income are put forward to explain the fact that some doctors are more at risk of burnout than others.[6] Factors associated with emotional exhaustion: 'having to deaden one's conscience', lack of time to provide needed care, work being so demanding that it influences one's home life, and not being able to live up to others' expectations.[7]

For psychiatric nurses: Unreciprocated giving, violent client population[8] leading to vicarious traumatization,[9] & frequency of on-calls.[10] High expressed emotion (evidenced by critical comments ± negative relationships) predicts depersonalization elements of burnout.[3]

For medical students: Impulsivity, depression, & money worries are predictive.[11]

Signs of burnout
• Stress and depression
• Fatigue
• Non-restorative sleep[2]
• Emotional exhaustion
• Motivation ↓; apathy ↑
• Libido ↓
• Insomnia
• Guilt or denial
• Paranoia/isolated
• Demoralization
• Amnesia
• Indecision
• Temper tantrums
• Low personal accomplishment
• Depersonalization
• Irritability/impatience

Management Some may respond to plans such as:
• Use the Copenhagen Burnout Inventory to measure work-related burnout.
• Diagnose and treat any depression (p. 710).
• Allow time for the person to recognize that there is a problem.
• More hobbies, and more nice holidays.
• Advice from wise colleagues in the specialty (regular follow-up). Mentoring consists of forming a supportive relationship with an independent colleague for the sole purpose of support.
• Return meaning and purpose to life via dialogue, self-transcendence, and a sense of connectedness with others (meaning-centred psychotherapy).[12]
• Learn new professional skills—or consider early retirement.
• Set achievable goals in work and leisure (eg protected time with family).

Prevention Strategies such as career counselling are said to be effective but really do no more than point a lollipop at a furnace.[13, n=171] *Reducing stress* is one (unproven) way of avoiding burnout. Psychiatrists have found their own 'stress busting' groups helpful—these entail problem-solving with airing of stresses—ideally accompanied by talking to colleagues for support and catharsis.

Having outside interests helps, as does getting support from family and friends, time management, and exercise.[14] On a more universal plane, ▶*we are all responsible for each other's burnout.* By being attentive to our own and others' feelings of troubled conscience we all have a role in preventing the burnout of our colleagues. We need opportunities to reflect on our troubled consciences. Appraisals (p. 872) and less formal routes to this awareness are becoming more accepted.[7]

'Bouncebackability' Iain Dowie, football manager.

Resilience The quality of being able to recover quickly or easily from, or resist being affected by, stressful events. It is derived from the Latin verb *'salire'* = to jump and the prefix 're-' = 'again'. Resilience is literally about jumping back. Resilient individuals demonstrate 6Cs:

• *Commitment:* Persistence in adversity.
• *Composure:* Low anxiety despite high-intensity situations.
• *Confidence:* Trusting your own feelings, judgements, and decisions.
• *Challenges:* The ability to manage challenges and make adversity meaningful.
• *Control:* Recognition of your own limits of responsibilities and power.
• *Coordination:* Predicting and planning for stress.

According to NHS England, a high level of resilience can be recognized in the following characteristics: • The ability to engage with and utilize others for your own support and development • The ability to manage negative emotions • The ability to assert influence but accept external controls • The ability to learn from past experience • The ability to seek and use supportive environmental factors • Practising the use of protective factors.

Being resilient maintains our health and well-being, increasing our compassion, empathy, and physical and mental health. It reduces burnout and helps us, as cynical doctors, to reconnect with the joy and purpose of our work. On a wider scale, staff resilience safeguards quality and sustainability of services. Where resilience is depleted, issues develop with slowing of work, sickness/absence, and ineffectual communication with teams and patients. Systemic issues within the NHS, such as understaffing, overworking, being under-resourced or poorly supported all contribute to burnout and it is important to acknowledge that even the most resilient of people may struggle when encountering issues they cannot directly address or control.

Resilience itself is not a stable trait but rather a dynamic state that can change between situations and over the lifespan. It can be learnt, practised, and shared. By now you will likely be thinking, 'How resilient am I?' This online resource is a good place to start: resiliencyquiz.com.

How do we develop resilience?

Be agile: Mental agility here hinges on the capacity to 'decentre' a stressor in order to efficiently handle it. This means responding to, rather than reacting to, a problematic event. 'Decentring' a stress doesn't ignore our feelings of being stressed; it allows us to pause, observe the experience from a neutral standpoint, and problem-solve. By pivoting attention from what we are feeling (the narrative experience) to what we are seeing, we can shift perspective, protect ourselves against being overwhelmed, and generate options. Upset toddlers are told 'use your words', because stopping and labelling emotions activates cognitive, rather than emotional, responses which are necessary to reflect and act.

Be (temporarily) detached: We have circadian (daily) rhythm and also ultradian (hourly) rhythms—times where our energy and productivity rises or falls. Mental focus cycles typically last 1–1.5 hours; outside these times, try to take a break just for a few minutes to 'reset' your motivation and regain drive. This can be tough, especially in a busy clinic or ward round, but even a brief time for detaching from an activity can promote increased energy and focus. This ultimately grows capacity for resilience throughout the course of the workday, preserving energy and preventing burnout over the longer term.

Be kind: This means to others and to yourself. Effectivity and kindness are mutually exclusive. Being compassionate helps increase cooperation and collaboration; in individuals it generates positive emotions and improves relationships. Stanford University's Centre for Compassion, Altruism and Research in Education (CCARE) runs 'Compassion training programs' which have demonstrated that practising kindness increases well-being and decreases stress. Develop your skills in treating challenging situations or disagreements as an opportunity to learn and potentially build a deeper relationship.

Be mindful: It is hard to describe 'mindfulness' in a medical textbook without it sounding fluffy and unscientific but there are clear evidence-based positive outcomes associated with using these techniques in clinical environments. At its root, mindfulness is simply focusing attention to the present moment—to your own thoughts and feelings, and to the world around you—to the exclusion of other thoughts, worries, or future planning. By reconnecting with our body and our sensations we can regain control over our thoughts. This feeling of control can boost resilience. Mindfulness needs to be practised but, once skilled up, it's easy to incorporate into daily life.

Be selfish: This means prioritizing your own health. Make sure your physical health is maintained: make sure you are engaging in the same high-quality preventive primary care that you would wish your own patients to receive. Check your mental health too, sometimes, withdrawing is protective. But it is also important to connect and give into personal relationships. We are more than technicians—take time each day to foster healthy relationships, with patients, colleagues, and friends.

Be regimented: We can't control the amount of information we receive—up to 11 million bits of information every second—but we can optimize how we process it. It may sound a little robotic, but try assigning tasks to different areas: work/family/relationships and then subdivide into activities—workplace-based activity eg ward tasks, research, etc. By compartmentalizing, it's easier to switch between tasks, make quality decisions, and stop thinking about other parts when you don't need to, increasing productivity. Even better, create dedicated times for specific activities (exclusively) as you would for a gym session or a favourite TV show. This is called 'serial monotasking'. It may feel overly regimented for some but it's worth a go.

☺ Bullying and harassment

Bullying can significantly increase job-induced stress leading to lowered self-confidence, anxiety, and depression. With this comes decreased job satisfaction and implications for recruitment and retention across the NHS.

Bullying in medicine is more common than we would like, particularly for junior doctors and students. Victims are often stereotyped as 'weak' but bullies are insecure and therefore target those who elicit jealous feelings: high-achievers and well-performing doctors. There is nothing to be ashamed of if you have been bullied.

The medical profession often uses hierarchical structures and traditional teaching methods, including intimidation and humiliation, which can result in a bullying cycle. This culture is analogous to 'abuse cycles' whereby those who experience it go on to abuse others when they take positions of power. There is no longer any value to the 'I was taught this way so it must be OK' approach.

If you feel you are being bullied, discuss it with someone. Talk to your predecessors—did they have similar difficulties? How did they handle it? Keep a diary of relevant events and witnesses. Speak to your consultant (or another trusted consultant if it is they who are the problem).

Trainees in difficulty

'A concern about a doctor's practice can be said to have arisen where an incident causes, or has the potential to cause, harm to a patient, staff or the organisation; or where the doctor develops a pattern of repeating mistakes, or appears to behave persistently in a manner inconsistent with the standards described in Good Medical Practice.' GMC, 2006

Any trainee can encounter difficulties during their education, for a variety of reasons: medicine is a highly pressured working environment with frequent job changes for junior doctors who may feel unsupported or socially isolated. For the majority, these difficulties are temporary blips which are usually resolved through supervision and support. As we move through training we are expected to take on more responsibility, which includes managing juniors. A good supervisor will support trainees and clearly identify the struggling minority so that they can receive additional support.

Performance problems are rarely straightforward. They often relate to interpersonal and personality difficulties which emerge during periods of stress. Poorly performing doctors and medical students often have problems in a range of different areas (known as 'a persistent pattern of poor performance'), each falling short of a serious enough problem for direct action. These doctors underperform in all domains, rather than being deficient in particular domains. Poor performance indicators may include the following:

- *The 'disappearing act':* Not answering bleeps; disappearing between clinic and ward; lateness.
- *Rigidity:* Poor tolerance of ambiguity; inability to compromise; inappropriate 'whistle blowing'.
- *Low work rate:* Slowness in doing procedures; clerking patients; dictating letters; making decisions.
- *'Ward rage':* Bursts of temper; real or imagined slights.
- *'Bypass syndrome':* Colleagues or nurses find ways to avoid seeking the doctor's opinion or help.
- *Career problems:* Difficulty with exams; lack of expected progression; uncertainty about career choice; disillusionment with medicine.
- *Insight failure:* Rejection of constructive criticism; defensiveness.

Trainees in difficulty often have a combination of the following factors:

- *Personality:* Anxious; overconfident narcissist; perfectionist/obsessional.
- *Situation:* Over-busy, under-supported; poor existing morale; weak team or poor team communication.
- *Personal:* Drug/alcohol misuse; relationship problems; mental health difficulties; change in jobs; exam stress.

Above all else, the strongest predictor of poor performance is *alexithymia*: a psychological concept that refers to an inability to connect with or be aware of one's own feelings or the feelings of others. Individuals may have alexithymia as a primary personality trait, or (more commonly) develop an induced alexithymia due to prolonged stress. ►This is burnout (see p. 863).

Early recognition and appropriate intervention, coupled with effective feedback and appropriate support for trainees in difficulty (and their supervisors) are essential. A supervisor should:

1 Ensure a positive, safe learning environment.
2 Deal with problems when they arise.
3 Clearly identify what the problem behaviour is with specific examples; identifying 'problem themes'.
4 Hear the trainee's point of view and encourage reflection.
5 Resist the temptation to 'pathologize' (but not miss health problems).

The hardest part is resisting the temptation to leave it for someone else to deal with or stop the process due to worries about counterclaims. Because of this, the GMC advises that supervisors take advice and seek support.

Over- and underperforming doctors

It would be nice for the public and the 'leaders' of our profession if there were a small number of underperforming doctors who could be retrained or removed from the GMC register. Things are rarely so simple, and we may have to accept that, for many reasons, including chance, training, and resilience, the performance of *all doctors* will, at times, be, or appear to be, suboptimal.

Could differences in data comparing doctors (even if that data were accurate, validated, and stratified for risk) occur by chance? Imagine a thought-experiment in which 4 equal doctors use different strategies for predicting whether a tossed coin will land heads or tails. One always chooses heads, one always chooses tails, and the other two alternate their choices out of synchrony with each other. When I did this experiment for a pre-decided 14 throws each (56 throws in total), the best doctor only had 2 'errors', whereas the worst had 7 errors—over 3 times the rate. The public would demand that this doctor be retrained or struck off. So, must we all be prepared to be sacrificial lambs? The answer is Yes, but there are certain steps that can be taken to mitigate our own and our patients' risk exposure.

- When we encounter doctors who are clearly underperforming (eg due to a health problem), we must speak out. This will encourage belief in the system.
- GMC guidance says *'All doctors have a duty to raise concerns where they believe that patient safety or care is being compromised by the practice of colleagues, or the systems, policies and procedures in the organisations in which they work. They must also encourage and support a culture in which staff can raise concerns openly and safely'.*[1]
- We should encourage an atmosphere of mutual support and trust—the sort of environment in which doctors feel safe to say 'All my cases of x seem to be going wrong—can anyone think why?' To stop this trust turning into cronyism we must be prepared to engage in, or be subjected to, audit (p.874).
- See also 'Trainees in difficulty', p. 866 & 'Whistleblowing', p.873.

Social media: professional use, personal use, or not at all?

It can be difficult to know how to use social media, and as doctors we have been given mixed messages. You might use social media solely in a professional or personal capacity, or a mix of the two, switching personas across different sites. Social media has many benefits—you can use it to learn, build relationships, network, provide peer support, influence debate, campaign, or simply use it for fun. As a doctor there are some risks to posting online—even if you do not identify yourself or post about medical matters, the ethical and legal standards expected of you still apply. What follows is some general advice from the BMA:

- Maintain a professional distance between you and your patients (there should be an overriding presumption against online interactions with people you only know from a doctor–patient context).
- Do not provide personalized health advice or discuss a patient's health via social media.
- Protect patient confidentiality. Even heavily anonymized information may allow a patient to be identified.
- Think before you post: don't post when angry, drunk, or emotionally upset.
- Don't say anything on social media that you would not want printed in a newspaper.
- The GMC recommends that if you identify yourself as a doctor online, it is best practice, but not mandatory, to also give your name.
- Declare any conflicts of interest.
- Manage your privacy settings and content. Whatever you choose, privacy cannot be guaranteed. Are you happy for a post to be shared wider than you originally intended?

BMA guidance (2018). *Social Media, Ethics and Professionalism* **and** *Social Media: Practical Guidance and Best Practice*. London: BMA.

1 GMC (2012). *Raising and Acting on Concerns about Patient Safety*, p5. London: GMC.

We have all been manipulated by our patients, and it is wrong to encourage in ourselves such stiffness of character and inflexibility of mind that all attempts by our patients to manipulate us inevitably fail. Nevertheless, a patient's manipulative behaviour is often counterproductive, and reinforces maladaptive behaviour. A small minority of patients are *very* manipulative, and take a disproportionate toll on your resources, and those of their family, friends, and colleagues. We are all familiar with these patients whom Madox Ford describes as being 'like fireships on a crowded lagoon, causing conflagration in their wake'.[15] After destroying their family and their home we watch these people cruise down the ward or into our surgeries with some trepidation. Can we stop them losing control, and causing meltdown of our own and our staff's equanimity? The first thing to appreciate is that these people *can* be communicated with, and you *can* help them.

Setting limits One way of avoiding becoming caught up in this web of maladaptive behaviour is to set limits, as soon as this behaviour starts. In a small minority of patients, the doctor may recognize that their needs for time, attention, sedation, and protection are, for all practical purposes, insatiable. Whatever a doctor gives, such patients come back for more and more, and yet in spite of all this 'input' they don't get any better. The next step is to realize that if inappropriate demands are not met, the patient will not become sicker (there may be vociferous complaints!). This realization paves the way for setting limits to behaviour, specifying just what is and is not allowed.

Take, for example, the patient who demands sedation, threatening to 'lose control' if it is not given immediately, stating that he cannot bear living another day without sedation, and that the doctor will be responsible for any damage which ensues. If it is decided that drugs do not have a part to play in treatment, and that the long-term aim is for the patient to learn to be responsible for himself, then it can be simply stated to the patient that medication will not be given, and that he is free to engage in destructive acts, and that if he does so this is his responsibility.

The doctor explains that in demanding instant sedation he undermines her professional role, which is to decide these matters according to her own expert judgement, and that this is not beneficial to anyone. If there is serious risk of real harm, admission to hospital may be indicated, where further limits may be set. If necessary, he is told that if he insists on 'going crazy' he will be put in a seclusion room, to protect others. Every person is responsible for the decisions they make, and if necessary, security can be asked to escort a patient out of the hospital, in line with hospital policies on abusive behaviour.

►Are you afraid of uncomfortable questions? Here are some asked by a very experienced psychotherapist.[2]

• Are you a saint? Or have you ever ...
  • Felt so bored and irritated by certain patients you want to quit?
  • Longed for the consultation to end, at any price?
• Can you say you have *never* felt a flicker of sexual interest in a patient?
• Have you never imagined the death of certain patients and the relief that would bring, not just to them but to us, their impotent carers?
• Have you never resented the demands of people for whom illness seems to have become a way of life?
• Whose thoughts have not sometimes drifted off towards their own concerns—to the need for sleep, food, or distraction or to some family, career, or future plans?

►The key to good doctoring is not regulation or revalidation, but

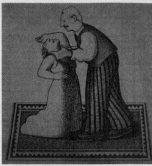

Fig 15.4 We may imagine doing all sorts of things to our patients. The crime is not the thought but the deed. The vital thing is to not bury these things but to know that they are just that: imaginings. Perhaps we can use them in the service of our work? If the stressed, isolated doctor had been aware of and able to voice his fantasies maybe he would not have ended up in custody or in bed with his sexually abused, vulnerable, and depressed patient.

fostering the ability to put ourselves in our patients' shoes. And we can use the feeling patients engender in us to understand how the patient's nearest and dearest are frustrated, perplexed, and deluded. For example, excessive worry about a patient may be the result of being infected by the patient's anxiety—beyond what is reasonable. This is known as *projective identification*.

Why does bad or harmful practice continue, despite GMC guidelines? It is because we are motivated by forces of which we are unaware (fig 15.4).

2 See Good doctor, bad doctor—a psychodynamic approach. *BMJ* 2002;325:722 by Jeremy Holmes (whom we thank for permission to quote from his excellent article).

Here is a list of some of the things pundits tell us we should be doing when we meet patients:[16]

1 *Listen*—no interrupting or taking control of the agenda (how often are we guilty of implying: 'Don't talk to me when I am interrupting you'?).
2 Examine the patient thoroughly (to establish the likelihood of competing diagnoses).
3 Arrange cost-effective incremental investigation.
4 Formulate a differential diagnosis in social, psychological, and physical terms.
5 Explain the diagnosis to the patient in simple terms (then re-explain it to relatives, and then try re-explaining it to the computer in terms *it* understands—ie searchable codes).
6 Consider additional problems and risk factors for promoting health.
7 List all the treatment options, and seek out relevant guidelines etc. (evidence-based bedside medicine).
8 Incorporate the patient's view on the balance of risks and benefits, harmonizing their view of priorities, with your own assessment of urgency.
9 Arrange follow-up and communicate with all of the healthcare team.
10 Arrange for purchase of all necessary care, weighing up cost implications for your other patients and the community, welcoming accountability for all acts and omissions, and for the efficient use of resources—with justifications based on explicit criteria, transparency, and principles of autonomy, non-maleficence, beneficence, and distributive justice.

The alternative Do your best.

The synthesis The alternative looks promising—even attractive, when compared with the 10 (im)possibilities just listed. But note that the alternative only looks attractive because it is vague. 'Do your best' is not very helpful advice—and once we start unpacking this 'best' we start to get a list like the 10 earlier points. *'Professionalism'* sums up *part* of what being a good doctor entails—ie: • Self-regulation • Self-actuating and self-monitoring of standards of care • Altruism • Commitment to service • Specialist knowledge and technical skills reflecting but not determined by society's values • Consistently working to high standards of probity and quality (no bribes, no favouritism, but a dynamic concern for distributive justice) • Self-determination—in relation to the range and pattern of the kinds of problems it is right to attempt to solve. For a further discussion, see *On Being a Doctor: Redefining medical professionalism for better patient care* (King's Fund, 2004) and fig 15.5.

Authenticity Trying to achieve authenticity is a meta-goal, and may be a better mast to nail your colours to than the 10 points listed earlier. Not because it is easier, but because paying attention to authenticity may make you a better doctor, whereas striving for all 10 of the points may make you perform less well (too many conflicting ideals). With *inauthentic consultations* you may be chasing remunerative activities, quality points, protocols, or simply be trying to clear the waiting room, at any cost, while the patient is trying to twist your arm into giving antibiotics or a medical certificate. *Authentic consultations* are those where there are no barriers; just two humans without status exploring and sharing hypotheses and beliefs and deciding what to do for the best (along the lines described in detail on pp. 790-1)—with no ulterior motives and no conflicts of interest. Authentic consultations know and tell the truth where possible, and where this is not possible, the truth is worked towards—diligently and fearlessly.

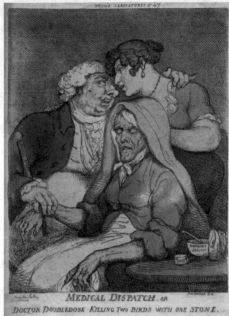

Fig 15.5 How *not* to be a good doctor: Rowlandson's Doctor Doubledose 'Killing Two Birds with One Stone' (1810). '*With one podgy hand the physician takes the pulse of the cadaverous senseless invalid, while throwing an arm around the neck of the nubile girl. The "Composing Draught" and opium pillbox on the table suggest the physician may be giving his patient a helping hand out of this world, so as to switch his medical ministrations to her maid.*'[17] Georgian anti-medical satire was designed to deflate, lampoon, and expose pretension in the profession. The standing of early modern medics was precarious—disease and death held sway and doctors prescribed violent and painful procedures. Threats to one's body were not just physical—Rowlandson's other works depict doctors gawping at and groping their patients in a most un-Hippocratic manner.[17] The 1841 Census estimated a third of all doctors were unqualified, with over 19 bodies regulating the medical profession—all using different tests for competence. There was no real way of saying who a doctor was until the GMC was established in 1858 allowing medical education and registration to be regulated.[18] Since then self-regulation has been replaced with professional regulation, and consequently we see a high public trust in doctors—one that must not be taken for granted, and one that is up to us to maintain and protect.

Appraisal All UK doctors practising medicine undergo a yearly appraisal. It has moved from being an informal chat with a peer to a formal structured review on which revalidation (see later) is based. The supporting information that doctors use at their appraisal falls into 4 broad categories:

1 *General information:* Giving context about what you do in all aspects of work.
2 *Keeping up to date:* How you maintain and enhance the quality of your work.
3 *Review of your practice:* Evaluating the quality of your professional work.
4 *Feedback on your practice:* How others perceive the quality of your work.

There are 5 types of supporting information that you need to provide and discuss at your appraisal:

1 *Continuing professional development (CPD):* CPD is the process of tracking and documenting knowledge and experience gained both formally and informally as you work + how you apply this to your work. CPD should be relevant to the current and emerging knowledge and skills required for your roles. You also need to reflect and evaluate on what you have learnt and how this improves your performance. 50 hours of CPD are required each year.
2 *Quality improvement activity:* Eg completion of an audit cycle or a case review. Currently this is only required once every 5-year revalidation cycle.
3 *Significant events:* Record any incidents or events ± any investigation or analysis of these, lessons learnt, and action taken/changes implemented.
4 *Feedback from colleagues and feedback from patients:* These are collected once every 5-year cycle using standardized questionnaires.
5 *Review of complaints and compliments.*

Appraisal is a supportive developmental process, to reflect on your work and consider developmental needs. 'By giving feedback on performance it provides the opportunity to identify any factors that adversely affect performance, and to consider how to minimize or eliminate their effects. It is an important building block in a clinical governance culture that *ensures* high standards and the best possible patient care.'[Chief Medical Officer][19]

There is a big question-mark over '*ensures*'. The effect of appraisal on patient care is unknown—but appraisal, it is hoped, can offer opportunities for interdependent support, self-education, self-motivation, and career development in the wider medical world. It may also be a catalyst for change and even a tonic against complacency.

Appraisal assumes doctors are professional, life-long learners (the 'move-&-grow' aspect of challenging appraisals). If this is not the case, the less cosy revalidation, performance management, assessment, and mediation will bite.

The *Annual Review of Competence Progression (ARCP)* is the appraisal and revalidation process for all specialty trainees, including general practice trainees, where a panel from the Deanery meet to consider the evidence/documentation provided by the trainee and assess their suitability to progress.

►If you decide not to work in a formal training programme (eg F3), you are responsible for organizing your appraisal and evidencing professional development in order to revalidate—this includes if you have been working overseas and wish to return to work in the UK.

Licence to practise To practise medicine in the UK, all doctors are required to be registered with the GMC and hold a licence to practise. This gives a doctor the legal authority to undertake certain activities in the UK, eg prescribing, signing death or cremation certificates, and working as a doctor in the NHS. Re-licensing occurs every 5 years by the process of revalidation.

Revalidation The process by which licensed doctors are required to demonstrate they are up to date and fit to practise. It is achieved by having annual appraisals and by providing the required 'supporting information' listed earlier. Revalidation occurs every 5 years but may be deferred if insufficient evidence is provided or there are unresolved concerns about a doctor's performance.

'Whistleblowing' and raising concerns

Whistleblowing is the term given when workplace concerns about serious safety or malpractice issues are raised in the public interest.[3] The GMC states that doctors have a professional duty to raise concerns where patient safety may be at risk. Employers should have a formal policy for raising serious concerns and no one should be victimized as a result of raising a concern.

Should a concern be raised? Ask yourself 'If this situation continues as it is, is it likely to result in harm to others?' If yes, something should be done. Concerns could include: • Poor quality of care • Systemic failings (eg inadequate equipment, poorly organized emergency procedures) • Illness or substance misuse affecting a person's ability to work • Negligence • Malpractice • Fraud. They do not include raising a personal complaint or grievance (ie concerns about the way in which an employer has acted towards you).

How to raise a concern Follow the procedure set out in your employer's policy and keep dated records and notes of the issues you are concerned about. If you need advice at any stage before or during the process of raising a concern you can contact the BMA or *Protect* (formerly *Public Concern at Work*): www.pcaw.org.uk. The NHS commits to 'support all staff in raising concerns about safety, malpractice or wrongdoing at work'.

Further reading

GMC (2019). *Supporting Information for Revalidation and Appraisal*. https://www.gmc-uk.org
GMC (2019). *The Licence to Practise*. www.gmc-uk.org/doctors/licensing.asp

3 BMA (2018). *Guide to Raising Concerns*. www.bma.org.uk/advice/employment/raising-concerns/guide-to-raising-concerns

Clinical governance *The framework through which NHS organizations are accountable for continuously improving the quality of their services and safeguarding high standards of care, by creating an environment in which clinical excellence will flourish.* It links continuing professional development, multidisciplinary learning, audit, risk management, and significant event reporting/analysis. It is about defining quality (eg standards set by NICE, CQC, Quality and Outcomes Framework (QOF)), assuring accountability, and improving quality (by monitoring standards).

Essential elements:
- *Risk avoidance*—risk management; clear protocols; safe environment.
- *Infrastructure*—access to evidence; time; training strategies; IT support.
- *Clinical effectiveness*—sharing good practice; significant event audit; evidence-based medicine.
- *Audit*—regular review of practice against quality standards (see later).
- *Education/training*—effective appraisal; performance feedback; targeted education.
- *Staff*—training; leadership; communication; common goals/teamwork.

What does clinical governance entail?: Individual doctors must consider their own professional development and educational needs. There must also be continuous review and appraisal of procedures and standards. Deficiencies in knowledge, skills, or experience must be acted upon through appropriate education and professional development. Resources should be provided to help develop clinical governance (eg protected time for audit, funding for courses and educational activities).

Significant event analysis All hospitals and GP practices should have systems for reporting and investigating incidents which have or could cause harm to a patient. This should be done in a systematic and detailed way to ascertain what can be learnt about the overall quality of care and to indicate changes that might lead to future improvements.

Audit The systematic critical analysis of quality of healthcare. Its purpose is to appraise current practice (*What is happening?*) by measuring it against preselected standards (*What should be happening?*) to identify and implement areas for change (*What changes are needed?*) and thus improve performance. Audit is a continual process and an integral part of clinical governance.

Aims of audit	
• Improved care of patients.	• Aid to administration.
• Enhanced professionalism of staff.	• Efficient use of resources.
• Aid to continuing education.	• Accountability to those outside medicine.

Criterion-based audit—the audit cycle The process of identifying areas of care to be audited, implementing necessary changes, and periodically reviewing the same issues is known as the audit cycle.
1 *Identify the issue.* This can be any practice matter—clinical or administrative. Make sure the topic is important, manageable, clearly defined, and data are available to assess the criteria chosen. Good starting points are significant events, QOF targets, complaints, clinical guidelines, or personal observations.
2 *Agree criteria.* These are specific statements of what should be happening.
3 *Setting standards.* These are the minimum levels of acceptable performance for a criterion (100% achievement is unusual). Set realistic standards. These can be based on previous audit, comparison with other trusts/practices, or guidelines (eg '90% of patients with iron deficiency anaemia should be screened for coeliac disease; British Society of Gastroenterologists 2005').

4 *Planning and preparation.* What data will you use? How will you search for it? What literature has been consulted?

5 *First data collection.* What is current practice (compared to standards set)? What changes are needed?

6 *Implement changes.*

7 *Second data collection.* Monitor the effects of change and compare data with the first round of data collection and against standards set.

8 *Summary of findings.*

Care Quality Commission (CQC)

The CQC is the independent regulator of health and adult social care in England. It inspects care providers to ensure patients are receiving safe, effective, compassionate, and high-quality care. Providers (eg hospital trusts, GP practices, ambulance trusts, or care homes/agencies) are required to provide evidence that they meet fundamental standards and legal requirements. Five questions are asked of all care services being inspected:

1 Is it safe?
2 Is it effective?
3 Is it caring?
4 Is it responsive?
5 Is it well led?

CQC reports give 1 of 4 ratings for each of the 5 areas: • Inadequate • Requires improvement • Good • Outstanding. If needed, care providers are given notices setting out what improvements must be made and by when.

Complaints

Complaints are a fact of life for most doctors. The most constructive and least stressful approach is to view them as a learning experience and a chance to improve risk management. Always contact your defence organization if you are directly implicated in a complaint. Patients who complain generally want:

• Their complaint to be heard and investigated promptly; and handled efficiently and sympathetically.
• To receive a genuine apology if mistakes have occurred; and to be assured that steps will be taken to prevent a recurrence.

Time limit for complaints NHS complaints can only be accepted <1yr after the incident which is the subject of complaint, or <1yr after the date at which the complainant became aware of the matter. There is a 3yr time limit placed on civil negligence cases.

Process Once a complaint is received, the complaints manager should acknowledge the complaint within 48h and advise the complainant of the right to use the *Independent Complaints Advocacy Service*. The complaints manager investigates the complaint, consulting all involved, and makes a written summary of the nature of the complaint, investigation findings, ± apology, ± actions to remedy the situation/prevent further occurrences. This must be completed <25 days after the original date of the complaint. If the complaint is not resolved at this point, the complainant can refer the matter to the NHS ombudsman.

Medicine is the art of managing uncertainty. Many patients present with problems or symptoms that are undifferentiated and unorganized and do not have an obvious diagnosis at presentation. Many symptoms are also medically unexplained (see p. 803). Almost any symptom can be made to seem fatal ('Is this lethargy due to cancer?'), even seemingly trivial problems ('This pain in my toe …'—could it be due to an embous or osteomyelitis?). Medicine is for gamblers (see later) and in order to survive we must learn to manage uncertainty and avoid lying awake at night worrying about the meaning of our patients' symptoms. (See also p. 793.)

Tips for dealing with uncertainty

Consider the differential diagnosis: A careful history and examination will allow you to consider the differential diagnosis. Making decisions when there is uncertainty and risk is difficult. Decisions are based not just on risk but also on possible outcome. High-risk problems should have a lower threshold for action (eg for possible MI or appendicitis).

Time as a tool: The skilful use of time (by reviewing a patient over a number of consultations across a period of time) can obviate the need for extensive investigation, or allow for incremental investigations as symptoms develop, or the results of initial investigations emerge.

Evidence-based medicine: When deciding on an investigation or treatment, consider what evidence exists for its use, how valid the evidence is, and if it is applicable to the patient you are seeing. No treatment is completely safe, entirely effective, or without side effects.

Sharing uncertainty: Sharing uncertainty with patients may increase trust and avoids deception. We can also share uncertainty with colleagues (eg discussing symptoms with another doctor or referring to a specialist—this is also useful if you think the source of your uncertainty might be a gap in your own knowledge).

Safety netting: Discuss a contingency plan with the patient by informing them what to do if things don't go to plan (eg seeking urgent review if red flags develop with back pain, or educating a parent about the signs to look for that should prompt review of a febrile child).

Gamble safely: Making decisions under conditions of uncertainty is a form of gambling. We cannot refer and investigate every problem, yet we still need to make decisions. Some of these decisions will be scientific and rational. Some will be based on subtle clues or feelings. Make sure you assemble sufficient evidence to maximize your chances of being lucky.

Clinical governance: No matter how carefully we practise, adverse events will occur. It is important to discuss, reflect, and learn from any errors and improve systems to try and prevent similar events (see pp. 874-5).

When decision analysts started observing consultations they were amazed at the number of decisions per minute, and the wide range of possible outcomes, such as 'no action', 'admit', or 'refer', or 'test a or b', 'prescribe x, y, and z, and stop q in a week ...'. The average decision analyst is disorientated by the sheer pace and apparent effortlessness of these decisions—so much so that doctors were often suspected of choosing plans almost randomly, until the idea of a 'perceptual filter' was developed.

Perceptual filters This is the internal architecture of our mind—unique to each doctor—into which we receive the patient's history.[20] It comprises our:
- Unconscious mental set: *tired/uninterested* to *alert, engaged, responsive*.
- Entire education, from school, to the last lecture we attended.
- Sum of all our encounters with patients. Ignore the fact that we can recall very few of these: this does not stop them influencing us strongly—does the rock recall each of those many, many waves which have sculpted it into extraordinary shapes, or which have entirely worn it away?
- Past specific, personal experience with this particular patient.
- Past specific, personal experience with the disease(s) in question.
- Non-personal subjective (eg 'endocarditis is the most dangerous and stealthy disease ...') or objective ideas (eg evidence-based medicine).

The mind's working space The perceptual filter achieves nothing on its own. What is needed is interpretation, rearrangement, comparison, and planning of executive action (fig 15.6). The abilities of our mental working space are determined by the number of items of data that can be integrated into a decision. There is evidence that this vital number is 3–8.

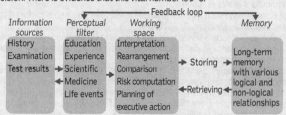

Fig 15.6 Consultation flowchart. After Sullivan.[20]

Thinking about thinking[4] [21–23] The rapid decision-making often required by doctors can be aided by *heuristics*—strategies that provide cognitive 'shortcuts' to quick decisions (conscious or unconscious) which are made without full information or analysis. Understanding how we use heuristics (ie by considering how a decision is made) can help us make effective choices, but there are pitfalls. Failed heuristics (biases) interfere with judgement and can lead to diagnostic error. Important examples include:
- *Anchoring:* A significant feature in the history is 'anchored' onto too early in the diagnostic process and is not adjusted for in light of later information. Adjusting probability by incorporating new information can help you become an intuitive thinker. Anchoring can be compounded by *confirmation bias*—the tendency to look for, notice, and remember information that fits with pre-existing expectations.
- *Availability:* Explains our tendency to judge something more likely if it readily comes to mind. A recent experience with a disease increases the likelihood of it being diagnosed—problematic if the disease is rare, or has not been seen for a while.
- *Representativeness:* A diagnosis is driven by the extent to which a patient resembles a classic case of a disease. When diagnosis is limited in this way, atypical variants can be missed.

4 This material was originally published in the *Oxford Handbook of Clinical Medicine* 9th edition by Longmore et al., and has been reproduced by permission of Oxford University Press.

All UK doctors should be registered with a *general practitioner*—your own GP can be a fantastic source of support and advice. There are few perks to working in the NHS and in general, doctors are keen to support and help their colleagues.

Doctors' Support Network is a confidential peer support network for doctors and medical students with concerns about their mental health: www.dsn.org.uk

DocHealth is a confidential, not-for-profit service giving doctors an opportunity to explore difficulties, both professional and personal, with senior clinicians. Self-referring doctors can access up to six face-to-face sessions. A fee structure is based on grade/circumstances. www.dochealth.org.uk

The NHS *Practitioner Health Programme* is an award-winning, free, and confidential service for doctors and dentists with issues relating to mental or physical health or addictions, in particular where these might affect their work. Any doctor in England can request a referral via their GP: www.php.nhs.uk

GP *Health Service* is a confidential NHS service for GPs and GP trainees in England. It aims to help doctors with issues relating to a mental health concern, including stress or depression, or an addiction problem, in particular where these might affect their work: www.gphealth.nhs.uk

RCPSYCH *Psychiatrists' Support Service* is a free, confidential support and advice service for psychiatrists at all stages of their career who find themselves in difficulty or in need of support: 020 7245 0412; pss@rcpsych.ac.uk

Health for Health Professionals Wales is a face-to-face counselling service for all doctors in Wales: 0800 058 2738.

BMA *Counselling* has a 24/7 telephone line and offers up to 6 structured telephone counselling sessions: 0330 123 1245.

BMA *Doctor Advisor Service* runs alongside BMA Counselling, giving doctors and medical students in distress or difficulty the choice of speaking in confidence to another doctor: 0330 123 1245.

BMA *Doctor Support Service* is for any doctor (you do not have to be a BMA member) who is facing a GMC investigation or licence withdrawal. Being subject to a GMC complaint can be uniquely and deeply stressful and this service offers emotional help from fellow doctors and functions independently of the GMC: www.bma.org.uk/advice/work-life-support/your-wellbeing

The Doctors Support Group aims to provide support and assistance to any medical professional or dentist facing suspension, exclusion, investigation of complaints, and/or allegations of professional misconduct: www.doctorssupportgroup.com

British Doctors and Dentists Group is a recovery group for doctors and dentists addicted to alcohol and/or drugs: www.bddg.org

The *Sick Doctors Trust* supports and helps doctors, dentists, and medical students who are concerned about their use of drugs or alcohol. 24/7 Helpline: 0370 444 5163. www.sick-doctors-trust.co.uk

---

Sources of financial support

Royal Medical Benevolent Fund www.rmbf.org

Royal Medical Foundation www.royalmedicalfoundation.org

BMA *Charities Trust Fund* info.bmacharities@bma.org.uk

Help me, I'm a doctor www.doctors help.org.uk

Useful apps

The apps and websites listed here were suggested by the contributing authors and are commonly used by doctors in the UK. Please note: OUP is not responsible for the content of external apps or websites.

- The *BNF/BNFC* app contains all the content from the *BNF* and the *BNFC* in one place, providing up-to-date information about the use of medicines and drug interactions for free. Essential!
- *Microguide* allows you to download your hospital's antimicrobial guidance, with easy-to-search first-line/alternative antibiotics listed by bodily system. Updated guidelines are automatically downloaded and the app works offline.
- *MDCalc* (other medical calculators are available!) contains all the widely used clinical calculators that help support decision-making and evidence-based care, from Apgar to VBAC (and many, many others in between).
- *Toxbase* is the clinical toxicology database of the UK National Poisons Information Service, providing advice on the features and management of poisoning/overdose. It is free if you sign up using an NHS.email address.
- Developed by NHS Blood and Transplant, the *Blood Components* app summarizes relevant national guidelines to act as a prompt to facilitate appropriate use of blood products. It is based on the National Blood Transfusion Committee Indication codes.
- The *Induction* app allows you to avoid dialling switchboard by viewing and dialling hospital extensions from your phone. You can also search who is paging you by entering the extension.

Other useful selected apps and websites

NHS Apps website: An updating list of NHS-approved apps for patients across a variety of specialties: www.nhs.uk/apps-library/

O&G: The RCOG *Green-top Guidelines* are aids to good clinical practice and are available to browse: www.rcog.org.uk/guidelines

Paediatrics:
- *NeoMate* is a free app for NICU staff and includes drug and fluid calculations, guides, and checklists for care.
- *BiliApp* helps you interpret and guide management of newborn jaundice based on NICE guidance.
- UK *Growth Charts* are available at www.rcpch.ac.uk/resources/growth-charts
- *Paediatric Care Online* (www.pcouk.org) is a decision-support tool on child health and safeguarding.

Dermatology:
- *DermNet NZ* (www.dermnetnz.org) is an A–Z of skin diseases and treatment with an excellent image library.
- The *British Association of Dermatologists* (www.bad.org.uk) also has a wealth of clinical information/patient leaflets.

ENT:
- www.ENT.org.uk (British Association of Otolaryngology) has published guidelines and patient leaflets.
- *Mimi Hearing Test* is an ios app calibrated for EarPods® and AirPods®.

Emergency medicine: Mersey Burns calculates burn area percentages.

Trauma & orthopaedics: OrthoFlow is a purchased app which helps you diagnose and manage orthopaedic trauma.

General practice:
- NICE *Clinical Knowledge Summaries* provide >300 summaries of current evidence and guidance on best practice for common/significant primary care presentations: https://cks.nice.org.uk
- *Patient.co.uk* and the NHS website (www.nhs.uk) have excellent information for patients on various illnesses and diseases.

Index

Note: syn. = syndrome; dis. = disease. Tables, figures, and boxes are indicated by an italic *t*, *f*, and *b* following the page number.